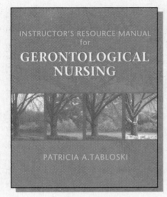

INSTRUCTOR'S RESOURCE MANUAL
ISBN: 0-13-094187-5
This manual contains a wealth of material that will help instructors plan and manage the gerontological nursing course. The manual includes learning objectives, concepts for lecture, detailed lecture outlines, MediaLinks, suggestions for classroom and clinical activities, a complete test bank, and more. The IRM also offers tips on how to use and assign the text-specific Companion Website, **www.prenhall.com/tabloski**, and the free CD-ROM that accompanies the textbook.

INSTRUCTOR'S RESOURCE CD-ROM
ISBN: 0-13-094188-3
This cross-platform CD-ROM provides a PowerPoint presentation with discussion points and illustrations from *Gerontological Nursing*. It also contains an electronic Test Item File, answers to the textbook critical thinking exercises, and animations from the Student CD-ROM. This supplement is available to faculty upon adoption of the textbook.

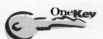

COMPANION WEBSITE SYLLABUS MANAGER
www.prenhall.com/tabloski
Faculty adopting this textbook have access to the online Syllabus Manager on the companion website, **www.prenhall.com/tabloski**. Syllabus Manager offers features that facilitate the students' use of the Companion Website and allows faculty to post syllabi and course information. For a demonstration of Syllabus Manager, please contact your Prentice Hall Sales Representative.

ONLINE COURSE MANAGEMENT SYSTEMS
OneKey is an integrated online resource that brings a wide array of supplemental resources together in one convenient place for both students and faculty. OneKey features everything you and your students need for out-of-class work, including interactive modules, text and image PowerPoints, animations, videos, case studies, and more. OneKey also provides course management tools so faculty can customize course content, build online tests, create assignments, enter grades, post announcements, communicate with students, and much more. Testing materials, gradebooks, and other instructor resources can be accessed by instructors only. OneKey content is available in three different platforms. For information about adopting a course management system to accompany *Gerontological Nursing*, please contact your Prentice Hall Sales Representative or go online to the specific website below and select "Courses," then "Nursing."
WebCT: http://cms.prenhall.com/webct/index.html/
BlackBoard: http://cms.prenhall.com/blackboard/indexs.html/
CourseCompass: http://cms.prenhall.com/coursecompass/

BRIEF CONTENTS

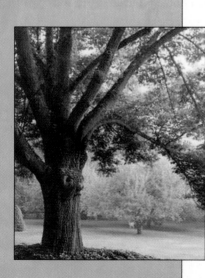

GERONTOLOGICAL NURSING

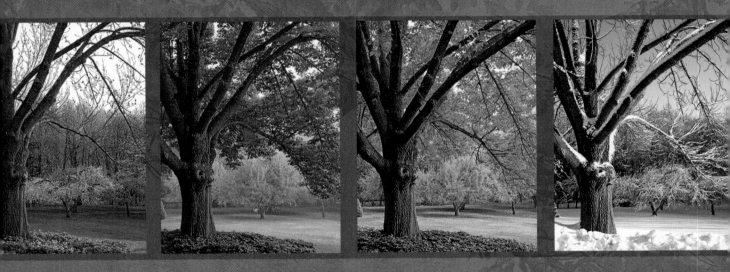

PATRICIA A. TABLOSKI

PhD, RNBC, GNP, FGSA
William F. Connell
School of Nursing at Boston College

PEARSON

Prentice
Hall

Upper Saddle River, New Jersey 07458

Library of Congress Cataloging-in-Publication Data

Tabloski, Patricia.
   Gerontological nursing / Patricia Tabloski.
     p. ; cm.
   Includes bibliographical references and index.
   ISBN 0-13-094155-7
   1. Geriatric nursing. I. Title.
   [DNLM: 1. Geriatric Nursing. WY 152 T113g 2006]
RC954.T33 2006
618.97′0231—dc22

                                        2005048863

Publisher: Julie Levin Alexander
Publisher's Assistant: Regina Bruno
Editor-in-Chief: Maura Connor
Acquisitions Editor: Pamela Fuller
Managing Development Editor: Marilyn Meserve
Development Editor: Elizabeth Garofalo
Editorial Assistant: Aline Filippone
Associate Editor: Michael Giacobbe
Director of Manufacturing and Production: Bruce Johnson
Managing Production Editor: Patrick Walsh
Production Liaison: Cathy O'Connell
Production Editor: Amy Gehl, Carlisle Publishers Services
Manufacturing Manager: Ilene Sanford
Manufacturing Buyer: Pat Brown
Design Director: Maria Guglielmo Walsh
Cover Designer: Vicky Kane
Interior Designer: Amanda Kavanaugh
Director of Marketing: Karen Allman
Marketing Coordinator: Michael Sirinides
Marketing Assistant: Patricia Linard
Media Product Manager: John Jordan
Media Production Manager: Amy Peltier
Media Project Manager: Tina Rudowski
Composition: Carlisle Publishers Services
Printer/Binder: Courier Kendallville
Cover Printer: Phoenix Color
Cover photograph copyright Nick Zungoli, The Exposures Gallery

Pearson Education Ltd.
Pearson Education Singapore, Pte. Ltd.
Pearson Education Canada, Ltd.
Pearson Education—Japan

Pearson Education Australia PTY, Limited
Pearson Education North Asia Ltd.
Pearson Educación de Mexico, S.A. de C.V.
Pearson Education Malaysia, Pte. Ltd.
Pearson Education, Upper Saddle River, New Jersey

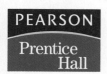

10 9 8 7 6 5 4 3
ISBN 0-13-094155-7

PATRICIA A. TABLOSKI, PhD, RNBC, GNP, FGSA

Patricia Tabloski possesses three degrees in nursing. She received her BSN from Purdue University, her MSN from Seton Hall University, and her PhD from the University of Rochester. As a gerontological nurse practitioner, Dr. Tabloski has provided primary care to older patients in a variety of settings, including acute care facilities, geriatric outpatient clinics, long-term care facilities, and hospice programs. She has taught graduate and undergraduate students about gerontology since 1981 and presently is a faculty member at the William F. Connell School of Nursing at Boston College. In 2002, Dr. Tabloski was honored as a Fellow in the Gerontological Society of America. She has numerous publications and presentations relating to gerontological nursing and has lectured internationally in Hungary, China, and the United Kingdom. Dr. Tabloski has chaired the Test Development Committee for the Gerontological Nurse Practitioner examination by the American Nurses Credentialing Center and is a member of the American Nurses Association, the Gerontological Society of America, the American Geriatrics Society, the National Organization of Nurse Practitioners Faculties, Sigma Theta Tau, and the Eastern Nursing Research Society. Dr. Tabloski is a federally funded researcher and conducts clinically based outcome studies relating to nonpharmacological interventions designed to improve sleep and ease agitation in older persons in community and institutional settings.

The 21st century heralds continuing dramatic changes in American health care. Advances in science, application in practice and new theories of care all contribute to a changing environment for the education and delivery of services. The profession of nursing is much a part of these changes. The challenges to nursing education and practice are great and huge and dominate the energies of all practitioners.

In this new century, the increasing age of the patient is well documented. The associated challenges to nursing educators and practitioners alike are complex and require new strategies and solutions in preparing future practitioners. Care to the older person is directly related to the above. This text offers the nursing professional a valuable direction in caring for life, especially as it is research-based and the applications of this knowledge is evidence based. The authors are experts in their fields and permit the reader to "be real" about their care. Dr. Tabloski is an eminent researcher and practitioner and has been a life-long advocate of responsible, considerate and expert nursing care for the older person. Along with her colleagues, they present challenges, solutions and sense about caring for our aging population. They make it fun to care for the aged and have influenced many nurses over the years toward that vision. The users of this text will discover that vision and will come to know the pleasure of caring and the pleasure of the older person.

Jean E. Steel, PhD, FAAN
Professor Emerita
MGH Institute of Health Professions
Boston, MA
August 4, 2005

We all need to address issues of aging and the study of human growth and development across the life span. As we experience the progression of human life through various stages, critical perspectives concerning life, death, growth, and relationships evolve. Like the seasons, we adapt.

This book is intended to guide the student in the care of persons in the winter of their lives. All patients, regardless of age, deserve expert and dignified nursing care, and our challenge is to encourage our patients to grow and evolve until the moment of death. The work of our hands and our hearts contributes much to the dialogue between nurses and patients and softens the sometimes harsh boundaries between humanity and technology.

The older population is the largest consumer of healthcare and nursing services. This population will present societal challenges to nurses and citizens as we plan to meet the healthcare needs of an increasingly diverse group with higher expectations regarding quality of life and health in old age. Nurses and other healthcare workers in a wide range of settings will find themselves caring for larger numbers of older persons with a variety of healthcare needs. Even those working in obstetrics and pediatrics will find themselves interacting with grandparents and multigenerational extended families during the course of their work. Additionally, we are all aging and encountering issues of aging within our own families, so there is a tremendous need for increased knowledge and preparation in gerontological nursing.

The new focus of research and healthcare for older persons involves "adding life to years" rather than a singular focus on "adding years to life." This new focus acknowledges that merely extending life without attention to the quality of life may lead to a life that is neither active nor fulfilling. This new focus calls for healthcare delivery within the context of a multidisciplinary team with recognition that nurses play a key and vital role in the function of this team. Highly specialized and expert healthcare is needed when caring for older adults, including emergency treatment of life-threatening illness; management of chronic health problems; primary health care services with emphasis on disease prevention and health promotion; support for professional and family caregivers; provision of culturally appropriate care to an increasingly diverse older population; removal of barriers to emotional, educational, and financial resources; and providing expert palliative and hospice care to frail older adults and those at the end of life. There are expert nursing faculty and graduate and undergraduate curricula available to instruct students, research-based journals and Websites with current information to assist clinicians, and a variety of specialized textbooks, such as this, designed to prepare the nurse to meet these crucial challenges.

The introduction of a new gerontological nursing text comes at a critical time in the evolution of our healthcare system. *Gerontological Nursing* is a comprehensive, research-based text to guide nursing students in their care of older adults. This text presents information related to the normal and pathological changes of aging, commonly encountered diseases of aging, and the broad psychosocial, cultural, and public health knowledge required to provide expert nursing care to older persons. The emphasis is to provide critical information needed to engage in the nursing process of assessment, diagnosis, planning, and evaluating outcomes of care.

The current emphasis on evidence-based practice and appropriate delivery of scarce healthcare resources are factors that have guided the development of this textbook. Several chapters provide information on "Best Practices" in the nursing care of older adults from the Hartford Institute of Geriatric Nursing at New York University. The nursing student of today will need to possess as much knowledge as possible regarding the care of the older person. It is no longer sufficient to utilize basic medical-surgical knowledge and modify it for use with the older person. The knowledge needed by the nurse caring for the older patient must be grounded in gerontology with emphasis on holistic assessment, setting realistic goals, use of appropriate pain assessment and pain management, recognition of cognitive impairment and frailty, and provision of end-of-life care. This text provides the comprehensive information that the nurse will use to practice safely, effectively, and appropriately when caring for the older patient in the home, hospital, long-term care, and hospice settings. Whether the goal is to return the older patient to his or her previous levels of health and function, improve precious levels of health and function, provide supportive care, or prepare for death by instituting palliative care, the nurse assumes a pivotal role on the interdisciplinary healthcare team and this text will provide crucial information in preparation for that role.

Organization of the Text

The text is organized to facilitate student learning. Unit One is composed of three chapters that form the foundations of gerontological nursing practice. In these chapters the principles of gerontology, identification of key gerontological nursing issues, and principles of geriatrics are covered. Unit Two describes the challenges of aging and the cornerstones of excellence in nursing care and includes information on cultural diversity, nutrition, pharmacology, psychological and cognitive function, sleep, pain management, violence and elder mistreatment, and care of the dying. Unit Three describes the physiological basis for nursing practice in gerontology with information on body systems, including the integument, the mouth/oral cavity, sensation, circulatory, respiratory, genitourinary, musculoskeletal, endocrine, gastrointestinal, hematologic, nervous, immune, and multisystem problems relating to care of the frail older adult.

The chapters in Units Two and Three begin with an overview of the content, describing the normal changes of aging, and the common diseases of aging, and move toward the assessment, diagnosis, management, and evaluation of nursing care. This framework allows the student to integrate the basic knowledge presented in Units One and Two with the clinical issues presented in Unit Three.

Throughout the text, issues related to cultural diversity are integrated into the discussions of disease and care. Increasingly large numbers of older adults will be from ethnically diverse cultures, and threats to healthy aging can vary according to cultural heritage.

Key Components of the Text

The following features will help students integrate the theoretical and clinical information essential to the understanding and practice of gerontological nursing.

Normal Changes of Aging – Each of the clinically based chapters covers the normal changes of aging as a basis for the nursing assessment and care to follow. Full-color illustrations and photographs complement the text, allowing for a more meaningful synthesis of information.

Common Diseases of Aging – Each clinical chapter emphasizes the common diseases (acute and chronic) that afflict older people, nursing implications of these diseases, atypical presentation of disease in older persons, functional implications of these diseases, pharmacological treatment, and evaluation of care. Etiology, risk factors, function, and complications are included.

Special Features

- **MediaLink,** at the beginning of each chapter, lists specific content, animations, anatomy and physiology review, NCLEX® review questions, tools, and other interactive exercises that appear on the Companion Website. Special MediaLink tabs appear throughout the chapter in the margins, encouraging the students to use the media supplements for special activities, applications, and resources. The purpose of the MediaLink feature is to further enhance the student's experience, build on knowledge gained from the textbook, prepare students for NCLEX®, and foster critical thinking.
- **Chapter Objectives** identify essential concepts and key issues addressed in the chapter.
- **Key Terms** are identified in bold and are defined in the audio glossary on the Companion Website.
- **Drug Alerts and Clinical Pearls** supply students with crucial information and call attention to key issues.
- The **Best Practices** feature presents a recommendation from the Hartford Institute of Geriatric Nursing for an assessment instrument, protocol, or nursing intervention that recommends the best practice for an older patient with the particular health problem under discussion.
- **NANDA** nursing diagnoses are suggested for each of the common diseases presented in order to help students categorize the nursing problems that accompany the medical diagnoses. Each nursing diagnosis forms the basis for the suggestions for nursing interventions that follow.
- **Patient and Family Teaching Guidelines** include sample questions and answers an older patient and his or her family may pose when receiving care for a particular problem. A rationale is given for each answer to assist the student to gain valuable insights into how best to provide succinct, focused answers to patient and family questions within the context of a busy and sometimes hectic clinical setting. When educating patients and families about a life-altering chronic illness such as diabetes, teaching priorities are described. The immediate teaching goal is what the patient needs to know to begin to manage the disease. This is followed by knowledge that is needed later to have more flexibility and control over situations that may arise in the future. This approach will help the student prioritize learning objectives and prevent the patient from feeling overwhelmed by the amount of knowledge to be absorbed immediately after diagnosis.
- **Care Plans** in each chapter are used to illustrate the nursing process. A case study is used to tie together content described in the chapter and provide an example of various nursing interventions and the planning and implementation of nursing care. Each case study presents an **ethical dilemma** in anticipation of the kinds of situations the student will encounter when delivering care to older persons. The case studies present the real-world experience of the author and contributors of this book and encourage the student to participate in the assessment and planning process. **Critical thinking exercises** follow the case studies, encouraging the student to engage in additional learning activities that stimulate and support learning. The exercises may be done individually or within a group setting. The insights

gained from the exercises will form the basis of individualized and empathetic nursing practice and widen the student's understanding of the older patient's situation. Answers to these exercises are found in Appendix B of this book.

- **Chapter Highlights** are listed at the end of each chapter. Students will find it helpful to read these highlights before reading the chapter in order to focus their attention. These are also a useful tool to quickly review the chapter content.
- **EXPLORE MediaLink,** at the end of each chapter, encourages students to use the CD-ROM and Companion Website to apply their knowledge of the chapter through additional case studies, practice NCLEX® questions, animation tutorials, and additional resources.

Complete Teaching/Learning Package

To supplement and facilitate active student learning and information provided in the text, a variety of student learning aids are included in a comprehensive supplement package.

FOR THE STUDENT

Companion Website – www.prenhall.com/tabloski. This *free* online study guide is designed to help students apply the concepts in the book. Each chapter-specific module features objectives, audio glossary, chapter summary for lecture notes, NCLEX® review questions, case studies, care plan activities, MediaLink Applications, MediaLinks, and nursing tools.

Student CD-ROM. This addition to the teaching/learning package is an interactive student program that contains videos, animations, NCLEX® questions, assessment tools, and case studies. This CD-ROM is packaged with every copy of the text and is free to students.

Clinical Handbook. Designed specifically for the nursing student to carry into the clinical setting, this pocket-sized handbook provides a succinct review of the instruments and nursing interventions described in the book. Each discussion includes the pathophysiology, nursing diagnoses and interventions, recommended assessment parameters, and outcome criteria for commonly encountered problems.

FOR THE INSTRUCTOR

Instructor's Resource Manual
ISBN: 0-13-094187-5

This manual contains a wealth of material to help faculty plan and manage the gerontology course. It includes chapter overviews, detailed lecture suggestions and outlines, learning objectives, a complete test bank, teaching tips, and more for each chapter. The instructor's manual also guides faculty how to assign and use the text-specific Website, **http://www.prenhall.com/tabloski**, and the free Student CD-ROM that accompany the book.

Instructor's Resource CD-ROM
ISBN: 0-13-094188-3

This cross-platform CD-ROM provides illustrations in PowerPoint from the textbook for use in classroom lectures. It also contains an electronic test bank and animations from the Student CD-ROM. This supplement is available to faculty free upon adoption of the book.

Companion Website Syllabus Manager
www.prenhall.com/tabloski
Faculty adopting this book have free access to the online Syllabus Manager on the Companion Website, **www.prenhall.com/tabloski**. Syllabus Manager offers a host of features that facilitate the students' use of the Companion Website, and allows faculty to post syllabi and course information online for students. For more information or a demonstration of Syllabus Manager, please contact a Prentice Hall sales representative.

Online Course Management Systems
Also available are online companions for schools using course management systems. The online course management solutions feature interactive modules, electronic test bank, PowerPoint images, animations, assessment activities, and more. For more information about adopting an online course management system to accompany *Gerontological Nursing*, please contact your Prentice Hall sales representative or go online to one of the following Websites and select "courses."

WebCT: http://cms.prenhall.com/webct/index.html/
Blackboard: http://cms.prenhall.com/blackboard/index.html/
CourseCompass: http://cms.prenhall.com/coursecompass/

ACKNOWLEDGMENTS

I wish to thank the many older patients and families I have worked with and cared for through the years. They have been wise teachers and provided the impetus for me to pursue my education, undertake my research, and write this text. I also wish to thank my students who have an insatiable desire to provide the highest quality nursing care possible and improve the quality of their patients' lives. The reviewers of this text have provided suggestions that have strengthened and improved the content, and I am most appreciative of their thoughtful suggestions. I also wish to express my appreciation to the expert contributors who generously agreed to share their knowledge and expertise even though they lead busy and overcommitted lives.

I especially want to thank the editorial and production staff of Prentice Hall, including Elisabeth Garofalo, Kim Wyatt, Pamela Fuller, Gosia Jaros-White, Carolin Hansa, Eileen Monaghan, Aline Filippone, Cathy O'Connell, Pat Walsh, and Carlisle Communications, especially Amy Gehl.

To the students with the clarity of vision to see beauty and strength in aging.

Text Contributors

Susan K. Chase, EdD, RNBC, FNP
Interim Assistant Dean, Doctoral Program
Christine E. Lynn College of Nursing
Florida Atlantic University
Boca Raton, Florida

Laurel Eisenhauer, RN, EdD, FAAN
Professor Emeritus
William F. Connell of Nursing at Boston College
Chestnut Hill, Massachusetts

Terry Fulmer, PhD, RN, FAAN
Professor and Associate Director of the Hartford Institute for Geriatric Nursing
Steinhardt School of Education
The Erline Perkins McGriff Professor &
Head, Division of Nursing
New York University
New York, New York

Gail A. Harkness, DrPH-RN, FAAN
Professor Emeritus,
University of Connecticut
Storrs, Connecticut

Rosalie Hentz, BS, RN
Gerontological Specialist and MDS Nurse
Beaumont Nursing Home
Westboro, Massachusetts

Ann C. Hurley, RN, DNSc, FAAN, FGSA
Executive Director
Center for Excellence
in Nursing Practice
Brigham and Women's Hospital
Boston, Massachusetts

Ellen K. Mahoney, RN, DNSc, FGSA
Associate Professor
William F. Connell School of Nursing at Boston College
Chestnut Hill, Massachusetts

Rita J. Olivieri, EdD, RN
Associate Professor
William F. Connell School of Nursing at Boston College
Chestnut Hill, Massachusetts

Rachel E. Spector, PhD, RN, FAAN
CultureCare Consultant
Needham, Massachusetts

Sheila Tucker, RD
Dietician and Part-time Faculty Member
Boston College
Chestnut Hill, Massachusetts

Ladislav Volicer, MD, PhD, FGSA, FAAN
Former Clinical Director
Geriatric Research Education and Clinical Center
ENR Memorial Veterans Hospital
Bedford, Massachusetts

Bridgette Maclaughlin Warnat, MS, RNBC, ANP
Framingham, Massachusetts

Gracie S. Wishnia, PhD, RN
Director of the Graduate Program
Spalding University
Louisville, Kentucky

Tamara Zurakowski, PhD, RNBC, GNP
Lecturer/Clinical Specialist
School of Nursing
University of Pennsylvania
Philadelphia, Pennsylvania

Supplement and Media Writers

Jo Anne Carrick, RN, MSN
Instructor
Penn State University
Sharon, Pennsylvania

Julieta Castaneda, RN, MSN
Instructor
University of Texas—El Paso
El Paso, Texas

Joan Dacher, PhD, RN, GNP
Director of Palliative Care
Community Hosptice, Inc.
Albany, New York
Assistant Professor
Sage Graduate School
Troy, New York

Vera Dauffenbach, RN, MSN, EdD
Bellin College of Nursing
Green Bay, Wisconsin

Julia A. Eggert, PhD, GNP-C, AOCN
Assistant Professor of Nursing
Clemson University
Clemson, SC

Joyce Hammer, RN, MSN
Lourdes College
Sylvania, OH

Hyacinth Martin, RN, MA, MSED
Borough of Manhattan Community College
New York, New York

Elizabeth M. Rash, PhD, ARNP-C
Adjunct Instructor
University of Central Florida
Orlando, Florida

Diane Weed, PhD, MSN, CRNP
Clinical Assistant Professor
University of Alabama at Huntsville
Huntsville, Alabama

REVIEWERS

Ann Bellar, PhD, APRN, BC
Assistant Professor
Wayne State University
School of Nursing
Detroit, Michigan

Nancy Blume, PhD, MSN, BSN, RN, BC ARNP-CNS
Associate Professor
Fort Hays State University
Department of Nursing
Hays, Kansas

Anna Brock, PhD, RN
Professor
University of Southern Mississippi
School of Nursing
Hattiesburg, Mississippi

Julia A. Eggert, PhD, GNP-C, AOCN
Assistant Professor
Clemson University
Clemson, South Carolina

Mary Golech, MSN, MAEd
Instructor
Kent State University
School of Nursing
Kent, Ohio

Polly Haigler, PhD, RN, BC
Clinical Associate Professor
College of Nursing, University of South Carolina
Columbia, South Carolina

Laurel Halloran, PLD, APRN
Professor
Western Connecticut State University
Danbury, Connecticut

Dorothy Herron, PhD, RN, CS
Associate Professor
University of Maryland
School of Nursing
Baltimore, Maryland

Linda M. Johnson, RN, BSN, MSN, MS
Instructor in Nursing
San Francisco Community College District
San Francisco, California

Roseann Kaminsky, MSN, BSN, BSEd
Associate Professor
Lorain County Community College
School of Nursing
Fairview Park, Ohio

Patricia Leary, MAEd, AEN
Allied Health Instructor
Ferris State University
School of Nursing
Lakeview, Michigan

Cheryl Lee, MSN, RN, CWO, CN
Associate Professor
Harding University
Cabot, Arkansas

Mary Hysell Lynd, PhD, MSN, BSN, RN
Associate Professor
Ohio University–Chillicothe
School of Nursing
Chillicothe, Ohio

Betty A. Maxwell, MSN, RN
Instructor
St. Clair County Community College
Port Huron, Michigan

Gail Moddeman, PhD, RN
Assistant Professor
Wright State University–Miami Valley College of Nursing and Health
Dayton, Ohio

Marsha K. Morton, MA, RN
Professor
Westminster College of School of Nursing
Salt Lake City, Utah

Maureen E. O'Rourke, RN, PhD
Associate Clinical Professor
University of North Carolina, Greensboro
Greensboro, North Carolina
Adjunct Assistant Professor of Medicine
Wake Forest University
School of Medicine

Sheila P. Patros, PhD, RN
Chairperson, Department of Nursing
Kentucky State University
Lexington, Kentucky

Debra Sanders, RN, MSN
Professor in Nursing
Bloomsburg University
Bloomsburg, Pennsylvania

Cheryl Ross Staats
University of Texas
Health Science Center at San Antonio School of Nursing
San Antonio, Texas

Stephanie Valdes, RN, MS
Professor, Assistant Chairperson
Black Hawk College
Moline, Illinois

Gracie Wishnia, PhD, MSN, RN
Associate Professor
Spalding University
School of Nursing
Louisville, Kentucky

How to use this textbook
to ensure your success in nursing...

Throughout each text chapter, the student CD-ROM, and the Companion Website, each feature is organized to facilitate your learning and to give you the theoretical and clinical foundation that you'll need to succeed in your future as a nurse.

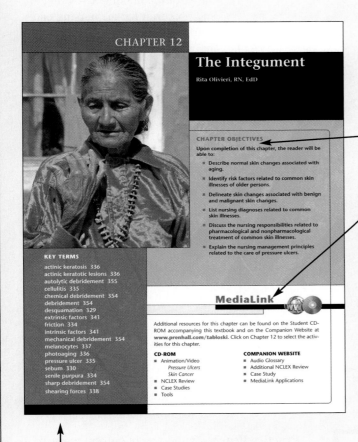

CHAPTER 12

The Integument

Rita Olivieri, RN, EdD

CHAPTER OBJECTIVES

Upon completion of this chapter, the reader will be able to:

- Describe normal skin changes associated with aging.
- Identify risk factors related to common skin illnesses of older persons.
- Delineate skin changes associated with benign and malignant skin changes.
- List nursing diagnoses related to common skin illnesses.
- Discuss the nursing responsibilities related to pharmacological and nonpharmacological treatment of common skin illnesses.
- Explain the nursing management principles related to the care of pressure ulcers.

KEY TERMS

actinic keratosis 336
actinic keratotic lesions 336
autolytic debridement 355
cellulitis 335
chemical debridement 354
debridement 354
desquamation 329
extrinsic factors 341
friction 334
intrinsic factors 341
mechanical debridement 354
melanocytes 337
photoaging 336
pressure ulcer 335
sebum 330
senile purpura 334
sharp debridement 354
shearing forces 338

MediaLink

Additional resources for this chapter can be found on the Student CD-ROM accompanying this textbook and on the Companion Website at **www.prenhall.com/tabloski**. Click on Chapter 12 to select the activities for this chapter.

CD-ROM
- Animation/Video
  Pressure Ulcers
  Skin Cancer
- NCLEX Review
- Case Studies
- Tools

COMPANION WEBSITE
- Audio Glossary
- Additional NCLEX Review
- Case Study
- MediaLink Applications

Chapter Objectives let you know what you can expect to learn by the end of the chapter.

MediaLink calls your attention to the additional learning tools for each chapter that are available on the CD-ROM and Companion Website that accompany your textbook.

Student CD-ROM
NCLEX-RN® Review—chapter-specific questions including the new test item features.
Case Studies—Based on the Best Practices feature, scenarios and critical thinking.
Animations & Videos—difficult concepts are brought to life.
Tools—Best Practices instruments from the text are available in printable format.

Companion Website
NCLEX-RN® Review—chapter-specific questions including the new test item features.
Case Studies—scenarios and questions
MediaLinks—content-related hyperlinks
MediaLink Applications—apply the information from the Web
Tools—useful instruments from the text are available in printable format.

Key Terms are defined for you in bold, black type in the book and also are pronounced in the audio glossary on the Companion Website.

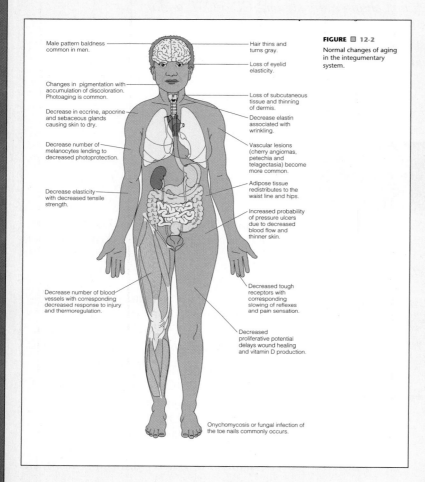

FIGURE ▪ 12-2

Normal changes of aging in the integumentary system.

Male pattern baldness common in men.

Hair thins and turns gray.

Loss of eyelid elasticity.

Changes in pigmentation with accumulation of discoloration. Photoaging is common.

Loss of subcutaneous tissue and thinning of dermis.

Decrease in eccrine, apocrine and sebaceous glands causing skin to dry.

Decrease elastin associated with wrinkling.

Decrease number of melanocytes lending to decreased photoprotection.

Vascular lesions (cherry angiomas, petechia and telagectasia) become more common.

Adipose tissue redistributes to the waist line and hips.

Decrease elasticity with decreased tensile strength.

Increased probability of pressure ulcers due to decreased blood flow and thinner skin.

Decrease number of blood vessels with corresponding decreased response to injury and thermoregulation.

Decreased tough receptors with corresponding slowing of reflexes and pain sensation.

Decreased proliferative potential delays wound healing and vitamin D production.

Onychomycosis or fungal infection of the toe nails commonly occurs.

Each of the clinically based chapters will highlight the **Normal Changes of Aging** as a basis for the nursing assessment and blueprint for the nursing care to follow. Full-color illustrations and photos clearly show you how these normal changes occur in each body system.

Practice Pearl

The area at risk for pressure sores should be washed gently with tepid water, with or without minimal soap. Soap removes natural oils from the skin, and cleaning the soap off may cause additional friction damage.

Practice Pearls remind you of helpful hints to facilitate clinical practice.

Drug Alert !

Older persons have a high rate of adverse reactions to corticosteroids and antihistamines, both of which are frequently prescribed for skin problems. Older persons should be reminded not to buy over-the-counter preparations of these drugs without specific instructions from their primary care provider. If these medications are prescribed, directions should be strictly followed and any unusual symptoms reported promptly.

Drug Alerts alert you to safety precautions to consider for providing safe care for older clients.

Best Practices prepare you for clinical success.

The **Best Practices** feature provides you with an assessment instrument or nursing intervention recommended by the Hartford Institute of Geriatric Nursing as the currently recognized best practice for care of an older patient.

Best Practices

Braden Scale for Predicting Pressure Sore Risk

The Braden Scale (Braden & Bergstrom, 1994) is a widely used tool that assesses mobility, activity, sensory perception, skin moisture, friction, shear, and nutritional status. Each dimension is rated from 1 to 4 on a Likert type scale, and the total score range is from 6 to 23. A score of 16 or less indicates a pressure sore risk and a need for a prevention plan. The Braden scale has been subjected to several validation studies and is considered the most valid of the available risk assessment tools. Once a risk assessment is completed, and a deficit exists, the nursing care plan should reflect on-going prevention as well as complete documentation of the older person's progress.

BRADEN SCALE FOR PREDICTING PRESSURE SORE RISK

Patient's Name _____ Evaluator's Name _____ Date of Assessment _____

SENSORY PERCEPTION ability to respond meaningfully to pressure-related discomfort	**1. Completely Limited** Unresponsive (does not moan, flinch, or grasp) to painful stimuli, due to diminished level of consciousness or sedation. OR limited ability to feel pain over most of body	**2. Very Limited** Responds only to painful stimuli. Cannot communicate discomfort except by moaning or restlessness OR has a sensory impairment which limits the ability to feel pain or discomfort over ½ of body.	**3. Slightly Limited** Responds to verbal commands, but cannot always communicate discomfort or the need to be turned. OR has some sensory impairment which limits ability to feel pain or discomfort in 1 or 2 extremities.	**4. No Impairment** Responds to verbal commands. Has no sensory deficit which would limit ability to feel or voice pain or discomfort.		
MOISTURE degree to which skin is exposed to moisture	**1. Constantly Moist** Skin is kept moist almost constantly by perspiration, urine, etc. Dampness is detected every time patient is moved or turned.	**2. Very Moist** Skin is often, but not always moist. Linen must be changed at least once a shift.	**3. Occasionally Moist:** Skin is occasionally moist, requiring an extra linen change approximately once a day.	**4. Rarely Moist** Skin is usually dry, linen only requires changing at routine intervals.		
ACTIVITY degree of physical activity	**1. Bedfast** Confined to bed.	**2. Chairfast** Ability to walk severely limited or non-existent. Cannot bear own weight and/or must be assisted into chair or wheelchair.	**3. Walks Occasionally** Walks occasionally during day, but for very short distances, with or without assistance. Spends majority of each shift in bed or chair	**4. Walks Frequently** Walks outside room at least twice a day and inside room at least once every two hours during waking hours		
MOBILITY ability to change and control body position	**1. Completely Immobile** Does not make even slight changes in body or extremity position without assistance.	**2. Very Limited** Makes occasional slight changes in body or extremity position but unable to make frequent or significant changes independently.	**3. Slightly Limited** Makes frequent though slight changes in body or extremity position independently.	**4. No Limitation** Makes major and frequent changes in position without assistance.		
NUTRITION usual food intake pattern	**1. Very Poor** Never eats a complete meal. Rarely eats more than ⅓ of any food offered. Eats 2 servings or less of protein (meats or dairy products) per day. Takes fluids poorly. Does not take a liquid dietary supplement OR is NPO and/or maintained on clear liquids or IV's for more than 5 days.	**2. Probably Inadequate** Rarely eats a complete meal and generally eats only about ½ of any food offered. Protein intake includes only 3 servings of meat or dairy products per day. Occasionally will take a dietary supplement OR receives less than optimum amount of liquid diet or tube feeding	**3. Adequate** Eats over half of most meals. Eats a total of 4 servings of protein (meat, dairy products) per day. Occasionally will refuse a meal, but will usually take a supplement when offered OR is on a tube feeding or TPN regimen which probably meets most of nutritional needs.	**4. Excellent** Eats most of every meal. Never refuses a meal. Usually eats a total of 4 or more servings of meat and dairy products. Occasionally eats between meals. Does not require supplementation.		
FRICTION & SHEAR	**1. Problem** Requires moderate to maximum assistance in moving. Complete lifting without sliding against sheets is impossible. Frequently slides down in bed or chair, requiring frequent repositioning with maximum assistance. Spasticity, contractures, or agitation leads to almost constant friction.	**2. Potential Problem** Moves feebly or requires minimum assistance. During a move skin probably slides to some extent against sheets, chair, restraints, or other devices. Maintains relatively good position in chair or bed most of the time but occasionally slides down.	**3. No Apparent Problem** Moves in bed and in chair independently and has sufficient muscle strength to lift up completely during move. Maintains good position in bed or chair.			

Copyright Barbara Braden and Nancy Bergstrom, 1988. All rights reserved.   Total Score

MediaLink Tabs appear wherever topics in the text are further explained visually on the Student CD-ROM or Companion Website as specific videos or animations.

MediaLink ● Pressure Ulcer Video

with pressure ulcers on a
dence of pressure ulcers i
rates were from 3.5% to 2
Prevalence rates increase
These include patients wi
admitted to the critical car
of the femur. In all patien
considered at high risk fo
66% of older people with
Paustian, 1999).

Definition and Stag
A pressure ulcer is defined
age to underlying tissue. I
a bony prominence, althou
sure for a length of time t

Practical features prepare you for career success.

Care Plan

A Patient With a Pressure Ulcer

Case Study

A registered nurse who works for a home health agency has been assigned to Mrs. Krebs, a 75-year-old patient with a chronic stage III ulcer on her heel that has not shown any progress in the last 3 months. The nurse notes that Mrs. Krebs has a smoking history of 40 pack years and has not followed her diet instruction. The supervisor of the home health agency has warned the nurse that if Mrs. Krebs does not improve, the insurance company will not continue to provide payment for the [care] and treatment. Mrs. Krebs has refused to be admitted to the hospital for ulcer [care] and feels the nurses and physician do not understand her situation.

Applying the Nursing Process

ASSESSMENT

On the first visit, the nurse did a complete assessment and discussed the p[atient's] history, which includes peripheral vascular disease and hypertension. Mrs. [Krebs's] physical examination showed blood pressure 140/82, pulse 76, respirations [16,] temperature 98°F. On examination of the heel ulcer, the nurse noted a 4 [×] 6 cm stage III ulcer with a minimal amount of serous drainage and no local s[igns of] inflammation.

Mrs. Krebs is eating poorly, mostly freezer and canned foods with little [protein] and high sodium. She admits that she is smoking and not following her di[et. She] states, "I lost my husband 6 months ago and have not been able to take care of [myself.] I tried to quit smoking but it only lasted 5 days. I have been smoking for 4[0 years] and it is just too hard to stop. I'm doing the best I can."

DIAGNOSIS

The current nursing diagnoses for Mrs. Krebs include the following:

- *Impaired skin integrity*, stage III ulcer, related to prolonged pressure, ina[dequate] nutrition, decreased vascular perfusion
- *Ineffective management of therapeutic regimen related to complex re[gimen,]* limited resources and impaired adjustment as manifested by patient['s self-]assessment of poor dietary intake, inability to rest and elevate foot, and [smok-]ing behavior
- *Risk for altered nutrition: less than body requirements* related to lack of [phys-]ical and economic resources, and increased nutritional requirements re[lated to] ulcer

A Patient With a Pressure Ulcer

EXPECTED OUTCOMES

The expected outcomes for the plan specify that Mrs. Krebs will:

- Describe measures to protect and heal the tissue, including wound care.
- Report any additional symptoms such as pain, redness, numbness, tingling, or increased drainage.
- Demonstrate an understanding of nutritional needs, including the need for supplemental protein drink and vitamins.
- Collaborate with the nurse to develop a therapeutic plan that is congruent with her goals and present lifestyle.

PLANNING AND IMPLEMENTATION

The following nursing interventions may be appropriate for Mrs. Krebs:

- Establish a trusting relationship with Mrs. Krebs.
- Begin to explore what the patient's goals are in relation to her healthcare.
- Determine her daily habits and schedule and find some small measures that can be started for health improvement.
- Begin to determine ways to work with Mrs. Krebs's family to motivate her toward a healthy lifestyle (i.e., nutrition, smoking, foot care).
- Set priorities of care that Mrs. Krebs will agree to such as (1) ulcer improvement, (2) diet adjustments, and (3) smoking reductions.

EVALUATION

The nurse hopes to develop a long-term relationship with Mrs. Krebs and make an impact on her health and well-being. The nurse will consider the plan a success based on the following criteria:

- Mrs. Krebs will develop a trusting relationship and develop a plan with the nurse to improve her health.
- A family member will agree to assist Mrs. Krebs with her wound care and shopping issues.
- Mrs. Krebs will begin a smoking reduction effort.
- Mrs. Krebs will agree that if the ulcer is not healing in 4 weeks, she will seek inpatient treatment.

Ethical Dilemma

The primary ethical dilemma that evolves from this situation is the conflict between the moral obligation of the nurse to respect the autonomy of the patient and the principle of beneficence. The patient has a right to self-determination, independence, and freedom. It is important to allow patients to make their own decisions, even if the healthcare provider does not agree with them. However, the nurse has a responsibility to "do good" and "do no harm" based on the principles of beneficence and nonmaleficence. These ethical obligations are outlined in the American Nurses As-

A Patient With a Pressure Ulcer *(continued)*

The nurse hopes to work with Mrs. Krebs and the supervisor to set new goals and priorities and make progress toward them. The nurse understands that the patient has a right to make any final decisions.

Critical Thinking and the Nursing Process

1. What are the intrinsic and extrinsic factors that can cause skin problems in elderly adults? Make a list with two columns and see how many factors you can identify.
2. How important is nutrition to the dermatological health of your skin?
3. What type of dressings do you see used in your clinical rotations with older people? Are they consistent with current guidelines and recommendations?
4. What positioning techniques have you seen used in your clinical rotations?

- Evaluate your responses in Appendix B.

Nursing Care Plans help you approach care from a nursing process perspective. A case study of a real-life patient scenario illustrates the content described in the chapter and provides an example of various nursing interventions and the planning and implementation of nursing care. Each case study presents an **Ethical Dilemma** in anticipation of those you may encounter when delivering care to older persons. **Critical Thinking Exercises** follow the case studies and encourage you to engage in additional learning activities that stimulate and support learning. You can find suggested responses to the critical thinking questions in Appendix B. You can find additional Care Plan activities on the Companion Website, *www.prenhall.com/tabloski*.

Patient–Family Teaching Guidelines include sample questions and answers an older patient and his/her family may pose when receiving care. Each answer gives a rationale, so you provide succinct, focused answers to patient and family questions.

Patient-Family Teaching Guidelines

EDUCATION GUIDE TO ORAL HEALTH

Being older does not necessarily mean wearing dentures and being toothless. Older patients should be urged to take these steps to protect their oral health and preserve their teeth.

1. What can I do to protect my teeth now that I am older?

Suggestions for good oral health include:

- Drink fluoridated water and use fluoridated toothpaste; fluoride provides protection against dental decay at all ages.
- Practice good oral hygiene. Brush teeth carefully twice a day and floss daily to reduce dental plaque and prevent periodontal disease. Use an egg timer to ensure that brushing is carried out for at least 3 minutes.
- Get professional oral healthcare, even if you have no natural teeth. Professional care helps to maintain the overall health of the teeth and mouth, and provides for early detection of precancerous or cancerous lesions. For patients with teeth, see the dentist and dental hygienist twice a year for evaluation, cleaning, and scaling. For the patient without teeth, see the dentist yearly for an oral cancer check.

RATIONALE:

Good oral self-care and professional care are needed to maintain oral health. Ongoing yearly or twice-yearly appointments augment self-care practices.

2. Are there substances I should avoid in my daily habits?

- Avoid tobacco. In addition to the general health risks of tobacco use, smokers have 7 times the risk of developing periodontal disease compared to nonsmokers. Tobacco used in any form—cigarettes, cigars, pipes, and smokeless (chewing) tobacco—increases the risk for periodontal disease, oral and throat cancers, and oral fungal infections.
- Limit alcohol. Excessive alcohol consumption is a risk factor for oral and throat cancers. Alcohol and tobacco use together greatly increase the risk.
- Get dental care before, after, and during cancer treatment with chemotherapy and radiation. Careful attention is needed to treat and prevent damage that can destroy teeth and oral tissues.

RATIONALE:

Many older patients and their families are unaware of how important oral health is to their overall health and function. Those without teeth or with dentures may feel that they need not worry about mouth care. By reinforcing these guidelines, older patients' oral health and general health can be improved (Centers for Disease Control, 2001).

Caregivers should attend to the daily oral hygiene of older people who cannot care for themselves. This includes older people with cognitive impairments and physical frailty. It is important to note effective techniques and provide a consistent approach.

NANDA Nursing Diagnoses are suggested for many of the common diseases presented in order to help you categorize the nursing problems that accompany the medical diagnoses.

NURSING DIAGNOSES

Nursing diagnoses appropriate to the older person with problems of the skin may include any of the following (North American Nursing Diagnosis Association, 2002):

- *Impaired skin integrity related to lesions and inflammatory response*
- *Risk for impaired skin integrity related to physical immobility*
- *Risk for impaired skin integrity related to decreased skin turgor*
- *Risk for impaired skin integrity related to the effects of pressure, friction, or shear*
- *Risk for impaired tissue integrity related to decreased circulation*
- *Risk for infection related to pressure ulcer*
- *Pain related to destruction of tissue due to pressure and shear*

The two major nursing diagnoses related to integumentary problems are risk for *impaired tissue integrity*, and *impaired skin integrity*.

Impaired tissue integrity is defined as "a state in which an individual experiences, or is at risk for damage to the integumentary, corneal, or mucous membrane tissues of the body." Defining characteristics (major) that must be present include "disruptions of integumentary tissue or invasion of body structure (incision, dermal ulcer)" (Carpenito, 2002, p. 696). *Impaired skin integrity* is defined as "a state in which the individual experiences, or is at risk for damage to the epidermal and dermal tissue" (Carpenito, 2002, p. 705). The major defining characteristic that must be present is disruption of epidermal and dermal tissue. There is both overlap and possible confusion as to when to use these diagnoses. According to Carpenito (2002), *impaired tissue integrity* is the broad category under which more specific diagnoses fall. *Impaired skin integrity*

EXPLORE MediaLink box reminds you to use the media resources. MediaLink will further enhance your learning experience, build upon knowledge gained from this textbook, prepare you for the NCLEX-RN®, and foster critical thinking processes.
www.prenhall.com/tabloski

 EXPLORE MediaLink

NCLEX review, case studies, and other interactive resources for this chapter can be found on the Companion Website at **www.prenhall.com/tabloski**. Click on Chapter 12 to select the activities for this chapter. For animations, video tutorials, more NCLEX review questions, and an audio glossary, access the accompanying CD-ROM in this textbook.

SPECIAL FEATURES

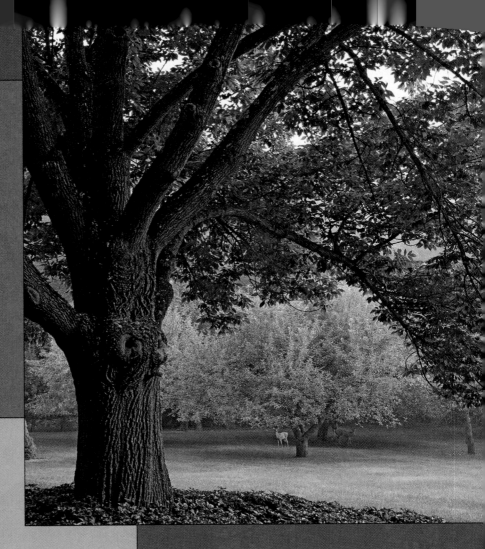
Foundations of Nursing Practice

CHAPTER 1

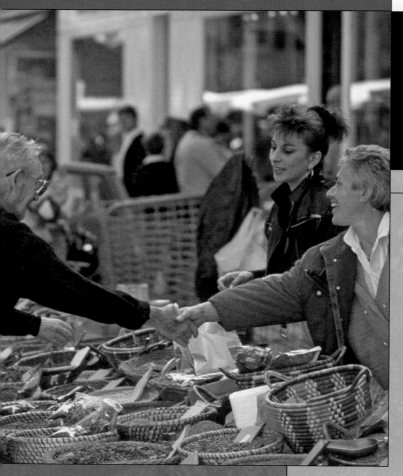

Principles of Gerontology

CHAPTER OBJECTIVES

Upon completion of this chapter, the reader will be able to:

- Identify mortality data according to race, gender, and age.
- Describe leading causes of disability among older adults.
- Identify common myths of aging.
- Describe the effects of chronic disease.
- Contrast several major theories of aging.
- Evaluate the natural history of disease using principles of epidemiology.

KEY TERMS

MediaLink

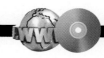

Additional resources for this chapter can be found on the Student CD-ROM accompanying this textbook and on the Companion Website at **www.prenhall.com/tabloski**. Click on Chapter 1 to select the activities for this chapter.

CD-ROM
- NCLEX Review
- Case Studies
- Tools

COMPANION WEBSITE
- Audio Glossary
- Additional NCLEX Review
- Case Study
- MediaLink Applications

The aging of America will trigger a huge demand for increased healthcare services. Nurses with skills in caring for older people will be especially in demand because of their understanding of the normal changes of aging and the ways that symptoms of illness and disease occur in the older adult. Gerontological nurses recognize that the presentation of disease and response to treatment differ in the older adult when compared to other groups of patients. The care of the frail older person, or the older person with multiple chronic conditions or comorbidities, presents a unique challenge. This book addresses the key issues involved in caring for the older person, with an emphasis on health problems encountered in the clinical setting.

The diverse health needs of an older person mandate diverse responses in the health delivery system. Older people receive nursing care in acute care hospitals, rehabilitation centers, long-term care facilities, assisted-living residences, home and community settings, ambulatory clinics, and a variety of other settings. The underlying core values and principles of **geriatrics** and gerontological nursing include health promotion, health protection, disease prevention, and treatment of disease, with emphasis on evidence-based best practices and current clinical practice guidelines. A well-educated and confident gerontological nurse is a vital member of the healthcare team and will bring improved health outcomes to older patients and their families by providing appropriate skilled nursing care and improving quality of life.

Aging is an inevitable and steadily progressive process that begins at the moment of conception and continues throughout the remainder of life. The life or aging process is artificially divided into stages and usually includes antepartum, neonate, toddler, child, adolescent, young adult, middle age, and older adult. The final stage of life, consisting of old age, can be the best or worst time of life and requires work and planning throughout all of the previous stages to be a successful and enjoyable period.

Most people do not consider the issues related to aging during their childhood and youth unless they have reason to contemplate certain milestones. For instance, some adolescents may anticipate reaching the age of 16 so that they may learn to drive an automobile. Perhaps others will anticipate turning 18 so they may enlist in the military. However, as we get older, we begin to dread our own aging because of the perception that disease, disability, and decline are inevitable consequences of the aging process. Many attitudes and myths about older people can be considered to be ageist or reflect negative stereotypes of aging. Box 1-1 lists myths of aging and why they are false.

Some people may say "you can't teach an old dog new tricks" when it comes to trying to change negative health behaviors such as smoking in older people. Others may think that everyone over 65 has lost the desire for sex and label an older man with a healthy sexual interest in another person a "dirty old man." While comments such as these can be hurtful and reflect poorly on the speaker, they do further damage by perpetuating stereotypes. Negative stereotypes of aging make it more difficult to recruit the best and the brightest nurses to work with older patients, limit the opportunities for rehabilitation and health promotion services offered to older people, and segregate older people from mainstream society.

The study of **gerontology** is a relatively new science. Congress created the National Institute on Aging in 1974 as part of the National Institutes of Health. In the 1950s and 1960s, little was known about aging. Much of the knowledge resulted from the study of diseases associated with aging. This practice resulted in the widespread idea that decline and illness were inevitable in old age (Dollemore, 2002). The focus of gerontology and gerontological nursing was to study, diagnose, and treat disease. However, in the last several years, the study of gerontology has moved beyond the disease focus to the improvement of health holistically, including physical, mental, emotional, and spiritual

Topic 1: Attitudes About Aging (E. Gould, C. Mariano, A. Sherman, M. Wallace)

Use the Facts on Aging Quiz (Palmore, 1998) to assess your attitudes and stereotypes of aging. Take it twice: once before beginning your clinical work with older persons and again several months later. Have you gained increased awareness of the concepts of ageism, myths, and successful aging, spirituality, and sexuality?

The Facts on Aging Quiz*

Instructions: Note which of the following statements are true and which are false.

1. The majority of old people (age 65+) are senile (have defective memory, are disoriented, or are psychologically challenged).
2. The five senses (sight, hearing, taste, touch, and smell) all tend to weaken in old age.
3. The majority of old people have no interest in nor capacity for sexual relations.
4. Lung vital capacity tends to decline in old age.
5. The majority of old people feel miserable most of the time.
6. Physical strength tends to decline in old age.
7. At least one-tenth of older adults are living in long-stay institutions (such as nursing homes, mental hospitals, homes for the aged, etc.).
8. Aged drivers have fewer accidents per driver than those under 65.
9. Older workers usually cannot work as effectively as younger workers.
10. Over three-fourths of older adults are healthy enough to carry out their normal activities without help.
11. The majority of older people are unable to adapt to change.
12. Older people usually take longer to learn something new.
13. Depression is more frequent among older adults than among younger people.
14. Older people tend to react slower than young people.
15. In general, old people tend to be pretty much alike.
16. The majority of old people say that they are seldom bored.
17. The majority of old people are socially isolated.
18. Older workers have fewer accidents than younger workers do.
19. Over 20% of the population are now age 65 or over.
20. The majority of medical practitioners tend to give low priority to the aged.
21. The majority of old people have incomes below the poverty line (as defined by the federal government).
22. The majority of old people are working or would like to have some kind of work to do (including housework and volunteer work).
23. Old people tend to become more religious as they age.
24. The majority of old people say they are seldom irritated or angry.
25. The health and economic status of old people will be about the same or worse in the year 2010 (compared to young people).

Answers to Facts on Aging Quiz: All odd numbers are false and all even numbers are true.

*The Facts on Aging Quiz, 2nd Edition, Palmore, E. B. Copyright © 1998, Springer Publishing Company, Inc., New York 10012. Used by permission.

	BOX
Myths of Aging and Why They Are False	**1-1**

- Myth: Being old means being sick.
  - Fact: Only 5% of older people live in nursing homes.
  - Fact: Some elderly people have chronic diseases but still function quite well.
- Myth: Older people are set in their ways and cannot learn new things.
  - Fact: Older people should be challenged to stay mentally active.
  - Fact: Older people who learn to play an instrument or learn a new language are less likely to get Alzheimer's disease.
- Myth: Health promotion is wasted on older people.
  - Fact: It is never too late to start good lifestyle habits like eating a healthy diet and engaging in exercise.
  - Fact: It is never too late to stop bad habits like smoking cigarettes or drinking too much alcohol.
- Myth: The elderly do not pull their own weight.
  - Fact: Older people contribute greatly to society by supporting the arts, doing volunteer work, and helping with grandchildren.
  - Fact: Paid employment is not the only measure of value and productivity.

Source: Adapted from Rowe, J., & Kahn, R. (1998). Breaking down the myths of aging. *Successful aging.* New York: Pantheon Books. Used by permission of Pantheon Books, a division of Random House, Inc.

---

well-being. The study of aging and health is imperative if older people are to enjoy quality of life in their final years. The enlightened nurse now knows that growing older is a privilege and the older person is biologically elite. Those who suffer from inherited illnesses, weak immune systems, and the inevitable damage from devastating poverty and substance abuse do not usually live to be old. Growing older is a reward and a time to be treasured and enjoyed. Some of the benefits of healthy aging are listed in Box 1-2.

The goal for nurses who provide healthcare to older people is not only to help them live longer, but also to help them live better. The healthcare needs of older patients are unique because of their stage of life, just as the health needs of children are different from those of adults. Most healthcare professionals do not receive the education and training necessary to respond to the unique and complex health needs of older adults (O'Neill, 2002). As a result, many older people receive inappropriate healthcare that may be harmful or limit their quality of life. Today, a nurse's typical patient is an older adult (Rosenfeld, Bottrell, Fulmer, & Mezey, 1999). Nursing educators must address

---

	BOX
Benefits of Healthy Aging	**1-2**

- Creativity and confidence are enhanced.
- Coping ability increases.
- Gratitude and appreciation deepen.
- Confidence increases with less reliance on the approval of others.
- Self-understanding and acceptance increase.

this issue by providing specialty courses with a gerontology focus and general content on aging during the basic nursing curriculum.

Demographics and Aging

Countries all over the world are facing demographic aging. In the United States, we often speak of "the graying of America," but all nations are or soon will be faced with important issues regarding the provision of healthcare to older persons. In 1997, approximately 10% (561 million) of the world's population was age 60 and older, and this level is projected to increase to 15% by 2025 (Gist & Velkoff, 1997). The U.S. population has more than tripled from 76 million in 1900 to 281 million in 2000.

Past fertility trends exerted the strongest influence on the U.S. age structure in the 20th century. Relatively high fertility at the start of the century, lower fertility in the late 1920s and 1930s, and higher fertility after World War II during the baby boom all affected the U.S. age composition. At the beginning of the 20th century, half of the U.S. population was younger than 22.9 years. At the century's end, half of the population was younger than 35.3 years, the country's highest median age ever (Hobbs & Stoops, 2002). The baby boomers, people born between 1946 and 1964, have had and will continue to exert a profound impact on American culture and demographics. In 2011, the first wave of boomers will turn 65 and this trend will continue for many years. Figure 1-1 ■ illustrates the changing age structure of the United States and projects the impact of the increased numbers of aging baby boomers.

Longevity and the Sex Differential

Prior to 1950, the male population outnumbered the female population. In 1950, this trend reversed. Women comprise the majority of the older population (55%) in all nations, and the majority of these women (58%) live in developing countries. Older women face different circumstances than men as they age. They are more likely to be widowed, to live alone, to be less educated, and to have fewer years of labor experi-

FIGURE ■ **1-1**

U.S. population age structure, 2000 and 2030 (projected).

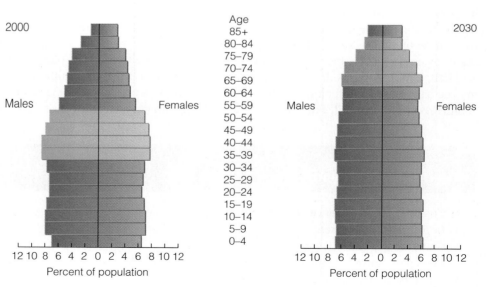

Baby-boom generation born between 1946 and 1964

Source: Centers for Disease Control, 2004.

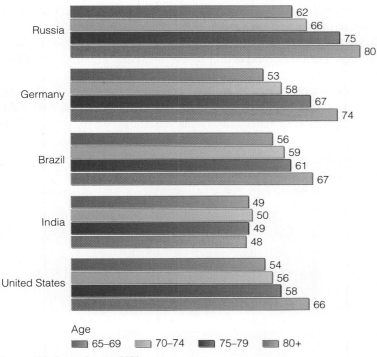

Source: U.S. Census Bureau, 2000.

FIGURE ■ 1-2

Percentage of females for older age groups, 2000.

ence, resulting in poverty (Gist & Velkoff, 1997). By 2025, nearly three quarters of the world's older women are expected to reside in what is known today as the developing world. The term *feminization of later life* describes how women predominate at older ages and how the proportions increase with advancing age (Arber, Davidson, & Ginn, 2003). In most countries, the relative female advantage increases with advancing age (U.S. Census Bureau, 2001) (Figure 1-2 ■).

Practice Pearl

Elderly women greatly outnumber elderly men in most nations. Therefore, the health and socioeconomic problems of the elderly are, to a large extent, the problems of elderly women (Kinsella & Gist, 1998).

Several observations can be made concerning the trends observed in developed countries. The differences between countries have narrowed over time. Male life expectancy has not improved as much as female life expectancy, and the differences between male and female longevity have widened over time (Kinsella & Gist, 1998). Some demographers predict that the gender gap will occur in developing countries as well over the next several years as women "catch up" to men in terms of educational and economic attainment.

The gender differences in **life expectancy** may be explained by the complex interaction between biological, social, and behavioral factors. Greater male exposure to **risk factors** such as tobacco, alcohol, and occupational hazards might negatively affect male life expectancy. If women begin to approach the rates of tobacco and alcohol use and face the same environmental hazards as men, the gender gap may narrow (Kinsella & Gist, 1998).

Human life expectancy has increased greatly in many parts of the world during the last century. Industrialized countries have made great progress in extending life expectancy at birth. Japan has the highest life expectancy of the world's major nations, with the average Japanese born today expecting to live 80 years. Figure 1-3 ■ illustrates life expectancy at birth for selected countries.

In the United States, there were nearly 35 million people over the age of 65 as documented in the 2000 census. The most rapid growth of the older population occurred in the oldest age groups. The population 85 years and over increased by 38% from 3.1 million

FIGURE ■ 1-3

Life expectancy at birth for selected countries, 1900–1998.

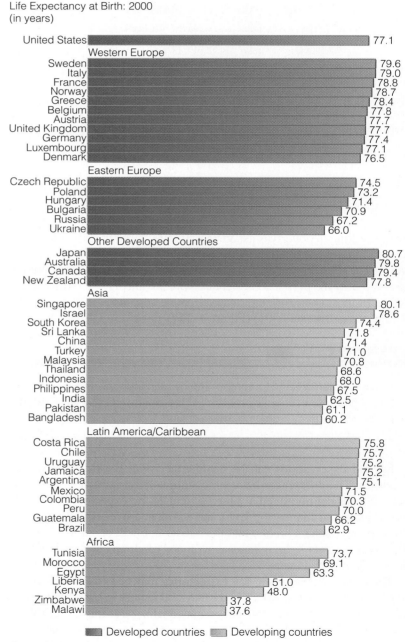

Life Expectancy at Birth: 2000
(in years)

Country	Years
United States	77.1
Western Europe	
Sweden	79.6
Italy	79.0
France	78.8
Norway	78.7
Greece	78.4
Belgium	77.8
Austria	77.7
United Kingdom	77.7
Germany	77.4
Luxembourg	77.1
Denmark	76.5
Eastern Europe	
Czech Republic	74.5
Poland	73.2
Hungary	71.4
Bulgaria	70.9
Russia	67.2
Ukraine	66.0
Other Developed Countries	
Japan	80.7
Australia	79.8
Canada	79.4
New Zealand	77.8
Asia	
Singapore	80.1
Israel	78.6
South Korea	74.4
Sri Lanka	71.8
China	71.4
Turkey	71.0
Malaysia	70.8
Thailand	68.6
Indonesia	68.0
Philippines	67.5
India	62.5
Pakistan	61.1
Bangladesh	60.2
Latin America/Caribbean	
Costa Rica	75.8
Chile	75.7
Uruguay	75.2
Jamaica	75.2
Argentina	75.1
Mexico	71.5
Colombia	70.3
Peru	70.0
Guatemala	66.2
Brazil	62.9
Africa	
Tunisia	73.7
Morocco	69.1
Egypt	63.3
Liberia	51.0
Kenya	48.0
Zimbabwe	37.8
Malawi	37.6

■ Developed countries ▨ Developing countries

Source: U.S. Census Bureau 2000.

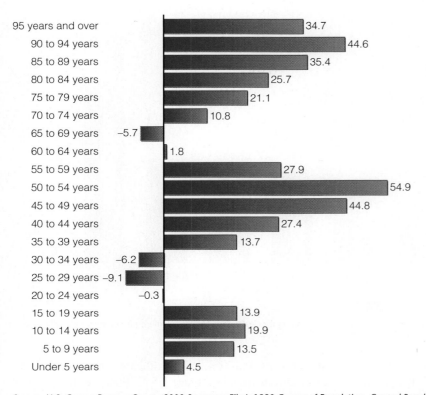

U.S. population percent change by age between 1990 and 2000.

Source: U.S. Census Bureau. Census 2000 Summary File I: 1990 Census of Population. *General Population Characteristics, United States* (1990 CP.1.13).

to 4.2 million. The implication of the rapid growth of the population over 85 (old-old) is that there will be larger numbers of older people with chronic illness and disabilities and a greater demand for preventive health services. Figure 1-4 ■ illustrates the rates of change by age between 1990 and 2000.

LIFE AFTER 65

Women who reach the age of 65 can expect to live another 19 years, while men can expect to live another 16. This increase in life expectancy has been attributed to improved healthcare, increased use of preventive services, and healthier lifestyles. Experts disagree as to whether this trend in life expectancy can continue without major treatment advances or even cures in heart disease and cancer, the major causes of death in the elderly (O'Neill, 2002). However, nurses should be aggressive in health promotion efforts and rehabilitation after surgery or illness, because the 65-year-old man or woman has the potential for 16 to 19 years of additional life. This is three to four times the traditional definition of the "cure" rate for cancer (5 years without recurrence) and can be a time of significant health or significant disability. Most older people would prefer to live out their final years independently and reside in their own homes, rather than living in extended care facilities and relying on others for care.

Chronic conditions usually develop over long periods and thus offer ample opportunity for nurses and other healthcare professionals to screen, detect, educate, and intervene. Using the principles of **epidemiology**, the study of health among populations, the stages of chronic disease have been documented to start at about age 20. The disease process may be altered or change course with a resultant increase or decrease in

FIGURE ☐ 1-5

Selected chronic conditions affecting U.S. adults age 70 or older.

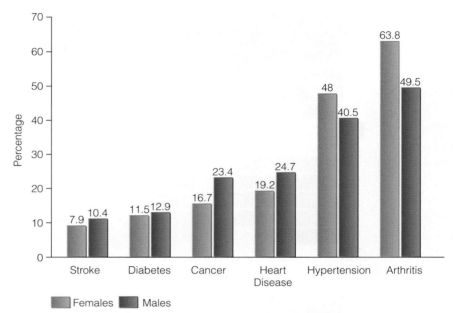

Source: Centers for Disease Control. National Center for Health Statistics. Supplement on Aging Study and Second Supplement on Aging Study. 1995.

symptoms. The actions that older persons, families, and healthcare professionals take can alter and change the course of a chronic illness. Figure 1-5 ☐ illustrates the chronic illnesses most commonly experienced by older persons in the United States.

During the many years it takes most chronic diseases to develop, nurses have the opportunity to intervene using the three levels of prevention designated as primary, secondary, and tertiary. Box 1-3 illustrates nursing interventions to promote health in older people.

The best strategy for the control of diagnosed chronic disease in the older adult is to employ tertiary prevention and attempt to slow the progression of the illness and prevent or reverse disabling loss of function. However, the nurse will have the opportunity to use primary and secondary prevention techniques in other areas of the older person's risk profile. For instance, when caring for an older patient after a surgical intervention to repair a broken wrist suffered in a fall, the nurse may avert a future stroke or myocardial infarction by carefully noting and reporting a consistently elevated blood pressure. Remembering that the person at age 65 has another 16 to 19 years of life expectancy, the nurse may employ all three levels of health prevention simultaneously even in the older person diagnosed with chronic illness.

In recent years, Medicare has expanded coverage of preventive services to encourage older people to stay healthy. Changes in coverage occur on an ongoing basis, and the gerontological nurse is urged to keep track of these changes by visiting Medicare or calling 1-800-MEDICAR (1-800-633-4227). At the present time, Medicare does not pay for routine physical examinations. However, Medicare Part B does cover the following preventive services:

- Screenings for breast, cervical, vaginal, colorectal, and prostate cancer
  - Fecal occult blood testing (once yearly)
  - Flexible sigmoidoscopy (once every 4 years)
  - Colonoscopy (once every 2 years for those at high risk)
  - Barium enema
  - Mammograms (routine screenings once yearly)

BOX 1-3

Nursing Interventions to Promote Health in Older People

Primary Prevention—Health Promotion
- Education
- Nutritional assessment and guidance
- Exercise prescriptions as appropriate
- Avoidance of tobacco
- Moderation of alcohol
- Limiting exposure or avoiding known carcinogens

Secondary Prevention—Early Diagnosis and Prompt Treatment
- Screening questions and health assessment (use of standardized assessment instruments appropriate for older adults, including function, cognition, mood, mobility, pain, skin integrity, quality of life, nutrition, neglect, and abuse)

- Referral for examination and testing
- Disease cure and aggressive treatment to limit disability and stop disease progression

Tertiary Prevention—Restoration and Rehabilitation
- Multidisciplinary rehabilitation (physical, occupational, speech, and recreational therapy)
- Short-term placement in rehabilitation facilities or aggressive in-home rehabilitation
- Appropriate services and aids to increase independence (walkers, canes, homemaker/home health aid, visiting nurse)

- Pap smears and pelvic examination (once yearly)
- Prostate-specific antigen (PSA) test (once yearly)
- Bone mass screening—once yearly for those at risk
- Diabetes monitoring—glucose monitors, test strips, lancets, and self-management training for those with diabetes
- Flu, pneumonia, and hepatitis B vaccinations—annual flu vaccine, pneumonia vaccine at the physician's discretion, and hepatitis B vaccine for those at medium to high risk for hepatitis

(Centers for Medicare and Medicaid Services, 2004)

As nurses and other healthcare professionals continue to work on closing the gap between **life span** and healthy life span, the older adult should be urged to assume more responsibility for healthy aging. About 70% of physical decline that occurs with aging is related to modifiable factors such as smoking, poor nutrition, lack of physical activity, injuries from falls, and failure to use Medicare-covered preventive services (CDC, 2004). Older people should be educated regarding the need to start exercise programs, stop smoking, and engage in other healthy behaviors (O'Neill, 2002). Nurses often interact with older patients when they are suffering an acute health problem or traumatic injury. This interaction can be an opportunity to achieve broader goals and improve the long-term health status of older people by reducing health risk behaviors.

Practice Pearl

The three major misconceptions about aging and health are that disease in old age is normal, older adults have no future and therefore health promotion efforts are wasted, and damage to health from poor diet and inactivity is irreversible (Kolcaba & Wykle, 1994).

BOX 1-4 Top 10 Causes of Death in the United States

1. Diseases of the heart
2. Cancer
3. Stroke
4. Chronic obstructive pulmonary disease (COPD)
5. Unintentional injury
6. Diabetes mellitus
7. Influenza and pneumonia
8. Alzheimer's disease
9. Nephritis and nephrosis
10. All other causes

Source: Centers for Disease Control, 2003.

LIVING LONGER OR LIVING BETTER?

In the 1990s, two of the three leading killers of older Americans (heart disease and stroke) declined by about one third. Box 1-4 notes the top 10 causes of death in the United States.

Five chronic diseases—heart disease, cancer, stroke, chronic obstructive pulmonary disease, and diabetes—cause more than two thirds of all deaths each year. The number of deaths alone, however, fails to convey the toll of chronic disease. More than 125 million Americans live with these diseases, and millions of new cases are diagnosed each year. Although treatable, these diseases are not curable. There is a great burden from the disability and diminished quality of life resulting from these diseases. Chronic, disabling conditions cause major limitations in activity for 1 of every 10 Americans, or 30 million people. Costs of caring for chronic illness are staggering both to older persons and their family members and to society. The cost of medical care for Americans with chronic illness was $470 billion in 1995, and these costs are projected to be as high as $864 billion in 2040 as the baby boomers continue to age (Centers for Disease Control, 2004). Box 1-5 lists the most common causes of disability in the United States.

BOX 1-5 Most Common Causes of Disability in the United States

- Arthritis or rheumatism
- Back or spine problems
- Heart trouble/hardening of the arteries
- Lung or respiratory problems
- Deafness or hearing problems
- Limb/extremity stiffness
- Mental or emotional problems
- Diabetes mellitus
- Blindness or vision problems
- Stroke

Source: Centers for Disease Control. (2004). *Chronic disease prevention, healthy aging: Preventing disease and improving quality of life among older Americans,* http://www.cdc.gov

Many people who have chronic conditions and disabilities lead active, productive lives, but some require assistance with activities of daily living (ADLs). About 41 million Americans with chronic conditions require assistance daily. In general, older people with lower incomes are more likely to have conditions that are difficult or costly to treat. African Americans are more likely than Caucasians to have limitations in ADLs when chronically ill. Older African American men and women with arthritis are more likely to have activity limitations than other older people (National Academy on an Aging Society, 1999). Nearly 60% of older African Americans report high blood pressure, and a growing number of older African Americans and Hispanics are reporting diabetes (O'Neill, 2002).

The number of Americans with chronic conditions is expected to increase significantly over the next several years. This will pose a challenge for nurses and other healthcare providers. The hospitalization rates are higher for those with arthritis and hypertension, two common chronic conditions of older people. Chronic conditions also affect emotional health. Women with chronic conditions are more likely to rate their health as poor, and older African American women provide the least positive assessment of their emotional well-being (National Academy on an Aging Society, 1999). The combined effects of poor health status with the negative impact of age and racial discrimination may be responsible for these assessments. With the cost of healthcare rising each year, the United States already faces the challenge of providing appropriate and accessible healthcare to all persons. In planning for the future, it will also be important to recognize that different groups of older and chronically ill persons have different healthcare needs.

Americans can improve their chances for a healthy old age by simply taking advantage of recommended preventive health services and by making healthy lifestyle changes. The challenge for nurses and other healthcare professionals is to encourage people at all stages of life to reduce their chances of disability and chronic illness by undertaking healthy lifestyle changes. This strategy will improve quality of life, delay disability, and increase the number of healthy years an older person is expected to live (O'Neill, 2002). Box 1-6 illustrates actions nurses and other healthcare professionals can take to improve older Americans' health and quality of life.

Healthy People 2010

Healthy People 2010 is the prevention agenda for the United States. It is a statement of national health objectives designed to identify the most significant preventable threats to health and to establish national goals to reduce these threats. The U.S. Department of Health and Human Services recently published this document with 28 specific areas for health improvement in 467 objectives. The two basic goals of this document are:

1. To increase quality and years of healthy life.
2. To eliminate health disparities.

The first goal signals the importance of quality of life as well as length of life. By placing emphasis on these two vital concepts in one goal, the link between the two is reaffirmed. The second goal, eliminating health disparities, addresses the growing problems related to access to quality healthcare and differences in treatment based upon age, race, sex, and insurance coverage. The goals of *Healthy People 2010* serve as a guide for healthcare research, practice, and policy, and set the

---

BOX 1-6 **Opportunities to Improve Older Americans' Health and Quality of Life**

Poor health and loss of independence are **not** inevitable consequences of aging. The following strategies have proven effective in promoting the health of older adults:

■ **Healthy lifestyles** Research has shown that healthy lifestyles are more influential than genetic factors in helping older people avoid the deterioration traditionally associated with aging. People who are physically active, eat a healthy diet, do not use tobacco, and practice other healthy behaviors reduce their risk for chronic diseases and have half the rate of disability of those who do not lead healthy lifestyles.

■ **Early detection of diseases** Screening to detect chronic diseases early in their course, when they are most treatable, can save many lives; however, many older adults have not had recommended screenings. For example, 60% of Americans over age 65 have not had a sigmoidoscopy or colonoscopy in the previous 5 years to screen for colorectal cancer, even though Medicare covers the cost.

■ **Immunizations** More than 40,000 people age 65 or older die each year of influenza and invasive pneumococcal disease. Immunizations reduce a person's risk for hospitalization and death from these diseases. Yet in 2002, 32% of Americans age 65 or older had not had a recent flu shot, and 37% had never received a pneumonia vaccine.

■ **Injury prevention** Falls are the most common cause of injuries to older adults. More than one third of adults age 65 or older fall each year. Of those who fall, 20% to 30% suffer moderate to severe injuries that decrease mobility and independence. Removing tripping hazards in the home and installing grab bars are simple measures that can greatly reduce older Americans' risk for falls and fractures.

■ **Self-management techniques** Programs to teach older Americans self-management techniques can reduce the pain and costs of chronic disease. For example, the Arthritis Self-Help Course, disseminated by the Arthritis Foundation, has been shown to reduce arthritis pain by 20% and visits to physicians by 40%. Unfortunately, less than 1% of Americans with arthritis participate in such programs, and courses are not available in many areas.

Source: Centers for Disease Control. (2004). *Healthy aging: Preventing disease and improving quality of life among older Americans,* http://www.cdc.gov

agenda for healthcare reform over the next 10 years. The focus areas pertinent to older people are listed in Box 1-7.

It is apparent when reviewing this list that nurses can intervene in most of these focus areas to promote health and wellness in older people. Many of the focus areas are linked to one another, and intervening in one area may stimulate a positive outcome in several other areas. For instance, by educating an older person about the benefits of a healthy nutritious diet, the nurse may decrease the chance of cancer, obesity, diabetes, heart disease, and stroke, and improve mobility to prevent falls. Further, the older person who eats a nutritious diet will probably have more energy to engage in social and recreational activities, thereby decreasing the chance of depression and social isolation.

To view the entire report, go to *Healthy People 2010.* Detailed information is provided regarding each focus area, and specific objectives are suggested for each age group.

MediaLink   *Healthy People 2010*

	BOX 1-7
Focus Areas in *Healthy People 2010* Applicable to Older Persons	

- Access to quality health services
- Arthritis, osteoporosis, and chronic back conditions
- Cancer
- Chronic kidney disease
- Diabetes
- Disability and secondary conditions
- Educational and community-based programs
- Environmental health
- Food safety
- Health communication
- Heart disease and stroke
- Human immunodeficiency virus

- Immunization and infectious diseases
- Injury and violence prevention
- Medical product safety
- Mental health and mental conditions
- Nutrition and obesity
- Occupational safety and health
- Oral health
- Physical activity and fitness
- Public health infrastructure
- Respiratory diseases
- Sexually transmitted diseases
- Substance abuse
- Tobacco use
- Vision and hearing

Source: *Healthy People 2010,* http://www.health.gov/healthypeople

Theories of Aging

The study of aging continues to grow and evolve, and new insights are uncovered daily as scientists make progress. The quest to understand aging, which began as the pursuit of one all-encompassing theory, has evolved to the knowledge that multiple processes can affect how humans age. These processes combine and interact on many levels, and individual cells, proteins, tissues, and organ systems are all involved. Some of the changes of aging are benign and superficial such as graying of the hair and wrinkling of the skin. Others, however, increase the risk of disease and disability, such as arteriosclerosis. Gerontologists prefer to use the term **senescence** when referring to the progressive deterioration of body systems that can increase the risk of mortality as an individual gets older.

The rate and progression of aging varies greatly from one individual to the next. Even identical twins that possess the same genetic makeup will age differently. If everyone aged at the same rate and in the same way, we would become more alike as we get older. However, just the opposite is true. When a group of older people gathers, there is a great variety in the way they look, express their attitudes, engage in recreational and social activities, and relate health problems. Notice the variety and differences in the older persons depicted in Figure 1-6 ■.

Generally, each body system is affected by aging. Some of the changes can begin in the 20s and 30s. "Plastic" or modifiable changes can be slowed by exercise, good nutrition, and other elements of a healthy lifestyle. For example, most people can avoid lung disease by not smoking and avoiding secondhand smoke exposure. There is a growing understanding of what is considered to be a disease or common problem of aging and what is considered as part of the "normal" aging process. Normal aging consists of those universal changes that occur in all older people. It is generally accepted that the level of organ reserve declines as we grow older. Longitudinal studies such as the Baltimore Longitudinal Study of Aging have supplied valuable information that can help to define normal aging. However, even within one person's organs and organ systems there are different rates of decline. Understanding these changes

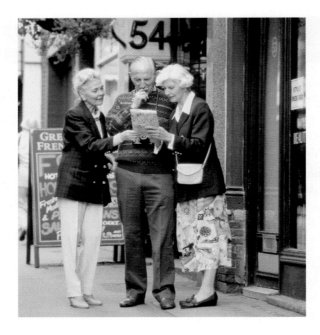

can help to distinguish chronological age (number of years from birth) from physiological age (degree of senescence experienced by each body system). Figure 1-7 □ illustrates normal changes of aging.

Normal aging includes the following changes:

1. **Heart.** Heart muscles thicken with age. The heart's maximum pumping rate and
   the body's ability to extract oxygen from blood diminish with age.
2. **Arteries.** Arteries tend to stiffen with age. The older heart has to beat harder to
   supply the energy needed to propel the blood forward through less elastic arteries.
3. **Lungs.** Maximum breathing capacity may decline by about 40% between the
   ages of 40 and 70.
4. **Brain.** With age, the brain loses some of the axons and neurons that connect with
   each other. Recent studies indicate that the older brain can be stimulated to produce
   new neurons, but the exact conditions that stimulate this growth are unknown.
5. **Kidneys.** Kidneys gradually become less efficient at removing waste from blood.
6. **Bladder.** Bladder capacity declines.
7. **Body fat.** Body fat typically increases until about middle age and then stabilizes
   until late life when weight tends to decline. When weight declines, older people
   lose both muscle and fat. With age, fat is redistributed to the deeper organs from
   the skin. Fat that is redistributed to the abdomen rather than the hips (being apple shaped rather than pear shaped) makes older men and women more vulnerable to heart disease.
8. **Muscles.** Without exercise, muscle mass declines 22% for women and 23% for
   men between the ages of 30 and 70. Exercise can slow this rate of loss.
9. **Bones.** Bone mineral is lost and replaced throughout life, but the loss outpaces
   the replacement for women at about age 35. This loss is accelerated at
   menopause. Regular weight-bearing exercise and high calcium intake can
   slow bone loss.

Normal changes of aging.

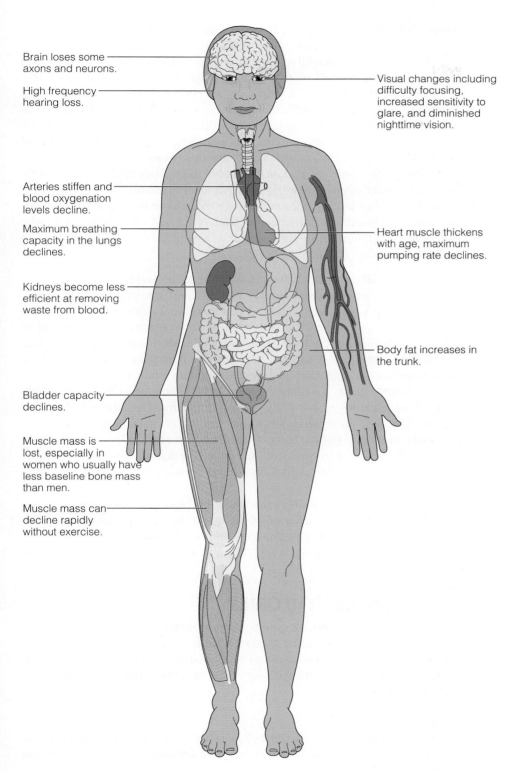

Brain loses some axons and neurons.

High frequency hearing loss.

Visual changes including difficulty focusing, increased sensitivity to glare, and diminished nighttime vision.

Arteries stiffen and blood oxygenation levels decline.

Maximum breathing capacity in the lungs declines.

Heart muscle thickens with age, maximum pumping rate declines.

Kidneys become less efficient at removing waste from blood.

Body fat increases in the trunk.

Bladder capacity declines.

Muscle mass is lost, especially in women who usually have less baseline bone mass than men.

Muscle mass can decline rapidly without exercise.

10. **Sight.** Difficulty focusing close up may begin in the 40s. After age 50, there is increased sensitivity to glare, greater difficulty in seeing at low levels of light, and more difficulty in detecting moving objects. Adapting to light changes and nighttime driving become more difficult. At age 70, ability to distinguish fine details begins to decline.

11. **Hearing.** It becomes more difficult to hear higher frequencies with aging. Even older adults with good hearing may have difficulty distinguishing vowels and understanding speech, especially in situations with high levels of background noise. Hearing declines more quickly in men than women.

12. **Personality.** Personality is remarkably stable throughout adult life, and rarely do healthy older people show signs of personality change during their final years. Personality usually does not change radically even as a result of major lifestyle changes such as retirement or death of a loved one. Older people who experience health problems, chronic illness, and pain are at risk for depression and social isolation (Dollemore, 2002).

The final result of all the normal changes of aging is the loss of organ reserve, or the ability of a given organ to react quickly and efficiently to physiological stress. When an individual is very young, the heart can increase its output during exercise sixfold, the kidneys can excrete efficiently if 80% of the nephrons are damaged or destroyed, and surgeons can remove a lung or three fourths of the liver without loss of life or function. The organ systems of the body combine their efforts and orchestrate a complicated set of responses designed to maintain equilibrium. This equilibrium consists of temperature, acid-base balance, body chemicals, and other vital life components. This tendency of the body toward maintaining equilibrium is called **homeostasis**. The loss of organ reserve that can occur with aging can lead to **homeostenosis**, or inability of the body to restore homeostasis after even minor environmental challenges such as trauma or infection. Therefore, an older person may die from pneumonia or influenza that may have been only a minor illness to a younger person (Mion, 2003).

Theories of aging fall into several groups, including biological, psychological, and sociological theories. A brief description of the major theories in each category follows; however, with the tools of biotechnology and new knowledge regarding aging, all-encompassing theories of aging are giving way to a more diverse perspective (Dollemore, 2002).

BIOLOGICAL AGING THEORIES

Biological aging theories fall into two groups: programmed theories and error theories. Programmed theories assert that aging follows a biological timetable and may represent a continuation of the cycle that regulates childhood growth and development. The error theories emphasize environmental assaults to the human system that gradually cause things to go wrong.

Programmed Theories

Programmed theories hypothesize that the body's genetic codes contain instructions for the regulation of cellular reproduction and death. The following are some of the most popular programmed theories.

Programmed Longevity. Aging is the result of the sequential switching on and off of certain genes, with senescence defined as the point in time when age-associated functional deficits are manifested. Persons who endorse this theory are interested in studying the human genome and genetic theories of aging.

Endocrine Theory. Biological clocks act through hormones to control the pace of aging. Proponents of this theory ascribe to the use of various natural and synthetic hormones, such as human growth hormone, to slow the aging process.

Immunological Theory. A programmed decline in immune system functions leads to an increased vulnerability to infectious disease, aging, and eventual death. Declines in immune system function can affect the outcomes of many illnesses such as postoperative infections, diabetes, urinary tract infections, and pneumonia. It is generally accepted that a healthy diet and lifestyle coupled with preventive health measures, such as a yearly flu shot and limiting exposure to pathogens, can support immune function in the older person.

Error Theories

The most popular error theories are listed below and hypothesize that environmental assaults and the body's constant need to manufacture energy and fuel metabolic activities cause toxic by-products to accumulate. These toxic by-products may eventually impair normal body function and cellular repair.

Wear and Tear Theory. Cells and organs have vital parts that wear out after years of use. Proponents of this theory believe that a "master clock" controls all organs and that cellular function slows down with time and becomes less efficient at repairing body malfunctions that are caused by environmental assaults. Abusing or neglecting one organ or body system can stimulate premature aging and disease (e.g., a person who drinks excessive amounts of alcohol may develop liver disease).

Cross-Link Theory. In this theory, an accumulation of cross-linked proteins resulting from the binding of glucose (simple sugars) to protein (a process that occurs under the presence of oxygen) causes various problems. Once the binding occurs, the protein cannot perform normally and may result in visual problems like cataracts or wrinkling and skin aging. The modern diet is often high in sugar and carbohydrates, and some nutritionists believe that low-carbohydrate diets can slow the development of cross-links (American Federation for Aging Research, 2004).

Free Radical Theory. Accumulated damage caused by oxygen radicals causes cells, and eventually organs, to lose function and organ reserve. The use of antioxidants and vitamins is believed to slow this damage.

Somatic DNA Damage Theory. Genetic mutations occur and accumulate with increasing age, causing cells to deteriorate and malfunction. Proponents believe that genetic manipulation and alteration may slow the aging process.

PSYCHOLOGICAL AGING THEORIES

Most psychological theories advance that various coping or adaptive strategies must occur for a person to age successfully. The triggers might be the physical changes of aging, issues of retirement, dealing with the death of spouse or friends, and perhaps declining health. Major psychological aging theories include Jung's theory of individualism and Erickson's developmental theory.

Jung's Theory of Individualism

This theory hypothesizes that as a person ages, the shift of focus is away from the external world (extroversion) toward the inner experience (introversion). At this stage of life, the older person will search for answers to many of life's riddles and try to find the essence of the "true self." To age successfully, the older person will accept past accomplishments and failures (Jung, 1960). Older persons subscribing to Jung's theory may spend a lot of time in contemplation and introspection.

Erickson's Developmental Theory

According to Erickson (1950), there are eight stages of life with developmental tasks to be accomplished at each stage. The task of the older adult includes ego integrity versus despair. Erickson advanced that during this stage the older adult will become preoccupied with acceptance of eventual death without becoming morbid or obsessed with these thoughts. If major failures or disappointments have occurred in the older person's life, this final stage may be difficult to accomplish because the older person may be despairing rather than accepting of death. Older persons who have not achieved ego integrity may look back on their lives with dissatisfaction and feel unhappy, depressed, or angry over what they have done or failed to do. Psychological counseling can help to resolve some of these issues.

SOCIOLOGICAL AGING THEORIES

Sociological theories of aging differ from biological theories because they tend to focus on roles and relationships that occur in later life. Each of the theories must be judged within the context of time that they were formulated. Major sociological theories of aging include disengagement theory, activity theory, and continuity theory.

Disengagement Theory

Introduced by Cummings and Henry in 1961, this controversial theory asserts that the appropriate pattern of behavior in later life is for the older person and society at large to engage in a mutual and reciprocal withdrawal. Thus, when death occurs, neither the older individual nor society is disadvantaged and social equilibrium is maintained. Mandatory retirement forces some older people to withdraw from work-related roles, accelerating the process of disengagement. In some cultures, older people remain engaged, active, and busy throughout their lives.

Activity Theory

This theory contradicts the disengagement theory by proposing that older adults should stay active and engaged if they are to age successfully (Havighurst, Neugarten, & Tobin, 1963). By staying active and extending the activities enjoyed in middle age, the older person has a better chance of enjoying old age. Happiness and satisfaction with life are assumed to result from a high level of involvement with the world and continued social involvement. According to this theory, when retirement occurs, replacement activities must be found.

Continuity Theory

This theory advances that successful aging involves maintaining or continuing previous values, habits, preferences, family ties, and all other linkages that have formed the basic underlying structure of adult life. Older age is not viewed as a time that should trigger major life readjustment, but rather just a time to continue being the same person (Havighurst et al., 1963). According to this theory, the pace of activities may be slowed. Activities pursued in earlier life that did not bring satisfaction and genuine happiness may be dropped at the discretion of the older person. For some, gaining relief from constant time pressures and deadlines is one of the bounties of old age.

Patient and Family Teaching

Gerontological nurses require skills and knowledge related to teaching patients and families about the key concepts of gerontology and the role of gerontological nurses. The patient-family teaching guidelines in the following feature will assist the nurse to assume the role of teacher and coach. Educating patients and families is critical so that older patients can assume a larger role in health promotion activities.

Patient-Family Teaching Guidelines

LEARNING ABOUT GERONTOLOGY

1. What is gerontology?

Gerontology is the study of aging. It involves all aspects of an older person's life, including physical, social, psychological, and spiritual function.

RATIONALE:

Many people including some healthcare professionals are unaware that gerontology is holistic, encompasses more than the medical model, and involves all aspects of an older person's life.

2. Why is this important to an older person like me?

With aging, an older person's health status can be affected by many factors. Gerontologists and geriatricians have extra training to become experts in the factors that can affect health status and function, including management of chronic illness, proper medication use, lifestyle changes to improve health, disease prevention and health promotion techniques, and early detection of diseases.

RATIONALE:

Nurses can educate older patients and their families regarding the many factors that contribute to maintaining and improving health status and function throughout the entire lifespan with emphasis on staying healthy in old age.

3. Is it too late for me to do anything to make myself healthier?

It is never too late to address behaviors and lifestyle choices that can contribute to premature death or disability. The top killers in the United States are heart disease, cancer, and stroke. Smoking, poor nutrition, and physical inactivity all can contribute to the formation and progression of these diseases.

RATIONALE:

The nurse should educate older persons and their families regarding the link between lifestyle choices and unfavorable health outcomes in an attempt to provide motivation and incentive for improving health behaviors.

4. Where should I go to get further information?

Many hospitals, community health agencies, and healthcare professionals can guide you to choose an appropriate source of information. Look for a specialty clinic with a geriatrician, advanced practice gerontological nurse,

RATIONALE:

Many older persons and their adult children are interested in learning more about staying healthy and seeking

(continued)

Patient-Family Teaching Guidelines, *cont.*

gerontological nurse, social worker, nutritionist, physical therapist, occupational therapist, and geropsychiatrist as part of a team to specialize in caring for older adults. These experts can address many common health problems of older people, including falls, medication side effects, pain, sleep disorders, memory problems, and urinary incontinence.

5. Should all older people be cared for by a team of geriatric experts?

There is great diversity in health needs of people over the age of 65. While it is generally agreed that all older people would benefit from receiving their healthcare from geriatric specialists, many older people are well cared for by primary care physicians, advanced practice nurses, and family physicians. Geriatricians are sought to provide care for frail older persons with complicated medical problems. Regardless of a person's age or healthcare status, a geriatric specialist should be consulted when placement in a long-term care facility is being considered for an older person, family members are feeling stressed or burdened, and the older person is not coping well with illness or disability.

resources specific to aging and geriatrics. The nurse can make a referral to a geriatric speciality clinic or specially trained healthcare professional in order to make the search easier.

RATIONALE:

There is great diversity in health needs of people over the age of 65. While it is generally agreed that all older people would benefit from receiving their healthcare from geriatric specialists, many older people are well-cared for by primary care physicians, advanced practice nurses, and family physicians, while geriatricians are sought to provide care for frail older persons with complicated medical problems. Regardless of a person's age or healthcare status, a geriatric specialist should be consulted when placement in a long-term care facility is being considered for an older person, family members are feeling stressed or burdened, or the older person is not coping well with illness or disability.

Care Plan

A Patient Who Experiences a Fall

Case Study

Mrs. Kane is a 78-year-old retired teacher. She was brought to the emergency department by ambulance after she fell and injured her right wrist. An X-ray reveals an acute problem of a fractured right wrist and notes the presence of significant osteoarthritis and osteoporosis (degenerative joint changes and thinning of the bones).

A Patient Who Experiences a Fall

Mrs. Kane lives independently and manages pretty well since the death of her husband about 8 years ago, although she gave up driving because she has difficulty seeing oncoming cars in intense sunlight or when headlights are on at night. She has a daughter who visits her often and helps with heavy cleaning and grocery shopping.

The patient reports she was bending over to feed some neighborhood stray cats when she lost her balance and reached out to break her fall. It was dark and she did not notice the loose rug on the back porch that may have contributed to her fall. Upon further questioning, she remembers that she may have fallen one or two times before both in the house and on the back porch during the last several months.

Applying the Nursing Process

ASSESSMENT

When an older person falls and experiences injury, the nurse should identify the factors of normal aging, disease, and environment that may have contributed to the fall. Just noting that an older person has fallen is an incomplete assessment. Further information is needed.

The nurse must recognize that a fall may be the result of an unfortunate accident (anyone can trip and fall, especially in a dark environment), but certainly Mrs. Kane's report of previous falls and visual impairment is a red flag. Further, the X-ray reveals the presence of osteoarthritis and osteoporosis, both of which can contribute to mobility problems and risk of serious injury. As the patient is 78 years old, she is experiencing many normal changes of aging including declines in neurological, cardiovascular, and musculoskeletal function that ultimately result in homeostenosis, or an inability of her body to maintain regular function under adverse conditions. Whereas a younger person might not have fallen at all or might have fallen without becoming injured, Mrs. Kane was unable to correct her balance and broke her wrist as a result of the fall. The nurse must think broadly and consider the fall the result of normal changes of aging, chronic disease processes, and environmental circumstances. A careful past medical history should include any diagnosed illnesses, significant health problems, surgeries or trauma, medications taken, health maintenance activities, name and address of her primary care provider, and baseline ADLs. This information is needed to gain a baseline understanding of Mrs. Kane and her health status.

DIAGNOSIS

Some appropriate nursing diagnoses for Mrs. Kane include the following:

- *Altered health maintenance* demonstrated by lack of adaptive behaviors to internal and external environmental changes (bending over in the dark with a loose scatter rug)
- *Inattention to home safety hazards* (as evidenced by recent falls)
- *Perceptual impairment* (related to visual problems)

(continued)

A Patient Who Experiences a Fall *(continued)*

- *Impaired physical mobility* (due to osteoporosis and degenerative joint disease)
- *Risk for falls, acute injury,* and *pain*

EXPECTED OUTCOMES

Expected outcomes for the plan of care specify that Mrs. Kane will:

- Become aware of the dangers of injury resulting from falling and institute appropriate safety measures in her home.
- Use appropriate visual aids to increase safety in the home.
- Develop a therapeutic relationship with the nurse and develop a mutually agreed upon plan for health and safety.
- Agree to a pharmacological and nonpharmacological pain management plan with assistance or temporary placement in a rehabilitation facility while her wrist is healing.
- Schedule medical appointments for ongoing treatment and assessment of her osteoporosis.

PLANNING AND IMPLEMENTATION

The following nursing interventions may be appropriate:

- Mrs. Kane requires pain management with appropriate pharmacological and non-pharmacological techniques.
- Her wrist will be set in a cast. She will require assistance from a home health aid or short-term placement in a rehabilitation center until she can safely cook, clean, and manage her own personal hygiene and ADLs.
- She requires further assessment of her health status and treatment and monitoring of her osteoporosis.
- She should be referred to an ophthalmologist and a low-vision clinic for further assessment of her vision and assessment of appropriate visual aids.
- Both Mrs. Kane and her daughter would benefit from counseling and education regarding appropriate levels of social involvement, balance training, reduction of environmental safety hazards, and health maintenance activities.

EVALUATION

The nurse hopes to work with Mrs. Kane over time and realizes the chronic nature of falls in older people. The nurse will consider the plan a success based on the following criteria:

- Mrs. Kane will not experience any more falls.
- She will accept temporary placement in a rehabilitation facility or assistance from a home health aid while her wrist heals.
- She will use appropriate visual aids to promote safety.
- Finally, Mrs. Kane will follow up and receive ongoing treatment for her chronic medical conditions.

A Patient Who Experiences a Fall

Ethical Dilemma

The nurse finds that Mrs. Kane's blood pressure is highly elevated, and an electro-cardiogram reveals significant cardiac ischemia with evidence of recent myocardial infarction. When questioned about the presence of cardiac symptoms, Mrs. Kane states, "Yes, I've had chest pain on and off but I didn't mention it to anyone. Honestly, I don't want to have cardiac surgery like my friend Louise. They cut her open and now she can't even walk across the room, because she is so weak. I just decided I'm not going to say a thing to anyone." What is the best course of action for the nurse to follow?

> *Mrs. Kane has the right to autonomy and to refuse medical interventions as she is cognitively intact and competent. However, she would benefit from education regarding pharmacological and behavioral techniques that can control blood pressure, prevent stroke, relieve the symptoms of chest pain, and improve the quality of life. As medical technology extends the options for older people, healthcare providers must function as patient educators and advocates so that appropriate care is provided to those who will benefit from these procedures. As the patient is generally healthy, she may be a good candidate for angiography and stent placement; both are minimally invasive techniques that have the potential to improve and maintain the quality of her life. The geriatric social worker should be consulted to talk with Mrs. Kane and her family (if she is willing). The conversation should be recorded in the confidential medical record.*

Critical Thinking and the Nursing Process

1. Imagine yourself at age 80. What will you be like? What will you like best about being older? What are your fears regarding your own aging?
2. Examine your lifestyle. Are you engaging in behaviors that will support and encourage healthy aging? Are you engaging in risky behaviors that might promote the development of chronic illnesses?
3. Think of older people you know who have aged successfully. What are some characteristics they possess that might have contributed to a healthy older age?
4. Examine the Website that describes your school of nursing. Is care of the older person mentioned? If not, do you think it should be?

■ Evaluate your responses in Appendix B.

EXPLORE MediaLink

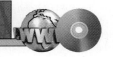

NCLEX review, case studies, and other interactive resources for this chapter can be found on the Companion Website at **www.prenhall.com/tabloski**. Click on Chapter 1 to select the activities for this chapter. For animations, video tutorials, more NCLEX review questions, and case studies, access the accompanying CD-ROM in this textbook.

Chapter Highlights

- The population of the world is aging. This trend is seen in all developed and most developing countries.

- Women comprise the majority of older people and outlive men by about 12 years. Older people are now more likely to suffer from chronic illnesses that have the potential to cause disability and limitations in ADLs.

- Nurses and other healthcare professionals have the opportunity to engage in health promotion activities at all stages of life, including old age. *Healthy People 2010* specifies goals for older Americans.

- With normal aging, there is loss of organ reserve that contributes to homeostenosis or narrowing of the zone of adaptation. Older persons with decreased organ reserve are unable to respond to physiological or psychological stress and need a more supportive environment to maintain function.

References

American Federation for Aging Research. (2004). *Biology of aging, theory of aging information center.* Retrieved August 11, 2004, from http://www.infoaging.org.

Arber, S., Davidson, K., & Ginn, J. (2003). *Gender and ageing: Changing roles and relationships.* Buckingham, England: Open University Press.

Census for Medicare & Medicaid Services (2004). Medicare Preventive Services. Retrieved August 16, 2004, from http://www.cms.hhs.gov.

Centers for Disease Control. (2004). *Chronic disease prevention. Healthy aging: Preventing disease and improving quality of life among older Americans.* Retrieved August 16, 2004, from http://www.cdc.gov.

Cummings, E., & Henry, W. (1961). *Growing old: The process of disengagement.* New York: Basic Books.

Dollemore, D. (2002). *Aging under the microscope: A biological quest.* Washington, DC: National Institute on Aging, U.S. Government Printing Office.

Erickson, E. (1950). *Childhood and society.* New York: W.W. Norton.

Fries, J., & Crapo, L. (1981). *Vitality and aging.* San Francisco: W.H. Freeman.

Gist, Y., & Velkoff, V. (1997). *Gender and aging. Demographic dimensions.* Washington,

DC: U.S. Department of Commerce, Bureau of the Census, U.S. Government Printing Office.

Havighurst, R., Neugarten, B., & Tobin, S. (1963). Disengagement, personality and life satisfaction in the later years. In P. Hanse (Ed.), *Age with a future.* Copenhagen, Denmark: Munksgoard.

Hobbs, F., & Stoops, N. (2002). *Demographic trends in the 20th century* (U.S. Census Bureau, Census 2002 *Special Reports,* Series CENSR-4). Washington, DC: U.S. Government Printing Office.

Jung, C. (1960). *The stage of life in collected works: Vol. 8. The structure and dynamics of the psyche.* New York: Pantheon Books.

Kinsella, K., & Gist, Y. (1998). *Gender and aging.* Washington, DC: U.S. Department of Commerce, Bureau of the Census, U.S. Government Printing Office.

Kolcaba, K., & Wykle, M. (1994). *Comfort theory and practice: A vision for holistic care and research.* New York: Springer.

Mion, L. (2003). Care provision for older adults: Who will provide? *Online Journal of Issues in Nursing, 8,* 2. Retrieved November 11, 2003, from http://www.nursingworld.org/ojin/topic21/tpc21_3.htm.

National Academy on an Aging Society. (1999). *Chronic conditions: A challenge for the 21st century.* Retrieved June 30, 2000, from http://www.agingsociety.org.

O'Neill, G. (2002). *The state of aging and health in America.* Washington, DC: Merck Institute of Aging & Health, Gerontological Society of America.

Palmore, E. B. (1998). *The facts on aging quiz.* New York: Springer.

R.W. Johnson Foundation. (1996). *Chronic care in America: A 21st century challenge.* San Francisco: Institute for Health and Aging.

Rosenfeld, P., Bottrell, M., Fulmer, T., & Mezey, M. (1999). Gerontological nursing content in baccalaureate nursing programs: Findings from a national survey. *Journal of Professional Nursing, 15*(2), 84–94.

Rowe, J., & Kahn, R. (1998). Breaking down the myths of aging. *Successful aging.* New York: Dell.

U.S. Census Bureau. (2000). *Data base news in aging. Federal interagency forum on aging-related statistics.* Washington, DC: U.S. Government Printing Office.

U.S. Census Bureau. (2001). *An aging world* (Series P95/01-1). Washington, DC: U.S. Government Printing Office.

CHAPTER 2

Gerontological Nursing Issues

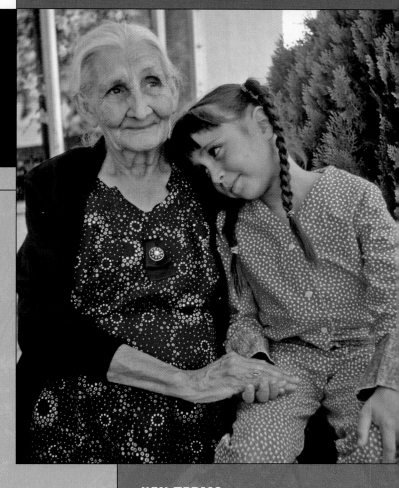

CHAPTER OBJECTIVES

Upon completion of this chapter, the reader will be able to:

- Discuss the nurse's role in caring for older adults.

- Identify appropriate educational preparation and certification requirements of the gerontological nurse generalist and specialist.

- Identify components of the long-term care system.

- Discuss the ANA standards and scope of practice for gerontological nursing.

- Identify the use of functional health patterns in the formulation of a nursing diagnosis.

- Describe the uses and need for gerontological nursing research as support for evidence-based practice.

- Describe effective communication techniques appropriate for use with the older adult.

KEY TERMS

advanced practice registered nurses (APRNs) 29
basic level nurse 28
certification 28
functional health patterns 34
geriatrics 28
gerontology 30
nursing diagnosis 34
scope of practice 28
standards 28

MediaLink

Additional resources for this chapter can be found on the Student CD-ROM accompanying this textbook and on the Companion Website at **www.prenhall.com/tabloski**. Click on Chapter 2 to select the activities for this chapter.

CD-ROM
- NCLEX Review
- Case Studies
- Tools

COMPANION WEBSITE
- Audio Glossary
- Additional NCLEX Review
- Case Study
- MediaLink Applications

In the 1920s, a few visionary nurses began to identify the need for a specialization in caring for older people. This need was based upon observations and evidence that older people responded differently to illness, disease, and treatments based upon their age and general state of health. These nurses also recognized that institutional settings such as old age homes or boarding houses were appropriate settings for gerontological nurses to deliver healthcare outside of the traditional acute care hospital. In 1925, **geriatrics,** the medical specialty focusing on aging, began to emerge. An anonymous column published in the *American Journal of Nursing* called for nurses to consider "yet another specialty" based upon the need for nursing services for larger numbers of older people and the trend toward increasing life expectancy.

The American Nurses Association (ANA) is responsible for defining the **scope** and **standards** of nursing practice. In 1966, the ANA established the Division of Geriatric Nursing Practice with the mission of creating standards for quality nursing care for aging persons in all settings. In 1976, the division's name was changed to the Division on Gerontological Nursing Practice to reflect the idea that nursing care of the older adult is holistic and emphasizes health as well as common diseases of old age. In 1970, the ANA published *A Statement on the Scope of Gerontological Nursing Practice* to define the nature and scope of current gerontological nursing practice and to address the concepts of health promotion, health maintenance, disease prevention, and self-care. This document was revised in 1981, 1987, 1995, 2000, and 2004.

The latest revision involves collaboration between the ANA and selected members from several national nursing organizations and is intended to be a guide to current practice in conjunction with other documents that articulate the values of professional nursing. While the *Scope and Standards of Gerontological Nursing Practice* (American Nurses Association, 2001) apply to all professional nurses, the gerontological standards contain specific criteria for defining expectations and competent care associated with basic and advanced clinical practice of gerontological nursing. These standards apply in all clinical practice settings, including acute care institutions, ambulatory treatment centers and clinics, home care, long-term care facilities, and adult day care centers. The ongoing revision and refinement of these standards reflect the rapid growth of the practice of gerontological nursing and the challenges that result from the evolving healthcare needs of older adults.

In 1973, the first gerontological nurses were certified by the ANA to provide tangible recognition of professional achievement in a defined functional or clinical area of nursing. **Certification** is defined as the formal process by which clinical competence is validated in a specialty area of practice (ANA, 2002). The certification process consists of a written examination developed and reviewed by nursing experts. Certification as a gerontological nurse assures the public, nursing colleagues, and the employer that the nurse possesses specialized skills and knowledge in providing care to older people. Certified nurses may be eligible for additional monetary compensation and promotion or advancement.

Nurses can become certified at the **basic or advanced practice levels** based upon their level of education and knowledge, skills, and experience. Nurses with associate, diploma, or baccalaureate degrees in nursing can seek certification as gerontological nurses if they are currently registered as a nurse in the United States or one of its territories, have practiced the equivalent of 2 years full-time as a registered nurse (RN), and have a minimum of 2,000 hours of clinical practice within the last 3 years (see the American Nurses Association Website for complete eligibility requirements). The generalist functions in a variety of settings and draws upon the expertise of the specialist. Generalists may coordinate services and manage care for older people. They may function as direct care providers, case managers, and nurse leaders and administrators within many settings of the healthcare system. Once certified, nurses may indicate their certification by signing their name and the initials BC (Board Certified).

Advanced practice nurses with master's degrees (clinical nurse specialists and nurse practitioners) may seek certification as gerontological specialists. Once certified, they may use the credentials RN, BC (board certified). The different credentials distinguish between levels of certification within the nursing profession, to other healthcare professionals, and to patients and their families. Advanced practice gerontological nurses serve as primary care providers and focus on health promotion, disease prevention, and long-term management of chronic conditions and their exacerbations that require prompt and intensive nursing interventions.

Scope of Practice

The American Nurses Credentialing Center (ANCC) supports the development and administration of the certification examinations based upon the ANA's scope and standards of practice. ANCC defines practice for the gerontological nurse as follows:

> Gerontological nurses specialize in the nursing care and the health needs of older adults. They plan, manage, and implement health care to meet those needs, and evaluate the effectiveness of such care. The nurse's primary challenge is to identify and use the strengths of older adults and assist them in maximizing their independence. Nurses actively involve older adults and family members as much as possible in the decision making process, which has an impact on the quality of their clients' everyday life. (ANCC, 2002, p. 2)

The responsibilities of the gerontological nurse include direct care, management and development of the professional and other nursing personnel, and evaluation of care and services for the older adult. All professional nurses practicing gerontological nursing need the basic knowledge and skills to perform the highest level of care. Box 2-1 lists the ANA-required knowledge and skills for gerontological nurses.

ADVANCED GERONTOLOGICAL NURSING

The advanced practice gerontological nurse is an RN who holds a master's, doctorate, or higher degree, and demonstrates advanced knowledge and clinical expertise in the care of the older adult. Currently, **advanced practice registered nurses (APRNs)** consist of clinical nurse specialists (CNSs) and nurse practitioners (NPs). APRNs function independently and in collaboration with other healthcare providers in a variety of healthcare settings. Gerontological nurse practitioners (GNPs) deliver primary care to older clients and have considerable autonomy addressing healthcare problems, often with prescriptive authority. CNSs provide direct and indirect care to patients and their families and serve as consultants to staff on complex issues of patient care. In some instances, the roles of the CNS and GNP are interchangeable, but often the GNP focuses more attention on the direct provision and evaluation of care while the CNS focuses more attention on the educator and consultative role. Advanced practice nurses play an important role in caring for older patients by preventing, recognizing, and treating common problems and illnesses that are major causes of morbidity and mortality in the older adult. Timely care in the nursing home setting has been shown to decrease inappropriate hospital admissions and transfers. Advanced practice nurses also work with nursing staff to provide palliative care to dying patients by providing pain and symptom control (Ruiz, Tabloski, & Frazier, 1995). They practice within the scope of their state's nurse practice act. Once they have fulfilled certification and licensure requirements, they may be authorized to prescribe medications, including controlled substances.

<table>
<tr><td>

BOX 2-1   **ANA Required Knowledge and Skills for Gerontological Nurses**

</td></tr>
</table>

1. Recognize the older adult may be competent, and allow him or her to make healthcare decisions.
2. Establish a therapeutic relationship with the older adult to facilitate his or her involvement in developing the plan of care, which may include family participation as needed.
3. Use current gerontological standards to initiate, develop, and adapt the older adult's plan of care while involving the patient, family, and other providers as needed.
4. Recognize age-related changes based on an understanding of physiological, emotional, cultural, social, psychological, economic, and spiritual functioning.
5. Collect data to determine health status and functional abilities in order to plan, implement, and evaluate care.
6. Participate and collaborate with members of the interdisciplinary team.
7. Participate with older adults, families if needed, and other health professionals in ethical decision making that is patient centered, empathetic, and humane.
8. Serve as an advocate for older adults and their families.
9. Teach older adults and families about measures that promote, maintain, and restore health and functional performance; promote comfort; and foster independence and preserve dignity.
10. Refer the older adult to other professionals or community resources for assistance as necessary.
11. Identify common chronic/acute physical and mental disease processes that affect the older adult.
12. Apply the existing body of knowledge in **gerontology** to nursing practice and intervention.
13. Exercise accountability to the older adult by protecting his or her rights and autonomy, recognizing and respecting their decisions about advance directives.
14. Facilitate palliative care and comfort during the dying process in order to preserve the older adult's dignity and provide a peaceful death.
15. Embrace the surviving spouse and family members, providing strength, comfort, and hope.
16. Engage in continuing professional development through participation in continuing education, involvement in state and national professional organizations, and certification.
17. Use the standards of gerontological nursing practice and collaborate with other healthcare professionals to improve the quality of care and quality of life of the older adult.

Source: American Nurses Association (ANA) (2001). *Scope and standards of gerontological nursing practice*, 2e. Washington, DC: American Nurses Publishing.

Standards of Gerontological Nursing

The *Standards of Clinical Gerontological Nursing Care* describe the necessary competencies of care for each step of the nursing process, including assessment, diagnosis, outcome identification, planning, implementation, and evaluation (Box 2-2). These competencies are the essential foundation of the actions taken by gerontological nurses when caring for their patients.

These standards enable the nursing profession to identify and meet the professional responsibility to deliver quality patient care to older persons. For further in-

MediaLink ◆ ANA: Scope and Standards of Gerontological Nursing Practice

---

ANA Standards of Clinical Gerontological Nursing Care

BOX 2-2

Standard I: Assessment. The gerontological nurse collects patient health data.

Rationale—Interviewing, functional assessment, environmental assessment, physical assessment, and review of health records enhance the nurse's ability to make sound clinical judgments. Assessment is culturally and ethnically appropriate.

Standard II: Diagnosis. The gerontological nurse analyzes the assessment data in determining diagnosis.

Rationale—The gerontological nurse, either independently or in collaboration with interdisciplinary care providers, evaluates health assessment data to develop comprehensive diagnoses that form the basis for care interventions.

Standard III: Outcome Identification. The gerontological nurse identifies expected outcomes individualized to the older adult.

Rationale—The ultimate goals of providing gerontological nursing care are to influence health outcomes and improve or maintain the aging person's health status. Outcomes often focus on maximizing the aging person's state of well-being, functional status, and quality of life.

Standard IV: Planning. The gerontological nurse develops a plan of care that prescribes interventions to attain expected outcomes.

Rationale—A plan of care is used to structure and guide therapeutic interventions and achieve expected outcomes. It is developed in conjunction with the older adult, significant others, and interdisciplinary team members.

Standard V: Implementation. The gerontological nurse implements the interventions identified in the plan of care.

Rationale—The gerontological nurse uses a wide range of culturally competent direct and indirect interventions designed toward health promotion, health maintenance, prevention of illness, health restoration, rehabilitation, and palliation. The gerontological nurse implements the plan of care in collaboration with the older adult and others. The gerontological nurse selects interventions according to his or her level of education and practice.

Standard VI: Evaluation. The gerontological nurse evaluates the older adult's progress toward attainment of expected outcomes.

Rationale—Nursing practice is a dynamic and evolving process. The gerontological nurse continually evaluates the older adult's responses to treatment and interventions. Collection of new data, revision of the database, alteration of nursing diagnoses, and modification of the plan of care are often essential. The effectiveness of nursing care depends on ongoing evaluation.

Source: American Nurses Association (ANA) (2001). *Scope and standards of gerontological nursing practice,* 2e. Washington, DC: American Nurses Publishing.

---

formation about the *Scope and Standards of Gerontological Nursing Practice,* go to the ANA Website. Performance standards are defined and each includes measurement criteria.

Working with older people is one of the most rewarding and challenging opportunities in the nurse's professional career. Sometimes seen as a difficult or depressing specialization, gerontological nursing offers unique joys and rewards. Many nurses enjoy working with older people because they enjoyed a special relationship with a grandparent. Those of us lucky enough to have laughed with and loved an older person know the joy of caring and the wisdom that can be gained in these relationships.

Nurses can be proud of a long history as leaders in public health and home care nursing as these systems address many needs of older people. Nurses provide valuable primary care to older people, seek out needed referrals, eliminate costly duplication of services, and provide continuity of care within a chaotic healthcare system. Nurses comprise the greatest number of healthcare providers to older people in hospitals, long-term care facilities, and community-based settings including home care. Of the 4.4 million workers employed in U.S. hospitals, 23% are RNs (American Hospital Association, 2000). There are approximately 2,694,540 persons holding licenses to practice as RNs, an increase of 62.2% since 1980. However, the years between 1996 and 2000 marked the slowest growth in the RN population over the 20-year period between 1980 and 2000. On average, the RN population grew only about 1.2% each year between 1996 and 2000 compared with average annual increases of 2% to 3% in earlier years. This slowdown reflects fewer new entrants to the nursing profession and larger numbers of nurses leaving the profession (Health Resources and Services Administration, 2000). By 2010, approximately 1 million new nurses will be needed to replace the nurses leaving the profession due to retirement (ANA, 2002). In 1980, 52.9% of the RN population was under the age of 40; in 2000, the average age of the RN population was 45.2 years. The nation's healthcare providers are reporting a shortage of nurses in a range of settings. There is a growing demand for nurses with skills to treat patients with complex health needs, and the shortage is expected to worsen as the aging population increases. Surveys indicate that nursing homes in some states have RN vacancy rates of about 15% (General Accounting Office, 2001).

A nursing shortage has serious implications for the quality of patient care. A recent study found a relationship between higher RN staffing levels and the reduction of certain negative hospital inpatient outcomes, such as urinary tract infection and pneumonia (Harvard School of Public Health, 2002). Another recent study found that inadequate RN staffing at mealtime is a barrier to adequate nutritional intake in nursing homes (see Chapter 5). ⊂⊃ Serious consequences related to poor nutrition include dehydration and aspiration leading to pneumonia (Kayser-Jones, 1997). A recent Health Care Financing Administration report to Congress found a direct relationship between nurse staffing levels in nursing homes and the quality of resident care. An analysis of three states' data demonstrated that, after controlling for case mix, there is a minimum nurse-staffing threshold below which quality of care may be seriously impaired (Health Care Financing Administration, 2002). The same report noted that approximately 30% of nursing homes surveyed reported that they were not staffed at the minimum RN staffing level.

Hospitals remain the major employer of nurses, although the number of nurses employed in other sectors has increased. In 2000, 59% of RNs worked in hospitals (down from 66% in 1980). Public and community health settings, ambulatory care, and other noninstitutional health settings increased RN employment by 155% during the same 20-year period. Hospital lengths of stay have decreased, and many older patients are now recuperating in long-term care facilities or at home. Consequently, nursing homes and home care nurses are caring for patients with a greater range of clinical needs (Hendrix & Foreman, 2001). The increasing diversity of the U.S. population, the growing number of vulnerable individuals, and the challenges of caring for increasing numbers of people with complex chronic illnesses call for revised thinking about the delivery of healthcare and the education of health professionals (National Academies of Practice, 2000). Nurse educators and policymakers are addressing the crucial issues of student recruitment and strengthening the infrastructures within the healthcare system to support healthcare and education of health professionals (Williams, 2001).

In the United States, there are approximately 20,000 nursing homes and 1.5 million to 2 million nursing home beds. Approximately 5% of the population age 65 and over lives in a nursing home, but the likelihood that a person will enter a nursing home at some time is about 43% (Mezey & Kovner, 2001). About 1.9 million older persons entered a nursing home in 2001. The average nursing home resident is frail, with 7.9% reported as bed bound, 23% with contractures, 7% with decubitus ulcers, 50% with urinary incontinence, and 15% with physical or chemical restraints (Harrington, Carrillo, Thollaug, & Summers, 1999). Given that nurses assist nursing home residents with bathing, dressing, eating, toileting, walking, and medications, staffing is a serious concern. In 1999, 21 states were considering legislation to increase staffing standards in nursing homes (National Citizens' Coalition for Nursing Home Reform, 1999). A 1998 survey showed that nurse staffing time averaged just 3.5 hours per resident per day (little more than 1 hour per shift) (Kovner & Harrington, 2000). There is cause for concern given the dangerously low RN staffing levels in nursing homes, the larger numbers of nursing home residents recuperating from acute illness, and the need for professional nursing judgment to monitor these residents for unpredictable healthcare events (Mezey & Kovner, 2001).

As the consistent caregivers in most healthcare settings, nurses assume responsibility for providing care and coordinating services throughout a 24-hour period. In addition to focusing on the physical health and function of their patients, gerontological nurses also address issues of access to healthcare services, quality and affordability of healthcare, and coordination of services by the interdisciplinary team. As healthcare continues to evolve, new roles will emerge for gerontological nurses. Strong linkages between nurse educators and practicing nurses will be vital to ensure appropriate education and inclusion of relevant clinical experiences in gerontology. This support for emerging clinicians will prepare them to play an important role in providing high-quality nursing care to patients and shaping the healthcare system throughout the remainder of the 21st century. In addition to the traditional role of clinical practitioner, the gerontological nurse may also serve in the role of patient advocate, nurse educator, nurse manager, nurse consultant, and nurse researcher. Key aspects of each role are listed as follows:

- **Advocate.** Advances the rights of older persons and educates others regarding negative stereotypes of aging.
- **Educator.** Organizes and provides instructions regarding healthy aging, disease detection, treatment of disease, and rehabilitation to older patients and their families. Also participates in in-service education, continuing education, and training of ancillary personnel as appropriate.
- **Manager.** Maintains current relevant information regarding federal and state regulations, and provides nursing leadership in a variety of healthcare settings.
- **Consultant.** Consults with and advises others who are providing nursing care to older patients with complex healthcare problems. Participates in the development of clinical pathways and quality assurance standards and the implementation of evidence-based practices.
- **Researcher.** Collaborates with established researchers in the development of clinically based studies, assists with data collection and the identification of appropriate research sites, communicates relevant research findings to others, and participates in the presentation of findings at gerontological conferences and publications.

Because they view patients holistically, nurses are in an ideal position to serve in these roles. Helping patients achieve their optimal level of physical, mental, and psychosocial well-being is the primary goal of the gerontological nurse.

Functional Health Patterns and Nursing Diagnosis

A systematic nursing assessment is necessary to provide holistic care to the older person (ANA, 2000). This nursing assessment must go beyond physical function and the diagnosis of disease (the medical model) by also focusing on the interaction of the older person with the environment. Gordon (1994) developed a set of health-related behaviors that form an assessment framework for nurses. This framework consists of 11 **functional health patterns** that can interact and form the basis for an older person's lifestyle. Although these functional health patterns were not specifically developed for use with older patients, they are ideally suited for use by gerontological nurses. An older person's functional status is a primary concern because it addresses key issues, including how the patient sees his or her present level of health, usual and preferred lifestyle and activities, demands of daily life and existing support systems, and functional ability. Each of the 11 functional areas guides the nurse to seek information about the older patient and forms a crucial foundation to the care-planning process and diagnosis of the patient's nursing needs.

The 11 functional health patterns include the following:

- **Health perception–health management.** The older individual's perceived health and well-being along with self-management strategies.
- **Nutritional-metabolic.** Patterns of food and fluid consumption relative to metabolic need and nutrient supply.
- **Elimination.** Patterns of excretory function and elimination of waste (bowel, bladder, etc.).
- **Activity-exercise.** Patterns of exercise and daily activity. Includes leisure and recreation.
- **Sleep-rest.** Patterns of sleep, rest, and relaxation.
- **Cognitive-perceptual.** Patterns of thinking and ways of perceiving the world and current events.
- **Self-perception–self-concept.** Patterns of viewing and valuing self (body image and psychological state, self-image, etc.).
- **Roles-relationships.** Patterns of engagement with others, ability to form and maintain meaningful relationships, assumed roles.
- **Sexuality-reproductive.** Patterns of sexuality and satisfaction with present level of interaction with sexual partners.
- **Coping–stress tolerance.** Patterns of coping with stressful events and level of effectiveness of coping strategies.
- **Values-beliefs.** Patterns of beliefs, values, and perception of the meaning of life that guide choices or decisions.

(Gordon, 1994)

Each of these patterns represents an expression of function within a whole individual and indicates the underlying physical, social, psychological, and spiritual foundations of the individual and his or her relationship with the environment (Gordon, 1994). By concentrating on these 11 crucial areas, the nurse can identify actual or potential health problems and each individual's health and life goals. When this information has been systematically gathered, the nurse can make a **nursing diagnosis.**

Nursing diagnosis is the naming of an individual's response to actual or potential health problems or life processes (Gordon, 1994; NANDA, 2003). Nursing diagnoses provide the basis for selection of interventions to achieve outcomes for which the nurse is accountable. The North American Nursing Diagnosis Association (NANDA) has developed standardized descriptions of human responses frequently encountered by nurses while providing healthcare to patients. Health problems are defined as dysfunctional patterns, and nursing's major contribution to healthcare is in preventing and treating these patterns (Gordon, 1994). A pattern is dysfunctional when it deviates from established norms or from an individual's previous condition or goals. These dysfunctional patterns may generate concern on the part of the older person, family members or significant others, healthcare professionals, or others knowledgeable of health promotion and health maintenance activities. Problems or dysfunctional patterns may be identified as actual or potential threats to health, allowing the nurse an opportunity to intervene.

For example, suppose an older man with type 1 diabetes mellitus has a long-established pattern of good control by careful and frequent blood glucose monitoring and appropriate administration of insulin. However, his wife notes that within the last 2 months he has tested his blood glucose less frequently, has failed to administer his premeal insulin bolus, and as a result has frequently recorded very high glucose levels. No actual harm has resulted as yet, but the nurse realizes that this behavior increases the patient's risk for complications of diabetes such as damage to the eyes and kidneys, and decreased immune function. Further, this behavior is a deviation from previously well-established patterns and indicates a potential health problem. Therefore, the nurse may suspect that something has changed in the patient's underlying physical, social, psychological, and spiritual foundation, and in his relationship to the environment. After systematic assessment in each of the 11 functional health patterns, the nurse may make the diagnosis of *impaired health maintenance*. The ability to formulate an accurate nursing diagnosis will depend on the nurse's adherence to a systematic approach, the application of relevant clinical skills, the nurse's experience, and the nurse's knowledge of the norms and presentation of disease in the older person.

Nursing diagnoses are constantly changing and evolving. The current list of nursing diagnoses can be found in Appendix A. ⊂▭⊃

Practice Pearl

A common omission made by gerontological nurses is to implement a nursing care plan without first obtaining an accurate diagnosis of the patient's problem. For instance, an older person may be placed on a liquid nutritional supplement to reverse weight loss without an understanding of why the person is losing weight. The patient may be depressed, have a developing cancer, or be unable to chew because of ill-fitting dentures. Appropriate nursing interventions would vary in each of these circumstances.

CARE PLANNING AND SETTING REALISTIC GOALS

After completing an assessment and reaching appropriate nursing diagnoses, the nurse formulates a plan of care. The goals of the care-planning process should be individualized to reflect the older adult's values. The overall goals of nursing care are to influence health outcomes, to improve or maintain the older person's health status, or to provide comfort care at the end of life. Gerontological nurses will often focus on improvement of the patient's quality of life, improvement of functional status, and promotion of well-being.

The clarity and achievability of the goals are critical to the development of an effective plan of care. Goals of nursing care should:

- Be linked to the nursing diagnoses.
- Be mutually formulated with the older adult, family, and interdisciplinary team whenever possible.
- Be culturally appropriate.
- Be attainable in relationship to available resources and the care setting.
- Include a time frame for attainment.
- Adequately reflect associated benefits and costs.
- Provide direction for continuity of care.
- Be measurable.

(ANA, 2000)

Beginning gerontological nurses are sometimes overwhelmed with the many problems identified by the older adult and the numerous nursing diagnoses generated from the assessment. One of the first steps is to assign priority to the problems diagnosed. Problems with high priority include those that have a potential for immediately impacting negatively on health status, those of concern to the older person and the family, and those that negatively affect function and quality of life. Other problems can be deferred and addressed at a later time. Patients can become overwhelmed when well-meaning healthcare providers attempt to do too much at one time.

For instance, imagine the situation in which Mr. Jones, 84 years old, visits a blood pressure screening clinic in a senior citizen center. During the encounter with the nurse, the patient relates he has not seen his physician for several years. He reports that his wife was very ill and he focused all his time and attention on the provision of her care. The nurse is alarmed that the patient has an elevated blood pressure, has not had his cholesterol checked in several years, has not had a screening colonoscopy, and has never received the pneumococcal vaccine. However, the nurse realizes that the most immediate need Mr. Jones has at this time is to visit his physician for further evaluation and treatment of his elevated blood pressure. The nurse advises Mr. Jones to phone his physician to request a problem-focused evaluation at this time and to follow up with an appointment for a full physical examination and screening at a later date. The nurse hopes to develop a trusting relationship with the patient, encouraging him to express his values and concerns, and to work with him over time on issues relating to his health. To increase the chance of success, the nurse will address one problem at a time (Prochaska, Velicer, Fava, Rossi, & Tsoh, 2001).

Mr. Jones's nursing diagnosis is *ineffective health maintenance.* Desired goals for Mr. Jones include the following:

1. Identifies positive beliefs regarding the benefits of taking action to seek medical attention to promote health and prevent illness.
2. Achieves a therapeutic relationship with a nurse at the senior center in order to develop a long-range plan to reduce risk of future illness or disease.
3. Identifies resources that will assist him to engage in appropriate action.

Nursing interventions appropriate to these goals might include the following:

1. Urge Mr. Jones to phone his physician or healthcare provider within the next 3 days to schedule a blood pressure evaluation.
2. Educate Mr. Jones regarding the immediate health risks associated with an elevated blood pressure.
3. Assess insurance status and availability of the patient's healthcare provider.
4. Assess need for transportation to and from the provider's office and identify community resources available to assist if needed.

5. Identify family members or significant others who may accompany the patient and provide comfort and support, if he so desires.
6. Schedule a follow-up appointment with Mr. Jones to return to the screening clinic next week.

Practice Pearl

Use measurable verbs when establishing goals of care. The nurse should use *states, performs, identifies, has an increase/decrease in, specifies,* and *administers.* The words *accepts, knows, appreciates,* and *understands* should be avoided as they are not measurable (Carpenito, 2003).

Assigning priority to problems is usually done with input from the patient and family as well as the interdisciplinary team. Some problems needing immediate attention can be resolved by nursing interventions, and some require referral to others, including family members, nursing colleagues, or interdisciplinary members of the healthcare team. A well-functioning interdisciplinary team demands that the participants take into account the contributions of other team members and communicate effectively in all phases of the care-planning process (Health Resources and Services Administration, 1996).

Practice Pearl

It is generally accepted that an interdisciplinary team can deliver the best healthcare to the older person. The complexity of problems and concerns common to the older person often require a team approach to practice. The gerontological nurse is a key member of the interdisciplinary healthcare team.

Another critical issue in goal formulation is the ability of the gerontological nurse to set realistic and achievable goals. When the nurse sets goals that are unattainable, the patient is set up for failure. Once older patients feel they have failed to meet the goals established by their healthcare providers, they may not keep follow-up appointments, they may become depressed and blame themselves for being weak or lazy, or they may manufacture excuses to protect themselves from criticism. For instance, a 74-year-old obese woman was informed by her healthcare provider that she must lose weight to ease her back pain and increase her mobility. The goal set by the provider was to lose 10 lb within the next month. This was extremely difficult for the patient as she was unable to exercise or move freely because of her back pain. At the end of the month she had only lost 5 lbs. She failed to return for her follow-up appointment, fearing she had disappointed her healthcare provider. If the provider had gained input from the patient and set a more realistic goal, the patient's weight loss could have been seen as a valuable first step in a long process toward achieving an ideal body weight.

Practice Pearl

Many health problems exhibited in older people are the result of lifestyle choices that take years to develop. It is unreasonable to think that these problems can be resolved within a short period of time. The nurse should work with older patients over time as they begin the journey toward lifestyle modification and activities aimed at reducing risk and promoting health.

IMPLEMENTATION OF THE NURSING CARE PLAN

After the goals of care have been carefully selected, the gerontological nurse will choose appropriate direct and indirect interventions in collaboration with the older adult, the family (if appropriate), and the interdisciplinary care team. The nursing profession must identify its unique focus and demonstrate accountability in terms of that focus. The nursing interventions identified on the nursing care plan demonstrate that accountability and communicate to the nursing staff the particular problems of the older patient and the prescribed interventions for directing and evaluating the care given (Carpenito, 2003). The interventions are selected on the basis of the needs, desires, and resources of the older adult and accepted nursing practice (ANA, 2000). Appropriate nursing interventions may include the following:

- Assisting the older patient to a higher level of function or self-care
- Identifying health promotion activities
- Identifying disease prevention and screening activities
- Health teaching
- Counseling
- Seeking consultation
- Collecting data on an ongoing basis and refining the initial nursing assessment
- Exploring treatment choices, including pharmacological and nonpharmacological options
- Implementing palliative care and holistic care of the dying or seriously ill patient
- Referring the patient to community resources
- Managing the patient's case
- Evaluating and educating ancillary caregivers and family

(ANA, 2004)

Nursing interventions will be selected based upon the following:

1. Linkage to the desired outcome
2. Characteristics of the nursing diagnosis
3. Strength of the research associated with the intervention
4. Probability of successfully implementing the intervention
5. Acceptability of the intervention to the older person and others involved in the plan of care
6. Assurance that the intervention is safe, ethical, culturally competent, and appropriate
7. Documentation of the intervention
8. Knowledge, skills, experience, and creativity of the nurse

(ANA, 2000; McCloskey & Bulechek, 2002)

The *Nursing Interventions Classification* (*NIC*) provides examples of nursing interventions based on theoretical or clinical perspectives (Iowa Intervention Project, 2000). Few nursing interventions have been extensively studied. Many are based upon tradition, anecdotal experience, practice protocols within the healthcare facility, literature searches, peer review, and professional judgment. Some institutions use standardized nursing care plans based upon specific medical and nursing diagnoses. However, these standardized care plans can always be modified to meet the individual needs of each patient. Care planning is not a "one size fits all" process.

Nursing interventions based upon clinical guidelines are sometimes published with a coding system that indicates the strength of the research associated with a particular recommendation. The gold standard for achieving the highest ranking is an intervention that has been tested in a randomized controlled clinical trial. Randomized controlled clinical trials are thought to have the strongest design and thus have the best chance of establishing a cause-and-effect relationship between a nursing intervention and the desired outcome of care. When the Agency for Health Care Policy and Research (now called the Agency for Healthcare Research and Quality) first published their clinical practice guidelines in 1993, the expert panel charged with developing the guidelines used a three-level coding system to indicate the strength of the available evidence on the recommended interventions. This system included:

A Good research-based evidence, with some panel opinion to support the guideline statement.

B Fair research-based evidence, with substantial panel opinion to support the guideline statement.

C Guideline statement based primarily on panel opinion, with minimal research-based evidence, but significant clinical experience.

Gerontological nurses choose appropriate nursing interventions based upon their knowledge of practice and the supports available in the practice environment. In the dependent role, the nurse will implement physician orders according to safe and acceptable standards of practice. Administration of treatments, medications, therapeutic diets, and preparation for diagnostic testing will usually be specified in writing for implementation by the nursing staff. In the independent role, the nurse will establish and implement nursing actions to carry out the nursing care plan. The goal of the nursing action is to direct individualized care to the older patient and prescribe care to prevent, reduce, or eliminate the actual or potential problem identified in the nursing diagnosis.

The nursing care plan also identifies nursing interventions that have proven successful based upon trial and error. These interventions when recorded can be helpful to nurses working other shifts, nurses "floating" to the unit who may not know the patient well, or agency or temporary nurses who do not know the patient at all. For instance, when nurses are attempting to increase fluid intake to an older patient who is at risk for fluid volume deficiency, a nursing intervention may be:

Goal: Increase fluid intake
1. Increase fluids to 2,500 ml/24 hours
   a. 1,500 ml on day shift
   b. 700 ml on evening shift
   c. 300 ml on night shift
2. Prefers apple juice or cool water
3. Offer fluids between meals with patient in sitting position
4. Record fluid intake on the intake/output sheet at patient's bedside

(Carpenito, 2003)

During implementation of the nursing intervention, the gerontological nurse will carefully monitor the patient's response, the response of others involved in the care delivery, achievement of the outcome, alternative interventions that may supplement or replace the specified interventions, the accuracy and safety of the intervention, the competency of others in delivering the care, and validation of the appropriateness of the intervention (Carpenito, 2003). Nursing interventions can be added, deleted, or modified as part of the ongoing process of providing individualized care.

EVALUATION

Evaluation is the final component of the nursing process, and the gerontological nurse will undertake a systematic and ongoing process to compare the patient's response to the activities identified in the nursing care plan to the established outcome criteria. The nurse will seek input from the patient, family, and others involved in the care. It is important to consider information from the physical, social, and psychological assessment of the patient; information from diagnostic testing; level of satisfaction with care; and documentation of the costs and benefits associated with the treatment. The initial assessment and nursing diagnosis may be revised with new goals and nursing interventions specified if appropriate. Either the problem has been resolved and the plan should be continued as specified, the problem has been resolved and the nursing interventions can be revised or discontinued, or the problem still exists. If the problem still exists despite implementation of the nursing care plan, that may indicate the interventions were not carried out as specified, the interventions were not effective in alleviating the problem, or there was an error or omission in the initial nursing assessment and diagnosis. At this point, the nurse has the opportunity to modify and revise the nursing care plan.

Some healthcare institutions routinely gather evaluation data as part of an ongoing quality assurance project. By gathering outcome data on large numbers of older patients, nurse managers and clinicians can identify opportunities for improvement. Quality assurance data will often focus on negative outcomes such as falls with injury, medication errors, unintentional weight loss, development of decubitus ulcers, and incidence of urinary tract infections. Should problems in these areas be identified, the gerontological nurse may become involved in the development of policies, procedures, and practice guidelines to improve quality of care and quality of life for the older adult (ANA, 2000).

RESEARCH AGENDA

Gerontological nurses interpret, apply, and evaluate research findings to inform and improve gerontological nursing practice (Standard VII, ANA, 2004). The gerontological nurse generalist participates by identifying clinical problems appropriate for study, gathering data, and interpreting findings to improve the nursing care provided to older adults. Additionally, gerontological nurses use research findings to provide evidence-based nursing interventions to their patients. The use of evidence-based practice is considered the best method for delivery of skilled and compassionate care to older adults.

Many gerontological nurses work as part of research teams and collaborate with nursing colleagues with advanced education and research training. Further, the gerontological nurse may serve on an institutional review board in order to give input on the protection of rights for research subjects involved in clinical research activities.

Nurses have long been recognized as direct healthcare providers, but the role of nurse as scientist is less recognized. In the United States, federal funding for nursing research began in the 1950s. It was not until 1986 that the National Center for Nursing Research, later to become the National Institute of Nursing Research (NINR), was established within the National Institutes of Health (NIH). NINR's mission is to support the science that advances the knowledge of nurses in order to:

- Understand and ease the symptoms of acute and chronic illness.
- Prevent or delay the onset of disease or disability, or slow its progression.
- Find effective approaches to achieving and sustaining optimal health.
- Improve the clinical settings in which care is provided.

(NINR, 2002)

Several private foundations (Robert Wood Johnson, Soros, Hartford Foundation, Research Retirement Foundation, American Association of Retired Persons) as well as federal agencies (National Cancer Institute, National Institute of Mental Health, National Institute on Aging) have lobbied for greater funding for gerontological nursing research. Nursing research efforts are needed to improve the delivery of healthcare to older adults. The demographics of an aging population make this imperative.

Over the past 10 years, knowledge regarding the aging process and the heterogeneity of older adults, as well as their special needs and strengths, has made gerontology a viable area of study and clinical practice. Many of the issues affecting older people have been traditionally managed by nurses. It is not surprising that much of the research in these areas has been done by nurse researchers and that findings from many nursing studies have been used by practicing nurses (Health Resources and Services Administration, 1996). Problems currently being studied by nurse researchers include urinary incontinence, bathing patients with Alzheimer's disease, positioning to prevent decubitus ulcers, and nonpharmacological ways to improve sleep in nursing home residents. Often, nursing research focuses on the development of noninvasive, cost-efficient behavioral techniques as alternatives or supplements to the usual care provided to older patients.

Nursing research can lead to broad policy and practice changes. For instance, studies by nurse researchers identified the problems that can result from the use of physical restraints in the clinical setting. Increases in agitation, falls, decubitus ulcers, and urinary and fecal incontinence were documented as harm that can result from physical restraints (Capezuti, Strumpf, Evans, & Maislin, 1999; Mion et al., 1999). As a result, the standard of practice and federal law now mandate that physical restraints be used only on an emergency basis when all other methods have been tried without success. This has improved the quality of life for many older patients.

The NINR is the lead institute at NIH in advancing the science of end-of-life care. A nurse researcher and her colleagues have studied the usefulness of advance directives and the barriers to having these available. Additional work done by the team has focused on pain management for dying hospitalized patients and other issues at the end of life (Tilden, Tolle, Garland, & Nelson, 1995; Tilden et al., 1999; Tilden, Tolle, Nelson, & Fields, 2001; Tolle, Tilden, Nelson, & Dunn, 1998).

The development of doctoral programs in nursing has played a major role in the production of gerontological research. Nursing research can address basic science and clinical questions. Gerontological nurse researchers have participated in and chaired many review panels across various institutes at NIH. Doctorally prepared nurse researchers now are urged to seek postdoctoral positions and funding.

Only a small percentage of NINR-funded research can be called basic or bench research (NINR, 2002). Most nurse investigators have a clinical background, and the problems they choose to study arise from their interactions with older patients.

Many nurse researchers present their findings at specialized nursing meetings and interdisciplinary conferences, and publish in nursing and interdisciplinary journals. The relationship between gerontological nursing practice issues and nursing research should be a dynamic one, with each informing the other. However, there is sometimes a lag between the dissemination of a research finding and the use of that finding in clinical practice. This may be the result of three factors:

1. Some nurses may have a natural reluctance to change the way things are done.
2. Many practicing nurses do not read research-based journals and therefore are unaware of the findings.

3. Many nurses may doubt the validity or generalizability of the findings and be unwilling to try new techniques in their clinical setting.

(NINR, 2002)

Nurse researchers continue to search for effective ways to inform and educate practicing nurses, older patients, and families about important research findings. Websites for specific diseases and problems are useful for those who have access to the Internet. Additionally, nurse researchers should publish important clinical findings in practice-based journals and popular magazines read by the general public. Making the research more accessible to the public will better serve patients and their families. In addition, increased media coverage would serve to further the status and credibility of nursing research while showing that nurses' professional knowledge can and does make a difference in the health of people (NINR, 2002).

Role by Setting

Gerontological nurses are employed in most healthcare settings. Approximately 60% of hospital patients, 80% of home care patients, and 90% of nursing home patients are over the age of 65 (Hartford Foundation, 1999). In the United States, the term *long-term healthcare delivery system* is now used to designate several types of non–acute care settings in which gerontological nurses have opportunities for practice. Patients requiring long-term care have varying degrees of difficulty in performing activities of daily living. They may have a mental impairment such as Alzheimer's disease, be physically frail, or both. Approximately 7 million elderly people needed assistance in 1999, with 1 million needing assistance with at least five activities of daily living (General Accounting Office, 2002).

Practice Pearl

Long-term care is different from acute healthcare. It encompasses services related to maintaining quality of life, preserving individual dignity, and satisfying preferences in lifestyle for someone with a disability severe enough to require the assistance of others in everyday activities (General Accounting Office, 2002).

About 64% of older people requiring assistance for a disability rely on unpaid care from family or other informal caregivers. Others rely on formal assistance from the long-term healthcare system. These sites of care include:

- **Skilled nursing facilities.** Skilled care is delivered by nurses and others to residents. Care may be subacute (Medicare reimbursed, short stay) or chronic (private pay or Medicaid) for frail elderly residents requiring help with activities of daily living.
- **Retirement communities.** Senior citizen retirement communities range in size and scope of services. Some are life care communities and offer coordinated indepen-dent living in apartments, assisted-living apartments, and nursing home care. Residents can move from one level of care to another as their situation demands. Some retirement communities offer a narrower range of services such as independent apartments only. Others have a clubhouse with activities; some have indoor or outdoor pools, dining rooms with optional meal services, healthcare facilities, and a range of housekeeping services. Usually the resident pays an admission fee and then a monthly fee for rent and services. Some communities have 24-hour supervision and concierge services.
- **Adult day care.** Adult day care is an option for frail elderly people who require daytime supervision and activities. Sometimes an older person lives with an adult child who may have to work during the day or otherwise be absent from the home. Some day care cen-

ters offer transportation and others do not. Usually the older person and family are offered options for attendance ranging from 1 or 2 days per week to daily attendance. Day care is usually paid for privately and not covered by insurance. Usually meals are served, planned activities are provided, and some health services (podiatry, immunizations, monitoring of blood pressure, blood glucose testing, etc.) may be offered on a private pay basis.

- **Residential care facilities.** Previously called rest homes, these facilities are sometimes large private homes that have been converted to provide rooms for residents who can provide most of their own personal care, but may need help with laundry, meals, and housekeeping. Supervision and health monitoring are usually provided.
- **Transitional care units.** Many acute care hospitals have established transitional care units to provide subacute care, rehabilitation, and palliative care health services to patients who no longer require acute care. Most of these patients are recuperating from major illness or surgery, have complex health monitoring needs, or require palliative care with pain and symptom control. Diagnostic and support services of the acute care facility support the care given on transitional care units as needed.
- **Rehabilitation hospitals or facilities.** Special facilities exist to provide subacute care to patients with complex health needs. These patients may be head injured or on ventilators, require aggressive rehabilitation after injury or surgery, or require the services and intensive treatments from specialists such as physical therapists, occupational therapists, dietitians, and physiatrists. Usually rehabilitation in these facilities is covered by the patient's private insurance or Medicare.
- **Community nursing care.** Visiting nurse services are an option for many older patients requiring skilled care in the home. The nurse may visit the patient on a regular basis to monitor vital signs, provide education or counseling, administer intramuscular injections, change a dressing and deliver wound care, and provide supervision to home health aids or homemakers. Usually home care is covered by Medicare for the time period when the need for skilled nursing services exists under the direction of a physician.

Many of the long-term care options previously listed are considered private pay and are not covered by insurance. Nationally, spending from all public and private sources for long-term care totaled about $137 billion in 2000, accounting for nearly 12% of all healthcare expenditures (General Accounting Office, 2000). Over 60% of expenditures for long-term care services are paid by public programs, primarily Medicaid and Medicare. About 25% is paid by patients and their families. Figure 2-1 ■ shows the major sources financing long-term care expenditures.

Medicaid, the joint federal and state program for low-income individuals, is the largest funding source for long-term care. To qualify for Medicaid, older persons must "spend down" their assets to cover the costs of long-term care. Nursing home care can be as high as $12,000 a month. In 2000, Medicaid covered about 57% of long-term care spending.

Medicare is a federal program for older people and younger disabled people with certain chronic conditions. At the time of this writing, a limited prescription drug benefit has been passed. Medicare recipients can purchase drug discount cards to help defray some of the cost of their prescription medications. Some older people are forced to choose between buying medicine or buying food. In the Northeast, some seniors charter buses to go to Canada where drug prices are much lower. Medicare spending accounted for 14% (about $19 billion) of total long-term care spending in 2000. Although Medicare primarily covers acute care, it can also pay for limited stays in subacute care units, rehabilitation hospitals, and home health care.

Currently, as a general requirement, an older person must have a 3-day qualifying stay in a hospital and require ongoing skilled care to receive Medicare reimbursement

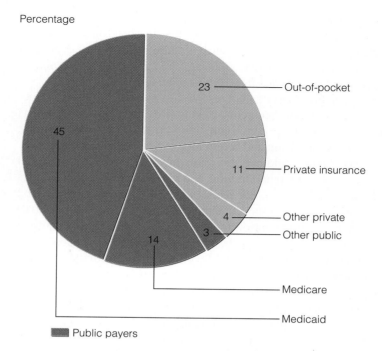

FIGURE ▨ 2-1

Major sources of financing for long-term care expenditures.

Note: Amounts do not include unpaid care provided by family member or other informal caregivers or expenditures for nursing home and home health services provided by hospital-based entitites.

Source: GAO analysis of 2000 data from the Centers for Medicare and Medicaid Services and The MEDSTAT Group.

Percentage

- 23 — Out-of-pocket
- 45
- 11 — Private insurance
- 4 — Other private
- 3 — Other public
- 14
- Medicare
- Medicaid
- ▨ Public payers

in a long-term care facility. With periodic recertification that documents the continued need for skilled care and the resident's progress toward established goals, 100 days of skilled care can be reimbursed per year.

Private insurance, which includes both traditional health insurance and long-term care insurance, accounted for 11% (about $15 billion) of long-term care expenditures in 2000. Less than 10% of the population age 65 and older and an even lower percentage of those age 55 to 64 have purchased long-term care insurance (General Accounting Office, 2002).

Trends in Financing Healthcare for Older Persons

The United States faces unprecedented demographic challenges with the aging of the baby-boom generation. As the share of the population 65 and over climbs, federal spending on older people will absorb a larger and ultimately unsustainable share of the federal budget. Federal spending for Medicare, Medicaid, and Social Security are expected to surge, nearly doubling by 2035, as people live longer and spend more time in retirement. Further, advances in medical technology and prescription drugs will likely keep pushing the costs of healthcare (General Accounting Office, 2002). A rational approach to these problems with input from gerontological nurses is needed.

It is impossible to predict what will happen in the future, but it is clear that larger numbers of nurses and other healthcare providers with specialized knowledge and training regarding caring for older persons will be needed. Gerontological nurse clinicians, researchers, and educators are needed to prepare the quantity and quality of nurses needed to meet the needs of the older person. Additional needs include more opportunities for ongoing continuing education regarding new nursing interventions and health promotion techniques appropriate for older persons.

Nurses should assume a leadership position in all debates and discussions regarding healthcare reform and financing relating to older people. Gerontological nurses recognize the benefits, burdens, and costs of informal caregiving and the need for respite services. Society has a responsibility to maintain a safety net for older people without resources, but the costs of this safety net may mean that choices and options are limited. Debate must ensue around the fundamental question of how much of the financing of long-term care should depend on the individual's own resources and how much is a societal responsibility. Everyone should be educated and urged to become personally prepared. One of the factors contributing to lack of preparation for long-term care is a widespread misunderstanding about what services Medicare will cover. Gerontological nurses can play a key role in this education process.

Gerontological nurses and others will face a changing healthcare system in the future that is likely to be:

- More managed with better integration of services and financing.
- More accountable to those who purchase and use healthcare.
- More aware of and responsive to the needs of the enrolled populations.
- Able to use fewer resources more efficiently.
- More innovative and diverse in how it provides for health services.
- More inclusive in the definition of health.
- More concerned with education, prevention, and care management, and less focused on treatment.
- More oriented to improving the health of the entire population.
- More reliant on outcomes data and evidence.

(Center for Health Professions, 2001)

Ethics

Gerontological nurses are required to provide nursing services and healthcare that are responsive to the public's trust and the older person's rights. This ethical practice is guided by the *Code for Nurses with Interpretive Statements* (ANA, 2001).

The gerontological nurse is concerned with the following ethical issues:

- Obtaining informed consent for research and clinical treatment
- Obtaining, clarifying, and carrying out advance directives
- Appropriateness of emergency treatment
- Provision of palliative care, including pain and symptom control, need for self-determination, quality of life, and treatment termination
- Elimination of the use of chemical and physical restraints
- Patient confidentiality including electronic records
- Surrogate decision making
- Access to complementary treatments
- Fair distribution of resources
- Economic decision making

(ANA, 2001)

The gerontological nurse follows all ethical principles in the roles of clinician, advocate, case manager, researcher, and administrator. Basic ethical principles include:

- **Beneficence/nonmaleficence.** To do good and not harm patients.
- **Justice.** To be fair and distribute scarce resources equally to all in need.
- **Autonomy.** To respect patients' needs for self-determination, freedom, and patient rights.

In addition, the nurse is required to follow federal, state, and local law governing aspects of gerontological nursing practice. For instance, suspected or actual abuse or neglect of elders must be reported as required by law. Additionally, the nurse's own value system will influence all clinical and ethical decision making. Each nurse has a unique set of values, morals, and life experiences. In a society with many divergent opinions regarding what can and should be done, the gerontological nurse may engage in ethical inquiry to determine the appropriate course of action. This decision-making process involves examination by the person facing a moral dilemma and often in the presence of conflicting opinions about the binding force of a specific ethical rule, attempting to discover where true professional and personal obligation lie (Edelman & Mandle, 2002). Advances in healthcare technology, changes in social and family systems, the advent of managed care, and an unlimited variety of healthcare choices have added to the complexity of caring for the older adult. While decisional authority may be ultimately the older patient's responsibility, the decision evolves within the therapeutic relationship with the nurse. The goal is to assist patients to identify and articulate genuine preferences and to make authentic choices.

Ethical decision-making competency involves the acquisition of knowledge and skills, knowledge application, and the creation of an environment that minimizes barriers to ethical practice (Reigle & Boyle, 2000).

- **Knowledge and skills.** Ethical theories, professional codes, professional standards, identification of issues, state and federal regulations.
- **Application.** Decision-making theory, mediation, facilitation of strategies to address ethical problems.
- **Ethical environment.** Support from nursing administration, role models, mentors, and a system to address and rectify barriers.

Our society is made up of individuals from diverse cultural and ethnic backgrounds. Cultural norms and practice are critical parts of any assessment of patients and families. Different subgroups respond to various situations in ways that do not always reflect the views of the dominant culture (Lapine et al., 2001). A conflict commonly encountered when caring for older people centers around the issue of disclosure. The family may request that the older patient not be told the diagnosis because of legitimate fears or anxiety about the patient's coping abilities. The healthcare providers may feel that the patient has a right to know. In many cultures (e.g., Asian and Native American), nondisclosure may be the norm (Lapine et al., 2001). (Refer to Chapter 4 ⊂▬⊃).

Important aspects of ethical decision making will include:

- **Assessment.** The older patient's condition, including medical problems, nursing diagnosis, prognosis, treatment goals, and treatment recommendations.
- **Relevant contextual factors.** Age, education, life situation, family relationships, setting of care, language, culture, religion, and socioeconomic factors.
- **Capability of the patient to make decisions.** Legally competent, clearly incapacitated, diminished capacity, fluctuating mental status, presence of drugs or illness to cloud capacity.
- **Patient preferences.** Understanding of condition, views on quality of life, values regarding treatment, and advance directives.
- **Needs of the patient as a person.** Psychic suffering, interpersonal dynamics, resources and coping strategies, adequacy of the environment for care.
- **Preferences of the family.** Competence as surrogate decision maker, judgment and evidence of knowledge of patient preferences, opinions on quality of life.
- **Competing interests.** Interests of family, healthcare providers, healthcare organization, and futile utilization of scarce resources.
- **Issues of power or conflict.** Between clinicians and family/patient, among family, among healthcare workers.

■ **Opportunity for all involved to speak and be heard.** Includes respect for opinions.

(Fletcher, Miller, & Spencer, 1997)

After completing the ethical assessment, the nurse should consider ethical standards and guidelines, analyze similar cases in the literature or practice environment, and identify morally acceptable options for resolving the dilemma. The nurse may consult with an ethics team if one is in place, a nursing mentor, or a trusted ethics advisor. All healthcare institutions should have access to an ethics committee. The purpose of the committee is to provide a forum for ethical reflection and discussion of values, to build a moral community, and to attempt to meet the needs of the patient and other affected individuals through group process and consensus. Ethics committees often validate or provide options regarding ethical dilemmas and support the care team in relation to already planned options (End-of-Life Nursing Education Consortium, 2003).

The interdisciplinary care team can also be convened to address the issue and assist in the process toward consensus. Often, the team can negotiate an acceptable plan of action. If satisfactory resolution cannot be achieved, the team may have to consider judicial review (Fletcher et al., 1997). If a satisfactory resolution is achieved and the plan of action is implemented, evaluation of the plan should be ongoing.

It is the gerontological nurse's responsibility to ensure that the patient and family fully understand treatment options in order to make informed decisions. The nurse also clarifies their wishes to others involved in the care. Gerontological nurses often engage in the process of ethical discernment, discourse, and decision making. Application of ethical principles can assist in the search for the best solutions to complex treatment problems of the older person. Gerontological nurses need to work closely with other disciplines to address ethical issues surrounding care of elderly patients.

Practice Pearl

When an ethical dilemma arises in a clinical practice, nurses should begin an ethical analysis and communicate with colleagues to seek a solution. The process is a way to seek balance, address issues, and understand the needs of all involved.

Communication

Communication is especially important to gerontological nurses. The lines of communication must be clear to develop an appropriate nursing care plan. Gerontological nurses need to communicate effectively with older patients with a variety of physical and cognitive impairments in order to develop a therapeutic relationship with each patient.

Communication is an ongoing, continuous dynamic process including verbal and nonverbal signals. Nonverbal communication is thought to make up 80% of the communication process and includes body language such as position, eye contact, touch, tone of voice, and facial expression. Nurses should follow these guidelines for verbal communication:

■ Do not yell or speak too loudly to patients. Not all older people are hard of hearing. If they are wearing a hearing aid, yelling can be disturbing.

■ Try to be at eye level with the patient. Sit down if the patient is sitting or lying down.

■ Try to minimize background noise as it can make it difficult for the patient to hear.

■ Monitor the patient's reaction. A puzzled look may mean the patient cannot hear but is ashamed to interrupt.

■ Touch the patient if appropriate and acceptable. Many older patients report that they are hardly touched by their caregivers and they appreciate the human contact.

- Supplement verbal instructions with written instructions as needed.
- Do not give long-winded speeches or complicated instructions to persons with cognitive impairment, anxiety, or pain.
- Ask how the patient would like to be addressed. Avoid demeaning terms like *sweetie, honey,* or *dearie.*

> ### Practice Pearl
>
> An elderly nursing home patient wears a button stating: "Touch me. Wrinkles aren't catching!"

An important part of communication involves attentive listening. Many healthcare providers try to anticipate what may be said and interrupt silent pauses. A careful listener will be rewarded with additional information. Open-ended statements will encourage the patient to talk. It is helpful to practice saying, "Tell me more about that . . . " or "How does this affect you?" The nurse should avoid misunderstandings by saying, "I'm not sure what you mean" or "On one hand you say . . . , but yet . . . "

Nurses should not be afraid to acknowledge their feelings. At times, a nurse may feel very sad when a patient is suffering and may even feel like crying. The older patient will probably not expect the nurse to have all the answers or know exactly what to do in all circumstances. The nurse may say, "I don't know how I can help you with this problem" or "I wish there was something I could do to make it better for you." Many times just the caring response and careful listening of the nurse will be a comfort to the patient.

Encouraging reminiscing is usually fruitful when communicating with older patients. It often gives comfort and reassurance to patients that they can talk about a time in their life when circumstances were better. It also allows the nurse to see the patient as an entire person with a life history and survival skills. If a patient cries, the nurse should offer a tissue, hold the patient's hand if appropriate, and wait a few minutes.

Communication barriers that can disrupt the process include:

1. Fear of one's own aging.
2. Fear of showing emotion or being around emotional patients.
3. Fear of missing something and feeling the need to write down every detail of the encounter.
4. Fear of being called upon to rectify every problem verbalized by the patient.
5. Lack of knowledge of the patient's culture, goals, and values.
6. Unresolved issues with aging relatives in the nurse's own family that can lead to insensitivity.
7. Feeling that professional distance must be maintained at all cost.
8. Being overworked, or overscheduled, and lacking proper time to communicate with older patients.

Many schools of nursing offer students the opportunity to role-play various patient encounters while being videotaped. This is a valuable learning experience. The student may say, "I can't believe I actually said that!" or "Why did I wrinkle my nose and look away when the patient brought that topic up?" Remember, practice makes perfect.

Patient and Family Teaching

Gerontological nurses require skills and knowledge related to teaching patients and families about the key concepts of gerontology and gerontological nursing. The guidelines in the following feature will assist the nurse to assume the role of teacher and coach.

Patient-Family Teaching Guidelines

LEARNING ABOUT GERONTOLOGICAL NURSING

1. What is gerontological nursing?

Gerontological nurses specialize in the nursing care and the health needs of older adults. They plan, manage, and implement healthcare to meet those needs, and evaluate the effectiveness of such care. They try to maximize independence and function by recognizing the strengths each older person has. Also, gerontological nurses actively involve older adults and family members as much as possible in the decision-making process, which has an impact on the quality of everyday life.

RATIONALE:

Educating the older person and his or her family regarding the goals of gerontological nursing helps to establish credibility and can form the foundation of a trusting and therapeutic relationship.

2. Why is this important to an older person like me?

With aging, an older person's health status can be affected by many factors. Gerontological nurses have extra training to become experts in the factors that can affect health status and function, including management of chronic illness, proper medication use, lifestyle changes to improve health, disease prevention and health promotion techniques, and early detection of diseases.

RATIONALE:

When older persons and their families begin to think of health in old age in a holistic manner, they can move beyond the medical model and begin to understand the importance of making appropriate lifestyle choices in order to stay healthy.

3. What are the factors that gerontological nurses consider important?

Gerontological nurses consider functional health patterns important. These are the key factors they consider when caring for older patients. These patterns include health management, nutrition, elimination, activity and sleep, cognition and self-perception, role, sexuality, values and beliefs, and coping and stress. The health of older people depends on all of these patterns, and nurses should consider them all.

RATIONALE:

The health of older people depends on all of these patterns and as nurses, we consider them all.

4. Where should I go to get further information?

Many hospitals, community health agencies, and clinics have hired and support nurses with special knowledge and expertise in caring for the older person. Ask your healthcare provider for a referral if you would like a visit or consultation with a gerontological nurse. Many gerontological nurse practitioners and clinical specialists work along with physicians and provide care to older people who want to stay healthy or recover after an illness.

RATIONALE:

Seeking information from geriatric specialists and specialty clinics can facilitate the search for resources and help ensure appropriate and accurate sources of information.

5. Should all older people be cared for by gerontological nurses?

There is great diversity in health needs of people over the age of 65. While all nurses caring for adults possess knowledge and skills in caring for older persons, sometimes a specialist is required. Regardless of a person's age or healthcare status, a gerontological nurse is helpful when placement in a long-term care facility is being considered for an older person, family members are feeling stressed or burdened, and the older person is not coping well with illness or disability.

RATIONALE:

Older persons with complicated health problems, frailty, families experiencing stress, or those who are at risk for entering a nursing home should receive care from a gerontological nurse. These elders at risk are the most likely to benefit from specialty care.

Care Plan

A Patient With a Cognitive Impairment

Case Study

Mrs. Kepler is an 85-year-old woman recovering from hip surgery. She smiles, nods her head, and looks away whenever any of the nursing staff tries to speak to her. Some staff members think the patient suffers from dementia and lacks the ability to stay focused long enough to carry on a conversation.

Applying the Nursing Process

ASSESSMENT

The nurse cannot assume the patient has a cognitive impairment based upon this information alone. Further assessment is clearly needed. Perhaps the woman is depressed, is in pain, or suffers from severe hearing loss. Many older patients will look away for fear that the nurse will ask a question that they cannot answer because they have not heard the question.

DIAGNOSIS

Possible nursing diagnoses for Mrs. Kepler include the following:

- *Impaired verbal communication*
- *Impaired social interaction*

The nurse's goal would be to begin a systematic assessment of all 11 functional health patterns in order to set realistic goals and devise a nursing care plan.

EXPECTED OUTCOMES

Expected outcomes for the plan of care specify that Mrs. Kepler will:

- Begin to make eye contact and appropriately respond to questions from the nurse.
- Make some effort to communicate level of comfort or presence of pain using verbal or nonverbal techniques.
- Begin to form a therapeutic relationship with the nursing staff and respond appropriately to nursing interventions designed to increase her security and comfort.

PLANNING AND IMPLEMENTATION

The following nursing interventions may be appropriate for Mrs. Kepler:

- Establish a therapeutic relationship.
- Avoid being frustrated or angry when she fails to respond to communication attempts.

A Patient With a Cognitive Impairment

- Encourage a family meeting to talk about health issues in general with Mrs. Kepler's permission.
- Begin a functional health pattern assessment to establish the underlying cause of the patient's communication problems.
- Observe the patient carefully for signs of pain, depression, or discomfort.

EVALUATION

The nurse realizes that it may take time to establish a trusting therapeutic relationship with Mrs. Kepler. The nurse will consider the plan a success based on the following criteria:

- Mrs. Kepler will progress through recuperation from her hip surgery with improving function and communication skills.
- A family meeting will be held to discuss the patient's overall health.
- Mrs. Kepler will use appropriate assistive devices such as hearing aids and eyeglasses to improve communication.
- She will communicate pain or discomfort to the nurses so that appropriate pharmacological and nonpharmacological pain control methods can be administered.

Ethical Dilemma

Other nurses on the floor state, "I never even try to talk to her anymore, because she just gives you that same silly smile in response. It's just more efficient to give her care without even trying to talk with her." How should the nurse respond?

By providing care without explanation, the principle of autonomy is being violated. Although the care is being delivered carefully and competently, the patient may feel anxiety and may not be prepared for what is about to happen to her. The patient may come to dread and fear nursing care and even become defensive or resistive to the care. It may be helpful to role-model appropriate verbal communication with the patient and the careful use of touch and nonverbal communication, consult with the patient's family if appropriate, and seek advice and consultation from others on the healthcare team.

Critical Thinking and the Nursing Process

1. Spend a day or two getting to know older people in your family, community, or church. Ask about their lives, struggles, successes, and regrets.
2. Try to discuss aging with colleagues from other professions such as social work, law, or premedicine. What is their view of gerontological nursing? Do they have accurate information and a good understanding of the nursing role?
3. Do you sometimes feel that nurses are underappreciated? Do your colleagues think of nurses as "pill pushers" and "Band-Aid appliers"? Try to educate them about the importance and autonomy of the nurse's role.
4. How does nursing diagnosis complement medical diagnosis? How does medical diagnosis complement nursing diagnosis?
5. What are the greatest assets the gerontological nurse can contribute to the multidisciplinary team?

- Evaluate your responses in Appendix B.

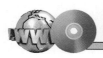

EXPLORE MediaLink

NCLEX review, case studies, and other interactive resources for this chapter can be found on the Companion Website at **www.prenhall.com/tabloski**. Click on Chapter 2 to select the activities for this chapter. For animations, video tutorials, more NCLEX review questions, and case studies, access the accompanying CD-ROM in this textbook.

Chapter Highlights

- While some would still like to "cure" old age and engage in an endless search for the fountain of youth, the prevailing view is now to search for ways to make aging more healthy and pleasant.

- Nurses are in an ideal position to encourage and support this new focus because of the variety of settings in which they encounter older people. All nurses will encounter older patients in their practice setting.

- With the percentage of older Americans increasing and the percentage of old-old growing the fastest, even nurses in pediatrics will be addressing the needs of caregiving grandparents, as well as giving advice to family and friends regarding issues of aging.

- Because aging is a progressive and universal process, it will happen to everyone. The nurse who is adequately prepared and educated to work with older people can face a long and enjoyable career.

References

American Hospital Association. (2000). *Hospital statistics*. Chicago: Author.

American Nurses Association (ANA). (2001). *Scope and standards of gerontological nursing practice*. Washington, DC: American Nurses Publishing.

American Nurses Association (ANA). (2001). *Code for nurses with interpretive statements*. Washington, DC: Author.

American Nurses Association (ANA). (2002). *ANCC certification*. Washington, DC: American Nurses Publishing.

American Nurses Association. (ANA) (2004). *Nursing: Scope and standards of practice*. Washington, DC: American Nurses Publishing.

Capezuti, E., Strumpf, N., Evans, L., & Maislin, G. (1999). Outcomes of nighttime physical restraint removal for severely impaired nursing home residents. *American Journal of Alzheimer's Disease, 1*(3), 1–8.

Carpenito, L. J. (2003). *Handbook of nursing diagnosis*. Philadelphia: Lippincott, Williams & Wilkins.

Center for Health Professions. (2001). *Critical challenges: Revitalizing the health professions for the twenty-first century*. San Francisco: University of California.

Congressional Budget Office. (2003). *Projections of expenditures for long term care services for the elderly*. U.S. Department of Health and Human Services. Retrieved November 20, 2003, from http://www.cbo.gov.

Edelman, C. L., & Mandle, C. L. (2002). *Health promotion throughout the lifespan*. St. Louis, MO: Mosby.

End-of-Life Nursing Education Consortium. (2003). *ELNEC graduate curriculum*. Retrieved June 19, 2003, from http://www.aacn.nche. edu/elnec.

Fletcher, J. C., Miller, F. G., & Spencer, E. M. (1997). Clinical ethics: History, content and resources. In J. Fletcher, P. Lombardo, M. Marshall, & F. Miller (Eds.), *Introduction to clinical ethics* (2nd ed., pp. 3–20). Frederick, MD: University Publishing Group.

General Accounting Office. (2000). *Nursing homes: Sustained efforts are essential to realize potential of the quality initiatives* (GAO-00-197).

General Accounting Office. (2001). *Nursing workforce. Recruitment and retention of nurses and nurse aides is a growing concern* (GAO-01-750T).

General Accounting Office (2002). *Long-term care: Aging baby boom generation will increase demand and burden on federal and state budgets* (GAO-02-544T).

Gordon, M. (1994). *Nursing diagnosis: Process and application*. St. Louis, MO: Mosby.

Harrington, C., Carrillo, H., Thollaug, S. C., & Summers, P. R. (1999). *Nursing facilities, staffing, residents, and facility deficiencies. 1991 through 1997.* San Francisco: University of California.

Hartford Foundation. (1999). *Best nursing practices in care for older adults. Incorporating essential gerontologic content into baccalaureate nursing education and staff development.* New York: John A. Hartford Foundation Institute for Geriatric Nursing.

Harvard School of Public Health. (2002). *Nurse staffing levels directly impact patient health and survival.* Retrieved December 1, 2002, from http://www.hsph.harvard.edu.

Health Care Financing Administration. (2002). *On-line survey certification and reporting data.* Washington, DC: Author.

Health Resources and Services Administration. (1996). *A national agenda for geriatric education: White papers.* Rockwell, MD: U.S. Department of Health and Human Services.

Health Resources and Services Administration, Bureau of Health Professions. (2000). *The registered nurse population: Findings from the national sample survey of registered nurses.* Retrieved September 14, 2001, from http://bhpr.hrsa.gov.

Hendrix, T., & Foreman, S. (2001). Optimal nurse staffing for minimal decubitus ulcer costs in nursing homes. *Nursing Economics, 19*(4), 164–175.

Iowa Intervention Project, J. C. McCloskey & G. M. Bulechek (Eds.). (2000). *Nursing interventions classification (NIC)* (3rd ed.). St. Louis, MO: Mosby.

Kayser-Jones, J. (1997). Inadequate staffing at mealtime: Implications for nursing and health policy. *Journal of Gerontological Nursing, 23*(8), 14–21.

Kovner, C., & Harrington, C. (2000). Nursing counts. *American Journal of Nursing, 100*(9), 53.

Lapine, A., Wang-Cheng, R., Goldstein, M., Nooney, A., Lamg, G., & Derse, A. R. (2001). When cultures clash: Patient and family wishes in truth disclosure for dying patients. *Journal of Palliative Medicine, 4*(4), 475–480.

McCloskey, J., & Bulechek, G. (2002). Nursing intervention classification (NIC). Overview and current status. In N. Oud (Ed.), *Proceedings of the special conference of ACENDIA in Vienna* (pp. 31–44). Bern, Switzerland: Verlag Hans Huber.

Mezey, M., & Kovner, C. (2001). *Nursing counts. Staffing issues.* Retrieved August 12, 2002, from http://www.nyu.edu/education/nursing.

Mion, L., Strumpf, N., Fulmer, T., Mezey, M., Ebersole, P., Foreman, M., et al. (1999). Use of physical restraints in the hospital setting. In I. Abraham, M. Bottrell, T. Fulmer, & M. Mezey (Eds.), *Geriatric nursing protocols for best practice* (pp. 159–172). New York: Springer.

National Academies of Practice. (2000). *Interprofessional education. Report of the expert panel.* Retrieved June 14, 2001, from http://nap.vcu.edu.

National Citizens' Coalition for Nursing Home Reform. (1999). *Federal and state minimum staffing requirements: Overview of law and regulations guidelines.* Retrieved March 19, 2003, from http://www.nccnhr.org.

National Institute of Nursing Research (NINR). (2002). *Making a difference. NINR research results.* Washington, DC: Author.

North American Nursing Diagnosis Association (NANDA). (2003). *NANDA nursing diagnoses: Definitions and classification 2003–2004.* Philadelphia: Author.

Prochaska, J., Velicer, W., Fava, J., Rossi, J., & Tsoh, J. (2001). Evaluating a population-based recruitment approach and a stage-based expert system intervention for smoking cessation. *Addictive Behaviors, 26,* 583–602.

Reigle, J., & Boyle, R. J. (2000). Ethical decision-making skills. In A. B. Hamric, J. A. Spross, & C. M. Hanson (Eds.), *Advanced nursing practice: An integrative approach* (2nd ed., pp. 349–378). Philadelphia: Saunders.

Ruiz, B., Tabloski, P. A., & Frazier, S. (1995). The role of gerontological advanced practice nurses in geriatric care. *Journal of the American Geriatrics Society, 43,* 1061–1064.

Tilden, V. P., Tolle, S.W., Garland, M. J., & Nelson, C.A. (1995). Decisions about life-sustaining treatment. *Archives of Internal Medicine, 155,* 633–638.

Tilden, V. P., Tolle, S. W., Nelson, C. A., Thompson, M., & Eggman, S. C., et al. (1999). Family decision making in foregoing life-sustaining treatments. *Journal of Family Nursing, 5*(4), 426–442.

Tilden, V. P., Tolle, S. W., Nelson, C. A., & Fields, J. (2001). Family decision-making to withdraw life-sustaining treatments from hospitalized patients. *Nursing Research, 5*(2), 105–115.

Tolle, S. W., Tilden, V. P., Nelson, C. A., & Dunn, P. M. (1998). A prospective study of the efficacy of the physician order form for life-sustaining treatment. *Journal of the American Geriatric Society, 46,* 1097–1102.

Williams, C. (2001). The RN shortage: Not just nursing's problem. *Academic Medicine, 76*(3), 218–220.

CHAPTER 3

Principles of Geriatrics

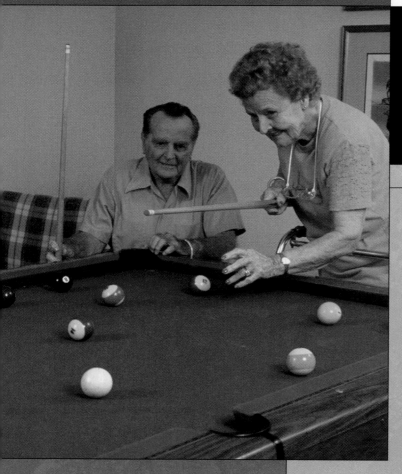

CHAPTER OBJECTIVES

Upon completion of this chapter, the reader will be able to:

- Define interdisciplinary geriatric assessment and terminology.

- Identify appropriate guidelines for health promotion and disease prevention.

- Identify the nurse's role in the geriatric assessment process.

- Describe the impact of culture and ethnicity on the assessment process.

- Identify ethical, legal, and public policy issues affecting care of the older patient.

KEY TERMS

comprehensive geriatric
  evaluation 55
functional assessment 55
interdisciplinary education 56
interdisciplinary teams 57

MediaLink

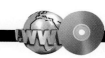

Additional resources for this chapter can be found on the Student CD-ROM accompanying this textbook and on the Companion Website at **www.prenhall.com/tabloski**. Click on Chapter 3 to select the activities for this chapter.

CD-ROM

- Animation/Video
    Initial Assessment
    Physical Examination
- NCLEX Review
- Case Studies
- Tools

COMPANION WEBSITE

- Audio Glossary
- Additional NCLEX Review
- Case Study
- MediaLink Applications

Comprehensive geriatric evaluation is essential to fully understand the health needs of an older person. A key part of the geriatric evaluation is the **functional assessment** or systematic evaluation of the older person's level of function and self-care. The comprehensive evaluation is usually interdisciplinary and multidimensional and will address function in the physical, social, and psychological domains. Key members of the interdisciplinary team are the gerontological nurse, the social worker, and the geriatric physician. Other healthcare professionals can be included in the evaluation or consulted depending on the needs and problems exhibited by the older patient. Sometimes physical therapists, occupational therapists, clinical pharmacists, psychologists, psychiatrists, podiatrists, dentists, and other professionals are called in to consult and evaluate an older patient with complex needs.

It is recommended that comprehensive geriatric evaluation be carried out on a regular basis, including:

1. After hospitalization for an acute illness.
2. When nursing home placement or a change in living status is being considered.
3. After any abrupt change in physical, social, or psychological function.
4. Yearly for the older person with complex health needs during the annual visit for routine health maintenance with the primary healthcare provider.
5. When the older patient or family would like a second opinion regarding an intervention or treatment protocol recommended by the primary care provider.

Not all older people will have access to trained interdisciplinary teams; however, the careful clinician can incorporate holistic assessment techniques and standardized instruments into routine evaluations. Gerontological nurses are in an ideal position to advocate for older patients who would benefit from holistic assessment and to urge them to seek the services of specialized geriatric assessment teams.

Research evaluating the clinical outcomes of comprehensive geriatric evaluation with older patients reveals reduced hospital use, reduced mortality rates, improved mental status, consumption of fewer medications, improved functional ability, and lower hospital readmission rates (Kane, Ouslander, & Abrass, 1999). The vision for the future is that every older person will have access to appropriate interdisciplinary healthcare and that every healthcare organization and setting providing care to older adults will have financial support for an interdisciplinary geriatric service or program (Health Resources and Services Administration, 1996). Not every older person would receive care from an interdisciplinary team, but the team would be available for those older patients whose needs require holistic evaluation.

The gerontological nurse requires a different perspective during the geriatric evaluation process, and special instruments are needed to gather appropriate data. The members of the team must not only be knowledgeable in the content area of gerontology and geriatrics, but also be educated regarding the issues of team dynamics. Essential skills in team dynamics include awareness of the roles and contributions of all team members, excellent communication skills in order to share information, conflict resolution skills, and the ability to see beyond "disciplinary ethnocentrism" that assumes only one's own discipline is competent to solve the problems of the older patient. Many schools of nursing and medicine offer interdisciplinary courses and educate students to work together and share knowledge to solve complex patient problems.

The Hartford Institute recommends the following instruments for use when assessing the function of older adults. These instruments have been used clinically for many years, are commonly referred to in practice, and are validated on large patient groups. They include:

1. Lawton Activities of Daily Living. Measures ability to perform tasks of personal care, including ambulation, transferring, dressing, bathing, toileting, and continence (Lawton, 1971).
2. Lawton Independent Activities of Daily Living. Measures abilities associated with living independently in the community, including cooking, cleaning, laundry, shopping, using the telephone, transportation, and managing finances (Lawton, 1971).
3. Pulses Profile. Measures general functional performance in mobility and self-care, medical status, and psychosocial factors.
   - P = physical condition
   - U = upper limb function
   - L = lower limb function
   - S = sensory components
   - E = excretory functions
   - S = support factors (Granger, Albrecht, & Hamilton, 1979)
4. SPICES. An overall assessment tool used to plan, promote, and maintain optimal function in older adults.
   - S = sleep disorders
   - P = problems with eating and feeding
   - I = incontinence
   - C = confusion
   - E = evidence of falls
   - S = skin breakdown

Source: Fulmer, 1991; Hartford Institute for Geriatric Nursing, 1999.

Collaboration implies the process of shared planning, decision making, accountability, and responsibility in the care of the patient (Hartford Institute, 1999). Reasons for collaborative care for older adults include the following:

- Older adults may face a multitude of complex problems requiring input and advice from various healthcare professionals.
- Assembling a group of knowledgeable providers can enhance problem solving and the delivery of healthcare.
- Coordination of services can be enhanced by various professionals working together.
- The patient will have access to a comprehensive and integrated care plan.
- Care can be more cost-effective and efficient.
- Healthcare professionals can feel supported and encouraged by the input and collaboration from other professionals. Interdisciplinary care has the potential to decrease feelings of "burnout" when caring for older patients with complex health needs.

(Hartford Institute for Geriatric Nursing, 1999)

The Veterans Administration (VA) system has provided funding to research and evaluate the geriatric evaluation process. In 1979, the Interdisciplinary Team Training in Geriatrics program was established to provide leadership in **interdisciplinary education** and training using a team approach to service delivery throughout the VA system. Approximately 50 clinical teams have been formed, and 5,000 VA personnel have been trained in the principles of teamwork. Geriatric Research, Education, and Clinical Centers have been formed to evaluate and meet the health needs of older veterans.

MediaLink • Initial Assessment and Physical Examination Video

The Health Resources and Services Administration has funded over 30 projects in underserved rural areas to educate health professionals in the principles of interdisciplinary education and patient care. In 1994, the Joint Commission on Accreditation of Healthcare Organizations (JCAHO) established standards that emphasize the importance of an interdisciplinary approach to providing patient care. Healthcare personnel working in JCAHO-approved healthcare facilities must possess the knowledge and skills to participate in **interdisciplinary teams** (JCAHO, 2004).

Geriatric evaluation can be conducted by teams within the acute care hospital setting, on an outpatient basis at an ambulatory clinic, or even in the home setting. Results of the assessment and recommendations can be implemented by the team or conveyed to the primary healthcare provider for implementation or follow-up as appropriate. Leadership of the team is based on expertise rather than discipline or authority. Gerontological nurses assume team leadership when the older patient's problems reside within the primary domain of nursing. Social workers assume leadership for social problems, and physicians assume leadership for the assessment and diagnosis of illness and disease.

Components of Comprehensive Geriatric Assessment

Despite variations in instruments, structure of the interdisciplinary team, and methods employed, several strategies have been proven to make the evaluation process more effective. These include the development of a close-knit interdisciplinary team with minimal redundancy in the assessments performed, the use of carefully designed questionnaires that reliable older patients or their caregivers can complete beforehand, and the effective use of assessment forms that are incorporated into computer databases (Kane et al., 1999).

There are three underlying principles of comprehensive geriatric assessment:

1. Physical, psychological, and socioeconomic factors interact in complex ways to influence the health and functional status of the older person.
2. Comprehensive evaluation of an older person's health status requires an assessment in each of these domains. The coordinated efforts of various healthcare professionals are needed to carry out the assessment.
3. Functional abilities should be a central focus of the comprehensive evaluation. Other more traditional measures of health such as medical diagnosis, nursing diagnosis, physical examination results, and laboratory findings form the basic foundation of the assessment in order to determine overall health, well-being, and the need for social services.

(Kane et al., 1999)

CONTEXTUAL VARIABLES AFFECTING HOLISTIC GERIATRIC ASSESSMENT

The interrelationships between the physical, social, and psychological aspects of aging and perhaps illness present a challenge to the gerontological nurse when beginning the geriatric evaluation. The gerontological nurse is often charged with the responsibility of obtaining the patient's past health history and history of the present illness. The following contextual variables should be considered.

Evaluation Environment

In order to make the older patient and family comfortable, environmental modifications should be made, if possible. Environmental modifications may include: adequate lighting, decreased background noise, comfortable seating for the patient and family, easily accessible restrooms, examination tables that can be raised or lowered to assist patients with disabilities, and availability of water or juice for patient use. Patient comfort will ease communication and improve the data-gathering process.

Accuracy of the Health History

Clear instructions should be provided to the patient and family beforehand regarding the parking arrangements and registration process. Many assessment clinics mail an information packet in advance so that the older patient can come prepared. This packet might include:

1. A past medical history form. This form can be completed at home and is helpful for patients with complicated medical histories. The dates of hospitalizations, operations, serious injuries or accidents, procedures, and so on can be ascertained beforehand to save time during the assessment appointment. The form would also include history of adverse drug effects or allergies.
2. Instructions to bring in all prescription and over-the-counter medications for review by the gerontological nurse.
3. Instructions to bring any medical records, laboratory or X-ray reports, electrocardiograms, reports of vaccination, and other pertinent health records that the patient or family may possess.
4. Instructions to write down and bring the names of all healthcare providers involved with the patient's healthcare, including primary care providers, specialists, and alternative medicine practitioners (e.g., acupuncturists, massage therapists, chiropractors).

The more information that the patient and family can organize ahead of time, the better and more efficient the assessment will be. Patience is a virtue when obtaining a history because many times the thought and verbal processes are slower in the older person. Patients should be allowed adequate time to answer questions and report information (Kane et al., 1999).

The history should include emphasis on the following:

- Review of acute and chronic medical problems
- Medications
- Disease prevention and health maintenance review: vaccinations, PPD (tuberculosis), cancer screening
- Functional status (activities of daily living)
- Social supports (family, caregiver stress, safety of living environment)
- Finances
- Driving status and safety record
- Geriatric review of symptoms (patient/family perception of memory, dentition, taste, smell, nutrition, hearing, vision, falls, fractures, bowel and bladder function)

(Stanford University Geriatric Education Resource Center, 2000)

Often, a standardized form is used to guide and direct the obtaining of the health history. The gerontological nurse should be aware of potential difficulties in obtaining health histories from older persons, including:

- **Communication difficulties.** Decreased hearing or vision, slow speech, and use of English as a second language have an effect on communication.
- **Underreporting of symptoms.** Fear of being labeled as a complainer, fear of institutionalization, and fear of serious illness can influence symptom reporting.

- **Vague or nonspecific complaints.** These may be associated with cognitive impairment, drug or alcohol use or abuse, or atypical presentation of disease.
- **Multiple complaints.** Associated "masked" depression, presence of multiple chronic illnesses, and social isolation are often an older person's cry for help.
- **Lack of time.** New patients scheduled for geriatric assessment should have the minimum of a 1-hour appointment with the gerontological nurse. Shorter appointments will result in a hurried interview with missed information.

(Kane et al., 1999)

Social History

Holistic evaluation is not complete without an assessment of the social support system. Many frail older persons receive support and supervision from family members and significant others to compensate for functional disabilities.

Key elements of the social history include the following:

- Past occupation and retirement status
- Family history (helpful to construct a family genogram)
- Present and former marital status, including quality of the relationship(s)
- Identification of family members, with designation of level of involvement and place of residence
- Living arrangements
- Family dynamics
- Family and caregiver expectations
- Economic status, adequacy of health insurance
- Social activities and hobbies
- Mode of transportation
- Community involvement and support
- Religious involvement and spirituality

If there is a social worker on the assessment team, the gerontological nurse may work closely to identify and address social problems. Older patients with inadequate health insurance can often be helped by accessing community services, hospital free care, hardship funds established for indigent patients by major drug companies, and referrals to community-based free clinics.

Psychological History

Another key component of the holistic geriatric assessment is evaluation of psychological and cognitive function. A significant proportion of older patients with mental illness remain unrecognized and untreated; when treated, the use of healthcare services decreases (Health Resources and Services Administration, 1996). The reported range of adults over the age of 65 with mental disorders, both in institutions and in the community, is estimated to be between 20% and 30%.

The older person is more likely to use general healthcare services than to seek specialized services with mental health professionals. Many older people are fearful of seeing a psychiatrist, psychiatric social worker, or psychiatric–mental health advanced practice nurse because they fear being labeled as "crazy." All healthcare workers working with older patients should be aware of the mental health problems common in the older adult, diagnostic instruments appropriate for screening and diagnosing mental health problems, and the resources for treatment and referral within their practice site. Mental and emotional problems are not a normal part of aging. When mental health problems manifest themselves in the older adult, they should be evaluated, diagnosed, and treated. By forming a trusting therapeutic relationship, the gerontological nurse can demonstrate caring, warmth, respect, and support for the older person who may be hesitant to verbalize feelings of low self-esteem, depression, bizarre thought patterns, or phobias and anxieties.

Key elements of the psychological history include:

- Any history of past mental illness.
- Any hospitalizations or outpatient treatments for psychological problems.
- Current and past stress levels and coping mechanisms.
- Current level of alcohol or recreational drug use.
- Medications taken for anxiety, insomnia, or depression.
- Identification of any problems with memory, judgment, or thought processing.
- Any changes in personality, values, personal habits, or life satisfaction.
- Identification of feelings regarding self-worth and hopes for the future.
- Feelings of appropriate emotions related to present life and health situation (feelings of sadness regarding losses, etc.).
- Presence of someone to love, support, and encourage the older patient.
- Feelings of hopelessness or suicidal ideation.

The accuracy of the health history and identification of problems depends on adequate mental and affective functioning. The higher the level of cognitive impairment, the more likely the older patient is to report inaccurate information. Problems with short-term memory can cause older people to forget to report adverse events such as falls, safety issues in the home, or other relevant problems that could influence the plan of care. Further, depressed older patients may score poorly on instruments used to assess psychological function because they do not have the energy or motivation to attend to or answer questions. The nurse should consider depression as a contextual variable when an older person continuously states, "I don't know" or "I couldn't tell you" when responding to questions.

There is benefit from interviewing the older person with and without the family or significant others present. Some older patients will confide difficulties to the gerontological nurse in private that they may be hesitant to report in the presence of family. These issues may encompass family dynamics, sexuality, matters relating to bowel and bladder function, or other personal issues. At times, family presence may assist in obtaining an accurate health history. Many gerontological nurses seek permission from the older patient to include the family to verify or gather additional information. An older patient with depression may feel demoralized and be unable to take part in rehabilitation or health promotion activities based upon lack of energy and motivation. Family members and involved caregivers are often in a position to report subtle changes in personality and function that may go undetected by others.

Instruments commonly used in clinical practice to assess psychological function include the following:

- Geriatric Depression Scale (Yesavage & Brink, 1983). The short form includes 15 questions and measures depression in the older adult.
- Mini-Mental State Examination (MMSE) (Folstein, Folstein, & McHugh, 1975). Ten questions measure orientation, memory, language, and writing ability.
- Life Satisfaction Index (Neugarten et al., 1961). Twelve open-ended questions assess the older person's life satisfaction.
- Philadelphia Geriatric Center Morale Scale (Lawton, 1971). A 17-question scale measures morale and associated problems with low morale.

Home Environment

Some geriatric assessment teams have the time and resources to visit the patient's home and conduct an assessment of the environment. While this direct observation is the best way to gather accurate and reliable data, it is time consuming and can be expensive. Therefore, many geriatric assessment teams question the older person and the family regarding the adequacy of the home environment and the available resources to maintain adequate levels of function.

Factors to be considered when assessing the home environment include:

- **Stairs.** Narrow stairs with poor lighting, inadequate railings, and uneven steps are fall risks. Does the older person have the strength and balance to climb stairs? If a wheelchair or walker is used, are there ramps present or space for them to be added?
- **Bathing and toileting.** Can the older person safely transfer on and off the toilet? Is a raised toilet seat needed? Are grab bars present? Is there an adequate bath mat in the tub? Is a shower seat needed? Is lighting adequate?
- **Medications.** Where are medications stored? Are there grandchildren in the home who are at risk because of open storage or nonreplacement of caps? Are old and outdated medications disposed of to prevent accidents? Are medications refilled on time to prevent on-off dosing patterns? Is there a list of medications available for use in emergencies?
- **Predetermined wishes.** Has the older person named a health proxy or established a living will? If so, does the family and primary care provider have a copy? Is the healthcare proxy knowledgeable regarding the patient's preferences? Is the proxy's number posted in an easily visible position (e.g., on the refrigerator)? Is the value quality of life or length of life specified?
- **Nutrition and cooking.** Is there adequate food in the home? Is there a stove or microwave to cook? Are any safety problems reported with the stove or microwave? If a gas stove, is it safe? Is the pilot functioning properly? Are there gas leak detectors? Is food storage adequate? Is spoiled food present? Is the food preparation environment clean? Who does the grocery shopping?
- **Falls.** Are the floors free of cords, debris, and scatter rugs? Is there adequate lighting? Are there night-lights? Are there pets who dart around quickly? If there is a history of falls, would the older person consider wearing an emergency alert system around the neck?
- **Smoke detectors.** Are there functioning smoke detectors? Are batteries changed yearly?
- **Emergency numbers.** Are emergency phone numbers posted or preprogrammed into the phone?
- **Temperature of home.** Is there adequate heat in the winter and cooling in the summer?
- **Temperature of water.** Is the hot water set below 120°F?
- **Safety of the neighborhood.** Can the older person venture outside without fear of becoming a crime victim? Are there adequate door locks and latches? How close is the nearest neighbor? Is there nearby help if it is needed?
- **Financial.** Are there piles of unpaid bills? Are services such as phone and electricity in good working order? Are there large amounts of cash hidden or stored around the house?

Culture and Education

The increasing need for healthcare providers to care for older adults from diverse backgrounds means that gerontological nurses must consider how assessment and development of a treatment plan are modified to avoid misunderstanding or ineffective care. Caution is urged when users of assessment instruments draw conclusions from test scores that are derived from patients of different cultures and various educational backgrounds (Gallo, Fulmer, Paveza, & Reichel, 2000). Some instruments such as the MMSE have developed and validated scoring norms based upon level of education. The examination has a component dependent upon reading a sentence and following instructions, writing a sentence, performing complex mathematical calculations, and spelling a word backwards. Older patients may be reticent to tell a healthcare provider that they are unable to read or write and may score poorly as a result. Low scores could falsely be attributed to cognitive impairment rather than low reading literacy. The gerontological nurse should always consider and assess educational level, language barriers, reading levels, and cultural background before using standardized instruments.

It is important to understand and elicit the beliefs, attitudes, values, and goals of older people relating to their lives, illness, and health states in order to provide culturally appropriate care. Cultural competence in healthcare consists of at least three components:

1. Knowing the prevalence, incidence, and risk factors (epidemiology) for diseases in different ethnic groups
2. Understanding how the response to medications and other treatments varies with ethnicity
3. Eliciting the culturally held beliefs and attitudes toward illness, treatment, and the healthcare system.

(Mouton & Espino, 2000)

There is heterogeneity within various ethnic groups, and the provision of culturally sensitive care dictates that each person be approached as a unique individual. Patient age, place of birth, where childhood was spent, and how the older person was socialized to American culture can all affect performance on standardized assessment instruments. Many of the instruments used by clinicians to assess older patients have not been validated for use with cultural minorities (Mouton & Espino, 2000). The members of some ethnic groups are less willing to report difficulty taking care of themselves and may fear admitting their dependence on others. Refer to Chapter 4 for a thorough discussion of culture.

MINIMUM DATA SET

Assessment of an older person for appropriate placement within the nursing home or within the long-term care system is done using the Minimum Data Set (MDS).

The MDS is a comprehensive multidisciplinary assessment that is used throughout the United States. It was devised and passed into law because of the belief that a better, more holistic patient assessment will facilitate improved patient care. The Omnibus Budget Reconciliation Act of 1987 (OBRA 87) contained a provision mandating that all residents of facilities that collect funds from Medicare or Medicaid be assessed using the MDS. The MDS is used for validating the need for long-term care, reimbursement, ongoing assessment of clinical problems, and assessment of and need to alter the current plan of care.

The MDS consists of a core set of screening, clinical, and functional measures. It is used with the Resident Assessment Protocols (RAPS), the Resident Utilization Guidelines (RUGS), and the Resident Assessment Instrument (RAI).

Categories of data gathered for the MDS include the following:

- Patient demographics and background
- Cognitive function
- Communication and hearing
- Mood and behavior patterns
- Psychosocial well-being

- Physical function and activities of daily living
- Bowel and bladder continence
- Diagnosed diseases
- Health conditions (weight, falls, etc.)
- Oral nutritional status
- Oral and dental status
- Skin condition
- Activity pursuits
- Medications
- Need for special services
- Discharge potential

Certain information gathered for the MDS such as functional decline or a poorly managed chronic disease may trigger the need for further assessment using the RAP. For instance, if information gathered for the MDS indicates that the nursing home resident has fallen, a RAP is triggered and indicates the need for direct gait assessment, medication review, and physical/occupational therapy evaluation. Table 3-1 indicates the RAP triggers and supplemental assessments.

The MDS can be viewed as a start in acquiring the broad base of clinical information necessary to provide quality long-term care. The gerontological nurse with excellent clinical skills will often be called upon to individualize the predetermined structured assessment and the interventions. For example, a nursing home resident with severe Alzheimer's

TABLE 3-1

RAP Triggers and Supplemental Assessments

RAP	Supplemental Assessment
Delirium	Medical assessment, attention measures, selected lab tests
Cognitive loss/dementia	Screening with MMSE
Visual function	Optometry evaluation
Communication	Speech therapist evaluation, hearing evaluation
Activities of daily living function loss	Performance-based assessment, physical/occupational therapy assessment
Urinary incontinence, use of indwelling catheter	Incontinence record, genitourinary, physical assessment
Psychosocial well-being	Social services assessment
Mood state	Clinical record review, depression screen, psychological evaluation
Behavioral symptoms	Behavior monitoring record, psychiatric evaluation
Activities	Social services assessment
Falls	Direct gait assessment, physical/occupational therapy evaluation
Nutritional status	Medical assessment, weight chart, dietary consult
Feeding tubes	Dietary evaluation, speech therapy evaluation
Dehydration/fluid maintenance	Dietary evaluation, intake/output record evaluation
Oral/dental care	Oral assessment/dental evaluation
Pressure ulcers	Braden scale, occupational therapy evaluation
Psychotropic drug use	Psychiatric evaluation, psychological assessment
Physical restraints	Medical assessment, physical/occupational therapy evaluation

Source: Centers for Medicare and Medicaid, 2000.

disease may be incontinent of urine. The probable cause of the incontinence is not a genitourinary problem, but rather the result of the older person's cognitive impairment and need to ask for help to get to the toilet (Teigland, 2000). Clinical experts in geriatrics and gerontology are working with federal regulators to develop a risk stratification system that would be better able to measure quality and trigger the need for further assessments based upon the risks associated with severe cognitive impairment.

HEALTH PROMOTION AND DISEASE SCREENING

Health for older adults is a complex interaction of physical, functional, and psychosocial factors. Clearly, it is not just the absence of disease, as many people diagnosed with a chronic disease consider themselves to be healthy. Health may be considered a state of physical, mental, and social functioning that realizes the potential of which a person is capable (Edelman & Mandle, 2002). The World Health Organization (1946) has defined health as "the state of complete physical, mental, and social well-being and not merely the absence of disease and infirmity."

Others speak of health and illness as opposite ends of a continuum with the midpoint forming the demarcation between illness and health (Figure 3-1 ■). The person is envisioned to move back and forth on the continuum in response to a variety of factors such as ability to function adequately, feelings of control of chronic illness, clinical markers, environmental supports, rate and degree of disease progression, and so on.

The goal of nursing interventions for persons with altered health maintenance is to facilitate:

1. Lifestyle changes.
2. Acquisition of new health-promoting thought patterns and behaviors.
3. Self-care in managing chronic health conditions or risks. (Maas et al., 2001).

These interventions are intended to move the older person along the continuum toward health and away from illness. The gerontological nurse would formulate indicators of movement on the health continuum by specifying markers, targets, and time intervals that are appropriate for assessing progress of the older patient.

The older person's health beliefs will indicate the motivational support and perceived benefits of action. Indicators of health beliefs include:

- Perceived importance of taking action.
- Perceived threat of inaction.
- Perceived benefits of action.
- Perceived internal control of action.
- Perceived control of health outcome.
- Perceived improvement in lifestyle from action.
- Perceived resources to perform action.
- Perceived absence of barriers to action.
- Perceived reduction of threat from action.

(Maas et al., 2001)

The older person who indicates strong health beliefs in these indicators will have a higher probability of being able to take positive action to move toward health on the continuum.

FIGURE ■ 3-1

The health continuum.

Illness   Midpoint   Health

According to Pender, Murdaugh, and Parsons (2002), health promotion is a "multi-dimensional pattern of self-initiated actions and perceptions that serve to maintain or enhance the level of wellness, self-actualization and fulfillment of the individual" (p. 9). Such behaviors often include:

- Engaging in regular physical activity.
- Engaging in challenging mental activity.
- Eating a healthy, balanced diet.
- Getting 8 hours of sleep a night.
- Having at least one friend to trust and confide in.
- Having some relaxing and pleasant activities to look forward to.
- Having the self-discipline to enjoy pleasant things in moderation.
- Trying to view things positively and have hopes for the future.

Health promotion for the older adult is not focused on disease or disability, but rather on strengths, abilities, and values of the individual. By maximizing strengths, identifying resources, and identifying values that guide behaviors, the gerontological nurse has the opportunity to greatly influence positive health behaviors in the older adult.

Healthy People 2010

The U.S. Department of Health and Human Services has developed guidelines for the nation's health, *Healthy People 2010: National Health Promotion and Disease Prevention Objectives* (2000). The overarching goals of this document are to:

1. Increase quality and years of healthy life.
2. Eliminate health disparities.

Both of these goals are appropriate for the older adult. The first addresses issues such as living longer and living better. The second goal addresses access to care without consideration of race, gender, ability to pay, place of residence, and so on.

HEALTH STATUS

To understand the health status of a population, it is essential to monitor and evaluate the determinants of health and their consequences. The health status of the United States is a description of the health of the total population, using information representative of most people living in this country. The goal of eliminating health disparities will necessitate improved collection and use of standardized data to correctly identify disparities among select population groups (*Healthy People 2010,* 2000).

Health status can be measured by birth and death rates, life expectancy, quality of life, morbidity from specific diseases, risk factors, use of ambulatory care and inpatient care, accessibility of health personnel and facilities, financing of healthcare, health insurance coverage, and many other factors. The information used to report health status comes from a variety of sources, including birth and death records, hospital discharge data, and health information collected from healthcare records, personal interviews, physical examinations, and telephone surveys (*Healthy People 2010,* 2000).

The leading causes of death are used frequently to describe the health status of the nation. Over the past 100 years, the United States has seen a great deal of change in the leading causes of death (Figure 3-2 ■). At the beginning of the 1900s, infectious diseases ran rampant in the United States and worldwide and topped the leading causes of death. A century later, with the control of many infectious agents and the increasing age of the population, chronic diseases top the list (*Healthy People 2010,* 2000).

FIGURE ■ 3-2

The leading causes of death as a percentage of all deaths in the United States, 1900 and 1997.

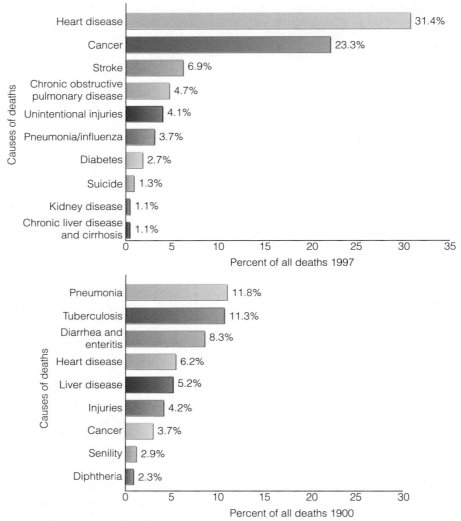

*Not all states are represented.

Source: Centers for Disease Control and Prevention, National Center for Health Statistics. National Vital Statistics System and unpublished data. 1997.

A very different picture emerges when the leading causes of death are viewed for various population groups. Unintentional injuries, mainly motor vehicle crashes, are the fifth leading cause of death for the total population, but they are the leading cause of death for people age 1 to 44 years. Similarly, HIV/AIDS is the 14th leading cause of death for the total population but the leading cause of death for African American men age 25 to 44 years (*Healthy People 2010,* 2000). In the older adult, the leading causes of death are heart disease, cancer, and stroke (Figure 3-3 ■).

The leading causes of death in the United States generally result from a mix of behaviors: injury, violence, and other factors in the environment; and the unavailability or inaccessibility of quality health services. Understanding and monitoring behaviors, environmental factors, and community health systems may prove more useful to monitoring and improving the nation's *true* health than the death rates that reflect the cumulative impact of these factors. This more complex approach has served as the basis for developing the leading health indicators.

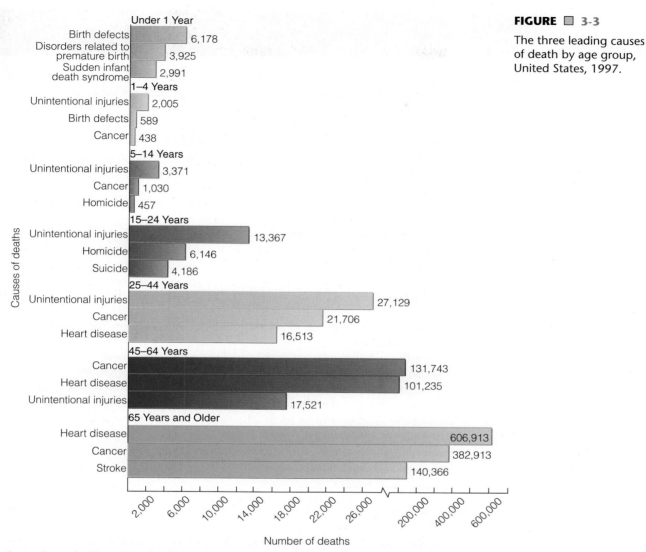

FIGURE 3-3

The three leading causes of death by age group, United States, 1997.

Source: Centers for Disease Control and Prevention, National Center for Health Statistics. National Vital Statistics System. 1999.

From the overarching goals of increasing quality and years of healthy life and eliminating disparities, specific goals have been developed that focus on increasing health promotion activities and decreasing morbidity and mortality in persons of all ages. To view the complete report, go to the *Healthy People 2010* website. Some of the goals that pertain to older adults are listed in Box 3-1.

The goals included in *Healthy People 2010* form the foundation of professional activities, influence the allocation of health resources, and direct clinical research activities over the next several years.

Many older adults are willing and eager to engage in health promotion activities. They may have seen their friends and relatives become ill, go to nursing homes, or die. As a result, they have come to realize how important it is to protect and maintain good health. Additionally, many older people fear they will become a burden on their children and therefore do everything they can to remain active, healthy, and independent. Health maintenance practices should also include regular visits to a primary

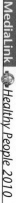

MediaLink ◈ *Healthy People 2010*

BOX 3-1	Selected Health Promotion Goals Applicable to Older People from *Healthy People 2010*

- Increase the proportion of persons with specific sources of ongoing care.
- Reduce hospitalization rates for uncontrolled diabetes and immunization-preventable pneumonia and influenza.
- Reduce the overall number of cases of osteoporosis.
- Reduce the number of vertebral fractures associated with osteoporosis.
- Increase the proportion of older adults who receive a colorectal cancer screening examination.
- Reduce the new cases of end-stage renal disease.
- Increase the proportion of persons with diabetes who receive formal diabetes education.
- Reduce the diabetes death rate.
- Reduce deaths from cardiovascular disease in persons with diabetes.
- Reduce the rate of lower extremity amputations in persons with diabetes.
- Increase the proportion of adults with diabetes who have an annual eye examination, foot examination, dental examination, and have glycosylated hemoglobin measurement.
- Increase the proportion of adults with diabetes who perform daily self-blood glucose measurement.
- Reduce the number of adults with disabilities who report feelings of sadness, unhappiness, or depression that prevents them from being more active.
- Increase the number of adults with disabilities who report sufficient emotional support.
- Increase the number of adults with disabilities who report satisfaction with life.
- Increase the number of older adults who have participated in at least one organized health promotion activity within the previous year.
- Reduce hospitalizations of older adults with heart failure.
- Reduce invasive pneumococcal infections.

care provider and appropriate diagnostic and screening tests as recommended. Table 3-2 lists recommended health screenings for older persons.

Additional recommendations include screening yearly for driving safety and capability, elder mistreatment, alcohol use, falls, and financial problems (Oakley, Duran, Fisher, & Merritt, 2003).

PAIN

Pain is an unpleasant sensory and emotional experience that can negatively impact the quality of life of older persons. Both acute and chronic pain are problems often assessed by gerontological nurses. It is estimated that 25% to 50% of community-residing older people and 45% to 80% of nursing home residents suffer significant undertreated pain (Hartford Institute, 1999). In the verbal patient, the most accurate evidence of pain and its intensity is based on the client's description and self-report. When assessing pain, the gerontological nurse should assess the intensity, quality, onset, duration, expression, aggravating and alleviating factors, and emotional response of the older person to the pain. In the nonverbal patient, the nurse should carefully assess vital signs, facial expression, resistance to movement, guarding of body parts, and sighing or moaning. Various measurement techniques used for pain assessment include visual analog scales, word descriptor scales, and numerical scales. (See Chapter 9 for further information.)

- Increase the numbers of older adults who are vaccinated annually against influenza and receive pneumococcal vaccine for the first time.
- Reduce hospitalizations from head injuries.
- Reduce pedestrian deaths on public roads.
- Reduce residential fire deaths.
- Reduce deaths from falls.
- Reduce hip fractures in older adults.
- Increase the number of primary care providers, pharmacists, and other healthcare professionals who routinely review with their patients age 65 years and older all newly prescribed and over-the-counter medications.
- Increase the proportion of older adults who are at a healthy weight.
- Increase the proportion of older adults who consume at least two daily servings of fruit, three daily servings of vegetables, six daily servings of grain, and less than 30% of calories from fat.
- Increase the number of persons who meet dietary recommendations for calcium.
- Increase the number of persons with chronic illness who receive counseling or education related to diet and nutrition.
- Reduce the number of older adults who have natural teeth extracted.
- Increase the number of older adults who receive annual dental care.
- Reduce the number of older adults who engage in no regular physical activity.
- Increase the number of adults who perform physical activities that enhance and maintain muscle strength, endurance, and flexibility.
- Reduce asthma deaths, hospitalizations, and emergency department visits.
- Reduce the number of adults with limited functional ability due to chronic obstructive pulmonary disease and breathing problems.
- Reduce the proportion of nonsmokers exposed to environmental secondhand smoke.

Source: *Healthy People 2010.* (2000). http://www.healthypeople.gov

Acute pain can be a warning sign for the presence of serious undiagnosed illness or injury and should be aggressively reported and investigated. Once the cause of the pain is known, the source can be treated and the pain alleviated. Chronic unrelieved pain is associated with hopelessness, depression, and suffering. Older patients with chronic unrelieved pain are less likely to engage in rehabilitation activities, have slower recoveries, manifest sleep disturbances, have decreased appetites, and contribute to increased healthcare costs (Hartford Institute, 1999).

Appropriate pain treatment strategies include systematic ongoing pain assessment and pain management using pharmacological and nonpharmacological techniques. Pain medication should be administered around the clock to provide baseline relief, with short-acting agents used to treat breakthrough pain. The least invasive route of administration should be used, doses should be carefully titrated, response to medication should be routinely monitored, and side effects should be minimized with aggressive nursing care plans. Acetaminophen, nonsteroidal anti-inflammatory drugs, opioids, and analgesics are all appropriate medications for treating pain in the older adult. Nonpharmacological techniques such as patient education, exercise, physical therapy, acupuncture, biofeedback, transcutaneous nerve stimulation, massage, heat and cold, Reiki, and spiritual healing are appropriate if they are within the older patient's value system.

TABLE 3-2

Recommended Health Screenings and Interventions for Older Persons

Screening/Intervention	Recommended Interval
For Primary Prevention	
Blood pressure	Yearly
Influenza immunization	Yearly
Height and weight measures	Yearly
Pneumonia immunization	Once at age 65 (consider repeating in 5 to 7 years)
Smoking cessation	Every health encounter
Tetanus booster	Every 10 years
Aspirin to prevent myocardial infarction	Daily
Cholesterol screening	Every 5 years
Diabetes mellitus screening	Yearly
For Secondary Prevention	
Skin examination	Yearly
Self-breast examination	Monthly
Bone densitometry	Baseline at menopause and then as determined by primary care provider
Cognitive impairment	Yearly
Thyroid-stimulating hormone	Yearly in older women
Prostate-specific antigen and/or digital rectal examination	Yearly in older men
Sigmoidoscopy/colonoscopy	Every 5 to 7 years
Fecal occult blood	Yearly
Mammography	Yearly
Hearing/vision screening	Yearly
Pap smears	Every 3 years

Source: U.S. Preventive Services Task Force. (1996). *Guide to clinical preventive services, periodic update* (3rd E.). Agency for Healthcare Research and Quality, updated 2004.

Practice Pearl

Pain is now considered the fifth vital sign. Assess pain early and often.

LEGAL ISSUES

Legal issues affecting older adults are increasingly common based on the number of people living longer, fuller lives. The gerontological nurse should be aware of all the rules, regulations, and standards that govern professional practice. When patients suffer injury or receive inappropriate care, patients or families may file a lawsuit seeking damages for personal injury. If a suit is filed, the care and treatment offered the patient will be compared with standards of care. Usually an expert witness will review the medical records and offer an opinion regarding whether the standard of care was met. Sources for establishing the nursing standard of care include the American Nurses Association, state nurse practice acts, nursing home regulation and standards, JCAHO, nursing journals, nursing textbooks, specialty Websites, and expert opinions.

OBRA 87 requires all states to operate long-term care ombudsmen programs and to notify patients about their rights. These programs provide trained people to investigate complaints made by residents and families about poor care or violation of patients' rights within the nursing home. If a violation is found, the ombudsman may seek administrative or legal action.

Older patients have the right to:

- Receive individualized care.
- Be free from abuse, neglect, and discrimination.
- Be free from chemical and physical restraints.
- Have privacy.
- Control their funds.
- Be involved in decision making.
- Raise grievances and make complaints.
- Vote.
- File lawsuits.
- Practice religion.
- Marry.
- Participate in facility and family activities.
- Have freedom to leave the facility.
- Make a will and dispose of property.
- Enter into contracts.

The healthcare facility is required to post the bill of rights in a conspicuous place and list the name and telephone number of the ombudsman so patients know who to contact if they feel that their rights have been violated.

All nurses should adequately prepare themselves for safe practice, question any action or physician's order that seems inappropriate or unsafe, and seek advice or guidance from their superior whenever they are unsure of the safety of an action. Additionally, all nurses are urged to purchase individual professional liability insurance to pay financial damages should they be the target of a lawsuit. Even if the healthcare facility where the nurse is employed offers liability coverage, the nurse should consider purchasing individual coverage to ensure that the individual nurse's professional interests will be defended as well as the nurse's interests as an employee of the institution.

Nursing care that violates the standards of practice can be considered malpractice. The legal definition of standard of care is to consider what a reasonable nurse would do if placed in a similar situation according to professional standards. When the nurse's performance does not meet that standard of care, malpractice can be charged. Situations that can lead to malpractice include:

- Not adequately assessing or monitoring patients as to change in condition.
- Not safeguarding the environment of a cognitively impaired patient.
- Not informing the physician that a patient is in need of medical care.
- Medication errors (wrong dose, wrong patient, wrong time, wrong route of administration).
- Incorrectly performing a nursing intervention that results in patient injury (placing a feeding tube in the lung, etc.).
- Failing to carry out positioning or treatment orders, resulting in patient injury (not offering fluids, changing dressing, repositioning the patient, etc.).

Careful documentation of nursing care is the best way to defend oneself should a legal suit be filed. Charting should be legible, accurate, timely, and specific enough to describe the care given. Nurses should follow these guidelines when documenting care:

- Write clearly and legibly so others can read the record without struggling or ambiguity.
- Record all significant nursing interventions and patient response.

- Record all significant nursing interventions withheld or deferred (e.g., laxative not given as patient has diarrhea).
- Record any unusual event or circumstances (falls, patient or family comments, concerns).
- Record routine and ongoing nursing care.
- Record conversations and phone calls to physicians, advanced practice nurses, families, diagnostic facilities, and so on.
- Record recommended actions or inactions (no new orders received) in response to phone calls and inquiries.
- When taking verbal medication orders by phone, request the physician repeat doses at least twice to verify accuracy. For example, "Dr. Jones, I would like to confirm that you ordered Compazine, 25 milligrams. Be given orally every 6 hours for complaint of nausea. Is that correct?"
- Ask the physician or advanced practice nurse to fax the information conveyed in the telephone order if possible, as an additional safeguard.
- Record thoughts when any actions are taken or not taken as the result of nursing judgments. For example, "Oral fluids withheld as patient lacks gag reflex and is at risk for aspiration. Dr. Jones notified by phone and IV fluid rate increased by 50 cc/hr to prevent dehydration."
- Do not scratch out, white out, enter notes later, or obliterate any part of the patient record. If an error is made, draw a single line through the entry and write "error, wrong chart" (or wrong patient, etc.) and sign your name.

When documenting an adverse event occurring in the clinical environment, the standard of practice is to record all circumstances surrounding the event. For instance, if a patient falls, the nurse should carefully document the circumstances of the fall, including:

- Time of day.
- Outcomes of the fall (injury, changes in vital signs, pain, deformity).
- What the patient said (I forgot my glasses!).
- Whether mechanical devices were involved (walkers, bed alarms, wheelchairs, etc.).
- Whether the nursing staff was aware of the fall risk.
- What fall-reducing measures (if any) were in place (placing the bed in the lowest to the floor position, scheduling of frequent observations, patient placed close to nurses' station, etc.).

Not all falls can be prevented, even with the highest quality nursing care. When frail elderly people move about on their own, falls will occur. The nurse can take steps to minimize the risks for fall and injury. See Chapter 18 for further information on patient falls.

At one time, physical restraints were routinely used in nursing homes and hospitals to prevent falls. Waist restraints, bed rails, vests, and lap belts were used to limit movement and keep patients confined to their bed or chair. However, since the passage of OBRA 87, restraints are now limited to short-term use (2 hours or less) and only with a physician's order in emergency situations. This is because nursing research illustrated the relationship between the use of physical restraints and many problems of immobility, including decubitus ulcers, fecal and urinary incontinence, increased agitation, and physical deconditioning. Now gerontological nurses are urged to develop alternatives to physical restraints such as addressing patient and environmental factors. Patient factors include making sure the resident is wearing eyeglasses and safe footwear, has discontinued all unnecessary medication, has supervision if it is required, has appropriate assistive devices such as canes and walkers, has frequently scheduled opportunities to use the toilet, and has the benefit of frequent nursing observation. Environmental factors include placing the bed in a low position, not using side rails to limit movement, having adequate environmental lighting, and reducing fall hazards such as dangling electrical cords, scatter rugs, and wet surfaces.

OBRA 87 also limits the use of chemical restraints, or the use of sedating psychotropic drugs to control behavior. It is now mandated that psychotropic drugs should be used only in circumstances where they will clearly benefit the older patient and improve the quality of the patient's life. They are not to be used in circumstances where behavior such as calling out is annoying to the nurses. See Chapter 6 for further information regarding OBRA 87 and medication regulation.

PATIENT CONFIDENTIALITY

The healthcare record and information regarding the care and treatment of the patient must be kept confidential. Patients have the right to view their medical record if they choose and to ask questions regarding information contained in the record. Patients can ask for copies of their medical records, and their request must be granted in a timely manner. Healthcare facilities must maintain medical records for at least 7 years. Each healthcare facility is required to develop policies and procedures to maintain the medical record and ensure confidentiality.

Healthcare providers should not discuss patients in elevators, cafeterias, or other public areas when they can be overheard. Even if patient names are not used, it is sometimes possible to determine who is being discussed by the clinical information provided in the conversation.

USE OF TECHNOLOGY IN ASSESSMENT

The use of technology in many healthcare facilities leads to additional problems with patient confidentiality and privacy. Computers should have passwords that limit access to authorized providers only. Healthcare providers must be reminded to log off after using a computer to access a patient's medical record so that an unauthorized person cannot come along and gain access to medical records.

E-mails and fax machines can also transmit confidential patient information that unauthorized persons may have access to. Fax machines should be used only when it is understood that the authorized provider is the only receiver or that the authorized receiver will "stand by" a shared fax machine to receive confidential information. When e-mail is used to transmit confidential information, only secure networks should be used. Larger healthcare facilities address this issue by offering private entry codes to authorized users. These codes are changed routinely, and caregivers are urged never to share them with others. Smaller facilities and individual providers should work with computer security consultants to ensure that their e-mail systems and networks are secure and that patients' records and communications cannot be read, deleted, or altered by unauthorized persons.

Patients must sign permission to authorize release of information before medical records can be copied, faxed, electronically transmitted, or released to others. Technology has the tremendous potential to enhance access to healthcare services for older patients, but extra efforts are needed to ensure privacy. The gerontological nurse should be informed of all regulations and restrictions governing emerging technologies and access to patient records.

HEALTH INSURANCE PORTABILITY AND ACCOUNTABILITY ACT

In 1996, the Health Insurance Portability and Accountability Act (HIPAA) was signed into law (Public Law 104-191) with the broad goal of improving the efficiency and effectiveness of the healthcare system. It is the first national legislation that protects every patient's health information through the establishment of standards and requirements for the electronic transmission of certain health information (eligibility, referrals, and claims). Healthcare providers were required to comply with privacy rules as of April 1, 2003.

Most larger healthcare institutions have developed HIPAA training and certification to educate their employees regarding the new requirements for the protection of patient privacy. The cornerstone of the training is that privacy and confidentiality are basic rights in our society and it is now the legal and ethical obligation of all healthcare providers to protect that right.

The following healthcare information is considered confidential:

- Patient-identifying information (name, medical record number)
- Health information relating to past, present, or future health status or condition
- Documentation regarding the provision of healthcare
- Past, present, or future payment for the provision of healthcare

During their initial visit to a healthcare provider, it is mandated that all patients will receive a privacy notice. The privacy notice is a written statement of how their healthcare information will be used and disclosed. The patient is asked to sign a form acknowledging receipt of the privacy notice.

If HIPAA standards are not followed and breaches in privacy occur, healthcare institutions can be held accountable for wrongful disclosures. Severe civil and criminal penalties will be brought forward, including fines and sanctions against business associates and workforce members in violation.

Examples of breaches or seemingly innocent activities that can lead to breaches include:

- Throwing test results or patient reports into the regular trash.
- Failing to log off after checking a patient record on the computer.
- Leaving a medical record open at the nurses' station, in the hallway, or in a conference room.
- Sending a patient report to be printed and forgetting to take it off the printer.
- Discussing patient information with a family member without the patient's permission.
- Failing to check the ID badge or reason for needing the chart when a coworker in scrubs or a lab coat asks for a patient chart.

Various policies have been developed to assist healthcare workers to practice safely and meet the new confidentiality legislations. Policies vary from institution to institution; however, the following guidelines are typical of the kinds of safeguards that can be instituted:

Computer Security

- Do not share passwords.
- Always log off after reviewing a patient record.
- Do not let others glance over your shoulder when you are reviewing a patient record at a computer workstation.
- Limit your viewing of patient records to only those patients for whom you are providing care or who are participating in a valid research study and have given informed consent.

Faxing

- Use caution with fax machines as they are the least secure of all technologies.
- When faxing information, always use a cover sheet with a confidentiality statement.
- Never leave fax machines sitting unattended.
- Always verify the fax number before faxing patient information, verify the receiver is available to immediately receive the fax, and verify patient permission to release the information before faxing.

E-mail

- When sending e-mail, never use a patient's name or medical record number in the subject line.
- Attach a confidentiality statement as part of your automatic signature. For example, "The information contained in this e-mail is intended only for the person to whom it is addressed and may contain confidential and/or privileged information. If you received this e-mail in error, please contact the sender and delete the material from your computer."
- E-mail of confidential patient information should not be sent over the Internet (public access), as security cannot be guaranteed. Use only Intranet secure systems (limited to use by authorized providers) to ensure privacy.

For more complete information on HIPAA and to follow the development and implementation of new regulations, visit the U.S. Department of Health and Human Services Website.

INFORMED CONSENT AND COMPETENCE

The Patient Self-Determination Act requires providers to seek informed consent from all patients before they receive healthcare or engage in a research protocol. Older patients are entitled to be told the full implications of their treatment or nontreatment and then have the freedom to make an independent decision, without coercion, whether or not to receive the care. Older persons have the right to make informed decisions about all care and treatment unless they have been determined to be incompetent (unable to make decisions) by a court of law. Failure to receive consent before a medical or surgical procedure is carried out can be considered assault and battery, a criminal offense.

Often, upon admission to a healthcare facility, the older person will sign a consent for routine care giving permission to others to provide care with bathing, dressing, feeding, and administration of medications. However, these general consent forms do not cover specialized procedures such as blood transfusions, electroshock therapy, experimental procedures, and invasive procedures.

For consent to be truly informed, the nurse must explain to the older patient in language that he or she can understand the benefits and burdens of the procedure being proposed. Benefits are considered to be outcomes of treatment that would improve the care or comfort of the patient. Burdens are considered to be any potential pain and suffering the patient may have to endure as a result of treatment. Ideally, treatments should offer benefits to the patient without overwhelming burdens. However, when burden is high and chance of benefit is low, the intervention may be considered medically futile. For instance, an older patient with widespread metastatic cancer may be offered one more surgery or one more round of chemotherapy, even though there is little chance of cure, remission, or improvement in quality of life. If the older patient and the family make an informed decision to receive this care after the risks and benefits are explained, the care may be considered legal but probably not ethical.

In order to feel comfortable gaining consent from older patients, the gerontological nurse will want to assess capacity for consent. To be considered capable of providing consent, older patients should have the ability to:

- Comprehend information (understand).
- Contemplate options (reason).
- Evaluate risks and consequences (problem solve).
- Communicate that decision (make their decision known).

While competence is a legal term, capacity is a clinical term. Gerontological nurses are called upon to assist in the determination of decisional capacity of older patients.

When a patient lacks decisional capacity because of severe illness, sedating drugs, or cognitive impairment, there are mechanisms and laws that dictate who may make a decision for the patient. If the patient has a living will, a healthcare proxy or surrogate decision maker, durable power of attorney, or involved family member, these persons or documents will be used to decide whether to proceed with the treatment or procedure in question (see chapter 22 for these documents). ⊂⊃ If an older person lacks decisional capacity and has no predetermined wishes, family, or healthcare proxy, the care facility may seek a court-appointed guardian. A guardian is appointed by a judge to act on behalf of a *ward* when the judge has determined that the ward is incapacitated and in need of a decision maker. Guardians may be relatives, friends, or strangers. Usually wards are people with advanced dementia, untreated mental illness, developmental disabilities, head injuries, strokes, or long-standing drug addictions (Johns & Sabatino, 2002).

Assessment of decisional capacity is an ongoing dynamic process. Patients have the right to make decisions that do not follow the recommendations of healthcare providers and to change their mind at any time. Even if patients have dementia or cognitive impairments, it does not mean that they should not be consulted regarding treatment decisions. Often, while true consent cannot be obtained from an older person, *assent* should be sought. If the older person does not assent to the care to be given, it ethically cannot be offered. For instance, if the healthcare proxy consents to a blood transfusion for an older patient with dementia, the patient may not agree to having the needle inserted into the arm and may violently resist the procedure. To avoid conflict and the risk of potential harm to the patient, assent for all procedures should be obtained from the older patient before beginning any treatment or procedure. Patients with dementia are assumed to be unable to participate in decision making, but current research indicates that this is an inaccurate assumption (Mezey, Teresi, Ramsey, Mitty, & Bobrowitz, 2000).

End-of-Life Issues

When the end of life is approaching, a variety of legal as well as ethical issues may emerge. (Chapter 11 provides a complete discussion of these issues.) ⊂⊃ An older patient who is approaching death may not be able to make ongoing treatment decisions. Confusion as to how to provide appropriate care may arise. If the person has named a healthcare proxy to make a decision or has an advance directive such as a living will, then healthcare professionals will have guidance through the decision-making process at the end of life. However, most older patients have not completed an advance directive or named a proxy. Barriers to the completion of an advance directive include the following:

- Inability to speak English
- Religious or ethnic beliefs
- Poor eyesight, cognitive impairment, hearing
- Standardized forms that are too technical or print that is too small to read
- Procrastination
- Dependence on family for all decisions
- Lack of knowledge about advance directives
- Belief a lawyer is necessary
- Fear of being written off or signing life away
- Acceptance of the will of God

(Ebersole & Hess, 2001)

Do-not-resuscitate (DNR) orders may appear on the charts of many frail older patients. They are written and signed by the physician or advanced practice nurse and are legally valid orders. Some healthcare facilities mandate that if a DNR order is not in place, then the older person should be a candidate for cardiopulmonary resuscitation (CPR). Unfortunately, CPR is not very successful in older people who experience cardiac arrest in the nursing home or community setting. Monitoring equipment, intravenous access, and equipment to reverse cardiac arrhythmias are usually not readily available and delays in treatment often occur. Older patients who survive the cardiac arrest may suffer brain damage or broken ribs and have an even poorer quality of life than they experienced before the cardiac arrest.

The gerontological nurse should consult the patient, the family, and advance directives when a patient's code status is being considered. All discussions with the patient and the family should be documented in the patient chart. If there are problems or disagreements within the family, the nurse should involve the social worker, clergy, or the ethics team.

Patient and Family Teaching

Gerontological nurses require skills and knowledge related to teaching patients and families about the key concepts of gerontology and gerontological nursing. The guidelines in the following feature will assist the nurse to assume the role of teacher and coach.

Patient-Family Teaching Guidelines

PRINCIPLES OF GERIATRICS

1. What should I look for when choosing a doctor?

Look for a doctor who is well trained, competent, and conveniently located. Additional things to consider include:

- Board certification. Choose a physician who is a specialist in geriatrics, internal medicine, or other area like cardiology to treat your specific problem.

- Type of insurance. Choose a physician who accepts Medicare or is in your managed care network.

- Hospital affiliation. Choose a physician who admits patients to a hospital you have faith in and is convenient to you and your family.

- Interdisciplinary team. Choose a physician who works with others who can help you to stay healthy, including gerontological nurses, social workers, nutritionists, physical therapists, and so on.

2. What type of doctor is best for me?

It is always good to choose a geriatrician, family practitioner, or internist for your primary care doctor. Some things to consider include the following:

- Family practitioners can treat a wide range of problems and do not specialize in any one area.

- Internists are physicians for adults. Some take extra training and specialize in a certain area like cardiology.

- Geriatricians focus specifically on problems of aging and are trained in family practice and internal medicine. Geriatricians usually work with a team of healthcare professionals.

RATIONALE:

Choosing a physician wisely is key to good healthcare. Older patients should benefit from having a physician who is convenient to see and accepts their insurance.

RATIONALE:

Talk to your family, friends, healthcare professionals, and neighbors when choosing a doctor. Ask how they chose their doctor and what they like and dislike about him or her. When a doctor is described consistently as "great," "friendly," "caring," "takes time to get to know you," you can feel confident in choosing this physician. When you need a specialist, get advice from a healthcare professional and be sure to pick someone who is knowledgeable and competent.

(continued)

Patient-Family Teaching Guidelines, *cont.*

3. How can I increase my chances of making an informed choice?

Here are some questions to ask the nurse or receptionist in the office of a physician you are considering.

- What age patients do you treat?
- Do you specialize in any areas like cardiology, dermatology, or orthopedics? (Choose areas to ask about that are of interest to you.)
- How long do I have to wait for an appointment?
- How long does the doctor spend with each patient?
- May I bring a family member with me?
- Is the doctor comfortable in including patients in healthcare decisions?
- Where are the laboratory tests and x-rays performed?

RATIONALE:

After asking these questions, the older person should meet with the physician and decide whether to proceed with the relationship.

4. What should I do to prepare for the first appointment?

During your first visit, your doctor and nurse will probably take a health history and ask you about your health. You can help by bringing a list of medications, medical diagnoses, tests and operations you have had, and any significant events like hospitalizations, accidents, and injuries. Make a list of any drug allergies or serious drug reactions you have had. During this visit, take time to ask questions and get comfortable with your new physician. Leave time to discuss how you wish to be treated should you become unable to make your own healthcare decisions. For example, do you want to have CPR if your heart stops beating? Would you want to have aggressive care like intravenous fluids if you had dementia or Alzheimer's disease? Discuss these issues with your new doctor and nurse and name a person whom you trust to make decisions if you are unable to make them yourself.

RATIONALE:

Finding a good doctor is just the first part of the caring process. The older patient should enter into an active partnership with the physician and nurse to solve health problems and improve function. Good communication is the key. Stay involved and advocate for your health and well-being!

Care Plan

A Patient With Multiple Diagnoses

Case Study

Mrs. Cooper is an 83-year-old woman who is admitted to the hospital for observation following a fall in her home. She lives alone with support from her daughter who visits once or twice a week to bring food and check up on her mom. Mrs. Cooper has several diagnoses including hypertension, nervous anxiety, macular degeneration, arthritis, and insomnia. Neither Mrs. Cooper nor her daughter can name all of the physicians and healthcare specialists she has seen in the last few years because she has received many referrals, has been evaluated by a variety of consultations, and does not have a stable primary care provider.

The patient reports she takes many medicines, most of which she cannot name. The daughter reports Mrs. Cooper does not eat very well and has lost weight recently. She worries that her mom has had other falls that she has not reported to anyone, because she is fearful of having to go to a nursing home.

Applying the Nursing Process

ASSESSMENT

The nurse should gain further information. Mrs. Cooper may have many physical, social, and psychological issues that could be influencing her health status. She needs a complete geriatric assessment with input from a variety of team members.

DIAGNOSIS

There are several that could be considered. The hospitalization and immediate problem is related to a fall. Therefore, *risk for falling* might be the most immediate problem. If the patient is released from the hospital without adequate assessment of her fall risks, she may suffer another fall with significant injury or even premature death. The immediate need is to assess fall risk and implement a fall-risk reduction program. Additional diagnoses to be considered might include the following:

- *Failure to thrive*
- *Ineffective coping resulting in anxiety or insomnia*
- *Ineffective health maintenance*
- *Knowledge deficit relating to medications and healthcare providers*
- *Imbalanced nutrition, less than body requirements*
- *Disturbed sensory perception (visual)*

EXPECTED OUTCOMES

Expected outcomes for the plan of care specify that Mrs. Cooper will:

- Become aware of the harmful effects of poor nutrition on health status and function.
- Use appropriate safety measures in the home to decrease falling.
- Develop a stable caring relationship with a primary healthcare provider to oversee and coordinate visits to specialists.
- Agree to establish a therapeutic relationship with the nurse and develop a mutually acceptable plan to work toward these outcomes.

PLANNING AND IMPLEMENTATION

The following nursing interventions may be appropriate for Mrs. Cooper:

- Establish a therapeutic relationship.
- Consult with nutritionist, social worker, and other members of the healthcare team.

(continued)

A Patient With Multiple Diagnoses *(continued)*

- Encourage a family meeting with the daughter present to talk about health issues in general with Mrs. Cooper's permission.
- Carefully assess all functional health patterns, noting strengths in order to maximize function.
- Begin a values clarification to establish long-term goals and facilitate end-of-life planning.

EVALUATION

Mrs. Cooper has several strengths, including a stable home environment, an involved daughter living close by, a history of adequate and appropriate self-care, and motivation to continue to live independently.

The nurse will consider the plan a success based on the following criteria:

- Improvement in functional ability and health status
- Reduction in risk for injury
- Identification of a stable primary care provider
- Improvement of trust in the healthcare system
- Reduction of possible feelings of strain and burden as verbalized by Mrs. Cooper's caregiver daughter

Ethical Dilemma

A second daughter from California pages the nurse at the hospital. She introduces herself and requests information regarding her mom's condition. The nurse asks why she has not spoken with her mom or her sister directly. She states she had a disagreement with them several years ago and is not on good terms, but wants to stay informed of her mom's condition. Because information cannot be shared with the daughter without the consent of the patient, the nurse can suggest she leave her phone number and have Mrs. Cooper give her a call if she is willing. The nurse could validate the daughter's concern and offer to share with Mrs. Cooper the fact that she phoned and is requesting information. HIPAA guidelines do not allow the sharing of confidential patient information with others (even families) without the consent of the patient. Violation of the regulations could result in fines and censure.

Critical Thinking and the Nursing Process

1. Imagine that you are caring for Mr. Turner, a hospice patient. He is dying of esophageal cancer and is cognitively intact. He asks you to make sure no one puts a tube down his throat when he is near death. His family is worried that when the end is near and he becomes short of breath, he may change his mind and will be unable to communicate his wishes. What strategies would you use to communicate and reassure this patient?
2. Imagine you are caring for Mrs. Lee. She lives alone and can no longer care for herself due to severe cognitive impairment. She has no family and refuses to discuss leaving her home. What is the best course of action to pursue?

A Patient With Multiple Diagnoses

3. You have a colleague who consistently forgets to log off from the computer when checking patient records. Once, you found a confidential psychiatric record clearly displayed on the computer terminal at the nurses' station. What action is appropriate?

■ Evaluate your responses in Appendix B. ⊂▭

EXPLORE MediaLink

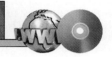

NCLEX review, case studies, and other interactive resources for this chapter can be found on the Companion Website at **www.prenhall.com/tabloski**. Click on Chapter 3 to select the activities for this chapter. For animations, video tutorials, more NCLEX review questions, and case studies, access the accompanying CD-ROM in this textbook.

Chapter Highlights

■ Providing holistic care to the older patient is a joy and a challenge. An interdisciplinary team can provide comprehensive evaluation to fully understand the health needs of an older person and to form the basis for the plan of care.

■ Standardized instruments are available to assist in the evaluation process, and the gerontological nurse is a key member of the interdisciplinary team.

■ A comprehensive geriatric assessment includes emphasis on physical, psychological, and socioeconomic factors, and input from various health professionals. Functional ability is the central focus of the examination.

■ Contextual variables such as the older person's culture and level of education can affect the assessment process and should be addressed to facilitate the gathering of accurate and complete patient information.

■ Health for older adults is a complex interaction of physical, functional, and psychosocial factors. The gerontological nurse can play a key role in the implementation of the goals of *Healthy People 2010*. The overarching goals for health promotion and disease prevention include increasing quality and years of healthy life and eliminating health disparities. Recommended health screenings and interventions for older persons can assist in meeting these goals.

■ Legal issues and the protection of patient privacy present challenges to gerontological nurses and other healthcare providers who often must seek or ask to share confidential patient information with others, obtain informed consent, and assist patients and families with end-of-life decision making. Guidelines for documentation, safeguarding confidentiality, and assessing decisional capacity are suggested.

References

Agency for Healthcare Research and Quality. (2004). *Guide to clinical preventive services* (3rd ed.). Periodic updates. Retrieved October 6, 2004, from http://www.ahrq.gov.

Centers for Disease Control and Prevention, National Center for Health Statistics. National Vital Statistics System and unpublished data. (1997). Mortality Data from the National Vital Statistics System. Retrieved September 8, 2004, from http://www.cdc.gov.

Centers for Disease Control and Prevention, National Center for Health Statistics. National Vital Statistics System. (1999). Fast Facts, Death/Mortality. Retrieved September 8, 2004, from http://www.cdc.gov.

Centers for Medicare and Medicaid Services. (2000). *Manuals—Minimum data set.* Retrieved September 14, 2001, from http://www. cms.hhs.gov.

Ebersole, P., & Hess, P. (2001). *Toward healthy aging: Human needs and nursing response* (5th ed.). St. Louis, MO: Mosby.

Edelman, C., & Mandle, C. (2002). *Health promotion throughout the lifespan.* St. Louis, MO: Mosby.

Folstein, M., Folstein, S., & McHugh, P. R. (1975). Mini-Mental State: A practical method for grading the cognitive state of patients for the clinician. *Journal of Psychiatric Research, 12,* 189–198.

Fulmer, T. (1991). The geriatric nurse specialist role: A new model. *Nursing Management, 22*(3), 91–93.

Gallo, J., Fulmer, T., Paveza, G., & Reichel, W. (2000). Handbook of geriatric assessment. Gaithersburg, MD: Aspen.

Granger, C., Albrecht, G., & Hamilton, B. (1979). Outcomes of comprehensive medical rehabilitation: Measures of PULSES profile and the Barthel index. *Archives of Physical Medicine and Rehabilitation, 60,* 145–154.

Hartford Institute for Geriatric Nursing. (1999). *Best nursing practices in care for older adults: Incorporating essential gerontologic content into baccalaureate nursing education and staff development.* New York: New York University.

Health Resources and Services Administration. (1996). *A national agenda for geriatric education: White papers* (Vol. 1). Washington, DC: U.S. Department of Health and Human Services.

Healthy People 2010. (2000). What are its Goals? Retrieved on June 14, 2000, from http://www.healthypeople.gov.

John A Hartford Foundation. (2002). Annual report. Retrieved on June 14, 2003, from http://www.jhartford.org.

Johns, A. F., & Sabatino, C. P. (2002). Wingspan—The second national guardianship conference recommendations. *Stetson Law Review, 31*(3), 595–609.

Joint Commission on Accreditation of Healthcare Organizations (JCAHO). (2004). *Provision of care, treatment and services. Standards for long-term care.* Retrieved August 14, 2004, from http://www.jcaho.org.

Kane, R., Ouslander, J., & Abrass, I. (1999). *Essentials of clinical geriatrics* (3rd ed.). New York: McGraw-Hill.

Lawton, M. (1969). Assessment of older people: Self maintaining and instrumental activities of daily living. *Gerontologist, 9,* 179–186.

Lawton, M. (1971). The functional assessment of elderly people. *Journal of the American Geriatrics Society, 19*(6), 465–481.

Maas, M., Buckwalter, K., Hardy, M., Tripp-Reimer, T., Titler, M., & Specht, J. (2001). *Nursing care of older adults: Diagnoses, outcomes and interventions.* St. Louis, MO: Mosby.

Mezey, M., Teresi, J., Ramsey, G., Mitty, E., & Bobrowitz, T. (2000). Decision-making capacity to execute a health care proxy: Developing and testing of guidelines. *Journal of the American Geriatrics Society, 48*(2), 179–187.

Mouton, C., & Espino, D. (2000). Ethnic diversity of the aged. In J. Gallo, J. Busby-Whitehead, P. Rabins, R. Silliman, & J. Murphy (Eds.), *Reichel's care of the elderly: Clinical aspects of aging* (5th ed., pp. 595–608). Baltimore: Lippincott Williams & Wilkins.

Neugarten, B. (1977). Personality and aging. In J. Birren & K. Schaie (Eds.), *Handbook of the psychology of aging* (pp. 626–649). New York: Van Nostrand Reinhold.

Neugarten, B., Havighurst, R., Tobin, S. (1961). The measurement of life satisfaction. *Journal of Gerontology, 16,* pp. 134–143.

Oakley, F., Duran, L., Fisher, A., & Merritt, B. (2003). Differences in activities of daily living motor skills of persons with and without Alzheimer's disease. *Australian Occupational Therapy Journal, 50*(2), 72–78.

Omnibus Budget Reconciliation Act (OBRA). (1987). Washington, DC: U.S. Department of Health and Human Affairs.

Pender, N. J., Murdaugh, C., & Parsons, M. A. (2002). *Health promotion in nursing practice* (4th ed.). Upper Saddle River, NJ: Prentice Hall Health.

Stanford University Geriatric Education Resource Center. (2000). *Tools for geriatric care.* Board of Trustees of the Leland Stanford Junior University. Retrieved October 3, 2004, from http://sugerc.stanford.edu/resources3.html www.geri-resources@lists.standford.edu.

Teigland, C. (2000, November). *Assessing quality of care for nursing home residents with dementia: The HCFA, QI's.* Presented at the Gerontological Society of America 53rd Annual Meeting, Washington, DC.

U.S. Preventive Services Task Force. (1996). *The guide to clinical preventive services.* Baltimore: Lippincott Williams & Wilkins.

World Health Organization. (1946). Preamble to the Constitution of the World Health Organization. Retrieved August 12, 2004, from http://www.who.int/about/definition/en/.

Yesavage, J. A., & Brink, T. L. (1983). Development and validation of a geriatric depression screening scale: A preliminary report. *Journal of Psychiatric Research, 17,* 37–49.

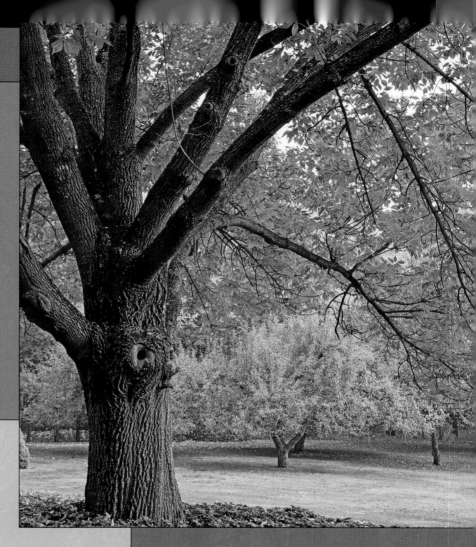

UNIT TWO

Challenges of Aging and the Cornerstones of Excellence in Nursing Care

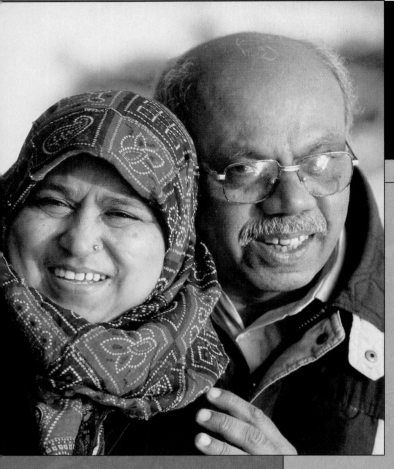

CHAPTER 4

Cultural Diversity

Rachel E. Spector, PhD, RN, CTN, FAAN
CulturalCare Consultant

CHAPTER OBJECTIVES

Upon completion of this chapter, the reader will be able to:

- Discuss the importance of culturally and linguistically appropriate services (CLAS) in healthcare.
- Describe the CulturalCare triad representing the complex interrelationships of the nurse, caregiver, and patient within community and institutional (home or residential) settings.
- Identify potential areas of conflict derived from the demographic, ethnocultural, and life trajectory variables of the people within the triad.
- Describe the value and process of heritage and life trajectory assessments of nurses, caregivers, and patients.
- Describe the integration of CulturalCare into the plan of care.

MediaLink

Additional resources for this chapter can be found on the Student CD-ROM accompanying this textbook and on the Companion Website at **www.prenhall.com/tabloski**. Click on Chapter 4 to select the activities for this chapter.

CD-ROM
- NCLEX Review
- Case Studies
- Tools

COMPANION WEBSITE
- Audio Glossary
- Additional NCLEX Review
- Case Study
- MediaLink Applications

Cultural diversity has significant implications for healthcare delivery and policy-making throughout the United States. The world's 210 nations are well represented in the United States, and the diverse cultures are continually being blended and merged. Given this sociodemographic phenomenon, the 2000 census allows for 66 different categories of racial and ethnic combinations. In addition, mobility is an ingrained feature of our society, and diversity is likely to continue to be an issue. Cultural diversity has clearly been expanding into all regions of the country—not just inner city and coastal areas, but throughout the Midwest, suburbs, and small towns of America (Office of Minority Health, 2001, p. 25).

In all clinical practice areas—nurse practitioner and doctor's offices, clinics, acute care settings, and long-term care settings—one sees this diversity every day. The need for culturally and linguistically competent healthcare services for diverse populations is attracting increased attention from health providers and those who judge their quality and efficiency. While certain providers, such as nurses, have struggled to deliver culturally appropriate services to diverse populations for many years, this has not been the case in many mainstream settings. Now, as the mainstream begins to treat a more diverse patient population as a result of demographic changes and participation in insurance programs, the interest in designing culturally and linguistically appropriate services that lead to improving nursing care outcomes, efficiency, and patient satisfaction has increased.

Cultural background and language have a considerable impact both on how patients access and respond to healthcare services and on how the caregivers work within the system. There are two main goals:

1. To develop cultural and linguistic competence by nurses and other healthcare providers
2. For healthcare organizations to understand and respond effectively to the cultural and linguistic needs brought by both patients and caregivers to the healthcare experience

This two-pronged phenomenon recognizes the diversity that exists among the patients, nurses, and caregivers. It is not limited to the changes in the patient population. It also embraces the members of the workforce—both the nurses who may be from other countries and the caregivers. Many of the people in the workforce are new immigrants or are from ethnocultural backgrounds that are different from that of the patients.

This chapter presents an overview of the salient content and complex processes necessary to enable professional nurses to develop knowledge and skills related to Cultural-Care and to integrate CulturalCare into their gerontological nursing practice and into the practice environment.

National Standards for Culturally and Linguistically Appropriate Services in Health Care

In 1997, the Office of Minority Health undertook the development of national standards to provide a much needed alternative to the patchwork that had been available in the field of cultural diversity. They developed the *National Standards for Culturally and Linguistically Appropriate Services in Health Care*. These 14 standards (Box 4-1) must be met by most healthcare-related agencies. The standards are based on an analytical review of key laws, regulations, contracts, and standards currently in use by federal and state agencies and other national organizations. They were developed with input from a national advisory committee of policymakers, healthcare providers, and researchers.

BOX 4-1	National Standards for Culturally and Linguistically Appropriate Services in Health Care

1. Health care organizations should ensure that patients/consumers receive from all staff members effective, understandable, and **respectful care** that is provided in a manner compatible with their cultural health beliefs and practices and preferred language.
2. Health care organizations should implement strategies to recruit, retain, and promote at all levels of the organization a diverse staff and leadership that are representative of the demographic characteristics of the service area.
3. Health care organizations should ensure that staff at all levels and across all disciplines receive ongoing education and training in culturally and linguistically appropriate service delivery.
4. Health care organizations must offer and provide language assistance services, including bilingual staff and interpreter services, at no cost to each patient/consumer with limited English proficiency at all points of contact, in a timely manner during all hours of operation.
5. Health care organizations must provide to patients/consumers in their preferred language both verbal offers and written notices informing them of their right to receive language assistance services.
6. Health care organizations must assure the competence of language assistance provided to limited English proficient patients/consumers by interpreters and bilingual staff. Family and friends should not be used to provide interpretation services (except on request by the patient/consumer).
7. Health care organizations must make available easily understood patient-related materials and post signage in the languages of the commonly encountered groups and/or groups represented in the service area.
8. Health care organizations should develop, implement, and promote a written strategic plan that outlines clear goals, policies, operational plans, and manage-

Accreditation and credentialing agencies can assess and compare providers of culturally competent services and ensure quality care for diverse populations. This includes the Joint Commission on Accreditation of Healthcare Organizations, the National Committee on Quality Assurance, professional organizations such as the American Medical Association and the American Nurses Association, and quality review organizations such as peer review organizations.

To ensure both equal access to quality healthcare by diverse populations and a secure work environment, nurses should "promote and support the attitudes, behaviors, knowledge, and skills necessary for staff to work respectfully and effectively with patients and each other in a culturally diverse work environment" (Office of Minority Health, 2001, p. 7). This is the first of the 14 standards for culturally and linguistically appropriate services (CLAS) in healthcare.

CulturalCare Nursing

CulturalCare is professional nursing care that is culturally sensitive, culturally appropriate, and culturally competent. CulturalCare nursing is critical to meet the complex nursing care needs of a given person, family, and community. It is the provision of nursing care across cultural boundaries and takes into account the context

ment accountability/oversight mechanisms to provide culturally and linguistically appropriate services.

9. Health care organizations should conduct initial and ongoing organizational self-assessments of CLAS-related activities and are encouraged to integrate cultural and linguistic competence-related measures into their internal audits, performance improvement programs, patient satisfaction assessments, and outcomes based evaluations.

10. Health care organizations should ensure that data on the individual patient's/consumer's race, ethnicity, and spoken and written language are collected in health records, integrated into the organization's management information systems, and periodically updated.

11. Health care organizations should maintain a current demographic, cultural, and epidemiological profile of the community as well as a needs assessment to accurately plan for and implement services that respond to the cultural and linguistic characteristics of the service area.

12. Health care organizations should develop participatory, collaborative partnerships with communities and utilize a variety of formal and informal mechanisms to facilitate community and patient/consumer involvement in designing and implementing CLAS-related activities.

13. Health care organizations should ensure that conflict and grievance resolution processes are culturally and linguistically sensitive and capable of identifying, preventing, and resolving cross-cultural conflicts or complaints by patients/consumers.

14. Health care organizations are encouraged to regularly make available to the public information about their progress and successful innovations in implementing the CLAS standards and to provide public notice in their communities about the availability of this information.

Source: National Standards for Culturally and Linguistically Appropriate Services in Health Care. (2001). *Final report.* Washington, DC: U.S. Department of Health and Human Services.

in which the patient lives as well as the situations in which the patient's health problems arise.

- **Culturally competent.** The nurse understands and attends to the total context of the patient's situation. It is a complex combination of knowledge, attitudes, and skills.

  For example, if the patient has dietary practices such as not mixing meat and dairy foods, food and beverage combinations that the patient prefers can be readily supplied. An exploration of dietary beliefs and practices will be inherent in the orientation of all nurses and assistive personnel.

- **Culturally appropriate.** The nurse applies the underlying background knowledge that must be possessed to provide a given patient with the best possible healthcare.

  For example, if the patient values modesty, the nurse will strive to have care provided by a person of the same sex and to protect the patient's personal privacy at all times. If the staff member is reluctant to provide care to a person of the opposite sex because of cultural or religious beliefs, the nurse will respect the beliefs and interpret them to the staff.

- **Culturally sensitive.** The nurse possesses some basic knowledge of and constructive attitudes toward the health traditions observed among the diverse cultural groups found in the practice setting.

For example, if a given patient does not desire adult immunizations, blood transfusions, or invasive procedures of any sort, the patient's, family's, or healthcare proxy's wishes will be granted and respected.

CulturalCare expresses all that is inherent in the development of nursing practice to meet the mandates of the **CLAS standards.** There are countless conflicts in the healthcare delivery arena that are predicated on cultural misunderstandings. Many of these misunderstandings are related to universal situations such as verbal and nonverbal language misunderstandings, the conventions of courtesy, sequencing of interactions, phasing of interactions, objectivity, and so forth. However, many cultural misunderstandings are unique to the delivery of nursing care. The necessity to provide CulturalCare demands that nurses be able to assess and interpret a given patient's health beliefs and practices and cultural needs. CulturalCare alters the perspective of nursing care delivery as it enables the nurse to understand the manifestations of the patient's cultural heritage and **life trajectory.** The nurse must serve as a bridge in the community and long-term care settings between the patient and the direct caregivers who are from different cultural backgrounds. This is accomplished by serving as a role model.

CulturalCare Triad

The delivery of CulturalCare to the elderly population is extremely complex. It grows from an understanding of the ethnocultural heritages and life trajectories of the people involved in the CulturalCare triad. The triad is set within the demographic change that has swept the United States over the past 30 years. It is composed of three distinct populations: the nurse, the patient, and the direct caregiver. Each of the populations enters into the patient care arena with different backgrounds that are predicated on their ethnocultural heritage and life trajectory; hence, the relationship between the parties is complex.

DEMOGRAPHIC CHANGE

The 2000 census of the United States indicates that the White, non-Hispanic majority is 69.1% of the population. It was 83.2% in 1980, and 75.6% in 1990. People of color are now over 30% of the population, and the numbers are growing. By the year 2020, it is predicted that people of color will be the majority population. In addition, millions of immigrants were admitted to the United States during the 1990s. The foreign-born population of the United States has grown from 8% in 1990 to 10% in 2000, the highest rate since 1930. The foreign-born population consists of 7.2 million people from Asian countries, 4.4 million people from Europe, and 14.5 million people from Latin America (Bernstein, 2002, pp. 1-2). The population proportions as depicted in the 2000 census are shown in Figure 4-1A ▣. The percentages displayed are those of Whites, non-Hispanic; Blacks, non-Hispanic; and Hispanics. The percentages of Asians and Native Americans are small and are not included in this figure.

THE NURSE

Of the nearly 2.2 million nurses in clinical practice in 2001, 93.1% were women, 9.9% were Black, and 3.4% were Hispanic (Figure 4-1B) (U.S. Department of Labor, 2002, p. 176). The registered nurse (RN), in general, is a White, non-Hispanic woman who is between the ages of 30 and 49 years, with an average age of 43 years. The majority of nurses (72%) are married, and more than half of all nurses (55%) have children. Approximately 10% of the nurses work in community health settings and are involved in delivering either primary or long-term care to the elderly population, and 7% of RNs

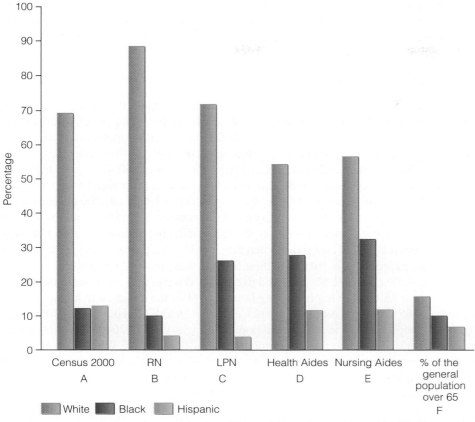

MediaLink   American Nurses Association

FIGURE ☐ **4-1**

A comparison of the population profiles of Whites, Blacks, and Hispanics from the Census of the United States, 2000.
A. The general population.
B. Registered nurses.
C. Licensed practical nurses.
D. Health aides.
E. Nursing aides.
F. The general population 65 and over as % of the general population.

Source: *A*, U. S. Census Bureau, 2001. B–E, Department of Labor, *Household data annual averages, 2001,* pp. 174, 176,177. *F*, U.S. Department of Commerce, 2001, *Current population survey, 2000,* released 2001.

work in nursing homes that include those based in hospitals, facilities for the mentally retarded, and retired home residences (American Nurses Association 2004). The demographic profile of professional nurses represents a significant variance from the overall demographic profile of the United States (see Figure 4-1B ☐). Licensed practical nurses are also highly represented by Whites, but there is a larger percentage of Blacks involved in this discipline (Figure 4-1C ☐).

THE CAREGIVER

In 2000, there were nearly 2.1 million people employed as nursing service providers, aids, attendants, and orderlies. Of these, 90.1% were women, 32.7% were Black, and 11.6% were Hispanic (U.S. Department of Labor, 2002, p.176). The proportions found in this demographic breakdown are not consistent with the overall demographic proportions of the United States. A greater percentage of Blacks are represented in these positions than are in the general population. Hispanics represent 12% of the general population and are slightly less in this workforce population. In many long-term care facilities, the setting may be one in which the nurses are White and the staff, especially certified nurses' aids, is composed of many people of color. Figure 4-1D and E ☐ illustrates the percentages of health aides and nursing aides. Many of the technical caregivers are over 20 years of age and earn minimal wages. A high school diploma is required in most settings; however, many of the caregivers are new immigrants and may have difficulty speaking and understanding English. The immigrants may well have limited understanding of the ethnocultural heritages and life trajectories of the patients and nurses, who in turn have a limited understanding of the immigrants' backgrounds.

THE PATIENT

The third party in the triad is the patient. The 2000 census required respondents to report their age and date of birth. The population of people 65 years and over has grown significantly since the 1990 census (Figure 4-1F ■). The elderly population of today was born shortly after the beginning of the 20th century. In 1900, the life expectancy at birth was 47.3 years; yet the number of people 100 years and over (50,454) is the highest it has ever been. California, New York, and South Dakota have the greatest number of centenarians (U.S. Census Bureau, 2001, p. 1). People born in 1930 had a life expectancy of 59.7 years. The generation of women born in 1910 was the first (58%) that lived to see their children become adults. In addition, the aging of the population may affect the way a given patient relates to a caregiver. When the caregiver is a person of color, some older patients may express prejudice that in their lifetime was seen as "acceptable."

In 2000, 4.5% of people 65 years and over were living in nursing homes, and 18.2% of people over 85 were living in nursing homes; 91% of the overall nursing home population was 65 years and older (National Center for Health Statistics, 2004). The population of people over 85 in the general population was 1.1% in 2000. The percentages broken down by race and ethnicity demonstrate that 1.4% of the White, non-Hispanic population was 85 and over, compared with 0.3% of the Hispanic population, 0.8% of the Black population, 0.2% of the Native American population, and 0.6% of the Asian Pacific Islander population (Centers for Disease Control, 2004).

Ethnocultural Heritage

A person's ethnocultural heritage is predicated on the concept of **heritage consistency,** which was developed by Estes and Zitzow (1980) to describe the degree to which a person's lifestyle reflects his or her respective tribal culture. The theory has been expanded in an attempt to study the degree to which a person's lifestyle reflects his or her traditional culture, whether European, Asian, African, or Hispanic. The values indicating heritage consistency exist on a continuum, and a person can possess value characteristics that are both heritage consistent (traditional) and heritage inconsistent (acculturated or modern). The concept of **heritage inconsistency** includes a determination of one's cultural, ethnic, and religious background (Spector, 2004, p. 8).

CULTURE

There is not a single definition of culture, and all too often definitions tend to omit salient aspects of culture or to be too general to have any real meaning. One definition of **culture** is that it is the thoughts, communications, actions, beliefs, values, and institutions of racial, ethnic, religious, or social groups (U.S. Department of Health and Human Services, 2001, p. 4).

Culture is a complex whole in which each part is related to every other part. The capacity to learn culture is genetic, but the subject matter is not genetic and must be learned by each person in the family and social community. Culture also depends on an underlying social matrix that includes knowledge, belief, art, law, morals, and custom (Bohannan, 1992, p. 13).

ETHNICITY

Cultural background is a fundamental component of one's ethnic background. The term **ethnicity** pertains to a social group within the social system that claims to possess variable traits such as a common religion or language. The term *ethnic* has for some time aroused strongly negative feelings and often is rejected by the general population. The upsurge in the use of the term may stem from the recent interest of people in discovering their personal backgrounds, a fact used by some politicians who overtly court "the ethnics." Paradoxically, in a nation as large as the United States and comprising as many different peoples as it does—with the American Indians being the only true native population—many people are still reluctant to speak of ethnicity and ethnic differences. Most foreign groups that came to this land often shed the ways of the "old country" and quickly attempted to assimilate themselves into the mainstream, or the so-called melting pot (Novak, 1973).

A phenomenon found in the 2000 census was that the numbers of people who listed their ancestry as European decreased 20%, while the numbers of sub-Saharan Africans rose 238% and Arabs rose 37%. The Latino population also increased in the declaration of ancestry (Rodriguez, 2001, p. A22).

RELIGION

The third major component of a person's heritage is **religion.** Religion is "the belief in a divine or superhuman power or powers to be obeyed and worshipped as the creator(s) and ruler(s) of the universe; and a system of beliefs, practices, and ethical values," and is a major reason for the development of ethnicity (Abramson, 1980, pp. 869–875). The practice of religion is revealed in numerous cults, sects, denominations, and churches. Ethnicity and religion are clearly related, and religion quite often is the determinant of a person's ethnic group. Religion gives a person a frame of reference and a perspective with which to organize information. Religious teachings about health help to present a meaningful philosophy and system of practices within a system of social controls having specific values, norms, and ethics. Adherence to a religious code is conducive to spiritual harmony and health. Illness is sometimes seen as punishment for the violation of religious codes and morals.

It is not possible to isolate the aspects of culture, religion, and ethnicity that shape a person's worldview. Each is part of the others, and all three are united within the person. When writing of religion, one cannot eliminate culture or ethnicity, but descriptions and comparisons can be made (Spector, 2004, p. 15).

SOCIALIZATION

Socialization is the process of being raised within a culture and acquiring the characteristics of that group. Education—be it elementary school, high school, college, or nursing—is a form of socialization. For many people who have been socialized within the boundaries of a "traditional culture" or a nonmodern culture (usually associated with the East or third and fourth world nations), modern "American," or Western, first world culture becomes a second cultural identity. Those who immigrate here, legally or illegally, from non-Western or nonmodern countries may find socialization into the American culture to be a difficult and painful process. As time passes, many people experience biculturalism, which is a dual pattern of identification and often of divided loyalty (LaFrombose, Coleman, & Gerton, 1993). Many people who have been socialized in cultures that use traditional healthcare resources may prefer this type of care even when residing in a modern cultural setting with modern healthcare resources.

Practice Pearl

Do not make assumptions about the way older patients have been socialized to their racial identities. Some older African Americans identify themselves as Black, persons of color, colored persons, or African Americans. Racial identity can vary by generation, geographical region of the country, and other subgroups.

Examples of Heritage Consistency

The following are the factors indicative of heritage consistency. These factors may determine the depth to which members of the CulturalCare triad identify with their traditional heritage:

1. Childhood development occurred in the person's country of origin or in an immigrant neighborhood in the United States of like ethnic group.

   For example, the person was raised in a specific ethnic neighborhood, such as an Italian, Black, Hispanic, or Jewish one, in a given part of a city and was exposed only to the culture, language, foods, and customs of that particular group.

2. Extended family members encouraged participation in traditional religious and cultural activities.

   For example, the parents sent the person to religious (parochial) school, and most social activities were church-related.

3. The individual engages in frequent visits to the country of origin or returns to the "old neighborhood" in the United States.

   The desire to return to the old country or to the old neighborhood is common; however, many people cannot return for various reasons. Those who came here to escape religious persecution or whose families were killed during World War II, during the Holocaust, in the killing fields of Cambodia, or in other recent massacres, may not want to return to their homelands. Other reasons why people may not return to their native country include political conditions or lack of relatives or friends in the homeland.

4. The individual's family home is within the ethnic community of which he or she is a member.

   For example, as an adult the person has elected to live in the ethnic neighborhood where the people are from a similar heritage.

5. The individual participates in ethnic cultural events, such as religious festivals or national holidays, sometimes with singing, dancing, and costumes.

   For example, the person is active in social and cultural groups and participates in festivities with family members.

6. The individual was raised in an extended family setting.

   For example, when the person was growing up, there may have been grandparents living in the same household, or aunts and uncles living in the same house or close by. The person's social frame of reference was the family.

7. The individual maintains regular contact with the extended family.

    For example, the person maintains close ties with family members of the same generation, the surviving members of the older generation, and members of the younger generation.

8. The individual's name has not been Americanized.

    For example, the person has restored the family name to its original European, or other national, name if it had been changed at the time the family immigrated or if the family changed the name at a later time in an attempt to assimilate to the dominant culture.

9. The individual was educated in a parochial (nonpublic) school with a religious or ethnic philosophy similar to the family's background.

    For example, the person's education plays an enormous role in socialization, and the major purpose of education is to socialize a given person into the dominant culture. Children learn English and the customs and norms of American life in the schools. In the parochial or private schools, they not only learn English but also are socialized in the culture and norms of the religious or ethnic group that is sponsoring the school.

10. The individual engages in social activities primarily with others of the same religious or ethnic background.

    For example, the major portion of the individual's personal time is spent with primary structural groups.

11. The individual has knowledge of the culture and language of origin.

    For example, the person has been socialized in the traditional ways of the family and expresses this as a central theme of life.

12. The individual expresses pride in his or her heritage.

    For example, the person may identify him- or herself as ethnic American and be supportive of ethnic activities to a great extent. (Spector, 2004, pp. 13–14).

Ethnocultural Life Trajectories

Generational differences have been described as deep and gut-level ways of experiencing and looking at the cultural events that surround us. "The differences between generations—and the determination of who we are—are more than distinct ways of looking at problems and developing solutions for problems" (Hicks & Hicks, 1999, p. 4). Changes in the past several decades have created cultural barriers that openly or more subtly create misunderstandings, tensions, and often conflicts between family members, coworkers, and individuals—and between patients and caregivers in the practice of gerontology. The cycle of life is an ethnocultural journey, and many aspects of this journey are derived from the social, religious, and cultural context in which a person is raised. Factors that imprint our lives are the characters and events that we interacted with at 10 years of age, more or less (Hicks & Hicks, 1999, p. 25).

People who reside in institutional settings may be cared for not only by people who are much younger but also by people who are immigrants and have limited knowledge as to what has been each patient's life trajectory. Figure 4-2 ▪ illustrates one ethnocultural heritage life trajectory model. The patient may also be an immigrant who experienced a much different life trajectory than others of the same age and the caregivers. Table 4-1 lists events over the past century that have had a profound impact on the lives of older patients as a cumulative experience. The later events have affected the nurses and caregivers. Depending on the heritage of the individuals, the experiences differ.

FIGURE ▨ **4-2**

Ethnocultural Heritage/Life
Trajectory Model: The
complex relationship of
nurse, caregiver, and
patient in community
and/or institutional
settings and commingling
variables.

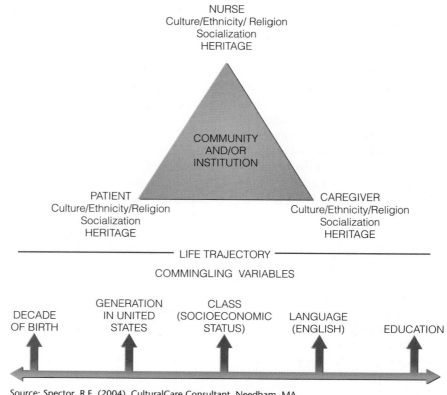

Source: Spector, R.E. (2004). CulturalCare Consultant. Needham, MA.

Several commingling variables relate to this overall situation as they may serve as potential sources of conflict. These include:

1. **Decade of birth.** One's life experiences will vary greatly depending on the events of the decade they were born and the cultural values and norms of the times. People who tend to be heritage consistent (i.e., have a high level of identification and association with a traditional heritage) tend to be less caught up in the secular fads of the time and popular sociocultural events.

2. **Generation in United States.** Worldviews differ greatly between the immigrant generation, subsequent generations, and people who score high as heritage consistent.

3. **Class.** Social class is an important factor among the elderly. It includes analysis of one's education, economics, and background. There are countless differences among people predicated on class. For example, the 2000 census found 54% of the foreign born were employed in service and skilled worker jobs and farm and manual labor as compared to 38% of the native people. The median household income of native-born people was $41,400 and for the foreign born it was $36,000 (DeNavas-Walt, Cleveland, & Webster, 2003).

4. **Language.** When people who are hard of hearing attempt to understand people with limited English speaking skills, many cultural and social misunderstandings can develop. There are also frequent misunderstandings when people who do not understand English must help and care for or take direction from English speakers.

TABLE 4-1

Selected Sociocultural and Healthcare-Related Events of the 20th Century Profoundly Impacting the Lives of Patients, Nurses, and Caregivers in the United States and World

Date	Cultural/Historical Events	Healthcare-Related Events
1900–1909	1903—Wright brothers' flight at Kitty Hawk 1906—San Francisco earthquake 1908—Model T Ford introduced 1909—NAACP organized	1900—Walter Reed—Mosquitoes transmit yellow fever 1900—Quinine used to cure malaria 1903—Radium used to treat cancer 1906—Pure Food and Drug Act; vaccine for plague 1907—Tuberculin testing begun
1910–1919	1914—Panama Canal opened 1914–18—World War I 1917—Russian Revolution 1918—Germany surrendered; Armistice signed 1919—Prohibition began	1914—Blood transfusions 1914—Ether developed 1914—Mayo Clinic opened 1915—Smallpox immunization mandatory 1916—Margaret Sanger and birth control 1917—Oxygen therapy introduced 1918–19—Influenza pandemic
1920–1929	1920—Women's suffrage 1920—First radio broadcast 1921—First Miss America 1925—Scopes trial 1927—Lindbergh flew from New York to Paris 1929—Stock market crash	1923—Dick test to determine susceptibility to scarlet fever 1923—Ethylene introduced as an anesthetic 1923—Mitral valve surgery introduced 1923—Peritoneal dialysis introduced 1924—BCG tuberculin test introduced 1924—Scratch test to determine susceptibility to diphtheria 1925—Exchange transfusions introduced 1929—Blue Cross begun
1930–1939	1930—Great southern drought 1931—Rise of Nazi Party in Germany 1932—F. D. Roosevelt elected president 1933—Prohibition ended 1935—New Deal and Social Security Act passed 1936—*Life* magazine born 1938—*Kristallnacht* in Germany 1939—The SS Saint Louis turned away from Cuba; Germany invaded Poland	1931–39—Pertussis immunization introduced 1932—Tuskegee syphilis experiment begun 1933—Tetanus toxoid immunization introduced 1933—Diphtheria immunization introduced 1933—Divinylether used 1934—Mumps virus isolated 1935—Sulfa drugs 1935—Insulin developed to treat diabetes 1936—Poliomyelitis virus isolated; cortisone developed 1937—First blood banks and blood transfusions; TB patch test developed 1938—Typhoid antiserum prepared
1940–1949	1940—London burned 1941—Pearl Harbor bombed; WW II; United States at war with Japan and then Germany. 1944—Normandy Invasion 1945—War ended in Europe 1945—Hiroshima—first use of atomic bomb 1946—Transistor discovered 1946—World's first electronic computer assembled	1943—Penicillin used to treat syphilis 1944—DDT insecticide introduced 1944—Hearing tests introduced Mid–1940s—Tetanus antitoxin developed 1944—Artificial kidney introduced 1945—Streptomycin used to treat TB 1947—Kolff-Brigham artificial kidney 1949—Cortisone discovered

(continued)

TABLE 4-1 *(continued)*

Selected Sociocultural and Healthcare-Related Events of the 20th Century Profoundly Impacting the Lives of Patients, Nurses, and Caregivers in the United States and World

Date	Cultural/Historical Events	Healthcare-Related Events
1950–1959	1953—Rosenberg trial 1953—Stalin died 1953—Television—*I Love Lucy* 1954—TV dinners 1955—Disneyland opened, Elvis Presley, Marilyn Monroe; Rosa Parks refused to give up her seat on a Montgomery, Alabama, bus and bus boycott ensued 1956—*Brown v. Board of Education*—desegregation of public schools 1957—Russians first in space with *Sputnik* 1959—Cuban Revolution	1952–53—Heart-lung machine perfected 1954—Salk vaccine for polio 1954—Antipsychotics and neuroleptics introduced 1954—First successful organ (kidney) transplant 1957—Valium introduced
1960–1969	1960—JFK elected president—Peace Corps begun; Bay of Pigs, Cuba; U.S. sent two helicopters to South Vietnam 1962—Berlin Wall; ballistic missiles in Cuba—standoff Kennedy/Khrushchev; the Beatles led the youthful, rebellion; Civil Rights Movement 1963—JFK assassinated; Vietnam War builds up; March on Washington with Martin Luther King Jr. 1965—Malcolm X assassinated; Robert Kennedy assassinated; Chicago riots; Civil Rights Act passed 1968—Martin Luther King Jr. assassinated 1965–68—Over 100 race riots in American cities 1969—Neil Armstrong walked on the moon; Woodstock	1961—External cardiac pacing 1961—Thalidomide disaster 1962—Rachel Carson, *Silent Spring* 1963—Liver transplant method developed 1963—Mumps live virus vaccine developed 1964—Surgeon General's report on smoking 1965—War on Poverty; Medicare/Medicaid passed 1966—Rubella vaccine developed 1967—First human heart transplant
1970–1979	1970—Kent State protest; My Lai massacre 1972—Watergate break-in; Nixon to China 1973–74—Oil embargo; Nixon resigned 1975—Vietnam Truce	1970—Earth Day; EPA founded; 1970s—Biotechnical explosion 1970s—Clotbusters introduced; interferon 1971—CT scans developed 1972—Tuskegee experiment ends; PSROs established; Clean Water Act 1973—Emerging infections identified 1973—*Roe v. Wade* decision legalized abortion 1978—First test-tube baby 1978—Love Canal; Hepatitis B (HBV) vaccine developed 1979—Three Mile Island
1980–1989	1981—Air Traffic Controllers' strike 1981—Tax cut—Reaganomics 1982—Vietnam Memorial Wall dedicated 1983—Recognition of HIV/AIDS epidemic 1986—*Challenger* explosion 1987—Black Monday—stock market crash; Glasnost 1989—Tiananmen Square; Berlin Wall down	1984—Bhopal, India—chemical leak 1984—Monoclonal antibodies 1985—Emergence of crack cocaine 1985—Retroviral oncogenes

TABLE 4-1

Selected Sociocultural and Healthcare-Related Events of the 20th Century Profoundly Impacting the Lives of Patients, Nurses, and Caregivers in the United States and World

Date	Cultural/Historical Events	Healthcare-Related Events
1990–1999	1991—Desert Storm; beating of Rodney King 1992—Los Angeles riots 1993—Assault on the Branch Davidians in Waco, Texas 1995—Million Man March; Oklahoma City bombing 1998—President Clinton impeached in the House of Representatives; Desert Fox	1992—Human Genome Project 1993—Family and Medical Leave Act 1993—Hantavirus pulmonary syndrome 1993–94—Failure of Health Reform 1996—Assisted suicide—Dr. J. Kevorkian 1997—Sextuplets born and survive 1998—Octuplets born—7 survive 1998—Stem cell cloning Medical events
2000–	September 11, 2001, Attack on the United States—the Pentagon and the World Trade Center with the subsequent collapse of the towers 2002—War in Afghanistan 2003—War in Iraq	

Source: Adapted from Jennings, P. (1998). *The century.* Copyright © 1998 by ABC Television Network Group, a division of Capital Cities, Inc. With permission.

5. **Education.** In the year 2000, the percentage of foreign-born high school graduates was 25 as compared to 34% of the native population in persons over 25 years of age. In addition, 53% of the native-born population over 25 were educated beyond high school, and 42% of the foreign born have had this educational experience (Bernstein, 2002). Many of the elders have experienced college and place an extremely high value on education (Spector, 2004, pp. 20–21).

Heritage Assessment Tool

A tool, or interview guide, has been developed to determine how deeply a given person identifies with a traditional heritage or is acculturated into the modern, dominant culture (Spector, 2004, pp. 321-323). Once a conversation begins and the person describes aspects of his or her cultural heritage, it becomes possible to develop an understanding of the person's unique health and illness beliefs and practices and cultural needs.

Figure 4-3 ■ depicts the questions to ask in the heritage assessment interview. The tool was developed to create a way of interviewing a given person about sociocultural background. It facilitates **communication** with patients and their families, staff members, and colleagues. The tool is designed to enhance the interviewing process to determine if a given person is identifying with a traditional cultural heritage (heritage consistent) or if the person has acculturated into the dominant culture of the modern society (heritage inconsistent). The tool may be used in any setting and both facilitates conversation and helps in the planning of CulturalCare. Many questions must be added regarding the person's life trajectory to integrate the cultural and historical events in the lives of each party into the work environment.

FIGURE ▫ 4-3

The Heritage Assessment tool.

1. Where was your mother born? _____

2. Where was your father born? _____

3. Where were your grandparents born?
   a. Your mother's mother? _____
   b. Your mother's father? _____
   c. Your father's mother? _____
   d. Your father's father? _____

4. How many brothers _____ and sisters _____ do you have?

5. What setting did you grow up in?
   Urban _____ Rural _____

6. What country did your parents grow up in?
   Father _____   Mother _____

7. How old were you when you came to the United States? _____

8. How old were your parents when they came to the United States?
   Father _____   Mother _____

9. When you were growing up, did you live in an extended family?
   (1) Yes _____   (2) No _____

10. Have you maintained contact with
    a. Aunts, uncles, cousins? (1) Yes _____   (2) No _____
    b. Brothers and sisters?   (1) Yes _____   (2) No _____
    c. Parents?   (1) Yes _____   (2) No _____
    d. Your own children?   (1) Yes _____   (2) No _____

11. Did most of your aunts, uncles, cousins live near your home?
    (1) Yes _____   (2) No _____

12. Approximately how often did you visit family members who lived outside of your home?
    (1) Daily _____   (4) Once a year or less _____
    (2) Weekly _____   (5) Never _____
    (3) Monthly _____

13. Was your original family name changed?
    (1) Yes _____   (2) No _____

14. What is your religious preference?
    (1) Catholic _____   (4) Other _____
    (2) Jewish _____   (5) None _____
    (3) Protestant _____
        Denomination _____

15. Is your spouse the same religion as you?
    (1) Yes _____   (2) No _____

16. Is your spouse the same ethnic background as you?
    (1) Yes _____   (2) No _____

17. What kind of school did you go to?
    (1) Public _____   (3) Parochial _____
    (2) Private _____

18. As an adult, do you live in a neighborhood where the neighbors are the same religion and ethnic background as you?
    (1) Yes _____   (2) No _____

19. Do you belong to a religious institution?
    (1) Yes _____   (2) No _____

20. Would you describe yourself as an active member?
    (1) Yes _____   (2) No _____

21. How often do you attend your religious institution?
    (1) More than once a week _____   (4) Special holidays only _____
    (2) Weekly _____   (5) Never _____
    (3) Monthly _____

22. Do you practice your religion in your home?
    (1) Yes _____ (if yes, please specify)
    (2) No _____
    (3) Praying _____
    (4) Bible reading _____
    (5) Diet _____
    (6) Celebrating religious holidays _____

23. Do you prepare foods special to your ethnic background?
    (1) Yes _____   (2) No _____

24. Do you participate in ethnic activities?
    (1) Yes _____ (if yes, please specify)   (5) Dancing _____
    (2) No _____   (6) Festivals _____
    (3) Singing _____   (7) Costumes _____
    (4) Holiday celebrations _____   (8) Other _____

25. Are your friends from the same religious background as you?
    (1) Yes _____   (2) No _____

26. Are your friends from the same ethnic background as you?
    (1) Yes _____   (2) No _____

27. What is your native language? (other than English)

28. Do you speak this language?
    (1) Prefer _____   (3) Rarely _____
    (2) Occasionally _____

29. Do you read your native language?
    (1) Yes _____   (2) No _____

Directions: Score one point for each positive answer except if a person has NOT changed his or her family name. That gets a point if negative. The greater the number of points, the greater the likelihood that the person identifies with a traditional culture and is not assimilated into the mainstream culture.

Source: Spector, R. E. (2004). *Cultural diversity in health and illness* (6th ed., pp. 321–323). Upper Saddle River, NJ: Prentice Hall.

Best Nursing Practices

The Hartford Institute for Geriatric Nursing (1999) has recommended recognition of cultural and religious beliefs, practices and life experiences of ethnic groups, and the influence of these on attitudes toward aging and healthcare. It is important for nurses to understand the following categories of belief from the perspective of their older patients:

- **Respect.** What does this person from another culture believe about the roles and responsibilities of older persons, children, doctors, nurses, and others?
- **Death and dying.** What are the cultural perspectives regarding death, life-sustaining treatments, treatment of the body after death, and funeral rituals?
- **Pain.** What is the cultural perspective toward pain? Is there a view that it is punishment for past behaviors? What are the socially accepted behaviors of a person in pain (e.g., crying, wailing, moaning, stoicism)?
- **Medicines and nutrition.** What is the role of folk and home remedies and caregiving practices?
- **Independence.** How does the culture value independence in old age? Are older people expected or encouraged to stay active in their healthcare and living arrangements?

The nurse is urged to discuss these key issues with the older patient and the family. It would be wrong to make assumptions based on stereotypes, so each person should be approached as a unique individual.

There are many ways that a given person's life trajectory can be discussed. The nurse can inquire about historical events that occurred during the person's lifetime. Did the person serve in the military? What was that experience like? What was school like when the person was young? What was it like without television? What was it like without a computer? Once people begin to recall life experiences, they generally feel free to discuss them. For many people, sharing experiences can also be painful. Talk of World War II, for example, can be difficult for people who are Holocaust survivors or who lost family in the military. People born before 1935 may not have had childhood immunization except smallpox. Vaccines did not become available until 1931 to 1939 for pertussis, and others came later. Table 4-1 illustrates the years when immunizations for various other illnesses were introduced.

Providing CulturalCare

There are several ways to develop and implement the knowledge and skills necessary to incorporate CulturalCare into nursing care. Professional nurses are the leaders and bridges in this sensitive endeavor. The knowledge and skills can be developed to the degree whereby a CulturalCare nursing environment can be established within the practice environment. This includes the following:

1. Development of cultural sensitivity
2. Determination of what care is culturally appropriate for a given patient
3. The steps involved in the process that leads to the development of cultural competency

CULTURAL SENSITIVITY

Sensitivity indicates a high level of awareness as to what is meaningful to the person. The assessment of heritage and ethnocultural life trajectory is important. How and when questions are asked requires both clinical judgment and sensitivity. The timing and phrasing of questions need to be adapted to the individual. Timing is important in introducing questions. Sensitivity is needed in phrasing questions and determining what questions are appropriate at a given time. Trust must be established before patients and caregivers can be expected to share sensitive information. The nurse needs to spend time with patients, their families, and the caregivers; introduce some social conversation; and convey a genuine desire to understand their values, beliefs, ethnocultural background, and life trajectories.

Before a cultural assessment begins, the nurse must determine what language the person speaks and the degree of fluency in the English language. It is also important to learn about the person's communications patterns and space orientation. This is accomplished by observing both verbal and nonverbal communication.

1. For example, does the person do the speaking or defer to another?
2. What nonverbal communication behaviors are exhibited (e.g., touching, eye contact)?
3. What significance do these behaviors have for the interaction between the nurse and the patient or caregiver?
4. What is the person's proximity to other people and objects within the environment?
5. How does the person react to the nurse's movement toward him or her?

It is vital to be culturally sensitive and to convey this sensitivity to patients, support people, and other healthcare personnel. Some ways to do so follow:

1. Always address patients, support people, and other healthcare personnel by their last names (e.g., Mrs. Cohen, Dr. Foley) until they give you permission to use other names. In some cultures, the more formal style of address is a sign of respect, whereas the informal use of first names may be considered disrespect. It is important to ask people how they wish to be addressed.
2. When meeting a person for the first time, introduce yourself by your full name, and then explain your role (e.g., My name is Lillian Cook and I am the nurse on this unit). This helps establish a relationship and provides an opportunity for patients, others, and nurses to learn the pronunciation of one another's names and their roles.
3. Be authentic with people, and be honest about the knowledge you lack about their ethnocultural heritage and life trajectory. When you do not understand a person's actions, politely and respectfully seek information.
4. Do not make any assumptions about the patient and your coworkers; always tactfully ask about anything you do not understand.
5. Respect the ethnocultural values, beliefs, and practices of others, even if they differ from your own or from those of the dominant culture.
6. Show respect for the patient's support people. In some cultures, males in the family make decisions affecting the patient, whereas in other cultures, females make the decisions.
7. Make a concerted effort to obtain the trust of patients and coworkers, but do not be surprised if it develops slowly or not at all. The heritage assessment and life trajectory interview takes time and usually extends over several time periods. Table 4-2 illustrates several examples of common cultural blunders, the potential consequences, and possible patient outcomes.

TABLE 4-2

Common Cultural Conflicts

Situation	Consequence	Patient Outcome
Linguistic barriers	Inadequate assessments (i.e., pain, needs, preferences)	Decreased quality of life
Dietary blunders	Refusal to eat specific foods, such as pork; and food combinations, such as milk and meat	Decreased oral intake Weight loss Dehydration
Missed cues	Inappropriate interventions Power struggles between nurses and family and patient	Withdrawal, depression, anger Loss of communication
Misunderstanding of religious or cultural beliefs and/or practices such as modesty	Avoid encounters Resist care Female refuses male caregiver or male refuses female caregiver	Fear Withdrawal Increased anxiety
Family dynamics	Controversies Confusion	Hostility Withdrawal
Violation of manners	Avoid encounters Resist touch	Withdrawal

CULTURAL APPROPRIATENESS

The determination of culturally appropriate care is necessary so that the comfort levels of both the patient and the caregivers are met and respected. The case study that appears later in this chapter describes a culturally appropriate response.

The provision of the recommended interventions demonstrates the level of sensitivity and responses necessary to meet the patient's needs. The skills necessary to incorporate CulturalCare into standard nursing require a broad base of knowledge about the different ethnocultural heritages and life trajectories a given patient, colleague, or caregiver comes from. It is an ongoing process, and both the skills and knowledge bases grow over time. As one's knowledge base grows, the ability to convey cultural sensitivity also grows.

STEPS TO CULTURAL COMPETENCY

The following are examples of the necessary steps:

1. Become aware of your own ethnocultural heritage.
   - Where were your parents and grandparents born?
   - What are examples of their ethnocultural life trajectories?
   - Do they value stoic behavior?
   - Are the rights of the individual valued over and above the rights of the family?

- What did they experience either as new immigrants or as children growing up in the United States?
- What do they see as seminal cultural events of their lifetime?
- Only by knowing one's own culture (values, practices, and beliefs) can a person be ready to learn about another's.

2. Become aware of the ethnocultural heritage and life trajectory described by both the patient and the caregivers.

   It is important to avoid assuming that all people of the same ethnic, religious, or national background have the same cultural beliefs and values. Similar questions as those previously listed may be asked in conversation. When there is knowledge of the patient's and caregiver's ethnocultural heritage and life trajectories, mutual respect between patient, caregiver, and nurse is more likely to develop. The triad can become more unified.

3. Become aware of adaptations the patient and caregivers made to live in the North American culture.

   During this part of the process, a nurse can also identify the patient's and caregivers' preferences in health practices, diet, hygiene, and so on.

4. Form a CulturalCare nursing plan with the patient and caregivers that incorporates their cultural beliefs regarding care.

   In this way, cultural values, practices, and beliefs can be incorporated with the necessary nursing care.

Implementing CulturalCare Nursing

CulturalCare nursing involves the presentation of culturally related customs and values into the life of a given setting. Recognizing the patient's and caregiver's viewpoints and finding mutually agreeable solutions requires expert communication skills. There must be an attempt to bridge the gaps between the perspectives of the people in the CulturalCare triad. During this process, the views of each party must be explored, acknowledged, and valued. If there are views that could lead to harmful outcomes or behaviors, there must be an attempt to shift the perspectives to an acceptable view. Every action must be taken to recognize potential conflict before the situation becomes irreversible. This may be all that is realistically possible to achieve. If a crisis develops, it may be possible to return to original care approaches.

CulturalCare nursing is challenging. It requires discovery of the meaning of the patient's or staff member's ethnocultural heritage and life trajectory, flexibility, creativity, and knowledge to adapt interventions. There must be a cumulative effort to learn from each experience. This knowledge and experience will improve the delivery of CulturalCare to future patients and staff members.

Patient and Family Teaching

Gerontological nurses require skills and knowledge related to teaching patients and families about the key concepts of gerontology and gerontological nursing. The patient-family teaching guidelines in the following feature will assist the nurse to assume the role of teacher and coach. Educating patients and families is critical so that nurses can interpret scientific data and individualize the nursing care plan.

CULTURAL COMPETENCE

The following are guidelines that the nurse may find useful when instructing older persons and their families about cultural competence in healthcare.

1. As a person from a different culture, what can I expect of my healthcare provider?

You can expect to receive culturally competent care. This means that you will be provided the highest quality of care, regardless of your race, ethnicity, cultural background, English proficiency, or literacy. Some common services provided may include:

- Interpreter services.
- Attempts to recruit persons from your culture (if possible) to work in health facilities in your area.
- Coordination with traditional healers.
- Respect for your values, beliefs, and traditions.
- Printed health information in your language and appropriate to your reading level.

(Georgetown University, 2004)

RATIONALE:

Many older persons and their families are not aware of the services that healthcare facilities are urged to develop in order to provide culturally competent care. Informing patients will empower them to be more proactive with their healthcare providers.

2. Why is culturally competent care important?

A culturally competent healthcare system can help improve health outcomes and quality of care, and can contribute to the elimination of racial and ethnic health disparities. It is both to your advantage and to the advantage of your healthcare providers to eliminate any barriers that stand in the way of improving your health and caring for you when you are ill.

RATIONALE:

Persons of color and ethnic minorities are burdened with a disproportionate amount of chronic illness and disability with aging. As the treatment of chronic illness is a long-term process requiring many lifestyle changes and adaptations, any barriers to effective communication should be removed to increase the odds of successful disease management.

3. What can I do to increase my chances of obtaining culturally competent healthcare?

Try to find a healthcare provider you can relate to. People who do not have a regular doctor or healthcare provider are less likely to obtain preventive services, or diagnosis, treatment, and management of chronic conditions. Health insurance coverage is also an important determinant of access to healthcare. People without healthcare insurance often wait longer to seek healthcare, delay treatment once diagnosed with an illness, and as a result suffer more serious health problems. Social workers and community clinics often have services for persons without health insurance and can direct you to receive free or low-cost care. Once you have located a healthcare provider, inform him or her about yourself and your culture. If your provider recommends an intervention that is not consistent with your beliefs, discuss this right away. Let your provider know if you cannot understand written material given to you, if verbal instructions contain too much medical jargon that you cannot understand, or if you are given forms to fill out that are inconsistent with your level of reading in English. Providing culturally competent healthcare is an ongoing learning process. Your healthcare provider will be grateful to hear your constructive comments and receive your support.

RATIONALE:

It is almost impossible to know everything about every culture. Training approaches that focus only on facts are best combined with the ongoing feedback from patients, families, and other healthcare providers. Curiosity, empathy, respect, and humility are some basic attitudes that can help the clinical relationship and yield useful information about the patient's beliefs and preferences. An approach that focuses on inquiry, reflection, and analysis throughout the care process is most useful for the healthcare provider who is attempting to provide culturally competent care.

Care Plan

A Patient Requiring CulturalCare

Case Study

Mrs. Rivera, a 79-year-old woman of Mexican heritage, was admitted to a long-term care facility and presented the following challenges for nurses, other health-care staff, caregivers, and the institution:

- She and her family could not read, speak, nor understand English.
- Her strong Catholic faith and Hispanic cultural traditions required modesty during physical examinations and when personal care was delivered.
- Her family had both religious and cultural reasons for not discussing end-of-life concerns or her impending death.

Applying the Nursing Process

ASSESSMENT

Mrs. Rivera will require a complete health assessment in order to provide her with culturally appropriate nursing care. The nurse should admit the patient to her room, make her comfortable, and begin to assess basic necessities such as dietary preferences, level of pain, safety, current medications taken, and strength and availability of the family support system. If the nurse does not speak Spanish, every attempt should be made to obtain an interpreter. If a bilingual family member is present, the nurse could rely on that person for establishing immediate communication, but it is advantageous to use a professional interpreter for ongoing communication with the patient.

DIAGNOSIS

Appropriate nursing diagnoses for Mrs. Rivera might include the following:

- *Imbalanced nutrition: less than bodily requirements* (if culturally appropriate foods cannot be provided)
- *Risk for injury* (if safety precautions cannot be communicated)
- *Impaired verbal communication*
- *Risk for loneliness* (if social interactions are precluded by language difficulties)
- *Spiritual distress* (if appropriate religious traditions are not heeded)
- *Decisional conflict* (if the care providers request the family and patient to discuss her impending death)
- *Pain* (if levels cannot be communicated)

(continued)

A Patient Requiring CulturalCare *(continued)*

EXPECTED OUTCOMES

Expected outcomes for the plan of care specify that Mrs. Rivera will:

- Accept nursing care and pain relief.
- Communicate her needs.
- Maintain adequate weight and levels of hydration.
- Carry out cultural and religious rituals as appropriate to Mexican culture.
- Have access to family, religious clergy, and healers as appropriate to her culture.
- Experience a peaceful death without suffering.

PLANNING AND IMPLEMENTATION

The nurse would develop a plan of care to include culturally and linguistically appropriate responses such as:

- Locating interpreter staff to not only translate but also explain the cultural meanings of beliefs and practices.
- Providing translated and understandable written materials at the reading level of the family.
- Providing sensitive and comprehensive explanations and discussions about treatment, informed consent, and advance directive forms.
- Locating clinical nursing and caregivers who know how and what to ask about perceived needs and recognized cultural issues.
- Obtaining appropriate food choices.
- Limiting caregivers to female care providers.

EVALUATION

The nurse hopes to work with the patient and her family over time to provide culturally appropriate care. The nurse will consider the plan a success based on the following criteria:

- Mrs. Rivera will accept nursing care and pain control interventions.
- The patient and family will be in agreement with the plan of care.
- Mrs. Rivera will suffer no adverse events (falls, decubitus ulcers, adverse drug events) while receiving care in the long-term care facility.
- She will experience a peaceful death with adequate pain control, family and religious support, and attention to cultural rituals.

Ethical Dilemma

One of the nurse's colleagues feels strongly that Mrs. Rivera should be told of her impending death. This colleague feels that truth telling is important and that patients should have access to all information regarding their condition. When this colleague attempts to tell Mrs. Rivera of her condition, the patient and family become very upset and ask the nurse to intervene. The nurse takes the colleague aside and urges the colleague to examine any personal beliefs or cultural bias that may

A Patient Requiring CulturalCare

be present and influencing this behavior. The colleague should be urged to attempt to meet the needs of Mrs. Rivera and her family rather than his or her own needs. The patient's right to know (or in this case, not to know) is overridden by the mandate to "do no harm." Blunt and inappropriate truth telling in this case is culturally insensitive and likely to cause harm to Mrs. Rivera and her family.

Critical Thinking and the Nursing Process

1. At your next clinical session, evaluate care plans you and others have devised for older patients for evidence of consideration of cross-cultural influences.
2. Interview a nurse who practices in your clinical setting. Ask him or her whether the age of the patient influences cultural aspects reflected in the planning or delivery of nursing care.
3. Pick a topic such as truth telling, and research the customs of different cultures related to that topic. Enlist the help of your fellow students.
4. Write a reflective narrative about how your ethnic and cultural background influences your values and beliefs regarding life, death, health, and aging.
5. Interview an older patient regarding his or her traditional cultural/native health practices and medicine.
6. How do family and community support systems vary by culture?

- Evaluate your responses in Appendix B. ⊂▭

EXPLORE MediaLink

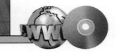

NCLEX review, case studies, and other interactive resources for this chapter can be found on the Companion Website at **www.prenhall.com/tabloski**. Click on Chapter 4 to select the activities for this chapter. For animations, video tutorials, more NCLEX review questions, and case studies, access the accompanying CD-ROM in this textbook.

Chapter Highlights

- The people residing in North America come from a variety of ethnic and cultural backgrounds, and each person has a unique ethnocultural heritage and life trajectory.
- Culturally and linguistically appropriate services in healthcare are now mandated by the federal government and regulating bodies.
- The CulturalCare triad represents the complex interrelationships of the nurse, patient, and caregivers within community and institutional (home or residential) settings.

- Many groups in North America may be living within their traditional heritage, or they may embrace their original ethnocultural traditional heritage and a North American, modern culture.

- There are potential areas of conflict derived from the demographic, ethnocultural, and life trajectory variables of the people within the triad.

- When assessing a patient, self, or caregiver, the nurse considers the patient's cultural values, beliefs, practices, and life trajectory.

- The integration of CulturalCare into the plan of care and workplace environment requires both thought and action.

References

Abramson, H. J. (1980). Religion. In S. Thernstrom (Ed.), *Harvard encyclopedia of American ethnic groups.* Cambridge, MA: Harvard University Press.

Balzer-Riley, J. W. (1997). *Communications in nursing: Communicating, assertively and responsibly in nursing: A guidebook* (3rd ed.). St. Louis, MO: Mosby.

Bernstein, R. (2002). *Census brief: Current population survey coming to America: A profile of the nation's foreign born (2000 update).* Washington, DC: U. S. Department of Commerce.

Bohannan, P. (1992). *We, the alien—An introduction to cultural anthropology.* Prospect Heights, IL: Waveland Press.

DeNavas-Walt, C., Cleveland, R., & Webster, B. (2003). Income in the United States, 2002, U.S. Census Bureau, Washington, DC: U.S. Government Printing Office.

Estes, G., & Zitzow, D. (1980, November). *Heritage consistency as a consideration in counseling Native Americans.* Paper presented at the National Indian Education Association Convention, Dallas, TX.

Georgetown University. (2004). *Cultural competence in health care: Is it important for people with chronic conditions?* Institute for Health Care Research and Policy, Issue Brief 5. Georgetown University Center for Research and Policy, Washington, DC.

Hartford Institute for Geriatric Nursing (1999). Try This: Best Practices in nursing care in older adults. Retrieved on June 14, 2003, from http://www.Hartfordign.org.

Hicks, R., & Hicks, K. (1999). *Boomers, Xers, and other strangers.* Wheaton, IL: Tyndale House.

LaFrombose, T., Coleman, L. K., & Gerton, J. (1993). Psychological impact of biculturalism: Evidence and theory. *Psychological Bulletin, 114*(3), 395.

National Center for Health Statistics. (2004). *Health, United States 2004,* U.S. Department of

Health and Human Services, National Center for Health Statistics, Washington. DC.

Novak, M. (1973). How American are you if your grandparents came from Serbia in 1888? In S. TeSelle (Ed.), *The rediscovery of ethnicity: Its implications for culture and politics in America.* New York: Harper & Row.

Office of Minority Health. (2001). *National standards for culturally and linguistically appropriate services in health care.* Washington, DC: U.S. Department of Health and Human Services.

Rodriguez, C. (2001, April 2). 1930 is window to the past. *Boston Globe,* p. B3; the unhyphenating of America. *Boston Globe,* (May 31), p. A1.

Spector, R. E. (2004). *Cultural diversity in health and illness* (6th ed.). Upper Saddle River, NJ: Prentice Hall.

Steinmetz, S., & Braham, C. G. (Eds.). (1993). *Random House Webster's dictionary.* New York: Ballantine Reference Library.

U.S. Census Bureau. (2001). *Profiles of general demographic characteristics 2000.* Washington, DC: U.S. Department of Commerce.

U.S. Department of Health & Human Services. (2001). *Member of the National Advisory Council for Nursing Research,* Jan 23-24, 2001, National Institutes of Health, Washington, DC.

U.S. Department of Labor, Bureau of Labor Statistics. (2002). *Quick Facts on Registered Nurses.* Washington, DC: U.S. Department of Labor.

Selected Bibliography

Anderson, J. M. (1990, May/June). Health care across the cultures. *Nursing Outlook, 38,* 136–139.

Baldonado, A. A. (1996). Transcending the barriers of cultural diversity in health care. *Journal of Cultural Diversity, 3,* 20–22.

Baldwin, D., Cotanch, P., Johnson, P., & Williams, J. (1996). *An Afrocentric approach to breast and cervical cancer early detection and screening.* Washington, DC: American Nurses Association.

Baye, A. L. (1995). A lesson in culture. *Minority Nurse,* Summer/Fall, pp. 35–38.

Bhimani, R., & Acorn, S. (1998, September). Managing within a culturally diverse environment. *Canadian Nurse, 94,* 32–36.

Crow, K. (1993). Multiculturalism and pluralistic thought in nursing education: Native American world view and the nursing academic world view. *Journal of Nursing Education, 32,* 198–204.

Doswell, W. M., & Erlen, J. A. (1998, June). Multicultural issues and ethical concerns in the delivery of nursing care interventions. *Nursing Clinics of North America, 33,* 353–361.

Eliason, M. J. (1993, September/October). Ethics and transcultural nursing care. *Nursing Outlook, 4,* 225–228.

Grossman, D., & Taylor, R. (1995, February). Working with people: Cultural diversity on the unit. *American Journal of Nursing, 95*(2), 64–67.

Kittler, P. G., & Sucher, K. P. (1990, March/April). Diet counseling in a multicultural society. *Diabetes Educator, 16,* 127–134.

Krakauer, E. L., Crenner, C., & Fox, K. (2002). Barriers to optimum end-of-life care for minority patients. *Journal of the American Geriatrics Society, 50,* 182–190.

Lea, A. (1994, August). Nursing in today's multicultural society: A transcultural perspective. *Journal of Advanced Nursing, 20,* 307–313.

Leininger, M. M. (1993, Winter). Towards conceptualization of transcultural health care systems: Concepts and a model. *Journal of Transcultural Nursing, 4,* 32–40.

Lipson, J., & Bauwens, E. (1988). Use of anthropology in nursing. *Practicing Anthropology, 10,* 4–5.

Lo, B., Ruston, D., Kates, L., Arnold, R., Cohen, C., & Faber-Langendoen, K., et al. (2002). Discussing religious and spiritual issues at the end of life. *Journal of the American Medical Association, 287*(6), 749–754.

Lynam, M. J. (1992, February). Towards the goal of providing culturally sensitive care: Principles upon which to build nursing curricula. *Journal of Advanced Nursing, 17,* 149–157.

Rosenbaum, J. N. (1991, April). A cultural assessment guide: Learning cultural sensitivity. *Canadian Nurse, 88,* 32–33.

Rosenbaum, J. N. (1995, April). Teaching cultural sensitivity. *Journal of Nursing Education, 34,* 188–189.

Smith, S. (1992). *Communications in nursing* (2nd ed.). St. Louis, MO: Mosby-Year Book.

Sprott, J. (1993). The black box in family assessments: Cultural diversity. In S. Feetham, S. Meister, J. Bell, & C. Gilliss (Eds.), *The nursing of families: Theory, research, education, practice* (pp. 189–199). Beverly Hills, CA: Sage.

Wenger, A. F. Z. (1993, January). Cultural meaning of symptoms. *Holistic Nursing Practice, 7,* 22–23.

Texts Authored by Nurses

The following texts have been authored by nurses and may be helpful in developing CulturalCare knowledge:

Boyle, J. S., & Andrews, M. M. (1995). *Transcultural concepts in nursing care* (2nd ed.). Philadelphia: Lippincott.

Galanti, G. (1991). *Caring for patients from different cultures.* Philadelphia: University of Pennsylvania Press.

Geissler, E. M. (1998). *Pocket guide cultural assessment* (2nd ed.). St. Louis, MO: Mosby.

Giger, J. N., & Davidhizar, R. E. (1995). *Transcultural nursing assessment and intervention* (2nd ed.). St. Louis, MO: Mosby.

Leininger, M., & McFarland, M. R. (Eds.). (2002). *Transcultural nursing: Concepts, theories, research, and practice* (3rd ed.). New York: McGraw-Hill.

Lipson, J. G., Dibble, S. L., & Minarik, P. A. (1996). *Culture & nursing care: A pocket guide.* San Francisco: UCSF Nursing Press.

National Center for Health Statistics Health of the United States. Retrieved October 13, 2004, from http://www.cdc.gov/ncs/hus.htm.

Purnell, L. D., & Paulanka, B. J. (1998). *Transcultural health care.* Philadelphia: F. A. Davis.

Spector, R. E. (2004). *Cultural diversity in health and illness* (6th ed.). Upper Saddle River, NJ: Prentice Hall Health.

Spector, R. E. (2004). *CulturalCare: Guides to heritage assessment and health traditions.* Upper Saddle River, NJ: Prentice Hall Health.

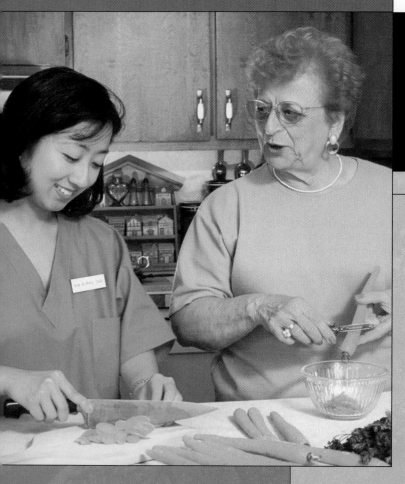

CHAPTER 5

Nutrition and Aging

Sheila Buckley Tucker, MA, RD, LDN
Part-time Faculty, Connell School of
Nursing & Lynch School of Education and
Executive Dietitian, Boston College

CHAPTER OBJECTIVES

Upon completion of this chapter, the reader will be able to:

- Describe the normal changes of aging in body composition and digestion, absorption, and metabolism of nutrients.
- Differentiate between normal and disease-related changes in risk factors for undernutrition in older persons.
- Identify normal nutrition requirements of the older person.
- Outline the causes and consequences of undernutrition in the older person.
- Identify tools and parameters used to assess nutrition status.
- Define appropriate nursing interventions and treatment for nutrition-related problems of the older person.
- Identify current dietary approaches to chronic disease in the older person.

KEY TERMS

MediaLink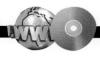

Additional resources for this chapter can be found on the Student CD-ROM accompanying this textbook and on the Companion Website at **www.prenhall.com/tabloski**. Click on Chapter 5 to select the activities for this chapter.

CD-ROM

- Animations
    Carbohydrates
    Protein
    Tube Feeding
- NCLEX Questions
- Case Studies
- Tools

COMPANION WEBSITE

- Audio Glossary
- Additional NCLEX Review
- Case Study
- MediaLink Applications

The biological process of aging proceeds at an individualized pace, yet predictable changes can place older persons at a disproportionate risk of **undernutrition**, or **malnutrition**, compared to younger adults. Both undernutrition and diseases associated with overnutrition, such as obesity, degenerative joint disease, hypertension, and type 2 diabetes, can adversely affect vitality and quality of life. Lifelong eating habits can help promote health maintenance into older personhood. Independent older persons may only require regular nutritional screening during routine health checks, whereas others may require intervention for unintentional weight loss or drug-nutrient interactions. Hospitalized or frail older persons in long-term care deserve additional nutritional consideration as they are at highest risk for malnutrition. The wide spectrum of well-being in the older person presents nutritional challenges along a continuum.

Normal Aging and Nutrition

The normal aging process can result in biological changes that may place the older person at risk of malnutrition. The effects of these normal changes should be considered even in a healthy individual.

CHANGES IN BODY COMPOSITION

Lean muscle mass diminishes with aging. The term **sarcopenia** refers to these age-related phenomena. Muscle loss occurs for a variety of reasons, including lessened physical activity, whether from disability or disease or related to a sedentary lifestyle; decreased anabolic hormone production (testosterone, growth hormone, dehydroepiandrosterone); increased cytokine activity; and decreased nutrition (Morley & Thomas, 2001). Regardless of the etiology, loss of muscle mass can lead to a spiral of negative physical and functional changes. Resting energy expenditure, or metabolic rate, is largely driven by lean body mass and will decrease with loss of muscle. The individual who continues with steady state calorie intake in the face of lessened muscle mass will most likely experience fat weight gain. This shift in body composition is not always apparent and cannot be discerned by measuring body weight alone. Such masked muscle loss has been demonstrated in healthy older persons (Gallagher et al., 2000).

Loss of muscle can lead to a functional decline as strength and endurance become affected by specific loss of type II muscle fibers (Evans, 1997). Physical activity then may decline with loss of strength, furthering the downward spiral with additional muscle loss and predisposing the older person to falls (Tinetti, 2003).

The loss of muscle leads to lower total body water in the older person. Total body water content in adults over 65 years drops to about 60% total body mass from about 72% as a younger adult (Chidester & Spangler, 1997).

Practice Pearl

Unintentional weight loss of 5% of body weight in one month or 10% in one year should not be considered a normal part of aging and requires intervention.

Bone mineral density commonly is lost with age in both men and women. Suboptimal bone growth in younger years, medications, and disease can cause pre-existing compromised bone density to which age-related bone losses are added. Bone loss puts women at risk for osteoporosis following menopause; men are at risk later in life (NIH Consensus Development Panel on Osteoporosis, 2001).

ORAL AND GASTROINTESTINAL CHANGES WITH AGING

Multiple changes may occur with age in the regulation of both appetite and fluid status. Additionally, gastrointestinal changes that may occur with aging can lead to altered dietary intake and eventually diminished nutritional status.

Dentition

By the age of 65 years, 33.1% of Americans suffer from **edentulism** (Hutton, Feine, & Morais, 2002). Poor dental health, missing or loose teeth, and ill-fitting dentures can affect the type and amount of food eaten and interfere with proper nutrition. Several studies have found an association between an edentulous state and poor intake of protein, vitamins, and minerals. Additionally, having fewer pairs of posterior teeth may result in less variety in the diet and higher fat intake (Hutton et al., 2002; Sahyoun, Lin, & Krall, 2003). Mandibular bone loss related to osteoporosis or periodontal disease can cause changes in structural tissue that affects chewing.

Xerostomia

Saliva production declines with age and can be further exacerbated by dehydration, medications, or disease. Lack of sufficient saliva production is termed **xerostomia**. Dry mouth can affect taste perception, hinder swallowing, and cause insufficient retention of poorly fitting dentures (Ship, 2002).

Atrophic Gastritis

In the stomach, decreases in size and number of glands and mucous membranes can lead to **atrophic gastritis**. Lack of hydrochloric acid production, or **achlorhydria**, is common in the aging process. Iron and vitamin B_{12} require an acid medium in the stomach to begin absorption; lack of adequate hydrochloric acid production can limit absorption of both nutrients.

Drug Alert ❗

Medications that alter gastric pH such as antacids, proton pump inhibitors, H_2 receptor blockers, and potassium salts may also alter iron and B_{12} absorption due to alkalinizing effects of these medications (White & Ashworth, 2000).

Gastric production of intrinsic factor, which is necessary for vitamin B_{12} absorption in the ileum, may also decrease.

Appetite Dysregulation

Cholecystokinin production increases with age and can cause early satiety as a result. Early satiation also occurs due to changes in gastric emptying and central neurotransmitters responsible for feeding drive. Studies have demonstrated continued diminished intake in older men compared to younger subjects following deliberate weight loss and refeeding, raising concerns about the effects of temporary weight loss becoming permanent in the older person. These physiological changes have been called the **anorexia of aging** (Chapman, MacIntosh, Morley, & Horowitz, 2002; De Castro, 1993; Morley & Thomas, 1999).

Constipation

Slowed intestinal peristalsis, inadequate intake of fluid and fiber, illness, medications, and a sedentary lifestyle are contributing factors to the prevalence of constipation in the older person.

Thirst Dysregulation

Aging blunts the thirst mechanism, and angiotensin production is impaired, increasing the risk of uncompensated dehydration in a population that already experiences lower total body water than in younger adults (Thomas & Morley, 2001). Symptoms of dehydration such as confusion or lethargy can go unrecognized while hydration status continues to worsen without a strong thirst response. Dehydration risk can be worsened by voluntary fluid restriction in the older person trying to cope with incontinence, nocturia, or the need for assistance with toileting. Individuals with cognitive or physical limitations may have inadequate access to free fluids in addition to thirst dysregulation. Refer to Box 5-1 for dehydration risk factors and symptoms.

SENSORY CHANGES

Age-related changes in vision, hearing, taste, and smell (see Chapter 14) can have a negative impact on nutrition. ⌘

Vision

Cataracts, macular degeneration, and general poor vision can make shopping, food preparation, and even eating a burden. Fine-print food labels and cooking directions are difficult to read; handling hot foods or using a stove can be a hazard. Dim or harsh lighting in the dining area can make it difficult to see a meal and reduce enjoyment associated with eating. Poor vision is associated with a decline in protein and energy intake in functional, community-dwelling older persons (Payette, Gray-Donald, Cyr, & Boutier, 1995).

Practice Pearl

Individuals with poor vision can benefit from mealtime assistance using the clock analogy with their dinner plate: "Your carrots are at two o'clock and the chicken is at six o'clock."

Hearing

Hearing losses that occur with age can make social dining a difficult experience. Some older persons may choose to dine alone rather than be embarrassed by not hearing well or frustrated trying to interact with others. Social isolation is considered a risk factor for undernutrition in the older person (Chia-Hui, Schilling, & Lyder, 2001).

BOX 5-1	Dehydration Risk Factors and Symptoms in the Older Adult

Dehydration Risk Factors

Physical changes of aging
- ↓ Lean body mass → ↓ total body water
- ↓ Thirst from aging, medication, or disease
- Impaired angiotensin production

Lack of free access to fluids
- Dependency on others
- Cognitive impairment
- Physical impairment

Voluntary fluid restriction to manage:
- Incontinence
- Nocturia
- Diuretic side effect
- Limited physical movement due to mobility or pain issues

Increased insensitive fluid losses
- Sweating from fever or climate
- ↑ Respiratory rate
- Vomiting
- Diarrhea
- Polyuria
- Exudative wound or fistula

Symptoms of Dehydration

Darkened urine

↓ Urine output

Confusion

Lethargy

Headache

Light-headedness

Sunken eyes

Dry mucous membranes

Dry axillae

Long tongue furrows

Postural changes in pulse and blood pressure

Taste and Smell

Olfactory and taste perceptions are intertwined. Both senses diminish with age in some, and the decline has been associated with reduced pleasure with eating (Bromley, 2000; Murphy et al., 2002). Medications are responsible for some taste alterations. ACE inhibitors, anticholinergics, antidepressants, and antihistamines can cause xerostomia and diminished taste perception. Dentures, zinc deficiency, smoking, and neurodegenerative disease, such as Parkinson's disease, are also associated with loss of taste (Bromley, 2000). Some older persons experience **dysgeusia**, or altered taste perception, and complain of metallic and chalky taste transmissions. Others report needing increased salt and sweet levels to perceive taste (Bromley, 2000; Mattes, 2002; Schiffman, 1997, 2000).

SOCIAL AND ECONOMIC CHANGES AFFECTING NUTRITION

Retirement from the workforce can lead to a more sedentary lifestyle for some older persons. The effects of decreased activity on body composition may involve muscle loss and fat gain. Social isolation, loneliness, loss of a spouse, or bereavement can in-

	BOX 5-2
Nutrition-Related Changes Associated With Aging	

- ↓ Lean body mass
- ↓ Metabolic rate
- ↓ Bone mineral density
- ↑ Cholecystokinin and early satiety
- ↓ Saliva production
- ↓ Thirst perception
- ↓ Taste and smell
- ↓ Production of gastric acid and fluids

troduce additional influences that can alter adequacy of diet. Changes in socioeconomic status may occur. Poverty or near poverty affects 19% of older persons and may force an individual to decide between paying bills, buying medications, or buying groceries. African American and Hispanic older persons are at disproportionate risk of poverty compared with White older persons (26.4%, 21%, and 8.9%, respectively). Women are twice as likely to live in poverty compared to men (Position of the American Dietetic Association, 2000). Many older persons have insufficient money for food, yet are not poor enough to qualify for government assistance (Wellman, Weddle, Krantz, & Brain, 1997). Box 5-2 outlines age-related nutritional changes in the body.

Nutritional and Disease-Related Health Changes

Many chronic diseases that affect older persons have nutritional implications of the disease and its treatment. Altered nutritional needs, therapeutic diets, and changes in nutrient utilization impact an individual's nutritional status. One example of this is cognitive impairment and mental illness, such as dementia, depression, or anxiety. Both the disease process itself and the medications used to treat these diagnoses can negatively impact appetite, taste, nutrient absorption, and metabolism; diminish saliva production; and cause gastrointestinal side effects. Numerous other diseases and medications have nutritional implications. Table 5-1 outlines some common medications with nutritional implications.

Nutritional Requirements and Aging

The older person has some unique nutritional requirements due to the physical and functional changes that occur with aging. While many older persons experience a decline in physical activity level and have lower calorie needs, there is not a decreased need for most vitamins and minerals with age. In fact, the dietary requirement for some nutrients increases with age. Obtaining a well-balanced diet while consuming fewer calories overall can present a challenge to many older persons.

There are several dietary standards that outline nutritional recommendations for older persons. The focus here is on recommendations that are unique to healthy older persons. The dietary reference intakes (DRIs) and the Food Guide Pyramid are two distinctly different approaches to providing nutritional recommendations that work well together as assessment and educational tools. These two standards are not intended to be guidelines for use when making recommendations for older persons at

TABLE 5-1

Medications With Nutritional Implications

Drug	Side Effect	Explanation
ACE inhibitors	Altered taste, dry mouth	Causes metallic taste/reduced taste perception
Alcohol	↓ Absorption and metabolism	Thiamin, folic acid, B_{12}, magnesium, B_6 affected
Antacids	↓ Absorption, constipation	Iron, B_{12} need acid pH
Antianxiety agents	Dry mouth	Affects taste and swallowing
Antidepressants and antipsychotics	↓ Intake and dry mouth	Affects taste, smell, swallowing
Antiparkinson agents	↓ Intake and dry mouth	Nausea, vomiting, taste changes
Colchicine	↓ Absorption	B_{12}, calcium, and iron affected
Corticosteroids	↓ Intake, ↓ nutrition	Nausea, vomiting; affects calcium, vitamin D, B_6, folate
Digoxin	↓ Intake	Anorexia and nausea
Isoniazid	Altered metabolism	Vitamin B_6 affected
KCl (potassium chloride)	↓ Intake, ↓ absorption	Nausea; B_{12} and iron affected
Metformin	↓ Intake, ↓ absorption	Anorexia; B_{12} affected
Methotrexate	↓ Intake, ↓ absorption	Nausea; folate, B_{12}, calcium affected
Narcotics and sedatives	↓ Intake, constipation	Nausea, vomiting, sedation
Penicillamine	↓ Intake, ↓ nutrition	Anorexia, B_6 affected
Phenytoin	↓ Intake, ↓ nutrition	Altered taste and smell; folate, B_6, vitamin D affected
Sulfasalazine	↓ Absorption	Folate and iron affected
Theophylline	↓ Intake, ↓ nutrition	Nausea, vomiting, anorexia; B_6 affected

Source: Adapted from Gazewood, J. D., & Mehr, D. R. (1998); Bromley, S. M. (2000); White, R., & Ashworth, A. (2000).

risk for undernutrition or those with illness. The DRIs provide specific nutrient recommendations and are the larger umbrella under which exist the recommended dietary allowances (RDAs) and the newer adequate intakes (AIs) and tolerable upper limits (TULs). The RDAs are researched to meet the needs of 97% to 98% of healthy people within specific age and gender groups. Recommendations for older persons are categorized in two age groups: 51 to 70 years and over 70 years. When insufficient data exist to establish an RDA for a nutrient, an AI recommendation is made instead. The newest vitamin D recommendation is an example of an AI and not an RDA. The TUL guidelines have been included in the DRI umbrella to provide guidelines for a safe upper limit of intake for a nutrient. The saying "if some is good, more must be better" does not hold for all nutrients as some have pharmacological action at high intakes. While a nurse can always refer to references for specific needs of random nutrients, knowledge of the unique nutritional needs and risk factors for the older person can be important to everyday practice. Knowledge of the TULs of commonly supplemented nutrients better allows a nurse to give crucial advice on supplement safety.

The U.S. Department of Agriculture (USDA) Food Guide Pyramid translates the scientific recommendations of the DRIs into recommendations for daily eating. The focus is on variety, balance, and moderation in all food groups while providing adequate nutrient intake. The Tufts University Modified Food Guide Pyramid for Older Adults is a modification of the USDA Food Guide Pyramid that is a useful complement to the DRIs when evaluating the nutritional history of an older person (Figure 5-1 ■).

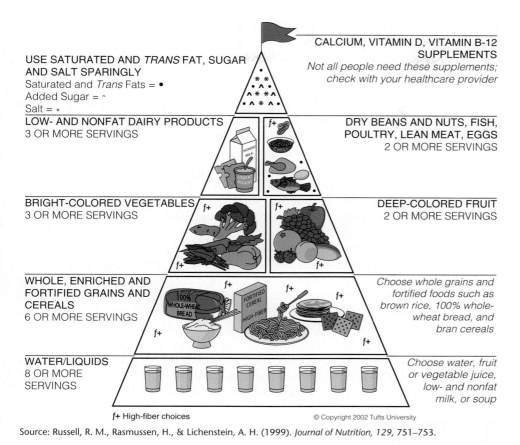

FIGURE ■ 5-1

TUFTS Modified Food Guide Pyramid for persons over 70 years of age.

CALCIUM, VITAMIN D, VITAMIN B-12 SUPPLEMENTS
Not all people need these supplements; check with your healthcare provider

USE SATURATED AND *TRANS* FAT, SUGAR AND SALT SPARINGLY
Saturated and *Trans* Fats = •
Added Sugar = ^
Salt = ⋆

LOW- AND NONFAT DAIRY PRODUCTS
3 OR MORE SERVINGS

DRY BEANS AND NUTS, FISH, POULTRY, LEAN MEAT, EGGS
2 OR MORE SERVINGS

BRIGHT-COLORED VEGETABLES
3 OR MORE SERVINGS

DEEP-COLORED FRUIT
2 OR MORE SERVINGS

WHOLE, ENRICHED AND FORTIFIED GRAINS AND CEREALS
6 OR MORE SERVINGS

Choose whole grains and fortified foods such as brown rice, 100% whole-wheat bread, and bran cereals

WATER/LIQUIDS
8 OR MORE SERVINGS

Choose water, fruit or vegetable juice, low- and nonfat milk, or soup

f+ High-fiber choices   © Copyright 2002 Tufts University

Source: Russell, R. M., Rasmussen, H., & Lichenstein, A. H. (1999). *Journal of Nutrition, 129,* 751–753.

UNIQUE NUTRIENT RECOMMENDATIONS

The DRIs for the general adult population and the older adult population are the same with the exception of vitamin D, calcium, vitamin B_{12}, vitamin B_6, and energy. There is some dispute about whether the older person should have an altered protein requirement due to the prevalence of sarcopenia, yet the current RDA for protein remains unchanged at 0.8 g/kg body weight with no unique recommendation for the older person (Institute of Medicine, 2002). The Modified Food Guide Pyramid recommends protein foods in the fourth tier of the pyramid with three dairy servings per day and at least two servings in the meat-poultry-fish-dry beans-eggs-nuts group.

Energy

The DRIs for energy, or estimated energy requirements (EERs), for all adults are based on gender, age, body mass index (BMI), and activity level. Individuals with higher lean body mass or higher activity levels require more energy than those at lower levels for any given age. The EER is adjusted for age to account for losses in lean muscle mass. Men are advised to adjust calorie intake downward by 7 cal/decade over 30 years of age; women adjust likewise by 10 cal/decade over 30 years of age (Trumbo, Schlicker, Yates, & Poos, 2002). The older person who maintains lean muscle mass through resistance training should not expect to see this drop in daily calorie requirements (Evans, 1997). The Modified Food Guide Pyramid makes overall recommendations for individual food groups to provide sufficient energy and nutrients together. Following the lowest daily recommended values for all the food groups will result in approximately 1,600 cal of energy. Use of this tool to guide energy recommendations is often more practical to the nurse and the client than calculating EER.

Vitamin D

Vitamin D is required for its role in maintaining bone mineralization and proper serum calcium levels. Inadequate vitamin D levels can lead to poor bone mineralization, rickets, and osteomalacia. The AI for vitamin D *triples* from young adulthood to age 71. Adults over age 70 require 600 IU (or 15 µg) of vitamin D compared with 200 IU (or 5 µg) for adults age 50 and under. The AI for adults 51 to 70 years of age is 400 IU (or 10 µg) (Institute of Medicine, 1997). Diminished endogenous synthesis of vitamin D with age, limited sun exposure, and potentially reduced absorption of vitamin D have guided these increased recommendations aimed at reducing bone loss and fracture risk.

Food sources of vitamin D include liver, fortified milk, and fish liver oils. Cheeses and yogurt are not mandated to be fortified with vitamin D and should not be considered good sources. In survey research, over 60% of older persons have intakes below recommended levels (Foote, Giuliano, & Harris, 2000). Others have reported an incidence in a Boston hospital of 57% of older persons with hypovitaminosis D (Thomas et al., 1998). Adults most at risk for poor vitamin D status include those who do not consume milk, have limited sun exposure, or take anticonvulsant medication or corticosteroids. The Modified Food Guide Pyramid recommends a supplement of vitamin D in addition to the three dairy servings per day recommended. The pyramid authors acknowledge the limited intake of good sources of vitamin D and limited endogenous

Drug Alert ❗

Fat-soluble vitamins A, D, E, and K are stored in the body in larger amounts than are water-soluble vitamins (vitamin C and all the B vitamins). Taking large amounts of some fat-soluble vitamins could lead to toxicity due to continued storage in adipose and other tissue. In many clinic or office settings, the nurse may be the only clinician who has the opportunity to assess supplement use. The nurse should pay particular attention to the TUL for vitamins A, D, and E (vitamin K has no TUL due to lack of data on toxicity). When assessing nutritional status, the nurse should ask about all dietary supplements and fortified foods, like breakfast cereals and meal replacement drinks and bars. Recent studies have brought to light the potentially increased risk associated with vitamin A intake at or near the TUL in the form of retinol, or increased plasma retinol levels, and hip fractures in older men and women (Denke, 2002; Feskanich, Singh, Willett, & Colditz, 2002; Michaelsson, Lithell, Vessby, & Melhus, 2003). The TUL of vitamin A as retinol is 3,000 µg/day (Institute of Medicine, 2001).

High vitamin E intake can interact with anticoagulant therapy as well as potentiate the antiplatelet effects of other supplements such as ginkgo biloba, ginger, ginseng, and garlic (Ang-Lee, Moss, & Yuan, 2001; Fairfield & Fletcher, 2002; Norred & Brinker, 2001). These herbs are among those most frequently used for self-treatment (Yoon & Horne, 2001). The TUL of vitamin E is 1,000 mg/day (Institute of Medicine, 2000).

Vitamin D has a TUL of 2,000 IU (or 50 µg), and reports have been made of accidental overdosing with dietary supplements (Koutkia, Chen, & Holick, 2001).

Food	Serving Size	Vitamin D Amount (IU)
Milk, vitamin D fortified	1 cup	127
Margarine, vitamin D fortified	1 tbsp	60
Egg yolk, large	1 ea	18
Beef liver, cooked	3.5 oz	30
Sardines with bones, canned, drained	3.5 oz	280
Salmon, cooked	3.5 oz	360
Cod liver oil	1 tbsp	1,360
Cereal, vitamin D fortified only	½ cup to 1 cup	~20 to 50 but varies—check label
Juice, vitamin D fortified only	1 cup	~20 to 50 but varies—check label
Soy milk or soy yogurt, vitamin D fortified only	1 cup	~100 to 150 but varies—check label

TABLE 5-2

Vitamin D Amounts of Common Food Sources*

*Note: Dairy sources such as cheese, yogurt, and ice cream contain calcium but are not good sources of vitamin D unless specifically fortified.

Source: Adapted from U.S. Department of Agriculture, http://www.nal.usda.gov/fnic/foodcomp National Institutes of Health Clinical Center, http://www.cc.nih.gov/ccc/supplements/vitd.html#food; and product labels.

vitamin D synthesis with aging (Russell, Rasmussen, & Lichtenstein, 1999). Table 5-2 outlines dietary sources of vitamin D. A thorough nutritional assessment of vitamin D food sources, including fortified foods and existing vitamin habits, should precede the recommendation of a supplement. It is not recommended to simply take two multivitamins to get the AI of 600 IU because of the risk of oversupplementation of vitamin A (Fairfield & Fletcher, 2002). The TUL of vitamin D is 2,000 IU or 50 μg (Institute of Medicine, 1997).

Calcium

Calcium in the diet is required for the maintenance of bone mineral density and plasma calcium levels. The majority of the body's calcium reserves are in bone and teeth with only 1% of total body calcium in plasma. The AI for calcium in adults over 50 years of age is increased to 1,200 mg compared to 1,000 mg for adults 19 to 50 years of age (Institute of Medicine, 1997). Some researchers recommend up to 1,500 mg daily due to the accelerated bone loss and risk of osteoporosis in this population (NIH Consensus Development Panel, 2001; Packard & Heaney, 1997). It is estimated that only 50% to 60% of older persons have a calcium intake of 1,000 mg to 1,500 mg per day (NIH Consensus Development Panel, 2001) and that between 26 million and 38 million U.S. adults have or are at risk for osteoporosis (Fuller & Casparian, 2001). Inadequate intake of calcium and vitamin D may contribute to the prevalence of osteoporosis among the older population (Dawson-Hughes, Harris, Krall, & Dallal, 1997). Low dietary intake of calcium is also indicative of periodontal disease risk, while adequate calcium intake has been associated with reduced incidence of alveolar bone loss in older men (Position of the American Dietetic Association, 2003). Box 5-3 lists risk factors for poor calcium nutrition.

The Modified Food Guide Pyramid urges three dairy servings daily as good calcium sources. See Table 5-3 for serving recommendations to meet the calcium needs of an older person. Recommendations are also given for lactose-intolerant or vegan individuals. The Modified Food Guide Pyramid also recommends consideration of a calcium supplement, denoted by a flag at the pinnacle of the pyramid. Calcium supplementation of 500 mg with concurrent vitamin D has been shown to reduce bone loss and

BOX 5-3	Risk Factors for Poor Calcium Nutrition

- Low or absent intake of dairy products, especially milk and yogurt
- Lack of fortified calcium products in diet (fortified juices, soy products, and cereals)
- Excessive protein or caffeine intake (causes urinary calcium losses)
- Medications that alter calcium absorption or metabolism: corticosteroids, colchicine, phenobarbital, methotrexate, cholestyramine
- Poor vitamin D status (need adequate vitamin D to absorb calcium)

reduce incidence of some fractures in older persons (Dawson-Hughes et al., 1997). The TUL for calcium is 2,500 mg (see Chapter 18).

The Dietary Approaches to Stopping Hypertension (DASH) initiative also recommends adequate dietary calcium intake in the form of three dairy servings daily because of the association between adequate calcium, potassium, and magnesium intake from foods and lowered blood pressure (National Institutes of Health, 2003).

Vitamin B$_{12}$

Vitamin B$_{12}$ (cyanocobalamin) is required in cell division and to maintain the myelin sheaths of the central nervous system. The RDA for vitamin B$_{12}$ is 2.4 µg. Exclusive to adults over the age of 50 years, both the DRI and the Modified Food Guide Pyramid recommend a vitamin B$_{12}$ supplement because of decreased absorption of the vitamin associated with atrophic gastritis and altered gastric pH (Institute of Medicine, 1998; Russell et al., 1999).

Practice Pearl

Vitamins D and B$_{12}$ and calcium are the only nutrients with routine consideration given to supplementation in the older person. The nurse should give careful consideration if an older person reports routine use of other supplements without medical need.

TABLE 5-3

Calcium Amounts of Common Food Sources

Food	Serving Size	Calcium Amount (mg)
Milk, 1% low fat	1 cup	300
Cheese, American	1 oz	174
Cottage cheese, low fat	½ cup	78
Yogurt, low fat	1 cup	345
Ice cream, hard	1 cup	176
Juice, calcium-fortified	1 cup	200-300
Soy milk, calcium-fortified	1 cup	300
Custard or pudding, avg	1 cup	297
Chowder or cream soup, avg	1 cup	180
Sardines, with bones	3 oz	371
Figs, dried	5 ea	134
Almonds, slivered	¼ cup	90
Spinach, cooked	½ cup	127

Source: Adapted from U.S. Department of Agriculture, http://www.nal.usda.gov/fnic/foodcomp

Decreased B_{12} stores are found in 12% of older persons (Willett & Stampfer, 2001). Vitamin B_{12} deficiency may be responsible for some cases of depression seen in older persons (Tiemeier et al., 2002). Supplemental B_{12} is not bound to protein, as it is in food sources, and hence does not require an acid medium to cleave the bond between the two nutrients. Vitamin B_{12} in fortified foods like breakfast cereals also is not bound to protein and therefore is more bioavailable than in natural food sources. Food sources include animal products like meats, fish, poultry, dairy, and eggs. Vegans must use nutritional yeast or consume fortified versions of foods like cereals and soy products to obtain B_{12} in the diet. There is no TUL published for B_{12}.

Supplemental forms of vitamin B_{12} generally are synthetic and acceptable to vegetarians and vegans. The B_{12} in plant-derived supplements, such as from algae, is not in a form that is bioavailable to humans and therefore is not an appropriate source to recommend (Position of the American Dietetic Association & Dietitians of Canada, 2003).

Symptoms of vitamin B_{12} deficiency include macrocytic anemia and neurological problems such as peripheral neuropathy, irritability, depression, and poor memory. In addition to those with atrophic gastritis, older persons at risk for poor B_{12} status include individuals who use antacids and other gastric pH–altering medications and have malabsorptive disease or gastric resection (B_{12} is absorbed in the ileum bound to intrinsic factor made in the stomach).

Practice Pearl

Folic acid supplementation can mask a B_{12} deficiency by treating the macrocytic anemia indices. However, neurological symptoms will continue to progress without adequate B_{12}. It is important not to dismiss memory loss, depression, or irritability as age associated. A B_{12} assessment should be part of any workup for these neurological symptoms or dementia (Eastley, Wilcock, & Bucks, 2000). The nurse should not recommend unopposed folic acid supplementation at doses approximating the TUL of 1 mg; B_{12} supplementation should be part of a folic acid regimen (Fairfield & Fletcher, 2002; Homocysteine Lowering Trialists' Collaboration, 1998).

Vitamin B_6

Vitamin B_6 (pyridoxine) is required as a coenzyme in metabolism of protein, fat, and other biochemical reactions. The DRI for B_6 in adults over 50 years of age is 1.5 mg per day for women and 1.7 mg per day for men. Younger adults require only 1.3 mg daily (Institute of Medicine, 1998). Neither the DRIs nor the Modified Food Guide Pyramid recommends a supplement of B_6 as it is widely available in the diet from meat, fish, poultry, legumes, and whole grains. A B_6 deficiency is unlikely to occur as a single event due to diet, but is more often found in combination with deficiencies of other B vitamins in chronic alcoholics. Medications that alter B_6 metabolism include isoniazid, theophylline, and penicillamine. Supplemental B_6 is routinely prescribed with isoniazid therapy (White & Ashworth, 2000). Symptoms of deficiency include an inflamed tongue and oral mucosa, called **glossitis and cheilosis**, depression, and confusion.

Drug Alert !

The TUL for B_6 is 100 mg. This dose is easily available over the counter. Toxicity can cause sensory neuropathy, which occurs with as little as 200 µg daily but diminishes when supplementation stops.

Fluid

Adequate fluid intake is important throughout the life cycle to ensure sufficient water is available to regulate body temperature, to provide a medium for biochemical reactions, and to eliminate waste products of metabolism and digestion. Blunted thirst perception, altered hormone response, and decreased total body water can predispose the older person to dehydration, especially when additional hydration stressors like fever or exudative wounds occur. The RDAs estimate general water requirements at 1.0 to 1.5 ml/cal of energy intake. Specific daily total water recommendations for adults older than 51 years, including water from all foods and beverages, are 3.7 L and 2.7 L for men and women, respectively (Institute of Medicine, 2004). This includes a recommendation that daily total water from beverages alone reach 13 cups for men and 9 cups for women.

Critics have faulted the water requirement being linked to energy intake by some recommendations as this could underestimate fluid needs for poor eaters. Other water requirement estimates have outlined the following:

- 30 ml/kg of body weight OR
- 100 ml/kg for the first 10 kg of weight + 50 ml/kg for the second 10 kg of weight + 15 ml/kg for the remaining weight
- WITH a minimum of 1,500 ml daily regardless of formula used unless medically contraindicated (Chidester & Spangler, 1997; Holben, Hassell, Williams, & Helle, 1999; Simmons, Alessi, & Schnelle, 2001)

The Modified Food Guide Pyramid emphasizes hydration by placing 8 cups of water as the foundation of the pyramid. Individuals may require increased fluid intake during increased activity or higher ambient temperature or due to medications such as diuretics. Other insensible fluid losses occur with fever, increased respiration, exudative wounds, and gastrointestinal losses. Increases in insensible losses over baseline should be accounted for when determining fluid needs. Alcohol and caffeine-containing beverages have a diuretic effect and should not be included in the fluid total (Russell et al., 1999). Older persons with poor renal function need their fluid requirements individually prescribed based on clinical parameters and urine output. A minimum of 1,000 ml is needed to compensate for insensible losses even with anuria.

The older person can benefit from drinking to a schedule rather than waiting until thirsty. A drinking schedule can be adjusted for individuals requiring assistance with toileting or hesitant about nocturia or incontinence. Cognitive adults with these symptoms may be voluntarily restricting fluid intake to manage symptoms and may already be at risk for dehydration. Adults with cognitive impairment should be offered fluids throughout the day, as altered thirst perception and ability to communicate thirst are not reliable. Box 5-1 on page 114 outlines risks and symptoms of dehydration.

Practice Pearl

Checking hydration by looking for "tenting" on the forearm is not a valid measure in the older person due to loss of skin elasticity. Instead, the nurse should check for tenting on the forehead or over the sternum. Additional symptoms felt to be better indicators of dehydration include darkened urine, confusion, lethargy, long tongue furrows, dry axillae, sunken eyes, and dry mucous membranes. Postural changes in pulse and blood pressure may exist with larger volume deficits (McGee, Abernethy, & Simel, 1999).

SUPPLEMENT SAVVY: BEYOND THE RDAS

Instead of taking dietary supplements to correct a nutritional problem, many consumers are swayed by early medical reports, the media, or their next-door neighbor to take a supplement for its purported disease-fighting or age-delaying properties. Gone are the days when supplements meant only vitamins, and minerals were just for preventing or correcting deficiencies. Current estimates report 30% of the U.S. population takes vitamin supplements (Willett & Stampfer, 2001); vitamins and minerals are the third largest over-the-counter drug category (Balluz, Kieszak, Philen, & Mulinaire, 2000), and 12.1% of adults in the United States had used an herbal medicine in the previous 12 months (De Smet, 2002). Others have reported even higher use of herbs and vitamins. One report found 45% of the older women studied took 2.5 herbal products in the previous 12 months (Yoon & Horne, 2001).

Many adults believe that because nutritional supplements are natural, they are nontoxic and well tested before being placed on the market. The Dietary Supplements and Health Education Act, which covers vitamins, minerals, herbals, weight loss products, and other dietary supplements, does not require manufacturers to seek pre-market approval from the Food and Drug Administration (FDA) for safety, purity, or product efficacy of any of these products. It is important to inquire about all dietary supplements in a nonjudgmental fashion as part of a client history to help guide individuals about safe choices regarding supplements. This area of nutrition has little peer-reviewed research to guide the clinician and requires constant vigilance to remain up to date.

Here are some common supplements that older persons may be taking for reasons other than prevention of deficiencies:

- **Folic acid, vitamins B_{12} and B_6 for hyperhomocysteinemia:** Homocysteine is an amino acid normally found in the body. High plasma levels of homocysteine concentration are associated with increased risk of cardiovascular disease and stroke (Homocysteine Studies Collaboration, 2002). Supplementation with both folic acid and B_{12} has been shown to lower high homocysteine plasma concentrations (Homocysteine Lowering Trialists' Collaboration, 1998). The same effect has been noted in the Framingham Offspring Study since government-mandated folic acid fortification of enriched grains in the United States began in 1996 (Jacques, Selhub, Bostom, Wilson, & Rosenberg, 1999). It remains to be proven whether lowering homocysteine in a high-risk population will result in decreased risk of cardiovascular disease. It has been shown that 1 mg folic acid, 400 µg vitamin B_{12}, and 10 mg vitamin B_6 supplementation decreases the rate of restenosis following coronary angioplasty (Schnyder et al., 2001).

  Hyperhomocysteinemia is also being researched for a potential association with increased risk of Alzheimer's disease and dementia. Reports to date have found elevated plasma homocysteine to be an independent risk factor for dementia and Alzheimer's disease (LeBoeuf, 2003; Seshadri et al., 2002). Similar associations are also being researched for Parkinson's disease (Miller, 2002).

  No area of research on hyperhomocysteinemia is conclusive enough to serve as a basis for primary prevention recommendations, but this has not stopped many individuals from taking supplements of these B vitamins already. The nurse should make sure clients are aware of the TUL for vitamin B_6 and the need for concurrent vitamin B_{12} with higher folic acid supplementation.

- **Vitamin E or ginkgo biloba and Alzheimer's disease:** High-dose vitamin E (2,000 IU) has been shown to delay the progress of existing Alzheimer's disease

(Sano, Ernesto, & Thomas, 1997). Subjects who took vitamin E delayed entry into a nursing home by 7 months compared to those who took a placebo. The dose of vitamin E given was twice the TUL.

The herb ginkgo biloba has been associated with slight cognitive improvements in patients with existing Alzheimer's disease (LeBars et al., 1997). The findings are consistent with others using ginkgo and are not considered clinically meaningful (Mayeux & Sano, 1999), yet have been captured by the popular press and consumers fearful of developing Alzheimer's disease. Combining vitamin E with ginkgo or any other supplement or medication with antiplatelet or anticoagulant effects could result in increased bleeding (Ang-Lee et al., 2001; Fairfield & Fletcher, 2002).

Practice Pearl

Supplements with antiplatelet effects include fish oils, garlic, ginseng, ginkgo biloba, evening primrose oil, fish oils, and vitamin E (De Smet, 2002; Norred & Brinker, 2001). Thoughtful analysis of supplement intake by the nurse should yield whether an older person is at risk for this form of polypharmacy and altered blood clotting. An assessment should also consider if such supplements are being used with medications that alter clotting, such as warfarin and aspirin.

■ **Antioxidants and age-related macular degeneration:** Age-related macular degeneration (AMD) is the most common cause of blindness in Americans over the age of 60 years. Nutrition-related research on AMD has focused on antioxidant and zinc supplementation. Findings thus far have reported that disease progress was reduced by 25% in persons with moderate to advanced AMD in one eye who were taking 80 mg zinc, 500 mg vitamin C, 400 IU vitamin E, and 15 mg beta-carotene (Hammond & Johnson, 2002). Results of supplementation with less advanced AMD yielded little change in disease progress. Other researchers believe different carotenoids called lutein and zeaxanthin play a role instead of beta-carotene (Bone, Landrum, Guerra, & Ruiz, 2003; Hammond & Johnson, 2002). Commercial equivalents to the supplements used in major AMD studies are now available to consumers. Most contain the carotenoids plus doses of vitamins above the individual RDAs but below the TULs with the exception of the mineral zinc. Zinc supplementation was studied at 80 mg, twice its TUL of 40 mg. Side effects from this amount could include diarrhea and cramping (Institute of Medicine, 2001). Carotenoids do not have daily requirements or known upper limits for safety. Little is known about the long-term efficacy of using supplements with lutein and zeaxanthin. Both are found naturally in food sources such as green leafy vegetables.

ALCOHOL AND VITAMINS

Chronic alcohol intake affects nutritional status in many ways. It is estimated that 2.5 million older persons are affected by alcohol abuse, and 10% of adults over age 65 are binge drinkers, having more than five drinks in a single sitting (Position of the American Dietetic Association, 2000). Older persons who ingest alcohol are at risk for deficiencies of thiamin, riboflavin, folate, vitamin B_6, and magnesium due to the direct negative effects of alcohol on gastric mucosa, nutrient absorption, metabolism, and excretion. When alcohol replaces food intake, additional effects of undernutrition occur.

The use of supplements continues as a widespread health behavior. These examples are indicative of more common choices of supplementation but are not exhaustive. Data from the Third National Health and Nutrition Examination Survey (NHANES III) illustrate that 30% to over 50% of older persons, particularly non-Hispanic White women and those with higher education levels, are using vitamin and mineral supplements (Balluz et al., 2000). At the same time, other large studies have reported dietary intakes below the RDA for vitamin D, vitamin E, folate, and calcium in over 60% of the older community-dwelling adults studied (Foote et al., 2000). The wide variance in nutrient intake, unpredictable use of dietary supplements, and unique nutritional needs of older persons reinforce the necessity of good nutritional assessment tools and sharp clinical judgment.

Nutritional Assessment

Both undernutrition and overnutrition in the older person can affect quality of life, morbidity, and mortality. Malnutrition is associated with adverse outcomes such as poor wound healing, skeletal muscle loss, functional decline, altered immune response, altered pharmacokinetics, and increased risk of institutionalization (Covinsky, 2002; Covinsky, Covinsky, Palmer, & Sehgal, 2002; Sullivan, Bopp, & Roberson, 2002). Overnutrition can also affect quality of life in the older person when it is manifested as obesity, degenerative joint disease, diabetes, hypertension, and cardiovascular disease. Excess weight and elevated cholesterol have less clinical significance in those over 70 years of age, but remain important individual psychosocial and functional considerations (Calle, Thun, Petrelli, Rodriguez, & Heath, 1999; Position of the American Dietetic Association, 2002).

There is no gold standard to define malnutrition nor is there a consensus on one tool or a set of tools to be used to assess nutritional status in the older person. Several validated screening tools exist and many more have been proposed. Although the parameters evaluated in each are different, assessment of nutritional risk factors for undernutrition should be standardly incorporated into the routine health screening of the older person.

NUTRITIONAL ASSESSMENT PARAMETERS

A comprehensive nutritional assessment reviews anthropometric measurements, laboratory values, and clinical findings from the physical examination and patient history.

Anthropometrics

Anthropometric measurements include any scientific measurement of the body. Height, weight and weight history, muscle mass, and fat mass measurements are included. Alternative techniques for obtaining anthropometric measurements may be necessary in the frail older person.

Weight. Current measured body weight and weight history are an important component of a good nutritional assessment. If an older person is unable to stand to be weighed, use of a chair scale or bed scale is indicated (Figure 5-2 ■). The nurse should not use verbal recall of current weight as a documented weight for anyone. Recorded weights on admission and at regular intervals are essential for hospitalized and long-term care patients. Individuals should be weighed with a minimum of clothing and after voiding. The nurse should note any presence of edema. A weight history that reveals unintentional weight loss of 5% body weight over a month or 10% over 6 months is clinically significant and

FIGURE ☐ 5-2

Nurse weighing patient on a bed scale.

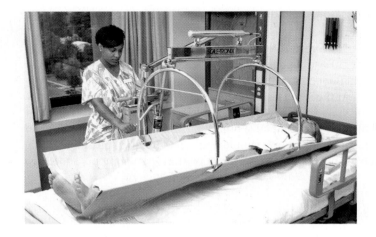

should trigger further investigation. The Centers for Medicare and Medicaid Services (2002) mandates further evaluation of long-term care patients with this history.

Height. Height can be measured using a standing measure or in a recumbent position. Recumbent measurements can be made with an individual lying flat and straight in bed with light pencil marks made on bed linens at head and heel to then be measured with a cloth tape. Generally bed height measurements are 1.5 in. longer than standing height (American Medical Directors Association, 2001). Indirect height measurement can be done measuring knee height and arm span estimations. Arm span or demi–arm span does not require any special calculations but does require some mobility on the part of the older person as either one or both arms and hands must be extended fully. Measurement is made from left hand fingertip to right hand fingertip; demi–arm span is made from fingertip to sternal notch and the value is doubled (American Medical Directors Association, 2001; Mini Nutritional Assessment Tool, 2003). Knee height is done with a sliding caliper that keeps the foot at a 90-degree angle to the leg during the measurement. A formula calculates height from the results (Chumlea, Roche, & Mukherjee, 1984). Impaired leg and foot flexibility can impede knee height measurement.

Body Mass Index. Body mass index is derived using measured height and weight with the following formula: BMI = weight (kg)/ height^2 (m). Parameters have been established to delineate underweight, normal weight, and overweight in the general population, but these generally are not applicable to the older person. Decreased BMI below 22 in the older person is predictive of undernutrition and associated with mortality (Sullivan et al., 2002). While a BMI over 25 is considered overweight and carries an increased mortality risk for the general population, the relative risk of death associated with being overweight decreases after age 65 (Calle et al., 1999; Stevens et al., 1998).

Body Fat Measurement. Tricep skinfold measures subcutaneous fat over the triceps muscle at the back of the upper arm using a caliper. Fat mass measurements are derived from a formula using tricep measurements. Reliable use of the calipers takes practice and should be done by an experienced person. Skinfold measurements can be done on other sites on the body such as subscapular, ileac crest, and thigh, but the tricep is most easily accessed.

Indirect measurement of body fat can be done with such technology as bioelectrical impedance, near infrared devices, and others. Such equipment requires proper hydration of the person or measurements will be inaccurate. Their use in the older population is largely for research purposes.

Muscle Mass Measurements. Loss of lean body mass, or muscle, occurs with aging and is more pronounced in the inactive person. This loss may be visible to the eye or when measuring body weight, but may also be masked due to increased fat mass or edema. Midarm circumference is a measurement used to derive lean body mass. Arm circumference is measured at the midarm using a cloth tape. The measurement and the tricep skinfold measurement are together incorporated into a formula to derive midarm muscle circumference and an estimate of lean muscle mass. Measurement of midarm circumference alone is of no clinical value.

Laboratory Values

Several laboratory parameters are used to assess nutritional status. No one parameter is unique in its sensitivity to malnutrition; each has confounding reasons for abnormal values. Laboratory measurements should be part of an overall nutritional assessment and not relied upon as a sole measurement of undernutrition. Recommendation of laboratory assessment should be in accordance with any advance directives for an individual. Box 5-4 outlines common laboratory measurements used in nutritional assessment.

Plasma Proteins. Albumin, prealbumin, and transferrin are all used to assess visceral protein status. An albumin ≤ 3.5 mg/dl is considered indicative of mild malnutrition. Some reports use ≤ 3.0 mg/dl as a cutoff for malnutrition (Chia-Hui et al., 2001). Albumin values can be affected by disease. Nephrotic syndrome causes increased urinary loss of albumin. Liver disease can lead to decreased albumin synthesis. Dehydration or overhydration will cause false albumin values. Additionally, albumin is an acute-phase reactant protein, and levels will diminish during inflammation or infection. Relying on serum albumin alone as a nutritional indicator may lead to discordance with clinical assessment (Covinsky et al., 2002). Using albumin in a nutritional assessment does not give the most current picture since the half-life of albumin is approximately 21 days.

Laboratory Values Used in a Routine Nutritional Assessment

BOX 5-4

- Albumin
- Retinol-binding prealbumin
- Transferrin
- Complete blood count (CBC) for:
  - Mean cell volume (MCV)
  - Hemoglobin
  - Hematocrit
- Serum folate and B_{12} assays

Prealbumin and transferrin have shorter half-lives than albumin (2 to 3 days and 8 days, respectively), so they give more current information on protein status. They are not generally part of routine blood work and thus are less often a component of an assessment. Prealbumin is an acute-phase reactant protein as well. Transferrin measurements are often derived from total iron-binding capacity and therefore would be affected by anemia states.

Folate and Vitamin B$_{12}$ Assessment. Evaluation of vitamin B$_{12}$ and folic acid status is particularly pertinent due to the effects of aging, disease, and medications on absorption and metabolism of both vitamins. A high red blood cell mean cell volume (MCV) should be followed up by assessments of plasma folic acid and vitamin B$_{12}$.

Cholesterol. It is debated whether low serum cholesterol concentration, defined as < 160 mg/dl, is an independent risk factor for malnutrition or just an indicator of an existing medical condition (Hu, Seeman, Harris, & Reuben, 2003; Volpato, Leveille, Corti, Harris, & Guralnik, 2001). Nevertheless, many still use hypocholesterolemia as an indicator of malnutrition (Azad, Murphy, Amos, & Toppan, 1999; Council for Nutrition Clinical Strategies in Long-Term Care, 2001; Gazewood & Mehr, 1998). The increased use of pharmacological interventions for elevated serum cholesterol may further complicate the usefulness of low cholesterol levels as a nutritional indicator. Low serum cholesterol due to pharmacological reduction is not believed to be associated with increased risk of mortality (Volpato et al., 2001).

Nursing Assessment

Even with limited resources, a nutritional assessment can be performed using sharp clinical observation and judgment. Examining the older person from head to toe can reveal significant findings that may indicate existing nutritional problems or risk factors for undernutrition. See Table 5-4 for indicators of possible nutritional problems.

The nursing assessment should focus on skin condition, including turgor, lesions, nonhealing ulcers, color variations, and excessive dryness or cracking. Additionally, the nurse should inspect the condition and distribution of the hair. The oral cavity is inspected for tooth or denture condition, oral lesions, hyperplasia of the gums, fissures around the lips, oral hygiene, and any coatings on the tongue. The abdomen should be palpated for firmness or tenderness. The bowel record should be checked for date of the last bowel movement, as constipation and fecal impaction will inhibit appetite. The nurse should observe the patient eating and drinking, note any swallowing difficulties or positioning problems, and consult with occupational therapy should adaptive tableware be needed to encourage independence and maximum nutritional intake.

It is important to assess pain levels and administer prn (as needed) medications 1 hour before mealtime if unrelieved pain appears to be a factor. The nurse should consult with the older patient and family regarding food preferences and timing, food dislikes, religious preferences, and cultural or ethnic traditions that could be negatively affecting nutritional intake.

Finally, the medication list should be reviewed for any medications (long-standing or newly prescribed) that could be causing anorexia or depression. Many medications have the side effects of early satiety, alterations of taste, lethargy, and appetite suppression. Common offenders are digoxin, diuretics, chemotherapy agents, some antibiotics, and some antidepressants. The older patient should be questioned regarding any feelings of depression as changes in appetite are often associated with depression in the older person. Nurses should ask, "Do you feel sad or blue?" as a screen-

TABLE 5-4

Nutritional Findings on Physical Examination of Older Adults

System	Area of Focus	Potential Physical Findings
Head	Mouth	Taste perception changes, swollen tongue, saliva production, angular lesions at lips, swollen gums, mouth sores
	Teeth	Loose or missing teeth, caries, dentures
	Chewing and swallowing	Pocketing food, drooling, note any complaints
	Hearing	Note alteration
	Vision	Note alteration
	Overall appearance	Note any temporal wasting
Trunk	Overall appearance	Note wasting of muscle or subcutaneous fat
	Skin turgor	Note presence of wounds, pressure ulcer
Extremities	Overall appearance	Note presence of edema, wasting of muscle or subcutaneous fat
Gastrointestinal tract		Note complaints of nausea, vomiting, diarrhea
Genitourinary tract		Note complaints of incontinence or nocturia with regard to voluntary fluid restriction
Neurological		Note tremors, neuropathy, depressive symptoms, impaired cognition
Functional capacity		Note ability to perform activities of daily living relative to eating

ing question that, if answered positively, could set in motion a complete depression assessment (Hartford Institute of Geriatric Nursing, 1999). (See Chapter 7 for further information on depression.)

It is also important to evaluate the eating environment. Some nursing home residents are assisted to the dining room over an hour before the meal is served. They may become restless, agitated, or bored and leave the dining room without eating. Many persons with dementia do better by eating smaller, more frequent meals. It helps to remove all unappetizing smells and provide a pleasant environment with music, small bouquets of flowers, and colorful tablecloths. Extra light should be supplied for older persons with visual limitations. The nurse should assist the older person with preparation for eating including opening straws and milk cartons, cutting meat, and so on. The food served to the residents should be warm (not too hot) and tasty. The family should be encouraged to dine with the resident if they are visiting. The same assessment parameters should be stressed for older patients living at home and being cared for by a family member or paid caregiver.

Practice Pearl

When serving food to an older person with dementia, it is best to serve one course at a time with the appropriate utensil. For instance, the nurse should serve the soup first with a spoon and then remove the soup and spoon before presenting the main meal. Supplying the appropriate utensil for the food will decrease frustration and encourage food intake.

Nutritional History

A careful nutritional history is part of a comprehensive assessment and can be accomplished in a variety of ways. Like other screening tools, reliance upon just one method will yield less valuable information than a combination of methods.

Diet Recall. A 24-hour dietary recall can be done during an office visit or as part of an admission interview. It is important to ask open-ended questions that make no assumptions. For example, if the nurse asks, "What did you have for lunch?" some older persons may be too embarrassed to divulge that they had nothing and may fabricate the answer they think the nurse is seeking. It is better to ask, "What was the first thing you had to eat today?" and then "When was the next time you ate something?" Asking questions about weekend eating, which may be different than weekday habits, improves the value of the recall information. The nurse should ask questions about intake of dietary supplements, all fluids including alcohol, therapeutic diet, food intolerances, grocery shopping, food preparation frequency and ability, and any religious or cultural influences on diet. The nurse can ask, "Do you follow any special food guidelines or traditions? Are there any foods that you avoid or include in your diet?" The nurse should also ask how food is prepared. Diversity exists among and within religious and cultural groups; it is important to obtain a personal history without assumptions. Interviewing a family member can yield a sample recall, but the accuracy is variable (Fryzek, Lipworth, Signorello, & McLaughlin, 2002). The 24-hour recall is only a snapshot in time and is not always indicative of normal habits.

Food Frequency. A food frequency assessment is an excellent tool to use with a 24-hour recall to fill in the gaps of missing information that occur with a one-day snapshot. Simple questions about each food group can be asked to determine daily, weekly, or less often consumption of foods. For example, while a 24-hour recall may list only one glass of milk and no other dairy intake, a food frequency may show that cheese and milk are consumed more regularly. The nurse should ask about all food groups including fluids and supplements. Table 5-5 is an example of a food frequency questionnaire.

Food Record. Having a cognitively intact older person record food intake for up to 3 days can provide a view of variable eating patterns. Recording 2 weekdays and 1 weekend day works best. Food records beyond 3 days length become cumbersome and may be filled out retrospectively right before being delivered.

SCREENING TOOLS

Nutritional screening and assessment tools exist to streamline the incorporation of nutritional status into routine healthcare processes. It is essential that any tool be used in the context for which it was developed and validated.

Nutrition Screening Initiative

The Nutrition Screening Initiative (NSI) was developed as a public health strategy. It consists of screening tools for use by individuals and healthcare providers to identify potential nutritional risk factors in community-dwelling older persons (Nutrition Screening Initiative, 2003). The DETERMINE checklist is a mnemonic outlining nine warning signs that are predictive of poor nutrition. The tool is scored and stratified according to nutritional risk. Suggestions are given for professional intervention if needed. See Figure 5-3 ■ for the NSI DETERMINE checklist. The checklist is used by

TABLE 5-5

Sample Food Frequency Quick Questionnaire

Food	Variety	Type	Amount per day	Amount per week	Amount or less
Fruit	Juice	Orange	4 oz		
	Fresh	None			
	Canned/frozen	Canned pears		1 cup	
Vegetables	Green	Varied		1–2×	
	Other	Carrots		1×	
Dairy	Milk	Low fat	2 cups		
	Cheese				1× month
	Yogurt	Never			
Protein	Animal	Poultry or fish	Each night		
	Plant	Hummus beans		1–2×	
Fats	Saturated	Butter	1–2 pats		
	Unsaturated				
Fluids	General	Water	4 oz 4× with meds		
	Caffeine	Tea	Each a.m.		
	Alcohol	Wine			1–2× month
Sweets and sugars		Cake or pie	After dinner		
Supplements		Multivitamin	One		

some as a clinical screening tool, but it has not been validated for this use (Sahyoun, Jacques, Dallal, & Russell, 1997).

Mini Nutritional Assessment and Subjective Global Assessment

Both the Mini Nutritional Assessment and Subjective Global Assessment tools have been validated as clinical tools for use in screening nutritional status in the older person (Covinsky et al., 2002; Persson, Brismar, Katzarski, Nordenstrom, & Cederholm, 2002; Sacks et al., 2000; Vellas et al., 1999). Each can be performed as a quick bedside or office visit assessment as part of a routine physical examination. The Mini Nutritional Assessment is a newer tool with extensive research published on its use in the older person (Mini Nutritional Assessment Tool, 2003; Vellas et al., 1999). See Figure 5-4 ■ for the Mini Nutritional Assessment.

Minimum Data Set

The Minimum Data Set (MDS) is a government-mandated component to the Resident Assessment Instrument used by all Medicare- or Medicaid-certified healthcare facilities. Assessments are done on admission, updated quarterly, and reassessed annually or whenever a significant change in resident status occurs. The MDS includes nutritional components that must be assessed for all residents (Centers for Medicare and Medicaid Services, 2002). A three-nursing-home study found two MDS nutrition-related criteria, weight loss and leaves 25% or more of food uneaten at most meals, predictive of malnutrition when considered with age, declining ability in activities of daily living, and psychiatric or mood disorder (Crogan, Corbett, & Short, 2002). See Box 5-5 for MDS nutrition-related criteria.

FIGURE ☐ 5-3

Nutrition Screening Initiative DETERMINE Checklist.
(The warning signs of poor nutritional health are often overlooked. Use this checklist to find out if you or someone you know is at nutritional risk.)

Read the statements below. Circle the number in the "yes" column for those that apply to you or someone you know. For each "yes" answer, score the number in the box. Total your nutritional score.

DETERMINE YOUR NUTRITIONAL HEALTH

	YES
I have an illness or condition that made me change the kind and/or amount of food I eat.	2
I eat fewer than 2 meals per day.	3
I eat few fruits or vegetables or milk products.	2
I have 3 or more drinks of beer, liquor or wine almost every day.	2
I have tooth or mouth problems that make it hard for me to eat.	2
I don't always have enough money to buy the food I need.	4
I eat alone most of the time.	1
I take 3 or more different prescribed or over-the-counter drugs a day.	1
Without wanting to, I have lost or gained 10 pounds in the last 6 months.	2
I am not always physically able to shop, cook and/or feed myself.	2
TOTAL	

Remember that Warning Signs suggest risk, but do not represent a diagnosis of any condition.

Total Your Nutritional Score. If it's-

0-2 Good! Recheck your nutritional score in 6 months.

3-5 You are at moderate nutritional risk. See what can be done to improve your eating habits and lifestyle. Your office on aging, senior nutrition program, senior citizens center or health department can help. Recheck your nutritional score in 3 months.

6 or more You are at high nutritional risk. Bring this Checklist the next time you see your doctor, dietitian or other qualified health or social service professional. Talk with them about any problems you may have. Ask for help to improve your nutritional health.

These materials are developed and distributed by the Nutrition Screening Initiative, a project of:

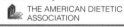

AMERICAN ACADEMY OF FAMILY PHYSICIANS   THE AMERICAN DIETETIC ASSOCIATION   THE NATIONAL COUNCIL ON THE AGING, INC.

The Nutrition Checklist is based on the Warning Signs described below.
Use the word DETERMINE to remind you of the Warning Signs.

Disease   Any disease, illness or chronic condition which causes you to change the way you eat, or makes it hard for you to eat, puts your nutritional health at risk. Four out of five adults have chronic diseases that are affected by diet. Confusion or memory loss that keeps getting worse is estimated to affect one out of five or more of older adults. This can make it hard to remember what, when or if you've eaten. Feeling sad or depressed, which happens to about one in eight older adults, can cause big changes in appetite, digestion, energy level, weight and well-being.

Eating poorly   Eating too little and eating too much both lead to poor health. Eating the same foods day after day or not eating fruit, vegetables, and milk products daily will also cause poor nutritional health. One in five adults skip meals daily. Only 13% of adults eat the minimum amount of fruit and vegetables needed. One in four older adults drink too much alcohol. Many health problems become worse if you drink more than one or two alcoholic beverages per day.

Tooth loss/mouth pain   A healthy mouth, teeth and gums are needed to eat. Missing, loose or rotten teeth or dentures which don't fit well, or cause mouth sores, make it hard to eat.

Economic hardship   As many as 40% of older Americans have incomes of less than $6,000 per year. Having less—or choosing to spend less—than $25-30 per week for food makes it very hard to get the foods you need to stay healthy.

Reduced social contact   One-third of all older people live alone. Being with people daily has a positive effect on morale, well-being and eating.

Multiple medicines   Many older Americans must take medicines for health problems. Almost half of older Americans take multiple medicines daily. Growing old may change the way we respond to drugs. The more medicines you take, the greater the chance for side effects such as increased or decreased appetite, change in taste, constipation, weakness, drowsiness, diarrhea, nausea, and others. Vitamins or minerals, when taken in large doses, act like drugs and can cause harm. Alert your doctor to everything you take.

Involuntary weight loss/gain   Losing or gaining a lot of weight when you are not trying to do so is an important warning sign that must not be ignored. Being overweight or underweight also increases your chance of poor health.

Needs assistance in self care   Although most older people are able to eat, one of every five have trouble walking, shopping, buying and cooking food, especially as they get older.

Elder years above age 80   Most older people lead full and productive lives. But as age increases, risk of frailty and health problems increase. Checking your nutritional health regularly makes good sense.

The Nutrition Screening Initiative • 1010 Wisconsin Avenue, NW • Suite 800 • Washington, DC 20007
The Nutrition Screening Initiative is funded in part by a grant from Ross Products Division of Abbott Laboratories, Inc.

Source: From *The Nutrition Screening Initiative.* Used by permission.

FIGURE ■ 5-4

Mini Nutritional Assessment®.

MINI NUTRITIONAL ASSESSMENT
MNA®

ID# _____

Last Name: _____ First Name: _____ M.I. _____ Sex: _____ Date: _____

Age: _____ Weight, kg: _____ Height, cm: _____ Knee Height, cm: _____

Complete the form by writing the numbers in the boxes. Add the numbers in the boxes and compare the total assessment to the Malnutrition Indicator Score.

ANTHROPOMETRIC ASSESSMENT

	Points
1. Body Mass Index (BMI) (weight in kg) / (height in m)^2 a. BMI < 19 = 0 points b. BMI 19 to < 21 = 1 point c. BMI 21 to < 23 = 2 points d. BMI ≥ 23 = 3 points	☐
2. Mid-arm circumference (MAC) in cm a. MAC < 21 = 0.0 points b. MAC 21 ≤ 22 = 0.5 points c. MAC > 22 = 1.0 points	☐.☐
3. Calf circumference (CC) in cm a. CC < 31 = 0 points b. CC ≥ 31 = 1 point	☐
4. Weight loss during last 3 months a. weight loss greater than 3 kg (6.6 lbs) = 0 points b. does not know = 1 point c. weight loss between 1 and 3 kg (2.2 and 6.6 lbs) = 2 points d. no weight loss = 3 points	☐

GENERAL ASSESSMENT

5. Lives independently (not in a nursing home or hospital) a. no = 0 points b. yes = 1 point	☐
6. Takes more than 3 prescription drugs per day a. yes = 0 points b. no = 1 point	☐
7. Has suffered psychological stress or acute disease in the past 3 months a. yes = 0 points b. no = 2 points	☐
8. Mobility a. bed or chair bound = 0 points b. able to get out of bed/chair but does not go out = 1 point c. goes out = 2 points	☐
9. Neuropsychological problems a. severe dementia or depression = 0 points b. mild dementia = 1 point c. no psychological problems = 2 points	☐
10. Pressure sores or skin ulcers a. yes = 0 points b. no = 1 point	☐

DIETARY ASSESSMENT

11. How many full meals does the patient eat daily? a. 1 meal = 0 points b. 2 meals = 1 point c. 3 meals = 2 points	☐

	Points
12. Selected consumption markers for protein intake • At least one serving of dairy products (milk, cheese, yogurt) per day? yes ☐ no ☐ • Two or more servings of legumes or eggs per week? yes ☐ no ☐ • Meat, fish, or poultry every day? yes ☐ no ☐ a. if 0 or 1 yes = 0.0 points b. if 2 yes = 0.5 points c. if 3 yes = 1.0 points	☐.☐
13. Consumes two or more servings of fruits or vegetables per day? a. no = 0 points b. yes = 1 point	☐
14. Has food intake declined over the past three months due to loss of appetite, digestive problems, chewing or swallowing difficulties? a. severe loss of appetite = 0 points b. moderate loss of appetite = 1 point c. no loss of appetite = 2 points	☐
15. How much fluid (water, juice, coffee, tea, milk, . . .) is consumed per day? (1 cup = 8 oz.) a. less than 3 cups = 0.0 points b. 3 to 5 cups = 0.5 points c. more than 5 cups = 1.0 points	☐.☐
16. Mode of feeding a. unable to eat without assistance = 0 points b. self-fed with some difficulty = 1 point c. self-fed without any problem = 2 points	☐

SELF-ASSESSMENT

17. Do they view themselves as having nutritional problems? a. major malnutrition = 0 points b. does not know or moderate malnutrition = 1 point c. no nutritional problem = 2 points	☐
18. In comparison with other people of the same age, how do they consider their health status? a. not as good = 0.0 points b. does not know = 0.5 points c. as good = 1.0 points d. better = 2.0 points	☐.☐

ASSESSMENT TOTAL (max. 30 points): ☐☐.☐

MALNUTRITION INDICATOR SCORE		
≥ 24 points	well-nourished	☐
17 to 23.5 points	at risk of malnutrition	☐
< 17 points	malnourished	☐

Ref: Guigoz Y, Vellas B and Garry PJ. 1994. Mini Nutritional Assessment: A practical assessment tool for grading the nutritional state of elderly patients. *Facts and Research in Gerontology.* Supplement #2: 15–59.

© 1994 Nestec Ltd (Nestlé Research Center)/Nestlé Clinical Nutrition

---

Source: Vellas, B., et al. (1999). The Mini Nutritional Assessment and its use in grading nutritional state of elderly patients. *Nutrition, 15,* 116–122. Used with permission from Elsevier.

BOX 5-5	**Pertinent Risk Factors for Malnutrition From MDS Criteria**

- Inability to feed oneself
- Chewing problems
- Swallowing problems
- Mouth pain
- Process: check mouth for food pocketing and abnormalities
- Weight loss
  - ≥ 5% in 1 month
  - ≥ 7.5% in 3 months
  - ≥ 10% in 6 months
- Altered taste
- Hunger complaints
- Leaves 25% or more of food uneaten at most meals
- Nutrition approaches: note parenteral/IV, tube feeding, mechanically altered diet, syringe feeding, therapeutic diet, supplement use, adaptive feeding equipment, or presence of weight gain program

Source: Adapted from CMS RAI Version 2.0 Manual Chapter 3 MDS Items G and K, http://www.cms.hhs.gov/medicaid/mds20/mds0900b.pdf

Other investigators have proposed different screening tools or edited versions of existing tools. Varying definitions and nutritional terminology among researchers and clinicians has contributed to confusion concerning the most appropriate screening tool (Lyne & Prowse, 1999). Until a consensus is reached on a gold standard for use in nutritional assessment, new screening tools will continue to be developed. Formal, validated, and quick screening tools are helpful reminders of the importance of including a nutritional assessment when caring for the older person.

Common Nutritional Concerns in the Older Person

Both undernutrition and overnutrition can affect morbidity and mortality in the older person. Undernutrition, such as that which occurs with unplanned weight loss, is an important concern and deserves attention.

UNINTENTIONAL WEIGHT LOSS

Adequate nutrition is an essential component for remaining autonomous into older personhood. Unfortunately, the prevalence of malnutrition in the older population is significant, affecting up to 60% of those who are hospitalized or under dependent care and up to 13% of community-dwelling older persons (Azad et al., 1999; Gazewood & Mehr, 1998; Sullivan, Sun, & Walls, 1999). Weight loss in nursing home residents is associated with a higher mortality rate than for those residents with stable weight (Gazewood & Mehr, 1998). Independent older persons have a lower prevalence of undernutrition but should not be overlooked since as many as two thirds of free-living elders are reported to consume inadequate diets and 18% consume less than 1,000 kcal daily (Thomas & Morley, 2001; Vozenilek, 1998). Malnutrition in the older person does not discriminate among economic, racial, or ethnic groups (Wellman et al., 1997).

**BOX
5-6**

Causes of Unintentional Weight Loss

Insufficient Intake

- Depression or bereavement/loneliness
- Medication side effects
- Social isolation
- Dependency on others
- Improper feeding assistance
- Pain
- Xerostomia
- Dehydration
- Food insecurity
- Sensory changes in smell, taste, vision, hearing
- Chewing or swallowing difficulty
- Cognitive impairment
- Therapeutic diet
- Lack of personal, cultural, or religious food preferences
- Iatrogenic

Nutrient Losses

- Malabsorptive disease
- Medications
- Diarrhea/ vomiting
- Alcoholism

Hypermetabolism

- Fever
- Infection or sepsis
- Wounds or pressure ulcers
- Bone fracture
- Tremors
- Disease, such as advanced chronic obstructive pulmonary disease

Etiology of Unintentional Weight Loss

The aging process alone is not the cause of unintentional weight loss. A complex assortment of contributing factors adds to the existing issues of the "anorexia of aging" and sarcopenia. Untreated malnutrition is followed by a sequela of negative consequences and poor outcomes that is difficult to stop (Chia-Hui et al., 2001). The known causes of unintentional weight loss fall into three general categories: insufficient intake of food and fluid, increased losses of nutrients, and hypermetabolism. Almost 25% of older persons with unintentional weight loss have no known cause for the loss (Huffman, 2002). Box 5-6 outlines possible causes of unintentional weight loss.

Insufficient Intake. Lack of adequate food and fluid intake occurs for multiple physical and psychosocial reasons.

Dehydration can be responsible for loss of weight. Lack of adequate fluid over time can cause a subtle and steady slip into hypovolemia. Dependence on others with lack of free access to fluids, altered thirst, and voluntary fluid restrictions for fear of incontinence or reliance on others for toileting can precipitate inadequate intake. Exudative wounds, fever, or gastrointestinal losses can lead to negative fluid balance if not compensated. Hydration risks and symptoms are outlined in Box 5-1.

Sadness and clinical depression are leading causes of unintentional weight loss in both community-dwelling and long-term care older persons (Gazewood & Mehr, 1998; Huffman, 2002; Wilson et al., 1998). Depression accounts for up to 36% of weight loss cases in long-term care (Thomas et al., 2000). Loneliness and bereavement are associated with dietary inadequacy and weight loss, especially in men (Chia-Hui et al., 2001; Gazewood & Mehr, 1998). Medications used to treat depression can diminish appetite and cause xerostomia, leading to poor taste perception and difficulty swallowing (Ship,

2002). Social isolation, even without a complaint of loneliness, is a risk factor for weight loss (Council for Nutrition Clinical Strategies in Long-Term Care, 2001).

Anorexia can be multifactorial. **Polypharmacy** is associated with undernutrition (Chia-Hui et al., 2001). Many medications can cause lack of appetite directly or from additional side effects, such as sedation. See Table 5-1 for specific medications contributing to anorexia. Twenty-three of the more frequently prescribed medications in long-term care have side effects such as anorexia or nausea, contributing to decreased intake (Position of the American Dietetic Association, 2002).

Pain from arthritis or chronic disease can dull the appetite or cause nausea. Pain medications may have sedative or gastrointestinal side effects, which further curb intake. (See Chapter 9 for a complete discussion of pain.) ▭

Chronic diseases such as chronic obstructive pulmonary disease and congestive heart failure can contribute to anorexia. Shortness of breath can cause **aerophagia** while eating, which results in bloating and early satiety from swallowing air. The physical effort of labored breathing can result in extreme fatigue with little energy left for the eating process. (See Chapter 24.) ▭

Practice Pearl

The nurse should discourage consumption of carbonated beverages, chewing gum, or use of straws in patients who complain of bloating as these contribute to aerophagia.

Other chronic diseases or symptoms such as cancer, constipation or fecal impaction, and alcoholism can cause direct loss of appetite.

Dysphagia can result from difficulty chewing or swallowing or both. Chewing difficulties contribute to declining intake and risk of aspiration. Poor oral health, loose or missing teeth, ill-fitting dentures, and xerostomia can make the eating process uncomfortable, time-consuming, and difficult. Generic texture-modified diets, often offered to those with chewing difficulties, are sometimes visually unattractive and can reduce interest in eating. (See Chapter 20 for more information on the gastrointestinal system.) ▭

Practice Pearl

Modification in diet texture runs along a continuum. For example, some older persons may be able to enjoy an apple if it is peeled and cut versus the usual applesauce. Texture-modified diets should be individualized. Collaborating with the registered dietitian (and speech pathologist if dysphagia is an issue) can often yield a more acceptable version of these diets.

Swallowing difficulties pose an immediate risk of aspiration and contribute to overall altered intake of both fluid and food. Dysphagia affects between 53% and 74% of residents in long-term care (Position of the American Dietetic Association, 2002). Pneumonia can result, especially if silent aspiration is occurring in those with insufficient coughing or cognitive impairment (Palmer, Drennan, & Baba, 2000). Dysphagia can occur as a result of neurological disease or events such as Parkinson's disease, multiple sclerosis, stroke, gastroesophageal reflux, cognitive impairment, esophageal motility disorders, cancer, and medications (Leslie, Carding, & Wilson, 2003). Box 5-7 outlines symptoms to monitor for dysphagia. Presence or absence of a gag reflex is not a defin-

BOX 5-7

Symptoms of Dysphagia

- Noticeable difficulty swallowing
- Coughing or throat clearing during swallowing process
- Complaint of food sticking or chest pain with swallow
- Multiple attempts to swallow single mouthful
- Pocketing food along gum line
- Inability to retain liquid bolus in mouth
- Drooling
- Voice changes
- Aspiration pneumonia
- Unexplained weight loss or dehydration

Source: Adapted from Leslie, P., Carding, P. N., & Wilson, J. A. (2003); Palmer, J. B., Drennan, J. C., & Baba, M. (2000); Farnell, Z. & O'Neill, D. (1999).

itive screening tool for aspiration risk or dysphagia (Palmer et al., 2000). Close observation for symptomatology and subsequent referral for clinical evaluation by a speech-language pathologist and a videofluoroscopic swallowing study or barium study are the recommended actions (Farrell & O'Neill, 1999; Palmer et al., 2000). Several bedside screening tools exist for nurses and other clinicians to assist with assessing symptoms (Farrell & O'Neill, 1999; Perry, 2001).

Dependency on others for feeding or eating-related activities is associated with a risk of undernutrition. Government data report that 28% of nursing home residents require assistance with eating and over 19% are totally dependent on others for feeding (Position of the American Dietetic Association, 2002). Additionally, 28% of older persons have difficulty with one or more of the instrumental activities of daily living, which include shopping and meal preparation (Chia-Hui et al., 2001). Much attention is being given to reports outlining poor feeding practices in long-term care. Inadequate length of time spent feeding patients, poor positioning, and inadequate supervision have been faulted. While it has been shown that older persons consume meals more slowly than younger adults (De Castro, 1993), findings have reported as little as 18 minutes per day to 9 minutes a meal spent feeding residents with dementia. This contrasts with 99 minutes per day spent feeding older persons with dementia living at home (Simmons, Lam, Rao, & Schnelle 2003; Thomas & Morley, 2001). It is estimated that 20 to 30 minutes is needed to feed a dependent nursing home resident (Position of the American Dietetic Association, 2000). Force-feeding has been observed (Porter, Schell, Kayser-Jones, & Paul, 1999). Lack of free access to fluid and food between meals adds to the risk of those who are dependent on others. Family members ranked "improved quantity and quality of feeding assistance" for their nursing home relative among their top choices of nutritional interventions to improve intake (Simmons et al., 2003).

Cognitive impairment is associated with unintentional weight loss. In addition to issues surrounding feeding dependency, cognitive impairment can impede the eating process. Diminished ability to recognize food, failure to respond to hunger cues, difficulty with chewing and swallowing, and behavioral issues such as agitation can lead to declining intake. Feeding cognitively impaired persons can present unique challenges to caregivers as it is often difficult to interpret aversive behaviors like clamping shut the mouth, expelling food, or turning the head. This can be interpreted as a desire to stop eating, but can also be dislike of the food, its temperature, or texture, or failure to recognize the eating process. A distracting environment, including too many foods on the plate, can also contribute to aversive behaviors during eating (Finley, 1997). Caregivers are faced with the dilemma of whether to continue feeding or stop when these behaviors occur. Nurses often come to different conclusions than one another when feeding the same patient (Pasman, The, Onwuteaka-Philipsen, van der Wal, & Ribbe, 2003). Poor eating manners such as drooling and expulsion of food can make the social dining experience unpleasant for others and lead to further social isolation of this population (Manthorpe & Watson, 2003). (See Chapter 22.) ▭

Sensory changes can make eating less pleasurable. Poor vision is associated with poor dietary intake (Payette et al., 1995). Poorly lighted dining areas and busy patterns on dishes make seeing the meal harder for those with poor vision. Hearing problems can remove the pleasure from social dining. Taste and smell changes occur with age, medications, and chronic disease. Full dentures obscure the soft palate affecting taste perception (Chia-Hui et al., 2001). Xerostomia, regardless of cause, contributes to reduced taste perception. Medications such as ACE inhibitors leave a metallic taste in the mouth (Bromley, 2000). Olfactory changes further contribute to taste changes as the two senses are intertwined (Murphy et al., 2002).

Improper diets can lead to diminished intake. Older persons in long-term care may be served unfamiliar foods after a lifetime of eating culturally familiar foods. Lack of food preferences and unpalatable textures can lead to lack of interest in eating.

Overzealous use of therapeutic diets may serve no clinical benefit if they are not eaten. Nursing home patients with evidence of malnutrition are often found to be on a therapeutic diet (Position of the American Dietetic Association, 2002). Many believe that use of a low-cholesterol diet after age 70 or a diabetic diet in long-term care has no clinical benefits (American Diabetes Association Task Force, 2002; Position of the American Dietetic Association, 2002; Tariq et al., 2001). Long-term care residents should be on liberalized diets unless deemed medically contraindicated following an individual assessment (Position of the American Dietetic Association, 2002).

Poverty and food insecurity can lead to poor nutritional health because of diminished intake. Lack of sufficient funds can result in both poor quality food intake as well as limited quantity. Food insecurity issues arise from lack of financial resources, but also from lack of access to adequate food because of mobility or transportation issues. All these factors can cause a decline in dietary intake.

Iatrogenic Practices. Iatrogenic practices can put an individual at risk for undernutrition. Polypharmacy and improper feeding practices are considered iatrogenic in nature. Other contributors include prolonged nothing-by-mouth (NPO) status, reliance on clear liquid diet or routine intravenous fluids for nutrition, and improper recording of consumption. As many as 21% of hospitalized older persons were found to have an average intake of less than 50% of their energy needs while in the hospital (Sullivan et al., 1999). Patients found to be below the 50% threshold were ordered NPO for 38% of their meals. The reason for this order was not clinically apparent 17% of the time, and 20% of the time there was unnecessary delay in returning to a normal diet.

Poor documentation of diminished intake has been observed in long-term care. The MDS mandates that a resident be reassessed if intake falls below 75% of a meal for 7 days (Centers for Medicare and Medicaid Services, 2002). Studies have noted that caregivers regularly overestimate documented consumption, with larger errors occurring with delayed reporting (Castellanos & Andrews, 2002; Shatenstein, Claveau, & Ferland,

2002). Subjective judgment as to what constitutes adequate intake and the perception that the amount a resident eats is indicative of caregiver job performance are theorized as reasons for the overestimation (Castellanos & Andrews, 2002). Nutritional risk can be wrongly underestimated because of such errors (Shatenstein et al., 2002).

Nutrient Losses. Nutrient losses during absorption or metabolism can lead to undernutrition even with adequate dietary intake. Malabsorption from disease or its treatment can alter nutrient absorption. Inflammatory bowel disease, high output ostomies, and radiation treatment to the abdominal area are such examples. Drugs, including alcohol, can alter nutrient status (see Table 5-1 for drug and nutrient interactions).

Hypermetabolism. Hypermetabolism warrants intake of increased energy and nutrients. When these increased needs are not met, undernutrition results. An older person with borderline nutritional status can easily be toppled into negative fuel balance by a hypermetabolic illness. Wounds, fever, infection, and fractures put difficult caloric and nutrient demands on an individual who may already be feeling and eating poorly. Cardiopulmonary disease can cause hypermetabolism due to the great physical effort of breathing when shortness of breath and diminished lung function occur. Tremors from neurological disease such as Parkinson's disease can increase metabolic rate due to increased physical movement (Thomas & Morley, 2001).

Consequences of Unintentional Weight Loss and Undernutrition

Undernutrition is associated with poor clinical outcomes, including mortality. Hospitalized malnourished older persons have twice the mortality rate 1 year after discharge from the hospital compared to well-nourished cohorts. Increased mortality rate remains up to 4 years after discharge (Persson et al., 2002; Sullivan & Walls, 1998). Malnutrition is associated with adverse outcomes such as poor wound healing, development of decubitus ulcers, skeletal muscle loss, functional decline, altered immune response, altered pharmacokinetics, and increased risk of institutionalization (Covinsky, 2002; Covinsky et al., 2002; Sullivan et al., 2002).

A BMI less than 21 is included as a trigger for decubitus ulcer assessment in the MDS for long-term care patients (Centers for Medicare and Medicaid Services, 2002). A direct relationship between number of existing risk factors for pressure ulcer development, including poor nutrition, dehydration, and weight loss, and prevalence of pressure ulcers has been reported (Coleman, Martau, Lin, & Kramer, 2002; Horn et al., 2002). Delayed wound healing in general occurs due to lack of nutritional substrates needed for each stage of tissue repair. Energy and protein deficits are often cited as limiting factors (Demling & DeSanti, 2001; Pontieri-Lewis, 1997; Rojas & Phillips, 1999). Vitamins A and C and zinc have also been cited as necessary for wound closure (Rojas & Phillips, 1999; Thomas, 2001). Altered immune response with increased susceptibility to infection puts the older person with malnutrition at further risk (Chia-Hui et al., 2001; Huffman, 2002).

Low levels of plasma proteins that occur in malnutrition can alter drug metabolism. Low serum albumin can lead to decreased binding of certain drugs and resultant increased circulating free fraction of those medications. Polypharmacy can lead to multiple drugs competing for diminished protein binding sites and increase the likelihood of adverse drug reactions. Altered drug binding can go on to upset the balance of drugs at the cellular enzyme level. Over-the-counter and herbal medications are to be included in this effect.

Treatment of Unintentional Weight Loss and Undernutrition

It is intuitive to treat undernutrition and weight loss by targeting the cause. However, as almost 25% of all cases of weight loss in older persons occur for unknown reasons, targeting the symptoms is inherent in the overall treatment. This nonspecific and sometimes slowly occurring weight loss in the older person is often called "the dwindles."

Developing a nutritional care plan for an older person with undernutrition first requires a conversation with the individual or a proxy to determine the extent of personal wishes, quality-of-life issues, and advance directives before any aggressive interventions are begun.

Altering the quality of feeding assistance, the physical environment, and the food itself can encourage sufficient intake of fluid and food. Restrictive diets should be liberalized in long-term care unless an individual clinical assessment finds it contraindicated. Collaborating with the registered dietitian will help to optimize and individualize the nutritional care plan. Offending medications should be evaluated for alternatives and overall efficacy. Nutritional assessment laboratory values should be assessed, including folic acid and vitamin B_{12}. Appropriate referrals should be made for adaptive feeding equipment, financial assistance, swallowing evaluation, or psychosocial issues. See Box 5-8 for more specific treatment recommendations targeting causes and symptoms of undernutrition. Figure 5-5 ◻ is an important clinical algorithm for use in long-term care.

It is essential that caregivers in long-term care receive proper training on feeding assistance and documentation. See Box 5-8 for guidelines on proper positioning and assistance while feeding. Documentation of mealtime consumption will have improved accuracy if performed while actively observing what was eaten versus delayed documentation of intake (Shatenstein et al., 2002). Training on interpretation of the MDS criteria for meal percentages is crucial.

Verbal prompting throughout the day has been shown to increase fluid intake by 78% in long-term care patients. Older persons who were cognitively intact improved their intake of fluids further when fluid preferences were available (Simmons et al., 2001). Increasing the volume of fluid given with each medication pass and snack is also beneficial.

Practice Pearl

Flagging the meal tray or door of long-term care patients at risk for dehydration can remind caregivers to provide extra prompting, and food service workers to leave unfinished beverages at the bedside, if safe to do so. Drinks can be provided in spillproof containers that can be left at bedside.

Social dining has been associated with a 44% increase in dietary intake over dining alone (Council for Nutrition Clinical Strategies in Long-Term Care, 2001). Congregate meals in the community and family-style dining in long-term care provide older persons with opportunities for social interaction during a meal. Buffet-style dining in a nursing home was found to increase energy and protein intake by 25% when residents could self-select types and amounts of food (Remsburg et al., 2001).

Alterations in the physical environment can benefit the older person with dementia. Music has been used to reduce agitated behavior and increase dietary intake (Lou, 2001). Limiting the amount of food presented at one time and the use of finger foods are suggested (Manthorpe & Watson, 2003). An optimized breakfast, lunch, and early snacks should be offered to the older person with dementia who experiences sundowning and may eat poorly later in the day (Finley, 1997).

BOX 5-8

Nutritional Interventions for Undernutrition

Enhanced Eating Environment

- Improve lighting
- Plain dishes for those with poor vision
- Play familiar music from older adults' youth
- Encourage social dining
- Use attractive place settings

Improved Taste Perception

- Avoid smoking
- Evaluate medication
- Add flavor enhancers to food
- Changes in texture to increase appeal
- Optimize aroma

Increase Nutrient-Dense Intake

- Liberalize restrictive diets if indicated
- Offer juices, milk, shakes vs. water as fluid
- Add nonfat milk powder to soup, pudding, scrambled eggs, recipes for extra protein, nutrients
- Offer liquid supplements > 1 hour from meals
- Add sauces, butter, gravy to foods
- Serve desserts made with eggs/ milk

Saliva Stimulation for Xerostomia

- Medication assessment for contributors
- Use sugar-free candy and gum
- Artificial saliva substitute available
- Serve fluids with meals
- Add sauces, butter, gravy to foods
- No overly hot foods or dry foods
- Maintain hydration
- Optimize aromas

Dysphagia Safety

- Clinical evaluation
- Gentle cough after each swallow
- Compensatory movements if prescribed
- Appropriately thinned or thickened foods
- Thin liquids or hard/dry/sticky foods only if prescribed since high aspiration risk
- Remain upright after meals

Hydration

- Offer fluids frequently
- Provide regular prompting to drink
- Provide beverage choices
- Do not wait for report of thirst to offer fluid

Alterations for Chewing Difficulty

- Dental consult if indicated
- Texture modification—individualize
- Find alternatives within food groups that are better tolerated (meat is hard to chew but tuna, eggs, hummus, beans, fish are easier to chew)
- Improve visual appeal of puree diet
  - Do not mix puree diets into mush on plate when assisting with feeding
  - Use attractive sauces, garnishes, molds

Improved Feeding Assistance

- Adequate unhurried time essential
- Proper posture: head and torso at 90-degree angle to lap
- Avoid head tipped back
- Avoid mixing foods together
- Offer finger foods where appropriate
- Avoid straws if aspiration risk
- For cognitively impaired:
  - Minimize amount of foods on plate at once
  - Remind to swallow/brush cheek gently
  - Play music to ease agitation
  - Cue throughout meal
  - Match appropriate utensil with each food introduced

FIGURE ▢ 5-5

Clinical guide to prevent
and manage malnutrition
in long-term care.

FOR NURSING STAFF AND DIETARY STAFF AND DIETITIANS (EVALUATE, DOCUMENT AND TREAT)

The American Dietetic Association supports the Clinical Guide to Prevent and Manage Malnutrition in Long-Term Care. Representatives from the American Dietetic Association were instrumental in its development.

These Guidelines were developed by the Council for Nutrition convened by Programs in Medicine under a grant from Bristol-Myers Squibb. A special committee of The Gerontological Society of America (GSA) served as critical reviewers and provided input and modification of the final Guidelines. While GSA does not endorse specific clinical measures, we support the principles underlying these Guidelines and their potential to improve nutrition in the nursing home.

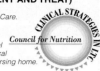

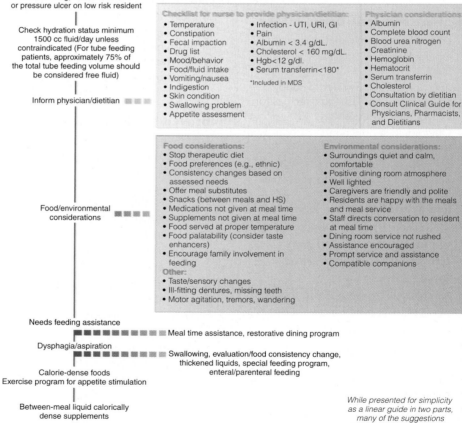

Trigger Conditions

Involuntary 5% weight loss in 30 days
or 10% in 180 days or less
or
BMI ≤ 21
or
Resident leaves 25% or more of food uneaten at two
thirds of meals (Assess over 7 days, based on 2000 cal/day)

This is a tool to assist in compliance. This is not an endorsement of the HCFA mandated criteria. It should be noted that because malnutrition in long-term care is multifactorial, any treatment that is initiated should be monitored for efficacy, and nursing interventions should proceed simultaneously with medical interventions.

Put on weekly weight
monitoring program/Proceed
with documentation
utilizing Nursing Nutritional
Checklist

Suggestions for family:
• Visit at meal time
• Help feed
• Discuss alternate food sources
• Review food preferences
• Recommend favorite foods or comfort foods
• Discuss quality of life issues and treatment goals

Quality indicator conditions:
•Fecal impactions, Infection (UTI, URI, pneumonia, GI)
•Tube feeding, decline in ADL's or pressure ulcer on low risk resident

Checklist for nurse to provide physician/dietitian:
• Temperature
• Constipation
• Fecal impaction
• Drug list
• Mood/behavior
• Food/fluid intake
• Vomiting/nausea
• Indigestion
• Skin condition
• Swallowing problem
• Appetite assessment

• Infection - UTI, URI, GI
• Pain
• Albumin < 3.4 g/dL.
• Cholesterol < 160 mg/dL.
• Hgb<12 g/dl.
• Serum transferrin<180*

*Included in MDS

Physician considerations:
• Albumin
• Complete blood count
• Blood urea nitrogen
• Creatinine
• Hemoglobin
• Hematocrit
• Serum transferrin
• Cholesterol
• Consultation by dietitian
• Consult Clinical Guide for Physicians, Pharmacists, and Dietitians

Check hydration status minimum
1500 cc fluid/day unless
contraindicated (For tube feeding
patients, approximately 75% of
the total tube feeding volume should
be considered free fluid)

Inform physician/dietitian

Food considerations:
• Stop therapeutic diet
• Food preferences (e.g., ethnic)
• Consistency changes based on assessed needs
• Offer meal substitutes
• Snacks (between meals and HS)
• Medications not given at meal time
• Supplements not given at meal time
• Food served at proper temperature
• Food palatability (consider taste enhancers)
• Encourage family involvement in feeding
Other:
• Taste/sensory changes
• Ill-fitting dentures, missing teeth
• Motor agitation, tremors, wandering

Environmental considerations:
• Surroundings quiet and calm, comfortable
• Positive dining room atmosphere
• Well lighted
• Caregivers are friendly and polite
• Residents are happy with the meals and meal service
• Staff directs conversation to resident at meal time
• Dining room service not rushed
• Assistance encouraged
• Prompt service and assistance
• Compatible companions

Food/environmental
considerations

Needs feeding assistance

Meal time assistance, restorative dining program

Dysphagia/aspiration

Swallowing, evaluation/food consistency change,
thickened liquids, special feeding program,
enteral/parenteral feeding

Calorie-dense foods
Exercise program for appetite stimulation

Between-meal liquid calorically
dense supplements

While presented for simplicity as a linear guide in two parts, many of the suggestions can be done simultaneously, and the order in which this approach is taken can be varied dependent on individual resident needs.

Consider other treatment options,
e.g., hospitalize or palliative care

Document reason

Source: Thomas, D.R., et al. (2000). Nutrition management in long-term care: Development of a clinical strategy. *Journal of Gerontology: Medical Sciences, 55*(A), M725–M735.

Practice Pearl

Some older persons with cognitive impairment may not recognize mealtime or the eating process and can benefit from cueing throughout the meal. Statements such as "here is your soup and the spoon to use to eat it" can help.

More aggressive intervention is indicated when other methods of improving nutritional status do not result in improvements. Such interventions should be in keeping with healthcare wishes and advance directives. Use of medications to promote weight gain is one consideration. Some medications used to treat depression may also lead to weight gain. Orexigenic medications, such as megestrol acetate, are sometimes considered, but no medication has yet to be approved by the FDA as an appetite stimulant for geriatric use (Council for Nutrition Clinical Strategies in Long-Term Care, 2001).

Commercial oral supplements have been prescribed to boost intake with mixed results. Some studies have found between-meal supplementation helps to increase overall intake while others have found that supplements simply replace food intake (Fiatarone et al., 1994; Payette, Boutier, Coulombe, & Gray-Donald, 2002).

Practice Pearl

Supplements should be liquid and not solid and should be given more than an hour before meals to minimize satiety (American Medical Directors Association, 2001; Huffman, 2002). Providing a 4-oz serving of liquid supplement instead of other fluids with four medication passes each day can provide almost 500 kcal.

Supplementation combined with a physical activity component has produced more results than supplementation alone (Fiatarone et al., 1994; Payette et al., 2002).

Alternative feeding routes can be considered when oral intake and supplementation fail following an earnest attempt at improving nutritional status via those routes. A nasogastric tube may be used for short-term feeding. A more permanent tube, such as a gastrostomy or jejunostomy tube, may be used for long-term feeding. Commercial enteral formulas provide between 1 cal and 2 kcal per ml. Most formulas that are 1 cal/ml are isotonic in nature, minimizing the osmotic draw of fluid into the gastrointestinal tract during feeding. Formulas with more than 1 cal/ml are generally hypertonic and need to be initiated at a dilute strength to minimize diarrhea. Full-strength delivery of these hypertonic formulas is reached gradually. Hypertonic formulas contain less free water than do isotonic formulas, warranting close monitoring of hydration status. A registered dietitian will generally make an assessment and recommendation for appropriate formula type and volume. Cognitively intact older persons who are not at risk for aspiration can receive several small bolus feedings while sitting upright, amounting to prescribed volume over the day. Bolus feedings are contraindicated in others. Continuous drip-feeding with the head of the bed or chair upright at least at a 30- to 45-degree angle is necessary when there is risk of aspiration. These guidelines are for all types of feeding tubes because aspiration risk is not eliminated with temporary or permanent feeding tubes (Li, 2002). Feeding tubes should be flushed both before and after giving medications to avoid clogging the tube with precipitate. Smaller bore tubes, such as a jejunostomy tube, will become easily clogged from lack of flushing. Pharmacists can give guidance on suitability of medications for delivery through a feeding tube and recommendations for liquid versions when available. While flushing may take extra time, it will save time and patient comfort when tube replacement is avoided. Table 5-6 outlines nursing interventions for common problems with tube feedings.

The decision as to whether continued nutritional support will improve clinical outcome and quality of life in a terminally ill older person needs to include an assessment of all risks and benefits as well as the emotional, religious, cultural, and ethical considerations of the patient (Position of the American Dietetic Association, 2002; Winter, 2000). Aspiration pneumonia and agitation resulting in self-extubation have been cited as prevalent in studies of nursing home patients receiving tube-feedings (Winter, 2000). A meta-analysis of tube-feeding use in patients with advanced dementia found no data suggesting improvement in clinical outcomes. Tube-feedings failed to stop weight loss. Median survival after placement of a percutaneous gastrostomy tube was 7.5 months, and the mortality rate was 50% or greater at 1 year (Finucane, Christmas, & Travis, 1999). A large-scale study of U.S. nursing home patients with advanced cognitive impairment found over one third had feeding tubes. Non-White nursing home residents living in urban locations or in larger and for-profit facilities as well as those lacking advance directives were more likely to have a feeding tube than other cognitively impaired residents. The presence of a dementia care unit in the facility or a nurse practitioner or physician assistant on staff lessened the likelihood of having a feeding tube in the same population (Mitchell, Teno, Roy, Kabumoto, & Mor, 2003). The independent influence of organizational and demographic variables on placement of feeding tubes deserves further study. The American Dietetic Association recognizes that "there is strong clinical, ethical and legal support for and against the administration of food and water when issues arise regarding what is or is not wanted by the patient and what is or is not warranted by empirical clinical evidence" and that when a conflict arises, patient-centered ethical deliberation is required to identify and clarify moral dilemmas (Position of the American Dietetic Association, 2002, p. 716).

MEDICAL NUTRITIONAL THERAPY FOR CHRONIC DISEASES

While liberalization of therapeutic diets is warranted for most older residents in long-term care, there are older persons for whom a therapeutic diet is beneficial. Obesity in older persons can have functional and psychosocial consequences due to impaired mobility and presence of comorbid conditions requiring intervention. It is estimated that 34% of women and 44% of men 65 to 74 years of age are overweight; an additional 27% of women and 24% of men are obese (Dausch, 2003). Women with BMI greater than 30 and men with BMI greater than 35 were 1.5 to 2 times more likely to report functional limitations in a population study (Davison, Ford, Cogswell, & Dietz, 2002). Older persons with sleep apnea and others with osteoarthritis experienced improvements following weight loss. Hypertensive adults 60 to 80 years of age were able to discontinue antihypertensive medications following weight loss and compliance with a moderate sodium restriction (Whelton et al., 1998). Supervised weight loss can be beneficial for some older persons, though prognostic value is not equivalent to that seen in younger adults (Dausch, 2003). A registered dietitian should be consulted to provide nutritional education and to ensure preservation of nutritional status. Acceptable levels of appropriate physical activity should be incorporated to help preserve lean muscle mass and increase metabolic rate. Quick weight loss and dietary supplements for weight loss are contraindicated.

NURSING DIAGNOSES

The following nursing diagnoses are appropriate for use in patient care plans when problems relating to nutrition are encountered by the gerontological nurse. *Imbalanced*

TABLE 5-6

Nursing Interventions
With Enteral
Nutritional Support

Problem List	Intervention
Potential for foodborne illness	• Wash hands before handling formula and equipment. • Wipe off top of formula container before opening. • Label, cover, and store open formula in refrigerator for not > 24 hours.
Aspiration	• Check for gastric residuals q4h. Hold for residual > ~100–150 cc and notify physician. • Ensure head of bed is elevated at least 30 degrees. • Avoid bolus feedings. • Consider smaller bore tube if nasally intubated. • Consider longer tube to reach duodenum or jejunum, if indicated. • Consider permanent feeding tube if on long-term feeding.

Clogged tube	• Administer feeding with pump vs. gravity drip.
	• Administer room-temperature feeding. High-temperature storage or heating of formula will cause protein content to coagulate.
	• Follow guidelines for medication administration.
	  1. Flush tube with 20-30 cc water before, between, and after each single medication.
	  2. Consult pharmacist re: suitability of crushing medication with a small amount of water and availability of liquid versions of medications.
	  3. *Note: If using longer feeding tubes, ensure medication absorption site is not bypassed by tube.*

Diarrhea	• Administer feeding at room temperature. Cold feeding may cause increased gut peristalsis. • Consider lactose-free formula. • Consider medications that can cause diarrhea: antibiotics, magnesium, potassium, digoxin among others. • Administer continuous drip vs. bolus. • Consider temporarily altering formula concentration or rate of delivery: consult registered dietitian. • Consider medical causes.
Constipation	• Consider formula with added fiber. • Monitor hydration. Ensure adequate intake. • Encourage ambulation as indicated. • Assess for contributing medications, such as narcotics and some antacids among others. • Consider obstruction/medical causes.
Dehydration	• Monitor hydration. • Ensure adequate free water intake. • Need 1,500 cc minimum with 1 kcal/cc. • Most formulas are 50%-75% free water (high calorie/protein formulas have less free water than 1 cal/cc formula).

nutrition: less than body requirements is appropriate when older persons do not consume enough calories to maintain their weight and are experiencing unintentional weight loss; are diagnosed with a malabsorption syndrome; are experiencing dysphagia or lower intestinal motility problems; or are lethargic or have a decreased level of consciousness. *Imbalanced nutrition: more than body requirements* is appropriate when older persons ingest more calories per day than needed or are unable to exercise and therefore experience weight gain. Older persons may also be diagnosed with *deficient knowledge related to diet* when they make poor nutritional choices based upon lack of education, cognitive impairment, or following fad diets or using dangerous weight loss products. *Noncompliance to diet* may be used when the older person is prescribed a therapeutic diet (low fat, 2 g sodium, etc.) and chooses not to follow recommendations.

Patient and Family Teaching Guidelines

Gerontological nurses require skills and knowledge related to teaching patients and families about the key concepts of gerontology and gerontological nursing. The patient-family teaching guidelines in the following feature will assist the nurse to assume the role of teacher and coach. Educating patients and families is critical so that nurses can interpret scientific data and individualize the nursing care plan.

Patient-Family Teaching Guidelines

The following are guidelines that the nurse may find useful when instructing older persons and their families about dietary supplements (adapted from NIH, 2000).

DIETARY SUPPLEMENTS

1. Do I need a dietary supplement?

Dietary supplements can consist of vitamins, minerals, fiber, herbs, hormones, or a variety of other substances. While it is generally accepted that taking a multivitamin daily is a good idea, great controversy exists surrounding the use of other supplements. Many supplement manufacturers promise that their product will keep you young, make you feel better, and help you live longer. As the FDA does not test or regulate these supplements, there is little evidence to back up these claims. In fact, some of these supplements can hurt you. Your best bet is to talk to your doctor, your nurse, or a dietitian about supplements if you are considering taking one.

RATIONALE:

Some older people think that supplements sold over the counter are safe and effective; however, many supplements can be dangerous and interact with prescription medications. It is always a good idea to consult with the physician, pharmacist, or dietitian about supplements. At best, they are harmless and a waste of money. At worst, they can be harmful and cause problems.

2. What about vitamins and minerals?

Vitamins and minerals are nutrients found naturally in food. The best way to get vitamins and minerals is by eating a balanced diet, not by taking supplements. Try to eat a variety of foods including meats, fruits, whole grains, and vegetables daily. Avoid foods that are low in fiber and high in fat and added sugar. If you occasionally skip meals or do not always eat right, taking a multivitamin may be a good choice for you. Remember:

RATIONALE:

Some older people think if a little is good, then a lot is better. The nurse should urge older patients to eat well and enjoy the nutritious foods they consume daily. Taking large doses can

Patient-Family Teaching Guidelines

- A regular multivitamin will do. It does not have to be a "senior" formula.
- Do not megadose or take large quantities of any vitamin or mineral supplement.
- Generally, store or generic brands are fine and equivalent to more expensive preparations.

3. What vitamins does my body need now that I am older?

Depending on your age and level of health you should take the following amounts of vitamins from food and supplements if needed:

- Vitamin B_{12}—2.4 µg. Some foods, like cereal, are fortified with B_{12}, but many older people cannot absorb the B vitamins from food.
- Calcium—1,200 mg. As you age, you need more calcium to keep your bones strong. Vitamin D helps calcium to be absorbed, so look for a calcium preparation with this vitamin.
- Vitamin D—400 IU daily up to age 70 and 600 IU daily after age 70. It is a vitamin stored in the body, so do not take over 2,000 IU each day.
- Iron—up to 8 mg daily. Normally older people do not lose blood (as do menstruating women) but if you are recovering from surgery or you are a blood donor, be sure to eat foods high in iron or take a supplement. Be careful; it can be constipating.
- Vitamin B_6—1.7 mg for men and 1.5 mg for women. Found in some whole grain products and fortified cereals.

4. How about herbal supplements?

You may have heard of ginkgo biloba, ginseng, echinacea, ephedra, St. John's wort, and black cohosh. These are herbal supplements that are harvested from certain foods and plants. Their ingredients will have some effect on your body, and they may interfere with medications you have been prescribed. Some herbal supplements can also cause serious side effects such as high blood pressure, nausea, diarrhea, constipation, fainting, headaches, seizures, heart attack, or even stroke. Play it safe. Check it out with your healthcare provider before you take any herbal supplement.

5. What is best for me if I am considering taking a dietary supplement?

If you are thinking of taking an herbal supplement for any reason, consider this advice:

- Talk to your doctor, nurse, pharmacist, or dietitian. Do not believe the manufacturer's claims. Be cautious and careful.
- Use only the supplement recommended by your healthcare professional. Treat it as you would a prescription medication with careful dosing, with monitoring for effect and side effects.
- If you decide to stop taking a supplement your doctor has recommended, make sure to let him or her know.
- Learn as much as you can about the supplement before taking it. Buy only from a reputable buyer. Avoid products sold over the Internet.
- If you are not sure, ask questions. Be an informed consumer.

be harmful depending on the patient's age, health, and dose. Some vitamins are stored and can reach toxic levels. Others are excreted in the urine and are a waste of money.

RATIONALE:

Some older people may not eat well for a variety of reasons. They may have problems chewing whole grain foods or fresh fruits and vegetables; they may buy prepackaged foods that have little nutritional value; they may have financial problems that limit their choices. The nurse should urge a balanced healthy diet that is acceptable to the older patient and the family. Older persons should use supplements as needed.

RATIONALE:

The safety and effectiveness of most herbals has not been documented by the FDA. Some herbals may be effective and others are not. The nurse should urge patients to consult with clinicians knowledgeable about herbal supplements to avoid problems.

RATIONALE:

Urging older patients to treat herbal supplements as they would prescription medications will underscore the seriousness and importance of safety and caution. Consult the Office of Dietary Supplements, National Institutes of Health Website for information and stay informed.

Care Plan

A Patient With Alterations in Nutrition

Case Study

Mrs. McGillicuddy is a 78-year-old woman admitted 2 weeks ago to a nursing home following a complicated hospital stay for a cerebrovascular accident. While hospitalized, she lost 10 lb in one month and developed a stage II decubitus ulcer. Her prior medical history was significant for hypertension managed with an ACE inhibitor and low-sodium diet.

On admission to the nursing home, she was found to weigh 115 lb and reported a height of 5′5″. Her albumin was 3.0 mg/dl and complete blood cell count was normal. Physical examination revealed residual right-sided weakness. Mrs. McGillicuddy reported that she had been feeding herself in the hospital and felt she could manage. A therapeutic 2-g low-sodium diet was ordered.

Now, 2 weeks later, it is discovered that she has lost another 4 lb. Her urine is dark in color and a mouth examination reveals dry mucosa and long tongue furrows. Pocketed food was noted along the gum line as well. Mrs. McGillicuddy's roommate has noticed that she now sounds "gravelly." Her decubitus ulcer is reportedly unchanged.

Upon further discussion with Mrs. McGillicuddy, it becomes apparent that she has been having difficulty with self-feeding and managing the utensils. Frequently, she spills food from the spoon or fork and feels embarrassed about this. She especially is having trouble with drinking liquids. It is difficult to hold the cup handle, and liquids seem to be spilling out of her mouth. This embarrasses her as well. Lately, she has just been moving the foods around on her plate to make it look like she has eaten. Her nursing care assistant has been recording her intake due to the report of weight loss on admission. The medical chart reports that 75% to 90% of food was eaten at most meals.

Mrs. McGillicuddy also reports that the food tastes too bland and she often has a bad taste in her mouth that reduces her appetite.

Applying the Nursing Process

ASSESSMENT

The nurse should think broadly and assess a variety of factors, including the following:

- **Physical.** Assess for signs or symptoms of dehydration—tongue furrows, dry oral mucosa; dysphagia symptoms—drooling, food pocketing, voice alterations, coughing during swallowing or afterwards. Reassess decubitus ulcer stage.

A Patient With Alterations in Nutrition

- **Diet.** Assess appetite; observe self-feeding and dietary intake, especially of calories and protein; note food textures that are difficult to swallow.
- **Laboratory.** Assess plasma levels for blood urea nitrogen, creatine, and sodium, and urine for sedimentation rate.

DIAGNOSIS

Appropriate nursing diagnoses for Mrs. McGillicuddy may include the following:

- *Alteration in nutrition:* less than body requirements related to increased need for nutrition with hypermetabolic state (decubitus ulcer) and decreased intake
- *Fluid volume deficit*
- *Risk for aspiration*
- *Impaired swallowing*

EXPECTED OUTCOMES

Expected outcomes for Mrs. McGillicuddy may include the following:

- Resident should safely consume adequate nutrients and fluid (consumes more than 75% of meal served at most meals) without aspiration.
- Decubitus ulcer should not increase in size and preferably reduce to stage I.
- Resident should report feeling improved self-feeding confidence.
- Resident's weight, hydration, and swallowing function should improve gradually without occurrence of adverse events.

PLANNING AND IMPLEMENTATION

The following nursing interventions may be appropriate for Mrs. McGillicuddy:

- Consult to speech language pathologist for possible dysphagia as evidenced by symptoms of hoarse voice, inability to maintain a fluid bolus in the mouth, and food pocketing.
- Consult to occupational therapy for adaptive feeding equipment if indicated.
- Nutritional consult to coordinate swallowing recommendations and increased nutritional needs into appropriate food. Resident food preferences as allowed.
- Consideration of an oral nutritional supplement if deemed safe for swallowing— may need texture alteration of supplement. Supplement must be given more than 60 minutes before meal.
- Consideration of a feeding tube if unable to consume adequate nutrition by mouth.
- Multivitamin and mineral supplement for adequate vitamins and minerals for wound healing.
- Adequate hydration—once swallowing consult indicates safety, put resident on fluid prompting program. Use adaptive cup to facilitate intake.
- Liberalization of low-sodium diet to improve intake.
- Medical and pharmacy evaluation of use of ACE inhibitor, which may be contributing to dry mouth, metallic taste residue and lack of taste perception of food, and difficulty swallowing.
- Reinforce nursing assistant training on recording accurate dietary intake.

(continued)

A Patient With Alterations in Nutrition *(continued)*

EVALUATION

The nurse hopes to work with Mrs. McGillicuddy over time and involve the interdisciplinary team in the plan of care. The nurse will consider the plan a success based on the following criteria:

- Mrs. McGillicuddy will exhibit improved function and social skills with decreased feelings of sadness.
- She will stop losing weight and eventually begin to gain weight.
- Her decubitus ulcer will begin to heal.
- She will report increased satisfaction with the taste and quality of the food served.
- She will have improved oral hygiene and hydration.

Ethical Dilemma

Mrs. McGillicuddy tells the nurse in confidence that there are several reasons why she thinks she is losing weight:

- She is feeling sad and has no desire to eat.
- The food tastes awful and is very unappealing to her.
- She does not want to "bother" the nurses by asking for additional help with her meals.

The nurse informs Mrs. McGillicuddy that these feelings are commonly reported, and many can be addressed or remedied. Mrs. McGillicuddy asks that the nurse not tell anyone of their conversation. The nurse weights the patient's request for privacy with the professional responsibility to assist the patient in her recovery. The nurse decides to consult with the physician and dietitian to see if Mrs. McGillicuddy can be placed on a regular, no-salt-added diet. This may make the food more appealing to her. Additionally, the nurse makes a note on the nursing care plan that the patient may not ask for assistance with meals but should be frequently observed to see if she needs assistance. Alerting others may alleviate some of Mrs. McGillicuddy's feelings of dependency as she will not have to ask for help cutting her meat, opening milk containers, and so on. Finally, the nurse urges the patient to talk with a social work colleague so that she can discuss her recovery in general. Since Mrs. McGillicuddy is not suicidal, there is no need for immediate referral with violation of her right to privacy. A skilled social worker will quickly pick up on her feelings of sadness and begin counseling her with referral to a geropsychiatrist if necessary.

Critical Thinking and the Nursing Process

1. Identify five or more risk factors for undernutrition in the older person. Pick three risk factors and outline appropriate nursing interventions for each factor. Which intervention would be a priority if all three factors were present in one person?

A Patient With Alterations in Nutrition

2. An older person is homebound with severe arthritis. What nutritional and hydration concerns should the nurse have?

3. An older person with cognitive impairment is admitted to a nursing home from the hospital with reports of inadequate dietary intake. The physician is contemplating insertion of a feeding tube. You note that there is no documentation in the hospital record on self- or hand-feeding. What nursing interventions might you consider before consideration of a feeding tube?

4. What are some possible nursing interventions for the long-term care resident at risk for dehydration?

5. An older person recently had multiple teeth extracted and now is wearing dentures. On a subsequent clinic visit you note weight loss. What other physical and nutritional findings should you assess that are related to the specific issue of the changes in dentition?

■ Evaluate your responses in Appendix B.

EXPLORE MediaLink

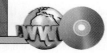

NCLEX review, case studies, and other interactive resources for this chapter can be found on the Companion Website at **www.prenhall.com/tabloski**. Click on Chapter 5 to select the activities for this chapter. For animations, video tutorials, more NCLEX review questions, and case studies, access the accompanying CD-ROM in this textbook.

Chapter Highlights

■ Physiological changes associated with aging can have negative effects on the nutritional status of the older person.

■ Older persons are at disproportionate risk for unintentional weight loss and malnutrition, especially those in the hospital and long-term care.

■ Nutritional screening and assessment should be an essential component of routine healthcare for the older person.

■ Prevention and treatment of malnutrition should focus on the common etiologies: insufficient intake, increased nutrient losses, and hypermetabolism.

■ Aggressive nutrition support in advanced disease states should be in accordance with the advance directives of the older patient and include a thorough evaluation of the risks, benefits, and ethical considerations.

■ Liberalization of therapeutic diets is urged for most long-term care residents.

References

American Diabetes Association Task Force. (2002). American Diabetes Association position statement: Evidence-based principles for the treatment and preventing of diabetes and related complications. *Journal of the American Dietetic Association, 102,* 109–118.

American Medical Directors Association. (2001). *Altered nutritional status: Clinical practice guideline.* Washington, DC: Author.

Ang-Lee, M. K., Moss, J., & Yuan, C. (2001). Herbal medicines and perioperative care. *Journal of the American Medical Association, 286,* 208–216.

Azad, N., Murphy, J., Amos, S. S., & Toppan, J. (1999). Nutrition survey in an elderly population following admission to a tertiary care hospital. *Canadian Medical Association Journal, 161,* 511–515.

Balluz, L. S., Kieszak, S. M., Philen, R. M., & Mulinaire, J. (2000). Vitamin and mineral supplement use in the United States. *Archives of Family Medicine, 9,* 258–262.

Bone, R. A., Landrum, J. T., Guerra, L. H., & Ruiz, C. A. (2003). Lutein and zeaxanthin dietary supplements raise macular pigment density and serum concentrations of these carotenoids in humans. *Journal of Nutrition, 133,* 992–998.

Bromley, S. M. (2000). Smell and taste disorders: A primary care approach. *American Family Physician, 61,* 427–436.

Calle, E. E., Thun, M. J., Petrelli, J. M., Rodriguez, C., & Heath, C. W. (1999). Body-mass index and mortality in a prospective cohort of U.S. adults. *New England Journal of Medicine, 341,* 1097–1105.

Castellanos, V. H., & Andrews, Y. N. (2002). Inherent flaws in a method of estimating meal intake commonly used in long-term care facilities. *Journal of the American Dietetic Association, 102,* 826–830.

Centers for Medicare and Medicaid Services. (2002). *Minimum Data Set manual, version 2.0.* Retrieved June 16, 2003, from http://www.cms.hhs.gov/medicaid/mds20/mds0900b.pdf.

Chapman, I. M., MacIntosh, C. G., Morley, J. E., & Horowitz, M. (2002). The anorexia of aging. *Biogerontology, 3,* 67–71.

Chia-Hui, C., Schilling, L. S., & Lyder, C. H. (2001). A concept analysis of malnutrition in the elderly. *Journal of Advanced Nursing, 36*(1), 131–142.

Chidester, J. C., & Spangler, A. A. (1997). Fluid intake in the institutionalized elderly. *Journal of the American Dietetic Association, 97,* 23–28.

Chumlea, W. C., Roche, A. F., & Mukherjee, D. (1984). *Nutritional assessment of the elderly through anthropometry.* Columbus, OH: Ross Laboratories.

Coleman, E. A., Martau, J. M., Lin, M. K., & Kramer, A. M. (2002). Pressure ulcer prevalence in long-term care nursing home residents since the implementation of OBRA '87. *Journal of the American Geriatrics Society, 50,* 728–732.

Council for Nutrition Clinical Strategies in Long-Term Care. (2001). Anorexia in the elderly: An update. *Annals of Long-Term; Care,* Supplement; 2–14.

Covinsky, K. E. (2002). Malnutrition and bad outcomes. *Journal of General Internal Medicine, 17,* 956–957.

Covinsky, K. E., Covinsky, M. H., Palmer, R. M., & Sehgal, A. R. (2002). Serum albumin concentration and clinical assessments of nutritional status in hospitalized older people: Different sides of different coins? *Journal of the American Geriatrics Society, 50,* 631–637.

Crogan, N. L., Corbett, C. F., & Short, R. A. (2002). The Minimum Data Set: Predicting malnutrition in newly admitted nursing home residents. *Clinical Nursing Research, 11,* 341–353.

Dausch, J. G. (2003). Aging issues moving mainstream. *Journal of the American Dietetic Association, 103,* 683–684.

Davison, K. K., Ford, E. S., Cogswell, M. E., & Dietz, W. H. (2002). Percentage of body fat and body mass index are associated with mobility limitations in people aged 70 and older from NHANES III. *Journal of the American Geriatrics Society, 50,* 1802–1809.

Dawson-Hughes, B., Harris, S. S., Krall, E. A., & Dallal, G. E. (1997). Effect of calcium and vitamin D supplementation on bone density in men and women 65 years of age or older. *New England Journal of Medicine, 337,* 670–676.

DeCastro J. M. (1993). Age-related changes in spontaneous food intake and hunger in humans. *Appetite, 21,* 255–272.

Demling, R. H., & DeSanti, L. (2001). *Protein-energy malnutrition and the nonhealing cutaneous wound.* Retrieved June 16, 2003, from http://www.medscape.com.

Denke, M. A. (2002). Dietary retinol—A double-edged sword. *Journal of the American Medical Association, 287,* 102–104.

De Smet, P. A.G. M. (2002). Herbal remedies. *New England Journal of Medicine, 347,* 2046–2056.

Eastley, R., Wilcock, G. K., & Bucks, R. S. (2000). Vitamin B-12 deficiency in dementia and cognitive impairment: The effects of treatment on neuropsychological function. *International Journal of Geriatric Psychiatry, 15,* 226–233.

Evans, W. (1997). Functional and metabolic consequences of sarcopenia. *Journal of Nutrition, 127,* 998S–1003S.

Fairfield, K. M. & Fletcher, R. H. (2002). Vitamins for chronic disease prevention in adults: Scientific review. *Journal of the American Medical Association, 287,* 3116–3126.

Farrell, Z., & O'Neill, D. (1999). Towards better screening and assessment of oropharangeal swallow disorders in the general hospital. *Lancet, 354,* 355.

Feskanich, D., Singh, V., Willett, W. C., & Colditz, G. A. (2002). Vitamin A intake and hip fractures among postmenopausal women. *Journal of the American Medical Association, 287,* 47–54.

Fiatarone, M. A., O'Neill, E. F., Ryan, N. D., Clements, K. M., Solares, G. R., & Nelson, M. E. (1994). Exercise training and nutritional supplements for physical frailty in very elderly people. *New England Journal of Medicine, 330,* 1769–1775.

Finley, B. (1997). Nutritional needs of the person with Alzheimer's disease: Practical approaches to quality care. *Journal of the American Dietetic Association, 97,* S177–S180.

Finucane, T. E., Christmas, C., & Travis, K. (1999). Tube feeding in patients with advanced dementia: A review of the evidence. *Journal of the American Medical Association, 282,* 1365–1370.

Food and Nutrition Board. (1989). *Recommended dietary allowances* (10th ed.). Washington, DC: National Academy Press.

Foote, J. A., Giuliano, A. R., & Harris, R. B. (2000). Older adults need guidance to meet nutritional recommendations. *Journal of the American College of Nutrition, 19,* 628–640.

Fryzek, J. P., Lipworth, L., Signorello, L. B., & McLaughlin, J. K. (2002). The reliability of dietary data for self- and next-of-kin respondents. *Annals of Epidemiology, 12,* 278–283.

Fuller, K. E., & Casparian, J. M. (2001). Vitamin D: Balancing cutaneous and systemic considerations. *Southern Medical Journal, 94,* 58–64.

Gallagher, D., Ruts, E., Visser, M., Heshka, S., Baumgartner, R. N., Wang, J., et al. (2000). Weight stability masks sarcopenia in elderly men and women. *American Journal of Physiology Endocrinology and Metabolism, 279,* E366–E375.

Gazewood, J. D., & Mehr, D. R. (1998). Diagnosis and management of weight loss in the elderly. *Journal of Family Practice, 47,* 19–25.

Hammond, B. R., & Johnson, M. A. (2002). The age-related eye disease study (AREDS). *Nutrition Reviews, 60,* 283–288.

Holben, D. H., Hassell, J. T., Williams, J. L., & Helle, B. (1999). Fluid intake compared with standards and symptoms of dehydration among elderly residents in a long-term care facility. *Journal of the American Dietetic Association, 99,* 1447–1450.

Homocysteine Lowering Trialists' Collaboration. (1998). Lowering blood homocysteine with folic acid based supplements: Meta-analysis of randomised trials. *British Medical Journal, 316,* 894–898.

Homocysteine Studies Collaboration. (2002). Homocysteine and risk of ischemic heart disease and stroke. *Journal of the American Medical Association, 288,* 2015–2022.

Horn, S. D., Bender, S. A., Bergstrom, N., Cook, A. S., Ferguson, M. L., Rimmasch, H. L., et al. (2002). Description of the national pressure ulcer long-term care study. *Journal of the American Geriatrics Society, 50,* 1816–1825.

Hu, P., Seeman, T., Harris, T.B., & Reuben, D. B. (2003). Does inflammation or undernutrition explain the low cholesterol-mortality association in high-functioning older persons? MacArthur studies of successful aging. *Journal of the American Geriatrics Society, 51,* 80–84.

Huffman, G. B. (2002). Evaluating and treating unintentional weight loss in the elderly. *American Family Physician, 65,* 640–650.

Hutton, B., Feine, J., & Morais, J. (2002). Is there an association between edentulism and nutritional state? *Journal of the Canadian Dental Association, 68*(3), 182–187.

Institute of Medicine, Food and Nutrition Board. (1997). *Dietary reference intakes for calcium, phosphorus, magnesium, vitamin D and fluoride.* Washington, DC: National Academy Press.

Institute of Medicine, Food and Nutrition Board. (1998). *Dietary reference intakes for thiamine, riboflavin, niacin, vitamin B-6, folate, vitamin B-12, pantothenic acid, biotin and choline.* Washington, DC: National Academy Press.

Institute of Medicine, Food and Nutrition Board (2000). *Dietary reference intakes for Vitamin C, Vitamin E, Selenium and Carotenolds.* Washington, DC: National Academy Press.

Institute of Medicine, Food and Nutrition Board. (2001). *Dietary reference intakes for vitamin A, vitamin K, arsenic, boron, chromium, copper, iodine, iron, manganese, molybdenum, nickel, silicon,vanadium and zinc.* Washington, DC: *National Academy Press.*

Institute of Medicine, Food and Nutrition Board. (2002). *Dietary reference intakes for energy, carbohydrates, fiber, fat, protein and amino acids (macronutrients).* Washington, DC: National Academy Press.

Institute of Medicine, Food and Nutrition Board. (2004). *Dietary reference intakes for water, potassium, sodium, chloride, and sulfate.* Washington, DC: National Academy Press.

Jacques, P. F., Selhub, J., Bostom, A. G., Wilson, P. W. F., & Rosenberg, I. H. (1999). The effect of folic acid fortification on plasma folate and total homocysteine concentrations. *New England Journal of Medicine, 340,* 1449–1454.

Koutkia P, Chen T. C., & Holick, M. F .(2001). Vitamin D intoxication associated with an over-the-counter supplement. *New England Journal of Medicine* 345, 66–67.

LeBars, P. L., Katz, M. M., Berman, N., Itil, T. M., Freedman, A. M., & Schatzberg, A. F. (1997). A placebo-controlled, double-blind, randomized trial of an extract of Ginkgo biloba for dementia. *Journal of the American Medical Association, 278,* 1327–1332.

LeBoeuf, R. (2003). Homocysteine and Alzheimer's disease. *Journal of the American Dietetic Association, 103,* 304–307.

Leslie, P., Carding, P. N., & Wilson, J. A. (2003). Investigation and management of chronic dysphagia. *British Medical Journal, 326,* 433–436.

Li, I. (2002). Feeding tubes in patients with severe dementia. *American Family Physician, 65,* 1605–1610.

Lou, M. (2001). The use of music to decrease agitated behaviour of the demented elderly person: The state of the science. *Scandinavian Journal of Caring Sciences, 15,* 165–173.

Lyne, P. A., Powse, M. A. (1999). Methodological issues in the development and use of instruments to assess patient nutritional statis or the level of risk of nutritional compromise. *Journal of Advanced Nursing, 30,* 835–842.

Manthorpe, J., & Watson, R. (2003). Poorly served? Eating and dementia. *Journal of Advanced Nursing, 41,* 162–169.

Mattes, R. D. (2002). The chemical senses and nutrition in aging: Challenging old assumptions. *Journal of the American Diabetic Assocation, 102,* 192–196.

Mayeux, R., & Sano, M. (1999). Treatment of Alzheimer's disease. *New England Journal of Medicine, 341,* 1670–1679.

McGee, S., Abernethy, W. B., & Simel, D. L. (1999). Is this patient hypovolemic? *Journal of the American Medical Association, 281,* 1022–1029.

Michaelsson, K., Lithell, H., Vessby, B., & Melhus, H. (2003). Serum retinol levels and risk of fracture. *New England Journal of Medicine, 348,* 287–294.

Miller, J. W. (2002). Homocysteine, folate deficiency and Parkinson's disease. *Nutrition Reviews, 60,* 410–413.

Mini Nutrition Assessment. (2003). *Tool and information on usage.* Retrieved June 16, 2003, from http://www.mna-elderly.com.

Mitchell, S. L., Teno, J. M., Roy, J., Kabumoto, G., & Mor, V. (2003). Clinical and organizational factors associated with feeding tube use among nursing home residents with advanced cognitive impairment. *Journal of the American Medical Association, 290,* 73–80.

Morley, J. E., & Thomas, D. R. (1999). Anorexia and aging: Pathophysiology. *Nutrition, 15*(6), 499–503.

Morley, J. E., & Thomas, D. R. (2001). Nutritional clinical strategies in long-term care:

Sarcopenia and vitamin and trace mineral deficiencies in the elderly. *Annals of Long-Term Care,* Supplement, 31–36.

Murphy, C., Schubert, C. R., Cruickshanks, K. J., Klein, B. E., Klein, R., & Nondahl, D. M. (2002). Prevalence of olfactory impairment in older adults. *Journal of the American Medical Association, 288,* 2307–2312.

National Institutes of Health. (2000). Age Page Dietary Supplements, http:www.niapublications. org downloaded May 14, 2002.

National Institutes of Health, National Heart, Lung, and Blood Institute. 2003. Facts about the *DASH eating plan.* Retrieved February 11, 2005, from http://www.nhlbi.nih.gov/health/public/ heart/hbp/dash/index.htm.

NIH Consensus Development Panel on Osteoporosis Prevention, Diagnosis and Therapy. (2001). Osteoporosis prevention, diagnosis and therapy. *Journal of the American Medical Association, 285*(6), 785–795.

Norred, C.L., & Brinker, F. (2001). Potential coagulation effects of preoperative complementary and alternative medicines. *Alternative Therapy Health Medicine, 7,* 58–67.

Nutrition Screening Initiative.. *Tool and information on usage.* Retrieved June 13, 2003, from http://www.aafp.org/nsi.xml.

Packard, P. T., & Heaney, R. P. (1997). Medical nutrition therapy for patients with osteoporosis. *Journal of the American Dietetic Association, 97,* 414–417.

Palmer, J. B., Drennan, J. C., & Baba, M. (2000). Evaluation and treatment of swallowing impairments. *American Family Physician, 61,* 2453–2462.

Pasman, H. R. W., The, B. A., Onwuteaka-Philipsen, B. D., van der Wal, G., & Ribbe, M. W. (2003). Feeding nursing home patients with severe dementia: A qualitative study. *Journal of Advanced Nursing, 42,* 304–311.

Payette, H., Boutier, V., Coulombe, C., & Gray-Donald, K. (2002). Benefits of nutritional supplementation in free-living, frail, undernourished elderly people: A prospective randomized community trial. *Journal of the American Dietetic Association, 102,* 1088–1095.

Payette, H., Gray-Donald, K., Cyr, R., & Boutier, V. (1995). Predictors of dietary intakes in a functionally dependent elderly population in the communities. *American Journal of Public Health, 85,* 677–683.

Perry, L. (2001). Screening swallowing function of patients with acute stroke. Part one: Identification, implementation and initial evaluation of a screening tool for use by nurses. *Journal of Clinical Nursing, 10,* 463–473.

Persson, M. D., Brismar, K. E., Katzarski, K. S., Nordenstrom, J., & Cederholm, T. E. (2002). Nutritional status using mini nutritional assessment and subjective global assessment predict mortality in geriatric patients. *Journal of the American Geriatrics Society, 50,* 1996–2002.

Pontieri-Lewis, V. (1997). The role of nutrition in wound healing. *Medsurg Nursing, 6,* 187–192, 221.

Porter, C., Schell, E. S., Kayser-Jones, J., & Paul, S. M. (1999). Dynamics of nutrition care among nursing home residents who are eating poorly. *Journal of the American Dietetic Association, 99,* 1444–1450.

Position of the American Dietetic Association and Dietitians of Canada: Vegetarian Diets. (2003). *Journal of the American Dietetic Association, 103,* 748–765.

Position of the American Dietetic Association: Ethical and legal issues in nutrition, hydration and feeding. (2002). *Journal of the American Dietetic Association, 102,* 716–726.

Position of the American Dietetic Association: Liberalized diets for older adults in long-term care. (2002). *Journal of the American Dietetic Association, 98,* 201–204.

Position of the American Dietetic Association: Nutrition, aging and the continuum of care. (2000). *Journal of the American Dietetic Association, 100,* 580–595.

Position of the American Dietetic Association: Oral health and nutrition. (2003). *Journal of the American Dietetic Association, 103,* 615–625.

Remsburg, R. E., Luking, A., Baran, P., Radu, C., Pineda, D., Bennett, R. G., & Tayback, M. (2001). Impact of a buffet-style dining program on weight and biochemical indicators of nutritional status in nursing home residents: A pilot study. *Journal of the American Dietetic Association, 101,* 1460–1463.

Rojas, A. I., & Phillips, T. J. (1999). Patients with chronic leg ulcers show diminished levels of vitamins A and E, carotenes and zinc. *Dermatologic Surgery, 25,* 601–604.

Russell, R. M., Rasmussen, H., & Lichtenstein, A. H. (1999). Modified food guide pyramid for people over 70 years of age. *Journal of Nutrition, 129,* 751–753.

Sahyoun, N., Lin, C., & Krall, E. (2003). Nutritional status of the older adult is associated with dentition status. *Journal of the American Dietetic Association, 103,* 61–66.

Sahyoun, N. R., Jacques, P. F., Dallal, G. E., & Russell, R. M. (1997). Nutrition screening initiative checklist may be a better awareness/educational tool than a screening one. *Journal of the American Dietetic Association, 97,* 760–764.

Sano, M., Ernesto, C., & Thomas, R. G. (1997). A controlled trial of selegiline, alpha-tocopherol, or both as treatment for Alzheimer's disease. *New England Journal of Medicine, 336,* 1216–1222.

Schiffman, S. S. (1997). Taste and smell losses in normal aging and disease. *Journal of the American Medical Association, 278,* 1357–1362.

Schiffman, S. S. (2000). Intensification of sensory properties of foods in the elderly. *Journal of Nutrition, 130,* 927S–930S.

Schnyder, G., Roffi, M., Pin, R., Flammer, Y., Lange, H., Eberli, F. R., et al. (2001). Decreased rates of coronary restenosis after lowering plasma homocysteine levels. *New England Journal of Medicine, 345,* 1593–1600.

Seshadri, S. S., Beiser, A., Selhub, J., Jacques, P. F., Rosenberg, I. H., D'Agostino, R. B., et al. (2002). Plasma homocysteine as a risk factor for dementia and Alzheimer's disease. *New England Journal of Medicine, 346,* 476–483.

Shatenstein, B., Claveau, D., & Ferland, G. (2002). Visual observation is a valid means of assessing dietary consumption among older adults with cognitive deficits in long-term care settings. *Journal of the American Dietetic Association, 102,* 250–252.

Ship, J. A. (2002). Diagnosing, managing and preventing salivary gland disorders. *Oral Diseases, 8,* 77–89.

Simmons, S. F., Alessi, C., & Schnelle, J. F. (2001). An intervention to increase fluid intake in nursing home residents: Prompting and preference compliance. *Journal of the American Geriatrics Society, 49,* 926–933.

Simmons, S. F., Lam, H. Y., Rao, G., & Schnelle, J. F. (2003). Family members' preferences for nutrition interventions to improve nursing home residents' oral food and fluid intake. *Journal of the American Geriatrics Society, 51,* 69–74.

Stevens, J., Cai, J., Pamuk, E. R., Williamson, D. F., Thun, M. J., & Wood, J. L. (1998). The effect of age on the association between body-mass index and mortality. *New England Journal of Medicine, 338,* 1–7.

Sullivan, D. H., Bopp, M. M., & Roberson, P. K. (2002). Protein-energy undernutrition and life-threatening complications among the hospitalized elderly. *Journal of General Internal Medicine, 17,* 923–932.

Sullivan, D. H., Sun, S., & Walls, R. C. (1999). Protein-energy undernutrition among elderly hospitalized patients. *Journal of the American Medical Association, 281,* 2013–2019.

Sullivan, D. H., & Walls, R. C. (1998). Protein-energy undernutrition and the risk of mortality within six years of hospital discharge. *Journal of the American College of Nutrition, 17,* 571–578.

Tariq, S. H., Karcic, E., Thomas, D. R., Thompson, K., Philpot, C., Chapel, D. L., & Morley, J. E. (2001). The use of no-concentrated-sweets diet in the management of type 2 diabetes in nursing homes. *Journal of the American Dietetic Association, 101,* 1463–1466.

Thomas, D. R. (2001). Improving outcome of pressure ulcers with nutritional interventions: A review of the evidence. *Nutrition, 17,* 121–125.

Thomas, D. R., Ashmen, W., Morley, J. E., Evan, W. J., & Council for Nutrition Strategies in Long-Term Care. (2000). Nutrition management in long-term care: Development of a clinical guideline. *Journal of Gerontology: Medical Sciences, 55*(A), M725–M734.

Thomas, D. R., & Morley, J. E. (2001). Nutritional strategies in long-term care: Anorexia and weight loss in elderly outpatients. *Annals of Long-Term Care,* supplement, 21–30.

Thomas, M. K., Lloyd-Jones, D. M., Thadhani, R. I., Shaw, A. C., Deraska, D. J., Kitch, B. T., et al. (1998). Hypovitaminosis D in medical inpatients. *New England Journal of Medicine, 338,* 777–783.

Tiemeier, H., van Tuijl, H. R., Hofman, A., Eijer, J., Kiliaan, A. J., & Breteler, M. M. B. (2002). Vitamin B-12, folate and homocysteine in depression: The Rotterdam study. *American Journal of Psychiatry, 159,* 2099–2101.

Tinetti, M. E. (2003). Preventing falls in elderly persons. *New England Journal of Medicine, 348* (1), 42–49.

Trumbo, P., Schlicker, S., Yates, A., & Poos, M. (2002). Dietary reference intakes for energy, carbohydrate, fiber, fat, fatty acids, cholesterol, protein and amino acids. *Journal of the American Dietetic Association, 102,* 1621–1630.

Vellas, B., Guigoz, Y., Garry, P. J., Nourhashemi, F., Bennahum, D., Lauque, S., & Albarede, J. L. (1999). The Mini Nutritional Assessment and its use in grading the nutritional state of elderly patients. *Nutrition, 15,* 116–122.

Volpato, S., Leveille, S. G., Corti, M., Harris, T. B., & Guralnik, J. M. (2001). The value of serum albumin and high-density lipoprotein cholesterol in defining mortality risk in older persons with low serum cholesterol. *Journal of the American Geriatrics Society, 49,* 1142–1147.

Vozenilek, G. (1998). Grandma eats like a bird: Helping caregivers improve the nutrition of older persons at home. *Journal of the American Dietetic Association, 98,* 1405.

Wellman, N. S., Weddle, D. O., Krantz, S., & Brain, C. T. (1997). Elder insecurities: Poverty, hunger and malnutrition. *Journal of the American Dietetic Association, 97,* S120–S122.

Whelton, P. K., Appel, L. J., Espeland, M. A., Applegate, W. B., Ettinger, W. H., Kostis, J. B., et al. (1998). Sodium reduction and weight loss in the treatment of hypertension in older persons. *Journal of the American Medical Association, 279,* 839–846.

White, R., & Ashworth, A. (2000). How drug therapy can affect, threaten and compromise nutritional status. *Journal of Human Nutrition and Dietetics, 13,* 119–129.

Willett, W. C., & Stampfer, M. J. (2001). What vitamins should I be taking, doctor? *New England Journal of Medicine, 345,* 1819–1824.

Wilson, M. M., Vaswani, S., Liv D., Morley, J. E., & Miller, D. K. (1998). Prevalence and causes of under nutrition in medical outpatients. *American Journal of Medicine, 104,* 56–63.

Winter, S. M. (2000). Terminal nutrition: Framing the debate for the withdrawal of nutrition support in terminally ill patients. *American Journal of Medicine, 109,* 723–741.

Yoon, S. L., & Horne, C. H. (2001). Herbal products and conventional medicines used by community-residing older women. *Journal of Advanced Nursing, 33,* 51–59.

CHAPTER 6

Pharmacology and Older Adults

Laurel A. Eisenhauer, RN, PhD, FAAN

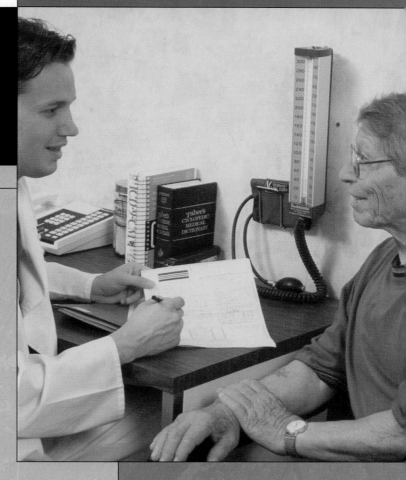

CHAPTER OBJECTIVES

Upon completion of this chapter, the reader will be able to:

- Explain the interaction between normal aging and responses to drug therapy in older people.

- Identify principles of safe medication management in a variety of patient care settings.

- Discuss measures to prevent and reduce polypharmacy in older patients.

- Describe assessments to monitor older patients for adverse drug effects and polypharmacy.

- Use teaching and nursing interventions to promote compliance and adherence to the medication regimen.

- Identify nonpharmacological therapies that may be useful as alternatives to medications.

- Discuss issues related to drug therapy in the older person.

KEY TERMS

adverse drug reactions (ADRs) 161
first-pass effect drugs 158
iatrogenesis 161
nonprescription medicines 156
over-the-counter (OTC)
   medications 156
pharmacodynamics 157
pharmacokinetics 157
polypharmacy 164

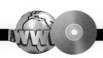

MediaLink

Additional resources for this chapter can be found on the Student CD-ROM accompanying this textbook and on the Companion Website at **www.prenhall.com/tabloski**. Click on Chapter 6 to select the activities for this chapter.

CD-ROM
- Drug Animations
- NCLEX Review
- Case Studies
- Tools

COMPANION WEBSITE
- Audio Glossary
- Additional NCLEX Review
- Case Study
- MediaLink Applications

The many advances in drug therapy have contributed to increasing longevity and the promotion of greater health of all adults. For example, medications have contributed to a 30% decline in cardiovascular disease over the past 30 years (Jordan & Robbins, 2000). The older person, however, uses a disproportionate amount of medications:

- Approximately 30% of all drugs prescribed are for the over-65 age group, who represent 12% to 15% of the population.
- Approximately 65% of nursing home residents over age 65 use an average of 5 to 8 medications a day (Schmucker & Vesell, 1999).
- Adults over 65 years use 30% of all prescription drugs and 40% of all **over-the-counter (OTC) medications** (Williams, 2003).
- Two thirds of adults over 65 use one or more drugs daily, and 25% use three or more drugs each day (Williams, 2003).
- The average older adult takes four to five prescription and two **nonprescription** (OTC) drugs each day and fills 12 to 17 prescriptions per year (Cusack & Vestal, 2005).

Drug therapy in the older person presents many challenges in ensuring the appropriate use of medications. Older persons have characteristics that affect the body's use of drugs; therefore, they are at a greater risk for adverse drug events than are younger persons. Aging impacts the body's ability to handle and respond to medications. Chronic diseases and the multiple drugs used to treat them affect the physiological and adaptive responses of the older person. Psychosocial variables and cognitive changes may also affect the ability of older persons to manage their medications safely.

Some adverse effects can be prevented to a great extent. The nurse is in a pivotal position in all clinical settings to promote the appropriate use of medications, to prevent or detect adverse drug events, and to prevent or reduce the need for drug therapy by the use of nursing interventions.

Although medications are used disproportionately by the older person, the effects of most drugs on older persons have not been studied extensively, especially those that have been on the market for many years. Since 1989 the U.S. Food and Drug Administration (FDA) has required that applications for the approval of new drugs show that they have been studied in the populations in which they will be used. A section called Geriatric Considerations is now included in the packet inserts for new drugs. Although larger numbers of older people have been included in clinical trials, there is concern that those included have tended to be the young-old (less than 75 years) and those with fewer medical problems that would be less likely to confound the study of a new drug. Therefore, the young-old persons may not represent the old-old (75+ years of age) with multiple conditions and multiple drug therapies who are most likely to receive the new drug after being approved by the FDA. However, biological age alone is a poor indicator of how an older person will react to a medication. More appropriate predictors of medication response include general state of health, number and types of other medications taken, liver and renal function, and presence of comorbidities or other diagnosed diseases.

Cultural Diversity and Medication Safety

Cultural diversity and ethnic background can affect the older person's beliefs about health, illness, medications, and physiological response to medications. Most Caucasian Americans are intolerant to pain and expect that their disease will be quickly cured. However, many Hispanics, Chinese, and Asians are cautious about American medicines and often initiate downward dosage adjustments to avoid even minor side effects. Some cultures will engage in extensive folk remedies and herbal preparations before they initiate treatment with American medications (Institute for Safe Medication Practices, 2003). The delay can result in the older person beginning treatment later in the disease process with a more advanced illness trajectory.

Ethnic beliefs can also affect adherence to instructions to take medications as prescribed. For instance, African Americans, Hispanics, and Native Americans often doubt the need for medications when symptoms ease and may discontinue drugs like antibiotics, oral hypoglycemics, and antidepressants prematurely. Women from Islamic and African cultures with vaginal yeast infections may prefer oral drugs to vaginally inserted medications due to cultural taboos restricting insertion of foreign bodies into the vagina. Vietnamese patients may take only one half of the prescribed dose, often fearing medication is too strong (Levy & Hawks, 1999).

Physiological response to medications may also depend on the race or ethnic background of the older person. Although this can be a sensitive subject and the nurse may fear offending patients, asking a person's racial and ethnic background can help to assess the risk of adverse drug events. For instance, Asians and Eskimos often require lower doses of anxiolytics than do Caucasians. Asians, Indians, and Pakistanis require lower doses of lithium and antipsychotic medications. African Americans' symptoms generally improve faster when taking neuroleptics and anxiolytics (Levy & Hawks, 1999). Hispanics often require lower doses of antidepressants than do Caucasians. African Americans receiving treatment for hypertension generally experience a better clinical response to diuretics and calcium channel blockers than to beta-blockers. Nurses and other health professionals should strive to bring effective healthcare to older patients within a context that is appropriate for culture and ethnic background (Institute for Safe Medication Practices, 2003). (See Chapter 4 for further information on the role of culture on illness, medications, and healing.) ⊂⊃

Practice Pearl

Older persons who are recent immigrants, live in ethnic enclaves, speak predominantly in their native language, and travel frequently to their country of origin are more likely to follow strongly held cultural beliefs (Institute for Safe Medication Practices, 2003).

Pharmacokinetic Alterations in the Older Person

As people age, they become increasingly complex and develop their own patterns of physiological and psychosocial responses. Each older person's response to medications is unique.

Alterations in physiological function resulting from normal processes of aging must be carefully considered in prescribing, administering, and monitoring medications. Older persons tend to have acute and chronic conditions that may alter **pharmacokinetics** (what the body does to the drug) and **pharmacodynamics** (what the drug does to the body). The impact of the concurrent drug therapy to treat these conditions can also affect a person's response to other medications.

Aging affects the body's ability to handle drugs. This requires consideration of the need for the dose of many medications to be less than that recommended for adults. As individuals age, a variety of physiological changes affect pharmacokinetics and pharmacodynamics. Many of these changes do not result in clinically significant changes in fit older persons because they have sufficient renal and hepatic adaptability to respond. However, frail older persons with multiple pathological alterations in function are less able to respond effectively.

With aging there is a decrease in body water (as much as 15%) and an increase in body fat. This could result in increased concentration of water-soluble drugs (e.g., alcohol) and more prolonged effects of fat-soluble drugs.

Hepatic blood flow may be decreased by as much as 50% in individuals over 65 years. This could result in increased toxicity when they take usual doses of "first-pass effect" drugs since less of these drugs would be detoxified immediately by the liver. **First-pass effect drugs** are significantly metabolized when they first flow through the liver (first pass into the liver). Liver mass and overall metabolic activity decrease with aging but are not usually clinically significant in relation to drug metabolism. The effect of aging on microsomal enzymes that regulate the rate of metabolism of drugs in the liver is believed to be minimal. Routine liver function tests, with the exception of a slight decrease in serum albumin, do not change significantly with age (Herrlinger & Klotz, 2001).

Practice Pearl

If a patient is receiving two or more drugs that are highly protein bound, the nurse should observe for drug interactions and variations in responses to each drug.

Decreases in serum albumin levels or binding capacity may result in increased serum levels of the "free" or unbound proportion of protein-bound drugs. This may result in toxic levels of highly bound drugs because more unbound drug is available to produce its effects. This is especially problematic in older patients with decreased liver or renal function.

Practice Pearl

Oral medications should be given with a nutritious liquid (e.g., juice) rather than water if a patient is anorexic or is likely to refuse to take a lot of liquid. This maximizes the nutritional values of liquids ingested.

The kidneys excrete most drugs. Renal function generally decreases with age and thus should always be considered in the choice of a drug, in judging the appropriateness of a dose, and in evaluating adverse drug reactions. Estimates of decline in renal function based on aging vary. After age 30, creatinine clearance declines an average of 8 ml/min/1.73 m^2 each decade (Beers & Berkow, 2005). Another estimate is that the glomerular filtration rate declines about 1 ml/min each year after age 40 (Repasy, 2003). However, individuals vary considerably in the degree of decline of renal function due to aging. Blood urea nitrogen (BUN) levels are poor indicators of renal function in the older person because of the decrease in muscle mass and other variables affecting BUN levels. Serum creatinine levels can be used to estimate creatinine clearance but are less reliable in older persons than in younger persons because older persons have less muscle mass, and creatinine is a product of muscle breakdown. The following formula (Cockcroft & Gault, 1976), which includes variables of age and for gender, is often used to estimate creatinine clearance:

$$\text{creatinine clearance} = \frac{(140 - \text{age}) \times \text{lean wt (kg)}}{72 \times \text{serum creatinine}} \times 0.85 \text{ for women}$$

Practice Pearl

Do not rely on BUN levels as an indicator of renal function in the older person. BUN is affected by muscle mass, level of hydration, and dietary intake of protein. Calculating the creatinine clearance provides a more accurate assessment of how the drug will be metabolized and cleared by the kidneys.

PHARMACODYNAMIC ALTERATIONS IN THE OLDER PERSON

Pharmacodynamic changes, which affect how the drug affects the body, can also occur because of the aging process. However, it is not always clear if changes in therapeutic responses are due to the pharmacodynamics or to the altered pharmacokinetics. Changes in pharmacodynamics in the older person may be due to decreases in the number of receptors, decreases in receptor binding, or altered cellular response to the drug-receptor interaction. An increased drug-receptor response can occur with benzodiazepines, opiates, and warfarin, resulting in increased sedation, increased analgesic effects and respiratory depression, and increased anticoagulation, respectively. The central nervous system, bladder, and heart tend to be more sensitive to medications with anticholinergic effects. (See later discussion of anticholinergic effects of medications.) Beta-blockers may have a less pronounced bradycardia in older patients. Older persons also have less tachycardia from isoproterenol (Bressler & Ball, 2003).

Practice Pearl

The rule of thumb for drug prescription in the older person is "start low; go slow." In other words, the drug should be administered at about one half the recommended adult dose, and the healthcare provider should wait twice as long as recommended in the literature before increasing the dose. This rule will help prevent toxic side effects and adverse drug reactions.

IMPACT OF CONCURRENT CONDITIONS AND THERAPY ON DRUG THERAPY

In addition to the alterations due to normal aging processes, older persons are more likely to have chronic pathological conditions that may affect responses to drugs. Only about 15% of those over the age of 65 have no disease or disability (Agency for Healthcare Research and Quality, 2001). The older person is more likely to be taking other drugs that may influence pharmacokinetics and pharmacodynamics. The increased emphasis on drugs to prevent conditions has also increased the use of medications in the absence of a pathological condition. Table 6-1 illustrates some of the alterations caused by the aging process, by pathological conditions, and by other concurrent drug therapy that may affect drug response in the older person.

TABLE 6-1

Effects of Aging and Concurrent Conditions and Other Drug Therapy on Drug Therapy

Physiological Changes of Aging	Effects on Drug Therapy	Examples of Pathological Conditions or Drugs Also Affecting Drug Therapy
Decreased gastrointestinal (GI) motility, decreased gastric acidity	Possible decreased or delayed absorption of acidic drugs; decrease in peak effect	Achlorhydria, malabsorption, diarrhea, gastric ulcers, pyloric obstruction or stenosis, pancreatitis, hypothyroidism, diabetic gastroparesis; antacids, H_2 blockers, proton pump inhibitors, anticholinergic drugs
Decrease in GI absorption surface of up to 20%	Effect on drug absorption believed to be minimal but possibly could decrease extent of absorption	
Dry mouth and secretions (xerostomia)	Difficulty in swallowing drugs	Dehydration
Decreased liver blood flow; decreased liver mass; decrease in microsomal enzymes	Delayed and decreased metabolism of certain drugs	Liver disease, fever, malignancy, congestive heart failure
Decreased lipid content in skin	Possible decrease in absorption of transdermal medications	
Increase in body fat (from 18% to 36% in men and 33% to 45% in women); decrease in body water	Possible increased toxicity of water-soluble drugs; more prolonged and possible increased effects of fat-soluble drugs	Obesity, dehydration, diuretic drugs
Decrease in serum proteins	Possible increased effect/toxicity of highly protein-bound drug; increased possibility of interactions of two or more highly protein-bound drugs	Malnutrition, burns, liver disease
Decrease in renal mass, blood flow, and glomerular filtration rate (decline of 50% between age 20 and 90, average of 35%)	Possible increased serum levels/toxicity of drugs excreted renally; NSAIDs may decrease renal blood flow and renal function	Renal insufficiency, CHF, hypovolemia, NSAIDs, use of drugs excreted by kidneys
Changes in sensitivity of certain drug receptors	Increase in drug effects: e.g., anticholinergics, antihistamines, barbiturates (paradoxical excitation), benzodiazepines, digitalis, warfarin Decrease in drug effects: e.g., amphetamines, beta-blockers, quinidine	
Visual and hearing changes	Interference with learning and/or safe administration of medications	Anticholinergic drugs (vision changes); loop diuretics, certain antibiotics (e.g., aminoglycosides) (hearing)

Source: Adapted from Eisenhauer & Murphy (Eds.), 1998. *Pharmacotherapeutics and advanced nursing practice.* New York: McGraw-Hill. Used with permission.

Drug Alert

The following drugs require special considerations for use in older patients:

1. Drugs that are widely used
2. Drugs that affect or are affected by a body system that is affected by changes of aging or disease
3. Drugs that act on the central nervous system
4. Drugs that have a low therapeutic to safety ratio and:
   a. are excreted largely by kidney
   b. are subject to large first-pass effect
   c. are metabolized by oxidative mechanisms
   d. generate significant metabolites
   e. are highly protein bound (Abrams, 1985)

ADVERSE DRUG REACTIONS AND IATROGENESIS

Adverse drug reactions (ADRs) are a particular problem in the older person. Symptoms of many adverse drug effects may be similar to those of other conditions affecting the older person and therefore may be overlooked or not attributed to the drug therapy. Difficulties in the activities of daily living may provide clues to the presence of ADRs in an older person.

Practice Pearl

Suspect an adverse drug effect if a patient has cognitive changes, falls, or experiences anorexia, nausea, or weight loss.

Older persons are more likely to have ADRs because of inappropriate drug or dosing, drug-drug interactions, polypharmacy, and noncompliance. Estimates of the occurrence of ADRs range from 3% to 69% (Herrlinger & Klotz, 2001). **Iatrogenesis** refers to harm from a therapeutic regimen. Iatrogenic risks and ADRs from drug therapy are related to age, the number of drugs taken, and complexity of pathophysiological alterations.

Various terms are used to describe drug side effects. A *side effect* is any effect other than the intended therapeutic effect; the intended therapeutic effect depends on the particular condition for which the drug is prescribed and the expected therapeutic outcome. Differences in terminology to describe side effects may reflect degrees of alteration produced. In some references, side effects are considered to be expected effects that need to be tolerated and treated only if they are bothersome to the patient or cause noncompliance. However, inability to tolerate the side effects of some drugs can result in the patient deciding not to continue to take the medication. The nurse often can assist the patient in reducing the impact of some side effects of drugs, therefore enhancing compliance. For example, promoting the adequate intake of bulk in the diet and an adequate fluid intake can help to offset drug-induced constipation. The administration of diuretics can be scheduled so that the peak diuretic effect does not interrupt activities important to the patient. Frequent intake of liquids or the use of lozenges can help with dry mouth caused by medications.

<table>
<tr><td>

BOX 6-1

Definitions of Adverse Drug Reactions or Adverse Drug Effects

- Serious adverse effects reportable to FDA MedWatch program: when the patient outcome is death, life threatening (real risk of dying), hospitalization (initial or prolonged), disability (significant, prolonged, or permanent), congenital anomaly, or required intervention to prevent permanent impairment of damage.
- A response to a medicine which is noxious and unintended, and which occurs at doses normally used in man (World Health Organization, 2002).
- Any response to a drug which is noxious and unintended, and that occurs at doses used in humans for prophylaxis, diagnosis, or therapy, excluding failure to accomplish the intended purpose.

</td></tr>
</table>

Source: Karch & Lasagna, 1975.

Adverse drug events (ADEs) or adverse drug reactions (ADRs) are terms that usually refer to drug side effects that are serious. An adverse drug event refers specifically to an injury resulting from an error in drug administration such as prescribing an incorrect dose. Definitions of an adverse drug reaction vary. Box 6-1 presents some definitions that are used.

A study of older outpatients found that more than 27% of adverse drug effects were preventable; 38% were serious, life threatening, or fatal, and 42% of these were considered to be preventable. The most common preventable adverse effects were related to cardiovascular drugs, diuretics, nonopioid analgesics, hypoglycemic agents, and anticoagulants. This study also found that drug-monitoring errors (failure to act on clinical or laboratory findings, inadequate laboratory monitoring) accounted for 60.8% of the preventable ADEs. Prescribing errors accounted for 58.4% of the preventable ADEs (Gurwitz et al., 2003).

In one study of nursing home residents, two thirds of those who experienced an ADR were taking an average of eight drugs for four conditions. The most common ADR-related hospitalizations were for gastropathy from use of nonsteroidal anti-inflammatory drugs (NSAIDs), falls from the use of psychotropics, oversedation from psychotropics, digoxin toxicity, and hypoglycemia from the use of insulin (Cooper, 2000).

Adverse drug reactions may manifest themselves differently in the older person. For example, digoxin side effects of amnesia, depression, nausea, vomiting, lethargy, confusion, and visual disturbances occur more often in older persons than in younger patients. Adverse drug effects may be mistaken for common syndromes in the older person. Falls have been associated with the use of psychotropic medications (Leipzig, 2001).

The potential for ADRs increases with increasing numbers of medications taken. There is a 6% risk of ADRs when two drugs are taken together, 50% when five drugs are taken together, and 100% when eight or more medications are taken together (Gurwitz et al., 2003). A study in nursing homes (Field et al., 2001) found those at greatest risk were those with multiple medications and those taking anti-infectives or psychoactive drugs. Older women have more adverse drug effects than men, probably due to their use of a greater number of medications or possibly because of their smaller size.

Multiple medication use by older patients is believed to be related to an estimated 51% of deaths and 32,000 hip fractures annually (Gurwitz et al., 2003). When multiple medications are used, there is a greater chance of drug-drug interactions, ADEs and ADRs, and errors of dosing (Hartford Institute for Geriatric Nursing, 1999).

Practice Pearl

Encourage the discontinuation of one drug when another is added to a drug regimen.

Drug therapy for older persons requires a careful assessment of each patient's physiological and psychosocial status, the need for the drug, and the risk of an adverse drug reaction.

REPORTING ADVERSE DRUG EFFECTS

Once the FDA releases a drug as new, there is no requirement that clinicians report side effects. However, both manufacturers and the FDA have initiated measures to encourage the reporting of suspected adverse effects of medications (drugs or biologicals), medical devices, special nutritional products, and other products regulated by the FDA. The MedWatch program provides a mechanism for the voluntary reporting of suspected problems; it is not necessary to have definitively established that the drug has caused the effect. The patient's name is held in strict confidence; the name of the person reporting the problem may be provided to the product's manufacturer unless requested otherwise.

Adverse effects that should be reported to MedWatch include serious events such as death, life-threatening events (real risk of dying), hospitalization (initial or prolonged), disability (significant, prolonged, or permanent), congenital anomaly, or required intervention to prevent permanent impairment of damage.

A copy of the MedWatch form can be found in the *Physicians' Desk Reference (PDR), FDA Drug Bulletin, AMA Drug Evaluations,* and other references. The forms also can be obtained 24 hours a day, 7 days a week by calling 800-FDA-1088 or from the FDA website.

Most patient care institutions have a system for reporting adverse drug events. Clinicians need to be aware of policies and procedures within their practice settings related to adverse drug events as well as medication errors (see Box 6-2 for a list of questions to determine if a symptom is caused by drug therapy).

MediaLink • FDA MedWatch

Determining If a Symptom Is Caused by Drug Therapy   **BOX 6-2**

The following questions may help to determine if the symptom is drug-related:

1. Is the observed symptom known to be a possible side effect of one or another drug that the patient takes?
2. Did the observed symptom develop shortly after the addition of a new drug to the regimen or a dosage increase for an existing drug in the regimen?
3. Did the observed symptom subside when a drug was discontinued or the dosage decreased?
4. Did the symptom reappear when a drug was reintroduced or the dosage increased?
5. What other factors might have led to or contributed to the observed symptom?
6. Has the patient had a similar symptom in the past in response to this drug or another one?

Source: Swonger & Burbank, 1995.

PREVENTION OF ADVERSE DRUG EFFECTS IN THE OLDER PERSON

Prevention of ADRs in the older person begins with appropriate prescribing. The most important problem to avoid is polypharmacy. The nurse may need to suggest to the prescribing clinician the possible need for reduced dosages of some medications, especially for a patient whose weight is less than average, who has decreased liver or renal function, or who is experiencing exaggerated responses to drugs that may reflect toxic levels.

The nurse has a major role in reducing the need for medications and in suggesting alternatives to their use. The nurse also should consider patient problems as having a possible basis in their drug therapy. Alternatives to the use of medications in certain circumstances are featured in Table 6-2.

Drug therapy should be used only if there is a specific diagnosis or clearly documented symptom or condition to be treated. The use of a drug to treat the side effects of another drug should be avoided. It is usually much better to change the offending drug or decrease the dose to decrease the side effects and avoid the need for another medication.

TABLE 6-2

Alternatives to Medications for Patient Problems

Medication	Patient Problem	Alternatives
Laxatives, cathartics	Constipation	Increase bulk in diet (e.g., apple, bran muffin), avoid cheese and excessive use of other calcium products (including calcium in antacids); encourage exercise, ensure adequate fluid intake.
Hypnotics	Insomnia	Suggest warm milk (contains natural tryptophan); adapt environment to promote sleep (e.g., decrease noise, light, use of music if soothing to patient). Keep patient awake and active during the day. Review medications for those producing altered sleep patterns, e.g., sedative-hypnotics, benzodiazepines, psychotropics, anxiolytics, diuretics (Giron et al., 2002).
Antacids	"Heartburn" Sour stomach	Help patient to identify foods that precipitate symptoms and avoid them; use of small frequent meals; keep in upright position for at least 30 minutes after taking oral medication.
Antianxiety agents	Anxiety	Suggest counseling, biofeedback and other stress reduction techniques, tai chi, yoga.
Analgesics	Pain	Suggest use of distraction, guided imagery, positioning (e.g., elevation of swollen limb), ice or heat, tai chi, or yoga.

Polypharmacy

Polypharmacy is defined as the prescription, administration, or use of more medications than are clinically indicated in a given patient. This can include the use of a medication that has no apparent indication, continuing use of a medication after a condition has been resolved, use of a medication to treat the side effects of another medication, use of an inappropriate dose, and use of duplicate medications because the same drug has been prescribed by more than one prescriber. Patients may not be aware of different names (e.g., generic and one or more brand names) that are used for the same medication. Polypharmacy may also occur when a patient self-medicates with OTC medications or herbal remedies to treat the same condition or to manage symptoms of an adverse drug effect. Some aspects of polypharmacy can be prevented by the use of the same pharmacy to fill all prescriptions so that the pharmacist can check for duplication or drug interactions. Patients should be encouraged to notify all prescribing clinicians about what other drugs they are taking.

Since more than one prescriber may treat a patient, the nurse should obtain a complete history of all drugs prescribed. Information about other drugs and remedies should also be elicited from the patient since they may be the basis for significant interactions with drug therapy. These include the use of vitamins, OTC medications, dietary supplements, and herbal remedies. Patients often do not think of these as medications when asked about their medication use.

ADVERSE DRUG EFFECTS OF CONCERN IN THE OLDER PERSON

Cognitive Effects

There are several adverse drug effects that are of particular concern to the older population. Cognitive impairment (e.g., delirium, dementia, depression) can be caused by a variety of medications. Delirium may be caused by drugs (including psychotropic medications) with anticholinergic effects. Changes in mood such as anxiety and depression can result from many types of drug therapy, such as antihypertensives (e.g., beta-blockers), antiparkinsonian agents, steroids, NSAIDs, narcotic analgesics, antineoplastic agents, central nervous system (CNS) depressants, and psychotropics (e.g., alcohol, benzodiazepines, and other antianxiety agents).

Cognitive changes from medications can lead clinicians to misinterpret these signs and possibly prescribe unnecessary medication to counteract them.

Cognitive changes also may interfere with the clinician's ability to accurately assess the patient. This might occur if patients are unable to describe symptoms such as the location or degree of any pain they may be experiencing, to request prn medications, or to describe side effects or changes in their well-being. Alterations in cognitive function can interfere with the patient's ability to manage the medication regimen as well as posing additional dangers to level of functioning and quality of life (Eisenhauer & Murphy, 1998).

Anticholinergic Syndrome

The use of drugs with anticholinergic effects presents a particular problem with the older person. This includes drugs classified as anticholinergics (e.g., atropine) as well as drugs in many pharmacological classifications that have anticholinergic side effects.

Many of the drug-related anticholinergic effects—both central and peripheral—can aggravate other conditions being experienced by the older person. Central anticholinergic effects include agitation, confusion, disorientation, poor attention, hallucinations, or psychosis. Peripheral effects include constipation, urinary retention, inhibition of sweating, decreased salivary and bronchial secretions, tachycardia, and mydriasis. Individuals with benign prostatic hypertrophy or other strictures of the urinary urethra may experience increased difficulty in initiating urine flow. Dryness of the mouth can slow the absorption of sublingual medications and may affect the ability to swallow

---

BOX 6-3	**Heuristic for Remembering Anticholinergic Effects**

Dry as a bone	Inhibition of secretions
Red as a beet	Flushing related to absence of sweating
Hot as a hare	Temperature elevation from absence of sweating
Blind as a bat	Cycloplegia and mydriasis
Mad as a hatter	Mental confusion, delirium

---

oral preparations. Drugs with anticholinergic effects may also affect vision. Anticholinergic effects on cardiac function may alter cardiovascular drug effects or lead to the possibly unnecessary prescription of cardiovascular drug therapy.

Atropine, a common medication given preoperatively to dry up secretions and prevent aspiration while the patient is under anesthesia, is often associated with anticholinergic side effects. These side effects include bradycardia, dry mouth, decreased sweating, tachycardia, dilated pupils, blurred near vision, decreased intestinal peristalsis, dysphasia, dysphagia, urinary retention, hyperthermia and flushing, ataxia, hallucinations, delirium, and coma. The risk of these side effects increases directly in response to increasing doses of the drug. The nurse should carefully observe older patients receiving large doses of these medications for extended periods of time and report any ADEs to the physician (Eisenhauer & Murphy, 1998). A useful heuristic to remember anticholinergic effects is in Box 6-3.

Since drugs with anticholinergic effects are also commonly found in frequently prescribed medications (including antidepressants, antihistamines, antiparkinsonian agents, antipsychotics, and quinidine), the nurse should check each drug for its anticholinergic profile. All drugs within a pharmacological classification may differ in the severity of their anticholinergic effects; therefore, a drug from a different class of medications or a different drug within the same class might be chosen for having less anticholinergic effects.

Gastric and Esophageal Irritation

Oral drugs that are swallowed but do not reach the stomach can result in esophageal obstruction or irritation of the esophageal lining. For example, it is important that enough water be taken with psyllium seed preparation (used to provide bulk to prevent constipation) to ensure that the medication reaches the stomach and does not swell in the esophagus and cause an obstruction. Box 6-4 provides strategies to prevent esophageal irritation from orally administered medications.

Gastric irritation can be caused by a variety of medications. This can lead to not only discomfort ("heartburn") but also gastric bleeding, which could be life threatening. Some drugs that have this effect are produced with an enteric coating that prevents the drug from dissolving until it reaches the alkaline environment in the duodenum. The coating of enteric-coated drugs (e.g., enteric-coated aspirin, erythromycin, oral bisacodyl tablets) may break down prematurely in the stomach if given with other drugs or foods that make the stomach alkaline; therefore, calcium, dairy products, and antacid should not be given with enteric-coated preparations or within 2 hours.

Commonly used medications of concern are aspirin and NSAIDs. These drugs not only cause irritation, but also block prostaglandin synthesis, which decreases resistance of the stomach lining to acid and other stomach contents. Additional effects of prostaglandin in-

---

Preventing Esophageal Irritation From Drug Therapy

BOX
6-4

- Patient should take medication while in an upright position and should remain upright for at least 30 minutes.
- Patient should swallow several sips of water to lubricate the throat and esophagus before taking the medication.
- Patient should not divide or break up tablets or capsules without consulting the pharmacist since some drugs may be enteric coated or compounded as a sustained-release preparation; breaking them apart could result in toxicity as more of the drug becomes immediately available for absorption.
- Patient should swallow medications one at a time with at least 8 oz of liquid.
- A dull aching pain in chest or shoulder after taking medication should be reported to the physician.
- A patient who has gastroesophageal reflux disorder should avoid use of medications that relax the lower esophageal sphincter and therefore would increase the reflux of stomach contents into the esophagus.

---

hibition include slowing of blood clotting, therefore increasing the danger of gastric bleeding from these drugs. Box 6-5 lists warning signs of NSAID-induced gastric irritation. However, gastric bleeding in an older person may occur with little or no prior symptoms.

Loss of appetite, nausea, and weight loss may be the result of drug therapy. Drugs that decrease peristalsis can cause decreased appetite. Nausea and loss of appetite may indicate toxic levels of drugs.

Warning Signs of NSAID-Induced Gastric Irritation*

BOX
6-5

- "Heartburn"
- Burning sensation in stomach or back
- Blood in stool or positive test for occult blood
- Bloody vomit
- Diarrhea

---

*In older adults, bleeding from NSAID-induced gastric irritation may occur with no warning signs.
Source: Adapted from Tolsoi, (2002).

Alternative and Complementary Medicine

Increasingly, people of all ages are using alternative or complementary medicine such as homeopathic and herbal medicines in addition to their routine medications. Homeopathic medications are well diluted and are not believed to interact with medications. Certain prescription medications (e.g., NSAIDs, antiulcer, and some pain medications), however, are considered by homeopathic practitioners to counteract the effectiveness of some homeopathic medicines. Herbal medicines have widespread use and availability today.

An estimated 30% of those over the age of 65 use at least one alternative medicine modality. Most commonly used are chiropractic (11%), herbal medicines (8%), high-dose or megavitamins (5%), and spiritual or religious healing (4%). Of concern is that most patients do not inform their physician about their use of alternative therapies (Foster, Phillips,

Hamel, & Eisenberg, 2000). The most common conditions for which patients use alternative medicine modalities are arthritis, back pain, heart disease, allergy, and diabetes. Therefore, it is especially important to ask patients with these conditions about their use of herbal medicines, vitamins, or food supplements.

Because the FDA does not regulate herbal medicines, there is no assurance or standardization of their ingredients, purity, dosage, potency, and so on. For most, there have not been sufficient clinical trials to demonstrate their effectiveness or appropriate dosage. Adverse effects may result from the herb itself as well as from contaminants in the preparation.

Herbs do interact with medications. Therefore, it is important to elicit from patients any herbs, home remedies, or dietary supplements that they take. If patients are to have anesthesia, it is important that they notify the anesthetist of what herbal remedies they have been using. Some herbs such as ginseng and ginkgo can inhibit platelet aggregation and increase bleeding time. Therefore, these drugs should be discontinued for several days before the anesthesia is given or surgery is scheduled. Table 6-3 highlights the uses and drug therapy concerns of some commonly used herbs.

TABLE 6-3

Common Herbal Preparations and Interactions With Drugs

Herbal Preparation	Use	Interactions/Precautions
Echinacea	Stimulation of immunity.	Counteracts effects of immunosuppressive drugs (e.g., cyclosporine).
Ephedra (ma huang) (no longer available in U.S.)	Promotion of weight loss, increasing energy, treatment of respiratory condition.	Sympathomimetic effects can cause elevated blood pressure, stroke, and death.
Garlic	Reducing risk of atherosclerosis by decreasing blood pressure, thrombin formation, and lipid and cholesterol levels.	Inhibits platelet aggregation and potentiates effects of platelet inhibitor drugs (e.g., indomethacin, dipyridamole).
Ginseng	Protection against effects of stress, helps to restore homeostasis.	Can cause bleeding problems and hypoglycemia.
Ginkgo	Enhancement of cognitive performance, treatment of peripheral vascular disease, age-related macular degeneration, vertigo, tinnitus, erectile dysfunction, altitude sickness.	Inhibits platelet-activating factor and can cause bleeding.
Kava	Anxiolytic and sedative.	Causes excessive sedation when used with other CNS depressants.
St. John's wort	Treatment of mild to moderate depression.	May cause excess levels of serotonin if taken with selective serotonin reuptake inhibitors (SSRIs). Can increase the metabolism of many drugs, resulting in reduced effectiveness.
Valerian	Sedative, hypnotic.	Withdrawal from valerian mimics acute benzodiazepine withdrawal syndrome. Potentiates sedative effects of barbiturates and anesthetics and anesthetic adjuvants.

Source: Adapted from Ang-Lee, Moss, & Yuan, 2001. Used with permission of the American Medical Association.

OVER-THE-COUNTER MEDICATIONS

Increasingly, more medications are being approved by the FDA for OTC use, allowing patients access to these drugs without a prescription. Although this provides easier access, it can increase the possibility of inappropriate medication use by the patient. There could be an increased risk of drug interactions with prescribed medications or overdosage by the use of an OTC drug identical or similar to a prescribed drug. The use of an OTC drug can result in increased out-of-pocket costs to patients since health insurance usually does not pay for OTC medications. An additional concern is that self-medication with OTC drugs may delay the timely medical diagnosis and prescription of more appropriate and effective therapy.

Patients' use of alcohol should be carefully assessed since alcohol is a CNS depressant, may cause gastric irritation, and interferes with the metabolism of certain medications such as acetaminophen. Ingestion of too much alcohol and acetaminophen can result in liver damage. Patients should be cautioned to use nonprescription drugs cautiously; some patients may think that these drugs are completely safe and that they can take as much as they want.

Table 6-4 provides examples of some common OTC drugs that can be associated with adverse drug effects if used inappropriately.

APPROPRIATE VERSUS INAPPROPRIATE PRESCRIBING PRACTICES

Inappropriate prescribing practices often are the basis for adverse drug effects in the older person. Appropriate prescribing may be defined as follows:

- The selection of a medication and instruction for its use that agree with accepted medical standards
- Use of appropriate dose and scheduling guidelines
- Agreement of the manufacturer's standards and FDA labeling guidelines, standard medication references, and interpretation of the scientific literature by drug therapy experts (Schmader et al., 1994)

A study of older adults living in the community showed that 23.5% over 65 (equivalent to 6.64 million Americans) were taking at least one of 20 drugs contraindicated for use in the older person; 20.4% were receiving two or more of these potentially harmful drugs (Willcox, Himmelstein, & Woolhandler, 1994). A more recent study showed similar results of 3% to 21% using a drug of concern (Curtis et al., 2004). Amitriptyline and doxepin accounted for 33% of the drugs of concern.

A study of nursing home residents found that 40% received at least one inappropriate medication. Inappropriate medications administered to these residents included prescriptions for drugs that should be avoided in the older person (e.g., long-acting benzodiazepines, dipyridamole, propoxyphene); long-term use of drugs that are to be used for short-term use only (e.g., histamine blockers, short-acting benzodiazepines, oral antibiotics); or high doses of drugs prescribed above dosage limitations (e.g., iron supplements, histamine blockers, antipsychotic agents) (Beers, Ouslander, Rollingher, Reuben, & Beck, 1991).

One of the most commonly used consensus criteria related to inappropriate medications in the older person is the "Beers criteria." These criteria, developed in 1997, were adopted in 1999 by the Centers for Medicare and Medicaid Services for the

TABLE 6-4

Examples of Interaction of OTC Drugs With Prescribed Medications

OTC Drug	Interactions
Acetaminophen	Inhibits liver metabolism of warfarin leading to an increase in the INR. Limit to six or fewer regular-strength tablets per week unless INR is carefully monitored or if stable dose of acetaminophen is taken and warfarin dose is regulated while taking steady doses of warfarin. Alert patient to other OTC or prescription medications (e.g., Percocet) that may contain acetaminophen as an ingredient. Alcohol can cause increased production of toxic acetaminophen metabolites that can result in irreversible liver damage. FDA-mandated labeling cautions against use of acetaminophen if a person takes three or more alcoholic drinks per day.
Alcohol	Pressor effects can increase blood pressure if a person takes more than 1 oz alcohol per day (the amount of alcohol in 2 oz whiskey, 8 oz wine, or 24 oz beer) (Neafsey & Shellman, 2001). The risk of gastric irritation and bleeding is increased when alcohol is consumed with NSAIDs; use of antacids may increase this risk even more. Bioavailability of alcohol is increased by the use of aspirin and H_2 antagonists within 2 hours due to inhibition of gastric alcohol dehydrogenase and more rapid gastric emptying.
Antacids and calcium supplements	Can cause premature dissolution of enteric-coated preparations (e.g., enteric-coated aspirin, erythromycin), resulting in premature dissolution of drug in the stomach and increased risk of gastric irritation. Should be taken 2 hours before or after these medications. Also can interfere with the absorption of ciprofloxacin, digoxin, levothyroxine, phenytoin, tetracyclines, thiamine, vitamin B_{12}, and zinc.
Cimetidine	Inhibits microsomal enzymes, which could result in higher than usual levels of other drugs whose metabolism is regulated by the microsomal enzymes.
Decongestants	Have pressor effects and may increase blood pressure and/or counteract effect of antihypertensives. Alert patient to decongestants to avoid in cough or cold remedies (e.g., pseudoephedrine, phenylpropanolamine).
NSAIDs (e.g., aspirin, ibuprofen)	May cause renal failure in individuals with decreased glomerular flow and pressure (e.g., age-related renal failure, heart failure, volume depletion from diuretics) (Neafsey & Shellman, 2001).
Vitamin A	May interfere with absorption of calcium.
Vitamin E	Doses above 400 IU per day may inhibit vitamin K synthesis and mimic warfarin activity. Lower doses (e.g., 100 IU) inhibit platelet aggregation in a manner similar to low-dose aspirin (Neafsey & Shellman, 2001).
Vitamin C	High doses acidify the urine and can affect the excretion of other medications.

regulation of nursing homes. These criteria have been updated recently by another consensus study (Fick et al., 2003), resulting in additions and deletions from the original list. Drugs added to the list independent of diagnoses of the patient include the following: ketorolac tromethamine, orphenadrine, guanethidine, guanadrel, cyclandelate, isoxsuprine, nitrofurantoin, doxazosin, methyltestosterone, mesoridazine, clonidine, mineral oil, cimetidine, ethacrynic acid, desiccated thyroid, ferrous sulfate, certain amphetamines, thioridazine, short-acting nifedipine, daily fluoxetine, stimulant laxatives, amiodarone, NSAIDs (naproxen, oxaprozin, piroxicam), reserpine (0.25 mg/d), and estrogens in older women. The 2003 criteria also indicate drugs that are inappropriate to use in patients with certain medical conditions. Table 6-5 lists drugs that are considered inappropriate to use in the older person based on the 1997 Beers criteria.

Drug Category	Drug
Analgesics:	meperidine, propoxyphene, pentazocine
Analgesics-NSAIDs:	indomethacin, phenylbutazone*
Antiarrhythmic:	disopyramide
Antidepressants:	amitriptyline and combinations, doxepin
Antihistamines:	chlorpheniramine, cyproheptadine, dexchlorpheniramine, diphenhydramine, hydroxyzine, promethazine, tripelennamine
Antihypertensives:	methyldopa or combinations, reserpine and combinations
Antiemetics:	trimethobenzamide
Dementia drugs:	ergoloid mesylates, cyclospasmol
Gastrointestinal antispasmodics:	belladonna alkaloids, dicyclomine, hyoscyamine, propantheline
Muscle relaxants/ antispasmodics:	carisoprodol, chlorzoxazone, metaxalone, methocarbamol
Oral hypoglycemics:	chlorpropamide
Platelet inhibitors:	dipyridamole, ticlopidine
Sedatives and hypnotics:	diazepam, chlordiazepoxide and combinations, flurazepam, meprobamate, all barbiturates (except pentobarbital)

TABLE 6-5

Drugs Inappropriate For Use in Older Patients Regardless of Dose, Duration, or Disease Condition

*Deleted from 2003 consensus criteria.

Source: Beers et al., 1991. Used with permission of the American Medical Association.

Appropriate Use of Psychotropics in the Older Person

The 1987 Omnibus Budget Reconciliation Act (OBRA 87) legislated the appropriate use of medications in institutionalized older persons, especially as their use may constitute chemical restraint, which is an important ethical, clinical, and regulatory concern.

OBRA 87 established guidelines for the appropriate use of psychotropic drugs in long-term care facilities. The guidelines can provide guidance to other clinicians prescribing for older persons in any setting. Similar regulations and monitoring of prescribing patterns and drug use also occurred as a result of Drug Use Review programs mandated by the 1990 OBRA (Eisenhauer & Murphy, 1998).

OBRA REGULATIONS AND INTERPRETIVE GUIDELINES

The following are provisions of OBRA 87 regulations as refined by OBRA 91 (Department of Health and Human Services, 2001):

- **Chemical restraint:** the use of a drug to control an individual's behavior and is legally permissible only to ensure the physical safety of residents or other individuals.
- **Unnecessary drug:** any drug when used in excessive dose (including duplicate therapy), or for excessive duration; or without adequate monitoring; or without adequate indication for its use; or in the presence of adverse consequences which indicate the dose should be reduced or discontinued; or without specific target symptoms.

USE OF ANTIPSYCHOTIC DRUGS

The facility must ensure that residents who have not used antipsychotic drugs are not given these drugs unless antipsychotic drug therapy is necessary to treat a specific condition, as diagnosed and documented in the clinical record. Residents who use antipsychotic drugs must receive gradual dose reductions, drug holidays, or behavioral programming, unless clinically contraindicated, in an effort to discontinue these drugs.

As-needed (prn) doses of neuroleptics are not to be used more than twice in a 7-day period without further assessment and are to be used only for the purpose of titrating dosage for optimal response or for management of unexpected behaviors that are otherwise unmanageable.

Conditions that are considered to be inappropriate as the sole basis for the use of antipsychotic drugs are wandering, poor self-care, restlessness, impaired memory, anxiety, depression (without psychotic features), insomnia, unsociability, indifference to surroundings, fidgeting, nervousness, uncooperativeness, or agitated behaviors that do not represent danger to the resident or others.

Long-acting benzodiazepines are strictly regulated and should not be used unless:

- There has been an attempt to use a shorter acting drug.
- The possible reasons for a resident's distress have been carefully assessed and treated if at all possible. For instance, a resident may be agitated because he or she is constipated and is experiencing abdominal pain and rectal pressure. It would be inappropriate to use an antianxiety agent in this situation. It would be much more appropriate to relieve the resident's constipation by use of increased fluids and laxatives and thus relieve the root cause of the anxiety rather than just treating the symptoms.
- The use of a long-acting agent results in maintenance or improvement in the resident's functional status.
- Daily use is less than 4 continuous months, and an attempt at gradual dose reduction has been tried without success.
- Daily use is less than or equal to the total daily doses in Table 6-6. If higher doses (as evidenced by the resident's response or the resident's clinical record) are necessary for the maintenance of or improvement in the resident's functional status, they may be cautiously used with the reasons documented in the medical record by the prescribing physician or advanced practice nurse.

TABLE 6-6

Maximum Daily Doses of Long-Acting Benzodiazepines

Generic Name	Brand Name	Maximum DAILY Oral Dosage
Chlordiazepoxide	Librium	20 mg
Clorazepate	Tranxene	15 mg
Clonazepam	Klonopin	1.5 mg
Diazepam	Valium	5 mg
Flurazepam	Dalmane	15 mg
Prazepam	Centrax	15 mg
Quazepam	Doral	7.5 mg

Generic Name	Brand Name	Maximum DAILY Oral Dosage for Elderly Residents
Short-Acting Benzodiazepines		
Alprazolam	Xanax	0.75 mg
Halazepam	Paxipam	40 mg
Lorazepam	Ativan	2 mg
Oxazepam	Serax	30 mg
Other Anxiolytics		
Buspirone	BuSpar	30 mg
Chloral hydrate	Many brands	40 mg
Diphenhydramine	Benadryl	50 mg
Hydroxyzine	Atarax, Vistaril	50 mg

TABLE 6-7

Maximum Daily Dosage of Anxiolytics in Elderly Residents

SHORT-ACTING BENZODIAZEPINES AND OTHER ANXIOLYTICS

OBRA 87 also regulated the use of short-acting benzodiazepines and other anxiolytics in residents of long-term care facilities.

Use of the anxiolytic drugs listed in Table 6-7 for purposes other than sleep induction should only occur when (1) evidence exists that other possible reasons for the resident's distress have been considered and ruled out; (2) use results in a maintenance or improvement in the resident's functional status; (3) daily use (at any dose) is less than 4 continuous months unless an attempt at gradual dose reduction is unsuccessful; (4) use is for one of the following indications as defined by the *Diagnostic and Statistical Manual of Mental Disorders,* 3rd ed. *(DSM-III)* or subsequent editions: generalized anxiety disorder, organic mental syndromes (including dementia) with associated states that are quantitatively and objectively documented and that constitute sources of distress or dysfunction of the resident or represent danger to the resident or others, panic disorder, or symptomatic anxiety that occurs in residents with another diagnosed psychiatric disorder (e.g., depression, adjustment disorder); and (5) use is equal to or less than following the listed total daily doses, unless higher doses as evidenced by the resident response or the resident's functional status.

Daily use of both long- and short-acting benzodiazepines should be limited to less than 4 continuous months unless an attempt at gradual dose reduction is unsuccessful; dose reductions should be considered after 4 months of continuous use.

EVALUATING APPROPRIATE PRESCRIBING OF MEDICATIONS

The following questions can guide the clinician in reviewing appropriateness of drug use and could help to assess compliance with OBRA 87 regulations:

1. Is the condition sufficiently problematic to require treatment?
2. Are there nursing or other nonpharmacological treatments that could alleviate the condition, prevent or delay use of a medication, or complement drug therapy?

3. If a drug is indicated for treatment of a specific condition, is the need for the medication documented in the medical record (e.g., an established or working diagnosis for which the drug is approved)?
4. Has informed consent for prescription been obtained from the patient or legally determined surrogate decision maker?
5. Is the prescription likely to be effective in achieving the prescriber's preset goals for therapy (i.e., objective measures of signs or symptoms)?
6. How long should the drug be used before decreasing dosage or discontinuing it? Will this be at a specific time or based on a change in the patient's condition?
7. Is there duplication of the specific drug with other drugs the patient is taking or overlap of therapeutic or adverse effects of other drugs being taken?
8. Are the dose and timing correct? Is the drug being administered correctly?
9. Are there potential drug-drug, drug-disease, or drug-nutritional interactions?
10. Is the patient being adequately monitored for common serious side effects (e.g., periodic blood levels, functional and mental status tests, movement disorder scales)?
11. If side effects are present, is there a positive balance of the risks and benefits? Are the negative effects of treatment outweighed by the positive aspects (e.g., improving, maintaining, or slowing decline of resident function or alleviating suffering)?

Practice Pearl

Before administering any medication to an older person, it is important to undertake a risk-benefit analysis. In consultation with the physician, patient, and family, the nurse should discuss the risks versus the benefit of the medication. If the risks are perceived to be too great, a nonpharmacological approach to the patient's problem should be considered.

Promoting Adherence and Compliance

Compliance with a prescribed regimen presumably leads to better patient outcomes. Noncompliance with medication regimens results in considerable costs to patients, employers, health insurers, and the healthcare system. Estimates of noncompliance range from 40% to 75%, depending on the definition of noncompliance used in the studies. It is estimated that 10% of hospital admissions are the result of medication nonadherence (Schlenk, Dunbar-Jacobs, & Engberg, 2004).

The nurse can be instrumental in promoting compliance and appropriate management of drug therapy by older patients or their caregivers in the home. Michaud (1996) found that community-dwelling older adults engaged in "intelligent noncompliance." These patients reduced their medication dosage or discontinued a drug when they experienced side effects that were bothersome or that they felt their prescriber did not address.

The use of the term *noncompliance* is objectionable to some patients and clinicians since it implies a patient must surrender to the orders of the clinician. Some prefer the term *adherence.* The following nursing diagnoses are useful for describing situations requiring nursing intervention to promote the effective use of medications by patients: *noncompliance (specify); therapeutic regimen management, effective; therapeutic regimen management, ineffective;* or *therapeutic regimen management, readiness for enhanced.*

The higher number of drugs usually prescribed for older persons makes drug regimens more complex. Cognitive changes resulting from aging processes, pathophysiological alterations, or drug therapy need to be carefully assessed (initially and on an ongoing basis) to determine if the patient is able to understand and remember instructions. Physical limitations may affect the patient's ability to open medication vials and packaging or to administer certain types of medications (Eisenhauer & Murphy, 1998).

Various levels of cognitive and physical skills are needed by the older person to safely take medications as prescribed. Depending on the drug and route of administration, the nurse should assess the following factors:

- Ability to read and comprehend main label (prescription)
- Ability to read and comprehend the auxiliary labels (e.g., warnings)
- Manual dexterity (open vials, remove correct number of tablets, recap medication) (Hartford Institute for Geriatric Nursing, 1999)

In a small study of frail older persons, more than 50% of both Hispanic and Anglo patients reported difficulty in reading drug labels, which were written in English (Lile & Hoffman, 1991). Additionally, the more complicated the dosing regimen, the more pills taken daily, and the more often pills must be taken, the greater the chance of error and adverse drug reactions (Gurwitz et al., 2003).

There have been efforts to develop measures to predict patients' capacity to comply with medications. The Regimen Adherence Capacity Tests (RACT) have been studied to determine their validity. It was found that while the Folstein Mini-Mental State Examination (MMSE) correlated fairly well with the RACT scores, it had less than desirable sensitivity and specificity and there would not be a good surrogate test for predicting capacity to comply (Fitten, Coleman, Siembieda, Yu, & Ganzell, 1995). Box 6-6 presents useful strategies for enhancing the older patient's compliance.

Measures to help older persons manage their medications correctly include:

- Simplifying the regimen by decreasing, to the extent possible, the number of drugs and the number of pills to be taken in a day.
- Establishing a routine for taking medications, such as preparing medications for the day in different containers.
- Scheduling medications at mealtime or in conjunction with other specific daily activities (e.g., before brushing teeth at night or before leaving for a daily activity such

---

BOX 6-6

Strategies for Enhancing Compliance

Enabling strategies: to prepare patient to be compliant
   Examples: counseling, patient education, simplifying regimens, increasing access to medical care and to prescriptions, prescription of less costly therapies

Consequence strategies: to reinforce compliant behavior
   Examples: teaching patients to maintain records of medication taking and rewards for compliance

Stimulant strategies: to prompt pill taking
   Examples: tailoring doses to daily rituals, use of reminder cards in prominent places in home, home visits to reinforce compliance, use of special drug package to help organize and prompt patient to take medications, medication reminder systems (e.g., phone calls, e-mail reminders)

Source: Adapted from McKinney, Munroe, & Wright (1992).

as exercise or card playing) unless contraindicated. When teaching a patient to take medications in relation to meals, it is important to determine if the patient does indeed have three meals a day and at what time of day to be sure the medication will be taken at the intended time interval.

■ Developing a method with the patient for remembering if he or she actually took the medication (e.g., moving the medication to another place).

■ Conducting a total assessment of all medications by asking the patient to bring in all medications he or she has at home, including OTC preparations. These can be checked for outdated preparations, unused or unfinished prescriptions, overlap, or duplication of medications.

■ Considering the use of telephone reminders (Fulmer et al., 1999) or computer-based or e-mail reminders.

Careful instruction should be given, providing written instructions in the language and at a reading level the patient can understand. An audiotape could be used for patients with visual impairments. Materials should be written at the fifth-grade level or lower. Instructions should include what adverse effects should be reported and to whom as well as what to do if a dose is missed. If possible, a family member or home caregiver should also receive instructions. An excellent resource for both clinicians and patients is the *USP Dispensing Information* (volume I for clinicians; volume II for patients). These publications identify signs and symptoms that should be reported immediately to a healthcare provider and those that do not need to be reported unless they are troublesome to the patient. This resource also indicates what to do if a dose is missed.

The U.S. Pharmacopeia (USP) website has a useful typology of medication counseling behaviors.

Encouraging patients to obtain all of their medications (prescription and OTC) from the same pharmacy will help the pharmacist to monitor medication use. Patients can request that prescribed drugs be dispensed without the childproof packaging or caps. However, one needs to consider possible dangers to children who might visit the patient's home.

It is important to determine any financial restraints that may affect the patient's ability to actually obtain the medication. Less expensive mail-order options may be available. Some states and the federal government may provide assistance to some older persons with high medication expenses. As of 2006, Medicare will offer prescription drug plans that can reduce the costs of prescription medications; individuals below certain income levels will not have to pay premiums or deductibles. For updated information, go to the Medicare Prescription Drug Plan website.

Practice Pearl

If a medication does not seem to be having the expected therapeutic effect in a patient, the nurse should investigate carefully. The patient may not be taking the medication at all or as prescribed because of cost and may be embarrassed to share this information.

In a poll conducted by the Associated Press, 33% of older persons stated they had trouble paying for prescription drugs. Many had to put off filling prescriptions because they could not afford the cost. Others stated that they had illegally purchased medications on the Internet or from foreign countries to obtain a better price (Institute for Safe Medication Practices, 2003). While these alternatives may work for some, drugs obtained via the Internet often are not safe. Many are counterfeit and contain little if any of the active ingredients found in the legitimate drug. When the nurse suspects that the older patient is not taking medications as prescribed because of financial difficulties, it is suggested that the following steps be initiated:

- Assess the patient's financial situation. It is not necessary to know the actual income of a patient, but rather ask questions such as, "Do you have enough money to buy food and medicine without difficulty? Do you sometimes put off refilling your medicine because of lack of money?"
- Consult with the physician and pharmacist to see if a generic brand of the medication or lower cost drug is an option.
- Seek advice from the geriatric social worker who may be aware of government-sponsored, pharmaceutical company–sponsored, and private patient assistance programs. Many of these programs offer medications at low cost, no cost, or significant discounts.

Practice Pearl

The nurse should inform older patients and families that medications bought on the Internet or illegally imported from other countries may be counterfeit, expired, or contaminated. Although credentialed Canadian pharmacies are generally safe, there are many bogus providers victimizing older Americans. These illegal drugs may cause more harm than good.

Some patients may experience difficulty in physically obtaining the prescriptions, especially if they are on multiple medications with frequent and different dates for refill. Coordination of refills with the prescribing clinician and the pharmacist may help to alleviate stress on the patient and family as well as help to ensure that the patient has an adequate supply of medications.

Assessing Older Patients' Appropriate Use of Medications

Nurses should assess the medications used by older patients in all settings: acute care, long-term care, or at home. Assessment of drug effects is a nursing responsibility whether or not the nurse administers medications to the patient. The nurse should follow these guidelines:

1. Review the patient's medical conditions and allergies. Ask about the use of grapefruit juice since this can dramatically increase the absorption of some medications. Ask for details about an allergy: "What happened when you took this drug?" Sometimes the patient uses the word *allergy* to describe an intolerance such as upset stomach. Be sure the patient's records have appropriate alerts warning of any allergies. Check patients for MedicAlert jewelry or cards indicating that they are taking certain medications or have certain allergies.
2. Review each drug. If patients are living at home, have them assemble all medications for review whether prescribed or OTC, including vitamins and herbal remedies. This is sometimes called a "brown bag" review because patients often bring their medications in a brown bag.
   a. Has it been prescribed? If not prescribed, does the physician prescribing other drugs for the patient know the patient is taking this OTC or herbal preparation? When was it prescribed? Has continued need for it been reviewed by the physician?

b. Is the drug considered to be inappropriate for use in older persons?

c. Is the patient taking it as prescribed: dose, route, frequency and timing in relation to food or other medications, method (e.g., with fluid or food), and duration?

d. Is the medication producing the intended therapeutic effect? Are appropriate observations or laboratory tests being used to determine this and are they documented in the patient record (e.g., blood pressure readings to evaluate effects of antihypertensives)?

e. Is the medication outdated? Is it being stored properly (e.g., refrigerated, away from sunlight or heat, away from reach of small children)?

f. Does the patient understand what condition the drug is treating and the signs and symptoms that should be reported to a physician immediately?

g. Does the patient have any cognitive or physical condition affecting the ability to safely administer the medication (i.e., remembering to take the medication, ability to read labels, ability to physically handle the medication and administer)?

h. Does the patient have financial resources for the costs of the medication? Is there a generic version of this drug (or another that is equally effective for the patient's condition) available that would be less expensive? Is the patient able to manage the obtaining and renewal of prescriptions?

i. Does the patient have any cultural or ethnic beliefs or practices that might impact compliance? A person from a culture that believes in balancing "hot" and "cold" or yin and yang may not take certain prescribed medications that do not fit these beliefs. Sometimes a different medication or another brand of the same medication is acceptable.

j. Does the patient have a family member or friend who can help with medication management on a regular basis if needed (e.g., if the patient becomes ill)?

k. Review each drug for:
   Interactions with other drugs.
   Interactions with herbal medicines.
   Interactions with vitamins or foods.
   Allergies.
   Duplicate therapy (from more than one prescriber or from patient's use of OTC medications containing the same or similar ingredients as prescribed medications).

Medication Management

The nurse has a major role in promoting the safe and effective management of medications, whether the patient is at home or in an institutional setting. This includes the correct storage, preparation, and administration (right patient, right drug, right dose, right route, and right time). The nurse also is responsible for promoting the intended therapeutic effect or reducing or eliminating the need for the medication (see examples in Table 6-2). It is also important to document indications that the therapeutic effect is or is not being achieved. Examples would be reduction of fever in a patient receiving anti-infectives or decrease in blood pressure in a patient receiving antihypertensives.

Monitoring for adverse effects is another important role. This includes observation of the patient for known adverse effects of a medication as well as more general symptoms that might be drug-related (e.g., nausea, loss of appetite, cognitive changes).

Monitoring laboratory tests such as potassium levels in patients receiving thiazide diuretics or international normalized ratio (INR) in patients on warfarin therapy is another important role. Prevention of adverse drug effects involves checking the patient's history for allergies and using knowledge of drug pharmacology to detect potential or actual interactions or contraindications.

In institutional settings, additional precautions are necessary to ensure the safe administration of medications. Institutional policies and practices need to be reviewed periodically to reduce medication errors. If patients are allowed to administer their own medications, policies should be in place that reflect applicable state laws and provide protection for patients. Computerized drug prescribing and the use of bar coding on medications is becoming the standard for reducing medication errors. Medication labels have bar codes similar to those used in grocery stores. When administering the drug, the nurse scans both the patient ID bracelet and the drug label. The computer then determines if the matches are correct in light of the physician's orders.

Identification of patients by ID bracelets is important, especially with older persons who may have hearing or cognitive deficits, and may not respond appropriately to their name being called.

Perhaps most important in any setting is to have an understanding of the older person's unique patterns of behavior and physiological functions so that the nurse can detect unusual responses that might result in the need to initiate or discontinue a medication.

HEALTHCARE FRAUD

Healthcare fraud is a major problem for the older person. Because many older persons have chronic conditions such as arthritis and cancer, they are more likely to be susceptible to claims of unproven remedies. In addition to wasting money, unproven remedies pose two major dangers: (1) from the preparation itself, which may be impure, toxic, or incompatible with the patient and ongoing therapy; and (2) from delay in or rejection of accurate diagnosis and treatment.

Clinicians should be able to answer questions patients may have about health products advertised in the media. They can provide guidelines to patients about how to evaluate claims. Some red flags to watch for include: celebrity endorsements, inadequate labeling, claims that the product works by secret formula, and promotion of the treatment only in the back pages of magazines, over the phone, by direct mail, in newspaper ads in the format of news stories, or in 30-minute infomercials (Kurtzweil, 1999). Other clues are claims that a product is all natural or effective for a wide variety of disorders (e.g., cancer, arthritis, and sexual dysfunction), or that it works immediately or completely, making visits to the doctor unnecessary.

COSTS OF MEDICATION

Medications can be costly for the older person. This is a major issue in healthcare. Some health insurance plans provide drug benefits; some states may help older persons with limited means to obtain prescription medications. Suggestions to patients to reduce costs of medications include the following:

- Ask the physician if the drug is really necessary or if there is a less expensive substitute.
- Ask the physician about free samples.
- Do not order large amounts of newly prescribed medications until you know that it is effective and that you can tolerate it.
- Ask if there is a generic version of the medication.

- Contact different pharmacies; shop around.
- Ask the pharmacist about store-brand substitutes for more expensive brand-name OTC medications.
- Ask for senior citizen discounts.
- Contact AARP or disease organizations for information about drugs that might be available at a discount.
- Go to the BenefitsCheckUpRx website at the National Council on the Aging to determine eligibility for help from community, state, or federal programs, or from drug companies.
- Try mail-order prescriptions.
- Try Internet pharmacies (see the following cautions).

USE OF INTERNET PHARMACIES

Medications can be purchased online from legitimate pharmacies. However, some Websites may be risky. Sites should require a prescription from a prescriber who is familiar with the patient and should have policies for verifying prescriptions. They also should have policies that ensure privacy and confidentiality. The legitimacy of a pharmacy can be checked by contacting the state board of pharmacy or the National Association of Boards of Pharmacy (NABP). If a website displays NABP VIPPS (Verified Internet Pharmacy Practice Site), this ensures that the site meets all applicable state and federal requirements.

UNSAFE MEDICATION PRACTICES

Older patients should be cautioned to avoid certain risky medication behaviors such as:

- **Sharing others' medications.** Sometimes older persons share their medications with each other. They should be cautioned that this practice is unwise and that they should take only medications prescribed for them.
- **Using imported medications.** The use of medication imported from or obtained in another country is controversial and is considered illegal. Some health professionals are concerned that imported medications may not meet the quality standards of drugs approved for use in the United States. Others claim that some drugs from other countries such as Canada come from the same drug manufacturers as the medications sold in the United States.
- **Using outdated medications.** The use of medications that are outdated is risky. The medications not only may be ineffective but also can actually cause injury to the heart, liver, or kidneys. It is unwise to use old medications in an attempt to save money.

Patient and Family Teaching

Gerontological nurses require skills and knowledge related to teaching patients and families about the key concepts of gerontology and gerontological nursing. The patient-family teaching guidelines in the following feature will assist the nurse to assume the role of teacher and coach. Educating patients and families is critical so that nurses can interpret scientific data and individualize the nursing care plan.

Patient-Family Teaching Guidelines

MEDICATIONS AND THE OLDER ADULT

The following are guidelines that the nurse may find useful when instructing older persons and their families about medications and drug safety.

1. I am taking a lot of medications prescribed by my doctor. How do I know if they are all safe?

Medications can be lifesaving and promote health and quality of life. However, you enter into a partnership with your doctor when you agree to take a medication he or she prescribes for you. Here are some suggestions for taking medication safely:

- Inform your doctor of all allergies, medical problems, drug reactions, over-the-counter medications, herbal remedies, and recreational drugs (including tobacco and alcohol) that you use.

- Ask about how to take the drug. Possible questions might include: Does "two tablets a day" mean two in the morning? One in the morning and one at night? Should it be taken with water? Should I sit up after taking the medication? Can I take it at the same time as my other medications? What should I do if I am ill and cannot take the medication?

- Ask about alternatives to the medication. Are there dietary or lifestyle changes that might decrease the need for or dose of the medication?

- What are the common side effects? What should be reported immediately?

- If you are on multiple medications, go over the schedule with your nurse. Write it down so you can keep the schedule in your wallet or pocketbook.

- Take the exact amount as prescribed.

- Do not share medications with others.

- Ask if you can drink alcohol. If so, ask how much is safe.

- Check for expiration dates on your medicine and throw away expired bottles. They may be unsafe to take.

- Take all medications as prescribed, even if you are feeling better. Check with your doctor or nurse before stopping a medication in the middle of the treatment.

- Adhere to lab tests, blood pressure checks, and ongoing monitoring so that your doctor can keep track of the effectiveness and safety of your medications.

RATIONALE:

Empowering the patient to ask questions and teaching about appropriate use of medications can help to decrease anxiety about prescribed medications and the therapeutic regimen.

2. As my nurse, how can you help me to take medications safely?

As your nurse, I would like to review your medications with you at every clinic visit. This should be done on a regular basis and after every acute care hospitalization because many medicines are changed when you go to the hospital. I will also make sure that you have not started taking any new over-the-counter medications or herbal remedies that could interact with your prescription medicine. I will ask you questions regarding dizziness,

RATIONALE:

Reviewing patients' medications can further enhance the nurse-patient relationship, provide opportunities for teaching, and can help the patient to see the nurse as a helpful resource.

(continued)

Patient-Family Teaching Guidelines, *cont.*

rashes, constipation, dry mouth, or other changes to make sure you are tolerating your medications without side effects. I will also let you know if there are any warnings or changes regarding the safety or interactions of your medications. If you would like, I will write out medication instructions for you after you have seen the doctor so that you can refer to the instructions at home if you have questions.

3. What is the pharmacist's responsibility?

Tell your pharmacist if you have trouble reading small labels or opening the childproof prescription bottles. If you request childproof bottles, store them in a safe place if grandchildren or neighborhood children are visiting your home. Try not to store medications in a bathroom medicine cabinet if you take long steamy showers. The humidity can cause the medication to break down and become ineffective.

Be sure to ask questions about the name of the medication, and go over instructions regarding dosage and how to take it. Check the label before you leave the pharmacy. Make sure you have the correct prescription. If the medication looks different, check with the pharmacist to verify there is no error. Medication safety is a team effort, and you and your family are the key players on the team. Remember, medicines that are strong enough to cure you can also hurt you if they are not used correctly. Do not be afraid to ask questions and advocate for your own safety.

RATIONALE:

Including the pharmacist as part of the therapeutic team provides the patient with an additional and valuable resource for help in medication management.

Care Plan

A Patient Experiencing a Possible Adverse Drug Reaction

Case Study

Mrs. Nash is a 75-year-old widow. She lives alone and has two children and five grandchildren ages 2 through 12 who visit regularly. Her prescribed medications are "baby aspirin," a beta-blocker, a thiazide diuretic, and warfarin. Her nonprescribed OTC medications are a multivitamin, vitamin C, vitamin E, calcium tablets, and Bayer PM for sleep. For an upset stomach she takes Tums, and for a headache either aspirin or acetaminophen. She also has been taking a laxative for some constipation she has developed recently. She is concerned about feeling "washed out,"

A Patient Experiencing a Possible Adverse Drug Reaction

sleeping poorly, and feeling chronic fatigue. Within the last 2 weeks, she has not been able to do her usual daily half-mile walk.

Her 24-hour diet recall revealed the following:

Breakfast: grapefruit juice, blueberry muffin, coffee with cream
Lunch: grilled cheese, tea
Late afternoon: glass of milk with cookies
Dinner: cheese with crackers and wine, broiled chicken, peas, carrots, mashed
    potato, butter, chocolate ice cream
Bedtime snack: coffee-flavored yogurt

Applying the Nursing Process

ASSESSMENT

Several factors may be contributing to Mrs. Nash's fatigue. A holistic assessment is needed. The nurse should consider malnutrition, constipation, depression, adverse drug effects, and polypharmacy.

Constipation may be a side effect of beta-blockers, and also can be caused by her calcium intake from calcium tablets, Tums, ice cream, yogurt, and cheese.

Beta-blockers can cause depression with long-term use and also may affect a person's ability to exercise due to a "braking" effect on cardiac response. Hypnotics could be causing a "hangover" effect. Mrs. Nash also may be experiencing hypokalemia from thiazide diuretics, especially since she has not had potassium-rich foods such as orange juice or bananas.

Her use of grapefruit juice may increase the absorption of some of her drugs, causing toxic effects. Vitamin C may be affecting the renal excretion of some of her medications.

She is on the oral anticoagulant warfarin, and a major concern would be the level of anticoagulation. It would be important to know when the last INR was checked and the results. It also would be important to check on whether she has been taking the correct dose. The nurse should assess Mrs. Nash for other indications of bleeding such as hematuria, blood in stools, decreased blood pressure, and postural blood pressure. The nurse should also inquire about recent headaches that might suggest bleeding.

Mrs. Nash is taking nonprescribed OTC medications that should be avoided in patients taking warfarin. She has been prescribed a small daily dose of aspirin, but on her own she has been taking aspirin for headaches and Bayer PM, which also contains aspirin. Vitamin E prolongs bleeding. Acetaminophen also can affect her INR reading. Many drugs that affect the INR of patients on warfarin can be used if they are given daily on a regular basis and the warfarin dosage is established while the patient is taking the same daily dose of the medications.

The patient's total caffeine intake (coffee, tea, and chocolate) should be reviewed and may be contributing to her sleeping difficulty. Caffeine should be avoided in the evening. The nurse can suggest that she use decaffeinated coffee and tea and that she have a glass of warm milk to produce a hypnotic effect from the natural tryptophan.

(continued)

A Patient Experiencing a Possible Adverse Drug Reaction (continued)

DIAGNOSIS

The current nursing diagnoses for Mrs. Nash include the following:

- *Sleep pattern disturbance*
- *Imbalanced nutrition: less than body requirements*
- *Altered activity levels*
- *Constipation*
- *Poisoning: risk for (through polypharmacy)*
- *Ineffective coping (possible depression)*

EXPECTED OUTCOMES

Expected outcomes for the plan of care specify that Mrs. Nash will:

- Become aware of the harmful effects of poor diet on overall health and function.
- Utilize sleep hygiene measures to improve sleep.
- Develop a more trusting relationship with her physician to schedule monitoring of her physical and psychological status (including monitoring her INR and dose adjustment of warfarin).
- Agree to establish a therapeutic relationship with the nurse and develop a mutually acceptable plan to work toward these outcomes.

PLANNING AND IMPLEMENTATION

The following nursing interventions may be appropriate for Mrs. Nash:

- Establish a therapeutic relationship.
- Educate Mrs. Nash regarding eating a balanced diet.
- Increase fluid and fiber intake to ease constipation. Measures to offset the constipation would be to decrease cheese intake, increase bulk in diet (e.g., bran muffins or cereal, adding a salad to her lunch and dinner), increasing fruit intake (e.g., apple), and increasing her fluid intake and level of exercise.
- Encourage Mrs. Nash to begin her daily walking regimen.
- Encourage a family meeting to talk about health issues in general with the patient's permission.
- Begin a sleep assessment to establish the underlying cause of Mrs. Nash's sleep disturbance.
- Begin a values clarification to establish long-term goals and facilitate end-of-life planning.

EVALUATION

The nurse hopes to work with Mrs. Nash over time and to form a therapeutic relationship with her. The nurse will consider the plan a success based on the following criteria:

- Mrs. Nash will continue to engage in her daily walk.
- A family meeting will be held to discuss her overall health.

A Patient Experiencing a Possible Adverse Drug Reaction

- Mrs. Nash will begin to report improved sleep based on relief of constipation and engagement in daily exercise.
- She will resume her normal bowel function with daily or every other day bowel movements that are passed without strain.
- She will visit her primary care provider and cooperate with monitoring her INR and titration of her daily warfarin dose.

Ethical Dilemma

Mrs. Nash's son (whom the nurse has not met) telephones and asks what his mother's last INR was and what dose of warfarin she has been taking. An important consideration in responding is the nurse's duty to protect the patient's privacy. This is an ethical issue as well as a legal one as evidenced by the Health Insurance Portability and Accountability Act (HIPAA) regulations. The nurse would need to establish that the caller is indeed the son and that Mrs. Nash has approved that her son have access to her medical information. The HIPAA regulations of the nurse's agency should be carefully followed.

The nurse also should explore with the son, once his right to know this information has been established, the basis for his concern.

Critical Thinking and the Nursing Process

1. Go to a local pharmacy or consult an online pharmacy and compute the cost of medications for one of your older patients who is taking five or more medications. Notice how the price varies from various sources. Discuss the difference in costs of medications with your classmates. Are you surprised by the degree to which prices vary? How does this affect your older patient?
2. Identify an older patient you are caring for in your clinical practicum. Review the number and types of prescription, OTC, and herbal medications that your patient is taking. Compare to the medical record. Are there differences? Is the record an accurate reflection of the patient's report?
3. Assess an older patient's knowledge about adverse and side effects of a medication he or she is taking on a regular basis. Analyze the patient's knowledge base and try to describe factors that increase or decrease an older person's knowledge about medication safety.
4. As a classroom exercise, purchase a large bag of colored M&M candies. Instruct your classmates to take four orange pills three times a day, two red in the morning, one blue at hour of sleep, and so on. Check with them the next day to see if they were able to follow your oral instructions without error.

- Evaluate your responses in Appendix B. ⊂⊃

Source: Adapted from Hartford Institute for Geriatric Nursing, *Best nursing practices in care for older adults,* 1999.

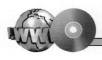

EXPLORE MediaLink

NCLEX review, case studies, and other interactive resources for this chapter can be found on the Companion Website at **www.prenhall.com/tabloski**. Click on Chapter 6 to select the activities for this chapter. For animations, more NCLEX review questions, and case studies, access the accompanying CD-ROM in this textbook.

Chapter Highlights

- Older persons receive considerable benefit from the many drugs available that can cure or control diseases and improve longevity and the quality of life.

- The medication needs of older persons pose special challenges to the nurse and other clinicians. Healthcare professionals should provide the appropriate type and dose of medication to optimize the intended therapeutic effects and avoid or reduce the possibility of adverse outcomes of drug therapy. The aging process and other characteristics of each older person dictate his or her unique drug regimen.

- The nurse can play a major role in the successful use of medications to enhance the quality of life of elderly adults in all settings.

References

Abrams, W. B. (1985). Development of drugs for use by the elderly. In S. R. Moore & W. Teal (Eds.), *Geriatric drug use—Clinical and social perspectives* (pp. 200–205). New York: Pergamon.

Agency for Healthcare Research and Quality. (2001). *Research activity: Pharmaceutical research and older Americans with chronic illness.* Retrieved October 19, 2004, from www.ahrq.gov/research.

Agency for Healthcare Research and Quality. (2002). *Research activity: Late referral to specialty care contributes to poor outcomes among patients with renal failure.* Retrieved September 18, 2004, from www.ahrq.gov/research.

Alliance on Aging Research. (1998). *When medicines hurt instead of help: Preventing medication problems in older persons.* Washington, DC: Author. Retrieved February 11, 2005, from www.agingresearch.org/brochure/medicinehurts/whenmedicinehurts.html.

Ang-Lee, M. K., Moss, K., & Yuan, C. S. (2001). Herbal medicines and perioperative care. *Journal of the American Medical Association, 286*(2), 208.

Beers, M. H., & Berkow, R. (Eds.). (2005). Pharmacokinetics, in Chapter 304 drug therapy in the elderly. *The Merck Manual.* Retrieved June 7, 2003, from www.merck-com/mrkshared/mmanual/home.jsp.

Beers, M. H. (1997). Explicit criteria for determining potentially inappropriate medication use by the elderly: An update. *Archives of Internal Medicine, 157,* 1531–1536.

Beers, M. H., Ouslander, J. G., Rollingher, J., Reuben, D., & Beck, J. C. (1991). Explicit criteria for determining inappropriate medication use in nursing home residents. *Archives of Internal Medicine, 151,* 1825–1832.

Bressler, R., & Bahl, J. J. (2003). Principles of drug therapy for the elderly. *Mayo Clinic Proceedings, 78:* 1564–1577.

Cockcroft, D. W., & Gault, M. H. (1976). Prediction of creatinine clearance from serum creatinine. *Nephron, 16,* 31.

Conn, V., Taylor, S. G., & Kelley, S. (1991). Medication regimen complexity and adherence among older adults. *IMAGE: The Journal of Nursing Scholarship, 23*(4), 231–235.

Cooper, J. W. (2000). Adverse drug reactions in geriatric nursing facility residents. *Medscape Pharmacotherapy, 2*(1), 2000. Retrieved June 7, 2003, from www.medscape.com/viewarticle/408590.

Curtis, L. H., Ostbye, T., Sendersky, V., Hutchison, S., Dans, P. E., Wright, A., et al. (2004). Inappropriate prescribing for elderly Americans in a large outpatient population. *Archives of Internal Medicine, 164*(15), 1621–1625.

Cusack, B. J., & Vestal, R. E. (2005). Clinical pharmacology. In M. H. Beers & R. Berkow (Eds.), *The Merck manual of geriatrics.* Whitehouse Station, NJ: Merck Research Laboratories. Retrieved February 12, 2005, from www.merk.com/mrkshared/mm_genstrics/home/sp.

Department of Health and Human Services Office of Inspector General. (2001). *Psychotropic Drug Use in Nursing Homes.* Retrieved February 12, 2005, from www.oig.hhs.gov/oei/reports/oei-02-00-00490.pdf.

Eisenhauer, L. A., & Murphy, M. A. (Eds.). (1998). *Pharmacotherapeutics and advanced nursing practice.* New York: McGraw-Hill.

Fick, D. M., Cooper, J. M., Wada, W. E., Waller, J. L., Maclean, J. R., & Beers, M. H. (2003). Updating the Beers criteria for potentially inappropriate medication use in older adults. *Archives of Internal Medicine, 163,* 2716–2724.

Field, T. S., Gurwitz, J. H., Avorn, J., McCormick, D., Jain, S., Eckler, M., et al. (2001). Risk factors for adverse drug events among nursing home residents. *Archives of Internal Medicine, 161*(13), 1629–1634.

Fitten, L. G., Coleman, L., Siembied, D. W., M., Yu, & Ganzell, S. (1995). Assessment of capacity to comply with medication regimens in older patients. *Journal of American Geriatrics Society, 43*(4), 361–367.

Foster, D. F., Phillips, R. S., Hamel, M. B., & Eisenberg, D. M. (2000). Alternative medicine use in older Americans. *Journal of the American Geriatrics Society, 48,* 1560–1565.

Fulmer, T., Feldman, P. H., Kim, T. S., Carty, B., Beers, M., Molina, M., & Putnam, M. (1999). An intervention study to enhance medication compliance. *Journal of Gerontological Nursing, 25*(8), 6–14.

Giron, M. S. T., Forsell, Y., Bernsten, C., Thorslund, M., Winblad, B., & Fastbom, J. (2002, April). Sleep problems in a very old population: Drug use and clinical correlates. *Journal of Gerontology: Biological Sciences and Medical Sciences, 57,* M236–M240.

Glazener, F. S. (1992). Adverse drug reactions: A critical review. In K. L. Melmon, H. F. Morelli, & B. B. Melmon (Eds.), *Clinical pharmacology: Basic principles in therapeutics* (3rd ed.). New York: McGraw-Hill.

Gurwitz, J. H., Field, T. S., Harrold, L. R., Rothschild, J., Debellis, K., Seger, A. C., et al. (2003). Incidence and preventability of adverse drug events among older persons in the ambulatory setting. *Journal of the American Medical Association, 289*(9), 1107–1116.

Hartford Institute for Geriatric Nursing. (1999). *Best nursing practices in care for older adults.* Retrieved October 17, 2003, from www.hartfordign.org.

Herrlinger, C., & Klotz, U. (2001). Drug metabolism and drug interactions in the elderly. *Best Practice & Research Clinical Gastroenterology, 15*(6), 897–918.

Institute for Safe Medication Practices. (2003). *Cultural diversity and medication safety.* Retrieved September 24, 2004, from www.ismp.org/MSAarticles/diversity.

Jordan, R.P., & Robbins, J. (2000). *The value of medicines: Yesterday, today, and tomorrow.* Meniscus Educational Institute. Retrieved August 28, 2004, from www.pharm.chula. ac.th/surachai/academic/ContEd/Value%20of%20medicines.pdf.

Karch, F. F., & Lasagna, L. (1975). Adverse drug reactions: A critical review. *Journal of the American Medical Association, 234,* 1236–1241.

Kurtzweil, P. (1999). How to spot health fraud. *FDA Consumer, 33*(6).

Leipzig, R. M. (2001). Keys to maximizing benefit while avoiding adverse drug effects. *Geriatrics, 56*(2), 30–40.

Levy, R., & Hawks, J. (1999). *Cultural diversity and pharmaceutical care.* Reston, VA: National Pharmaceutical Council.

Lile, J. L., & Hoffman, R. (1991). Medication-taking by the frail elderly in two ethnic groups. *Nursing Forum, 26*(4), 19–24.

McKinney, J. M., Munroe, W. U. P., & Wright, J. T. (1992). Impact of electronic medication compliance aid on long-term blood pressure control. *Journal of Clinical Pharmacology, 32,* 277–283.

Melmon, M. D., Morelli, H. F., Hoffman, B. B., & Nievenberg, D. W. (Eds.). (1992). *Clinical pharmacology: Basic principles in therapeutics* (3rd ed.). New York: McGraw-Hill.

Michaud, P. L. (1996). *Independent older persons managing medications at home: A grounded theory.* Unpublished doctoral dissertation, Boston College, Chestnut Hill: Massachusetts.

National Pharmaceutical Council. (1992). *Noncompliance with medicine regimens: An economic tragedy with important implications for healthcare reform.* Reston, VA: Author.

Neafsey, P. J., & Shellman, J. (2001). Adverse self-medication practices of older adults with hypertension attending blood pressure clinics. *Internet Journal of Advanced Nursing Practice, 5*(1). Retrieved June 19, 2003, from www.ispub.com/ostia/index.

Repasy, A.B. (2003). *Pharmacotherapy in Geriatrics Resource Guide.* Retrieved February 11, 2005, from www.galter.northwestern. edu/geriatrics/chapters/pharmacotherapy.cfm.

Schmader, K., Hanlon, J. T., Weinberger, M., Landsman, P. B., Samsa, G. P., Lewis, I., et al. (1994). Appropriateness of medication prescribing in ambulatory elderly patients. *Journal of the American Geriatrics Society, 42,* 1241–1247.

Schlenk, E. A., Dunbar-Jacobs, J., & Engberg, S. (2004). Medication non-adherence among older adults: A review of strategies and interventions for improvement. *Journal of Gerontological Nursing, 30*(7), 33–43.

Schmucker, D. L., & Vesell, E. S. (1999). Are the elderly underrepresented in clinical drug trials? *Journal of Clinical Pharmacology, 39,* 1103–1108.

Swonger, A. K., & Burbank, P. M. (1995). *Drug therapy and the elderly.* Boston: Jones & Bartlett.

Tolsoi, L. G. (2002). Drug-induced gastrointestinal disorders. *Medscape Pharmacotherapy, 4*(1). Retrieved June 7, 2003, from www.medscape.com/viewarticle/437034.

Willcox, S. M., Himmelstein, D. U., & Woolhandler, S. (1994). Inappropriate drug prescribing for the community-dwelling elderly. *Journal of the American Medical Association, 272*(4), 292–296.

Williams, R. D. (2003). *Medications and older adults.* FDA publication. Retrieved June 6, 2003, from www.pueblo.gsa.gov/cic_text/health/meds4old/697_old.html.

World Health Organization. (2002). *Safety of medicines. A guide to detecting and reporting adverse drug reactions.* Geneva, Switzerland: Author.

CHAPTER 7

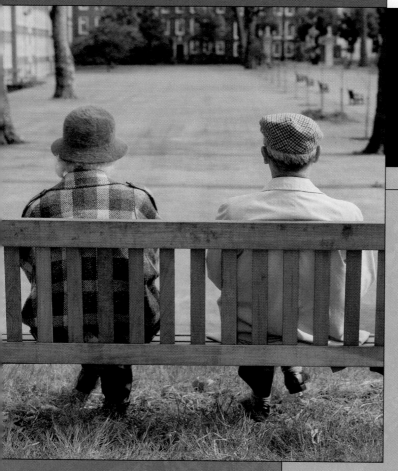

Psychological and Cognitive Function

CHAPTER OBJECTIVES

Upon completion of this chapter, the reader will be able to:

- Describe age-related changes that affect psychological and cognitive functioning.
- Explain the impact of age-related changes on stress and coping.
- Identify risk factors for high levels of stress, poor coping, and impaired mental health, including alcoholism, stress-related disorders, and depression.
- Examine risk factors that influence cognitive functioning in older adults.
- Define appropriate nursing interventions directed toward assisting the older adult to develop coping resources, use effective coping mechanisms, and minimize the functional consequences of stress.
- Identify means to strengthen social support groups and healthy aging.
- Identify interventions directed toward alleviating risk factors for late-life depression, treating depression in older adults, and preventing suicide.

KEY TERMS

MediaLink

Additional resources for this chapter can be found on the Student CD-ROM accompanying this textbook and on the Companion Website at **www.prenhall.com/tabloski**. Click on Chapter 7 to select the activities for this chapter.

CD-ROM
- Animation
  Tardive Dyskinesia
- NCLEX Review
- Case Studies
- Tools

COMPANION WEBSITE
- Audio Glossary
- Additional NCLEX Review
- Case Study
- MediaLink Application

The well-being of older adults is a major concern to healthcare providers in the United States and to society in general. Undiagnosed and untreated mental disorders such as **depression** can lead to increased disability, premature death, increased morbidity, increased risk of institutionalization, and a significant decrease in an older person's quality of life (Morris, 2001). Healthcare professionals, including nurses, should aggressively work to improve the quality of mental health services delivered to older adults in order to meet the goals established in *Healthy People 2010,* including increasing the quality of years of healthy life and eliminating health disparities (U.S. Public Health Service, 2000).

Older people evidence fewer diagnosable psychiatric disorders than younger persons, excluding cognitive impairment. Major population-based surveys find that the overall prevalence of mental disorders for older adults is lower than for any other age group. Only cognitive impairments such as Alzheimer's disease show a definite age-associated increase (American Psychological Association, 1998). Yet, when older adults experience mental health problems, they may be denied access to mental health services for a variety of factors, including missed diagnosis of psychological problems and the perceived stigma many older persons attach to having a psychological problem. Their **competence** or ability to care for themselves and make decisions may be questioned. An older adult whose competence is questioned may suffer losses of autonomy and independence such as having a legal guardian appointed or being prematurely institutionalized in a nursing home or long-term care facility.

Older adults can evidence a variety of psychological problems, including almost all of those experienced by younger adults. Some of these problems may be new onset, the result of late-life **stress** or neuropathology, and others may be recurrences of psychological problems experienced in earlier life. As with physical problems, the older adult may experience multiple psychological symptoms or syndromes that make recognition and diagnosis challenging for the gerontological nurse. Additionally, psychological problems can result from and coexist with physical problems. For instance, an older person with congestive heart failure may complain of symptoms of lethargy, inability to eat, and falling. This older person may be taking several medications. These symptoms may be the result of a drug-drug interaction, a physical response to chronic illness, a new-onset psychological problem, or a combination of all of these factors. The expanding older population will place increasing demands on mental health services and create greater demands for mental healthcare (Morris, 2001).

Racial and ethnic minorities bear a greater burden from unmet mental health needs and thus suffer greater losses that negatively impact their overall health and productivity at all ages. Most minority groups are less likely than Whites to use services, and they receive poorer quality mental healthcare, despite having similar community rates of mental health problems. Especially at risk are racial and ethnic minorities and older gay men and lesbians. Similar prevalence, combined with lower utilization and poorer quality of care, means that minority communities have a higher proportion of individuals with unmet mental health needs. Because of preventable disparities in mental health services, a disproportionate number of minority older persons are not fully benefiting from the opportunities that others have to enjoy their older years. The major barriers include the cost of care, societal stigma, and the fragmentation of services. Additional barriers include healthcare providers' lack of awareness of cultural issues, bias, or inability to speak the older person's language, and the older person's fear and mistrust of treatment (U.S. Surgeon General, 2003).

The older population is highly heterogeneous and includes a diverse mix of immigrants, refugees, and multigenerational Americans with vastly different histories, languages, spiritual practices, demographic patterns, and cultures. Generations within the same minority family may represent different racial or cultural orientation, religious affiliation and practices, societal values, and attitudes toward the larger society. Minority elders may be considered especially vulnerable and at risk for mental health problems because of **ageism** (negative stereotypes toward elderly adults) and cultural bias.

Psychological changes and chronic illness associated with older adulthood may affect a person's functional abilities; however, the psychosocial changes are often the most challenging and demanding. Some of the psychosocial challenges arise from physical changes, but many are attributable to changes in roles, relationships, losses, and living environments. Like many age-related psychological changes, some psychosocial changes are inevitable and somewhat predictable. Therefore, older adults can prepare for and respond to psychosocial changes by developing and using effective coping strategies. With each day that passes, the opportunity for change, both positive and negative, presents itself. A rich full life usually encompasses joyous and sad events. Older people experience multiple and significant losses as they age. The positive **coping mechanisms** a person developed and used earlier in life may be inadequate in later life, and depression or another serious mental health problem may result from inadequate coping ability. Although older adults suffer from major depressive disorders less often than younger adults, 27% of older adults experience depressive symptoms (Hartford Institute for Geriatric Nursing, 1999).

Depression in older adults is often undetected and untreated. Therefore, it is difficult to determine prevalence rates. Primary healthcare providers are often not vigilant or consistent in their diagnosis of depression and may fail to make the diagnosis. One approach is to distinguish between the psychiatric diagnosis of major depression and the depression-related affective disturbances (minor depression) of daily life. Using these categories, the rate of major and minor depression in community-living older adults is approximately 13%, and 43% among institutionalized older persons. The symptoms of depression are often associated with chronic illness and pain.

Practice Pearl

Most older adults successfully adjust to the challenges of aging, but be alert for symptoms of depression that will present differently in the older person. Vague physical decline and somatic complaints may be the only clues of underlying depression.

Cognition is a complicated process by which information is learned, stored, retrieved, and used by the individual. Cognitive processing supports reasoning, problem solving, remembering, interpreting, and communicating. Normal, healthy aging is not characterized by cognitive and mental disorders (U.S. Department of Health and Human Services, 2001). Some cognitive abilities may decline with age, some may improve, and some stay relatively stable. These changes are highly variable from one person to another as they age and may even vary within a given person over time. Most older people will not suffer a significant memory impairment, but many may experience mild problems with word finding and remembering names. Usually, however, these problems are mild in scope and the older person can compensate for these deficits. (For a complete discussion of Alzheimer's disease, see Chapter 22.)

Drug Alert !

Certain medications like sleeping pills, tranquilizers, and some pain medications can cause symptoms similar to dementia (confusion, lack of interest, memory impairment) but are not true dementia. These symptoms are called false or pseudodementia.

Educational attainment within the older population has increased significantly. In 1993, 34% of those 65 years and older had graduated from high school and 12% had a college degree. In 2030, 83% of older adults will have completed high school and 24% will have at least a bachelor's degree. Higher levels of education are associated with increased travel, recreation, income, and opportunities for personal growth and development. However, even though older people share similar generational experiences, there may be considerable diversity among them. Life experiences, health status, race, culture, sexual orientation, and a variety of other factors can make an older person who is a high school dropout think and act more like a college professor and vice versa.

Positive mental health is a necessary component of successful aging. Box 7-1 lists the key components of mental health as defined by the Surgeon General of the United States. Positive mental health can last a lifetime and support growth, creativity, sense of humor, and zest for life until the moment of death. For instance, Georgia O'Keeffe and Pablo Picasso painted into their 90s and were considered by many to do their best work in their old age. Jeanne Calment of Arles, France, took up fencing lessons at the age of 85 and rode a bicycle at age 100. At Mme. Calment's 120th birthday party, a journalist hesitantly told her, "Well, I guess I'll see you next year." Instantly she shot back, "I don't see why not. You look to be in pretty good health to me!" Her life ended on August 4, 1997, at age 122 years, 5 months, and 14 days. She is believed to have lived longer than any person in recorded history (National Institute on Aging, 2002).

Mental Health: Themes From the Surgeon General's Report (2003)	BOX 7-1

- Mental health is fundamental to health.
- Mental illnesses are real health problems.
- The efficacy of mental health treatments is well documented.
- Mind and body are inseparable.
- Stigma is a major obstacle preventing older people from getting help.

Source: U.S. Surgeon General's Report. (2003). Washington, DC: U.S. Department of Health and Human Services.

Normal Changes With Aging

Normally, an older person's mental health and cognition remain relatively stable. For those functions that do change, usually the change is not severe enough to cause significant impairment in daily life or social ability. Severe changes and sudden loss of **cognitive function** are usually symptoms of a physical or mental illness such as

Alzheimer's disease, stroke, or serious depression. Some general cognitive changes considered to be normal age-related changes include the following:

- Information-processing speed declines with age, resulting in a slower learning rate and greater need for repetition of information.
- The ability to divide attention between two tasks shows age-related decline.
- The ability to switch attention rapidly from one auditory input to another shows age-related decline (visual input switching ability does not change significantly with age).
- Ability to maintain sustained attention or perform vigilance tasks appears to decline with age.
- Ability to filter out irrelevant information appears to decline with age.
- Short-term or primary memory remains relatively stable.
- Long-term or secondary memory exhibits more substantial age-related changes, with the decline greater for recall than for recognition. (Cueing improves performance of long-term memory.)
- Most aspects of language are well preserved, such as use of language sounds and meaningful combinations of words. Vocabulary improves with age. However, word finding, naming ability, and rapid word list generation decline with age.
- Visuospatial task ability such as drawing and construction ability declines with age.
- Abstraction and mental flexibility show some age decline.
- Accumulation of practical experience, or wisdom, continues until the very end of life.

(American Psychological Association, 1998)

Practice Pearl

Normal healthy older persons who forget where they put the egg beater can be assured there is no significant memory problem. But if they forget what an egg beater is or how to use it, they should be referred for further evaluation and treatment.

Decrements in intellectual function are generally greater in older people who develop disease and disability than in those who remain healthy. Many decrements in cognitive capacity, mood, and performance that formerly were attributed to "normal aging" are now known to be associated with psychiatric illness or physical disease. Contrary to the stereotype of increasing rigidity and inflexibility with age, healthy older people maintain stable personalities and psychological adaptation throughout their lives. **Personality** stability across the second half of the adult life span may be stronger than across the first half.

Life satisfaction does not usually decrease as one ages. A positive life satisfaction is associated with good health, an adequate income, reciprocal social relationships, and a sense of control over one's life (American Psychiatric Association, 2000). Significant changes in mood, cognitive ability, and personality should never be dismissed as normal aging, but always aggressively assessed and referred for treatment.

Late adulthood is no longer seen as a period of growth cessation and arrested cognitive development, but rather a continued period of growth with the opportunity for development of unique capacities (Ebersole, Hess, & Lugfen, 2004). Education, pulmonary health, general health, and activity levels all influence cognitive activity in later life. Older adults often have a positive outlook and seek challenges and activities that maintain their well-being. Many older people take classes, participate in elder hostels, exercise, study new subjects, travel, and maintain healthy interpersonal and sexual relationships.

Older adults cope with normal aging changes in a variety of ways. Since most changes of aging are gradual in onset, the older person gradually adjusts to the changes. Methods for coping with age-associated cognitive changes include:

- Making lists, posting appointments on calendars, and writing "notes to self."
- Memory training and memory enhancement techniques (for instance, when meeting a new person for the first time, trying to link his or her name to a common object or easily remembered item).
- Keeping the mind challenged and mentally active (reading daily, completing a crossword puzzle, playing bridge, etc).
- Using assistive devices such as pill boxes and reliance on habit such as preprogrammed telephones, parking in the same place in the mall parking lot, and so on, to reduce chances of forgetting vital information.
- Seeking support and encouragement from others.
- Staying positive and hopeful for the future, including laughing at oneself when appropriate. ("You won't believe what I did today. I showed up for my doctor's appointment with one brown and one black shoe! Oh well, at least I'm not a slave to fashion!")

Older adults must be able to monitor their cognitive abilities and adapt to changes in their memory skills to function safely in their everyday lives. Some people with severe cognitive deficits may continue to engage in behaviors that are unsafe for them such as driving, cooking, and trying to live independently. Others with good memories may continuously live in fear that they are developing Alzheimer's disease whenever they forget a name or an appointment. It is difficult to predict whether an older person who has mild problems with memory will go on to develop more severe memory loss. Some older people try to hide or cover up memory problems because they fear restrictions on their freedoms and living situation. Memory changes may result from a variety of causes, including Alzheimer's disease, depression, underlying psychiatric illness, physical illness, medications, vitamin deficiencies, and sensory impairments. Any alteration or concerns over cognitive abilities should be assessed to identify reversible causes of memory loss and institute appropriate safety measures in a supportive environment.

Personality and Self-Concept

Erik Erikson's original theory (1963) about the eight stages of life has been used widely in relation to older adulthood. Erikson defined the stages of life as trust versus mistrust, autonomy versus shame and doubt, initiative versus guilt, industry versus inferiority, identity versus identity diffusion, intimacy versus self-absorption, generativity versus stagnation, and ego integrity versus despair. Each of these stages presents certain conflicting tendencies that must be balanced before the person can move successfully from that stage. In 1982, when Erikson was 80 years old, he described the task of old age as balancing the search for integrity and wholeness, thus avoiding a sense of despair. He believed that successful accomplishment of this task, achieved primarily through life review activities, would result in wisdom.

Havighurst (1972) concentrated his studies of developing life course theories on middle or later adulthood. He defined tasks of later life as (1) adjusting to decreased physical strength and health, (2) adjusting to retirement and reduced income, (3) adjusting to death of a spouse, (4) establishing an explicit association with one's group, (5) adapting to social roles in a flexible way, and (6) establishing satisfactory physical living arrangements.

These and many other personality type theories attempt to question whether personality changes or remains the same throughout the life course. Although most researchers agree that personality remains relatively stable over the life span, they disagree about the extent and causes of personality change. Neugarten and colleagues (1976) conducted studies and identified three basic personality characteristics occurring in older people: (1) a change of focus from the outer world to the inner world, (2) a movement from active mastery of the environment to a more reactive or accommodating approach, and (3) patterns of isolation from the outside world. This last group included people with psychological problems, those with irrational behavior, and those who failed to cope with the demands of daily living.

When rigidity and excess cautiousness are apparent in an older person, the underlying explanation may be generational or cohort differences rather than a normal change of aging. Older people have been brought up with different expectations, have had different life experiences, and possess different generational values. As a result, they may be hesitant to make decisions in areas where they feel less comfortable and the outcome is uncertain. For instance, some older people may be hesitant to invest in the stock market, preferring instead to put their money into low-interest-rate bank accounts or safety deposit boxes. Others may prefer to invest their money in riskier ventures to gain higher returns and may even become victims of scam artists and others who take advantage of older adults. Like younger people, older people assess risk in very different ways.

Self-concept is a component of personality (American Psychological Association, 1998) that can be viewed as an attitude toward the self. An older person's self-concept can be eroded or enhanced over time as a result of circumstance and life experiences. Additionally, an older person's personality influences self-concept and adaptation to role transitions, such as widowhood or retirement. Research related to personality traits and self-concept indicates that individuals can maintain continuity and coherence in the course of adult life. People do not necessarily become depressed, isolated, and rigid with older age, and well-adjusted and happy individuals are likely to remain so in late life. Those who are less happy with themselves can take steps such as counseling or engage in empowerment groups to improve their self-concept and change their lives.

Practice Pearl

Ask your older patients to tell a short story about themselves or a significant event in their life. By analyzing the content of the story, the nurse can learn if an older patient is a survivor, a victim, or a person who relies on the help and guidance of others. This brief story can reveal a lot about the older person's self-concept.

Personality Disorders

The incidence and prevalence of most personality disorders decline with age. Narcissistic, borderline, histrionic, and antisocial personality disorders generally peak in the younger years. However, personality disorders may present differently in the older adult. Any selfish or impulsive behavior toward family or caregivers should be carefully investigated and referred for treatment if indicated.

Psychiatric symptoms that should be investigated and not written off as normal changes of aging include:

- **Memory and intellectual difficulties. Pseudodementia** or cognitive changes due to underlying **anxiety**, depression, or other potentially treatable psychiatric disorders can masquerade as Alzheimer's disease.

- **Change in sleep patterns.** Drastic changes in sleep patterns such as early morning awakening, declines in total sleep time, and increased sleep latency (longer time to fall asleep) may be signs of underlying anxiety of depression. Physical problems such as pain, respiratory disease, and cardiac disease can also interfere with sleep. Underlying psychiatric problems can exaggerate and intensify sleep disturbances in the older adult.
- **Changes in sexual interest and capacity.** Healthy older adults with a history of and interest in normal sexual function should be evaluated when sudden changes in sexual interest and capacity occur. In men, erectile dysfunction can have physical and psychological correlates. In women, libido and ability to reach orgasm can likewise be affected by a variety of factors. Common medical causes, medications, and underlying psychiatric problems can all contribute to sexual dysfunction in both genders. See Chapter 17 for further information on the evaluation of sexual dysfunction. ⟳
- **Fear of death.** For healthy older people, fear of death is uncommon. While older people do think about death and their own mortality, excessive focus on death and high death anxiety is uncommon. When older people focus excessively on death, they may be exhibiting signs of depression or anxiety, or they may be attempting to cope with a diagnosis of a terminal illness.
- **Delusions**. **Delusions** are false beliefs that persist and exert a negative influence on behavior or attitude (e.g., the belief that all food is poison and eating food will cause death).
- **Hallucinations**. **Hallucinations** are false perceptions and sensations such as hearing voices or seeing people who are not there.
- **Disordered thinking.** Disordered thinking is characterized by lack of logical thought processes. As a result, thoughts and communications become disorganized and fragmented. Serious problems such as legal situations can result from poor judgment and inability to communicate basic needs and safety concerns.
- **Problems with emotional expression.** Sudden or prolonged gradual loss of emotional responsiveness and expression may indicate the presence of psychiatric illness in the older adult. Failure to show emotion, laugh, cry, or make eye contact, or withdrawal from opportunities for human interaction, may be signs of severe depression. This is sometimes called the **flat affect** (Journal of the American Medical Association, 2000; *Merck Manual of Geriatrics,* 2001).

Elder Abuse or Mistreatment

Some older adults are vulnerable to mistreatment by spouses, adult children, or other caregivers. Elder abuse is more likely to occur when the older person is emotionally, physically, or cognitively impaired and vulnerable. Sexual abuse is the most underreported form of abuse among older adults. Older women who have been sexually abused will often refuse perineal care or be resistant to pelvic examination in an attempt to hide physical signs of abuse or because they fear further pain or invasion of the vagina.

The physical manifestations of elder abuse include unexplained bruises and trauma, signs of physical or psychological neglect, excessive anxiety, and excessive withdrawal or fear when questioned about abuse. Persons who abuse older people often have problems with substance abuse and may have diagnosed or undiagnosed psychological problems themselves. Elder abuse occurs at all economic levels and among all age groups. All states require mandatory reporting of known or suspected elder abuse, and an attempt is made to provide services and support to end the abusive situation and allow the older person to live safely and free from abuse (see Chapter 10 for further information on elder abuse and mistreatment). ⟳

Psychotic Disorders

Schizophrenia rarely occurs for the first time in old age. Only about 10% of people with diagnosed schizophrenia experience the onset of symptoms after the age of 40 (American Psychological Association, 1998). Therefore, it is likely that the older person with schizophrenia will have a long history of hospitalization and psychotropic drug use. Some symptoms of schizophrenia such as hallucinations and delusions appear to decline with age, but other symptoms such as apathy and withdrawal may place the older person at high risk for social isolation and neglect.

The most common form of psychosis in later years is paranoia (American Psychological Association, 2003). Hearing loss may place older persons at risk for developing paranoia as they may misinterpret casual conversation of others and believe they are the focus of the conversation. Other risk factors include social isolation, underlying personality disorder, cognitive impairment, and delirium. Older persons with early dementia may blame others for hiding or stealing their belongings when, in reality, they have simply forgotten where they have been left. These delusions can be hurtful to family and friends who are attempting to assist the older person and may result in increased social isolation.

Life Satisfaction and Life Events

Life satisfaction is an attitude toward one's own life; it may be defined as a reflection of feelings about the past, present, and future. Life satisfaction and morale are closely related to well-being. George et. al. (1985) posited that life satisfaction is the cognitive assessment of well-being, and happiness is the affective assessment. The two major components of well-being are affect (happiness) and satisfaction (realized expectations). These components may reflect a changing balance with age. Thus, age-related declines in positive affect may be countered by increases in the sense of satisfaction with life accomplishments (Maddox, 1994). Fewer than one third of older people report feelings of boredom or loneliness, and they express more life satisfaction when their social networks include friends as well as relatives (National Institute on Aging, 2004). Some researchers have found that greater independence in instrumental activities of daily living and greater perceived control of events significantly attenuate the adverse effects of stress on psychological well-being.

Life events demand an emotional adjustment on the part of the person experiencing the event, and different challenges are likely to occur during different periods in life. Some of these life events might be unexpected, unwanted, or feared. Others, such as coping with the loss of a spouse, might be more or less expected. Some examples of common events requiring psychological adjustments in older adults are widowhood, confronting negative attitudes of aging, retirement, chronic illness, functional impairments, decisions about driving a car, death of friends and family, and relocation from home to assisted living or long-term care. The longer a person lives, the more likely it is that events will occur that require coping and adaptation. Older adults may encounter losses of significant magnitude, losses of people or objects that have been part of their lives for many decades. Older adults with troubled pasts are less likely to adjust to losses and may develop chronic health problems and experience negative feelings such as anxiety or powerlessness. For example, people who fled from Europe to escape persecution before and during World War II, people who suffered great losses such as fires or other natural disasters, or people who have been victims of serious crime may be at risk for anxiety or depression when attempting to cope with an adverse life event. These older people may experience pain and loss much differently than the older person who has had a stable life without major trauma or fear. It is always valuable to consider how the events of history and past experience can affect the orientation and personality of the older person.

ADJUSTMENT DISORDER

The most common stressor that leads to adjustment disorder in later life is physical illness. Other stressors that may precipitate adjustment disorders among older adults include forced relocation, financial problems, family problems, and lengthy hospitalizations (American Psychological Association, 1998).

BEREAVEMENT

Most older adults experience the loss or death of loved ones, including spouse, family members, and friends. While bereavement is considered a normal reaction to loss and death, pathological grief may occur in some older adults. Symptoms of pathological grief among older adults are essentially the same as those of younger adults. They include preoccupation with death, extensive guilt, an overwhelming sense of loss and worthlessness, marked psychomotor retardation, and functional impairment. The length of time spent in grieving is culturally determined and is also a function of the individual's resources and the circumstances of death. In the United States, grief in the older adult is considered normal within a 2-year time frame, and grief persisting longer than 2 years is considered pathological. However, establishing preconceived time frames and judging others according to various theories quickly becomes problematic. In some cultures, bereavement lasts for the lifetime of the survivor. Traditional Greek widows wear black for the rest of their lives. The professional standard of care regarding the grieving older person should not be time related, but rather focus on the prevention of grief-related psychiatric disorders, medical illness, and social incapacitation (Parkes, 1999).

Factors that can affect the duration and course of grieving include:

Centrality of the loss. If the person who has died occupied a central place in the survivor's life (either physically or emotionally) the loss will be harder to bear. An older person with psychological attachments to others will receive support and assistance with grieving after the loss.

Health of the survivor. An older person with robust mental and physical health will be better able to cope with loss of a loved one and complete the work of grieving. Unresolved issues from the past, feelings of ambiguity toward the one who has died, and unresolved or incomplete coping with previous losses can all complicate the grieving process and prolong the time required to perform the grief work.

Survivor's religious or spiritual belief system. Personal religion or spirituality can be deeply integrated into the older person's perspective and positively influence the grieving process. When an older person believes a loved one has lived a meaningful life and has passed into the care of a Higher Power, a sense of selfworth and acceptance of the death may occur. However, the gerontological nurse should be aware that older persons who are religious are not necessarily spiritual, and vice versa. Some people attend churches or temples for the social or recreational opportunities and can find very little comfort from their religion when it is most needed. Other older people may have grown away from organized religion but still may possess a deep and abiding faith in God and the meaning of life.

History of substance abuse. Older people who have used drugs or alcohol to cope with unpleasant life events and serious losses in the past may experience a desire to use these substances again. Careful monitoring and support of these older adults is warranted.

Nature of the death. Sudden deaths that are a result of trauma, natural disaster, or violent acts may be more difficult to bear and prolong the grieving process. These deaths, in addition to the great personal loss felt by the survivor, may also trigger more symbolic losses such as loss of trust, security, and control. These older persons may experience the double psychological burden of bereavement and posttraumatic stress reaction. Symptoms include feelings of shock, horror, and numbness. Recurrent violent and frightening dreams may disrupt sleep and cause daytime anxiety. These older adults may focus exclusively on retelling the horrific events of the death, return to the scene of the old crises, overidentify with the deceased, and focus on pictures and objects. The gerontological nurse can assist older persons with their grief work and to gain mastery and control over the trauma by urging them to seek mental health services and counseling. (See Chapter 11 for a further discussion of grief and grieving.) ⊂▭

Stress and Coping

Stress is a universal phenomenon that all people experience in their daily lives. Stress is the response to demand or pressure. However, excessive and persistent stress has been linked to the development of illness (Selye, 1965). Gerontological nurses should recognize and understand stress and its influence on older persons. Chemically, stress mimics the fight-or-flight response that can preserve life in the short term, but threaten life if allowed to persist for long periods of time. The fight-or-flight response stimulates epinephrine release and increases in pulse, blood pressure, blood glucose, and muscle tension. The person may feel alarm, and thinking usually becomes narrow and concrete, focusing on the threat at hand. Ability to communicate decreases as all the emphasis is on mobilization of body defenses. If left untreated, persistent stress can result in exhaustion, adrenal cortex hormone depletion, and even death.

Risk factors that influence psychosocial functioning are categorized according to Miller (1996) into two subgroups: those that contribute to high levels of stress and poor coping, and those that may impair mental health in older adulthood. Risk factors for high levels of stress and poor coping are diminished economic resources, immature developmental level, unanticipated events such as death of a spouse, many hassles at the same time in one day, and many major life events occurring in a short period of time. Unrealistic appraisal of a situation also may increase risk for poor coping because the individual has to recognize the need for change in a given situation. High levels of stress and poor coping can cause mental and physical health impairments.

Stressors are highly individual. The event that one older person perceives as challenging may be stressful for another. Stressors may be physical, emotional, biological, or developmental. One older person may dread the thought of moving into an assisted-living facility. He or she may fear loss of privacy or independence, loss of cherished possessions, or even separation from loving memories of family events. Another older person may eagerly anticipate the move and feel joy at the thought of living in a secure environment with proximity to others. He or she may have felt lonely in a large family home and inadequate to cope with the demands of maintaining the home and yard. How the older person appraises an event depends on the individual's personality, values, and past experiences. With aging comes diversity as persons reflect their past histories, their present circumstances, and their hopes for the future.

The way an older person copes with excessive stress has been associated with poor health outcomes. Higher rates of heart disease, cancer, and other illness have been cited in the literature (McCance & Huether, 2001). Symptoms that indicate the older person may be suffering negative effects of stress include the following:

■ Sleep problems and insomnia
■ Chronic high anxiety levels

- Use or abuse of alcohol, prescription or recreational drugs, or tobacco
- Jumpiness and inability to remain still for long periods of time
- New-onset hypertension, tachycardia, tremors, or irregular heartbeat
- Depression, chronic fatigue, or lack of pleasure in life
- Chronic pain or physical complaints

Nurses working with older persons with high stress levels sometimes start to feel stressed themselves. It is important to understand the concept of stress and to break the cycle before long-term negative effects can occur. Suggested nursing actions include:

- Assisting older persons to identify stressors and rate their levels of stress.
- Educating the older person and family about stress theory and the stress cycle.
- Helping the older person identify successful coping mechanisms used in the past during periods of high stress.
- Assisting the older person to examine current coping mechanisms and behaviors and to alter or eliminate negative or maladaptive mechanisms.
- Reinforcing and strengthening positive coping mechanisms.
- Investigating community resources, support groups, stress-reduction clinics, and other stress relievers that may be useful to the older person.

Alternative therapies to relieve stress may be used in conjunction with traditional treatment approaches and counseling. Alternative therapies have been shown to be effective for older persons. Biofeedback, the process where a person learns to monitor and control body responses such as heart rate, blood pressure, and muscle tension, can be a useful technique for older people. Massage therapy can relieve muscle strain and tension, relieve pain, aid relaxation, and improve sleep. Progressive muscle relaxation can be used to induce the relaxation response. These exercises involve consciously contracting and then relaxing groups of muscles, starting at the head and working downward to the toes. They often assist older people to reduce stress levels and increase feelings of well-being. Audiotapes can be purchased or borrowed from local libraries that provide instruction for the older person learning the exercises. In addition to muscle relaxation, the older person is urged to concentrate on slow, deep breathing and to visualize a pleasant scene from childhood or youth that will induce feelings of happiness and relaxation. Exercises such as yoga, t'ai chi, and walking may reduce stress levels in addition to promoting cardiovascular health and may be appropriate for some older persons. In addition, stress-reducing techniques used in the past such as listening to music, reading a book, or watching a movie may be appropriate for coping with the current problems related to stress.

Depression

Depression is the mental health problem of greatest frequency and magnitude in the older population. Depression is defined as a clinical syndrome characterized by low mood tone, difficulty thinking, and somatic changes precipitated by feelings of loss or guilt. Clinically depressive symptoms range from 8% to 15% among community-dwelling older persons and as high as 30% in institutionalized elderly adults. Symptoms of depression are often associated with chronic illness and pain. While the rates of major depression are lower in the older population, 27% of older adults experience some depressive symptoms (Hartford Institute for Geriatric Nursing, 1999).

The economic cost of this disorder is high, but the cost in human suffering associated with caregiver burden and distress is significant. The burden of illness with depression is thought to cost the United States $43.7 billion per year. This cost includes lost productivity, the cost of direct treatment and medications, household and social difficulties, and limitation in functional ability (Tangelos & Wise, 2003). Serious depression can destroy family life as well as the life of the ill person.

Depression is best understood as a group of disorders with variable severity. Depression can include mild sadness over long periods of time, brief periods of sadness, intense reaction to loss, severe psychotic depression with hallucination and bizarre behavior, or the profound regression of pseudodementia where the older person "tunes the world out" and appears to be cognitively impaired. During the early phases of dementia, the older person may be aware that something is wrong. These feelings may trigger the onset of depressive symptoms, and depression and dementia may coexist. These patients may barely cooperate with mental status testing. When asked questions, they may respond, "I don't know." They often appear hopeless and respond slowly. They may have a flat affect and put little effort into performing any requested task. Referral to a skilled clinician (neuropsychologist, geriatric psychiatrist, or gerontological mental health nurse) is usually indicated to diagnose and treat these complicated coexisting morbidities.

Some older people may have persistent mild feelings of sadness called **dysthymia,** yet may not meet the criteria for diagnosis of clinical depression with few accompanying physical symptoms. This less severe type of depression involves long-term, chronic symptoms that do not disable, but instead keep the older person from functioning well or from enjoying life to the fullest. Many older people with dysthymia also experience major depressive episodes at sometime in their lives. Older people with dysthymia may benefit from increased socialization and involvement with others. They are less likely to benefit from traditional psychotherapy. However, they require close monitoring to ensure they do not develop symptoms of major depression.

Symptoms of depression may be emotional and physical. Emotional symptoms include sadness, diminished ability to experience joy in life, inability to concentrate, recurrent thoughts of death, and excessive guilt over things that happened in the past. Physical symptoms can include body aches, headaches, pain, fatigue, change in sleep habits, and weight gain or loss.

The major clues to depression in the older person include multiple somatic complaints and reports of persistent chronic pain. Many older people with depression tend not to consider themselves depressed and therefore complain more of physical symptoms than emotional ones. There is a stigma among many older people toward the diagnosis or acknowledgment of mental illness or psychiatric problems. Some older people find it more socially acceptable to seek advice and support from a physician or nurse for a physical reason rather than a psychological reason. Only about 20% of older depressed patients seek advice and counseling from a mental health professional. Only 12% of older people will take medication to treat depression, whereas more than 70% will take medication for headache (Jenike, 1999).

The criteria for diagnosis of a major depression as manifested by the *Diagnostic and Statistical Manual of Mental Disorders–IV–TR* (American Psychiatric Association, 2000) include the following:

- Depressed mood or loss of interest or pleasure
- Duration of symptoms for at least 2 consecutive weeks that represent a change from previous functioning
- At least five of the following (**SIG E CAPS**):
  1. Depressed mood
  2. (**S for Sleep**) Insomnia or hypersomnia (excessive sleepiness)
  3. (**I for Interest**) Diminished interest or pleasure
  4. (**G for Guilt**) Feelings of guilt or worthlessness

5. (**E for Energy**) Energy loss or fatigue
6. (**C for Concentration**) Lack of ability to concentrate
7. (**A for Appetite**) Appetite or weight change (gain or loss)
8. (**P for Psychomotor**) Psychomotor retardation or agitation
9. (**S for Suicide**) Suicidal thoughts or attempts, or recurrent thoughts of or desire for death with or without a plan

Another type of depression is bipolar disorder, also called manic-depressive illness. This disorder is not as prevalent as other forms of depressive disorders in the older person. Bipolar disorder is characterized by cycling mood changes with severe highs (mania) and lows (depression). Sometimes the mood switches are dramatic and rapid, but most often they are gradual. When in the depressed cycle, an individual can have any or all of the symptoms of a depressive disorder (Sanacore, 2003). The individual in the manic cycle may be overactive and have a great deal of energy. Mania often affects thinking, judgment, and social behavior in ways that cause serious problems and embarrassment. The symptoms of mania in bipolar depression are listed in Box 7-2.

Some types of depression appear to be familial and occur generation after generation. However, depression can also occur in older people who have no family history of the disorder. Depressive disorders are often associated with changes in brain structure or brain function. People who have low self-esteem, who consistently view themselves and the world with pessimism, or who are readily overwhelmed by stress are prone to depression. In recent years, researchers have shown that physical changes in the body can be accompanied by mental changes as well. Physical illnesses such as stroke, heart attack, cancer, and Parkinson's disease can be accompanied by disabling symptoms of depression. These symptoms can cause older persons to be apathetic and unwilling to care for their physical needs, thus prolonging the recovery period. It has been estimated that up to 57% of patients with Alzheimer's disease, 25% to 50% of patients with Parkinson's disease, 30% to 60% of those who have had a stroke, and 50% of those with Huntington's disease suffer from disabling symptoms of major depression (Jenike, 1999). Additional physical diagnoses associated with depression include endocrine disorders (hypo- and hyperthyroid), neoplastic disorders (brain tumors, pancreatic cancer, metastatic bone cancer), epilepsy, multiple sclerosis, congestive heart failure, vitamin B_{12} deficiency, and viral illness.

Symptoms of Mania in Bipolar Depression   **BOX 7-2**

- Abnormal or excessive elation
- Unusual irritability
- Decreased need for sleep
- Grandiose notions
- Increased talking
- Racing thoughts
- Increased sexual desire
- Markedly increased energy
- Poor judgment
- Inappropriate social behavior

Source: National Institutes of Health. (2000). http://www.nimh.nih.gov/publicat/depression.cfm

Serious losses, difficult relationships, financial problems, and unwelcomed stressors such as changes in life patterns can trigger depressive episodes. Changes in social roles require adjustment and can affect the identity of the older person involved. Retirement, widowhood, or an unplanned move from the home may precipitate a role change that can be perceived as positive or negative by the older person. If much of the older person's identity is based on the lost role, coping problems and depression can follow. For instance, if the older woman primarily thinks of herself as Mrs. John Smith or the wife of John Smith, the death of her husband may be more difficult and more likely to negatively affect her mental health.

Women experience depression about twice as often as men (Blehar & Oren, 1997). Although men are less likely to suffer from depression, 3 million to 4 million men in the United States are affected by the illness. Men are less likely to admit to depression, and doctors are less likely to suspect it. Gender differences in the prevalence of depression may be explained by social risk factors. More than 50% of older women live alone compared to 25% of older men. Older women may be more prone to loneliness, financial difficulties, and loss of independence due to functional disability. Marriage has been shown to be protective against the development of depression, and married older persons have a lower suicide rate than others. Further, older women are more likely to be institutionalized in a nursing home. Stress and coping styles may differ by gender with older women developing depression in response to a stressful life event at a rate three times higher than older men (Nelson, Lavretsky, & Burke, 2003).

Some people have the mistaken idea that depression is a normal occurrence in older adults. However, most older people feel satisfied with their lives. When depression develops, it is sometimes dismissed as a normal part of aging. Undiagnosed depression in the older person causes unnecessary suffering for the family and for the individual. Depressive symptoms can be side effects of medications the older person is taking for a physical problem; therefore, it is important for the nurse to become familiar with medications that can cause or exacerbate symptoms of depression. Patients with symptoms of depression taking these medications should be urged to seek consultation with their primary care provider to see if the medication can be safely discontinued or switched to another medication without this troubling side effect. Box 7-3 lists some of the medications that can cause depressive symptoms.

NURSING ASSESSMENT OF DEPRESSION

Various instruments are used to assess depression in the older adult. Each instrument has advantages and limitations. The symptoms of depression can be so vague and unique to each individual that the gerontological nurse is urged to use various methods and multiple observations when assessing depression. Sometimes after spending time with a depressed older patient, the nurse will also feel a little down. Because nurses are caring and empathetic individuals, they pick up on subtle cues the patient is transmitting and become aware of the patient's sadness. Careful and systematic assessment can lead to a definitive diagnosis and early treatment.

The Geriatric Depression Scale (GDS) is a screening instrument used in many clinical settings to assess depression in older people. The GDS is a 30-item (long version) or 15-item (short version) instrument with questions that can be answered "yes" or "no." An older person can complete the GDS alone by circling the correct answer, or it can be read to an older person. When tested in various groups of older people, the GDS was found to successfully distinguish between depressed and nondepressed older

BOX 7-3

Medications That Can Cause Symptoms of Depression

Analgesics
   Narcotics (codeine, morphine, etc.)
   Nonsteroidal anti-inflammatory agents (ibuprofen, naproxen, indomethacin)
Antihypertensives/Cardiac
   Clonidine, methyldopa, propranolol, reserpine, thiazide diuretics, digitalis
Antipsychotics
   Chlorpromazine, fluphenazine, haloperidol, thioridazine, thiothixene
Anxiolytics
   Chlordiazepoxide, diazepam, lorazepam, oxazepam
Chemotherapeutics
   L-asparaginase, cisplatin, tamoxifen, vincristine
Sedative-Hypnotics
   Ethchlorvynol, flurazepam, pentobarbital sodium, phenobarbital, secobarbital sodium, temazepam, triazolam
Other
   Antiulcer medications—cimetidine, ranitidine hydrochloride
   Corticosteroids—dexamethasone, prednisone
   Alcohol

Source: Adapted from Epocrates.com, 2003; Wynne, Woo, & Millard, 2002; Youngkin et al., 2005.

people (Yesavage et al., 1983). The GDS can be used for screening physically healthy, or ill individuals, and those with cognitive impairment (Mini-Mental State Examination [MMSE] score above 15) (Hartford Institute for Geriatric Nursing, 1999). Older people scoring above 10 should be referred for further assessment. The Cornell Depression Scale (CDS) can be used to screen for depression in older adults with severe cognitive impairments (MMSE below 15). The CDS does not rely on patient responses, but rather observations of behaviors and functional measures. People who score 12 or above on the CDS should be referred for further assessment. Because the CDS requires patient observations, it takes slightly longer to administer than the GDS. See the Best Practice feature on page 214 for the GDS.

SUICIDE

Older persons age 65 and over have the highest suicide rates of all age groups (Bille-Brahe & Andersen, 2001). A major risk factor for suicide is depression. Older Caucasian men have the highest death rates from suicide of all groups of older people. Older men, but not women, with serious neurological, vascular, and heart diseases were found to be at increased risk for suicide (Waern et al., 2002). Approximately 70% of older adults who commit suicide had visited their primary care physician within the previous month (U.S. Department of Health and Human Services, 2001).

Gerontological nurses can play a key role in the identification and referral of those older people who are depressed and at risk for suicide. When the gerontological nurse is interacting with an older patient who seems sad or depressed, the nurse should ask about suicidal intent. Many nurses are hesitant to do this because of fear of placing the idea in the older person's mind. However, this is rarely if ever the case. Most older people, when asked this question gently by a caring nurse, will respond openly and appreciate the gesture. The nurse may ask, "Mr. Jones, you seem sad today. Do you ever think of hurting yourself or ending your life?" If the older person answers affirmatively, this threat must be taken seriously and immediately reported to a physician or mental health professional.

In the older population, the ratio of attempts to completed suicides is 4 to 1. An older person who contemplates suicide is more likely to complete the act than a younger person. There are several reasons for this fact. First, elderly people often employ lethal methods when attempting suicide. Second, older people experience greater social isolation (Oslin & Mellow, 2000). Finally, elderly people generally have poorer recuperative capacity, which makes them less likely to recover from a suicide attempt.

A direct relationship exists between alcoholism, depression, and suicide. Studies indicate that the risk of suicide in alcoholics is 50% to 70% greater than in the general population. Studies show that individuals suffering from a major affective disorder have a greater than 50% higher suicide rate than the general population. Lifetime risk for suicide in the general population is 1%, compared with 15% for persons suffering from depression and 15% for alcoholics. Studies of alcoholics reveal that between 30% and 60% suffer from depression, and a significant proportion of alcoholics have other persons in their families suffering from depression.

Risk factors for suicide that may be determined from the past health history include a previous suicide attempt, alcohol or substance abuse, presence of a psychiatric illness, history of a psychiatric illness, presence of auditory hallucinations (hearing voices commanding action), and living alone (Jenike, 1999). Older men are more likely to have access to and use guns as a means to suicide, whereas older women are more likely to overdose on medications. Once the suicide intent is verbalized, the means to carry out the plan should be assessed. Older patients who have the means to carry out a suicide attempt should be immediately referred for evaluation. Those perceived to be at risk for suicide will probably be hospitalized for a short period to protect their lives and provide for intensive observation and treatment.

Patients hospitalized with suicidal ideation will be placed on "suicide precautions" that include one-to-one monitoring by an observer, locked window, and removal of items that have potential for self-harm such as belts, sharp knives, medications, and so on. Therapy and treatment of the underlying depression will most often improve the older patient's situation. By providing a safe and supportive environment and listening therapeutically to the older patient, the nurse has the opportunity to prevent suffering and the needless loss of human life.

Some nurses confuse an older patient's desire to have a natural death with suicidal intent. A seriously ill patient who cries and states "I'm ready to go when God calls me" is probably not expressing suicidal thoughts. Any patient who receives bad news of serious illness or failed treatment has the right to be sad and overwhelmed. An older person who is diagnosed with a life-threatening illness may begin the work of preparing for death, and the gerontological nurse provides palliative care. Encounters that allow for exploring areas of meaning, fears and hopes, guilt, grief, and relatedness to others can facilitate mental health in older patients with serious illness (Coward & Reed, 1996). However, patients who request assistance from the nurse with suicide and active euthanasia should be informed that the nurse will not participate as these acts are in direct violation of the American Nurses Association (2001) Code for Nurses. Active euthanasia or "mercy killing" means that someone other than the patient commits an action with the intent to end the patient's life. Mercy killing is immoral and illegal, even when a suffering patient requests assistance from the nurse to hasten death. An example may be the injection of a lethal dose of morphine into a patient, not to relieve suffering, but to end life. Active euthanasia is distinguished from assisted suicide in that with active euthanasia someone not only makes the means of death available, but also serves as the direct agent of death. The American Nurses Association statement advances that assisted suicide and active euthanasia are inconsistent with the code for nurses and are ethically unacceptable. There are many ways to support older patients and their families at the end of life without participating in assisted suicide or active euthanasia. Gerontological nurses should aggressively investigate depression and advocate for effective pain control to prevent needless suffering at the end of life (see Chapter 11 for further information on end-of-life care). ▭

ALCOHOL ABUSE

The prevalence of alcohol abuse and dependence in older adults ranges from 2% to 5% for men and about 1% for women. There is a decline in substance abuse for older adults after the age of 60. There are several reasons, however, why drinking alcohol may negatively impact the physical and mental health of the older person. Age-related physical changes, diagnosed physical illness, and prescription drugs can combine with relatively low levels of alcohol to produce negative outcomes in older people. Older persons experience higher blood levels per amount of alcohol consumed due to decreased lean body mass and total body water. Older patients are hospitalized as frequently for alcohol-related problems as they are for heart attacks (Scott & Popovich, 2001). As the number of older people increases, so will the absolute number of older people who have alcohol abuse problems.

Risk factors for alcohol abuse include genetic predisposition, being male, limited education, poverty, and a history of depression (American Psychological Association, 2003). Men over 65 are five times more likely to suffer from alcoholism than their female counterparts; however, older women with drinking problems are more likely to go undetected (Copley News Service, 1999). Older women are more likely to become dependent on prescription drugs, such as benzodiazepines, than their male counterparts (Hays, Olson, & Blow, 1999). Older widowers have the highest prevalence rates of alcohol abuse among older adults (American Psychological Association, 2003). Problems related to excessive or regular alcohol consumption include:

- **Malnutrition.** Failure to prepare and eat an adequate diet.
- **Cirrhosis of the liver.** One of eight leading causes of death for the older person.
- **Osteomalacia.** Thinning of the bones.
- **Decreases in gastric absorption.** Failure to absorb key minerals and vitamins from ingested food.
- **Decline in cognitive function.** Impairment of memory and information processing.
- **Interactions with medications.** Interaction with benzodiazepines greatly increases risk of falls and hip fractures.

(American Psychological Association, 1998; Scott & Popovich, 2001)

Unlike other psychoactive drugs, alcohol has a generalized effect on the central nervous system. Alcohol seems to impair learning and memory because of its ability to inhibit acetylcholine action. Judgment and reasoning are also adversely affected, with degree of impairment related to blood alcohol level or duration of consumption. Additionally, alcohol can lead to loss of social inhibition and problems in regulation of emotion. Higher levels of consumption lead to drowsiness, stupor, and motor coordination problems (Wiscott, Kopera-Frye, & Seifert, 2001). Alcohol consumption in excess of three drinks per day increases the risk of hypertension, some cancers (esophagus and breast in women), and possibly injury (World Health Organization, 2001). Alcohol may interact with certain drugs and cause adverse systemic effects. These drugs include antihypertensives, nonsteroidal anti-inflammatory drugs (NSAIDs), H_2 blockers, sedatives, and antidepressants (Reuben et al., 2002).

The *DSM-IV-TR* criteria for possible **alcohol dependence** include three or more of the following:

- Tolerance (requiring more alcohol to get effect)
- Withdrawal or drinking to ease withdrawal
- Drinking in larger quantities or for longer periods of time than expected
- Persistent desire to drink or unsuccessful efforts to control drinking
- Spending a lot of time obtaining or using alcohol, or recovering from effects
- Giving up important social or recreational activities to pursue drinking
- Drinking despite persistent or recurrent physical or psychological problems caused by alcohol

The *DSM-IV-TR* criteria for possible **alcohol abuse** include one or more of the following:

- Drinking resulting in the failure to fulfill major obligations
- Drinking in situations where it is physically hazardous
- Alcohol-related legal problems
- Continued drinking despite social problems caused or worsened by alcohol

Screening for alcohol use not only is a means for detection, but also provides the opportunity for intervention to reduce adverse consequences (Moore, Seeman, Morgenstern, Beck, & Reuben, 2002). The CAGE (acronym for Cut down, Annoyed by criticism, Guilty about drinking, Eye-opener drink) questionnaire has been validated in the older adult (Reuben et al., 2002). One positive answer to the CAGE questionnaire suggests the older person is a problem drinker. Additional questions that may provide valuable information to supplement the CAGE include:

- How many days do you drink per week?
- How many drinks do you have per day?
- What is the maximum number of drinks you have per day?
- What type of alcohol do you drink (beer, wine, liquor)?
- What is "a drink"?

More than two drinks per day for women or three for men is considered potentially harmful, depending on the older person's tolerance, physical health, medication use, and living situation (Reuben et al., 2002).

It is recommended that older persons consume no more than one drink per day after the age of 65. Red wine consumed in small to moderate amounts has been shown to decrease risk of cardiovascular disease.

Older persons who are dependent on or abusing alcohol should be referred for further evaluation and treatment. The gerontological nurse plays a key role in educating the older person about the potential health problems associated with continued alcohol use. Self-help groups such as Alcoholics Anonymous, professional counseling, social support, and drug therapy have all been shown to be effective in treating alcohol problems in older people. Disulfiram (Antabuse) is not recommended for use in older people because of the potential for serious cardiovascular side effects and multiple drug interactions (Reuben et al., 2002).

Older persons who are hospitalized or institutionalized in long-term care facilities may become delirious during acute alcohol withdrawal. Acute agitation and hallucination may occur (delirium tremors). Nonpharmacological measures to protect patient safety include keeping the room as quiet as possible, avoiding excessive light and stimulation, encouraging family visitation for comfort and reassurance, providing orientation to time and place, communicating directly and succinctly, and providing frequent observation and monitoring of vital signs. Usually the physician will prescribe lorazepam (Ativan) 0.5 to 2.0 mg every 4 to 6 hours to prevent alcohol withdrawal seizures. Adequate hydration and nutrition will ease the withdrawal process (Reuben et al., 2002).

BASIC PRINCIPLES RELATING TO PSYCHOLOGICAL ASSESSMENT IN OLDER ADULTS

Because of the physical and sensory changes of aging, the testing environment must be appropriate to ensure optimal performance by the older adult. Specially trained psychologists can administer a battery of neuropsychological tests to provide specific and detailed information about the older person's cognitive and psychological status. The gerontological nurse may be the first to notice signs and symptoms of psychological change and recommend the referral to the geriatric mental health specialist. Psychological testing should be done under the following circumstances:

- When considering admission to a geropsychiatric inpatient unit
- When considering need for and benefit of outpatient geropsychiatric services
- To assist in the diagnosis of dementia versus depression
- To provide information for the legal determination of competency
- When evaluating sudden or severe changes in mood, personality, or psychological function
- To evaluate and monitor response to therapy or psychotropic medication

The nurse's interpersonal skills will facilitate the clinical interview and the gathering of information in an individualized, comprehensive, holistic assessment. Some suggestions for improving the quality of information gathered at the clinical interview include the following:

- Make sure the older patient is not in pain, has been to the bathroom, and has water or juice to sip on during the assessment. If the person wears glasses or hearing aids, make sure they are in place and functioning.
- Educate the older adult about the purpose and procedure for the testing. The nurse may say, "I'm going to ask you some questions about your mood. Some of these may seem silly to you, but we ask these questions of most of our clinic patients." Older adults may not be used to testing procedures and may need some reassurance.
- Try to make the testing environment as quiet as possible. Turn off the overhead page and any beepers. Make sure there is adequate lighting.
- Speak slowly and clearly. Make sure the older adult understands the testing instructions. If vision is impaired, use a magnifying lens or large-print testing materials.
- Observe the older patient carefully. If the patient becomes tired and has difficulty concentrating, take a break and resume testing at another time.
- If English is the second language for the older patient, request assistance from a translator rather than asking a family member to translate. The translator has been trained in the precise use of medical terminology.

The gerontological nurse should assess the older patient's current mental status and obtain informed consent before beginning mood testing. The older patient's education, culture, ethnicity, religion, health status, and comfort should form the context for the nurse's assessment. The older person's social context should also be considered. Financial stressors, active grieving, living situation, family support, and degree of loneliness will greatly affect the older person's responses. Mood is evaluated by observation of the patient (e.g., facial expressions, posture, speed of movements, and thoughts) and of verbal content. Although patients often spontaneously express feelings of helplessness, hopelessness, worthlessness, shame, or guilt, they should be asked directly about such feelings (e.g., "Do you feel that you are a good person?" "Do you feel guilty about things you have done?") and about mood (e.g., "How are your spirits?" or "How is your mood?"). Questions such as "How does the future look?" and "Do you feel you have unusual talents or abilities?" may detect excessive optimism or overconfidence.

Current and past medical history is needed to assess the impact of physical illness on psychological status. Chronic pain is a known correlate of depression, and a careful pain assessment should be done whenever depression is suspected. The patient should be asked about changes in energy, appetite, or sleep that are related to mood disturbances. Additional assessment information includes use of prescription and over-the-counter medication, as well as current and past use of alcohol, tobacco, and recreational drugs. The nurse should ascertain whether the older patient is taking the medication as directed, whether the prescription is current and not expired, and whether the conditions under which the medication is taken are appropriate (on an empty stomach, before bed, only when needed, etc.). It is important to pay special attention to sudden changes in mood or personality, as these may be signs of delirium related to recent changes in medication, onset of undetected illness, or exacerbation of chronic illness. When the older patient's cognitive status appears to be impaired, the nurse should request the patient's permission to include a family member or caregiver in the assessment to supplement and verify the information reported by the patient.

Depression in elderly adults may manifest itself as a sense of dread or impending doom, as apathy, or as irritability without a specific cause. Depression may also be suggested by complaints of pain, tiredness, or other physiological changes; by slow speech; by anxiety (sometimes as panic attacks with shortness of breath, palpitations, and sweating); by phobias, obsessions, or compulsions; or by abnormal perceptions (e.g., delusions, hallucinations). When the nurse suspects an underlying anxiety disorder, the patient should be asked about phobias or irrational fears of particular places, things, or situations.

Older patients should also be asked about obsessions (recurrent, unwanted ideas that cannot be resisted, although they may seem unreasonable) and compulsions (repeated, unwanted behaviors such as hand washing or rechecking a locked door). Obsessions in the older person are usually due to severe depression, whereas compulsions often result from an obsession. Obsessions can be elicited by asking, "Do you have thoughts that keep coming to your mind and are difficult to get rid of? Are the thoughts reasonable, or do they sometimes seem silly?" Compulsions can be elicited by asking, "Must you do certain things (e.g., wash your hands) repeatedly, more than you need to?"

It is important to differentiate depressive signs from delusions. Delusions are false, fixed, and idiosyncratic ideas. Patients may reveal delusional thoughts when questioned (e.g., "Are people treating you kindly? Is anyone trying to harm you?"). Delusions of harm (e.g., of food poisoning) or of harassment may occur in elderly persons with paranoid schizophrenia or *paraphrenia* (late-life schizophrenia). Delusions also occur in 40% of persons with dementia. Delusions of poverty or of fatal illness may occur in depressed persons, who may verbalize multiple somatic complaints and become overly focused on body functions. *Delusions of persecution* (e.g., belief that someone is out to get them) or of *misidentification* (e.g., belief that family members are strangers or that persons long dead are alive) may occur in persons with cognitive impairment. Delusions should be differentiated from *overvalued ideas* (emotionally laden preoccupations or hobbies that override other activities or concerns), from culturally determined suspicions, and from religious beliefs. Furthermore, the nurse should be able to detect hallucinations in the form of false visual, auditory, olfactory, or tactile perceptions. The presence of visual or auditory hallucinations may be elicited by asking, "Do you hear voices or see visions? If you hear voices, are they similar to my voice in your ear?" Further questioning is needed to determine whether the phenomena are really perceived (e.g., "Do you hear the voices even when you do not see anyone talking? Do you hear them through your ears, or are they in your thoughts? Do you hear them as clearly as you hear me now?"). The nurse should respond with sympathy (e.g., "That must have frightened you"), not with surprise or disbelief. Visual and tactile hallucinations are prominent in delirium, and auditory hallucinations may occur when the older person is cognitively impaired and in paraphrenia. Auditory hallucinations (e.g., hearing one's name called) also may occur in late-life depression. Hallucinations may occur in persons with sensory deficits, especially profound blindness, at which time the condition is called Charles Bonnet syndrome. In addition, hallucinations may occur during bereavement, when the patient sees or hears the deceased person.

When all the information from the older patient has been gathered, the nurse and other members of the healthcare team will integrate the findings with relevant social and health variables. Strengths and weaknesses should be identified so the gerontological nurse can begin to formulate nursing interventions that build on areas of strength and compensate for areas of weakness. Older patients in acute psychological distress such as those who are severely agitated, depressed, or in danger of harming themselves or others should be referred to a mental health professional for psychotherapy or psychotropic medication. If underlying health problems are thought to be negatively influencing psychological function, a referral to an internist or geriatrician may greatly benefit the older person. Complete assessment of health problems includes a head-to-toe physical examination and a variety of laboratory tests, including a complete blood count (CBC), a chemistry panel (SMA-18), test of thyroid function (TSH), and assessment of serum levels of medications taken on a regular basis (digoxin, warfarin, etc.). Additional testing may be needed based upon the older patient's unique personal and health history.

Cultural Considerations

The older population is becoming more culturally and ethnically diverse in the United States. Currently, the typical older person is a Caucasian; however, by the middle of this century the number of older African Americans will triple, increasing their proportion of the total older adult population from 8% to 10%. The number of older Hispanics will increase from less than 4% to nearly 16% of the older population (American Psychological Association, 1998). The unique life experiences, values, and beliefs of these minority elders may be very different from those of the larger cohort of older adults.

In order to reach the *Healthy People 2010* goal of equal access to healthcare, the mental health needs of minority elders, who are at highest risk of death and disability, should be addressed. Poor income and low literacy, often associated with minority status, are important risk factors for major chronic illness (American Psychological Association, 1998). Several factors should be acknowledged regarding health status and minority aging:

- The onset of chronic illness is usually earlier than in Caucasian older adults.
- There are frequent delays in seeking health treatment.
- Health problems may be underreported because of lack of trust in healthcare workers.
- Mental health services are underutilized.

- There are higher rates of treatment dropout and medical noncompliance.
- Although longevity for African American men is shorter than that for Caucasian men, African American men and women surviving to the age of 75 live longer than Caucasians.
- There is a higher incidence of obesity and type 2 diabetes mellitus.
- A large number of minority elders possess no health insurance.

Factors contributing to poor mental health include poverty, segregated and disorganized communities, poor quality education, few role responsibilities, sporadic and chronic unemployment and underemployment, stereotyping, discrimination, and poor healthcare (American Psychological Association, 1998). The use and refinement of culturally sensitive instruments to assess mental status, depression, dementia, and pain is encouraged.

Nursing Interventions

Treatment of mental health problems in the older person can use nonpharmacological approaches, pharmacological approaches, or a combination of the two. Information on these techniques follows.

NONPHARMACOLOGICAL TREATMENTS

Many older adults referred for psychological services will feel embarrassed or ashamed of the need for psychotherapy or psychotropic medication. The gerontological nurse can reassure the older person and the family that mental health problems can be effectively treated. This treatment will enhance the chances of returning to former levels of psychological function.

No single psychological intervention is preferred for older adults. The treatment of choice is guided by the nature of the problem, therapeutic goals, preferences of the older adult, and practical considerations (American Psychological Association, 1998). Both individual and group psychotherapy have been shown to be effective in treating the older adult's psychological problems. Family or couples therapy may be appropriate when marital or family relationship problems occur within the context of late-life illness or stress. Often, a family member may feel stress by the burden of caring for a spouse or parent and may need support and respite from the responsibility of care. Behavior modification, self-help groups, educational sessions, and changes in the social or physical environment may lead to improved emotional health and functioning.

Some older people find it beneficial to engage in reminiscence or a "life review" of the present, the past, and the future. Both successes and failures should be considered in an effort to identify the older person's life themes with the goal of attaining greater psychological integration and emotional strength. Geriatric social workers and advanced practice psychiatric–mental health nurses can greatly assist with this process.

Support group attendance can help the older person and the family cope with problems by identifying with others who are in the same situation. The Alzheimer's Association, the American Cancer Society, and other groups focusing on specific illnesses in late life (Parkinson's disease, arthritis, cardiac or lung problems, etc.) provide a forum for conversation, social interaction, education, and problem solving. Grief or bereavement groups can also assist the older person dealing with multiple or serious losses or unresolved grief. Additional helpful interventions include travel with senior citizens' groups, taking classes at the local college, elder hostels, volunteer work, regular exercise, hobbies and crafts, and increased family involvement.

For older persons experiencing caregiver stress, attendance at self-help groups can be especially helpful. There are an estimated 25 million family caregivers in the United

States who deliver care to a frail older person (spouse, parent, sibling), including help with daily activities and around-the-clock supervision. Caregivers can experience enormous stress from the added responsibility of caring for a loved one and may become depressed or anxious, or develop physical illness as a result of the stress of caregiving. In addition to concrete suggestions to improve safety in the home, education about stress-reducing techniques emphasizes mutual support and caring. The following suggestions for caregivers may help to reduce stress:

- Share the responsibility for care. Do not take on more than you can handle, and involve others who can help out.
- Meditate, listen to music, or take a brief walk every day. Caregivers who do not care for themselves will be of no use to anyone.
- Set priorities. Work on one problem at a time. Trying to do too much will cause you to feel distracted, frustrated, and "at loose ends." Make a list and cross one problem off before moving to the next.
- Maintain your own physical health. Get regular checkups, take medications, eat nutritious meals, avoid alcohol and caffeine, and get regular exercise. Should something happen to you, your loved one may be at risk for institutionalization.
- Seek love and support from your family, friends, clergy, and others. Do not be afraid to seek additional help and recognize when professional counseling is needed to cope with difficult decisions.
- Educate yourself about your loved one's condition. Knowledge is power.
- Join a local support group. Contact your local aging resource center for phone numbers.
- Accept yourself for what you are. Do not strive for perfection. You are a human being doing the best you can to cope with a difficult situation. Self-acceptance and nurturing will go a long way.

Light therapy has been shown to be effective for older patients diagnosed with **seasonal affective disorder**, a cyclic depression that occurs when hours of daylight are short, usually in the fall and early spring. Older patients who respond to light therapy will sit before specially designed lights for several hours during the shortened daylight periods. Biochemical changes are thought to be stimulated in the brain by various blue and red hues in the spectrum of light. Medications can also be used to augment light therapy in older patients with seasonal affective disorder.

Older persons with substance abuse problems (drug or alcohol) may attend Alcoholics Anonymous meetings. They may benefit from professional treatment and counseling or age-specific inpatient or outpatient treatment during the withdrawal period. Many late-life mental health problems are recurrent. The goals of treatment should be flexible and emphasize improving function, managing disabling symptoms, preventing relapse, and building a safety net for quick recognition of recurring problems.

Pharmacological Treatments

When the older patient experiences only a partial response or no response at all after 6 to 12 weeks of therapy and nonpharmacological interventions for depression, use of antidepressant medication is usually warranted. As with all drugs prescribed to an older person, the risks and benefits should be carefully analyzed. Many antidepressant drugs, especially the tricyclic antidepressants, have troublesome anticholinergic side effects and can cause orthostatic hypotension.

As many of the antidepressants take 6 to 12 weeks to achieve therapeutic effects and ease depression, the older person and the family should be patient and realistic in their expectations regarding antidepressant therapy. For mild, moderate, or severe depression, the duration of therapy should be at least 6 to 12 months following remission for older patients experiencing their first depressive episode. Most older patients with a history of major depression require lifelong antidepressant therapy (Reuben et al., 2002). As with all medications, the initial dose should be about one half the usual adult dose, in order to decrease the severity of any adverse side effects. Careful monitoring is needed during the first few days of treatment so that any adverse side effects can be quickly noted and the medication changed or discontinued if needed. Falls, sedation, urinary retention, constipation, drowsiness, visual changes, appetite changes, tachycardia, and photosensitivity have all been reported as side effects of antidepressants and may pose a significant health and safety risk for older adults. Some antidepressants can increase the therapeutic effects and interact with warfarin, anticholinergics, antihistamines, opioids, antihistamines, and sedative-hypnotics. Older patients taking warfarin should be closely monitored during the first few weeks of the initiation of antidepressant therapy.

Antidepressants can decrease the effects of certain drugs, including some anticonvulsant medications (phenytoin) and some antihypertensives. Postural blood pressure should be carefully monitored during the first few weeks of antidepressant therapy in older patients with hypertension. Older patients should be strongly urged to avoid alcohol while taking antidepressant medications.

Because many of the tricyclic antidepressants (TCAs) are associated with anticholinergic side effects such as constipation, urinary retention, dry mouth, hypotension, and tachycardia, some geriatricians prefer to use the selective serotonin reuptake inhibitors (SSRIs) as first-line drugs for many older patients, especially those with the following conditions:

- Heart conduction defects or ischemic heart disease
- Benign prostatic hypertrophy
- Difficult-to-control glaucoma

In general the SSRIs are well tolerated in the older person. Side effects include nausea, diarrhea, headache, erectile dysfunction, insomnia, or somnolence. Table 7-1 lists the SSRIs commonly used with older people.

The TCAs have been most widely used in the older population. In general, those who respond best to these medications are older people with loss of appetite, psychomotor agitation or retardation, history of previous use and response to TCAs, and family history of depression that responded to TCA treatment (Kane, Ouslander, & Abrass, 2000). All the tricyclics have the potential of producing bothersome and potentially dangerous side effects. Careful nursing assessment is indicated during the initial dosing period. Divided dosages can help minimize side effects. For older patients with sleep disturbances, a single bedtime dose can be used to take advantage of the sedative side effects; however, these patients are

TABLE 7-1

SSRIs Used for Older Adults

Drug	Initial Dose	Usual Dose	Comments
Citalopram (Celexa)	10 mg	20–30 mg qd	Hyponatremia in renal failure
Fluoxetine (Prozac)	5 mg	10–50 mg q a.m.	Long half-life; raises levels of haloperidol, diazepam, valproate, aprazolam, and carbamazepine
Sertraline (Zoloft)	25 mg	50 mg q a.m.	Short half-life; raises levels of warfarin
Paroxetine (Paxil)	5 mg	10–20 mg qd	Short half-life; raises levels of digoxin

Source: Adapted from epocrates.com, 2003; Jenike, 1999; Reuben et al., 2002..

at risk for postural hypotension and may fall if they get out of bed to use the bathroom in the middle of the night. Many prescribers avoid the use of imipramine and amitriptyline because they can cause severe orthostatic hypotension, placing the older person at risk for fall and injury. To decrease the development of symptoms of tardive dyskinesia like dystonia and parkinsonism, amoxapine should be avoided. Table 7-2 lists the TCAs commonly used in older people.

Additional drugs sometimes used to treat depression in the older person include bupropion (Wellbutrin). This drug may lower seizure threshold and is contraindicated in older patients with seizure disorders. It is usually started at 37.5 mg bid and titrated to 75 to 100 mg bid. It has been used successfully in some older patients who have failed to respond to SSRI and TCA therapy (Reuben et al., 2002). Although bupropion has not been well studied in older people, initial results indicate that there are no known anticholinergic effects and it does not induce postural hypotension (Jenike, 1999). Methylphenidate (Ritalin), a stimulant, has been used in some older people who exhibit marked psychomotor retardation and apathy. It is recommended only for short-term use with careful monitoring of cardiovascular side effects. It is usually dosed at 5 to 10 mg once or twice a day (Jenike, 1999).

Lithium carbonate has been used to treat recurrent bipolar illness. The half-life of lithium is prolonged in the healthy older person (more than 36 hours) and greatly prolonged in older persons with chronic renal failure. Side effects include bradycardia, hypothyroidism, tinnitus, tremor, ataxia, nystagmus, mental status changes, and seizures (Jenike, 1999). This drug must be used with caution, and blood levels and patient function must be carefully monitored during the initial dosing period.

Monoamine oxidase inhibitors (MAOIs) are sometimes used in older people with dementia and depression and in those who have not responded to other drug therapies. Orthostatic hypotension is common and peaks 4 to 5 weeks after beginning therapy (Jenike, 1999). Because these drugs inhibit the metabolism of norepinephrine, hypertensive crisis can occur if they are administered with other drugs or food that raise blood pressure such as anticholinergics, stimulants, and foods containing tyramine (red wine, cheese, etc.). These restrictions apply during use and for 14 days following discontinuation of the MAOIs. Older patients and their families should be well informed about the adverse effects and drug and dietary restrictions necessary for safe administration.

Electroconvulsive therapy (ECT) is indicated in older patients who do not respond to other antidepressant medications, are diagnosed with delusional depression, or have life-threatening behaviors (suicidal ideation, catatonic, etc.). ECT involves the use of a brief, controlled electrical current to produce a seizure within the brain. This seizure activity is believed to bring about certain biochemical changes that may cause an older person's symptoms to diminish or even disappear. A series of seizures, generally 6 to 12, given at a rate of 3 per week is required to produce such a therapeutic effect (Maki, 2003). The ECT process has been improved greatly since the 1950s, and the ECT procedure is relatively

TABLE 7-2

Commonly Used TCAs in Older People

Drug	Initial Dose	Usual Dose	Comments
Amitriptyline (Elavil)	10 mg hs	25–100 mg hs	Anticholinergic, sedating, hypotension
Desipramine (Norpramin)	10 mg a.m.	50–100 mg a.m.	Activating agent
Nortriptyline (Pamelor)	10 mg hs	75–100 mg hs	Long half-life

Source: Adapted from epocrates.com, 2003; Jenike, 1999; Reuben et al., 2002.

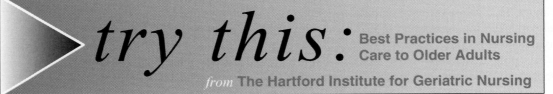

> *try this:* Best Practices in Nursing Care to Older Adults
> *from* The Hartford Institute for Geriatric Nursing

Issue Number 4, May 1999   Series Editor: Meredith Wallace, PhD, RN, MSN, CS

The Geriatric Depression Scale (GDS)
By: Lenore Kurlowicz, PhD, RN, CS

WHY: Depression is common in late life, effecting nearly five million of the 31 million Americans aged 65 and older. Both major and minor depression are reported in 13% of community dwelling older adults, 24% of older medical outpatients and 43% of both acute care and nursing home dwelling older adults. Contrary to popular belief, depression is not a natural part of aging. Depression is often reversible with prompt and appropriate treatment. However, if left untreated, depression may result in the onset of physical, cognitive and social impairment as well as delayed recovery from medical illness and surgery, increased health care utilization and suicide.

BEST TOOL: While there are many instruments available to measure depression, the Geriatric Depression Scale (GDS), first created by Yesavage et al., has been tested and used extensively with the older population. It is a brief questionnaire in which participants are asked to respond to the 30 questions by answering yes or no in reference to how they felt on the day of administration. Scores of 0 - 9 are considered normal, 10 - 19 indicate mild depression and 20 - 30 indicate severe depression.

TARGET POPULATION: The GDS may be used with healthy, medically ill and mild to moderately cognitively impaired older adults. It has been extensively used in community, acute and long-term care settings.

VALIDITY/RELIABILITY: The GDS was found to have a 92% sensitivity and a 89% specificity when evaluated against diagnostic criteria. The validity and reliability of the tool have been supported through both clinical practice and research.

STRENGTHS AND LIMITATIONS: The GDS is not a substitute for a diagnostic interview by mental health professionals. It is a useful screening tool in the clinical setting to facilitate assessment of depression in older adults especially when baseline measurements are compared to subsequent scores.

MORE ON THE TOPIC:
Koenig, H.G. Meador, K.G., Cohen, J.J. Blazer, D.G. (1988). Self-Rated Depression Scales and Screening
    for Major Depression in the Older Hospitalized Patient with Medical Illness. *Journal of the American
    Geriatrics Society, 699-706.*

Kurlowicz, L.H., & NICHE Faculty (1997). Nursing Stand or Practice Protocol: Depression in Elderly Patients.
    Geriatric Nursing, 18, 192-199

NIH Consensus Development Panel. (1992). Diagnosis and Treatment of Depression in Late Life.
    JAMA, 268, 1018-1024.

Sheikh, R.L. & Yesavage, J.A. (1986). Geriatric Depression Scale (GDS). Recent Evidence and Development
    of a Shorter Version. *Clinical Gerontologist*, 5, 165-173.

Yesavage, J.A., Brink, T.L., Rose, T.L., Lum, O. Huang, V., Adey, M., Leirer, V.O. (1983). Development
    and Validation of a Geriatric Depression Screening Scale: A Preliminary Report. *Journal of Psychiatric
    Research*, 17, 37-49.

Patient _____ Examiner _____ Date _____

Directions to Patient: Please choose the best answer for how you have felt over the past week.

Directions to Examiner: Present questions VERBALLY. Circle answer given by patient. Do not show to patient.

1. Are you basically satisfied with your life? . . . . yes   **no (1)**
2. Have you dropped many of your activities and interests? . . . . **yes (1)**   no
3. Do you feel that your life is empty? . . . . **yes (1)**   no
4. Do you often get bored? . . . . **yes (1)**   no
5. Are you hopeful about the future? . . . . yes   **no (1)**
6. Are you bothered by thoughts you can't get out of your head? . . . . **yes (1)**   no
7. Are you in good spirits most of the time? . . . . yes   **no (1)**
8. Are you afraid that something bad is going to happen to you? . . . . **yes (1)**   no
9. Do you feel happy most of the time? . . . . yes   **no (1)**
10. Do you often feel helpless? . . . . **yes (1)**   no
11. Do you often get restless and fidgety? . . . . **yes (1)**   no
12. Do you prefer to stay at home rather than go out and do things? . . . . **yes (1)**   no
13. Do you frequently worry about the future? . . . . **yes (1)**   no
14. Do you feel you have more problems with memory than most? . . . . **yes (1)**   no
15. Do you think it is wonderful to be alive now? . . . . yes   **no (1)**
16. Do you feel downhearted and blue? . . . . **yes (1)**   no
17. Do you feel pretty worthless the way you are now? . . . . **yes (1)**   no
18. Do you worry a lot about the past? . . . . **yes (1)**   no
19. Do you find life very exciting? . . . . yes   **no (1)**
20. Is it hard for you to get started on new projects? . . . . **yes (1)**   no
21. Do you feel full of energy? . . . . yes   **no (1)**
22. Do you feel that your situation is hopeless? . . . . **yes (1)**   no
23. Do you think that most people are better off than you are? . . . . **yes (1)**   no
24. Do you frequently get upset over little things? . . . . **yes (1)**   no
25. Do you frequently feel like crying? . . . . **yes (1)**   no
26. Do you have trouble concentrating? . . . . **yes (1)**   no
27. Do you enjoy getting up in the morning? . . . . yes   **no (1)**
28. Do you prefer to avoid social occasions? . . . . **yes (1)**   no
29. Is it easy for you to make decisions? . . . . yes   **no (1)**
30. Is your mind as clear as it used to be? . . . . yes   **no (1)**

TOTAL: Please sum all bolded answers (worth one point) for a total score. _____

Scores: 0–9 Normal 10–19 Mild Depressive 20–30 Severe Depressive

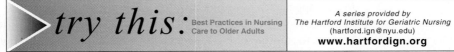

try this: Best Practices in Nursing Care to Older Adults

A series provided by
The Hartford Institute for Geriatric Nursing
(hartford.ign@nyu.edu)
www.hartfordign.org

quick and simple. In most cases the patient is responsive in 15 minutes, and fully recovered and ready for discharge within 1 to 2 hours. Patients should avoid driving, operating heavy machinery, and drinking alcohol during the treatment period. Short-term memory loss is common for up to 2 weeks after the treatment, so older patients should forgo making important decisions during this period. ECT is contraindicated for patients with increased intracranial pressure, space-occupying brain lesions, severe heart disease, recent myocardial infarction, and aortic aneurysm because of the increased risk of arrhythmia and death (Maki, 2003). The mortality rate is low (less than 1 in 10,000) and the relapse rate is 50% to 70% without maintenance with antidepressant drugs. With antidepressant drug use, the relapse rate drops to 10% to 20% (Jenike, 2003).

BEST PRACTICES

The Hartford Institute for Geriatric Nursing (1999) presents the overview of treatment for depression including use of the GDS. See the Best Practice feature on pages 214-15.

As always, the process begins with a careful diagnosis and ongoing assessment of treatment with adjustments as needed.

NURSING DIAGNOSIS

Gerontological nurses soon come to recognize the cardinal symptoms of depression in the older person. Older people who look sad, experience functional decline, and seem to have no enjoyment in life will alert the nurse to carry out a complete depression assessment and evaluation. Physical diagnoses that may be used based on somatic symptoms related to depression include *constipation, fatigue, social isolation, altered nutrition, self-care deficit, disturbed sleep pattern,* and *impaired communication.* Nursing diagnoses addressing the older person's psychological state may include *anxiety, ineffective individual coping, self-esteem disturbance, dysfunctional grieving, powerlessness, hopelessness, impaired adjustment, caregiver role strain, spiritual distress,* and *risk for suicide.* Some experts recommend that NANDA develop a nursing diagnosis for depression based on the *DSM-IV-TR* criteria, etiologies, and defining mood characteristics so that advanced practice nurses can be reimbursed for psychiatric services (Maas et al., 2001). The nurse should be familiar with the *DSM-IV-TR* criteria published and regularly updated by the American Psychiatric Association, as these criteria provide for a categorical approach to the diagnosis and treatment of depression.

The following nurse-sensitive outcomes are identified in the *Nursing Outcomes Classification (NOC)* (Iowa Outcomes Project, 2000):

- **Suicide self-restraint.** Indicated by establishing and maintaining a contract to not harm him/herself, seeks help with feeling self-destructive tendencies, maintains connectedness in social relationships; expresses feelings in therapeutic counseling.
- **Mood equilibrium.** Exhibits appropriate affect, maintains self-care including grooming and hygiene, complies with medication regimen, reports adequate sleep, shows interest in surroundings.
- **Hope.** Expresses optimism, looks forward to and plans future events, expresses joy in life, appears to have inner peace.
- **Coping.** Identifies and uses effective coping strategies, modifies lifestyle with behaviors to minimize stress, seeks out and uses social and professional support, reports decreased severity and number of stress-related physical symptoms.

As all older patients are different and unique in their mental health needs, the nurse should choose the most appropriate nursing outcomes to establish the effectiveness of the nursing care plan.

Patient and Family Teaching

Gerontological nurses require skills and knowledge related to teaching patients and families about the key concepts of gerontology and gerontological nursing. The patient-family teaching guidelines in the following feature will assist the nurse to assume the role of teacher and coach. Educating patients and families is critical so that nurses can interpret scientific data and individualize the nursing care plan.

Patient-Family Teaching Guidelines

Many older people think it is normal to have a variety of physical and mental problems. However, mental health problems, including depression and anxiety, are not part of the normal aging process. If you, a family member, or friend experience a sudden change in mood, the way you think, or your memory, see your healthcare professional as soon as possible.

MENTAL HEALTH AND THE OLDER ADULT

1. What causes mental health problems?

Some mild memory or mood problems can occur in healthy older adults, but serious problems can be a sign of underlying mental health disease.

RATIONALE:

Chronic unrelieved pain, some physical illnesses, problems with eyesight and hearing, certain medications, and use of alcohol can cause mental health problems. To further complicate things, serious physical illnesses can cause delirium or acute mental status changes that will usually resolve when the underlying cause is treated. Late-life psychosis or paraphrenia is a serious mental condition in which a person loses touch with reality and has difficulty telling fact from fantasy.

2. What tests are needed to tell if I have a serious mental health problem?

Your healthcare provider will probably conduct a complete physical examination, ask about your daily function, survey your medications (prescription and over the counter), and obtain some laboratory tests to make sure you are not anemic, to make sure you have adequate levels of B_{12} and folate, or to determine if you are having trouble with your thyroid. Your healthcare provider will also ask a lot of questions about your mood and memory. Sometimes a CT scan of the brain or other tests such as MRI are necessary to detect the source of mental health problems. If further information is needed, you may be referred to a neuropsychologist for more in-depth testing that can give more detailed information about your memory and mood. The results of this test can help your healthcare provider decide if additional testing is needed to diagnose your mental health problem.

RATIONALE:

Mental health problems in the older person can be caused by a variety of factors. A complete holistic assessment of physical, social, and psychological function is indicated.

(continued)

Patient-Family Teaching Guidelines, *cont.*

3. How do I know if I have depression?

If you experience feelings of sadness, fatigue, lack of enjoyment of life, sleep problems, feelings of being helpless and hopeless, loss of interest in sex, or difficulty concentrating and making decisions, you may be depressed. Some older people say that they just do not feel like their old self. Others gain or lose weight because they change the way they eat. Others may avoid going out to social events and prefer to stay home alone. Everyone is different, so it is important to think broadly and look for a variety of symptoms.

RATIONALE:

Recognition of depression in the older person is a key skill for every clinician working with elderly patients. Depression is a treatable disease and may masquerade as a symptom of illness or be falsely attributed to normal aging.

4. Is suicide a problem with older people?

Yes, some groups of older people (especially older White men) have high suicide rates. If you have persistent thoughts of death or harming yourself or others, seek help immediately. There are mental health professionals who are available to protect your life and help you return to mental health. Do not risk ending your life prematurely.

RATIONALE:

Older people with suicidal ideation need immediate help and preventive services. Inform your patients and their families that help is available if needed.

5. Is treatment available and effective for older people with mental health problems?

Yes, there are a variety of pharmacological and nonpharmacological methods to treat mental health problems. The newer antidepressants have fewer side effects and are just as effective in treating depression in older people as they are in treating middle-aged and younger people, so do not be afraid to try them if your doctor thinks it will help you. Mental health professionals such as social workers, psychologists, psychiatrists, and psychiatric–mental health nurses can also provide counseling to help you identify the source of and appropriate intervention for your mental health problems. Nonpharmacological ways to ease depression include exercise, increased social activity, alcohol avoidance, light therapy, and a variety of other methods unique to each older person.

RATIONALE:

Many older people and their families are afraid to acknowledge a mental health problem. They may see it as a sign of weakness, or be fearful of institutionalization in a mental hospital. Be sure to stress the benefits and possibilities of treatment for mental health problems.

Care Plan

A Patient With Depression

Case Study

Mrs. Drew is an 80-year-old woman who lives alone in a senior citizens' housing project. She is quite functional and manages very well with the assistance of a weekly homemaker and her daughter. Mrs. Drew has several stable chronic illnesses such as type 2 diabetes mellitus, hypertension, age-related macular degeneration, insomnia,

A Patient With Depression

and mild depression. She had a myocardial infarction several years ago and had a stent inserted in a partially occluded coronary artery. Since then she has done quite well and engages in social activities with her family and friends in her housing complex.

Recently, Mrs. Drew began to complain to her physician and nurse that she has been increasingly irritated with her upstairs neighbor. She relates, "She stomps around all night. I think she was rearranging furniture the other night at 2 a.m. I've called the apartment manager to complain but they don't do a thing. Now my neighbor doesn't speak to me and I think she's telling everyone who lives in our complex." In addition, the nurse notes that Mrs. Drew's blood pressure is elevated, her blood sugar is higher than normal, and she looks disheveled. Normally she is well dressed and well groomed. Mrs. Drew reports that she has not bothered to refill her blood pressure medication. When asked about this she just sighs and says, "Why should I bother to fix up and take so many pills? I just sit in my apartment all day. No one really cares about me anyway."

Applying the Nursing Process

ASSESSMENT

Mrs. Drew is exhibiting a change in function and mood. While she has been mildly depressed in the past, she has always cared for herself and exhibited an enjoyment of life. Recently, she has become more irritable and has become noncompliant in taking her medications. Should the trend continue, she could suffer another heart attack, further complications from uncontrolled diabetes, and increasing social isolation. The nurse should carefully assess Mrs. Drew's current situation and determine the following:

- Has any recent event or significant loss occurred?
- Has there been any change in financial situation or family structure?
- Has any significant decline in her physical condition or chronic illnesses occurred that could be causing or exacerbating this mood disorder?
- Does she ever think of harming or killing herself?
- Does she have insight into her situation and have any ideas as to why she is feeling hopeless?

The complete nursing assessment should include the following:

- Cognitive testing—the MMSE
- Depression screen—the GDS
- Suicide screen—to rule out the risk of suicide
- Further assessment of physical condition—assessment of all vital signs, pain screen, and physical examination
- Medication survey—review of all prescribed and over-the-counter medications, compliance with medications, and presence or absence of medication side effects

DIAGNOSIS

Appropriate nursing diagnoses for Mrs. Drew may include the following:

- *Social isolation*
- *Sleep deprivation*

(continued)

A Patient With Depression (continued)

- *Situational low self-esteem*
- *Risk for loneliness*
- *Ineffective health maintenance*

EXPECTED OUTCOMES

Short-term goals might include that Mrs. Drew will:

1. Return to taking medications as ordered by the physician.
2. Have normal blood pressure and blood sugar levels at her next scheduled clinic visit.
3. Return to daily self-care and grooming activities.

Long-term goals might include that Mrs. Drew will:

1. Resume former sleep patterns and social activities.
2. Comply with recommendations for antidepressant medication, counseling, or nonpharmacological recommendations to improve her mood and ease her symptoms of depression.
3. Identify and appraise past adaptive coping mechanisms and implement them to maintain her mood improvement and prevent further depressive episodes.

PLANNING AND IMPLEMENTATION

The following nursing interventions may be appropriate for Mrs. Drew:

- Establish a therapeutic relationship.
- Assess ability to obtain and pay for needed medications.
- Consult with the social worker colleague for information on socialization and community linkages that may increase Mrs. Drew's daily contact with other persons and are appropriate for someone with limited vision.
- Establish a schedule to monitor her ability to manage her chronic illnesses and care for herself.
- Begin a values clarification to establish long-term goals and facilitate end-of-life planning.

Mrs. Drew has a history of appropriate self-care and independence. She has family support and is cognitively intact (scored a 28 on the MMSE). Her score on the GDS was 8, indicating her mild depression has progressed in severity. She is nonsuicidal and expresses faith in God and a reason for living. Her physical illnesses appear to be stable, and her blood pressure and blood sugar should return to normal limits when she begins to take her medication.

EVALUATION

The nurse hopes to work with Mrs. Drew over time and realizes the chronic nature of mood problems in older people. The nurse will consider the plan a success based on the following criteria:

A Patient With Depression

- Mrs. Drew will resume attending social activities within her capabilities and exhibit improved function and social skills.
- She will resume taking medications to manage her health problems.
- She will engage in counseling and take antidepressant medications if indicated and report improved sleep and mood as a result of these interventions.

Ethical Dilemma

Mrs. Drew informs the nurse that she is suspicious that her homemaker, Ms. Miller, is stealing money and jewelry from her apartment. Within the last few weeks she has been unable to find her bankbook, some gold jewelry, and some coins she has saved for her great-grandchildren. When the nurse asks Mrs. Drew if she has reported this to the agency providing the homemaker's services, she replies, "Oh no. I don't want her to get fired. I'm afraid she would try to get back at me if I did that." What are appropriate nursing actions?

Mrs. Drew should be encouraged to seek her family's assistance to carry out a systematic search and ascertain the items are truly missing and not merely misplaced. As Mrs. Drew has macular degeneration and a visual impairment, she may be unable to see clearly into the back of drawers or other poorly lighted storage areas. If the items are truly missing, persons other than Ms. Miller (if any) should be identified. If it is fairly clear that Ms. Miller is a potential thief, Mrs. Drew should be encouraged to report this to the agency. Although she may not have her items returned, she may be able to stop Ms. Miller from stealing from others and causing further distress. Further investigation as to why Mrs. Drew is afraid of retribution is needed. Has she ever been threatened or intimidated by Ms. Miller? If so, it may constitute elder abuse and should be reported and investigated by state officials. The principle of Mrs. Drew's autonomy (she is cognitively intact and expressing clearly her wishes) is weighed against the principle of justice (doing the right thing to prevent Ms. Miller from hurting others) and beneficence (the nurse's desire to do the right thing and help Mrs. Drew to report Ms. Miller's crime).

Critical Thinking and the Nursing Process

1. List the 10 major causes of depression in the older person from your perspective.
2. Describe how common sensory impairments can cause an older person to have delusions or become paranoid.
3. What factors make alcohol use and abuse more difficult to detect in an older person?
4. In your opinion, what factors make the assessment and treatment of an older person with mental health problems challenging for the gerontological nurse and other members of the healthcare team?
5. What actions can society take to improve the mental health of all Americans and older people in particular?

- Evaluate your responses in Appendix B. ⊂⊃

EXPLORE MediaLink

NCLEX review, case studies, and other interactive resources for this chapter can be found on the Companion Website at **www.prenhall.com/tabloski**. Click on Chapter 7 to select the activities for this chapter. For animations, more NCLEX review questions, and case studies, access the accompanying CD-ROM in this textbook.

Chapter Highlights

- The gerontological nurse can educate other professionals about the facts regarding normal aging, mental health problems the older adult may encounter, and the various options for addressing those problems.

- Education takes place not only in the classroom, but also at professional meetings, at community gatherings, and by serving as a role model to other nurses in the workplace.

- Gerontological nurses should seek out opportunities to volunteer and consult with self-help groups because 80% of long-term care is provided by family members (American Psychological Association, 2003). Many older persons, families, and even healthcare professionals are unaware of the issues involved with the assessment and treatment of mental health problems in the older adult.

- Although depression is not necessarily more common in the older adult, the presence of functional disability, numerous losses, and physical illness all predispose the older person to develop depressive symptoms that if left untreated may progress to a major depression. Older persons suffering from major depression are more likely to develop serious illness, are less likely to recover and cooperate with rehabilitation after illness, and have a lower life expectancy.

- Gerontological nurses along with other healthcare providers can engage in a wide variety of advocacy efforts on behalf of older adults in need of mental health services. Providing local and state lawmakers with information about the mental health needs of older people can facilitate the development of public policy to support and encourage appropriate mental health services.

- The nurse can support and augment the efforts of professional nursing organizations to advocate and encourage legislation and policy to improve the intellectual, social, and emotional well-being of older adults.

References

American Nurses Association. (2001). *Code of ethics for nurses with interpretive statements.* Washington, DC: Author.

American Psychiatric Association, Committee on Nomenclature and Statistics. (2000). *Diagnostic and statistical manual of mental disorders* (4th ed., text revision) (*DSM-IV-TR*). Washington, DC: Author.

American Psychological Association. (1998). What practitioners should know about working with older adults. *Professional Psychology: Research and Practice, 29*(5), 413–427.

American Psychological Association. (2003). What practitioners should know about working with older adults. *Professional Psychology: Research and Practice, 29*(5), 413–427.

Bille-Brahe, U., & Andersen, K. (2001). Suicide among the Danish elderly. In D. De Leo (Ed.), *Suicide and euthanasia in older adults: A transcultural journey* (pp. 47–56). Seattle, WA: Hogrefe & Huber.

Blehar, M., & Oren, D. (1997). Gender differences in depression. *Medscape Women's Health Journal, 2*(1). Retrieved on June 14, 2000, from www.medscape.com/urewartich/408844.

Copley News Service. (1999, February 18). Alcoholism among senior citizens: A hidden epidemic. *Hoosier Times*, p. 11.

Coward, D., & Reed, P. (1996). Self-transcendence: A resource for healing at the end of life. *Issues in Mental Health Nursing, 17*(3), 275–288.

Ebersole, P., Hess, P., & Lugfen, A. (2004). *Toward healthy aging: Human needs and nursing response* (6th ed.). St. Louis, MO: Mosby.

Epocrates.com. (2003). Retrieved October 4, 2003, from Drug Information www.epocrates.com.

Erikson, E. H. (1963). *Childhood and society.* New York: Norton.

George, L., Okun, M., & Landerman, R. (1985) Age as a moderator of the determinants of life satisfaction. *Research on Aging, 7,* 209–233.

Hartford Institute for Geriatric Nursing. (1999). *Best nursing practices in care for older adults.* New York: New York University.

Hartford Institute for Geriatric Nursing, Division of Nursing, New York University. (1999). The Geriatric Depression Scale. Try this: Best pracices in nursing care to older adults. M. Wallace, ed. 1(6). Retrieved October 3, 2004, from http://www.hartfordign.org.

Havighurst, R. J. (1972). Nurturing the cognitive skills in health. *Journal of Health, 42*(2), 73–76.

Hays, L., Olson, D., & Blow, F. (1999, December). *Substance use disorders in the elderly: Prevalence, special considerations, and treatment.* Presented at the American Academy of Psychiatry 10th Annual Meeting and Symposium, New York.

Iowa Outcomes Project. M. Johnson, M. Maas, & S. Moorhead (Eds.). (2000). *Nursing outcomes classification (NOC)* (2nd ed.). St. Louis, MO: Mosby.

Jenike, M. (1999). *Depression in the elderly. Geriatric medicine.* Boston: Harvard Medical School, Division on Aging.

Journal of the American Medical Association. (2000). *JAMA Patient Page: Psychiatric illness in older adults, 283*(21), 2886.

Kane, R., Ouslander, J., & Abrass, I. (2000). *Essentials of clinical geriatrics.* New York: McGraw-Hill.

Maddox, G. (1994). Lives through the years revisited. *Gerontologist, 34*(6), 764–767.

Maki, R. (2003). Electroconvulsive therapy. *Advances for Nurses, 3*(19), 14–16.

McCance, K., & Huether, S. (2001). *Pathophysiology. The biologic basis of disease in adults and children.* New York: Mosby.

Merck manual of geriatrics. (2001). Rahway, NJ: Merck Sharp & Dohme Research Laboratories.

Miller, R. (1996). The aging immune system: Primer and Perspectives. *Science, 273,* 70–74.

Moore, A., Seeman, T., Morgenstern, H., Beck, J., & Reuben, D. (2002). Are there differences between older persons who screen positive on the CAGE questionnaire and the Short Michigan Alcoholism Screening Test–Geriatric Version? *Journal of the American Geriatrics Society, 50,* 858–862.

Morris, D. (2001). Geriatric mental health: An overview. *Journal of the American Psychiatric Nurses Association, 7*(6), S2–S7.

National Institute on Aging. (2002). *Aging under the microscope: A biological quest* (NIH Publication No. 02-2756). Bethesda, MD: National Institutes of Health.

National Institute on Aging. (2004). *Clinician's handbook* (NIH Publication No. 04-0487). Bethesda, MD: National Institutes of Health.

National Institutes of Health. (2000). *Depression in the older person.* Retrieved October 16, 2003, from www. ninh.nih.gov/publicat/depression.cfm.

Nelson, J., Lavretsky, H., & Burke, W. (2003). Managing mood disorders in older patients: A focus on depression and anxiety. *Supplement to Annals of Long-Term Care and Clinical Geriatrics,* June, 1–9.

Neugarten, B., & Hagestad, G. (1976). Age and the life course. In R. Binstock & E. Shanas (Eds.), *Handbook of aging and the social sciences* (pp. 35–57). New York: Van Nostrand Reinhold.

Oslin, D., & Mellow, A. (2000). Neurotransmitter-based therapeutic strategies in late-life alcoholism and other addictions. In E. S. L. Gomberg, A. Hegedus, & R. Zucker (Eds.), *Alcohol problems and aging* (NIH

Publication No. 4163). Bethesda, MD: National Institutes of Health.

Parkes, C. M. (1999). *Bereavement: Studies of grief in adult life.* London: Tavistock.

Reuben, D., Herr, K., Pacala, J., Potter, J., Pollock, B., & Semla, T. (2002). *Geriatrics at your fingertips.* Malden, MA: Blackwell. American Geriatrics Society.

Sanacore, F. (2003). *Pharmacotherapies for depression and other conditions.* Retrieved August 12, 2003, from www.drugtopics.com.

Scott, C., & Popovich, D. (2001, January). Undiagnosed alcoholism & prescription drug misuse among the elderly. *Caring Magazine, 20*(1), 20–25.

Selye, H. (1965). *The stress of life.* New York: McGraw-Hill.

Tangelos, E., & Wise, T. (2003). Mood disorders in the older adult. *Supplement to Annals of Long-Term Care and Clinical Geriatrics, 11*(07), 2–9.

U.S. Department of Health and Human Services. (2001). *In harm's way: Suicide in America.* National Institute of Mental Health. Retrieved October 16, 2001, from www.nimh.nih.gov/publicat/harmaway.cfm.

U.S. Public Health Service. (2000). *Healthy people 2010.* Washington, DC: U.S. Department of Health and Human Services.

U.S. Surgeon General. (2003). *Executive summary. Mental health: Culture, race and ethnicity.* U.S. Department of Health and Human Services, U.S. Public Health Service. Retrieved September 27, 2003, from www.surgeongeneral.gov.

Waern, M., Rubaenowitz, E., Runeson, B., Skoog, I., Wilhelmson, K., & Allebeck, E. (2002). Burden of illness and suicide in elderly people: Case control study. *British Medical Journal, 324,* 1355–1357.

Wiscott, R., Kopera-Frye, K., & Seifert, L. (2001). Possible consequences of social drinking in the early stages of Alzheimer disease. *Geriatric Nursing, 22*(2), 100–105.

World Health Organization. (2001). *Brief intervention for hazardous and harmful drinking. A manual for primary care.* Retrieved September 16, 2003, from www.euro.who.int.

Wynne, A., Woo, T., & Millard, M. (2002). *Pharmacotherapeutics for nurse practitioner prescribers.* Philadelphia: F.A. Davis.

Yesavage, J., Brink, T., Rose, T., Lum, O., Huang, V., Adey, M., & Leirer, V. (1983). Development and validation of a geriatric depression screening scale: A preliminary report. *Journal of Psychiatric Research, 17,* 37–49.

Youngkin, E., Sawin, K., Kissinger, J., & Israel, D. (2005). *Pharmacotherapeutics: A primary care clinical guide* (2nd ed.). Stamford, CT: Appleton & Lange.

CHAPTER 8

Sleep and the Older Adult

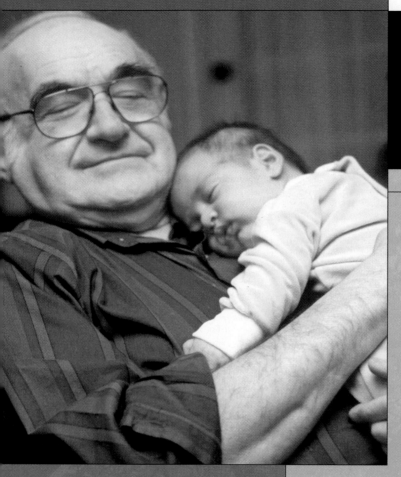

KEY TERMS

MediaLink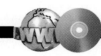

Additional resources for this chapter can be found on the Student CD-ROM accompanying this textbook and on the Companion Website at **www.prenhall.com/tabloski**. Click on Chapter 8 to select the activities for this chapter.

CD-ROM
- Video
  - *Sleep Apnea*
- NCLEX Review
- Case Studies
- Tools

COMPANION WEBSITE
- Audio Glossary
- Additional NCLEX Review
- Case Study
- MediaLink Applications

Sleep complaints are common among older people, and the incidence of sleep problems increases with age. Older adults experience age-related changes in the nature of their sleep, including greater difficulty falling asleep, more frequent awakenings, decreased amounts of nighttime sleep, and more frequent daytime napping. Proper **sleep architecture** and adequate total sleep time are necessary for proper functioning. In order for sleep to be restful and restorative, the sleeper must progress through non-rapid eye movement (NREM) stages of slow wave sleep and about every 90 minutes throughout the night cycle into rapid eye movement (REM) stages. Most people sleep in the dark portion of the 24-hour cycle and carry out activities during the light portion. Sleep and wakefulness fall into a circadian pattern of periodicity meaning about one cycle per 24-hour period. This sleep-wake distribution pattern is regulated by the suprachiasmatic nucleus located in the hypothalamus and forms the basis for **circadian rhythms**. This rhythmic pattern can be disrupted by isolation from the normal light-dark cycle, isolation from environmental stimuli, and rapid travel to differing time zones (jet lag).

The exact purpose of sleep is unclear, but sleep deprivation can result in harmful physical and psychological changes, including daytime fatigue, irritability, impaired learning ability, delayed healing, and visual and auditory hallucinations. Sleep disturbances can exacerbate behavioral problems in older persons with Alzheimer's disease and other cognitive impairments.

In order to assist persons with sleep disturbances, nurses need scientific knowledge about sleep. The North American Nursing Diagnosis Association (NANDA, 2001) recognizes sleep pattern disturbance as an alternation in an individual's habitual pattern of sleep and wakefulness that causes discomfort or interferes with a desired lifestyle. Defining characteristics according to NANDA criteria include the following:

- Complaints of difficulty falling asleep (sleep latency greater than 30 minutes)
- Awakening too early in the morning
- Three or more nighttime awakenings
- Changes in behavior and function, including lethargy, listlessness, and irritability
- Decreased ability to function
- Dissatisfaction with sleep and not feeling well rested
- Presence of related factors including:
  - Physical discomfort/pain
  - Psychological discomfort
  - **Sleep hygiene** problems
  - Environmental factors

Sleep problems can be classified as transient (short term), intermittent (on and off), and chronic (constant). Transient sleep problems may be caused by short-term health problems, stress, worry related to a situational event like a move to a new residence, or changes in sleep schedules such as those due to travel and jet lag. Intermittent sleep problems may be related to exacerbations of chronic illness or recurrent anxiety. **Insomnia** is chronic if it occurs on most nights and lasts a month or more (National Institutes of Health, 2000).

Sleep Architecture

For sleep to be restorative and restful, the sleeping person must cycle through several sleep stages. Normal sleep physiology is composed of four distinct stages when measured by electroencephalography. Sleep ranges from stage 1 (light sleep) to stage 4 (deep sleep) and can be classified as either REM sleep or NREM sleep (Figure 8-1 ■).

FIGURE ▨ 8-1

Sleep stages. A. Electroencephalograph tracings of awakeness, REM, and non-REM sleep. B. Sleep cycles during nighttime sleep.

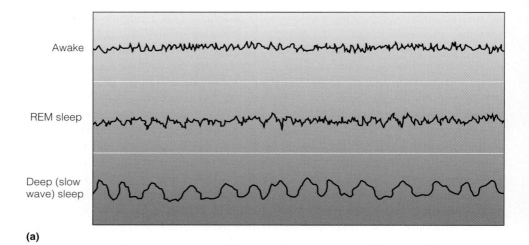

(a)

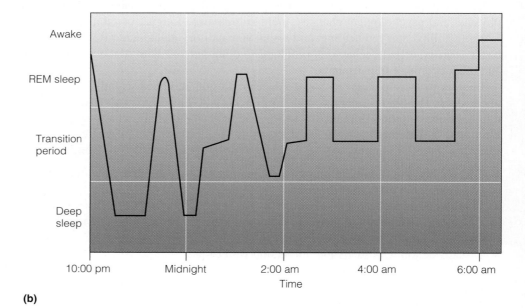

(b)

During NREM sleep, growth hormone, prolactin, and thyroid-stimulating hormones are released, aiding in physiological restoration. Deep sleep appears to stimulate physical restoration through the release of growth hormone while decreasing blood pressure and respiratory function (McCance & Heuther, 2001). With aging, the amount of time spent in deep sleep decreases as the night progresses. In a healthy older adult, deep sleep comprises 33% of the first sleep cycle, 17% of the second, 6% of the third, 2% of the fourth, and 1% of the fifth. Stage 1 is light sleep in which persons feel as if they are drifting in and out of sleep and can be accompanied by a feeling of falling with sudden muscle contractions. In stage 2, brain waves slow and eye movements stop. Stage 3 sleep is characterized by slowing brain waves and sleep spindles, which are bursts of electrical activity. In stage 4, the brain produces mostly delta waves characterized by large, slow patterns of brain activity. During stages 1 and 2, persons are easily aroused from sleep, whereas persons in stages 3 and 4 sleep are more difficult to arouse. Brief awakenings normally occur throughout the night (Beers & Berkow, 1999). As the sleep

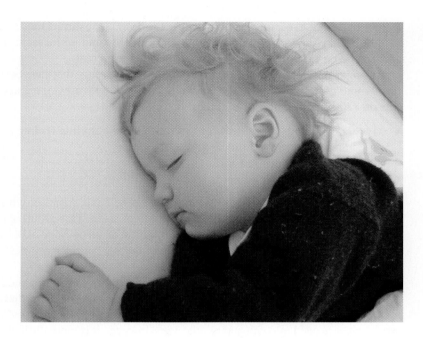

FIGURE 8-2

The deepest slow wave sleep occurs in childhood.

stages progress, it becomes increasingly difficult to awaken the sleeper, and the more frequent nighttime awakenings observed in older people may be related to the reduced amount of slow wave sleep in this cohort. This process of slow wave sleep reduction begins at about age 20 with the deepest sleep occurring in childhood (Figure 8-2). The abundance of slow wave sleep in childhood lends support to the expression "sleeping like a baby."

REM sleep is characterized by intense brain activity resulting in small, brief muscle contractions. REM sleep is accompanied by an increase in heart rate and blood pressure. Breathing is irregular and shallow, eyes dart quickly from side to side, and limbs become temporarily paralyzed. REM sleep is sometimes referred to as "dream sleep" because dreaming occurs during REM sleep and is thought necessary for psychological restoration. REM sleep is necessary for learning, memory consolidation, and daytime concentration. REM sleep occurs cyclically every 90 to 120 minutes throughout the night. As the night progresses, sleep becomes lighter and the person spends more time in REM sleep.

Normal Sleep and Aging

Age-related changes in the nervous system can affect sleep. These changes may be at the chemical, structural, and functional levels and may result in a disorganization of sleep and disruption of circadian rhythms (Jao & Alessi, 2004). The neuromechanisms for sleep are distributed in the brain stem, basal forebrain, and subcortical and cortical regions. Neurotransmitters such as serotonin and norepinephrine keep some parts of the brain on alert during sleep. Sensory inputs such as loud noises and bright lights can stimulate the reticular activating system and cause an older person to awaken. Other neurons at the base of the brain send signals to disregard stimuli that would normally keep a person awake. Normal sleep depends upon the integrity of these complex mechanisms. Declines in the cerebral metabolic rate and cerebral blood flow, reductions of neuronal cell counts, and structural changes such as neuronal degeneration and atrophy can all occur with aging (National Institute of Neurological Disorders and Stroke,

2003). The amount of time spent in deeper levels of sleep diminishes with aging. There is an associated increase in awakenings during sleep and an increase in the total time spent in bed trying to sleep as sleep becomes less efficient.

Abnormal sleep behaviors are a category of events that can occur at any time throughout the life cycle but become more common with advancing age. According to Merritt (2000), this category includes the following:

- Myoclonus or sudden contractions of muscles and tingling feelings in the legs, also called "restless leg syndrome"
- Sleepwalking or sleep terrors
- Sleep-related epileptic seizures

Older persons exhibiting these sleep problems will experience daytime sleepiness as a result of poor quality and insufficient quantity of sleep. This group of abnormal sleep behaviors requires evaluation from neurologists or sleep specialists and is usually treated with medications such as antianxiety agents, benzodiazepines, and dopamine agonists (Merritt, 2000).

Some healthy older adults continue to have satisfactory sleep throughout advanced age (Figure 8-3■). A common myth held by many nurses and laypersons is that a person's need for sleep decreases with age. In general, the amount of sleep needed in old age is about the same as was needed in youth and middle age. However, it is more difficult for many older persons to obtain the quality and quantity of sleep that supports health and well-being.

Most older adults require 6 to 10 hours of sleep nightly. Less than 4 or more than 9 hours of sleep is associated with higher mortality rates than those sleeping 8 hours (Chesson, 2000). Often, the time it takes to fall asleep serves as a good indicator of whether a person is getting enough sleep. Those who fall asleep almost immediately upon placing their head on the pillow may be sleep deprived. When an older person's sleep requirements are not met, a sleep deficit accumulates with resulting loss of overall daytime function. A decrease in sleep of about 1.5 hours can reduce daytime alertness by 33%, and drowsiness may contribute to as many as 30% of all traffic accidents (Laube, 1998; National Highway Traffic Safety Administration, 1998). Further, lack of sleep can lead to loss of initiative, memory lapses, emotional instability, and decreased daytime function (Merritt, 2000).

Older persons may nap more often during the day, thus further disrupting normal circadian patterns. While one or two "cat naps" (naps under 50 minutes) a day were found

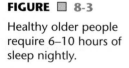

FIGURE ☐ 8-3

Healthy older people require 6–10 hours of sleep nightly.

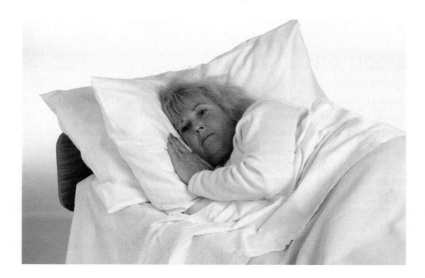

not to disrupt the nighttime sleep of older people, more frequent daytime napping can be disruptive (Floyd, 1999). If an older person normally requires 8 hours of sleep in a 24-hour period and 2 to 3 hours of sleep occur during the daytime hours, the person cannot expect to enjoy 8 hours of uninterrupted sleep at night. The older person may toss and turn, become frustrated with the inability to sleep, and suffer further disruption in the sleep-wake patterns. For good sleepers, the bed and bedroom are strong cues for drowsiness and sleep; for poor sleepers, these places signal alertness, frustration, and sleeplessness.

Practice Pearl

Changing problematic sleep behaviors is a long-term process. Goals that are set too high or too quickly will discourage the nurse and the patient. Realistic goals are the key to success.

Health Problems and Sleep Disruption

Approximately 5 million older persons in the United States have a serious sleep disorder (Jao & Alessi, 2004). Sleep problems in older persons may result from personal characteristics, environmental characteristics, or a combination of these factors. Personal characteristics include advanced age (generally considered over 60), female gender, and history of depression (National Institutes of Health, 2000). Further, older women are more likely than older men to take longer to fall asleep, wake more frequently after the onset of sleep, and stay awake longer during these nighttime awakenings (Floyd, 1999).

Various health problems and the medications used to treat them are associated with sleep disruption in older persons. Pulmonary disease, heart disease, arthritis, dementia associated with Alzheimer's disease, and depression may cause sleep disruption. Diseases of the cardiac and respiratory system are often associated with orthopnea and shortness of breath. Persons with congestive heart failure are often asked "the pillow question" as an indicator of the stability and progression of their disease. The nurse should ask, "How many pillows do you sleep with at night? Is this your usual number of pillows?" Older persons with severe congestive heart failure may find it necessary to sleep sitting nearly upright to allow the lungs to clear fluid and breathe, but this position may not offer adequate support for the back and the head during deep sleep (Figure 8-4■).

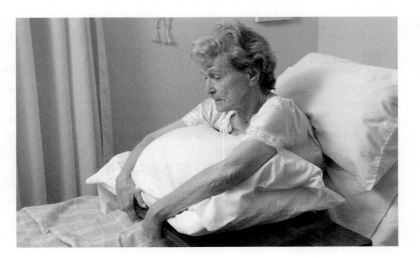

FIGURE ■ 8-4

Sleep may be difficult for older persons with heart and lung disease.

FIGURE ■ 8-5

Sleep disturbances in institutional settings are common.

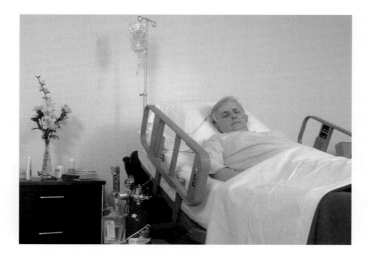

Physical discomfort or pain can be a major deterrent for sleep. Older people with pain take longer to fall asleep and have an increased number of nighttime awakenings. Pain makes it difficult to achieve a comfortable sleeping position, may cause tension and muscle spasms, and may keep an older person awake during the night if pain medication wears off (Jao & Alessi, 2004). A common source of pain in older persons is the chronic pain resulting from osteoarthritis. This disease often results in chronic pain of the knee or hip and was reported to disrupt sleep in one third of the respondents of the National Survey of Self-Care and Aging Study (Wilcox et al., 2000). Further, older adults who experience chronic pain may also limit daytime activities, resulting in physical inactivity, deconditioning, and further disruption of the sleep-activity cycle. Acutely ill hospitalized patients may also experience pain from surgical incisions, pain from the trauma or injury that was the cause of the hospitalization, or discomfort from intravenous tubing, indwelling urinary catheters, or other instrumentation (Figure 8-5■).

Sleep Disruption

Sleep disruption is common in older persons with psychosocial problems. Life stresses when combined with predisposing emotional factors such as depression and anxiety may be related to the onset of sleep problems (Jao & Alessi, 2004). Many studies identify anxiety, stress, and depression as a major deterrent to falling and staying asleep in people of all ages (Floyd, 1999). One study of older women found that worries about health, family, and finances interfered with sleep (Floyd, 1999).

At least 90% of patients with depression report sleep problems (Howcroft & Jones, 1999). Sleep problems identified in depressed older people include difficulty in falling asleep, increased frequency of early morning awakenings, and frequent daytime napping. For some older women, sleep problems began during menopause. Menopause, the cessation of menstruation resulting from declines in estrogen levels, is associated with a variety of behavioral changes, including hot flashes and mood swings. Hot flashes that occur routinely during sleep can lead to fatigue, irritability, and chronic sleep disruption, establishing a poor sleep pattern that persists into old age for many women (Burgess & Dawson, 1999). Older depressed persons are more likely to report somatic complaints like sleep problems and changes in appetite rather than feeling "sad" or "blue." Younger people are more likely to acknowledge the connection between sleep disturbances and emotional problems; therefore, the nurse should be aware of this connection.

DEMENTIA

Older persons with dementia endure even more sleep disruptions than other older persons. Sleep disruptions common in dementia such as those with Alzheimer's disease include breakdown of the normal sleep-wake cycle with short periods of fragmented sleep occurring throughout a 24-hour period, reduced stage 3 and REM sleep, and no stage 4 sleep (Jao & Alessi, 2004). Older persons with dementia may suffer other problems as a result of their impairment such as social isolation, boredom, nursing home placement, excessive daytime napping, and periods of agitation or restlessness throughout the evening or night. Sleep disturbances in older persons with dementia cause caregiver stress, increase the potential for nursing home placement, and cause serious problems for those providing care in the nursing home or home environment. These behaviors may contribute to caregivers' complaints about their own disrupted sleep, daytime sleepiness, and fatigue (Riccio, Knight, & Cody, 1999). If nighttime wandering occurs, serious safety problems can result such as older persons leaving their homes, becoming disoriented, and wandering into heavy traffic or remote wooded areas. Every year, there are news reports of older people who die or suffer serious trauma from exposure when they are found several days after wandering from home. The Alzheimer's Association has started a "safe return" program that encourages older persons with Alzheimer's disease to register with the local police department. In an attempt to promote more normal sleep patterns in those with dementia, psychotropic medications may be administered. These medications are usually indicated for short-term use only. When used for chronic sleep problems, the side effects may become problematic. Typical side effects of hypnotic drugs include falls, swallowing difficulties, constipation, dizziness, and daytime sleepiness (Tabloski, Cooke, & Thoman, 1998). Additionally, most psychotropic medications alter sleep architecture, including decreases in REM sleep, decreased levels of arousal, and increases in slow wave sleep. The older person habitually taking these medications may report feeling "hung over" or lethargic during the daytime as a result of these changes in sleep architecture. For a thorough discussion of dementia in older persons, refer to Chapter 22.

SNORING

Many older people consider snoring a minor annoyance, but it can signal a potentially serious condition known as **sleep apnea**, or temporary interruption of breathing during sleep. For those affected by sleep apnea, there can be many temporary interruptions in breathing, each lasting about 10 seconds throughout the sleep period. These interruptions in breathing can occur as often as 20 to 30 times per hour (Pace, Lynn, & Glass, 2001). Symptoms of sleep apnea include the following:

- Heavy snoring, usually on inspiration
- Choking sounds or struggling to breathe during sleep
- Delays in breathing during sleep (usually with a reduction in blood-oxygen saturation), followed by a snort when breathing begins
- Excessive daytime sleepiness
- Morning headaches
- Difficulty with concentration and staying awake during driving or other tasks

Older persons who repeatedly suffer repetitive hypoxemic events may be more prone to sudden death, stroke, angina, and worsening hypertension (Jao & Alessi, 2004). Bed partners are very helpful in providing information about snoring and nighttime breathing

FIGURE ■ 8-6

Structures of the mouth, the pharynx, and the esophagus.

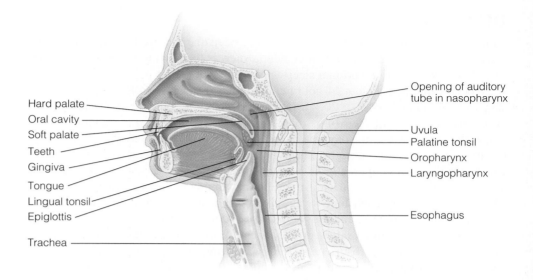

Hard palate
Oral cavity
Soft palate
Teeth
Gingiva
Tongue
Lingual tonsil
Epiglottis

Trachea

Opening of auditory tube in nasopharynx

Uvula
Palatine tonsil
Oropharynx
Laryngopharynx

Esophagus

difficulties. For older persons living alone, a portable tape recorder may be placed by the bed at bedtime. The nurse can later play the recording to hear any snoring or breathing problems on the audiotape.

SLEEP APNEA

Sleep apnea can be caused by problems with the central nervous system and the brain or may be caused by partial obstruction of the airway when the muscles in the throat, soft palate, and tongue relax during sleep (Pace et al., 2001). This can lead to partial or complete collapse of the airway, making breathing labored (Figure 8-6■). Apneic episodes are terminated by brief awakenings, which usually occur without the sleeper's knowledge (Merritt, 2000). If the older person does not fully experience deep sleep, the REM stage will not occur. On waking, the older person with sleep apnea will complain of fatigue and daytime sleepiness (Brown, 1999). Risk factors for sleep apnea include obesity (body mass index >30), hypertension, and anatomical abnormality to the upper respiratory tract. Obstructive sleep apnea is more common in older persons than in younger persons and in older men than in older women (Phillips & Ancoli-Israel, 2001).

If sleep apnea is suspected, the older person should be referred to a sleep center for an overnight sleep study using polysomnography, a specialized method of sleep testing that measures brain and body activity during sleep. The polysomnogram includes the following:

- Electroencephalograms to monitor brain waves and identify sleep stages
- Electro-oculograms to measure eye movement so that REM sleep can be distinguished from NREM sleep
- Facial and leg electromyograms to measure muscle tone and movement
- Electrocardiograms to monitor cardiac activity
- Measurement of chest movement and oxygen saturation

Unfortunately, many older persons find it difficult to sleep with all the wires and monitors attached to them and often must return a second night to achieve any sleep at all (Figure 8-7■).

Treatment for sleep apnea may begin with simple interventions designed to keep the airway open such as weight reduction for the obese, encouraging sleep on the side rather

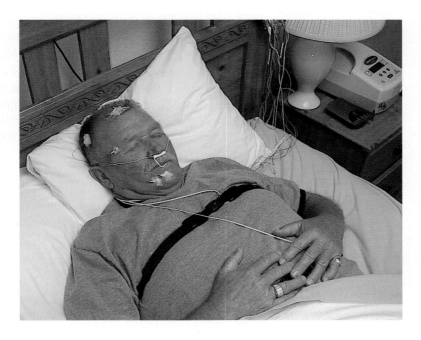

Polysomnography measures brain and body activity during sleep.

than the back by wearing a tennis ball in a pocket sewn on the back of a nightshirt, avoiding sleeping pills and alcohol before sleeping, and avoiding smoking (Pace et al., 2001). For those with anatomical abnormalities of the upper airway, surgery may be required to restore normal structure and function. The surgery, known as uvulopalatopharyngoplasty, is usually performed to the pharyngeal walls or the base of the tongue to enlarge the pharyngeal air space (Merritt, 2000). However, the most common medical treatment for sleep apnea is continuous positive airway pressure (CPAP). CPAP is a noninvasive treatment administered through a nasal mask (Figure 8-8☐). The pressure keeps the airway open, preventing its collapse and allowing the patient to breathe more normally.

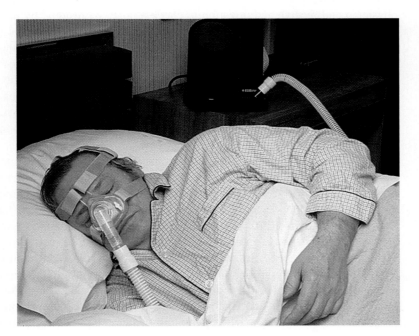

FIGURE ☐ 8-8
Continuous positive airway pressure (CPAP) is a noninvasive method for treatment of sleep apnea.

Usually, between 5 and 20 cm of CPAP is needed to prevent apnea and maintain adequate oxygen saturation (Merritt, 2000). Some older persons have difficulty finding a mask that is comfortable during sleep and may discontinue treatment. Nurses should be aware that sedative-hypnotic medications are contraindicated in patients with untreated sleep apnea, because they raise the arousal threshold to the extent that the patient does not awaken when apneic. Older persons with sleep apnea should inform healthcare providers of their apnea before any surgical procedure because of the danger of severe apnea after preoperative medications are administered (Jao & Alessi, 2004).

> ### Drug Alert
>
> Older persons with untreated sleep apnea should not use alcohol or sedative-hypnotic medications because of their potential to increase the severity of apneic episodes.

URINARY PROBLEMS

Older persons may be awakened from sleep because of the need to urinate. Common age-related alterations in urinary tract function include urinary frequency, nocturia, and incontinence (Miller, 2000). These alterations result from changes in the renal and hormonal systems that control urine production and from decreases in the reservoir capacity of the bladder. In youth, there is a circadian pattern to urine production with nighttime urine production less than daytime production; with aging, nighttime urine flow rates may equal or exceed daytime rates. Voiding frequency, nocturia, and urinary urgency have been shown to increase with age (Miller, 2000). Many older persons take diuretics, which increase urinary output. Older men may suffer from benign prostatic hypertrophy, which inhibits complete emptying of the bladder and may be associated with the sensation of always feeling the urge to void. Nurses who suspect urinary retention in older men with benign prostatic hypertrophy are encouraged to consult with the physician and receive authorization to check a postvoid residual by inserting a urinary catheter immediately after the patient voids to ascertain the amount of urine that is retained in the bladder. Older men who retain more than 50 cc of urine should be referred to a urologist for urological evaluation or cystoscopy and cystometric studies. Many older persons suffer from recurrent urinary tract infections. Older persons who report urgency, frequency, burning on urination, foul odor, and cloudy urine should seek medical evaluation. Sometimes treatment with a simple antibiotic such as sulfamethoxazole trimethoprim (Bactrim DS) can ease the symptoms of urinary tract infection and help restore restful sleep.

For those who are institutionalized in a hospital or nursing home, nurses may do frequent nighttime checking on those with urinary incontinence in order to prevent skin breakdown. Almost 50% of nighttime awakenings in the nursing home are caused by the staff's incontinence care routines or other activities (Endeshaw, Johnson, Kutner, Ouslander, & Bliwise, 2004). Because sleep is so fragmented in those frail, elderly residents, many of whom have dementia, intensive interventions to improve continence at night may disrupt sleep further. The nurse must individualize nighttime care in this population with the goal of minimizing sleep disruption while maintaining skin integrity and the dignity of the older person (Endeshaw et al., 2004). An alternative approach might involve frequent rounding to observe the nursing home resident or hospitalized patient, but providing care only when the patient appears to be awake or moving about in the bed. For patients who appear to be deep in sound sleep or REM sleep, the nurse may wish to return in 30 minutes to ascertain if the patient requires incontinence care.

SLEEP PROBLEMS IN HOSPITALS AND NURSING HOMES

When older persons are hospitalized, they frequently complain of sleep disruption. Studies of sleep in the acute care setting indicate that patients have extremely fragmented and disturbed sleep regardless of their diagnosis (Jao & Alessi, 2004). The lack of restful sleep can slow an older person's recovery to health. Stressors identified by patients in a critical care unit include noise, lack of sleep, enforced mobility, pain from procedures, and poor communication with staff members (Ely, Siegel, & Inouye, 2001). Additionally, many older persons report the hospital environment is too hot (or cold), the bed may be uncomfortable (hard plastic surface), a sleeping partner or comfort item (cat or dog) may be missed, or nighttime rituals may be disrupted. It is often difficult to distinguish between sleep pattern disturbances caused by the hospital environment and those caused by the illness itself (Redeker, Tamburri, & Howland, 1998).

Practice Pearl

When older persons are institutionalized in the hospital or nursing home, sleep problems are common and the environment may be part of the problem. Nurses should ask themselves, "Would I like to sleep here tonight? What would bother me if I were sleeping here?" Some care rituals cannot be avoided, but they can be timed to coincide with awakenings naturally occurring during the patient's sleep cycle. Waking a patient from deep sleep to provide routine care can result in sleep deprivation, which can delay healing and recovery.

ALCOHOL AND CAFFEINE

Although many older persons use alcohol to promote sleep, alcohol is a potent disrupter of REM sleep due to its sedative effect on the central nervous system (Brown, 1999). Further, many older persons are on medications with the potential for serious interactions with alcohol (Tabloski & Church, 1999). Cardiac medications, diuretics, sedative-hypnotic drugs, and painkillers can have their therapeutic effects heightened and reach toxic levels when combined with alcohol. After alcohol ingestion equivalent to just one to two drinks, awaking from intense dreaming occurs with regularity (Floyd, 1999). Additionally, caffeine and nicotine can affect the older adult's ability to initiate and maintain sleep. Nicotine extends the time it takes to fall asleep and reduces total sleep time and REM sleep (Brown, 1999). Both caffeine and nicotine increase the number of nighttime awakenings and the length of time it takes to fall back to sleep. Because alcohol, caffeine, and nicotine are typically used in conjunction with one another, the sedating and arousal effects frequently interact, creating multiple sleep disturbances.

SLEEPING MEDICATIONS

Prescription drugs have also been shown to affect sleep. It is generally agreed that long-term administration of hypnotics is an inadequate treatment strategy for chronic insomnia in the older adult (Cheng, Umland, & Muirhead, 2000). Hypnotic medications are generally recommended for short-term use: about 2 weeks or less. Long-term use will blunt the effect of these medications. For those with long half-lives, steady states or relatively high constant blood levels will occur, which can cause excessive daytime sleepiness. Older persons may also use over-the-counter (OTC) sleep aids without seeking medical advice or attention. The major ingredient in OTC sleep aids is antihistamines, especially diphenhydramine (Benadryl). These drugs have a number of side effects, including daytime sleepiness, dizziness, and blurred vision. These effects can exacerbate an older person's risk of fall and injury.

Drugs used to treat mood disorders such as depression can also affect sleep. Some drugs are sedatives and should be given in the evening, whereas others are stimulants and are best taken in the morning. Sedating antidepressants best taken in the evening include the following:

- Amitriptyline (Elavil)
- Doxepin (Sinequan)
- Nortriptyline (Pamelor)

Stimulating antidepressants best taken in the morning include the following:

- Desipramine (Norpramin)
- Sertraline hydrochloride (Zoloft)
- Paroxetine hydrochloride (Paxil)

Benzodiazepines, even those with short half-lives like lorazepam (Ativan), should be used with caution in older persons. They can exacerbate sleep apnea, suppress deep sleep, increase the likelihood of falling, and cause increased confusion (Tabloski & Church, 1999).

Drug Alert !

Some benzodiazepines carry a high risk of addiction. Diazepam (Valium) and alprazolam (Xanax) are not recommended for routine use with older persons.

When the nurse is asked to advise an older person regarding the discontinuation of sleep medication, the following rule is advised: If the medication has been used at least 5 nights a week for greater than 2 weeks, a taper and withdrawal schedule should be followed. By using a gradual withdrawal schedule (one half the dose for 1 week prior to discontinuation), the chances of inducing rebound insomnia and other withdrawal symptoms are lessened (Tabloski et al., 1998).

Practice Pearl

It is difficult to ask an older person to give up part of a nighttime ritual. If taking a sleeping pill is a longtime habit, the nurse can suggest substituting a vitamin pill as an alternative.

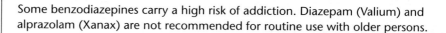

Nursing Assessment

Nursing assessment of sleep problems in older persons should utilize a holistic approach. Because of the multifactorial causes of sleep problems in the older person, a thorough evaluation should precede any nursing intervention. The components of a sleep assessment should include a health history, a physical examination, daily sleep diaries, and polysomnography testing if sleep apnea is suspected. Key assessment areas are as follows:

Health History

- Diagnosed acute or chronic illness
- Current medications (including OTC)
- Chronic pain or pruritus
- Psychological problems
- Change in living conditions or sleep routines
- Current stressors or worries
- Nicotine, alcohol, or caffeine use
- Last complete medical examination

Practice Pearl

Sleep problems arise from a variety of causes. It is poor nursing practice to suggest or offer a therapeutic solution without a complete nursing assessment. A Band-Aid approach may cover up and mask serious underlying problems.

Best Practices

The Philadelphia Sleep Quality Index (PSQI) is an effective instrument used to mea-sure the quality and patterns of sleep in the older adult (Hartford Institute for Geriatric Nursing, 1999). It differentiates "poor" from "good" sleep by measuring seven areas: subjective sleep quality, sleep latency, sleep duration, habitual sleep efficiency, sleep disturbances, use of sleeping medication, and daytime dysfunction over the last month. Scoring of answers is on a 0 to 3 scale, with 3 reflecting the negative extreme. A total score of 5 indicates a "poor" sleeper. See the Best Practices feature on the following page.

Nursing Interventions

The nurse is in an ideal situation to intervene with older persons with sleep problems. Nursing interventions for sleep promotion should be grounded in an understanding of the relationship between mind and body (Jao & Alessi, 2004). Sleep disturbances caused by underlying medical problems should be referred for treatment. Nighttime pain should be investigated for cause and treated. Depression and anxiety disorders likewise require medical intervention and treatment.

Sleep hygiene should be encouraged in any older person with a sleep problem. Emphasis is placed on individual sleep requirements and on changes in the nature and quality of sleep associated with aging (Beck-Little & Weinrich, 1998). Inadequate sleep hygiene refers to daily activities that interfere with the maintenance of good quality sleep and daytime alertness. Environmental problems should be corrected if possible. If the nighttime environment is too hot or cold, portable air conditioners or heaters may be appropriate. Earplugs may ease nighttime noise. The timing of medications should be examined for appropriateness. Dietary and lifestyle changes should be recommended after the older person is appropriately educated regarding the harmful effects of nicotine, caffeine, and alcohol on sleep. Activities, hobbies, and special interests should be pursued, and multiple long naps should be avoided because excessive daytime sleep and boredom may interfere with nighttime sleep (Jao & Alessi, 2004). Appropriate exercise

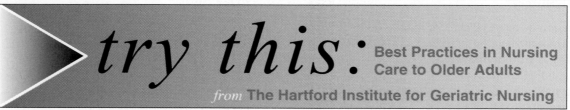

try this: Best Practices in Nursing Care to Older Adults

from The Hartford Institute for Geriatric Nursing

Issue Number 6, November 1999   Series Editor: Meredith Wallace, PhD, RN, MSN, CS

The Pittsburgh Sleep Quality Index (PSQI)

By: Carole Smyth, RNC, MSN

WHY: Sleep is a necessary part of life. However, normal aging changes, medical problems, psychiatric problems, and psychosocial issues can alter the pattern and quality of sleep as one grows older, and thus affect the quality of life in the older adult. Assessment of sleep patterns enables the nurse to intervene immediately by implementing interventions with the client, or by referring the client for further assessment.

BEST TOOL: The Pittsburgh Sleep Quality Index (PSQI) is an effective instrument used to measure the quality and patterns of sleep in the older adult. It differentiates "poor" from "good" sleep by measuring seven areas: subjective sleep quality, sleep latency, sleep duration, habitual sleep efficiency, sleep disturbances, use of sleeping medication, and daytime dysfunction over the last month. The client self-rates each of these seven areas of sleep. Scoring of answers is based on a 0 to 3 scale, whereby 3 reflects the negative extreme on the Likert Scale. A global sum of "5" or greater indicates a "poor" sleeper. Although there are several questions that request the evaluation of the client's bedmate or roommate, these are not scored (not reflected in attached instrument). Refer to "More on the Topic", Buysse et al., 1989, for these questions.

TARGET POPULATION: The PSQI can be used for both an initial assessment and ongoing comparative measurements with older adults across all health care settings.

VALIDITY/RELIABILITY: The PSQI has internal consistency and a reliability coefficient (Cronbach's alpha) of 0.83 for its seven components. Numerous studies using the PSQI have supported high validity and reliability.

STRENGTHS AND LIMITATIONS: The PSQI is a subjective measure of sleep. Self-reporting by clients can empower the client, but can reflect inaccurate information if the client has difficulty understanding what is written, or can not see or physically write out responses. Moreover, the scale is presented in English. The scale can be adapted to enable the client to respond verbally to items on the scale by having the nurse read the statements to the client.

MORE ON THE TOPIC:

Beaton, S.R., Voge, S.A. (1998). Measurements for Long-Term Care (pp.169-170). Thousand Oaks, CA: Sage Publications.

Beck-Little, R., Weinrich, S.P. (1998). Assessment and Management of Sleep Disorders in the Elderly. *Journal of Gerontological Nursing,* 24(4), 21-29.

Buysse, D.J., Reynolds III, C.F., Monk, T.H., Berman, S.R., Kupfer, D.J. (1989). The Pittsburgh Sleep Quality Index: a New Instrument for Psychiatric Practice and Research. *Journal of Psychiatric Research,* 28 (2), 193-213.

Instructions: *The following questions relate to your usual sleep habits during the past month only. Your answers should indicate the most accurate reply for the majority of days and nights in the past month. Please review all questions.*

During the past month,

1. When have you usually gone to bed? _____

2. How long (in minutes) has it taken you to fall asleep each night? _____

3. When have you usually gotten up in the morning? _____

4. How many hours of actual sleep did you get that night? (This may be different than the number of hours you spend in bed) _____

5. During the past month, how often have you had trouble sleeping because you . . .	Not during the past month (0)	Less than once a week (1)	Once or twice a week (2)	Three or more times a week (3)
a. Cannot get to sleep within 30 minutes				
b. Wake up in the middle of the night or early morning				
c. Have to get up to use the bathroom				
d. Cannot breathe comfortably				
e. Cough or snore loudly				
f. Feel too cold				
g. Feel too hot				
h. Have bad dreams				
i. Have pain				
j. Other reason(s), please describe, including how often you have had trouble sleeping because of this reason(s):				
6. During the past month, how often have you taken medicine (prescribed or "over the counter") to help you sleep?				
7. During the past month, how often have you had trouble staying awake while driving, eating meals, or engaging in social activity?				
8. During the past month, how much of a problem has it been for you to keep up enthusiasm to get things done?				
	Very good (0)	Fairly good (1)	Fairly bad (2)	Very bad (3)
9. During the past month, how would you rate your sleep quality overall?				

Component 1 #9 Score C1 _____

Component 2 #2 (Score (≤15 min (0), 16–30 min (1), 31–60 min (2), >60 min (3))
+ #5a Score (if sum is equal 0 = 0; 1–2 = 1; 3–4 = 2; 5–6 = 3) C2 _____

Component 3 #4 Score (>7(0), 6–7(1), 5–6(2), <5 (3)) C3 _____

Component 4 (total # of hours asleep)/(total # of hours in bed) × 100
>85% = 0, 75%–84% = 1, 65%–74% = 2, <65% = 3 C4 _____

Component 5 # sum of scores 5b to 5j (0 = 0; 1–9 = 1; 10–18 = 2; 19–27 = 3) C5 _____

Component 6 #6 Score C6 _____

Component 7 #7 score + #8 score (0 = 0; 1–2 = 1; 3–4 = 2; 5–6 = 3) C7 _____

Add the seven component scores together _____ **Global PSQI Score** _____

Source: Reprinted from Buysse, D. J., Reynolds III, C. F., Monk, T. H., Berman, S. R., & Kupfer, D. J. The Pittsburgh Sleep Quality Index: A new instrument for psychiatric practice and research, *Journal of Psychiatric Research, 28*(2), 193–213. Copyright 1989, with permission from Elsevier Science.
Try This: Best Practices in Nursing Care to Older Adults. A series from the Hartford Institute for Geriatric Nursing, **www.hartfordign.org.**

like walking and stretching should be recommended, but not just before bedtime. Sleep hygiene measures such as limiting time spent in bed to 8 hours a night, avoiding daytime napping, and using the bed only for sleep and sex have been found to be an effective intervention (Beck-Little & Weinrich, 1998).

ADDITIONAL NONPHARMACOLOGICAL MEASURES

Sleep restriction therapy is based on the theory that many older persons with sleep problems spend too much time in bed trying to get 8 hours of satisfactory sleep. Therefore, the nurse can assist the older person to identify how many hours of sleep are needed to feel rested and refreshed in the morning. Prompts can include: "How many hours of nighttime sleep is normal for you?" or "Name a time in your life when you thought your sleep was good. How many hours were you sleeping then?"

After the nurse and the older person have identified an appropriate goal, a schedule is established for time to bed and time to arise. For instance, if an older person wishes to obtain 8 hours of quality sleep and wishes to go to bed at 11 p.m., he or she must arise at 7 a.m. At first, older people with sleep problems will be sleep deprived because they will be spending time in bed trying to sleep, but this helps to consolidate sleep (Beck-Little & Weinrich, 1998). Gradually, older persons will increase their sleep efficiency as their bodies learn to become more sleep efficient. Additional rules to be followed in sleep restriction therapy include:

- Use the bed only to sleep. No reading, TV watching, or eating in bed is allowed. Sexual activity is the only exception to this rule.
- If you are unable to sleep, get up and go to another room. Watching the clock is not recommended. When you are sleepy, go back to bed. The goal is to learn to associate the bed with restful sleep.
- Get up at the same time every day, regardless of the amount or quality of sleep obtained the night before.
- Do not nap during the day.

Older persons who vigorously adhere to the provisions of sleep restriction therapy may find improved quality and quantity of sleep.

Cognitive therapy focuses on changing the older person's expectations about sleep. Many older persons worry about their inability to sleep and become anxious "trying" to sleep. With instruction and support from the nurse, the older person with sleep problems may be taught to understand that everyone has a sleep problem from time to time and that daytime fatigue usually follows a circadian pattern and can be managed with short rest periods. **Bedtime rituals** such as progressive relaxation exercises, nature tapes, praying, reading a few pages of a novel, or other relaxing activities may assist the older person who is anxious at bedtime to sleep. The hour before the older person will go to bed should be considered a "transition" hour in which the daytime cares and activities begin to shut down and the body and mind begin to prepare for the onset of sleep. Loud or violent television programs should be avoided. Even the nightly news can be upsetting to some older people if shootings, car crashes, fires, and other disasters are reported in detail. Once a satisfactory nighttime ritual is established, it should be maintained to ease the transition from wakefulness to sleep.

Unfortunately, the nonpharmacological interventions mentioned above are not appropriate for the older person with dementia. Because the central nervous system is unable to maintain 8 hours of consolidated sleep in the older person with dementia, sleep fragmentation occurs. Environmental noise, light, and care routines can disrupt sleep in many cases. The following recommendations are made to nurses working in long-term care facilities (Schnelle, Alessi, Al-Samarrai, Fricker, & Ouslander, 1999):

- Establish consistent nighttime routines, which signal to both staff and residents that sleep is to be facilitated.
- Reduce noise and light disruption throughout the night.
- Turn down televisions and radios and ringers on phones.
- Avoid using intercoms and beepers during sleep hours.
- Turn night-lights on at the hour of sleep and turn off overhead lights.
- Keep residents busy and occupied during the daytime with exercise and recreational programs so that long naps are avoided.
- Do not put residents to bed immediately after supper. Try to provide restful evening activities like music or group readings so that gastrointestinal problems such as gastroesophageal reflux disease are avoided.
- If residents are awake and noisy during the night, assist them from bed to a lounge or recreation area where they will not disturb other residents. When they become sleepy, they can return to their beds.

A multifaceted intervention to improve sleep hygiene can successfully be implemented in the nursing home setting to improve sleep and overall well-being for many of the residents (Schnelle et al., 1999).

PHARMACOLOGICAL TREATMENTS FOR ALTERED SLEEP PATTERNS

A variety of prescription and nonprescription medications as well as herbal remedies are taken by older persons for sleep. When behavioral interventions are not helpful, pharmacotherapy may be indicated. Many older persons with sleep problems are chronic users of sleep medication. Sleep medication use is more prevalent among older adults, particularly older women (National Institutes of Health, 2000).

Studies have shown that most benzodiazepines are effective for promoting sleep on a short-term basis. However, the nurse should be aware of the lack of evidence that these drugs are effective for long-term use.

Drug Alert !

Benzodiazepine therapy is recommended for short-term use not to exceed 2 weeks. If used long term, it is to be given in intermittent courses.

Daytime residual effects include tolerance, psychological dependence, rebound insomnia on discontinuation, and impairment of psychomotor and cognitive performance. It is important to avoid using benzodiazepines with longer half-lives such as alprazolam and diazepam. These drugs are associated with abuse potential, daytime sedation and falls, and memory impairment (Cheng et al., 2000). Shorter acting benzodiazepines (half-life 6 hours) like lorazepam are suggested to be the better choice for elderly adults. These drugs have the best effect profile and raise the fewest safety concerns (Cheng et al., 2000). These preparations are metabolized in the kidneys and are less likely than other agents to cause liver damage (Brown, 1999).

Sedating antidepressants may also be used if the older person exhibits signs and symptoms of depression. Amitriptyline, doxepin, and nortriptyline may be used cautiously. The nurse must carefully monitor the older person for postural hypotension and other anticholinergic side effects such as constipation, dry mouth, tachycardia, and changes in cognitive status. Generally, lower doses of tricyclic antidepressants are needed for sleep disorders than are needed to treat depression, thereby lessening the risk of adverse side effects (Cheng et al., 2000).

Antihistamines such as diphenhydramine (Benadryl) should not be used because of the anticholinergic side effects and the potential to decrease respiratory drive. Barbiturates, sedatives, hypnotics, opiates, and antipsychotics should not be used for the routine treatment of sleep disorders. The use of barbiturates has fallen out of favor because of the potential for abuse, overdose, and severe withdrawal symptoms (Cheng et al., 2000). Additionally, movement disorders such as tardive dyskinesia are common with antipsychotics.

Chloral hydrate is an old-fashioned sleep remedy that is still used. It has less hangover effect than some of the benzodiazepines and most barbiturates. However, as with other sleep aids, tolerance quickly develops within 2 weeks of use and the drug can cause gastric irritation as well as renal, hepatic, and cardiac toxicity (Cheng et al., 2000).

A newer drug, zolpidem (Ambien), has been used in low doses for older persons. Unlike other classes of sleep-inducing drugs, this drug does not adversely affect sleep architecture and has not been associated with harmful side effects. However, as with all newer drugs, caution is recommended until long-term safety and efficacy have been established (Cheng et al., 2000). Daytime sedation and decreased cognitive performance have been reported in older persons, especially when the medication is taken in the middle of the night and the older person does not remain in bed for a full 8 hours of sleep. Many older persons also use herbal or natural remedies. Melatonin is a hormone produced in the pineal gland and plays a role in the regulation of sleep. Melatonin is sold in many pharmacies and health food stores and is effective for some older persons with sleep disturbances due to decreased levels of melatonin. Doses of 0.5 to 3 mg have been suggested for sleep (Huebscher, 1999). It should be taken approximately 2 hours before bedtime. Melatonin has been found to significantly improve sleep in older persons with insomnia and can even help older persons who are "benzodiazepine addicted" withdraw from these drugs. Because melatonin has a short half-life (about 40 minutes), a controlled-release formulation is recommended to maintain sleep throughout the entire sleep cycle (Garfinkle, Zisapel, Wainstein, & Laudon, 1999).

Additional natural remedies include herbal chamomile tea (if no allergies to ragweed or daisies), hops, lemon balm, and valerian (Huebscher, 1999). Valerian root has been used in Europe for the past several years, and a dose of 400 to 450 mg of the extract will shorten sleep latency similar to a short-acting benzodiazepine (Brown, 1999). Larger doses are not recommended, because they are associated with morning drowsiness. As with all herbal remedies, older persons should be cautioned that the U.S. Food and Drug Administration does not regulate valerian, and the amount of active ingredients and purity may vary from preparation to preparation. Sometimes a small evening snack such as a glass of milk or a turkey sandwich may promote sleep onset because of the natural tryptophan contained in these foods.

Practice Pearl

When developing interventions to improve sleep it is important to include the patient. Priorities should be set according to the patient's wishes. It may be difficult for older persons to change their diet, exercise more, avoid caffeine, limit daytime napping, and so on. Making all of these changes at once may be nearly impossible. Approaching each individual behavior with a reasonable plan and appropriate goal setting is key to success.

Patient-Family Teaching Guidelines

INSOMNIA OR SLEEP PROBLEMS

The following are guidelines that the nurse may find useful when instructing older persons and their families about sleep problems (adapted from National Institutes of Health, 2000).

1. What is insomnia or disordered sleep?

These disorders are characterized by the perception or complaint of inadequate or poor quality sleep because of:

- Difficulty falling asleep (longer than 20 minutes is considered a problem).
- Waking up often during the night and being unable to fall quickly back to sleep.
- Waking up too early in the morning and staying awake.
- Waking up in the morning without feeling refreshed.

RATIONALE:

Insomnia is not defined by the number of hours of sleep a person gets or tries to get or even how long it takes to fall asleep. Insomnia is the older person's perception and complaint about either the quality or the quantity of sleep.

2. What causes sleep problems?

Certain conditions make some older persons more likely to have sleep problems than others. Examples of these conditions include the following:

- Age over 60
- Female gender
- History of or current diagnosis of depression
- Certain medications (diuretics or long-term use of sleep medications)
- Daytime loneliness or boredom with long naps
- Chronic illness with components of pain or difficulty breathing
- Diagnosis of Alzheimer's disease or other neurological problems
- Situational events like moving to a new home or loss of a loved one

RATIONALE:

Everyone has transient sleep problems from time to time. In general the amount of sleep needed remains stable throughout the lifetime, but periods of stress, illness, travel, or other change in life events can precipitate sleep problems. The goal is to quickly retrain the body and brain to regain normal sleep.

3. What seems to make sleep problems worse?

The following behaviors seem to perpetuate sleep problems and make them more likely to become chronic:

- Worry about sleep and expecting to have problems every night
- Drinking too much caffeine
- Drinking alcohol before bedtime
- Smoking cigarettes before bedtime
- Sleeping longer than 50 minutes during the day
- Being told by a sleep partner that you are snoring and gasping during sleep
- Not seeking medical attention for pain, urinary problems, nighttime gastroesophageal reflux disease, or tingling sensation in the legs

RATIONALE:

These behaviors may prolong transient insomnia or sleep problems or be responsible for causing the problem initially. Stopping these behaviors and investigating the cause of others early on may eliminate the problem completely.

(continued)

Patient-Family Teaching Guidelines, *cont.*

4. Where should the older person go for evaluation and treatment?

An older person who does not have a current healthcare provider should seek evaluation from a primary care physician, geriatrician, or gerontological nurse practitioner. Underlying acute and chronic health problems should always be investigated and ruled out or treated optimally. These providers can then make referrals for polysomnography and sleep laboratory testing if appropriate. It is helpful to keep a sleep diary for a week or so before the medical appointment because this valuable information will encourage better decision making by the healthcare provider.

RATIONALE:

The older person should not be labeled as having insomnia or chronic sleep problems without a thorough evaluation and physical examination. Some older persons are automatically given sleeping pills that can mask the symptoms of underlying health problems such as untreated or diagnosed pain, cardiac disease, or psychological disorders and have the potential for harmful side effects.

5. How are sleep problems treated?

Some sleep problems are transient and intermittent and will resolve spontaneously. For instance, jet lag may last only a few days. Pain from a fractured bone may resolve within a week or 10 days. The strangeness of moving to a new home may resolve within a few weeks. For long-term sleep problems, the treatment will depend on the cause. A thorough assessment of sleep problems will guide the competent clinician toward appropriate treatment.

RATIONALE:

It is important to avoid taking over-the-counter sleep medications or prescription sleep aids for extended periods of time. They suppress normal sleep architecture, perpetuate sleep problems, and have the potential for harmful side effects.

Care Plan

A Patient With a Sleep Problem

Case Study

A nurse working at an adult day care center notices that Mrs. Johnson, an 84-year-old woman who has attended the center regularly for 1 year, is lethargic, disinterested, and constantly nodding off to sleep during activities. Other clients at the center have begun to complain about her and have asked the nurse to speak with her and tell her to "stay home if she wants to sleep all day."

A Patient With a Sleep Problem

Applying the Nursing Process

ASSESSMENT

Mrs. Johnson has recently had a complete physical examination and health history, and there is no apparent medical reason for her sleep problems. The nurse requests permission from Mrs. Johnson to visit her at home and she agrees. The next day during the home visit the nurse notices a liquor bottle on the counter. When asked about this, Mrs. Johnson replies, "Oh yes. I take a nip or two every night because I can't sleep at all without it. Don't tell my son because he wouldn't approve and I'm afraid he would think I'm an alcoholic or something like that." She appears angry and defensive as she makes this statement.

DIAGNOSIS

The current nursing diagnoses for Mrs. Johnson include the following:

- *Sleep pattern disturbance*
- *Potential for substance abuse*
- *Altered activity levels*

EXPECTED OUTCOMES

The expected outcomes for the plan of care specify that Mrs. Johnson will:

- Become aware of the harmful effects of alcohol on quality and quantity of sleep.
- Use sleep hygiene measures as an alternative to alcohol.
- Develop a more trusting and open relationship with her son regarding her health status.
- Agree to establish a therapeutic relationship with the nurse and develop a mutually acceptable plan to work toward these outcomes.

PLANNING AND IMPLEMENTATION

The following nursing interventions may be appropriate for Mrs. Johnson:

- Establish a therapeutic relationship.
- Avoid being judgmental or using "scare" tactics.
- Encourage a family meeting with the son present to talk about health issues in general with Mrs. Johnson's permission.
- Begin a sleep assessment to establish the underlying cause of her sleep disturbance.
- Begin a values clarification to establish long-term goals and facilitate end-of-life planning.

EVALUATION

The nurse hopes to work with Mrs. Johnson over time and realizes the chronic nature of sleep problems in older people. The nurse will consider the plan a success based on the following criteria:

(continued)

A Patient With a Sleep Problem *(continued)*

- Mrs. Johnson will continue to attend the day care center with improved function and social skills.
- A family meeting will be held to discuss her overall health.
- Mrs. Johnson will begin to decrease her alcohol consumption at bedtime and report improved sleep based upon positive behavioral changes.

Ethical Dilemma

The ethical dilemma that emerges in this case is the conflict between the nurse's obligation to patient autonomy and confidentiality versus beneficence. Mrs. Johnson is physically frail but cognitively intact. The nurse cannot share confidential information with others who may wish to assist Mrs. Johnson to improve her health status. This includes her family, her physician, and other healthcare providers. However, the nurse wishes to meet her moral and professional obligation to assist this patient to regain her previous function and vigor and realizes the addictive and harmful effects of alcohol use in older people.

Critical Thinking and the Nursing Process

1. What is the physiological basis for Mrs. Johnson's poor quality of sleep after alcohol consumption?
2. Explain possible reasons in addition to alcohol consumption for this patient's poor sleep.
3. Outline a teaching plan with behavioral interventions designed to improve Mrs. Johnson's sleep.
4. Suggest a nursing action if Mrs. Johnson continues to increase her alcohol consumption and still refuses to accept family or professional help for her drinking.
5. Suppose that Mrs. Johnson asks if sleeping medication may be appropriate for her to use. How should the nurse respond?

- Evaluate your responses in Appendix B. ⊂▭⊃

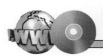

EXPLORE MediaLink

NCLEX review, case studies, and other interactive resources for this chapter can be found on the Companion Website at **www.prenhall.com/tabloski**. Click on Chapter 8 to select the activities for this chapter. For animations, more NCLEX review questions, and case studies, access the accompanying CD-ROM in this textbook.

Chapter Highlights

- Older persons often report sleep problems. Some are transient in nature, but many are chronic. These problems may be the result of age-related changes, physical or mental health problems, medication use or abuse, or lifestyle issues.

- In order to be restful and restorative, sleep must cycle through stages and phases. Normal changes of aging and some medications suppress the cyclic changes, making restful sleep harder to achieve.

- Older persons in nursing homes and hospitals may have even more disrupted sleep because of noise and light interruptions from nursing staff and other residents. Every attempt should be made to minimize nighttime awakenings so that restful sleep may be achieved.

- Alzheimer's disease and other kinds of dementia can further disturb sleep. These disruptions may lead to institutionalization if caregivers become fatigued by their inability to achieve restful sleep.

- Sleep apnea can be a significant problem for older people. Those at high risk—including persons who snore, have hypertension, are obese, or have central nervous system problems—should seek polysomnography testing in a sleep laboratory.

- Prescription and OTC sleep aids can have dangerous side effects when taken by older persons. These drugs should be used in the smallest doses for the shortest period of time.

- Nurses should carry out a complete sleep history before recommending an intervention for an older person with sleep problems. Sleep problems may result from a variety of causes, and the nursing intervention should be appropriately based upon the cause.

References

Beck-Little, R., & Weinrich, S. (1998). Assessment and management of sleep disorders in the elderly. Journal of Gerontological Nursing, 24(4), 21–29.

Beers, M. H., & Berkow, R. (Eds.). (1999). *The Merck manual of diagnosis and therapy* (17th ed.). Whitehouse Station, NJ: Merck Research Laboratories.

Brown, D. B. (1999). Managing sleep disorders. *Clinician Reviews, 9*(10), 51–71.

Burgess, H., & Dawson, D. (1999). Melatonin: Its physiological effects and clinical applications (invited review). *Journal of British Menopause Society,* September 5(3), 122–126.

Cheng, C., Umland, E., & Muirhead, G. (2000, June 15). New and old drugs to treat insomnia.

Patient Care, 34–43. Retrieved March 12, 2001, from http://www.patientcareonline.com.

Chesson, A. (2000). Practice parameters for the evaluation of insomnia. *Sleep, 23*(4), 237–241.

Cohen-Mansfield, J., Werner, P., & Freedman, L. (1995). Sleep and agitation in agitated nursing home residents: An observational study. *Sleep, 18*(8), 674–680.

Ely, W., Siegel, M., & Inouye, S. (2001). Delirium in the intensive care unit: An under-recognized syndrome of organ dysfunction. *Seminar in Respiratory Critical Care Medicine, 22*(2), 115–126.

Endeshaw, Y., Johnson, T., Kutner, M., Ouslander, J., & Bliwise, D. (2004). Sleep-disordered breathing and nocturia in older

adults. *Journal of the American Geriatrics Society, 52*(6), 957–960.

Floyd, J. (1999). Sleep promotion in adults. *Annual Review of Nursing Research, 17*(6)27–56.

Garfinkle, D., Zisapel, N., Wainstein, J., & Laudon, M. (1999). Facilitation of benzodiazepine discontinuation by melatonin. *Archives of Internal Medicine, 159*(20), 1–11.

Hartford Institute for Geriatric Nursing, Division of Nursing, New York University. (1999). The Pittsburgh Sleep Quality Index. Try this: Best practices in nursing care to older adults. M. Wallace, ed. 1(6). Retrieved June 14, 1999, from www.hartfordign.org.

Howcroft, D., & Jones, R. (1999). Sleep, older people and dementia. *Nursing Times, 95*(33), 54–56.

Huebscher, R. (1999). Natural, alternative, and complementary therapies for sleep. *Nurse Practitioner Forum, 10*(3), 117–119.

Jao, D., & Alessi, C. (2004). Sleep disorders. In C. Landefeld, R. Palmer, M. Johnson, C. Johnston, & W. Lyons (Eds.), *Current geriatric diagnosis and treatment.* New York: Lange Medical Books/McGraw-Hill.

Laube, I. (1998). Accidents related to sleepiness. *Switzerland Medical Journal, 128*(40), 1487–1499.

McCance, K., & Huether, S. (2001). *Pathophysiology: The biologic basis for disease in adults and children.* New York: Mosby.

Merritt, S. (2000). Putting sleep disorders to rest. *RN, 63*(7), 26–30. Retrieved March 12, 2001, from www.rnweb.com.

Miller, M. (2000). Nocturnal polyuria in older people: Pathophysiology and clinical implications. *Journal of the American Geriatrics Society, 48,* 1321–1329.

National Heart, Lung and Blood Institute Working Group on Insomnia. Insomnia: Assessment and Management in Primary Care. (1999). *American Family Physician, 59,* 3029–3039.

National Highway Traffic Safety Administration. (1998). Drowsy driving and automobile crashes. National Center on Sleep Research, retrieved on June 14, 2000, from www.NHLBI.NIH.gov/health/prof/sleep/drsy_drv.pdt.

National Institutes of Health. (2000). *National Center on Sleep Disorders Research, Test your sleep IQ* (Publication No. 00-3797). Washington, DC: U.S. Government Printing Office.

National Institute of Neurological Disorders and Stroke. (2003). *Brain basics: Understanding sleep.* Retrieved June 19, 2003, from www.ninds.nih.gov.

North American Nursing Diagnosis Association (NANDA). (2001). *Nursing diagnoses: Definitions & classification 2001-2002.* Philadelphia: Author.

Pace, B., Lynn, C., & Glass, R. (2001). Breathing problems during sleep. *Journal of the American Medical Association, 285*(22), 2936.

Phillips, B., & Ancoli-Israel, S. (2001). Sleep disorders in the elderly. *Sleep Medicine, 2*(2), 99–114.

Redeker, N., Tamburri, L., & Howland, C. (1998). Prehospital correlates of sleep in patients hospitalized with cardiac disease. *Research in Nursing & Health, 21,* 27–37.

Riccio, P., Knight, B., & Cody, M. S. (1999). Medication use with implications for sleep in elderly dementia caregivers. *Home Health Care Managed Practice, 12*(1), 42–49.

Schnelle, J., Alessi, C., Al-Samarrai, N., Fricker, R., & Ouslander, J. (1999). The nursing home at night: Effects of an intervention on noise, light and sleep. *Journal of the American Geriatrics Society, 47,* 430–438.

Tabloski, P., & Church, O. M. (1999). Insomnia, alcohol and drug use in community-residing elderly persons. *Journal of Substance Use, 3*(4), 147–154.

Tabloski, P., Cooke, K., & Thoman, E. (1998). A procedure for withdrawal of sleep medication in elderly women who have been long-term users. *Journal of Gerontological Nursing, 24*(9), 20–28.

Wilcox, S., Brenes, G., Levine, D., Sevick, M. A., Shumaker, S. A., & Craven, T. (2000). Factors related to sleep disturbance in older adults experiencing knee pain or knee pain with radiographic evidence of knee osteoarthritis. *Journal of the American Geriatrics Society, 48,* 1241–1251.

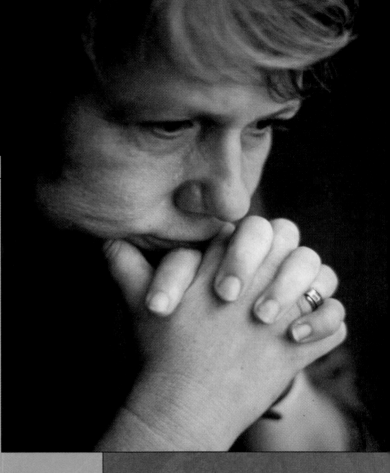

CHAPTER 9

Pain Management

CHAPTER OBJECTIVES

Upon completion of this chapter, the reader will be able to:

- Define pain and the outcomes of pain in the older adult.
- Identify appropriate pain assessment techniques, including those to use with dementia.
- Describe pharmacological and nonpharmacological approaches useful in treating pain in the older adult.
- Identify the nurse's role in treating pain in the older adult.
- Describe patient-family teaching guidelines for pain management.

MediaLink

Additional resources for this chapter can be found on the Student CD-ROM accompanying this textbook and on the Companion Website at **www.prenhall.com/tabloski**. Click on Chapter 9 to select the activities for this chapter.

CD-ROM
- NCLEX Review
- Case Studies
- Tools

COMPANION WEBSITE
- Audio Glossary
- Additional NCLEX Review
- Case Study
- MediaLink Applications

KEY TERMS

acute pain 250
adjuvant drugs 253
central pain 250
chronic pain 250
hyperalgesia 251
neuropathic pain 250
nociceptive pain 250
pain 250
pain management 250
tolerance 255
visceral pain 251

Pain is a common negative sensation experienced by all human beings during the process of living. The **nociceptive pain** sensation can be protective and is designed to provide a signal that tissue damage or inflammation is occurring somewhere in the body. For example, persons with diabetes who have peripheral neuropathies are at risk for development of foot ulcers since they cannot feel the sensation of pain to alert them of the developing injury. Although acute pain can be protective, chronic pain can become an intolerable burden (Thomas, Flaherty & Morley, 2001).

Undertreatment of **acute** and **chronic pain** is a serious problem relating to care of the older adult. Despite the fact that safe and effective pharmacological and non-pharmacological techniques are available to treat pain, many older adults live with untreated pain on a daily basis. A study of 13,625 cancer patients in nursing homes reported that up to 40% of these patients were in pain every day and 25% of them received no pain medications at all (Bernabei et al., 2002). Further, this study found that older patients and minorities were even less likely to receive pain medications than younger White patients. The authors of the study speculated that this may be because these older and minority patients were less likely to complain or reveal that they were suffering. Studies of both community-residing and nursing home elderly adults have revealed that 45% to 80% have substantial pain that is undertreated (Helme & Gibson, 1999). This is not surprising because many older persons have been diagnosed with multiple medical problems that can be a source of both **neuropathic and central pain**. Box 9-1 lists conditions that are associated with pain in older adults.

There is increased emphasis on the assessment and treatment of pain, and patients and their families are becoming more aware of the need to treat both acute and chronic pain. Barriers to effective **pain management** include lack of knowledge of the care providers, persistent misperceptions regarding addiction to pain medication, and state and federal regulation of the prescribing of opioid analgesics (American

BOX 9-1	Conditions Associated With Pain in Older Adults

- Degenerative joint disease
- Rheumatoid arthritis
- Chronic back pain
- Osteoporosis (with and without spinal fracture)
- Neuropathic pain (with diabetes mellitus and postherpetic neuralgia)
- Gastroesophageal reflux disease
- Peripheral vascular disease
- Poststroke syndromes
- Immobility, contractures
- Headache
- Oral problems and gum disease
- Amputation
- Pressure ulcers
- Angina and other cardiac disease
- Cancer pain and pain from resulting treatment

Source: Adapted from Thomas et al., 2001.

Pain Society Quality of Care Committee, 1995). Further, many older people and their families believe that pain is a normal part of aging and fear that complaining is a sign of weakness.

In a literature review of eight textbooks for geriatric nurses in which over 5,000 pages were examined, researchers found only 18 pages addressing the subject of pain alleviation (Volicer & Hurley, 2003). Pain treatment in elderly adults is considered a neglected phenomenon (Warden, Hurley, & Volicer, 2003). The high prevalence of dementia in the nursing home, the effect of multiple sensory impairments, and disability in many older persons make assessment and management of pain more difficult (American Geriatrics Society [AGS], 2002).

Pathophysiology of Pain

Pain and pain transmission involve both the peripheral receptors and sensory pathways and synaptic contacts in the spinal cord and brain stem. Processes within the dorsal horn are essential elements in modulating and facilitating pain transmission and initiating efferent responses (Sinatra, 2002).

The nociceptors in the peripheral nervous system respond to stimuli that threaten or produce damage to the organism. Figure 9-1 ■ illustrates the configuration of the brain, spinal cord, and peripheral receptors. With untreated pain, these nociceptors become sensitive and more responsive to stimuli with a lowered pain threshold. This can lead to **hyperalgesia** or an increase in pain production and intensity (Willis, 1998). This sensitization can cause an exaggerated pain response to stimuli that usually cause only discomfort or mild pain such as administration of injections, starting an intravenous (IV) line, or even taking a blood pressure. Nurses and other healthcare providers may become impatient with older persons exhibiting this exaggerated pain response and feel that it is out of proportion to the procedure being carried out. The older person may be labeled as a "hypochondriac," and further complaints of pain may not be taken seriously.

Few studies have examined the relationship between pain perception and aging. The few studies that have enrolled older persons have found that with the exception of skin sensation, nociception appears not to change with age, although pain tolerance decreases (Gloth, 2001). Certain types of **visceral pain** may be less severe in the older adult, and that may explain the higher incidence of silent myocardial infarction and the less dramatic presentation of surgical abdomen. The younger adult experiencing myocardial infarction will most often report severe, crushing chest pain, often with radiation down the left arm, sweating, and tremor. However, the older person may report vague complaints of pain that can be attributed to heartburn or sour stomach, the presence of nausea and vomiting, or unexplained fatigue or falls.

The Art and Science of Pain Relief

The goal of ideal pain management is to relieve both acute and chronic pain with appropriate pharmacological and nonpharmacological techniques while minimizing side effects. Nurses often assume responsibility for the assessment of pain, administration of medications, and assessment of the effectiveness of the pain management plan. Each older patient is a unique individual and will respond differently to analgesic medications and other pain control techniques. Therefore, individually tailored pain management plans are necessary for each patient. This requires careful titration of analgesic drugs and consistent monitoring of therapeutic and adverse effects by the nurse and other members of the healthcare team. Patients with severe pain require more rapid titration to get symptoms under control. This is often better accomplished in the acute care setting where

FIGURE ☐ 9-1

The brain, spinal cord, and peripheral pain receptors.

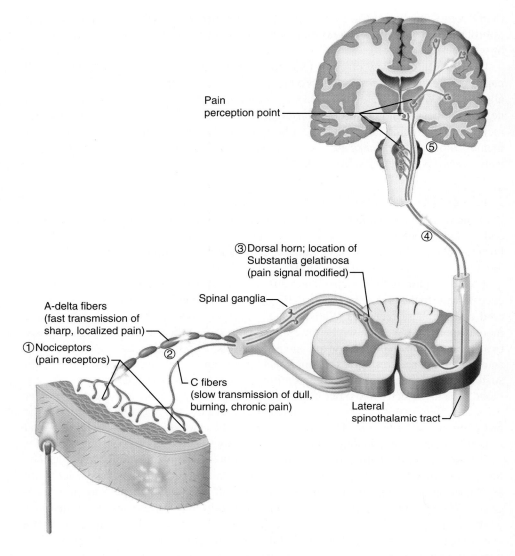

Pain perception point

⑤

④

③ Dorsal horn; location of Substantia gelatinosa (pain signal modified)

Spinal ganglia

A-delta fibers (fast transmission of sharp, localized pain)

① Nociceptors (pain receptors)

②

C fibers (slow transmission of dull, burning, chronic pain)

Lateral spinothalamic tract

nurses can carefully monitor function, vital signs, and renal and hepatic function (AGS, 2002). Older patients are generally more susceptible to adverse drug reactions, but analgesic drugs can be safely and effectively used with proper monitoring. Older patients are generally more sensitive to opioid analgesics, and most often these patients are started on smaller doses to avoid toxicity. The dose is then titrated upward until effective pain relief is achieved without adverse effects. The titration process may take several days or even longer, especially when drugs with longer half-lives are used.

Greater reductions in pain are seen when pharmacological and nonpharmacological techniques are combined (AGS, 2002). The nurse should assess the older patient's beliefs and willingness to use relaxation techniques, heating pads or cold compresses, biofeedback, music, therapeutic touch, or other methods to enhance or replace analgesic drugs. Additionally, the nurse should question the patient as to use of over-the-counter (OTC) medications or herbal remedies that may interact with every additional drug taken as part of the pain management plan. Ineffective drugs or drugs that cause troubling side effects should be tapered or discontinued because they do not contribute to a positive therapeutic outcome.

Dying patients have special pain and symptom control needs that mandate respectful and responsive care. Concern for the patient's comfort and dignity should guide all aspects of care during the final stages of life. The Joint Commission on Accreditation of Healthcare Organizations (JCAHO, 2003) has proposed the following standards for healthcare organizations providing end-of-life care:

- Providing appropriate treatment for any primary and secondary symptom, according to the wishes of the patient or the surrogate decision maker
- Managing pain aggressively and effectively
- Sensitively addressing issues such as autopsy and organ donation
- Respecting the patient's values, religion, and philosophy
- Involving the patient and, where appropriate, the family in every aspect of care
- Responding to the psychological, social, emotional, spiritual, and cultural concerns of the patient and the family

Effective pain management is appropriate for all patients, not just the dying; however, preventing needless pain and suffering at the end of life is a key aspect of the nurse's role, no matter what the age of the patient. Given nursing's ongoing presence and care of the dying at the bedside, the nurse has the opportunity not only to assess and manage pain, but also to educate, support, serve as patient advocate regarding end-of-life preferences, and collaborate with others to develop systems-level policies and procedures related to implementation of advance directives. Management of pain in terminal conditions usually calls for higher doses of opioids, regardless of the secondary effects on respiration and resulting length of life (Tolle, Tilden, Nelson, & Dunn, 1998). (See Chapter 11 for further discussion of death and dying.)

Pharmacological Management

In most cases, it makes sense to progress from non-opioid analgesics such as acetaminophen to anti-inflammatory drugs, neurotransmitter-modulating and membrane-stabilizing drugs, and opioids to balance the risk and benefits of treating more severe pain (AGS, 2002). Table 9-1 provides information on pharmacotherapeutic agents that may be used to treat chronic pain in elderly patients.

ADJUVANT DRUGS FOR OLDER PATIENTS WITH PAIN

Adjuvant drugs (antidepressants and anticonvulsants) are not typically considered pain medicines, but they may relieve discomfort and potentiate the effect of pain medications to reduce the side effect burden. Examples of adjuvant drugs that nurses may see used in the clinical setting include:

1. **Antidepressants and anticonvulsants (tricyclics, selective serotonin reuptake inhibitors, carbamazepine, gabapentin)**—helpful for diabetic neuropathy, trigeminal neuralgia, and postherpetic neuralgia.
2. **Topical analgesics (capsaicin, menthol methylsalicylate, EMLA cream, lidocaine gel)**—helpful for chronic arthritis pain, herpes zoster, and diabetic neuropathy; may be used in anticipation of painful procedures such as venipuncture for blood draws, IV insertion, and so on.
3. **Muscle relaxants (baclofen, diazepam, carisoprodol)**—helpful when there is significant muscle spasm component to pain; to be used in addition to, not in place of, analgesic medications.
4. **Antianxiety medications (diazepam, doxepin, oxazepam)**—helpful when patient is anxious or agitated.

TABLE 9-1

Pharmacotherapeutic Agents and Dosing Suggestions for Management of Persistent
Pain in the Older Person

Drug	Starting Dose	Titration	Comments
Non-Opioids			
Acetaminophen	325 mg q4h	After 4–6 doses	Maximum dose 4 g/24 hr. Reduce dose with hepatic disease or history of alcohol abuse.
Ibuprofen	400–600 mg q6h	After 2–3 days	Take with food to reduce risk of GI distress.
Corticosteroids	5 mg qd	After 2–3 doses	Use lowest possible dose to avoid chronic steroid side effects.
Tricyclic antidepressants	10 mg hs	After 3–5 days	Significant risk of anticholinergic side effects.
Anticonvulsants			
Carbamazepine	100 mg qd	After 3–5 days	Monitor LFTs, CBC, BUN/creatinine, electrolytes.
Gabapentin	100 mg hs	After 1–2 days	Monitor sedation, ataxia, edema.
Opioids			
Morphine sulfate	10–20 mg q4h	After 1 day	Start low and titrate to comfort. Anticipate and treat side effects.
Oxycodone Hydrocodone	5–10 mg q4h	After 1–2 days	Start low and titrate to comfort. Anticipate and treat side effects.
Hydromorphone	1.5 mg q4h	After 1–2 days	Start low and titrate to comfort. Anticipate and treat side effects.
Transdermal fentanyl	25 μg q72h	After 3 days	Apply to clean, dry skin. Peak effects of first dose take 24 hr, so cover with oral meds the first day of application.

5. **Medications to dry secretions (scopolamine, glycopyrrolate)**—helpful when patient has thick secretions that require frequent suctioning.
6. **Antipruritics (diphenhydramine, hydroxyzine)**—helpful when patient has pruritus secondary to liver disease or other conditions that are itchy and result in scratching.
7. **Diuretics (furosemide, hydrochlorothiazide)**—helpful to ease discomfort from ascites from liver cancer or cirrhosis.
8. **Magic mouthwash (diphenhydramine elixir/Maalox/viscous lidocaine)**—helpful when patient has mucositis secondary to chemotherapy. Add nystatin if there is evidence of thrush (Thomas et al., 2001; Woods-Smith, Arnstein, Rosa, & Wells-Federman, 2002).

SPECIAL PHARMACOLOGICAL ISSUES REGARDING PAIN MANAGEMENT IN THE OLDER PERSON

It is becoming more acceptable for physicians and others to manage persistent non-cancer pain with the use of opioid analgesics (AGS, 2002). Although true addiction (drug craving to achieve euphoria) to opioid medication in elderly patients is rare, physical dependency is an inevitable consequence over time, especially when patients experience relief from chronic, debilitating pain. Studies indicate that **tolerance** (the need for more drug to get the same therapeutic effect) is slow to develop in the face of stable disease (AGS, 2002). Nurses should urge patients to seek further diagnostic testing and evaluation of chronic illnesses when the need for opioid medication increases suddenly rather than assuming that tolerance to opioids is the underlying issue. Concerns over drug dependency and addiction do not justify the failure to relieve pain (AGS, 2002). Because of the serious misuse and abuse of oxycodone, it has become difficult for many patients with significant pain to obtain legitimate prescriptions for this opioid. Nearly 300 oxycodone overdose deaths occurred nationally during the year 2000. Nurses are urged to counsel their patients to store the drug securely away from children and others in a locked cabinet, to notify the pharmacy 24 hours in advance of needed refills, and to count and track tablets if they feel someone in or around their residence may be diverting and misusing medication for pleasure (Gelfand, 2002).

When mixed drugs containing opioids and acetaminophen or aspirin are used to control pain (acetaminophen with codeine, oxycodone with aspirin, aspirin with codeine), the nurse should be aware that doses are limited by the toxic effect that can occur as a result of high salicylate or acetaminophen levels. Acetaminophen is hepatotoxic above 4 g/day, and aspirin can cause gastric bleeding and abnormal platelet function at doses above 4 g/day. Special caution is advised in older patients with decreased renal and hepatic function and those currently using alcohol or possessing a history of alcohol abuse.

Propoxyphene is not recommended for treatment of persistent pain in the older person (AGS, 2002). The efficacy is similar to that of aspirin or acetaminophen alone, but propoxyphene carries the added burden of serious side effects caused by the accumulation of toxic metabolites. These metabolites can cause delirium, ataxia, and dizziness. Other drugs are suggested for the treatment of persistent pain in the older person.

PHARMACOLOGICAL PRINCIPLES FOR SUCCESSFUL PAIN MANAGEMENT

Pain medication given by mouth is the preferred way to control pain in the older person. Even patients who cannot swallow can be given concentrated liquid morphine drops by the sublingual or buccal route. It is the safest, least expensive, and easiest route. When pain medication is given via the IV route, the older person may have restricted movement because of the IV apparatus and needle placement in the arm. Additionally, should the needle be displaced or the solution infiltrate, the IV must be discontinued and restarted, causing the patient to experience some period of time without medication. This may be insignificant in the acute care setting where many nurses are available to restart IVs, but delays may occur in the nursing home, community, and hospice settings if trained nurses are not immediately available.

Pain medication works best when it is administered around the clock. The nurse should be familiar with the duration of action of analgesics and give the medication routinely to prevent the return of pain. Patients avoid the needless suffering and mental anguish that can occur when medication is given on a prn (as needed) basis. These techniques require patients to wait until they experience pain, request pain medication, and then wait for the medication to relieve their pain. The use of long-acting or sustained-release forms of medication (MS Contin) has improved management of chronic pain conditions (Thomas et al., 2001). Once-daily dosing with these medications can control chronic pain very effectively, and immediate-release, short-acting preparations (Roxanol) can be used for breakthrough pain or pain associated with activity or procedures.

Practice Pearl

Avoid the use of prn medication for pain control as the patient will learn to expect the return of pain, suffer psychologically and spiritually by dealing with recurrent pain, and need more medication to relieve the recurrent pain.

If the patient experiences breakthrough pain on a consistent basis, the nurse should notify the physician so that the dose of the long-acting, sustained-release preparation can be increased to more effectively control the pain. The dose may be increased by up to 25%. If the nurse notes that pain is effectively relieved for a period of time but recurs at the end of the dosing interval, end-of-dose failure should be suspected. In this case, the analgesic medication should be dosed more frequently, if possible, depending on the product. For instance, a medication administered every 12 hours may be changed to an every 8-hour schedule to provide more sustained coverage. Medication should be available as needed for breakthrough pain for optimal pain control. The nurse can educate the patient and the family to monitor the pain sensation and intensity during the course of treatment to provide ongoing assessment of the success of the pain treatment plan.

Drug Alert

Warn patients that crushing or chewing sustained-release preparations of analgesics destroys their controlled-release properties and causes rapid absorption of the entire dose, resulting in overdosage (AGS, 2002).

The use of placebos, inert medications, sham injections, and other pain control methods known to be ineffective is considered to be unethical in clinical practice for management of acute or persistent pain (AGS, 2002). The use of placebos should be limited to research protocols where patients have given informed consent and are aware of the fact that they may receive an inert medication as part of the research protocol.

Patients who experience a poor response to a well-developed pain management plan should be encouraged to speak with their physician regarding referral to a pain management clinic. These specialty clinics may be housed in larger teaching hospitals and usually utilize the services of pain specialists and a well-trained multidisciplinary team. An integrated approach to pain management and access to a wide variety of treatment options have been shown to be effective for patients with persistent pain (Wells-Federman, 1999).

Nonpharmacological Methods to Manage Pain in the Older Person

Nonpharmacological methods to control pain can be effective as stand-alone treatments and adjuncts to pharmacological interventions with the potential to lessen dosages of medications and thus reduce the odds of adverse drug reactions. Nurses can assess older patients' preferences and attitudes toward nonpharmacological methods to relieve pain and encourage them to use methods appropriate for their needs. Nonpharmacological methods of pain control include pain education programs, socialization or recreation programs (movies, art therapy, therapeutic use of music), behavior modification (imagery, hypnosis, relaxation), physical therapy (massage, ultrasound, exercise, hot and cold packs), and neurostimulation (acupuncture, transcutaneous nerve stimulation) (Thomas et al., 2001).

Drug Alert

Opioid analgesics should be titrated slowly, and mild sedation and impaired cognitive function should be anticipated until tolerance develops (Thomas et al., 2001).

Consequences of Unrelieved Pain

Unfortunately, chronic pain has become a label associated with negative images and stereotypes of long-standing psychiatric problems, futility in treatment, malingering, or drug-seeking behavior (AGS, 2002). Further, uncontrolled or poorly controlled pain can result in serious physiological responses, including hypertension, tachycardia, and even coronary ischemia in patients with underlying cardiac disease (Sinatra, 2002). Depression, anxiety, decreased socialization, sleep disturbance, impaired ambulation, and increased healthcare costs have all been found to be associated with the presence of pain in older people (AGS, 2002). Older patients suffering the psychological burden of pain are less likely to participate in rehabilitation and self-care activities, thus making their care more difficult and potentially slowing recovery from illness while lowering their quality of life.

Some older people are hesitant to report pain or seek pain medication. They may fear addiction or side effects of pain medication, going to the hospital or clinic for invasive testing, being labeled as a complainer, or that their pain may be associated with serious underlying disease such as cancer. Therefore, nurses need to be proactive in screening for and assessing pain.

Practice Pearl

Be alert for patients who report that their pain level is tolerable and that it only hurts when they move. These patients are likely to suffer the negative effects of long-term immobility such as decubitus ulcers, aspiration pneumonia, deep vein thrombosis, dehydration, and constipation. Effective pain relief should be provided to encourage movement and participation in rehabilitation activities.

When older people are actively involved in the assessment and management of their pain, the nurse has a better chance of implementing an effective plan for pain relief. The Pain Foundation has developed a Pain Care Bill of Rights for persons with pain (Box 9-2).

Practice Pearl

Many older persons and some healthcare providers believe pain is a normal part of aging. When caring for an older person with unrelieved pain, the nurse should be persistent in assessing and establishing a pain management plan. Effective pain management will allow the patient to maintain dignity, functional capacity, and quality of life (AGS, 2002).

BOX 9-2	Pain Care Bill of Rights

As a person with pain, you have:

- The right to have your report of pain taken seriously and to be treated with dignity and respect by doctors, nurses, pharmacists, and others.
- The right to have your pain thoroughly assessed and promptly treated.
- The right to be informed by your doctor about what may be causing your pain, possible treatments, and the benefits, risks, and costs of each.
- The right to participate actively in decisions about how to manage your pain.
- The right to have your pain reassessed regularly and your treatment adjusted if your pain has not been relieved.
- The right to be referred to a pain specialist if your pain persists.
- The right to get clear and prompt answers to your questions, take time to make decisions, and refuse a particular type of treatment if you choose.

Although not required by law, these are rights persons with pain should expect and if necessary demand for quality pain care.

Source: American Pain Foundation, 2001. Pain care bill of rights, retrieved August 14, 2002, from www.painfoundation.org. Used with permission.

In order to change the mindset and culture regarding pain control that exists in some hospitals and nursing homes, JCAHO developed new standards for institutional pain assessment that went into effect on January 1, 2001. An expert JCAHO panel developed the Seven Commandments of Pain Management as listed in Box 9-3.

ACUTE PAIN IN ELDERLY ADULTS

Acute pain is pain occurring from a time-limited illness, a recent event such as surgery, medical procedures, or trauma (Agency for Health Care Policy and Research, 1995). When acute pain occurs, it is important for the nurse to adequately identify the source of the pain and facilitate treatment of the underlying disease or trauma whenever possible. Conditions that cause acute pain in older persons include exacerbations of degenerative joint disease; flare-ups of chronic conditions such as gout or rheumatoid arthritis; trauma from falls including muscle strain, bone fractures, bumps, and bruises; skin problems such as burns, decubitus ulcers, and skin tears; presence of infection such as urinary tract infection; pleuritic pain in pneumonia and the neuropathic pain of herpes zoster; constipation; and postoperative pain from surgical intervention.

Ideally, the nurse should conduct a baseline patient assessment prior to a known painful event such as surgery, an invasive medical procedure, or a planned rehabilitation event such as postoperative physical therapy. This baseline assessment will allow the nurse to (1) investigate pain terminology typically used by the patient and the patient's attitudes toward pain medication and pain relief techniques, (2) identify sociocultural variables that may influence pain behaviors and expression, (3) obtain a health history that can identify accompanying chronic conditions that could contribute to the anticipated pain experience, (4) investigate past methods of pain relief, (5) identify pain medications used effectively in the past and any medication allergies and intolerance, and (6) select an appropriate pain scale and measurement technique for later use (Titler & Mentes, 1999).

BOX
9-3

The Seven Commandments of Pain Management

Commandment I

Recognize the right of patients to appropriate assessment of pain management. (Think of pain as the fifth vital sign to be routinely included in all patient assessments.)

Commandment II

Assess the existence and, if present, the nature and intensity of pain in all patients.

Commandment III

Record the results of the assessment in a way that facilitates regular reassessment and follow-up.

Commandment IV

Determine and assure staff competency in pain assessment and management, and address pain assessment and management in the orientation of all new staff.

Commandment V

Establish the policies and procedures that support the appropriate prescription or ordering of effective pain medications.

Commandment VI

Educate patients and their families about effective pain management.

Commandment VII

Address patient needs for symptom management in the discharge planning process.

Source: JCAHO, 2003.

If the patient is unable to communicate effectively because of language differences, cognitive impairment, or expressive aphasia after a stroke, the nurse may wish to obtain information from a family member or significant other about the baseline function and pain level of the patient. There is no reason to believe that the cognitively impaired patient is insensitive or indifferent to pain. If no family member is present to provide such information, the nurse may wish to observe the patient carefully during the baseline period and document the information in the patient care plan. Important indicators are baseline vital signs; ability to walk, stand, or move about in bed; baseline agitation level; appetite and eating pattern; sleep patterns; elimination habits; and cognitive function and mood. Postoperative or postprocedure assessments can then focus on noting and treating changes from baseline and the identification of new behaviors that may be pain-related such as grimacing, moaning, guarded movements, and bracing. Researchers have documented that the most frequently seen behavioral symptoms associated with discomfort and pain are tense body language, sad facial expression, fidgeting, persistent verbalizations, and verbal outbursts (Kovach et al., 1999). It is important to use both self-report and nonverbal measures when assessing pain in the frail elderly population.

If the nurse first encounters the patient at a time when he or she is experiencing acute pain, such as in the emergency department after a trauma, the first priority after life-sustaining care is provided is to relieve pain through the administration of analgesics. The safe administration of analgesics in the older person is complicated by a number of factors, including potential drug interactions with underlying chronic disorders, potential drug-drug interactions, presence of underlying nutritional deficiencies, and altered pharmacokinetics. Older persons generally have higher peak levels and longer duration of action from analgesics than younger persons; therefore, dosing should be initiated at lower levels (usually one half the adult dosage) and titrated upward carefully (Young-McCaughan & Miaskowski, 2001). Emergency relief of pain may best be provided by administration of analgesics by the intravenous or intramuscular route. Slowed intramuscular absorption of analgesics in older patients may result in delayed or prolonged effect, altered analgesic serum levels, and potential toxicity with repeated injections.

The use of patient-controlled analgesia for intravenous analgesics may be less effective in elderly patients, especially those with cognitive impairment. The nurse should carefully monitor the patient during the immediate posttrauma or postoperative period. If acute confusion develops, it is important to assess for other contributing factors such as unrelieved pain before discontinuing analgesic medication. Bowel function should be carefully monitored and a constipation protocol put in place to prevent fecal impaction and ileus related to narcotic analgesics (Agency for Health Care Policy and Research, 1992, 1995). The nurse should monitor urinary output and assess for urinary retention and renal function.

CHRONIC PAIN IN THE OLDER PERSON

Chronic pain that continues over a prolonged period of time affects one in five persons age 65 and older. Chronic pain in older persons results from spine disorders (spinal stenosis, osteoporosis with compression fractures, osteoarthritis, degenerative disk disease, arthritis and related disorders), cancer, and neuropathic disorders. Other conditions include back pain and the ischemic pain of vascular disease. Pain can be defined as chronic when it persists after the tissue has healed and the pain is no longer serving a protective function and when it is nonresponsive to medical treatment (Wells-Federman, 1999). All older persons suffering from chronic pain are candidates for pharmacological therapy (Partners Against Pain, 2002).

Approximately 80% of nursing home residents, who often have a variety of physical ailments, are estimated to be in substantial pain that is often undertreated (AGS, 2002). Although good coping mechanisms and family support can lower pain levels, depression can exacerbate pain levels. It is recommended that nurses routinely screen for depression when working with older patients with chronic pain. A comprehensive pain treatment plan is needed to treat the biopsychosocial needs of the older patient. A vicious chronic pain cycle can occur with negative consequences, including inactivity, withdrawal from daily life, fatigue, sleep disturbance, irritability and physical deconditioning, and other signs of stress and depression (Wells-Federman, 1999).

PAIN ASSESSMENT TECHNIQUES

Pain is measured subjectively according to the patient's self-report or by careful observation in the nonverbal or severely cognitively impaired patient. Older people who feel that their reports of pain will be taken seriously are more likely to be open and honest during the pain assessment process. Even patients with mild to moderate cognitive impairments can be assessed with simple questions and screening tools (AGS, 2002). Many cognitively impaired residents can report pain accurately at the time of interview but have difficulty reporting intensity and duration of previous episodes. The nurse may have to do more frequent assessments to obtain an accurate pain assessment for the patient with a cognitive impairment.

See the Best Practice feature on the following page for the Hartford Institute for Geriatric Nursing pain assessment recommendation for older adults.

The Hartford Institute for Geriatric Nursing (1999) recommends the Geriatric Pain Assessment instrument for use with older patients as an example of a medical record form that can be used to summarize pain assessment in older persons. This form is ideal for clinical use because it is brief and objective. It summarizes pertinent information and quantifies mood, sleep, bowel habits, exacerbating and relieving factors, and a plan for pain relief. A copy of the instrument is included here.

GERIATRIC PAIN ASSESSMENT

Date: _____   Medical Record Number: _____

Patient's Name: _____

Problem List: Medications:

_____   _____
_____   _____
_____   _____
_____   _____
_____   _____

Pain Description

Pattern: Constant   Intermediate   Pain Intensity:
Duration: _____   0 1 2 3 4 5 6 7 8 9 10
Location: _____   None   Moderate   Severe
Character:
Laminating   Burning   Stinging   Worst Pain in Last 24 Hours:
Radiating   Shooting   Tingling   0 1 2 3 4 5 6 7 8 9 10
                                                 None   Moderate   Severe
Other Descriptors:

_____   Mood: _____
_____
_____   Depression Screening Score: _____
_____
                                                 Gait and Balance Score: _____
Exacerbating Factors: Impaired Activities:
_____   _____
_____   _____
                                                 _____
Relieving Factors: _____
_____   Sleep Quality: _____
_____   Bowel Habits: _____
                                                 _____

Other Assessments or Comments: _____
_____
_____

Most Likely Cause of Pain: _____

Plans: _____
_____
_____

Source: Clinical Practice Guidelines. The Management of Chronic Pain in Older Persons. American Geriatrics Society. (1998). *Journal of the American Geriatrics Society, 46*(5), 635–651. Used with permission

For those unable to verbally communicate their pain experience, the nurse should carefully question the family or a consistent caregiver who can report any changes in function such as changes in gait, recent falls, new-onset withdrawn or agitated behavior, moaning, groaning, crying, changes in eating or drinking patterns, or any other changes in baseline behavior that could be interpreted as nonverbal pain behaviors. Persistent pain can affect all aspects of an older person's life and can adversely impact all body systems. Additional behaviors to assess include wandering, fidgeting, repetitive verbalization, tearfulness, delusions, sad or frightened facial expressions, noisy breathing, tense body language, repeated nighttime awakenings, and hallucinations (Kovach et al., 1999). Reports from caregivers are valuable in assessing pain in the nonverbal older adult.

Practice Pearl

Patients with late-stage dementia are unable to advocate for improved treatment. Nurses in long-term care should be expert in providing effective pain control to this population (Kovach et al., 1999).

Box 9-4 illustrates sample questions that may be included in a pain interview. After completing the pain assessment, the nurse should list and prioritize each pain complaint. This valuable information will guide the physician in the design of a pain management plan that targets the individual needs of the patient. The nurse should also indicate when the next pain assessment will occur and how often pain should be assessed. For patients in severe pain, the reassessment should occur within 24 hours. The nurse can provide continuity of care and an empathetic attitude in order to reassure the patient and build a trusting relationship.

Additional information may be gathered by asking the patient to complete graphic rating scales such as the pain intensity scales illustrated in Figure 9-2■.

Practice Pearl

Pain intensity and relief must be assessed and reassessed at regular intervals.

When assessing pain in the older person, the guidelines in Box 9-5 are useful.

ANALYSIS OF THE PAIN MANAGEMENT PLAN

When pain persists despite the administration of analgesics, the pain treatment plan can be analyzed to refine the treatment and successfully manage the pain for most individuals. The nurse may follow these steps:

1. Review the initial pain assessment. Was anything missed? Was any area incomplete? Where is further information needed?
2. Analyze the alignment of the intensity of pain with the analgesia provided. Are mild analgesics being prescribed for severe pain? Is the patient taking the medication properly? If prn medications are available, have they been appropriately administered?
3. Determine the patient's medication requirement. Has partial response been achieved at a certain dose? Have side effects occurred?

Sample Pain Interview Questions

BOX 9-4

1. **Pain history.** When did the pain start? Use alternative words such as "discomfort" or "pressure" or "ache." Consult with a family member to gain their perspective, with the patient's permission. Try to pinpoint the onset of the pain.

2. **Distinguish acute from chronic pain.** Can you describe your pain? Is it burning, stabbing, throbbing, aching? How does the pain in your hip affect your headache? Older patients in chronic pain are sometimes more sensitive to acute pain and chronic pain can be exacerbated by new onset acute pain. Try to sort out the relationship between pain and the meaning of pain for that patient.

3. **Location.** Where is the pain? Many patients have pain in multiple sites. Pain from systemic diseases like rheumatoid arthritis may be felt all over the body. Pain also may be referred from one site to another.

4. **Frequency.** Does the pain occur every day? Does it come and go? Is there a constant level of baseline pain? Is breakthrough pain present and predictable? Many patients will report a pain pattern with pain levels consistently higher or lower at various times of the day.

5. **Intensity.** On a 1 to 10 scale with 10 being the worst pain ever, can you rate your pain? How does the rating vary during the day or night? How does the pain impact your life and mental health? For the cognitively impaired patient, observe moaning, limitation of movement, grimacing, physical distress illustrated by increased blood pressure or respiratory rate.

6. **Alleviating and aggravating factors.** What makes it better? What makes it worse? What have you tried that seems to relieve your pain? What seems to make your pain worse? Consider non-pharmacological approaches as well including exercise, massage, warm baths, heat pads, ice packs, topical rubs, acupuncture, and other alternative therapies.

7. **Associated symptoms.** Do you have other symptoms with your pain? Are you having any nausea, vomiting, chills, cramps, or loss of appetite? Many patients report that nausea is more difficult to deal with than pain because nausea may be unpredictable, limits food enjoyment and intake, may cause painful vomiting, and is frightening to others.

8. **Response to previous and current analgesic therapy.** Are you taking pain medication now? Have you ever taken pain medication before? Was it effective? Any medication allergies or intolerances? Is the patient reluctant to take pain medication? Is cost of the medication a barrier? Are their side effects like nausea, constipation, or lethargy that are associated with the medication regimen? Do you have trouble swallowing pills? Are there important or anticipated events that may occur during a typical day that may interfere with medication dosing? Many older patients and their families are concerned that they will become "drug addicts" or "hooked on narcotics." Reassurance, education, and treatment of side effects may be needed to achieve effective pain relief.

9. **Meaning of the pain.** What does the pain mean to you? How does your culture and religion influence the meaning of pain for you and your family? Some older patients and their families see pain as punishment for previous deeds while others may feel pain is to be expected and courage and fortitude are needed to be a strong person. Refer issues you are uncomfortable dealing with to a priest, minister or rabbi, social worker, or spiritual advisor.

Source: Data from Wells-Federman, 1999; American Pain Society (1999). *Principles of analgesic use in the treatment of acute pain and cancer pain* (4th ed.). Glenview, IL: American Pain Society: McCaffery, M., & Pasero, C. (1999). *Pain: Clinical Manual* (2nd ed.). St. Louis, MO: Mosby.

FIGURE ☐ 9-2

Example of pain intensity scales.

Source: Adapted from AGS Panel on Chronic Pain in Older Persons, (1998). The management of chronic pain in older persons. *Journal of the American Geriatrics Society, 46*, 635–651. Used with permission.

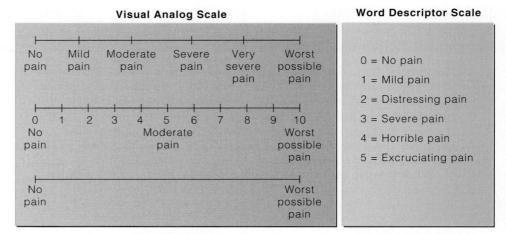

Visual Analog Scale

No pain | Mild pain | Moderate pain | Severe pain | Very severe pain | Worst possible pain

0 1 2 3 4 5 6 7 8 9 10
No pain — Moderate pain — Worst possible pain

No pain — Worst possible pain

Word Descriptor Scale

0 = No pain
1 = Mild pain
2 = Distressing pain
3 = Severe pain
4 = Horrible pain
5 = Excruciating pain

Graphic Scale

Verbal Scale

"On a scale of 0 to 10, with 0 meaning no pain and 10 meaning the worst pain you can imagine, how much pain are you having now?"

4. Provide feedback and documentation as needed to refine the plan. Are there indications that stronger medications are needed? Are dosing changes indicated? Should more effective relief of breakthrough pain be available? Are there indications that dosing intervals should be shortened?

5. Use nondrug techniques to complement the analgesic regimen. Have heat and cold packs been tried? Have patients had access to social or recreational activities?

6. Use all available resources in the clinical setting. Have pain experts, if available, been consulted? Are there other members of the interdisciplinary team who can offer insight? Are there unaddressed spiritual or religious issues?

(Adapted from Woods-Smith et al., 2002)

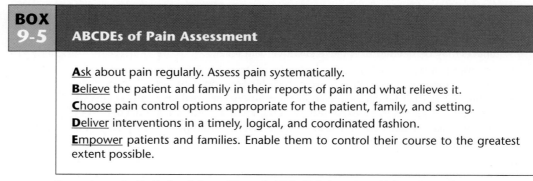

BOX 9-5 **ABCDEs of Pain Assessment**

Ask about pain regularly. Assess pain systematically.
Believe the patient and family in their reports of pain and what relieves it.
Choose pain control options appropriate for the patient, family, and setting.
Deliver interventions in a timely, logical, and coordinated fashion.
Empower patients and families. Enable them to control their course to the greatest extent possible.

Source: Agency for Health Care Policy and Research, 1995. Clinical practice guidelines, Acute pain management clinical guide. Retrieved June 14, 2002, from www.AHRQ.gov.

Patient and Family Teaching

Gerontological nurses require skills and knowledge related to teaching patients and families about the key concepts of gerontology and gerontological nursing. The patient-family teaching guidelines feature will assist the nurse to assume the role of teacher and coach. Educating patients and families is critical so that nurses can interpret scientific data and individualize the nursing care plan.

Patient-Family Teaching Guidelines

DEALING WITH CHRONIC PAIN

1. What is chronic pain?

Persistent or chronic pain is discomfort that continues for an extended time. Some conditions that cause pain can come and go over a period of years. In addition to pain, you can also suffer from depression, insomnia, problems walking, and difficulty healing from disease. There are treatments for pain that can make you feel better.

RATIONALE:

Many older people do not report their symptoms of pain because they are afraid to be labeled as complainers. By validating their situation and pain, the nurse gives the older person permission to discuss the pain and the implications it has on health and well-being.

2. How can I tell my doctor and nurse about my pain?

Persistent pain can be reported to your healthcare providers. Be as specific as you can to accurately convey your situation. Keep a diary or pain log for a few days before your visit. Here are things to jot down:

- Where it hurts
- How often it hurts
- What the pain feels like (burning, stabbing, shooting, dull ache, etc.)
- What makes it worse
- What makes it better
- What medications you have tried that work and don't work
- How the pain affects your life

RATIONALE:

Helping the older patient organize his or her thoughts about pain will help the healthcare provider appreciate the unique situation the patient is in. A pain diary is a good place to start.

3. Will over-the-counter remedies help?

Acetaminophen (Tylenol) is a good choice for mild to moderate pain caused by osteoarthritis. Check with your healthcare provider about the dose if you take it for more than a few days. Nonsteroidal anti-inflammatory drugs (NSAIDs) such as aspirin and ibuprofen work well also, but are associated with the risk of side effects like stomach upset and ulcer formation. Take NSAIDs with food for a short period of time. If you have or have had ulcers, avoid NSAIDs altogether. The new COX-2 inhibitors are more selective in treating pain without side effects, but their safety is being debated and the cost is high. Vioxx has been withdrawn from the market because of its association with stroke and heart attack, and Celebrex is being studied to establish its safety for long-term use.

RATIONALE:

Older patients should be carefully and completely informed about the nature of the medications they are taking for chronic pain because in all probability they will be taking them for years. Careful monitoring and support is needed to prevent adverse drug reactions.

(continued)

Patient-Family Teaching Guidelines, *cont.*

4. Will I get addicted to my pain medicine?

Most older people take painkillers, even narcotics, safely without becoming addicted. It is important not to drive or engage in tasks requiring your full attention (such as babysitting) when you start a new pain medication.

RATIONALE:

Many older people are fearful they will turn into "drug addicts" and therefore do not take prescribed pain medications. Reassurance is required.

5. Once my pain is treated, will I be back to my old self again?

In addition to treating your pain, you may also need treatment for accompanying conditions such as depression. People with chronic pain often complain of feeling blue, and these feelings sometimes hang on even when the pain is gone. Antidepressants can help older people to deal with certain kinds of pain (from nerve diseases or nerve injury) and treat the depression that can result from living with pain. Using a second medication may allow your healthcare provider to prescribe a lower dose of pain medication, thus lessening the risk of side effects.

RATIONALE:

The older patient should be prepared to think beyond the immediate pain and issues of pain relief. Even though the pain is treated, the underlying chronic illness remains and that may be a cause of concern for the patient. Patients with complicated pain or severe depression should seek a referral to a geropsychiatrist or pain clinic for specialized care.

Care Plan

A Patient With Chronic Pain

Case Study

Mr. Adams is a 79-year-old man who suffers from chronic pain in his knees. The physician has diagnosed Mr. Adams with osteoarthritis of both knees and has advised him to take acetaminophen (Tylenol) for the pain. He reports he has been taking it "on and off" with some relief.

Mr. Adams lives by himself in senior citizen housing and has an apartment on the second floor. Recently, he has been unable to walk up the stairs without experiencing severe pain. The building does not have an elevator.

He reports that after walking and stair climbing, the pain is an 8 on a 10-point scale. He usually shops for groceries every other day, but now in order to avoid the stairs, he has been shopping once a week. Additionally, Mr. Adams used to play bridge once or twice a week with friends, but he has stopped that to "conserve energy." He has a daughter to help him out, but she works full-time and has three young children.

A Patient With Chronic Pain

Applying the Nursing Process

ASSESSMENT

Mr. Adams recently had a complete physical examination and health history and was found to have a chronic degenerative process causing pain in both of his knees. He is at risk for malnutrition and depression because of his inability to get up and down the stairs without experiencing severe pain. It is unlikely that he would be able to shop only once a week and carry the needed groceries up the stairs to his apartment.

It appears that the patient's attempts to manage his pain are ineffective. He reports that after walking and climbing stairs, his level of pain increases. This is unfortunately a common occurrence with many older people, and the natural response is to limit movement. The nurse needs more information about his baseline level of pain, level of pain with other activities, ability to care for himself, and perception of his situation. By limiting his socialization and bridge playing with his friends, he is at risk for social isolation and depression. The nurse should conduct a complete functional health pattern assessment.

DIAGNOSIS

The current nursing diagnoses for Mr. Adams include the following:

- *Risk for loneliness*
- *Impaired physical mobility*
- *Altered activity levels*
- *Chronic pain*
- *Risk for imbalanced nutrition: less than body requirements*

EXPECTED OUTCOMES

Expected outcomes for the plan of care specify that Mr. Adams will:

- Keep a pain diary and record pain levels several times a day, systematically noting the effectiveness of acetaminophen on his pain and identifying any nonpharmacological ways to treat his pain that might be appropriate for him.
- Request help from family and friends to assist in obtaining groceries and needed supplies.
- Agree to a physical therapy consultation for strengthening exercises and assistive aids to decrease pain.
- Agree to establish a therapeutic relationship with the nurse and develop a mutually acceptable plan to work toward these outcomes.

PLANNING AND IMPLEMENTATION

The following nursing interventions may be appropriate:

- Establish a therapeutic relationship.
- Explore alternative living situations or other supports.

(continued)

A Patient With Chronic Pain (continued)

- Encourage a family meeting to talk about health issues in general with Mr. Adams's permission.
- Begin an in-depth pain assessment of the effectiveness of pharmacological and nonpharmacological techniques to treat pain.
- Begin a values clarification to establish long-term goals and facilitate end-of-life planning.

Generally, osteoarthritis pain responds well to heating pads, OTC topical creams, and mild exercise and physical therapy. Mr. Adams should be educated about the issues involved with treating chronic pain and the need to take medication on a regular basis. Mr. Adams should be informed that acetaminophen is not habit forming and can be very effective in controlling the pain of osteoarthritis. He should be informed about side effects and dosing recommendations to avoid medication-related problems. If a trial of acetaminophen twice or three times a day for several days does not help to control his pain, he should return to the physician for further advice and evaluation of his osteoarthritis.

EVALUATION

The nurse hopes to work with Mr. Adams over time and realizes the chronic nature of pain in older people. The nurse will consider the plan a success based on the following criteria:

- Mr. Adams will report improved function and social skills.
- A family meeting will be held to discuss his overall health.
- Mr. Adams will report decreased levels of pain based upon pain management techniques.
- He will continue to be well nourished and hydrated by obtaining groceries through the help of family and friends.

Ethical Dilemma

As the nurse gets to know Mr. Adams better, he reports in confidence that his friend has told him the best way to make his knees feel better is to drink a glass of wine with his acetaminophen. He asks the nurse not to tell his daughter about this habit. How should the nurse respond?

Taking acetaminophen with alcohol is a very risky behavior and can cause liver damage. Mr. Adams should be informed that if this practice continues, he is placing himself at risk for premature institutionalization or injury from falls. Once he is informed of the risk and develops a trusting relationship with the nurse, he may stop taking alcohol with his medication. If he does not, the nurse should recommend that he speak with his physician regarding this practice. Perhaps the physician can prescribe a more effective medication that does not need wine to boost its analgesic effects.

A Patient With Chronic Pain

Critical Thinking and the Nursing Process

1. What is the physiological basis for Mr. Adams's pain?
2. Explain possible reasons for this patient's pain in addition to degenerative joint disease.
3. Outline a teaching plan with behavioral interventions designed to improve Mr. Adams's level of pain.
4. Suggest a nursing action if Mr. Adams continues to consume alcohol while taking acetaminophen.

■ Evaluate your responses in Appendix B. ⊂▭▭

EXPLORE MediaLink

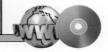

NCLEX review, case studies, and other interactive resources for this chapter can be found on the Companion Website at **www.prenhall.com/tabloski**. Click on Chapter 9 to select the activities for this chapter. For animations, video tutorials, more NCLEX review questions, and case studies, access the accompanying CD-ROM in this textbook.

Chapter Highlights

■ With aging, the probability that the patient will develop a condition that can cause pain increases.

■ Many healthcare professionals who care for older patients have not had sufficient education regarding pain control in older persons. Common errors or omissions include inadequate pain assessment and reluctance by clinicians to use appropriate pain medications including opioids with elderly patients.

■ Older people will often not report pain because they fear hospitalization, worsening of their disease, or being labeled a chronic complainer.

■ When a patient has unrelieved pain, many negative effects occur such as depression, anxiety, insomnia, problems of immobility, and nutritional problems. All of these conditions can slow healing and rehabilitation, placing the older person at risk for complications and premature institutionalization.

■ In addition to the traditional pain assessment methods, when the patient is nonverbal or suffers from severe dementia, the nurse should gather information from caregivers and behavioral observations.

■ The general rule for analgesic medications is to start low and go slow. When analgesic medications are started, the nurse should carefully monitor the patient for adverse events, educate the patient regarding the pain management plan, implement nonpharmacological methods as appropriate to the patient, and keep the lines of communication open through periodic and regular reassessment of the patient's pain.

References

Agency for Health Care Policy and Research. (1995). *Acute pain management: Operative or medical procedures and trauma* (AHCPR Publication No. 92-0032). Rockville, MD: U.S. Department of Health and Human Services.

American Geriatrics Society (AGS) Panel on Chronic Pain in Older Persons. (2002). The management of persistent pain in older persons. *Journal of the American Geriatrics Society, 50,* S205–S224.

American Pain Society Quality of Care Committee. (1995). Quality improvement guidelines for the treatment of acute pain and cancer pain. *Journal of the American Medical Association, 274,* 1874–1880.

Bernabei, R., Gambassi, G., Lapane, K., Landi, F., Gatsonis, C., Dunlop, R., et al. for the SAGE Study Group. (1998). Management of pain in elderly patients with cancer. *Journal of the American Medical Association, 279,* 1877–1882.

Effects of integrating therapeutic touch into a cognitive behavioral pain treatment program: Report of a pilot clinical trial. *Journal of Holistic Nursing, 20,* 367–387.

Gelfand, S. (2002). The pitfalls of opioids for chronic nonmalignant pain of central origin. *Medscape Rheumatology, 4*(1). Retrieved April 12, 2002, from www.medscape.com/viewarticle/425468.

Gloth, F. (2001). Pain management in older adults: Prevention and treatment. *Journal of the American Geriatrics Society, 49,* 188–199.

Hartford Institute for Geriatric Nursing. (1999). Best nursing practices in care of older adults, *Try this assessing pain in older adults,* Retrieved November 14, 2004, from www.hartfordign.org.

Helme, R., & Gibson, S. (1999). Pain in Older People. In I. Crombie, (Ed), *Epidemiology of Pain* pp. 103–112. Seattle, WA: IASP Press.

Joint Commission on Accreditation of Healthcare Organizations. (2003). *Improving the Quality of Pain Management through Measurement and Action.* Oakbrook Terraa, IL: Department of Publications, Joint Commission Resources.

Kovach, C., Weissman, D., Griffie, J., Matson, S., & Muchka, S. (1999). Assessment and treatment of discomfort for people with late-stage dementia. *Journal of Pain and Symptom Management, 18*(6), 412–419.

Partners Against Pain. (2002). *Senior care: The management of persistant pain in older persons.* Retrieved June 14, 2003, from www.partnersagainstpain.com.

Sinatra, R. (2002). *Changing paradigms of pain management: The evolving role of coxibs.* Plainsboro, NJ: MultiMedia HealthCare/Freedom.

Thomas, D., Flaherty, J., & Morley, J. (2001). The management of chronic pain in long-term care settings. *Supplement to the Annals of Long-Term Care,* November. Newtown Square, PA: MultiMedia HealthCare/Freedom.

Titler, M., & Mentes, J. (1999). Research utilization in gerontological nursing practice. *Journal of Gerontological Nursing, 25*(6), pp. 6–9.

Tolle, S., Tilden, V., Nelson, C., & Dunn, P. (1998). A prospective study of the efficacy of the physician order form for life-sustaining treatment. *Journal of the American Geriatrics Society, 46*(9), 1097–1102.

Volicer, L., & Hurley, A. (2003). Management of behavioral symptoms in progressive degenerative dementias. *Journal of Gerontology, 58A*(9), 837–845.

Warden, V., Hurley, A. C., & Volicer, L. (2003). Development and psychometric evaluation of the Pain Assessment in Advanced Dementia (PAINAD) scale. *Journal of the American Medical Directors Association, 4*(1), 9–15.

Wells-Federman, C. (1999). Care of the patient with chronic pain: Part I. *Clinical Excellence in Nursing Practice, 3*(4), 192–204.

Willis, W. (1998). The somatosensory system. In R. Berne & M. Levy (Eds.), *Physiology.* New York: Mosby.

Woods-Smith, D., Arnstein, P., Rosa, K., & Wells-Federman, C. (2002). Effects of integrating therapeutic touch into a cognitive behavioral pain treatment program: *Report of a pilot clinical trial. Journal of Holistic Nursing, 20,* 367–387.

Young-McCaughan, S., & Miaskowski, C. (2001). Definition & Mechanism of opioid—induced Sedation. *Pain Management Nursing, 2,* 84–97.

CHAPTER 10

Violence and Elder Mistreatment

Annemarie Dowling-Castronovo, APRN-BC
Lisa Guadagno, MPA
Terry Fulmer, PhD, RN, FAAN

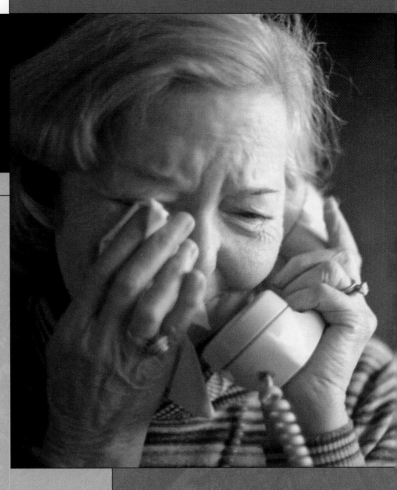

CHAPTER OBJECTIVES

Upon completion of this chapter, the reader will be able to:

- Discuss current trends in elder mistreatment, including incidence and prevalence.

- Review key reasons why elder mistreatment occurs.

- Conduct clinical assessment for screening and detection of elder mistreatment.

- Create a nursing care plan for the ongoing well-being of older patients.

- Summarize key resources for elder mistreatment information.

MediaLink

Additional resources for this chapter can be found on the Student CD-ROM accompanying this textbook and on the Companion Website at **www.prenhall.com/tabloski**. Click on Chapter 10 to select the activities for this chapter.

CD-ROM
- NCLEX Review
- Case Studies
- Tools

COMPANION WEBSITE
- Audio Glossary
- Additional NCLEX Review
- Case Study
- MediaLink Applications

KEY TERMS

abandonment 272
adult protective services
  (APS) 272
domestic violence 272
elder mistreatment 272
exploitation 272
guardianship 284
neglect 272
physical abuse 273
self-neglect 273
sexual abuse 273

This chapter will explore the nursing role in identifying and managing **elder mistreatment**. It is important to have an awareness of a larger issue, **domestic violence**.

Domestic violence affects a significant proportion of the U.S. population either as direct victims or as witnesses of abuse directed toward spouses or intimate partners, children, and elders. Child maltreatment affects nearly 3 million children annually and results in the death of more than three children every day. Between 2 million and 4 million women are physically battered each year by partners or former partners. The mistreatment of elders is estimated to afflict between 700,000 and 1.1 million individuals annually (Pillemer & Finkelhor, 1988). The National Research Council *Report on Elder Mistreatment* estimates even higher rates (2003).

Elder mistreatment is the least addressed and least reported form of domestic violence. Anecdotally identified in the 1970s as "granny battering," elder mistreatment is still a poorly understood phenomenon that often goes unrecognized by healthcare providers (Walshe-Brennan, 1977). Elder mistreatment is the outcome of abuse, **neglect**, **exploitation**, or **abandonment** of older adults and represents some of the most tragic behavior in the area of family violence. Nurses are in key positions to screen, assess, and intervene for older adults subjected to elder mistreatment (Lachs & Pillemer, 1995).

National Incidence and Prevalence of Elder Mistreatment

The National Elder Abuse Incidence Study, conducted in 1996, provides the best national estimate to date (Thomas, 2002). Over 1.5 million older adults experience abuse or neglect in domestic settings. Approximately 50% of the cases identified by this study were neglect, while 35% were psychological abuse, 30% were financial exploitation, and 25% were physical abuse.

Furthermore, cases of domestic elder mistreatment were shown to be largely unreported, with only 21% of cases being reported and substantiated by APS agencies (National Center on Elder Abuse at the American Public Human Services Association, 1998). In an earlier population-based prevalence study, Pillemer and Finkelhor used structured interviews to screen for physical abuse, psychological abuse, and neglect among a sample of noninstitutionalized persons 65 years and older in the Boston area. Yearly prevalence in this study was estimated to range from 700,000 to 1.2 million older adults or a rate of 3.2% (Pillemer & Finkelhor, 1988). The number of cases of elder mistreatment nationwide is overwhelming, and the detrimental outcomes that elder mistreatment has upon older adults warrant the attention of every healthcare clinician.

LEGAL ISSUES

Every state in America has mechanisms for reporting elder mistreatment, and **adult protective services (APS)** programs exist in each state. Amendments to the Older Americans Act in 1987 included federal definitions of elder abuse. State to state variations do exist (Capezuti, Brush, & Lawson, 1997). Nursing homes' standards for care are based on policy stipulated in the Nursing Home Reform Act of 1987 (Omnibus Budget Reconciliation Act, 1987). This law was set forth to prevent substandard care and mistreatment of older adults. Many states currently have mandatory reporting laws for elder mistreatment, in which nurses and other healthcare practitioners are required by law to report suspected cases. In some states, failure by clinicians to report suspected incidents of mistreatment is a misdemeanor, punishable by fine or penalty (Capezuti et al., 1997).

CATEGORIES OF ELDER MISTREATMENT

One challenge of understanding elder mistreatment is that the literature proposes a variety of definitions and categories. There are three basic categories of elder mistreatment:

1. Domestic mistreatment generally occurs within the older adult's home dwelling at the hand of significant others (i.e., child, spouse, in-law).
2. Institutional mistreatment occurs when an older adult has a contractual arrangement and suffers abuse (i.e., long-term care facilities, assisted-living facilities, rehabilitation facilities, hospitals).
3. **Self-neglect** occurs when older adults who are mentally competent enough to understand the consequences of their own decisions engage in behaviors that threaten their own safety.

INSTITUTIONAL MISTREATMENT

Most of the elder mistreatment research to date focuses on mistreatment in the domestic setting, and there is a dearth of information about mistreatment in nursing homes and other residential care facilities. Research that does exist suggests abuse and neglect of nursing home residents may be a widespread phenomenon. The types of mistreatment that occur in nursing homes likely mirror those that occur in domestic settings, such as **physical abuse**, **sexual abuse**, neglect, financial abuse, and psychological abuse. One survey of nursing home staff members revealed that 36% had witnessed at least one incident of physical abuse by another staff member in the previous year, and 81% had observed at least one incident of psychological abuse. Ten percent of the staff members reported actually committing an act of physical abuse against a resident in the previous year, and 40% admitted to having committed an act of psychological abuse (Pillemer & Moore, 1989). Pillemer and Moore (1989) have found that patient aggressiveness is a predictor of physical and psychological abuse by staff members and that abusers are more likely to be younger than nonabusers. Researchers have also speculated that shortages of staff, inadequate training of staff, and staff burnout may be precipitating factors in mistreatment of nursing home residents.

A recent federal report revealed large delays in the reporting of incidents of elder mistreatment in nursing homes (U.S. General Accounting Office, 2002). One of the issues highlighted in this report is that there currently exists no federal law requiring criminal background checks of nursing home employees, although many states do require them. Furthermore, although the U.S. Centers for Medicare and Medicaid Services requires that incidents of abuse and neglect be promptly reported to law enforcement or state survey agencies, approximately 50% of the notifications to state survey agencies reviewed in the report had been submitted 2 or more days after the alleged incident occurred. In addition, great delays were reported in the length of time it takes for state survey agencies to follow up and make determinations about reports of mistreatment. A 1999 review of nurse aid registry records in Pennsylvania revealed that a large number of determinations took 10 months or more. These delays hamper efforts of state survey agencies to collect evidence and, ultimately, put other nursing home residents at risk of being mistreated by nursing home staff members against whom complaints have been made (U.S. General Accounting Office, 2002). Burgess, Dowdell, and Prentky (2000) reported several reasons for delay in reporting incidents of mistreatment in nursing homes. Residents may be afraid of retribution, and family members may fear having to find a new nursing home for the resident. Staff members may fear losing their jobs or facing recrimination by other staff members and management if they report abuse. Finally, managers of nursing homes may want to avoid adverse publicity.

DEFINITIONS OF ELDER MISTREATMENT

The majority of evidence-based research on elder mistreatment is in the domestic setting; therefore, the remaining part of this chapter will address this area. There is a lack of consensus on the definitions of elder mistreatment. The Panel to Review Risk and Prevalence of Elder Abuse and Neglect (2002) defined physical abuse, sexual abuse, emotional/psychological abuse, neglect, abandonment, financial/material exploitation, and self-neglect. These definitions along with other terms defined in the literature are found in Table 10-1. This chapter will use *elder mistreatment* as an umbrella term and cite more specific types as indicated.

TABLE 10-1

Types of Elder Mistreatment

Type	Definition	Examples	Signs and Symptoms
Physical abuse	Intentional infliction of physical injury or pain	Hitting, shaking, pushing, improper use of physical restraints	Bruises, black eyes, bone fractures, injuries in various stages of healing
Psychological/ emotional abuse	Infliction of anguish, pain, distress	Yelling, swearing, name-calling	Emotional upset or agitation, extreme withdrawal
Sexual abuse	Any form of nonconsensual sexual intimacy	Rape, molestation, sexual harassment	Genital bruising, unexplained sexually transmitted disease
Financial exploitation	Taking advantage of an older person for monetary or personal benefit	Unexplained monetary expenditures, lack of money for personal necessities	Unexplained inability to pay bills or purchase necessity items such as food
Caregiver neglect	Intentional (active) or unintentional (passive) failure to meet needs necessary for elder's physical and mental well-being	Failure to provide adequate food, clothing, shelter, medical care, hygiene, or social stimulation	Dehydration, malnutrition, unattended or untreated health problems, listlessness, decubitus ulcers, urine burns, history of being left alone
Self-neglect	Personal disregard or inability to perform self-care	Poor hygiene, unkempt home environment	Malnutrition, fungal skin and nail infections, insect and rodent infestation in the home
Abandonment	Desertion or willful forsaking of an elder	Dropping off an older adult in the emergency department	An older adult left inappropriately alone
Institutional mistreatment	When older adult has a contractual arrangement and suffers abuse or neglect	May be any combination of the aforementioned	See above column entries

CHARACTERISTICS OF OLDER ADULTS AT RISK

A completely clear picture of those at risk of elder mistreatment has been difficult to obtain; however, several characteristics are more common among victims. Risk factors for elder mistreatment include sex, age, race, low socioeconomic status, low educational level, impaired functional or cognitive status, and a history of domestic violence, stressful events, and depression (Dyer, Pavlik, Murphy, & Hyman, 2000; Pillemer & Finkelhor, 1989). Older adults who are victimized are more likely to be old-old (75+ and above), to be female (Dunlop, Rothman, Condon, Hebert, & Martinez, 2000), and to live with their abusers (Lachs, Williams, O'Brien, Hurst, & Horwitz, 1997; Pillemer & Finkelhor, 1988). Moreover, older adults who suffer from chronic, disabling illnesses that impair function and create care needs that exceed their caregiver's capacity to meet these needs are at higher risk of being mistreated (Fulmer & O'Malley, 1987). See Table 10-2.

CHARACTERISTICS OF PEOPLE WHO MISTREAT OLDER ADULTS

Studies have shown that abusers are more likely to be male and suffer from impairments such as substance abuse, mental illness, or dementia (Brownell, 1999). Moreover, abusers are more likely to lack strong social support networks and to be more dependent on the care recipient for financial or other needs (Reis & Nahmiash, 1998; Wolf & Pillemer, 1997). See Table 10-2. In a majority of cases, family members have been shown to be the abusers (National Center on Elder Abuse at the American Public Human Services Association, 1998). Caregivers of older adults should be assessed for caregiver stress, substance abuse, and a history of psychopathology (Swagerty, 1999).

CULTURAL PERCEPTIONS OF ELDER MISTREATMENT

Definitions of the different subtypes of elder mistreatment need to be examined in the context of cultural considerations. Researchers and clinicians have documented differences in the way that people from different cultural groups define elder mistreatment as well as in

TABLE 10-2

Elder Mistreatment Characteristics

Older Adult Characteristics	Abuser Characteristics
Over 75 years old*	Mental illness
Dependent functional status*	Substance abuse
Poor social network (less than three significant others)*	History of family violence
Poverty+	Legal or financial issues
Minority+	Poor social network
Cognitive impairment+	Dependency on older adult
Living with one individual+	
Less than eighth-grade educational level	
Female	
Older adult living alone or living with abuser	
History of family violence	

(*) Lachs, Berkman, Fulmer, & Horwitz. (1994). A prospective community-based pilot study of risk factors for the investigation of elder mistreatment. *Journal of the American Geriatrics Society, 42*(2), 169–173.

(+) Lachs, Williams, O'Brien, Hurst, & Horwitz. (1996). Older adults. An 11-year longitudinal study of adult protective service use. *Archives of Internal Medicine, 156*(4), 449–453.

the behaviors that they perceive as abusive or neglectful (Moon & Benton, 2000). Other researchers have found that members of minority groups may not define abusive behavior the same way that professionals do (Hudson, Armachain, Beasley, & Carlson, 1998; Hudson et al., 2000). These discrepancies across cultural and ethnic subgroups may be linked to the fact that these subgroups have different expectations about the responsibility that grown children and other relatives have for caring for older adults (Tomita, 1999). Some researchers speculate that cultural-specific approaches to interventions based on these differences in perception would be more effective than a general approach (Moon & Benton, 2000). However, the findings from research studies on elder mistreatment and culture are less than conclusive, and no studies examining different interventions for cultural subgroups have been completed to date. At the very least, nurses and other clinicians should be aware of the possibility of differences in perceptions about what constitutes mistreatment based on culture, and should take this into account during assessment and care planning. The Institute of Medicine stresses the importance of clinicians understanding the physical, cultural, and community environments of their patients in order to adequately address family violence. Cultural and linguistic competences are important for successful intervention in cases of elder mistreatment (Institute of Medicine, 2002).

THEORIES OF ELDER MISTREATMENT

Six leading theories or conceptual frameworks are used to examine the etiology of elder mistreatment. The first is *psychopathology of the abuser,* which refers to caregivers who have pre-existing conditions that impair their capacity to give appropriate care. For example, a caregiver who has mental retardation or alcohol dependency may not be able to exercise appropriate judgment in caregiving of older adults. This can ultimately lead to abuser neglect (Lachs & Fulmer, 1993). The next framework is referred to as *transgenerational violence.* Elder mistreatment is thought to be a part of the family violence continuum, which may begin with child abuse and end with elder mistreatment. Little work has been done to obtain empirical evidence to support this theory; however, selected case studies indicate this could be important to the study of elder mistreatment. Another aspect of transgenerational violence relates to adult children who have had a long-standing, contentious relationship with an older parent. For example, a child who is abused by the parent and grows up to be the caregiver may ultimately become aggressive and abusive toward the elderly person. Finally, transgenerational violence has been explained in terms of a *learning theory* in that a child who observes violence as a coping mechanism may learn it and bring it to adult life.

The next theory is *situational theory,* which is also referred to as *caregiver stress.* As care burdens multiply, they outweigh the caregiver's capacity to meet the needs of the older adult; therefore, caregiver stress can overwhelm the situation. Elder mistreatment can be the outcome (Steinmetz, 1990). The *isolation theory* espouses that mistreatment is prompted by a dwindling social network. According to the National Elder Abuse Incidence Study (National Center on Elder Abuse at the American Public Human Services Association, 1998), about 25% of all elderly persons live alone and even more interact only with family members and have little social interaction with the outside world. Isolated older adults are at particular risk because there are no outsiders watching out for them, and they may not be identified by the healthcare system or reporting agencies until it is too late. According to Godkin, Wolf, and Pillemer (1989), it is difficult to determine whether isolation is the result of mistreatment (family members or caregivers may be trying to hide the mistreatment from the outside world) or a precipitating factor of mistreatment. Table 10-3 lists the various measures used to assess elder mistreatment

TABLE 10-3

Elder Mistreatment Measures

Measures/Author	Characteristics	Source
Adult Protective Service Reports (APS)	No specific format. Intake forms used to document calls of suspected elder mistreatment from public hotlines and state agencies.	Varies from state to state.
AMA Assessment Protocol	Checklist to use if abuse is suspected.	American Medical Association. (1992). *Diagnostic and treatment guidelines on elder abuse and neglect.* Chicago: Author.
Brief Abuse Screen for the Elderly— BASE	Five standard questions.	Reis, M., Nahmiash, D., Shrier, R., & Senneville, C. (1995). When seniors are abused: An intervention model. *Gerontologist, 35*(5), 666–671.
Case Detection Guidelines	Reference list of risk factors and physical findings.	Rathbone-McCuan, E., & Voyles, B. (1982). Case detection of abused elderly parents. *American Journal of Psychiatry, 139*(2), 189–192.
Conflict Tactic Scale (CTS)	A 19-item self-report, e.g., "Has anyone threatened you with a knife or gun?" Perception of upsetting and injurious circumstances in a person's life.	Straus, M. A. (1978). The Conflict Tactic Scale. Reprinted in J. Touliatos, B. Perlmutter, & M. Straus (Eds.), *Handbook of family measurement techniques.* Newbury Park, CA: Sage.
Elder Abuse and Neglect Protocol	Comprehensive outline describing an approach to abuse.	Tomita, S. (1982). Detection and treatment of elderly abuse and neglect: A protocol for health care professionals. *Physical Therapy and Occupational Therapy in Geriatrics, 2*(2), 37–51.
Elder Assessment Instrument (EAI)	A 40-item screening tool with both subjective and objective items to determine if an older person should be referred for suspected elder mistreatment. Provides information to clinicians to better inform judgments about risk of elder mistreatment.	Fulmer, T., Street, S., & Carr, K. (1984). Abuse of the elderly: Screening and detection. *Journal of Emergency Nursing, 10*(3), 131–140.
Fulmer Restriction Scale (FRS)	A 34-item scale designed to elicit information regarding unnecessary restriction of the older adult. Assessment of physical, psychological, and financial restriction of older adults.	Fulmer, T., & Gurland, B. (1996). Restriction as elder mistreatment: Differences between caregiver and elder perceptions. *Journal of Mental Health and Aging, 2,* 89–98.
Health Attitudes to Aging & Living Arrangements Finances (H.A.L.F.)	Checklist requiring interview and period of observation.	Ferguson, D., & Beck, C. (1983). H.A.L.F.—A tool to assess elder abuse within the family. *Geriatric Nurse, 4*(5), 301–304.
Hwalek-Sengstock Elder Abuse Screening Test (H-S/EAST)	A 15-item assessment screen for detecting suspected elder abuse and neglect. Assessment of physical, financial, psychological, and neglectful situations.	Neale, A., Hwalek, M., Scott, R., Sengstock, M., & Stahl, C. (1991). Validation of the Hwalek-Sengstock Elder Abuse Screening Test. *Journal of Applied Gerontology, 10*(4), 406–418. Hwalek, M., & Sengstock, M. (1986). Assessing the probability of abuse of the elderly: Towards the development of a clinical screening instrument. *Journal of Applied Gerontology, 5,* 153–173.

(continued)

TABLE 10-3 *(continued)*

Elder Mistreatment Measures

Measures/Author	Characteristics	Source
Indicators of Abuse Screen (IOA)	A 29-item set of indicators for use by social service agency practitioners to identify elder mistreatment. Developed specifically for use by social service agency practitioners likely to visit the older adult in the home.	Reis, M., & Nahmiash, D. (1998). Validation of the indicators of abuse (IOA) screen. *Gerontologist, 38*(4), 471–480.
Pathophysiological signs and symptoms	Subjective and objective clinical observations as documented by healthcare clinicians. Uses items such as unexplained bruising, dehydration, urine burns, and fractures.	Fulmer, T. (1984). Elder abuse assessment tool. *Dimensions of Critical Care Nursing, 3*(4), 216–220. Lachs, M. S., & Fulmer, T. (1993). Recognizing elder abuse and neglect. *Clinical Geriatric Medicine, 9*(3), 665–681. Dyer, C. B., Pavlik, V. N., Murphy, K. P., & Hyman, D. J. (2000). The high prevalence of depression and dementia in elder abuse or neglect. *Journal of the American Geriatrics Society, 48*(2), 205–208. Haviland, S., & O'Brien, J. (1989). Physical abuse and neglect of the elderly: Assessment and intervention. *Orthopedic Nursing, 8*(4), 11–19. O'Brien, J. G. (1986). Elder abuse and the physician. *Michigan Medicine, 85*(11), 618, 620.
Screening Protocols for the Identification of Abuse and Neglect in the Elderly	Checklist requiring interview and period of observation.	Johnson, D. (1981). Abuse of the elderly. *Nurse Practitioner, 6*(1), 29–34.
Screening Tools and Referral Protocol Stopping Abuse Against Older Ohioans: A Guide for Service Providers—STRP	A combination of several tools; includes a referral protocol.	Anetzberger, G. J., Palmisano, B. R., Sanders, M., Bass, D., Dayton, C., Eckert, S., & Schimer, M. R. (2000). A model intervention for elder abuse and dementia. *Gerontologist, 40*(4), 492–497.
The QUALCARE Scale	A 53-item observational rating scale designed to quantify and qualify family caregiving. Assessment of six areas: physical, medical management, psychosocial, environmental, human rights, and financial.	Phillips, L. R., Morrison, E. F., & Chae, Y. M. (1990). The QUALCARE Scale: Developing an instrument to measure quality of home care. *International Journal of Nursing Studies, 27*(1), 61–75. Phillips, L. R., Morrison, E. F., & Chae, Y. M. (1990). The QUALCARE Scale: Testing of a measurement instrument for clinical practice. *International Journal of Nursing Studies, 27*(1), 77–91.

Source: Adapted from Fulmer, T. (2002). Elder mistreatment. In J. Fitzpatrick, P. Archbold, B. Stewart, & K.S. Lyons (Eds.), *Annual review of nursing research: Focus on geriatric nursing* (Vol. 20, pp. 369–394). New York: Springer.

and the organizations and authors that have developed these measures. The various definitions and measures used in clinical practice make the problem of elder mistreatment more difficult to detect, substantiate, and report.

Assessment

Screening for domestic violence has been recommended by the American Medical Association (Aravanis et al., 1993) for over a decade. A sample elder assessment instrument is included in the Best Practices feature on page 280. An interdisciplinary team's comprehensive geriatric assessment of the older adult's cognitive and psychosocial function is essential in identifying elder mistreatment, and the nurse's role is of utmost importance. The nursing history should entail asking older adult patients about the presence of violence in their lives. Sample screening questions are listed in the case study on page 289. Research has demonstrated that nurses can accurately identify elder mistreatment cases in busy emergency department settings (Fulmer, Paveza, Abraham, & Fairchild, 2000).

Ideally, the patient and the suspected abuser should be interviewed separately, which may reveal inconsistencies. Maintaining a nonjudgmental environment will enable the nurse to obtain more accurate data. A caregiver's refusal to allow for separate interviews should increase suspicion of elder mistreatment.

Assessing caregiver stress and burden allows for a more complete assessment. Various caregiver assessment questionnaires are available (Zarit, Reever, & Bach-Peterson, 1994). An example includes the Caregiver Strain Index, which is a simple screening instrument as shown in Figure 10-1 ■ (Robinson, 1994). Caregivers should be asked to complete this questionnaire. A score of 7 or more indicates the presence of significant caregiver strain and the need for support and additional services. Demonstrating empathetic communication with the caregiver may disclose existing or potential elder mistreatment scenarios that may be prevented or resolved with nursing and social service interventions.

PHYSICAL EXAMINATION

The physical symptoms of elder mistreatment are often difficult for clinicians to discern because older adults may suffer from chronic and acute illnesses that mask the presence of mistreatment. Cognitively impaired older adults provide an additional challenge. Their subjective reporting may be questioned for accuracy or they may be unable to express the mistreatment situation due to amnesia, *aphasia* (total or partial loss of ability to speak or understand language), *agnosia* (inability to recognize common persons and things), and *apraxia* (inability to perform simple tasks), which commonly occur with dementia. It is often difficult to determine whether the older adult's worsening physical condition is a result of the natural progression of illness or mistreatment on the part of a caregiver. Because some frail older individuals are prone to underlying conditions that give rise to trauma, such as instability of gait and poor vision resulting in falls, it may be difficult for clinicians to differentiate accidental from willful injuries. The presence of both fresh and healing injuries may suggest ongoing episodes of trauma and represent the need for further investigation to determine whether abuse or neglect may be a contributing factor. Examples include fractures, bruising, and burns (Lachs & Pillemer, 1995).

The Hartford Institute for Geriatric Nursing (1999) recommends the Elder Assessment Instrument (EAI) for use in the clinical setting. Screening can facilitate accurate assessment, risk categorization, referral for services, and ultimately protection of the older person who is being mistreated or abused.

Various screening instruments have been developed that aid nurses and other clinicians in undertaking a thorough mistreatment assessment. The EAI (Fulmer & Cahill, 1984; Fulmer, Street, & Carr, 1984) assesses signs and symptoms of elder mistreatment. The nurse should first assess general appearance. An older adult appearing disheveled with poor hygiene warrants further investigation. Common signs of abuse include bruising, malnutrition, burns, excoriations, and fractures. Common clinical manifestations of neglect include dehydration, malnutrition, decubitus ulcers, and contractures. Other signs and symptoms of elder mistreatment include delays between the injury or illness and the seeking of medical treatment, frequent visits to the emergency department, and diagnostic testing results inconsistent with the history given (Lachs & Pillemer, 1995).

I. General Assessment	Very Good	Good	Poor	Very Poor	Unable to Assess
1. Clothing					
2. Hygiene					
3. Nutrition					
4. Skin integrity					
5. Additional Comments:					

II. Possible Abuse Indicators	No Evidence	Possible Evidence	Probable Evidence	Definite Evidence	Unable to Assess
6. Bruising					
7. Lacerations					
8. Fractures					
9. Various stages of healing of any bruises or fractures					
10. Evidence of sexual abuse					
11. Statement by elder re: abuse					
12. Additional Comments:					

III. Possible Neglect Indicators	No Evidence	Possible Evidence	Probable Evidence	Definite Evidence	Unable to Assess
13. Contractors					
14. Decubiti					
15. Dehydration					
16. Diarrhea					
17. Depression					
18. Impaction					
19. Malnutrition					
20. Urine burns					
21. Poor hygiene					
22. Failure to respond to warning of obvious disease					
23. Inappropriate medications (under/over)					
24. Repetitive hospital admissions due to probable failure of health care surveillance					
25. Statement by elder re: neglect					
26. Additional Comments:					

IV. Possible Exploitation Indicators	No Evidence	Possible Evidence	Probable Evidence	Definite Evidence	Unable to Assess
27. Misuse of money					
28. Evidence of financial exploitation					
29. Reports of demands for goods in exchange for services					
30. Inability to account for money/property					
31. Statement by elder re: exploitation					
32. Additional Comments:					

V. Possible Abandonment Indicators	No Evidence	Possible Evidence	Probable Evidence	Definite Evidence	Unable to Assess
33. Evidence that a caretaker has withdrawn care precipitously without alternate arrangements					
34. Evidence that elder is left alone in an unsafe environment for extended periods of time without adequate support					
35. Statement by elder re: abandonment					
36. Additional Comments:					

VI. Summary	No Evidence	Possible Evidence	Probable Evidence	Definite Evidence	Unable to Assess
37. Evidence of abuse					
38. Evidence of neglect					
39. Evidence of exploitation					
40. Evidence of abandonment					

VII. Comments: _____

_____

_____

_____

_____

_____

NB: There is no "score." A patient should be referred to social services if the following exists:
    1) if there is any evidence (±) without sufficient clinical explanation,
    2) whenever there is a subjective complaint by the elder of EM
    3) whenever the clinician deems there is evidence of abuse, neglect, exploitation, abandonment

Source: Adapted from Fulmer, T., & Cahill, V. M. (1984). Assessing elder abuse: A study. *Journal of Gerontological Nursing, 10(12),* 16–20; Fulmer, T., Street, S., & Carr. K. (1984). Abuse of the elderly: Screening and detection. *Journal of Emergency Nursing, 10(3),* 131–140.

FIGURE ☐ **10-1**

The Caregiver Strain
Index.

Source: Robinson, B. (1994).
Validation of a Caregiver Strain
Index. *Journal of Gerontology, 38,*
344–348. Copyright (c) The
Gerontological Society of America.
Reproduced by permission of the
publisher.

The Caregiver Strain Index: I am going to read a list of things that other people have found to be difficult. Would you tell me if any of these apply to you? (Give examples)

	Yes = 1	No = 0
Sleep is disturbed (e.g., because _____ is in and out of bed or wanders around at night)		
It is inconvenient (e.g., because helping takes so much time or it's a long drive over to help)		
It is a physical strain (e.g., because of lifting in and out of a chair, effort or concentration is required)		
It is confining (e.g., helping restricts free time or cannot go visiting)		
There have been family adjustments (e.g., because helping has disrupted routine; there has been no privacy)		
There have been changes in personal plans (e.g., had to turn down a job; could not go on vacation)		
There have been other demands on my time (e.g., from other family members)		
There have been emotional adjustments (e.g., because of severe arguments)		
Some behavior is upsetting (e.g., because of incontinence; _____ has trouble remembering things; or _____ accuses people of taking things)		
It is upsetting to find _____ has changed so much from his/her former self (e.g., he/she is a different person than he/she used to be)		
There have been work adjustments (e.g., because of having to take time off)		
It is a financial strain		
Feeling completely overwhelmed (e.g., because of worry about _____ ; concerns about how you will manage)		
TOTAL SCORE (Count yes responses. Any positive answer may indicate a need for intervention in that area. A score of 7 or higher indicates a high level of stress.)		

Practice Pearl

If you suspect elder mistreatment or abuse, a complete visual examination of the older person without clothing is necessary. Abusers may strike where clothing hides the resulting bruises. You can protect privacy by viewing the older person's body one area at a time from head to toe.

Laboratory findings that support the presence of dehydration and malnutrition without medical causes also increase suspicion for elder mistreatment. The nurse may anticipate the need for diagnostic studies such as a complete blood count to evaluate for anemia; chemistry studies for dehydration, vitamin B_{12}, folate, total protein, and albumin to evaluate nutritional status; and toxicological screening to assess for evidence of illicit drug use. If sexual abuse is suspected, the nurse may be needed to assist with a pelvic examination that will likely include a Papanicolaou test (Pap smear) and cultures for sexually transmitted diseases. Radiological testing may also be anticipated if there is suspicion of fractures or internal injuries (Wagner, Greenberg, & Capezuti, 2002).

NURSING DIAGNOSES

Elder mistreatment may be addressed by the following nursing diagnoses from the North American Nursing Diagnosis Association (NANDA , 2001):

- Caregiver role strain
- Coping, ineffective family: compromised
- Coping, ineffective family: disabling
- Coping, ineffective individual
- Protection, altered
- Rape-trauma syndrome
- Self-care deficits
- Self-esteem deficits
- Social isolation
- Violence, risk for

These nursing diagnoses do not specifically address elder mistreatment, with the exception of *rape-trauma syndrome*. Cowan (2001) has suggested the need for research and practice to further develop specific classifications for elder mistreatment to facilitate data collection and interpretation in data sets. Doing so may assist in tracking elder mistreatment trends to facilitate policy initiatives.

INTERVENTIONS

Healthcare staff working with older adults must be aware of local elder mistreatment reporting laws. As previously mentioned, many states have mandatory reporting laws, and healthcare professionals must report suspected cases. Nurses and other healthcare professionals should make themselves familiar with the contact information for local departments on aging and APS agencies. State contact numbers

Practice Pearl

When beginning employment in a new clinical agency, it is important to ask about the reporting of elder mistreatment. Identify members of the interdisciplinary team who can be of assistance, identify and record appropriate phone numbers, assemble forms that should be completed in the reporting process, and familiarize yourself with any other institutional procedures involved in the reporting process. Later on, you can report suspected mistreatment in an accurate and timely manner if the situation should arise.

for reporting suspected elder abuse cases are available online at the National Center on Elder Abuse website.

Elder mistreatment requires an interdisciplinary team approach. Some forms of elder mistreatment, such as caregiver neglect, may benefit from interdisciplinary interventions. Educational interventions that may assist a stressed informal caregiver include disease management, aging changes, maximizing healthcare services, respite services, behavioral management, or caregiver support groups. Learning about Medicaid benefits and home care services can often alleviate caregiver burden (Parks & Novielli, 2000).

In cases where abuse is suspected, an older adult may benefit from a hospital admission to allow the healthcare team to carefully assess and formulate a plan of care. Some institutions have employed elder mistreatment teams, comprising interdisciplinary members, to assist staff in evaluating elder mistreatment cases. These types of teams, which may consist of a geriatrician, nurse, social worker, and perhaps representatives from APS agencies, have been very effective in managing cases of elder mistreatment (Wolf & Pillemer, 1994). Researchers and clinicians recognize the need to incorporate an interdisciplinary team approach into APS systems to use comprehensive geriatric assessment to best identify and serve mistreated older adults (Dyer & Goins, 2000). Anecdotally, other institutions have utilized the ethics committee in assisting to evaluate elder mistreatment cases. This strategy may be particularly helpful if legal action, such as seeking **guardianship** for an older adult, is necessary.

For the older adult living in longer term care facilities, *the California Advocates for Nursing Home Reform* (2002) recommend the following steps in preventing elder abuse in long-term care settings:

- Residents and significant others should join or form a resident's council.
- Residents and their significant others must stay informed by being active participants in care plan meetings and monitoring care.
- Significant others should stay connected to long-term care residents and visit at varied times.

DOCUMENTATION

The nurse must clearly provide objective documentation. Documentation that focuses on the older adult's reactions when the suspected abuser is present must be provided in an unbiased manner. Physical indicators of elder mistreatment that are clearly documented will assist interdisciplinary members in discussing and planning goals of patient care. Photo-documentation is especially warranted in cases where there is evidence of physical or sexual abuse.

IMPLICATIONS FOR GERONTOLOGICAL NURSING PRACTICE

The Joint Commission on Accreditation of Healthcare Organizations recommends the American Medical Association's *Diagnostic and Treatment Guidelines on Elder Abuse and Neglect* (American Medical Association, 1992). These guidelines are presented in Figure 10-2A and B■.

Screening and assessment for elder mistreatment should follow a routine pattern. Assessment of each case should include the following:

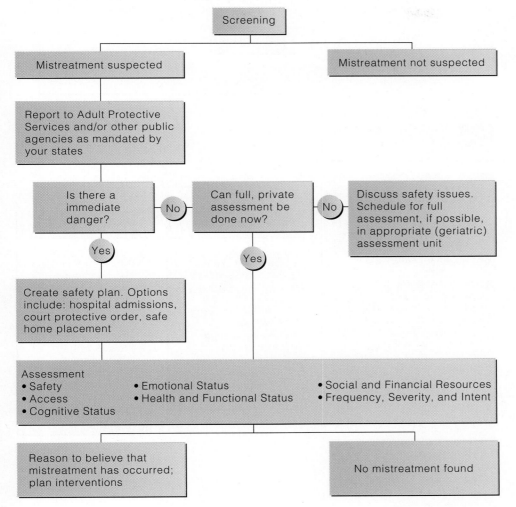

FIGURE 10-2A

Intervention and case management: Part 1.

Source: Reprinted with permission of the American Medical Association. (1992). *Diagnostic and treatment guidelines on elder abuse and neglect,* 13.

Future Considerations

Identified elder mistreatment and self-neglect cases significantly impact older adult mortality (Lachs, Williams, O'Brien, Pillemer, & Charlson, 1998). Barriers to detecting and treating elder mistreatment include the fact that victims may try to hide the mistreatment suffered, cultural issues, and inadequate educational preparation of healthcare professionals (Clarke & Pierson, 1999). There is a lack of evidence-based interventions to offer victims and their families (Fulmer, 2002). Future research focusing on the effectiveness of healthcare interventions is needed. The patient-family teaching guidelines in the following feature will assist the nurse to assume the role of teacher and coach in detecting elder mistreatment.

FIGURE ▢ 10-2B

Intervention and case
management: Part 2.

Source: Reprinted with permission
of the American Medical
Association, (1992). *Diagnostic and
treatment guidelines on elder abuse
and neglect,* 14.

Case management should be guided by choosing the alternatives that least restrict the patient's independence and decision-making responsibilities and fulfill state-mandated reporting requirements. Intervention will depend on the patient's cognitive status and decision-making capability and on whether the mistreatment is intentional or unintentional.

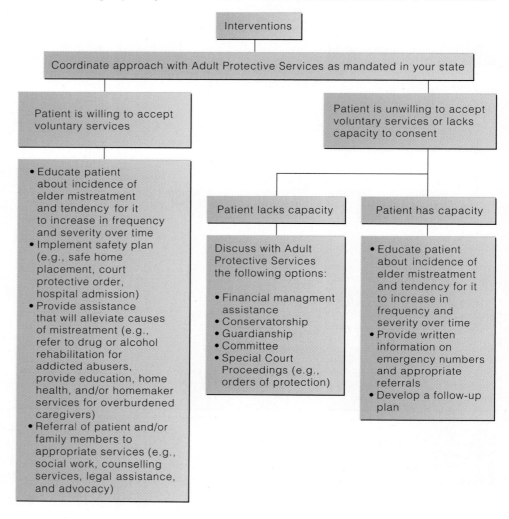

Patient-Family Teaching Guidelines

EDUCATING ABOUT ELDER MISTREATMENT

The following are guidelines that the nurse may find useful when instructing older persons and their families about elder mistreatment.

1. I am worried about my older aunt who may be being abused by her son. What is elder mistreatment?

Any action or inaction that harms or endangers the welfare of an older adult may be considered elder mistreatment. There are approximately 1.2 million cases of elder mistreatment in the United States each year.

Types of abuse:

- Physical abuse is an intentional infliction of physical injury or pain such as slapping or hitting.
- Psychological or emotional abuse is infliction of anguish such as repeatedly scolding an older individual who cannot perform personal hygiene tasks.
- Sexual abuse is any form of nonconsensual sexual intimacy.
- Financial exploitation is when an older individual is taken advantage of for monetary or personal benefit.
- Neglect may be on the part of a caregiver who intentionally or unintentionally does not provide adequate care or services for an older adult (i.e., not seeking healthcare when needed or withholding prescribed medications). Neglect may also be on the part of the older adult (self-neglect) who exhibits personal disregard or inability to perform self-care.
- Institutional mistreatment occurs when an older adult has a contractual arrangement and suffers abuse or neglect.
- Abandonment is desertion or willful forsaking of an older person. An example of this is when an older individual is dropped off and left at the emergency department.

RATIONALE:

Most people are unaware of the broad definition and scope of caregiver activities that are legally considered abuse, neglect, and mistreatment of older people. A complete description is needed when abuse is suspected.

2. If she is being abused, how can I help? I am only a niece.

If you suspect elder mistreatment, contact your local adult protective services office or the department of human services in your state, county, or local jurisdiction. A case worker will visit your aunt and assess the situation. If help and support for her caregivers is needed, additional services will be brought into the home and the situation will be monitored to protect your aunt's safety.

RATIONALE:

Many people are unsure of how to proceed when they suspect abuse or mistreatment of an older person. Education and identification of resources will empower them to act responsibly.

3. What if abuse or neglect of my aunt is found? Will she be put in a nursing home?

The goal of the caseworker's first assessment is to identify if your aunt is in immediate danger. Older people in immediate danger from abuse are removed from the home and temporarily protected in hospitals or safe havens with the authority of a court order. If the abuser needs mental health treatment or detoxification from drugs or alcohol, this will be facilitated. The goal is to improve the situation if possible and return the older person to the home environment when safe. If your aunt is not in immediate danger, resources will be brought into the home to ease the caregiver strain and improve your aunt's safety.

RATIONALE:

Many people are hesitant to make referrals regarding possible abuse as they fear the older person will be placed permanently in a long-term care facility. Reassurance and education regarding all of the possible outcomes is needed.

Care Plan

A Patient With Signs of Self-Neglect

Case Study

Mrs. Baker is brought to the emergency department by ambulance attendants. Her mail carrier noticed that her mail had not been collected for 2 days and called 911. She is in a diabetic coma.

Mrs. Baker's past medical history is significant for heart failure, hypertension, diabetes, peripheral vascular disease, and depression.

A review of her social history reveals that Mrs. Baker is a 70-year-old widow whose only living relatives are her 95-year-old mother who lives in a nursing home 500 miles away and a daughter who lives 70 miles away. She lives alone in a lower-middle-class neighborhood in a modest but run-down home. She has a protective services caseworker who has tried to arrange help, but Mrs. Baker refuses. Her usual routine consists of eating an occasional meal (soup, a sandwich, or cereal), smoking two packs of cigarettes a day, drinking a pint of alcohol every 2 days, and lying on the sofa watching television. She rarely sees her neighbors and does not respond to her physician's request to see him. On occasion, she may answer her telephone or doorbell. Last year she was the victim of fraud by two men claiming to protect her home from termites and water damage. She realizes she cannot fully maintain her home or herself on her own, but she refuses in-home assistance and is determined to stay in her home, manage her own money and affairs, and die there.

Mrs. Baker remains in the emergency department, receives her insulin, and is stabilized for admission. The nurse is unable to get an accurate history of her medications and cannot tell what she is taking. She refuses to answer any questions about a caregiver. She says she is completely independent and refuses to discuss her financial support. She denies being left alone for long periods of time and says she has all the contact she wants. She says she is able to express her needs and have them met.

Mrs. Baker's vital signs are as follows:

- Temperature: 98°F, oral
- Pulse: 70, regular
- Respiratory rate: 20
- Blood pressure: 210/100

Applying the Nursing Process

ASSESSMENT

A complete assessment of Mrs. Baker's health status and self-care is needed. Some appropriate questions the nurse may ask include:

A Patient With Signs of Self-Neglect

Do you feel safe where you live?

Has anyone ever tried to hurt you in any way?

Do you ever feel afraid?

If there is suspected physical evidence of abuse (i.e., bruise, fracture):

What happened?

When did _____ occur? *(i.e., bruise, injury, fracture, not having personal necessities)*

Did anyone do this to you?

Has this ever happened before?

How do you manage your finances?

(Wagner, Greenberg, & Capezuti, 2002)

DIAGNOSIS

The current nursing diagnoses for Mrs. Baker might include the following:

- *Caregiver role strain (possible)*
- *Coping, ineffective family: compromised or disabling*
- *Coping, ineffective individual*
- *Protection, altered*
- *Self-care deficits*
- *Self-esteem deficits*
- *Social isolation*
- *Risk for poisoning: alcohol and tobacco abuse*
- *Violence, risk for*

EXPECTED OUTCOMES

The expected outcomes for the plan of care specify that Mrs. Baker will:

- Become aware of the harmful effects of alcohol and tobacco on overall health status.
- Identify family and community supports that might allow her to return home and achieve her goal of spending the rest of her life there.
- Develop a more trusting and open relationship with her physician regarding her health status.
- Agree to establish a therapeutic relationship with the nurse and develop a mutually acceptable plan to work toward these outcomes.

PLANNING AND IMPLEMENTATION

The following nursing interventions may be appropriate:

- Establish a therapeutic relationship.
- Avoid being judgmental or using scare tactics.

(continued)

A Patient With Signs of Self-Neglect *(continued)*

- Encourage a family meeting with the daughter present to talk about health issues in general with Mrs. Baker's permission.
- Begin a mental status and mood assessment to establish the underlying cause of Mrs. Baker's self-neglect.
- Begin a values clarification to establish long-term goals and facilitate end-of-life planning.

EVALUATION

The nurse hopes to work with Mrs. Baker over time and realizes the sensitive nature of self-neglect in older people. The nurse will consider the plan a success based on the following criteria:

- During hospitalization, Mrs. Baker's condition will become stable and physical indicators of health status will improve (dehydration, nutrition, skin integrity, etc.).
- A family meeting will be held to discuss Mrs. Baker's overall health and values.
- She will accept counseling and discuss beginning to decrease her alcohol and tobacco consumption.
- Ongoing assessment of Mrs. Baker's cognitive status, mood, and resources will be conducted as her condition stabilizes.
- Appropriate discharge planning will take place, and safe living arrangements will be identified and used at the time of hospital discharge.

Ethical Dilemma

On physical examination, the nurse notes Mrs. Baker is 5'5", 101 lb. Her MMSE score is 20, she is extremely dirty, and she has evidence of greater than 15% dehydration. She has a small blister on her left thigh, which looks like a burn. She also has a sacral pressure ulcer 2 cm in diameter. She has no bruising, contractures, diarrhea, impaction, or urine burns.

Mrs. Baker says the burn is from a cigarette and that she often falls asleep while smoking on the couch. She asks the nurse not to inform the others on the team that she has burned herself. Ignoring the older person's request not to share information with others is usually considered a violation of the right to privacy; however, Mrs. Baker is at immediate and high risk for injury due to self-neglect. Her dehydration, pressure ulcers, uncontrolled diabetes, low body weight, and impaired cognitive status are all indicators that her situation must be reported to a caseworker for investigation. The nurse is bound by law and ethics to intervene on behalf of this patient and advocate for her safety. A report should be filed immediately.

Critical Thinking and the Nursing Process

1. What is your emotional response to the thought of caring for an older person who has been mistreated?
2. Can you identify some unique reasons for elder mistreatment in your community?

A Patient With Signs of Self-Neglect

3. Have you ever witnessed elder mistreatment during your clinical experiences as a student nurse?

4. Identify actions that can help relieve stress in family caregivers.

■ Evaluate your responses in Appendix B. ⊂⊃

EXPLORE MediaLink

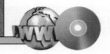

NCLEX review, case studies, and other interactive resources for this chapter can be found on the Companion Website at **www.prenhall.com/tabloski**. Click on Chapter 10 to select the activities for this chapter. For animations, video tutorials, more NCLEX review questions, and case studies, access the accompanying CD-ROM in this textbook.

Chapter Highlights

■ Elder mistreatment is a general term for both abuse and neglect.

■ The prevalence of elder mistreatment is difficult to ascertain since many cases go unreported.

■ Family violence is a significant public health issue for all of society, and the rates of elder mistreatment are expected to increase in the coming years.

■ Elder mistreatment may include physical abuse or neglect, psychological abuse or neglect, financial or material abuse or neglect, or self-abuse or neglect.

■ Indicators of mistreatment are subtle and vary according to the situation. Complete assessment of possible mistreatment and contributing factors is needed.

■ Nearly all states require designated healthcare professionals, including nurses, to report suspected elder mistreatment to a state authority. Calls are confidential.

References

American Association of Colleges of Nursing. (2001). *Position statement on violence as a public health problem.* Washington, DC: Author.

American Medical Association. (1992). *Diagnostic and treatment guidelines on elder abuse and neglect.* Chicago: Author.

Aravanis, S. C., Adelman, R. D., Breckman, R., Fulmer, T., Holder, E., Lachs, M. S., et al. (1993). Diagnostic and treatment guidelines on elder abuse and neglect. *Archives of Family Medicine, 2*(4), 371–388.

Brownell, P. (1999). Mental health and criminal justice issues among perpetrators of elder abuse. *Journal of Elder Abuse and Neglect, 11*(4), 81–94.

Burgess, A.W., Dowdell, E. B., & Prentky, R. A. (2000). Sexual abuse of nursing home residents. *Journal of Psychosocial Nursing, 38*(6), 10–18.

California Advocates for Nursing Home Reform. (2002). *Elder abuse: What can you do to prevent elder abuse.* Retrieved November 10, 2004, from www.canhr.org/abuse/ abuse_prevent.htm.

Capezuti, E., Brush, B. L., & Lawson, W. T. (1997). Reporting elder mistreatment. *Journal of Gerontological Nursing, 23*(7), 24–32.

Clarke, M. E., & Pierson, W. (1999). Management of elder abuse in the emergency department. *Emergency, 17*(3), 631–644, vi.

Cowan, P. S. (2001). Elder mistreatment. In M. L. Mass, K. C. Buckwalter, M. D. Hardy, T. Tripp-Reimer, M. G. Titler, & J. P. Specht (Eds.), *Nursing care of older adults: Diagnoses, outcomes, & interventions.* St. Louis, MO: Mosby.

Dunlop, B., Rothman, M. B., Condon, K. M., Hebert, K. S., & Martinez, I. L. (2000). Elder abuse: Risk factors and use of case data to improve policy and practice. *Journal of Elder Abuse and Neglect, 12*(3/4), 95–122.

Dyer, C. B., & Goins, A. M. (2000). The role of the interdisciplinary geriatric assessment in addressing self-neglect of the elderly. *Generations,* 23–27.

Dyer, C. B., Pavlik, V. N., Murphy, K. P., & Hyman, D. J. (2000). The high prevalence of depression and dementia in elder abuse or neglect. *Journal of the American Geriatrics Society, 48*(2), 205–208.

Fulmer, T. (2002). Elder mistreatment. *Annual Review of Nursing Research, 20,* 369–395.

Fulmer, T., & Cahill, V. M. (1984). Assessing elder abuse: A study. *Journal of Gerontological Nursing, 10*(12), 16–20.

Fulmer, T., & O'Malley, T. (1987). *Inadequate care of the elderly: A health care perspective on abuse and neglect.* New York: Springer.

Fulmer, T., Paveza, G., Abraham, I., & Fairchild, S. (2000). Elder neglect assessment in the emergency department. *Journal of Emergency Nursing, 26*(5), 436–443.

Fulmer, T., Street, S., & Carr, K. (1984). Abuse of the elderly: Screening and detection. *Journal of Emergency Nursing, 10*(3), 131–140.

Godkin, M., Wolf, R. S., & Pillemer, K. A. (1989). A case-comparison analysis of elder abuse and neglect. *International Journal of Aging and Human Development, 28*(3), 207–225.

Hartford Institute for Geriatric Nursing. (1999). *Best practices in nursing care to older adults.* New York: New York University Division of Nursing.

Hudson, M. F. (1989). Analyses of the concepts of elder mistreatment: Abuse and neglect. *Journal of Elder Abuse and Neglect, 1*(1), 5–25.

Hudson, M. F., Armachain, W. D., Beasley, C. M., & Carlson, J. R. (1998). Elder abuse: Two Native American views. *Gerontologist, 38*(5), 538–548.

Hudson, M. F., Beasley, C., Benedict, R. H., Carlson, J. R., Craig, B. F., Herman, C., & Mason, S. C. (2000). Elder abuse: Some Caucasian-American views. *Journal of Elder Abuse and Neglect, 12*(1), 89–114.

Institute of Medicine. (2002). *Confronting chronic neglect: The education and training of health professionals on family violence.* Washington, DC: National Academy Press.

Lachs, M. S., & Fulmer, T. (1993). Recognizing elder abuse and neglect. *Clinical Geriatric Medicine, 9*(3), 665–681.

Lachs, M. S., & Pillemer, K. A. (1995). Abuse and neglect of elderly persons. *New England Journal of Medicine, 332*(7), 437–443.

Lachs, M. S., Williams, C., O'Brien, S., Hurst, L., & Horwitz, R. I. (1997). Risk factors for reported elder abuse and neglect: A nine-year observational cohort study. *Gerontologist, 37*(4), 469–474.

Lachs, M. S., Williams, C. S., O'Brien, S., Pillemer, K. A., & Charlson, M. E. (1998). The mortality of elder mistreatment. *Journal of the American Medical Association, 280*(5), 428–432.

Moon, A., & Benton, D. (2000). Tolerance of elder abuse and attitudes toward third-party intervention among African American, Korean American and White elderly. *Journal of Multicultural Social Work, 8*(3/4), 283–303.

National Center on Elder Abuse at the American Public Human Services Association (formerly the American Public Welfare Association) in collaboration with Westat. (1998). *The National Elder Abuse Incidence Study; final report: September 1998.* Washington, DC: National Aging Information Center.

National Research Council. (2003). *Elder mistreatment: Abuse, neglect, and exploitation in aging America.* Washington, DC.

North American Nursing Diagnosis Association (NANDA). (2001). *Nursing diagnoses: Definitions and classification, 2001–2002.* Philadelphia: Author.

O'Malley, T. A., Everitt, D. E., O'Malley, H. C., & Campion, E. W. (1983). Identifying and preventing family-mediated abuse and neglect of elderly persons. *Annals of Internal Medicine, 98*(6), 998–1005.

O'Malley, T. A., O'Malley, H. C., Everitt, D. E., & Sarson, D. (1984). Categories of family-mediated abuse and neglect of elderly persons. *Journal of the American Geriatrics Society, 32*(5), 362–369.

Omnibus Budget Reconciliation Act. (1987). *Public Law 100-203. Subtitle C: Nursing home reform.* Washington, DC: U.S. Department of Health and Human Services: 52 Fed. Reg. 38582, 38584.

Panel to Review Risk and Prevalence of Elder Abuse and Neglect. (2002). R.J. Bonnie & R.B. Wallace (Eds.), *Elder mistreatment: Abuse, neglect, and exploitation in an aging America.* Washington, DC: Division of Behavioral and Social Sciences and Education, National Research Council, National Academy Press.

Parks, S. M., & Novielli, K. D. (2000, December 15). *A practical guide to caring for caregivers. American Family Physician.* Retrieved June 14, 2002, from www.aafp.org.

Pillemer, K. A., & Finkelhor, D. (1988). The prevalence of elder abuse: A random sample survey. *Gerontologist, 28*(1), 51–57.

Pillemer, K. A., & Finkelhor, D. (1989). Causes of elder abuse: Caregiver stress versus problem relatives. *American Journal of Orthopsychiatry, 59*(2), 179–187.

Pillemer, K. A., & Moore, D. W. (1989). Abuse of patients in nursing homes: Findings from a survey of staff. *Gerontologist, 29*(3), 314–320.

Reis, M., & Nahmiash, D. (1998). Validation of the indicators of abuse (IOA) screen. *Gerontologist, 38*(4), 471–480.

Robinson, B. C. (1994). Caregiver Strain Index. In J. Fischer & K. Corcoran (Eds.), *Measures for clinical practice: A sourcebook* (2nd ed., Vol. 2). New York: Free Press.

Steinmetz, S. K. (1990). Elder abuse by adult offspring: The relationship of actual vs. perceived dependency. *Journal of Health and Human Resources Administration, 12*(4), 434–463.

Swagerty, D. L. (1999). Elder mistreatment. *American Family Physician, 59*(10), 2804–2808.

Thomas, C. (2002). The first national study of elder abuse and neglect: Contrast with results from other studies. *Journal of Elder Abuse and Neglect, 16*(2).

Tomita, S. (1999). Exploration of elder mistreatment among the Japanese. In T. Tatara (Ed.), *Understanding elder abuse in minority populations* (pp. 119–139). (CANE File No. N4672-13). New Zealand: MacMillan.

U.S. General Accounting Office, Report to Congressional Requesters. (2002). *Nursing homes: More can be done to protect residents from abuse* (GAO-02-312). Washington, DC. Retrieved February 18, 2005, from www.gao.gov/new.itemsd02312.pdf.

Wagner, L., Greenberg, S., & Capezuti, E. (2002). Elder abuse and neglect. In V. T. Cotter & N. E. Strumpf (Eds.), *Advanced practice nursing with older adults clinical guidelines.* New York: McGraw-Hill.

Walshe-Brennan, K. (1977). Granny bashing. *Nursing Mirror, 145*(25), 32–34.

Wolf, R. S., & Pillemer, K. A. (1994). What's new in elder abuse programming? Four bright ideas. *Gerontologist, 34*(1), 126–129.

Wolf, R. S., & Pillemer, K. A. (1997). The older battered woman: Wives and mothers compared. *Journal of Mental Health and Aging, 3*(3), 325–336.

Zarit, S. H., Reever, K. E., & Bach-Peterson, J. (1994). Caregiver's Burden Scale. In J. Fischer & K. Corcoran (Eds.), *Measures for clinical practice: A sourcebook* (2nd ed., Vol. 2). New York: Free Press.

CHAPTER 11

Care of the Dying

Rosalie Hentz, BS, RN
Patricia Tabloski, PHD, GNP

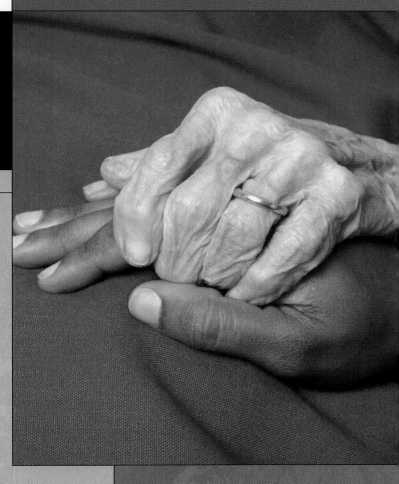

CHAPTER OBJECTIVES

Upon completion of this chapter, the reader will be able to:

- Describe the role of the nurse in providing quality end-of-life care for older persons and their families.
- Recognize changes in demographics, economics, and service delivery that require improved nursing interventions at the end of life.
- Describe how pain and presence of adverse symptoms affect the dying process.
- Identify the diverse settings for end-of-life care and the role of the nurse in each setting.
- Explore pharmacological and alternative methods of treating pain.
- Identify the signs of approaching death.
- Describe appropriate nursing interventions when caring for the dying.
- Describe postmortem care.
- Discuss family support during the grief and bereavement period.

MediaLink

Additional resources for this chapter can be found on the Student CD-ROM accompanying this textbook and on the Companion Website at **www.prenhall.com/tabloski**. Click on Chapter 11 to select the activities for this chapter.

CD-ROM
- Animation/Video
  Massage for the Terminally Ill
  Morphine
- NCLEX Review
- Case Studies
- Tools

COMPANION WEBSITE
- Audio Glossary
- Additional NCLEX Review
- Case Study
- MediaLink Applications

KEY TERMS

Nurses are uniquely qualified to provide comprehensive, effective, compassionate, and cost-effective care to persons at the end of life because of their unique holistic focus. As members of the largest healthcare profession, nurses have long advocated for attention to quality of life. To achieve that goal, nurses have provided competent, caring, professional nursing care. Nursing's social policy statement indicates that nurses attend to a full range of human experiences and responses to health and illness. Nurses are present in every setting where Americans receive healthcare (American Nurses Association, 1995). The Hospice and Palliative Nurses Association (HPNA) (2003) has issued a position statement declaring that professional nursing care is critical to achieving the patients', families', and communities' goals of care at the end of life and that support of hospice and palliative care research and education is necessary to ensure that care is evidence based, effective, and appropriate.

Nurses spend more time with patients and their families at the end of life than any other member of the healthcare team. When faced with a serious illness, people turn to their nurse for education, support, and guidance. Nurses are intimately involved in all aspects of end-of-life care. They are the primary team members who coordinate, assess, direct, and evaluate patient care needs that arise during the illness experience. With their knowledge about the physical, psychosocial, and spiritual dimensions of life-limiting and terminal illness, nurses are central in ensuring the comfort, autonomy, and healing of patients and families. The professional nurse is also a key player in moving the healthcare team toward recognition of end-of-life care situations and the comfort care and psychological support that are required. Professional nursing at the end of life is grounded in keeping the positive traditions of past practices while shaping care for the future that will meet the evolving needs of the sick and dying. The professional nurse establishes and supports the methods and means to ensure these outcomes are met (HPNA, 2003).

Death is as natural a part of life as is birth. Although birth is embraced with joy and celebration, death is frequently denied and often prolonged for the sake of the living. Nurses, by nature of their work with the ill and older persons, have a unique opportunity and an obligation to help patients and their families through the dying process. Student nurses learn to do this by confronting their own feelings about death and seeking guidance and mentorship when confronting death during clinical experiences. The student learns how to acknowledge and accept death as part of life, and realizes that the nurse grieves the loss of patients. Viewing death as a natural process, and not a medical failure, is of utmost importance. The nurse who helps the patient die comfortably and with dignity provides the following benefits of good nursing care:

- Attention to pain and symptom control
- Relief of psychosocial distress
- Coordinated care across settings with high-quality communication between healthcare providers
- Preparation of the patient and family for death
- Clarification and communication of goals of treatment and values
- Support and education during the decision-making process, including the benefits and burdens of treatment

(National Consensus Project [NCP] for Quality Palliative Care, 2004)

To achieve these goals, the nurse must be well educated, have appropriate supports in the clinical setting, and develop a close collaborative partnership with palliative care service providers and hospice programs.

The social and scientific changes in recent years have helped to make dying a medical process. Although medicine can cure many illnesses and extend the lives of those with serious illnesses, an unintended consequence of these interventions may be the prolongation of the dying process instead of the extension of a life with quality. Dying occurs in hospitals, hospices, and long-term care settings more than in the familiar home setting. Because of medical technology, sometimes the timing of death is less a natural event and more a human decision. This can result in a "negotiated" death that follows a long period of invasive treatments that exhaust and demoralize patients, families, and nurses (Tilden, 1998).

Nurses must be confident in their clinical skills when caring for the dying, and aware of the ethical, spiritual, and legal issues they may confront while providing end-of-life care. Many feel that the first step in the process is confronting their own personal fears about death and dying. By addressing their own fears, nurses are better able to help patients and families when they are confronted by impending death. The nurse can then more objectively recognize and respect the patient's and family's values and choices that guide their decisions at the end of life.

Facing one's own mortality can help to clarify beliefs and values. As death nears, the meaning of hope shifts from striving for cure to striving for relief of pain and suffering. There is no "right" or "correct" way to die, and each person will face death in his or her own unique and individual way. In order to prepare to work with the dying, the student nurse may wish to consider the questions in Table 11-1. The purpose of this exercise is to increase nurses' awareness of their own feelings about death and dying so that they are better prepared to comfort and care for others.

By coming to terms with their own feelings surrounding death, nurses can better meet the emotional, spiritual, social, and physical needs of the patient. Often it is the caregiver who forms the bonds with the dying patient and is present when the last breath is taken. The nurse provides a presence as a way of expressing compassionate caring. In this way, nurses enter into another's reality and use all of their skills of

TABLE 11-1

Questions and Critical Thinking in Preparation to Care for Dying Patients

Question for Consideration	Critical Thinking Application
Have I ever seen a dead body?	Identify and overcome feelings regarding the lifeless body of another.
What are my own views of death?	Recognize feelings that death indicates a failure of the medical model.
Have I experienced the death of a close friend or relative?	By contemplating the death of a loved one, different emotions emerge, including feelings of sadness and perhaps relief or joy for a life well lived.
How would I like to be remembered by my family and friends?	The way we hope to be remembered often adds purpose and meaning to our lives.
What age do I think I will be when I die?	Death in old age is often seen as a natural end to a long and productive life.
How do I think I will die?	The fear of death is often accompanied by fear of pain, suffering, and isolation from family and friends. These fears may be greater than the fear of death itself.

FIGURE ▢ 11-1

Providing compassionate and holistic end-of-life care allows the nurse to apply a wide range of skills.

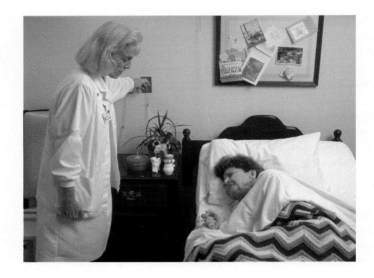

compassionate care. This is a humbling and beautiful privilege. It too is a celebration of a life lived (Figure 11-1▢).

The Changing Face of Death

Many older people grew up with death as a real and inevitable part of life. Some may have cared for their parents or grandparents for extended periods of time and remember holding wakes or funerals in the living room of the home where death occurred. During the middle 1900s, technological advances dictated that sick people should go to hospitals where they could safely receive high-tech care. Surgery, antibiotics, and advanced testing techniques became the focus of healthcare, shifting away from the provision of care to the pursuit of cure (Corr, 1998). Table 11-2 illustrates the changing demographic and social trends surrounding the cause of death in the years 1900 and 2000.

TABLE 11–2

Cause of Death and Demographic/Social Trends

	1900	2000
Focus of care	Comfort	Cure
Primary cause of death	Infectious diseases—e.g., pneumonia, influenza	Chronic illnesses—e.g., heart disease, cancer
Average life expectancy	50 years	76 years
Number of older persons (>65)	3.1 million	Approximately 35 million
Place of death	Home	Institutions
Caregivers	Family	Professional healthcare providers
Disease trajectory	Short, downward trend	Prolonged, variable, peaks and valleys
Functional decline at the end of life	Short term—expected and surprise	Lingering expected—frailty

Source: Adapted from Administration on Aging, 2000; Field & Cassel, 1997. Lunney, Lynn, Fole, Lipson, & Guralnik, 2003.

The 10 leading causes of death accounting for 80% of all death in the United States in 2000 include, in rank descending order, heart disease, malignant neoplasms, cerebrovascular disease, chronic lower respiratory disease, accidents, diabetes mellitus, influenza and pneumonia, Alzheimer's disease, renal disease, and septicemia (End-of-Life Nursing Education Consortium [ELNEC], 2003). Many times, the exact cause of death is difficult to determine in an older person. For instance, an older person with Alzheimer's disease may fall and break a hip, and die shortly after the injury. However, the actual cause of death may have been a myocardial infarction that was not detected by the physician. The cause of death on the death certificate may indicate a fall or Alzheimer's disease while the cause of death was actually the myocardial infarction.

Most Americans, regardless of age, would prefer to die in their own homes rather than institutions. However, about 50% of Americans die in hospitals, 25% in nursing homes, 20% at home or the home of a loved one, and 5% in other settings, including inpatient hospices (NCP, 2004). Almost half the population age 65 and older will spend some time in a nursing home prior to death, more than half of the persons over age 85 die in a nursing home, and 43% of persons over age 65 reside in a long-term care facility at some time before they die. Data from numerous studies demonstrate high degrees of symptom distress in hospitalized and nursing home patients, high use of burdensome nonbeneficial technologies among the seriously ill, caregiver burden on families, and problems with communication between patients, families, and caregivers about the goals of care and medical decisions that should follow (Last Acts, 2002; NCP, 2004; Quill, 2000; Steinhauser & Christakis, 2000; SUPPORT, 1995).

When a national survey asked how the current healthcare system does in caring for dying people, only 3% of respondents answered excellent, 8% said very good, 31% said good, 33% said fair, and 25% said poor (Last Acts, 2002). When viewing these results, most professionals agree that there is much room for improvement.

Possible barriers to the provision of excellent end-of-life care include failure of healthcare providers to acknowledge the limits of medical technology, lack of training about effective means of controlling pain and symptoms, the unwillingness of providers to be honest about a poor prognosis, discomfort telling bad news, and lack of understanding about the valuable contributions to be made by referral and collaboration with comprehensive end-of-life programs such as hospice or **palliative care** services (Kyba, 1999). All healthcare providers, including nurses, are challenged to address and overcome these barriers to improve the quality of care provided to the dying and their families.

Practice Pearl

Although not all deaths involve pain and suffering, there are deficiencies in the way end-of-life care is currently provided in the U.S. healthcare system. Barriers include lack of knowledge regarding pain and symptom control. Challenge yourself to develop expert skills in these areas to improve the dying process for their patients.

Palliative Care

The goals of palliative care are to prevent and relieve suffering and to support the best possible quality of life for patients and their families, regardless of the stage of the disease or the need for other therapies. Palliative care is both a philosophy of care and an organized, highly structured system for delivery of that care. Palliative care transcends the traditional disease-model medical treatments and includes the goal of enhancing quality of life for patient and family, optimizing function, helping with decision making, and providing opportunities for personal growth. It can be delivered concurrently with life-prolonging care or as the main focus of care (NCP, 2004). Although palliative care can be delivered to patients of any age, including children, it is especially appropriate when provided to older people who have:

- Acute, serious, life-threatening illness (such as stroke, trauma, major myocardial infarction, and cancer where cure or reversability may or may not be a realistic goal but the burden of treatment is high).
- Progressive chronic illness (such as end-stage dementia, congestive heart failure, renal or liver failure, and frailty).

Palliative care may take place in hospitals, in outpatient clinics, in long-term care facilities, or in the home. The patient and family are supported during the dying and **bereavement** process. The care provided emphasizes quality of life and living as full a life as possible up until the moment of death.

Hospice Care

The hospice movement began in the United States in the 1970s. Since 1974, over 7 million patients and families have received end-of-life care at home as well as in nursing homes and hospitals through hospice programs, with escalating use in recent years (NCP, 2004). Nursing pioneers in palliative care such as Florence Wald, Cicely Saunders (also a physician), and Jeanne Quint Benoliel have emphasized that those in need of care at the end of life merit competent, expert, evidence-based care provided in a way that embodies compassion, respect for dignity, and an appreciation for the whole person and the family. In 1962, registered nurse Harriet Goetz published an approach to care for the dying that focused on open communication with the patient and family and symptom management techniques such as atropine for secretions and environmental adjustments (such as making the room pleasant, soft lighting, and so on) to provide comfort. The work of these nurse leaders forged the way toward the current standard practice for comprehensive and compassionate care at the end of life (HPNA, 2003).

Hospice care can be defined as the support and care for persons in the last phase of an incurable disease so that they may live as fully and comfortably as possible (National Hospice and Palliative Care Organization, 2000). The Medicare hospice benefit was designed to support dying patients with less than 6 months to live. It is often difficult to predict with accuracy how long a patient will live, especially when the diagnosis is chronic renal failure, congestive heart failure, cancer, or progressive dementia. Many hospices are expanding service options so that patients and families can receive palliative care long before the last 6 months of life to meet the needs of patients dying from chronic illnesses (Dembner, 2004).

When there is no cure, and the dying person and family are comfortable with the knowledge that death is impending and have agreed to accept palliative care, hospice is often sought. Hospice care focuses on the whole person by caring for the body, mind, and spirit. Since end-of-life care deeply affects the family, support is also provided to family and caregivers. Hospice care is centered on the patient living the last days as fully as possible.

A multidisciplinary team of physicians, nurses, therapists, home health aids, pharmacists, pastoral counselors, social workers, and trained lay volunteers assist the family in providing care at home. The hospice nurse assumes the role of specialist in the management of pain and the control of symptoms. Hospice care may be provided at home if someone is available to safely provide care. The hospice nurse assesses the patient's and family's coping mechanisms, the available resources to care for the patient, the patient's wishes, and the support systems in place.

There are also freestanding hospices that provide a homelike atmosphere in which care is provided by trained staff at the facility. Hospitals may have affiliated hospices, or some home health agencies may also promote their home care hospices. Reimbursement for hospice services is provided by Medicare, Medicaid, private health insurances, and some health maintenance organizations. Some hospices accept donations for care, some have a sliding scale, and some may have access to foundations to help with payment. Hospice personnel may work with staff and patients in nursing homes, other long-term care settings, and hospitals. All hospices encourage family involvement and promote death with dignity. Supportive care continues for the family after the death of the loved one.

There are many misconceptions and myths concerning hospice care. Table 11-3 illustrates common myths and facts regarding hospice.

STAGES OF THE DYING PROCESS

Elisabeth Kübler-Ross, a psychiatrist at the University of Chicago, was also a pioneer. Her research helped support the early hospice movement. Kübler-Ross interviewed hundreds of dying patients and published her findings in *On Death and Dying: What*

TABLE 11-3

Myths and Facts Regarding Hospice

Myth	Fact
Medicare provides only 6 months of hospice care, so enrollment should be delayed as long as possible.	Medicare law does not limit the hospice benefit, but Medicare regulations often discourage a longer length of stay. Patients may enroll when their physician judges their life expectancy to be 6 months or less.
All hospice care is the same.	Hospices vary widely in the services they provide. Visit and observe services before choosing or recommending one for care.
Patients cannot receive curative treatments while on hospice.	Although Medicare requires beneficiaries to forego curative treatment, some hospices accept patients into special programs where they continue receiving therapies directed toward reversing disease and controlling complications of illness.
Hospice means giving up hope. Hospices help people die.	Hope for comfort and relief of pain is always present. Hospice workers do not hasten death.
Hospice helps only when advice is needed regarding pain medication.	Hospice care is holistic and goes beyond traditional medical care.
You cannot keep your own doctor on hospice.	Most hospices have working relationships with the referring physician.
Hospice is only for cancer patients.	Hospice is available to all patients with a variety of diagnoses, including those with cancer and heart and lung diseases.
Hospice is only for the sick family member.	Hospice supports all family members during the illness and supports the family for 1 year after the death.
Hospice is a place, so you must leave home to go there.	Most hospice care is delivered in the home, although inpatient care is available to those with no in-home caregiver or to those whose families are overwhelmed by providing the care.
Hospice is expensive.	In general, hospice costs less than traditional hospital or nursing home care.

Source: Adapted from Labyak, 2001.

BOX 11-1 Kübler-Ross Stages of Dying

- **Denial.** They must have the wrong patient or lab results. I can't be dying, I feel so well.
- **Anger.** I can't believe this. I always took care of others and this is my reward? Why not someone else instead of me?
- **Bargaining.** OK, doctor. I'll give chemotherapy another try if you can guarantee that I'll live for another year. If God lets me live until my grandson graduates from college, I'll make a large donation to my church.
- **Depression.** Why should I bother taking my medicine? I'm helpless to fight this cancer. It's stronger than I am and getting the best of me.
- **Acceptance.** OK. I'm going to die, so I'd better get my act together. I'd like to leave a few pieces of jewelry to my daughter and my books to my son. I hate to think of leaving this world, but I've had a good life and now my time has come. I'll face this final act with all the dignity and courage I can pull together.

the Dying Have to Teach Doctors, Nurses, Clergy and Their Own Families (1969). It was through her efforts that healthcare providers began to understand the needs of dying patients. Pain relief for the terminally ill was another of her successful crusades. Stages of dying were created and are still used as guidelines today (Box 11-1). It must be remembered that a dying person may not exhibit all of these stages, or may move through a stage, only to return to it at a later time.

Today not all researchers agree with Kübler-Ross and some claim that her research cannot be replicated. Death and dying is a unique experience, and each person and family progresses through the process differently. The nurse should remain objective and not quickly jump to conclusions that "one size fits all" is the best approach. Depending on circumstance, a patient may enter the acceptance stage and quickly revert to the denial stage. Since each person lives differently, each will die differently (Knox, 2001).

Complementary and Alternative Care

Besides hospice care, the patient or family member may seek other alternative care. Traditional medicine may share the spotlight with acupuncture, massage therapy, Reiki therapy, chiropractors, or herbal medicine. Healthcare reimbursement may be a problem for some of these nontraditional forms of medicine. Patients must check their health insurance provider for coverage. Many plans allow for a designated number of paid or copaid visits per year, after which the patient must pay privately. Credentials of all healthcare providers should be checked. Each state requires various qualifications of its practitioners. In 1998, the National Institutes of Health initiated the National Center for Complementary and Alternative Medicine (NCCAM).

NCCAM is dedicated to exploring complementary and alternative healing practices in the context of rigorous science, training complementary and alternative medicine researchers, and disseminating authoritative information to the public and professionals. Use of alternative therapies has great potential when integrated into traditional medical practices used by healthcare professionals.

Within the context of quality end-of-life care, the unique needs of each older patient and family (including significant others who may or may not be related to the patient) are respected, and the patient and family constitute the unit of care. Nurses who regularly assist patients and families to understand changes in their health status and the implications of these changes can alleviate many commonly held patient fears. The common fears and concerns of the dying include the following:

- Death itself
- Thoughts of a long or painful death
- Facing death alone
- Dying in a nursing home, hospital, or rest home
- Loss of body control, such as bowel or bladder incontinence
- Not being able to make decisions concerning care
- Loss of consciousness
- Financial costs and becoming a burden on others
- Dying before having a chance to put personal affairs in order

The nurse can assist the older patient to address some of these fears by ensuring patient comfort and support. Often, the nurse is present for the patient and family and can communicate compassion through caring acts. For instance, the small act of adjusting the patient's position in bed and fluffing the pillow can be greatly appreciated by the patient and family. When one is diagnosed with a serious illness, life still proceeds for an indefinite period of time. The time of death cannot be accurately predicted, and many older patients live much longer than their prognosis. It is essential that each person have the opportunity to live life fully each day and engage in living until the moment of death rather than engaging in a long, tedious dying trajectory. Therefore, accurate and timely deliverance of nursing care and addressing potential problem areas is of prime importance. The nurse's assessment frequently guides the interdisciplinary team in providing the individualized care, combined with respect for the patient's wishes. The goal of the nurse is to achieve the best possible quality of life through relief of suffering, control of symptoms, and restoration of functional capacity while remaining sensitive to personal values, cultural practice, and religious beliefs (Last Acts, 2002).

Practice Pearl

Collaboration of team members is essential for providing end-of-life care to older patients and their families. Effective sharing of information, active listening, and ongoing clarification of the patient's goals and values are critical communication skills.

The Nurse's Role

The nurse providing quality end-of-life care to an older person and his or her family will assume the roles of clinician. As an expert clinician, the nurse will carry out a complete physical, psychological, social, and spiritual assessment, and design a plan of care (in collaboration with the patient, family, and interdisciplinary team) to meet the needs of the older patient. Many validated instruments are available for use by healthcare professionals, including instruments for the assessment of pain and symptoms, mental health and mood, meaning in life and spirituality, functional assessment, quality of life, and caregiver strain. See the Toolkit of Instruments to Measure End-of-Life Care (TIME) for online copies and instructions for use of these various instruments.

Core principles for the care of patients at the end of life include the following:

- Respecting the dignity of patients, families, and caregivers
- Displaying sensitivity and respect for patient and family wishes
- Using the most appropriate interventions to accomplish patients' goals
- Alleviating pain and symptoms
- Assessing, managing, and referring psychological, social, and spiritual problems
- Offering continuity and collaboration with others
- Providing access to therapies (including complementary therapies) that may improve the quality of the patient's life
- Providing access to palliative care and hospice services
- Respecting the right of patients and families to refuse treatment
- Promoting and supporting evidence-based clinical practice research

(Adapted from Cassell & Foley, 1999)

PAIN RELIEF AT THE END OF LIFE

Merciful relief of pain is essential to the provision of quality care to the dying older patient. Pain is feared and dreaded by many as they approach the end of life. However, the nurse plays a vital role in the treatment of pain by providing the initial and ongoing assessment of levels of pain, administration of pain medication, and evaluation of the effectiveness of the pain management plan.

Pain is a distressing sensation that is described as acute or chronic. Assessment of pain has been called the fifth vital sign and must be routinely carried out when other vital signs such as temperature, pulse, respiration, and blood pressure are assessed (Joint Commission on Accreditation of Healthcare Organizations, 2000). Pain has the potential to hasten death and is associated with needless suffering at the end of life. People in pain do not eat or drink well, do not move around, cannot engage in meaningful conversations with others, and often become isolated from the world in order to save energy and cope with the pain sensation. (Refer to Chapter 9 for more information on pain.)

Although efforts are under way to improve end-of-life care, there is growing evidence that improvements are not being experienced by all groups of patients. For instance, some older patients may be unable to report their pain. At the end of life, many patients cannot communicate due to delirium, dementia, aphasia, motor weakness, language barriers, and other factors. Minority patients have been identified as being at high risk for inadequate end-of-life care. Possible barriers for these patients include disparities in access to many treatment options at the end of life, insensitivity to cultural differences in attitudes toward death and end-of-life care, and mistrust of the healthcare system due to the history of racism in medicine (Krakauer, Crenner, & Fox, 2002). Several studies report that lower doses of analgesia are used for severely ill African American cancer patients with pain (Phillips et al., 1996). Additionally, one study showed that African Americans preferred aggressive life-sustaining treatments such as cardiopulmonary resuscitation more than did Mexican American, Korean American, or European American senior citizens in Los Angeles (Blackhall et al., 1999). The provision of culturally sensitive care is a necessary component of effective and comprehensive end-of-life care.

Pain in a patient with dementia may be expressed by a change in behavior. The patient with a cognitive impairment may not be aware of the sensation of pain actually causing a problem. The nurse, family members, and other staff are the reporters for the non–cognitively intact resident. A family member will often notice increased agitation, restlessness, grimacing, crying, withdrawal from normal activity, a change in function such as loss of appetite, moaning, repeated verbalizations, or other signs. When dealing with patients with dementia, the nurse needs to consult the family because the patient may not be able to self-report accurately. This group would seem to be at risk for undertreatment of pain because of lack of verbal communication skills. More than 60% of nursing home residents experience some type of dementia. The nurse should acknowledge the family as valuable in providing needed information and accurate assessments. They possess long-standing knowledge of their family member, have intimate knowledge of the patient's usual personality and level of function, and will be the first to notice differences from usual patterns.

Pain is acknowledged to be a subjective experience. Self-report is the gold standard for measuring pain. When an older person cannot speak or is so cognitively impaired that he or she cannot report the level of pain, in addition to questioning significant others, the nurse should carefully observe the patient for the following signs:

- Moaning or groaning at rest or with movement
- Failure to eat, drink, or respond to the presence of others
- Grimacing or strained facial expression
- Guarding or not moving parts of the body
- Resisting care or noncooperation with therapeutic interventions
- Rapid heartbeat, diaphoresis, or change in vital signs

Factors that may render an older person unable to report pain include delirium, language barriers, expressive aphasia, excessive fatigue and weakness, and profound depression. If a patient has a potential reason for pain at the end of life, the nurse should assume it is present until proven otherwise (American Pain Society, 1999).

Accurate pain assessment is the basis of pain treatment and should be done in a systematic and ongoing manner. The elderly patient and family members should be questioned as to a person's usual reaction to a painful situation.

Helpful questions may include:

- Do you usually seek medical help when you believe something is wrong with you?
- Where does it hurt the most?
- How bad is the pain (may use the facility pain indicator such as smiley face, or rate the pain on a scale of 1 to 10)?
- How would you describe the pain (e.g., sharp, shooting, dull)?
- Is the pain accompanied by other troublesome symptoms like nausea or diarrhea?
- What makes the pain go away?
- Are you able to sleep when you are having the pain?
- Does the pain interfere with your other activities?
- What do you think is causing your pain?
- What have you done to alleviate the pain in the past?

(ELNEC, 2003)

Refer to Chapter 9 for further information regarding the Geriatric Pain Assessment instrument ⊂⊃ and additional tools to assess pain.

PAIN DURING THE DYING PROCESS

Acute pain is associated with sudden onset and often may be correlated with a single cause or event. For instance, an older person may fall and break a hip, resulting in acute-onset bone pain. Often this pain is treated relatively easily, and correction of the underlying pathology or trauma will result in pain resolution. Appropriate analgesia can be used while the healing process is occurring.

Chronic pain is associated with long-term illness designated by a disease or condition that shows minor change, progresses slowly, or is of long-standing duration. The pain is always present to some degree and may worsen at times. As years pass, a pain tolerance becomes a way of life, yet everyone would like to be pain-free, and so medical help is sought. Age affects pain when it is related to past life experiences. Chronic pain is associated with depression, poor self-care, and decreased quality of life. When persons with chronic pain achieve relief through effective pain management techniques, their quality of life is greatly improved and they will begin to smile, move about more often, eat a more balanced diet, and engage in social and recreational activities.

Neuropathic pain occurs when the nerves have been damaged. Diabetic neuropathies and neuralgias are frequently seen in elderly adults. The pain associated with these conditions is often referred to as burning, electrical, or tingling. The pain may be deep and severe and is often very difficult to relieve with routine pain relief medications. At times, anticonvulsants, antidepressants, and opioids are used for pain relief. Cutting of the nerves is a radical technique that may be necessary for complete relief of uncontrolled neuropathic pain.

Nociceptive pain occurs in 70% of nursing home patients and is treated first with generalized pain relievers via titration of the drugs. To treat pain, clinicians will use acetaminophen usually as the first choice, and progress to non-steroidal anti-inflammatory drugs (NSAIDs) followed by opioids. Nociceptive pain is the signal the brain imparts when there is tissue inflammation or damaged tissue. Cardiac ischemia or arthritis and its variations are examples of nociceptive pain (Chamberlain, 2002). See Chapter 9 for a more complete discussion of pain.

EFFECTS OF UNRELIEVED PAIN DURING THE DYING PROCESS

Inadequate pain relief hastens death by increasing physiological stress, potentially diminishing immunocompetency, decreasing mobility, worsening risk of pneumonia and thromboembolism, and increasing the work of breathing and myocardial oxygen requirements. Older adults are often less likely to admit to having pain because of fear of addiction or loss of control. Pain may often present as confusion or agitation in the older person with cognitive impairments. Further, obtaining good pain relief in the older adult is often complicated by the prescriber's lack of knowledge in pain management and fear of prescribing opioids (ELNEC, 2003). Unrelieved pain at the end of life can cause psychological distress to the patient and family and is often associated with negative outcomes such as suffering and spiritual distress.

PRINCIPLES OF PAIN RELIEF DURING THE DYING PROCESS

Various methods of pain control may be used to control pain in the older person. Pharmacological methods require close collaboration between the nurse, the physician, and the pharmacist to use the correct medication, dosing regimen, and route of administration. The World Health Organization (1990) has initiated a model for pain relief that is frequently the basis for the pharmacological approach to pain management (Figure 11-2■). It advocates a stepped approach for pain treatment based on the presence of mild, moderate, and severe or unrelenting pain. Mild pain (patient rated as 1 to 3 on the 0 to 10 scale) should be treated with non-opioid medications with **adjuvant drugs** (antidepressants or muscle relaxers) if the patient has neuropathic pain. Moderate pain (4 to 6 on the pain scale) is treated with low doses of opioids; the use of non-opioids and adjuvants may be continued at this stage. If the pain is severe (7 to 10), higher opioid doses are used. Patients presenting with severe pain should be started at higher doses rather than risking prolonged periods of uncontrolled pain while medications are titrated up from lower doses. Medications should be titrated based on patient goals, requirements for supplemental analgesics, pain intensity, severity of undesirable or adverse drug effects, measures of functionality, sleep, emotional state, and patient's or caregiver's report of the impact of pain on quality of life (ELNEC, 2003).

Studies suggest that many older persons, including long-term care residents, are being undertreated for chronic and end-of-life pain (McClaugherty, 2002). Whatever drugs are chosen, it is important to administer them routinely and not on a prn or as-needed basis in order to prevent the unpleasant experience of the patient perceiving pain and then waiting for pain relief. Long-acting drugs (sustained-release formulations) are ideal because they provide consistent pain relief. Short-acting or immediate-release agents are excellent prn medications and should only be used to control **breakthrough pain**. Breakthrough pain is a sudden worsening of pain that may occur with increased movement or emotional stress, or pain occuring for no apparent reason before the next dose of regularly scheduled medication. Breakthrough pain should be treated promptly to avoid the fear or memory of pain, and to prevent decreased functional ability. Older patients who consistently experience breakthrough pain should have the dosage of their regularly scheduled medications increased to prevent further exacerbations.

Anticipate and treat adverse effects such as nausea and constipation. Most patients on opioids will require laxative/stool softener combinations.

PHARMACOLOGICAL APPROACH TO PAIN MANAGEMENT DURING THE DYING PROCESS

After conducting a complete pain assessment, the nurse shares the information with other members of the healthcare team including the physician, advanced practice nurse, pharmacist, and others. This collaboration is essential to achieve adequate pain control.

The following are types of drugs used to control pain at the end of life:

- **Non-opioids.** Common types of drugs in this category include acetaminophen and NSAIDs. These drugs are very effective for the treatment of mild to moderate pain. They may be used alone or in combination with other medications to enhance their effect. Cautions: Acetaminophen use should be limited to 4 g daily or less in patients with normal liver function to avoid liver damage. It is essential to use with caution in those with liver disease or in heavy drinkers of alcohol. NSAIDs can cause gastric irritation by inhibition of prostaglandin formation. Decreased prostaglandin synthesis results in thinning of the mucous lining that protects the stomach. This may result in gastrointestinal bleeding, especially in the older person. A new class of NSAIDs selectively block the cyclooxygenase-2 (COX-2) enzymes, and there appears to be less risk of gastrointestinal bleeding with these drugs; however, these drugs have been linked to increased risk of heart

FIGURE ☐ **11-2**

World Health Organization three-step analgesic ladder.

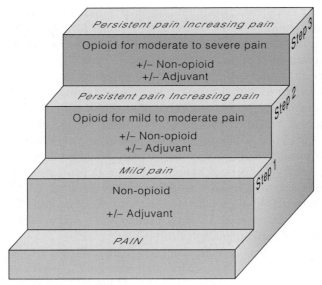

Source: World Health Organization, 1990.

attack and stroke at high doses. The FDA has withdrawn several of these drugs, while others continue to be used with caution.

- **Opioids.** These drugs block the receptors in the central nervous system and prevent the release of chemicals involved in pain transmission. Examples are codeine, morphine, hydromorphone, fentanyl, methadone, and oxycodone. Morphine is considered the gold standard by the World Health Organization for the relief of cancer pain. Adverse effects are rare, and the one most often cited is respiratory depression. This rarely occurs at the end of life. Most often when the respiratory rate is slowed, it is the result of the dying process and not the medication. Constipation and sedation are two troublesome symptoms that are often associated with opioid use. Meperidine and propoxyphene are not recommended for use in the older person because of their ineffectiveness in treating pain and their association with the serious side effects of seizure, delirium, and tremor caused by the accumulation of toxic metabolites.

- **Adjuvant analgesics.** These drugs are given for other reasons. Their effect may be to enhance the effectiveness of other classes of drugs, thus allowing effective treatment of pain at lower doses and less chance of side effects. They may be used at any step of the "analgesic ladder" developed by the World Health Organization (1990), as presented in Figure 11-2. Medications in this class include muscle relaxers, corticosteroids, anticonvulsants, antidepressants, and topical medications.

Routes of Administration

Usually the oral route of administration is preferred because it is the easiest and most comfortable for the patient. However, at times alternative routes of administration offer benefits over the oral route. Pain medication may be administered by the following routes:

- **Oral.** Tablets, liquids, and capsules are administered orally to control pain. Long-acting or sustained-release tablets can control pain for up to 24 hours. Patients who can swallow can use this method until very close to the time of death. Liquid medications can be mixed in juice, and capsules may be opened and the contents mixed with applesauce. Usually a higher dose of medication is needed when given orally because of the first-pass effect or deactivation that occurs when medication passes through the liver. Oral routes may become difficult to utilize near the very end of life when the older person may be unable to swallow.

- **Oral mucosa.** Highly concentrated liquids such as morphine may be given by dropper into the oral or buccal mucosa. The medication can be delivered even when the patient can no longer swallow because the medication is absorbed from the mucosa and swallowing is not necessary. The medication may need to be administered more frequently because of a short half-life and duration of action.
- **Rectal.** Some medications come in suppository form, and the rectal route may be used when the patient can no longer swallow or has problems with nausea and vomiting. The rectal route is invasive. If the patient cannot move easily, the positioning required for suppository insertion may be difficult.
- **Transdermal.** The fentanyl patch may be placed on the skin every 72 hours for relief of pain. Because of changes in blood flow, metabolism, and fat distribution, some patients do not achieve or maintain stable drug levels and adequate pain relief. Peak onset may be delayed up to 24 hours necessitating coverage with short-acting agents during the initial day of treatment.
- **Topical.** Topical capsaicin and local anesthetics (EMLA) can be used for pain associated with herpes and its aftermath, for arthritis pain, and before invasive procedures such as insertion of intravenous medication or injections. Topical medications usually have little systemic absorption when applied as recommended in small amounts to confined areas.
- **Parenteral.** The intravenous, intramuscular, and subcutaneous routes are used when the patient cannot swallow. Usually pain is associated with these methods of administration. If the intravenous route is used, it is important to use the appropriate fluid delivery system and use the smallest amount of fluid possible to minimize excess secretions that require suctioning and cause difficulty breathing.
- **Epidural or intrathecal.** The administration of drugs into or around the spinal cord is reserved for those patients who cannot achieve pain control in any other manner. There is increased cost and risk of infection when these techniques are used.

Addiction need not be feared when treating end-of-life pain. The nurse need not be concerned with the physical dependence problem. However, the patient can build up a tolerance for drugs. What once was effective may no longer be so, especially when the disease worsens. It is important not to undertreat pain. Instead, the reason for the increased pain should be explored, the patient should be medicated promptly, response to medication should be monitored, and other team members should be informed about the effectiveness of the pain relief plan. Family members may express concern about their perception that opioids and other analgesics will cause addiction or mean that death is imminent. Reassurance and explanations concerning the difference between physical dependence and addiction may need to be explored. The goal is to eliminate pain and improve the quality of life. Otherwise, the patient's suffering hinders the quality of life. *The Study to Understand Prognoses and Preferences for Outcomes and Risks of Treatment* (SUPPORT, 1995) showed that more than 50% of people dying in hospitals suffered from uncontrolled pain, and that decisions were inappropriately timed (von Gunten, 2002). Use of opioids requires careful monitoring. They may be used for chronic, nonmalignant pain with the proper diagnosis and care.

> **Drug Alert** !
>
> Dying patients may need more pain medication than the normal range for the prescribed drug. Organic changes are occurring rapidly and systems are closing down, thus, absorption levels of drugs are also diminishing.

Management of Adverse Reaction

By establishing a pain log to determine when the patient's pain is most severe, the nurse may find that the patient needs a different class of medication, an adjuvant drug, or a different dosing schedule. Many drugs will slow the intestinal tract and result in poor bowel elimination. Constipation can be responsible for much pain in older patients, and it is extremely important that the nurse monitor the bowels carefully. Circulation of older adults is often impaired, and drugs may contribute to or help the problem. Extra warmth of lightweight blankets may make the patient comfortable and decrease the pain response. Listen to what the patient tells you when you ask questions to help the patient describe how the pain feels, when the pain occurs, and what might relieve it. The log may indicate the need for other interventions or other types of comforting responses such as a glass of warm milk to promote sleep, a back rub, a change of position, a favorite peaceful musical selection, spending time listening to the patient, and visits from a priest, minister, or rabbi to meet spiritual needs.

NURSING CARE AT THE END OF LIFE

Personal hygiene needs to remain a top priority when providing terminal care. Oral hygiene is crucial. Mouth care should be provided several times a day and whenever the mouth has a foul smell or is uncomfortable for the patient. The nurse may instruct family members to use oral swabs or moistened cloths to help provide oral comfort. Products that have perfume or alcohol can be irritating and drying, and their use is discouraged. Soothing ointments or petroleum jelly may be applied to the lips to help keep them from cracking or drying out. Often, the dying patient relies upon mouth breathing, and the oral mucosa becomes dry and painful. This in turn causes a swallowing problem and impedes clear speech. It is often too uncomfortable for the patient to wear dentures, and thus the facial features change in appearance. Lack of dentures makes speech and swallowing difficult. The disease process itself may contribute to halitosis and even mouth sores. Oral thrush may appear and should be treated. Ice chips to relieve the feeling of dryness may be offered as long as the swallowing reflex is present. To prevent aspiration, the nurse should remind caregivers not to give oral fluids when the patient can no longer swallow. The nurse may choose to use the buccal mucosa route for drop medications or tiny ice chips.

Eye care is provided to promote comfort. Artificial tears or ophthalmic saline solutions may be used to prevent drying of the eyes. Opened or half opened eyelids dry and become irritated. Seeing the eyes half open, red, or puffy may be disturbing to family members.

Anorexia and dehydration are common and normal with the terminal patient. If the patient chooses to refuse food and drink and believes it is time to die, consider this a rational decision and offer emotional and psychological support. A benefit of dehydration is decreased lung congestion, which prevents noisy or labored respirations. If the patient is suffering from multiple tumors, the tumors are less pressured. Oliguria (less than 15 cc of urine produced per hour) is another favorable outcome because the patient does not have to be positioned to use the bedpan or urinal frequently. The patient and family can be reassured that anorexia may result in ketosis and that can lead to a peaceful state of mind and decreased pain. If intravenous fluids are administered, it may be helpful to administer drugs with anticholinergic side effects (atropine) to prevent noisy respirations. By eliminating noisy respirations, the patient is deemed more comfortable and quiet breath sounds eliminate anxiety for the family members.

Skin integrity should be monitored carefully to prevent complications. Edema, bruising, dryness, and venous pooling may appear. A complete bed bath may be impractical and could be given in a divided time frame. The family may feel comfortable applying body lotion to the back or hands of their loved one. The patient may be repositioned by using lift sheets, being careful to avoid shearing forces. Positioning on the side or in a semiprone position may also alleviate noisy respirations, as well as afford a comfortable change of position.

Bowel and bladder incontinence are frequent occurrences at the end of life. Seepage from body orifices may be uncontrolled and it becomes necessary to have protective pads or briefs. It is extremely important to prevent decubitus ulcers from forming at this time since the healing process does not occur. Barrier creams and change of position may also help maintain skin integrity. It is important to avoid the use of indwelling urinary catheters if at all possible because they often are associated with urinary tract infections that can be distressing and painful to the older patient.

Side effects of certain pain medications affect the status of the bowels. Constipation needs to be treated with stool softeners to prevent further pain or bowel discomfort. Nonverbal patients need to be monitored by the nurse. Facial grimacing, moaning, restlessness, or splinting of the abdomen may indicate gastrointestinal problems.

Pharmacological interventions are frequently sought for relief of anxiety. Side effects may include delirium, hallucinations, or increased agitation. It is best to decrease the use of medications not needed for comfort at the end of life. Pain medication and other medication used for comfort measures should be given freely, however.

Visual or auditory hallucinations at the end of life sometimes occur. These hallucinations are usually not frightening to the patient, but the family may be upset if they witness the event. The patient may refer to this as a dream or a strange occurrence.

Eventually, neurological changes occur and the patient slips from a lethargic state into an unconscious state, which may include periods of lucidness, then coma, and finally death. Family members frequently ask how much longer their loved one will live. The anxiety level and general distress of family and friends at this time seems insurmountable. Waiting for death is not an easy task, and time can seem to be an enemy. The exact time of death cannot be predicted any easier than the time of birth. This can be frustrating to those who are at the bedside.

It is prudent to assume that the patient can hear what is being said. It is believed the sense of hearing is intact in obtunded and comatose patients. Those present must not say anything they would not want the patient to hear. The nurse can encourage family members to "let go" and give the terminal patient permission to die. Family members can assure their loved one that they will be OK and thank the person for loving them. Appropriate affection should be encouraged and privacy provided. Table 11-4 summarizes suggested strategies for the management of common symptoms in older patients at the end of life.

Practice Pearl

Read a poem, tell a joke, listen to a past story, sing a song, report on a recent news happening, linger for a moment, or provide a hug. The nurse should be creative and individualize the care for each patient.

TABLE 11–4

Suggested Strategies for the Management of Common Symptoms in Older Patients at the End of Life

Problem	Suggested Nursing Intervention
Constipation	Stimulant such as prune juice, senna, or lactulose. Avoid bulking agents (psyllium) in patients with inadequate fluid intake to avoid impaction. Monitor bowel function. Do not allow the patient to go longer than 3 days without a bowel movement. A mineral oil enema may be necessary to prevent impaction.
Delirium	Treat underlying cause if possible (fever, urinary tract infection, pain). Avoid use of physical restraints, sleep disruption, excessive medications. Urge family to remain with the patient, and have staff frequently visit and speak to and touch the patient. Use alternative interventions like massage and music.
Dyspnea	Treat underlying cause if known (bronchospasm, hypoxia). Administer opioids to slow respiratory rate. Maintain the patient in a sitting position if possible. Minimize exertion by spacing out interventions and treatments. Provide humidified oxygen for comfort. Use alternative interventions like massage and music.
Decubitus ulcers	Use appropriate positioning techniques, changing position every 2 hours. Keep the patient's skin clean and dry. Use special mattress pads to relieve pressure.
Cough	Assess and treat underlying cause such as postnasal drip or obstruction. Use chest physical therapy, cool humidified air, elevate head of the bed, and suction secretions as necessary. Cough suppressants may be used for comfort.
Anorexia and cachexia	The etiology of cachexia is rarely reversible in advanced disease, and aggressive nutritional treatment does not improve survival or quality of life and may create discomfort for the dying patient whose body is shutting down. Provide excellent mouth care. Treat oral problems such as candidiasis (thrush). Treat constipation, nausea, and vomiting if present as underlying causes. Assess the room for problem odors and try to minimize as much as possible. Appetite stimulants such as megestrol acetate (Megace) may improve intake. Generally, parenteral or enteral nutrition is useful only for patients with appetite who cannot swallow. Offer the patient's favorite food and fluids as the patient tolerates.
Nausea and vomiting (N & V)	N & V occurs in up to 70% of patients at the end of life. Causes include metabolic disturbances, visceral disturbances, vestibular problems, medication side effects, emotional upset, and radiation. Assess cause and treat if possible (i.e., remove offending medication). Medications used to treat N & V include anticholinergics, steroids, benzodiazepines, and antinausea drugs (ondansetron and granisetron). Anticipate N & V and administer medications if needed before symptoms occur. Position the patient to prevent aspiration. Use complementary therapies such as music, relaxation, hypnosis, and acupuncture.
Fatigue	Fatigue may be disease related, treatment related, or psychological. If tolerated, exercise can improve function and sleep. Frequent rest periods and transfusions for very anemic patients may improve quality of life.
Anxiety	Anxiety may be a side effect of many medications such as stimulants and corticosteroids, or a paradoxical reaction to analgesics. Antidepressants and benzodiazepines may be beneficial.

Source: ELNEC, 2003; Ross & Alexander, 2001.

NURSING DIAGNOSES AT THE END OF LIFE

Nursing diagnoses (North American Nursing Diagnosis Association, 2002) at the end of life vary according to the unique and individual circumstances surrounding the death of each older person. The following nursing diagnoses may be appropriate for use with older patients in certain situations:

■ *Death anxiety* (for those patients with apprehension, worry, or fear related to death or dying)

- *Imbalanced nutrition: less than body requirements* (for those patients with anorexia and cachexia)
- *Constipation*
- *Urinary/bowel incontinence*
- *Ineffective airway clearance*
- *Risk for aspiration*
- *Impaired oral mucous membrane*
- *Impaired skin integrity*
- *Social isolation*
- *Caregiver role strain*
- *Acute/chronic pain*
- *Nausea*

POSTMORTEM CARE

The nurse's views, knowledge, emotional development, and cultural background help determine how effectively he or she may deal with the death process. Witnessing a death is a privilege. Caring for the dying requires sensitivity to their needs and the needs of the family. Accepting and facing one's own mortality helps to deal with the death of others. The fear or horror of watching death needs to be conquered to prevent those responses from being transmitted to the patient. Death eventually comes to everyone and is an important part of life.

Before death actually occurs, there are many body changes. Mottling of the lower extremities can take place days or hours before the actual death. The so-called death rattle or noisy respirations may appear. This is caused by the buildup of secretions from the nose and mouth. Cheyne-Stokes respirations may announce the impending death. Skin may look dusky or gray, and feel cold or clammy. Eyes may appear discolored, deeper set, or bruised. Watching the body changes can be disturbing to family members. The nurse's approach and explanations of the death process are reassuring to those present. It is extremely difficult to assure the patient or family that death will happen within a certain time frame. Some family members may want to be present when death happens, and others may want to be nearby but not physically present. It is important that the nurse support whatever decision is comfortable for the family and patient. It is not unusual for the dying person to want to be alone and to die quietly with no one present. It can be difficult for the dying person to have loved ones near. Others find it a comfort to have family or staff present. The dying process is as individual as living.

When respirations cease and the stethoscope does not detect breath sounds or heart sounds, the nurse should use the stethoscope or manually check the patient's carotid pulses. Next, the nurse should check the eyes for pupillary light reflex. If there is none of the above, the patient can be pronounced dead. Note the time you observed the occurrence of death and chart appropriately, notify the attending physician of the death, and chart the time of notification as well as any directions. There are certain settings when a nurse may make the death pronouncement. Notify family members of the death and express your condolences. Even if the family is expecting the death, the actual notification of the death comes as a shock and needs to be handled gently and with empathy. If the family is present, they should be allowed sufficient time to spend with the deceased before having the body removed.

One of the most difficult but essential parts of nursing is providing the actual **postmortem care**. It needs to be done promptly, quietly, efficiently, and with dignity. If possible, before death occurs the limbs should be straightened and the head placed on a pillow. If the death is suspicious or occurs outside of a healthcare facility, the coroner may request the body be left undisturbed until an autopsy can be performed. However, most deaths of older people who die in their own homes, hospitals, hospices, and long-term care facilities are not investigated by the coroner.

After the pronouncement, the nurse should glove, remove all tubes, replace soiled dressings, pad the anal area in case of drainage, and gently wash the body to remove any discharges. The body is placed on the back, with head and shoulders elevated on the pillow. The nurse should grasp the eyelashes and gently pull the lids down. Dentures should be inserted. It is important not to tie or secure any body parts as this may cause skin indentations. The nurse should place a clean gown on the body and cover with a clean sheet up to the shoulders. When the body is moved or the extremities repositioned, the body may produce respiratory-type sounds or the chest may appear to rise and fall. This can be alarming, but it is only the sound of air leaving the lungs. The nurse may want to check for respiration sounds again in order to be reassured that the patient is dead. The nurse should gather eyeglasses and prepare necessary paperwork for the removal of the body from the facility; call the funeral home, morgue, or other personnel for the removal of the body; and note the time in the chart as well as who was called and again chart when the body was released and to whom. It is advisable to also note if eyeglasses, dentures, or any personal artifacts were released with the body and to whom they were given. If the facility has a policy to identify the body with an identification tag, it must be secured properly.

DESIGNATIONS OF LEVEL OF CARE

Frail older patients and their families face difficult decisions when nearing the end of life. For some patients, medical treatments offer little or no benefit and at the same time may be painful or increase the burden of living. Nurses, physicians, social workers, clergy, and others may counsel patients and families to make decisions regarding the type and level of care they wish to receive for the remainder of their lives. After the decision has been reached, it is usually noted in the patient's chart so that the entire healthcare team will be aware of the patient's wishes.

- An older patient may be designated to receive **comfort measures only (CMO).** CMO is the preferred choice when the time comes to think of less aggressive treatment and the self-deception of immortality fades. The use of life-sustaining technologies should be reviewed with the seriously ill older patient. If the patient is in an intensive care unit, palliative care and comfort measures may be emphasized. Older persons have a higher comorbidity rate and increased likelihood of having a form of dementia that complicates and makes aggressive care less effective (Baggs & Mick, 2000). Older patients designated as CMO may receive traditional hospice care with all of the efforts of the healthcare professionals focused on quality of life rather than length of life.

The CMO status is usually ordered by the physician or advanced practice nurse when the patient, family, and staff are in agreement that the best care for the patient is not to prolong the dying process, but to keep the patient as comfortable as possible. This does not mean that nursing care or treatments are stopped. Alterations of skin, hydration, continence, activities of daily living, behaviors, and pain control are assessed and treated on a daily basis. Provision of excellent nursing care at the end of life can be a challenge, especially when the family has been told by the physician that "nothing more can be done." The designation of a patient as CMO does not signal the end of care, but rather shifts the focus of care from aggressive treatment of the disease to aggressive nursing interventions to improve function, comfort, and quality of life.

ADVANCE DIRECTIVES

Many Americans are fearful of death and hesitate to discuss end-of-life preferences with their families and significant others. This can be problematic when the older person becomes very ill or incapacitated and the family is consulted for medical decision making. People of all ages should begin to discuss these issues with others who may be called upon to make decisions if serious illness or injury should occur. This should be done in a noncrisis situation when the older person has time to discuss the issue in depth, ask questions, and think about the risks and benefits of various interventions. Some state laws mandate the use of living wills. Others mandate the designation of healthcare proxies. Living wills are documents in which older persons describe their wishes regarding treatment at the end of life. This document must be copied and shared with others to be effective. The physician, nurse, family members, and significant others should have copies of the living will and indicate their willingness to comply with the terms stated therein. Many older people lock the living will in their safety deposit box where it is not accessible by others, and thus the document is not known and cannot be honored. A **healthcare proxy** is a designation of another person (and a backup if the primary proxy is not available) to make decisions for the older person. The older person should then discuss his or her wishes with the proxy to ensure appropriate end-of-life care. The healthcare proxy is only responsible for healthcare decisions should the older person be unable to make the decisions. The healthcare proxy does not have legitimate input into any other areas of the older person's affairs (including financial). Multiple copies of the proxy form should be made and kept by healthcare providers and family members (including the proxies) for easy access if needed.

> **Practice Pearl**
>
> Advance care planning is less traumatic to think about when one is in good health, but is often overlooked. Provide your older patients the opportunity to discuss their end-of-life preferences.

Personal values, past experiences, cultural beliefs, religious preferences, medical knowledge, family orientation, and life experiences all help in determining the end-of-life preferences and formation of **advance directives**. Each older person and his or her family should provide input into treatment decisions based on goals of care, assessment of risk and benefit, best evidence, and personal preferences. A sample healthcare proxy form is provided in Figure 11-3■.

Decision making around the time of death raises legal and ethical questions. Public debate and scrutiny help shape the ethical outcome of medical dilemmas. Healthcare professionals must work within the limits of the law and their professional standards of practice. Established ethical principles and moral norms play a vital role in determining healthcare issues.

In 1976, the Karen Ann Quinlan case brought life-sustaining medical treatment to the forefront of the U.S. legal system. A medical intervention, procedure, or administration of medicine to prevent the moment of death is seen as life sustaining. This includes cardiopulmonary resuscitation (CPR), renal dialysis, use of ventilators, insertion of feeding tubes, total parenteral nutrition, chemotherapies, and other life-prolonging interventions.

FIGURE ■ 11-3

A sample health care proxy form.

Health Care Proxy

(1) I, _____

hereby appoint

_____

(name, home address and telephone number)

_____

_____

as my health care agent to make any and all health care decisions for me, except to the extent that I state otherwise. This proxy shall take effect only when and if I become unable to make my own health care decisions.

(2) **Optional: Alternate Agent**

If the person I appoint is unable, unwilling or unavailable to act as my health care agent, I hereby appoint

_____

(name, home address and telephone number)

_____

_____

as my health care agent to make any and all health care decisions for me, except to the extent that I state otherwise.

(3) Unless I revoke it or state an expiration date or circumstances under which it will expire, this proxy shall remain in effect indefinitely. *(Optional: If you want this proxy to expire, state the date or conditions here.)* This proxy shall expire *(specify date or conditions):*

_____

_____

(4) **Optional:** I direct my health care agent to make health care decisions according to my wishes and limitations, as he or she knows or as stated below. *(If you want to limit your agent's authority to make health care decisions for you or to give specific instructions, you may state your wishes or limitations here.)* I direct my health care agent to make health care decisions in accordance with the following limitations and/or instructions *(attach additional pages as necessary):*

_____

_____

In order for your agent to make health care decisions for you about artificial nutrition and hydration *(nourishment and water provided by feeding tube and intravenous line),* your agent must reasonably know your wishes. You can either tell your agent what your wishes are or include them in this section. See instructions for sample language that you could use if you choose to include your wishes on this form, including your wishes about artificial nutrition and hydration.

(5) **Your Identification** *(please print)*

Your Name _____

Your Signature _____ Date _____

Your Address _____

FIGURE ■ **11-3** *(continued)*

Health Care Proxy (continued)

(6) **Optional: Organ and/or Tissue Donation**

I hereby make an anatomical gift, to be effective upon my death, of: (check any that apply)

☐ Any needed organs and/or tissues

☐ The following organs and/or tissues _____

_____

☐ Limitations _____

If you do not state your wishes or instructions about organ and/or tissue donation on this form, it will not be taken to mean that you do not wish to make a donation or prevent a person, who is otherwise authorized by law, to consent to a donation on your behalf.

Your Signature _____ Date _____

(7) **Statement by Witnesses** *(Witnesses must be 18 years of age or older and cannot be the health care agent or alternate.)*

I declare that the person who signed this document is personally known to me and appears to be of sound mind and acting of his or her own free will. He or she signed (or asked another to sign for him or her) this document in my presence.

Date   Date

_____   _____

Name of Witness 1   Name of Witness 2

(print) _____   *(print)* _____

Signature _____   Signature _____

Address _____   Address _____

_____   _____

Source: New York State, 2003.

When questions regarding the initiation, ongoing use, and removal of life-sustaining technologies arise and there are no advance directives in place, ethical and emotional issues will arise. Many hospitals and long-term care facilities have formed ethics committees to address these issues and provide guidance and advice to the clinician, patient, and family. If the patient lacks a responsible family member, the courts may appoint a legal guardian. This is a cumbersome and difficult process and may be avoided by naming a healthcare proxy or completing a living will.

In 1990, the U.S. Supreme Court declared that all Americans have a right to make healthcare decisions. Even if a patient is deemed incompetent or unable to make his or her own decisions, the patient's previous wishes become the determining factor concerning care. The Patient Self-Determination Act became a federal law in 1991. This act states that the patient must be informed that medical treatment, care, procedures, medicines, and other similar acts may be refused. It also states that patients are to be informed of their right to prepare advance directives.

Most healthcare institutions have developed policies concerning self-determination that comply with specific state laws. It is necessary that the interdisciplinary team form a collaborative relationship with the patient and family in providing proper care as determined by the state statutes. When the patient is unable to make decisions, the healthcare team must consider the patient's diagnosis, the benefit or burden of treatment, the effect on the prognosis, and expressed verbal patient preference. The healthcare team must determine if there are family members or other concerned individuals or surrogates to include in the decision-making process. Reevaluation must be ongoing as the patient's situation changes throughout the entire course of treatment. Although a patient's decision-making capacity may be fluctuating or limited, the nurse should seek input from the patient whenever possible and the family if appropriate. The patient at times may be able to understand some of the medical situation and even provide or express preferences through nonverbal communication.

USE OF FEEDING TUBES FOR ARTIFICIAL NUTRITION

Patients with life-limiting, progressive illness often experience a decline in appetite, loss of interest in eating and drinking, and weight loss. Some patients may experience dysphagia, which also decreases oral intake. At some point in the illness trajectory, most patients will be unable to take food and fluids by mouth or will refuse food, including their favorite foods. These changes can cause distress, especially for families and other caregivers, and raise questions about artificial nutrition and hydration.

The decision to implement artificial nutrition and hydration should consider probable benefits and burdens of the therapy. Artificial nutrition and hydration has traditionally been used to meet several therapeutic goals: (1) prolong life, (2) prevent aspiration pneumonia, (3) maintain independence and physical function, and (4) decrease suffering and discomfort at the end of life. However, these goals are not supported in the literature. Artificially delivered nutrition does not protect against aspiration and in some patient populations may actually *increase* the risk of aspiration and its complications. Finally, research has shown that artificial nutrition and nutritional supplements do not enhance frail elders' strength and physical function (ELNEC, 2003; Hallenbeck, 2002; HPNA, 2003).

Many families are fearful that their loved ones are hungry and are "starving to death." Contrary to expectations, however, most actively dying patients do not experience hunger even if they have inadequate caloric intake. Collaboration with other healthcare professionals like nutritionists and speech therapists is indicated to explore alternatives to artificial nutrition techniques.

Older patients who feel strongly that they do not want tube-feedings should inform their healthcare proxies of this fact and specify this in their living wills. Administration of artificial nutrition and hydration is considered a medical treatment and thus can be accepted or rejected by the patient. This right reflects respect for patient autonomy.

Cardiopulmonary resuscitation (CPR) is administered to a person who is suffering cardiac or respiratory arrest. It is seen as a very acceptable form of intervention, and there are even portable defibrillators available to the public in malls and on airplanes. The decision to designate an older person with a do not resuscitate (DNR) order is usually made by the older person, his or her family, the nurse, physician, and others on the healthcare team. In most facilities, the physician or primary healthcare provider must write the DNR order in the chart for it to be a legal order. In many facilities if no order is written, by default CPR must be administered if the need arises. However, CPR offers no medical benefits to the patient who is terminally ill. It can be very upsetting for the nurse to provide CPR to the ill older adult, and the patient may suffer injury from anoxia, broken ribs, and aspiration.

When the nurse approaches the older patient and the family for clarification of the patient's code status, it is best to discuss the issue fully and as objectively as possible. Facts should be presented with empathy and by conveyance of the idea that the nurse will support whatever reasonable decision is made. Emphasize that making someone a

DNR is *not* condemning that person to die. Rather, you are helping the person decide if in the final moments of life, medical involvement *might* reverse the death process and even prohibit a peaceful death. The letting-go process may be painful for both the patient and the family. Hope is not being taken away when one decides to choose DNR status, since CPR is often a futile, invasive act that offers little chance of success for the older patient.

MERCY KILLING OR EUTHANASIA

Mercy killing, or euthanasia, is presently not legal in any state, but there are frequent bills by legislators and much public debate concerning this issue. Oregon does allow physician-assisted suicide. Other states may approve of the physician helping the patient intentionally take his or her life. The American Nurses Association does not endorse the concept of or participation of nurses in the process of euthanasia, mercy killing, or assisted suicide (American Nurses Association, 1994).

There are rare occasions when a medication given for pain relief may have the unintended consequence of shortening the patient's life span. This is not considered mercy killing. The intent was the relief of pain, not to hasten death, as occurs with euthanasia.

CULTURAL ISSUES

The United States is composed of people from various cultural and ethnic backgrounds. Sensitivity and empathy are essential when caring for a dying person from another culture. Although the cultural preferences may influence the needs of the dying patient, the family, and the caregivers themselves, each older person is a unique individual with specialized needs. (See Chapter 4 for a thorough discussion of culture.) ⸛

Cultural preferences and economics may influence the patient's choices of where and when to seek care. Some older people may choose to die at home; others may choose to die in hospitals, long-term care settings, or hospices on the basis of cultural preferences. Some family members may hope to provide care to their loved one, but finances, inability to cope with the responsibility of caregiving, or family obligations may hinder the decision. All settings should provide support, comfort, and privacy for the dying patient. Provisions should be made for family members to stay at the bedside if they so choose and if the patient is comfortable with the family being there. Some patients prefer to die alone and are uncomfortable with others hovering about them.

Several cultures accept hospitalization for end-of-life care, but there is mistrust of the healthcare system in general. Krakauer et al. (2002) reported a fear of denial of care and racism by minority patients. Older African American patients and their families often choose more aggressive life-prolonging treatment such as feeding tubes and CPR out of fear of being denied healthcare similar in scope to that of Caucasians.

Religion plays an important role in the forming of beliefs and practices that are paramount when death is imminent. Feelings of guilt, remorse, comfort, or peacefulness may all be related to religious beliefs. Religious customs are extremely important to many dying patients, and concerns may be intensified. It is helpful to know the religious preference of an individual, but each patient's spiritual reactions to situations will be different. Requests by family or patients to seek spiritual counseling should be met with respect. Many healthcare facilities have chaplains, clergy, social workers, and others to assist staff. Spiritual care should be individualized and made available to the terminal patient.

At times, the religious belief may help the patient in determining the type of end-of-life care to request. Nurses must be aware of concerns the patient may have and respond therapeutically. The age-old question of why this is happening may take on religious tones or thoughts. Punishment, atonement, God's will, or hope for a miracle may all be discussed or alluded to by the patient. Follow the patient's lead in determining spiritual needs and beliefs. Serious illnesses frequently bring a search for life's meaning. Questions arise as to the individual's purpose in life. Even the emotional response to pain may be influenced by religious or spiritual beliefs.

When discussing religion or spirituality with the patient, it is important to assist the patient to seek meaning. Nurses who feel unable to assist older patients in discussions of spirituality should make referrals to others on the team with skills and knowledge in this area. Spiritual care interventions that may be chosen by the older person to affirm life and hope include renewal of vows, faith readings, guided meditation, receiving sacraments, spiritual life review, and discussion of spiritual pain (ELNEC, 2003).

It is common for one of Catholic faith to wish to receive the Sacrament of the Sick to give spiritual strength and prepare for death. A religious item such as a rosary or medal may bring comfort. The Jewish believer may want to see a rabbi and participate in prayers. Burial is performed as soon as possible and before the Sabbath. Muslims prefer that a family member be notified as soon as death occurs. It is best to wait for the member since there are special washing and shrouding procedures. Islam believers also prefer that the family wash the body. The body is then placed in a position that faces Mecca. If there is no family member to prepare the body, the staff may do so provided that gloves are worn. Cremation is not accepted, and burial of the body takes place as quickly as possible. Table 11-5 summarizes some religious beliefs and rituals practiced at the end of life.

PREPARING FOR DEATH

The knowledge or presumption that death is imminent may cause anxiety for the staff, family, and patient. Watching the patient decline and the body itself starting to shut down life processes can bring feelings of helplessness and anxiety. The nurse must help alleviate the fears and anxiety of the patient and the family. Questions of an afterlife, unresolved emotional or social issues, concerns centered around family members and their acceptance of death, and financial matters are common problems. Nurses must also remember to support themselves through this difficult period and may need to recognize and accept personal feelings. Feelings are neither good nor bad but are simply part of each person. The nurse may need individual support as well as team support from outside the healthcare facility in order to express true feelings and accept them. By doing this, burnout may be prevented.

Hope should never be taken away from the dying patient and family. It is difficult to leave the only life one knows and is certain of. Hoping to be cured or to "get better" is not unusual for both the patient and family members. The patient may hope for small things to make the present situation more tolerable. It is not unusual for patients to hope to speak with or see certain people before they die. The will to live is extremely strong in many older patients, especially when confronting death and unfinished business in life. Older patients sometimes need reassurance from their families and caregivers that all is well and it is OK to let go.

GRIEF

Although death may be expected, it is usually met with shock by those left behind. Rationalizations (e.g., he lived a long life) may help ease the initial numbness of the actual death. Relief statements, such as the person is no longer in pain, may help the bereaved to cope with the immediate loss. The grieving process is considered diffi-

TABLE 11-5

Religion and End-of-Life Care

Religion	Belief	Ritual
Christian	Christians believe in an afterlife and the resurrection of Jesus Christ.	Catholic • Anointing the sick by a priest. • Reconciliation and communion. • Funeral held 2 to 3 days after death. Protestant • No last rites. • Anointing of the sick by some. Others • Mormons will administer a sacrament. • Jehovah's Witnesses will not receive blood transfusions. • Some sects have hands-on healing techniques.
Judaism	Death confers meaning to life.	Euthanasia is prohibited. Burial usually takes place within 24 hours. The funeral or shiva is held after the burial. Autopsy, organ donation, and cremation are not allowed. A rabbi is usually called when death is near.
Muslim	Muslims believe in an afterlife. The purpose of worldly life is to prepare for eternal life.	As death approaches, the patient is positioned supine facing Mecca. The room is perfumed, and anyone who is unclean leaves the room. Prayer occurs five times a day. Discussion of death and grief counseling are discouraged. Euthanasia is not allowed by law. Organ donation is allowed. Autopsy is discouraged.
Buddhist	Belief in the afterlife through the pursuit of perfection in worldly life.	End-of-life decisions are made with much family consultation. Families often do not want the patient to know diagnosis in order to hide bad news. The elderly do not talk about funeral arrangements and often defer to physicians to make treatment decisions for them.

Source: Kirkwood, 1993; Ross, 2000; Cheng, 1997.

cult work that lasts for years, and it truly is hard to endure at times. Past death experiences, emotional health, religious beliefs, and support of friends and family all are factors that may help to ease the grief process. Bereavement is the process one undergoes after a loss. **Grief** is the emotion felt after the loss. The recovery from the loss is referred to as the period of **mourning**.

A child views the death process differently than an adult. The death of a grandparent may be the child's first exposure to personal death. A young child may not understand the permanence of death. Allowing the child to express fears or ask questions will help with the grief process. The child may need to visit and interact with the dying person. The nurse may need to encourage positive interaction to help the child begin the grief process (Krohn, 1998). Young children may not understand that death is permanent, but view death as a temporary state. It may be necessary for the parents to show a young child that when something dies it does not come back. Children may see an actor die in a television show, only to be seen on a different channel in a new feature. Thus, death may be misunderstood, as well as the feelings associated with it.

The child from age 5 to 9 years may personify death. Fears and nightmares may occur. The understanding that death is final appears around age 7 to 8. By the time the child reaches 10 or 11, there is understanding of illness, accident, congenital diseases, and similar things that are often viewed as a normal occurrence by the child. Helping the child to understand that death is a natural part of life is extremely important. Leo Buscaglia's book, *The Fall of Freddie the Leaf,* may help prepare the child and adult for the actual death. Reading non frightening stories about death may prove beneficial for all. The question of the actual existence of ghosts may also need to be discussed with children. This is an opportunity to discuss religious beliefs and family values. Children's fears, such as is this going to happen to them when they become ill, need to be addressed. The child may feel abandoned by a favorite relative. Reassure the child it is good to remember the deceased and encourage him or her to express feelings. Reminiscence therapy provides outstanding support for all ages.

The widow or widower experiences grief for many years. Phases of grief include:

First phase: numb shock. The widow cannot believe the spouse's death occurred. This phase is marked by a restless behavior that includes stupor and withdrawal. It may include physical characteristics such as nausea or insomnia. One wants to protect self from the feeling of loss.

Second phase: emotional turmoil. Alarm or panic-type reactions occur. Anger, guilt, or longing for the deceased take place.

Third phase. When the full effects of widowhood set in, so do regret, self-doubt, and at times, despair. Life's purpose becomes confusing and mood swings are prevalent. Being alone in the house may be a major problem.

Fourth phase: reorganization. Eventually takes place and coping strategies and positive outlooks emerge (Hegge & Fischer, 2000).

CARING FOR THE CAREGIVER

Most nurses enter the profession to make a difference in others' lives. However, to prevent feelings of stress and burnout, those caring for the dying need support and an opportunity to express emotional responses and grief. A periodic self-assessment might be beneficial to the nurse providing end-of-life care. Some questions may include:

- What have I done to meet my own needs today?
- Have I laughed today?
- Did I eat properly, rest enough, exercise, and play today?
- What have I felt today?
- Do I have something to look forward to?

Caring for oneself prevents anger, frustration, and anxiety. It makes it possible to continue to be a sensitive caregiver. It is important not to neglect personal needs.

The art of healing requires knowing and nourishing oneself. Giving to others, treating patients with dignity and respect, and being compassionate to them are trademarks of a nurse. Patients give these same gifts back, and help instruct the nurse how to care. The partnership of caring and receiving becomes gifts given and received.

Patient and Family Teaching

Gerontological nurses require skills and knowledge related to teaching patients and families about the key concepts of gerontology and gerontological nursing. The patient-family teaching guidelines in the following feature will assist the nurse to assume the role of teacher and coach. Educating patients and families is critical so that nurses can interpret scientific data and individualize the nursing care plan.

Patient-Family Teaching Guidelines

CHOICES AT THE END OF LIFE

The following are guidelines that the nurse may find useful when instructing older persons and their families about their choices at the end of life.

1. I am seriously ill. My physician has recommended a palliative care program. Does that mean I am dying?

No, not at all. Palliative care is a program of care that can be delivered to any person who is seriously ill. Palliative care programs have been developed to provide for pain and symptom control, to help with patient-centered communication and decision making, and to coordinate care across settings. Aggressive care and palliative care can be delivered at the same time by your healthcare provider, thus ensuring your comfort during the treatment process.

RATIONALE:

Older patients and their families may require reassurance when they are considering choosing palliative care programs as they are relatively new and may not be completely understood. The principles of palliative care should be clearly delineated to prevent misunderstanding and confusion.

2. How is palliative care delivered?

The main approach is the management of pain and distressing symptoms like nausea, bowel function, sleep, and nutrition. A team of healthcare experts will address your needs, including physicians, nurses, social workers, nutritionists, pharmacists, chaplains, and others. Because a person with serious illness has a variety of needs, it takes a team of experts to deliver quality care.

RATIONALE:

Older patients and their families may be unfamiliar with the roles and expertise of various persons on the healthcare team. A coordinated team approach with good communication between members is essential to the provision of palliative care.

3. Does my insurance cover palliative care?

Many insurance programs do cover the delivery of palliative care, and more are beginning to examine the payment of this service as a benefit for patients and families. In the long run, it may actually decrease costs to the healthcare system because it has the potential to decrease hospitalization for many things that can be prevented by the palliative care focus such as pain, dehydration, infections, constipation, and other symptom problems.

RATIONALE:

Potential payment sources for palliative care services can include Medicare, Medicaid, private insurance, out-of-pocket payment, and community funds for uninsured patients. It is important check with social worker colleagues to ensure that patients have accessed all possible funding sources for palliative care.

4. What is the difference between hospice and palliative care?

Generally, hospice programs accept patients who are near the end of life and are no longer receiving aggressive disease interventions like chemotherapy and radiation. However, many hospice programs are expanding services and accepting patients who are not near the end of life but may benefit from the principles of palliative care, including the emphasis on pain and symptom control, while they are still receiving aggressive treatment for their illness. Most palliative care programs will help you and your family to receive the care you need in a variety of settings, including your home, the hospital, the nursing home, or a hospice if you need that kind of care.

RATIONALE:

The healthcare system is dynamic and complex. The patient and family may move in and out of various care settings as their condition changes over time. The integration of a palliative care program into a coordinated system is a big plus for patients and families. Most palliative care programs can make referrals to other care providers and coordinate services and movement between settings. These settings may include acute care hospitals, palliative care programs, home care agencies, and hospice programs.

Care Plan

An Older Person at the End of Life

Case Study

Mrs. Lodge is a 79-year-old woman who is admitted to the nursing home after a 6-day hospitalization for pneumonia and weight loss. She had previously lived at home alone. Her hospital discharge record notes that she has lost 15 lb over the last 6 months and had complained of abdominal pain while in the hospital. A computerized tomograph (CT) scan noted a pancreatic mass, which was thought to be cancer of the pancreas. Other chronic conditions include hearing loss, type 2 diabetes, cataracts, and osteoarthritis. Today, Mrs. Lodge is lethargic and appears withdrawn. Her 58-year-old daughter is present and seems anxious about her mother's condition. Mrs. Lodge's daughter would like to take her home when her condition improves.

Applying the Nursing Process

ASSESSMENT

Mrs. Lodge has been diagnosed with a very aggressive form of cancer that usually carries a high treatment burden and a poor prognosis. In addition to her age, she has diagnoses that indicate frailty, including cataracts, weight loss, osteoarthritis, and diabetes. Based on this information, she could be considered a candidate for palliative care services or a hospice referral (depending on her physician's assessment of her prognosis).

DIAGNOSIS

The current nursing diagnoses for Mrs. Lodge include the following:

- Imbalanced nutrition: less than body requirements
- Pain: chronic (osteoarthritis) and acute (pancreatic cancer)
- Altered activity levels
- Fatigue
- Compromised family coping

EXPECTED OUTCOMES

Expected outcomes for the plan of care specify that Mrs. Lodge will:

- Achieve satisfactory pain relief.
- Be free from disabling symptoms associated with the end-of-life trajectory, including constipation, nausea, and disturbed sleep.

An Older Person at the End of Life

- Overcome her fatigue and lethargy as much as possible so that she has the opportunity to engage in discussion with her healthcare providers, daughter, significant others, and clergy (if appropriate) regarding her end-of-life decisions.
- Receive a hospice referral (if appropriate) so that services can be provided to allow Mrs. Lodge to die in her daughter's home if this is consistent with Mrs. Lodge's wishes.

PLANNING AND IMPLEMENTATION

The following nursing interventions may be appropriate:

- Establish a therapeutic relationship.
- Conduct initial and ongoing pain assessment with use of pharmacological and nonpharmacological relief measures.
- Encourage a family meeting with daughter and other family members present to discuss end-of-life planning and care with Mrs. Lodge's permission.
- Consult with other members of the interdisciplinary team to evaluate safety, nutrition, spiritual needs, psychological status, and other key parameters.
- Begin a values clarification to establish goals and facilitate end-of-life planning.

EVALUATION

The nurse will consider the plan a success based on the following criteria:

- Mrs. Lodge will achieve pain and symptom relief.
- A family meeting will be held to discuss her overall health.
- Mrs. Lodge will have access to appropriate services and family support in order to achieve a peaceful death in the setting of her choice.

Ethical Dilemma

As you are preparing to institute a hospice referral, another daughter who lives in a distant state telephones you and says that she feels her mother should receive aggressive chemotherapy to fight the cancer and possibly extend her life. The oncologist has agreed to begin chemotherapy, although he advises that the regimen will be quite toxic with little chance of success. Mrs. Lodge and her daughter who is involved in her care are unsure of what to do, but based on the advice of the palliative care nurse, and others on the healthcare team, they decide to refuse further chemotherapy. The nurse and the palliative care team are supporting the decision to refuse treatment based on the oncologist's recommendation and Mrs. Lodge's preferences. She is competent to make her own decisions regarding treatment, and her refusal of treatment is appropriate to her unique circumstance and immediate family situation.

Critical Thinking and the Nursing Process

1. Speak to nurses and nursing assistants who work in one of your clinical rotations about the assessment of pain in the older patient. What factors do they identify as important?

(continued)

An Older Person at the End of Life *(continued)*

2. Explain possible reasons caring for older patients at the end of life may be difficult. Tell a story in a small group of fellow students and observe their reactions.
3. Keep a clinical journal of your feelings and experiences as you begin to become proficient in providing end-of-life care to older people and their families.
4. Identify a few key people in your life who can help you as you struggle to become proficient in the provision of end-of-life care.

■ Evaluate your responses in Appendix B. ⊂▭

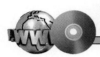

EXPLORE MediaLink

NCLEX review, case studies, and other interactive resources for this chapter can be found on the Companion Website at **www.prenhall.com/tabloski**. Click on Chapter 11 to select the activities for this chapter. For animations, video tutorials, more NCLEX review questions, and case studies, access the accompanying CD-ROM in this textbook.

Chapter Highlights

■ Studies have documented that the American healthcare system has substantial shortcomings in the care of seriously ill patients and their families.

■ Many older patients die in pain or suffering from adverse symptoms.

■ Aggressive care that carries a high burden of treatment is often delivered inappropriately to older people because of communication barriers and lack of planning.

■ The gerontological nurse can play a key role on the interdisciplinary team and serve as patient advocate, educator, care provider, and planner of quality end-of-life care.

■ Pain and symptom control are crucial to the delivery of quality end-of-life care.

■ Cultural and ethnic variations are key factors to be considered when providing end-of-life care.

■ Palliative care and hospice programs can assist the nurse in the delivery of quality end-of-life care to older patients and their families.

■ Families often rely on the nurse for support and assistance during the dying process and afterwards in the mourning and grieving period.

References

Administration on Aging. (2000). *Older population by age: 1900 to 2050*. Retrieved January 15, 2001, from www.aoa.dhhs.gov.

American Geriatrics Society. (1998). The management of chronic pain in older persons. *Journal of the American Geriatrics Society, 46*(5), 635–651.

American Nurses Association. (1994). *Position statement: Assisted suicide*. Retrieved April 14, 2002, from http://nursingworld.org.

American Nurses Association. (1995). *Social policy statement*. Washington, DC: Author.

American Pain Society. (1999). *Principles of analgesic use in the treatment of acute pain and cancer pain*. Glenview, IL: Author.

Baggs, J., & Mick, D. (2000). Collaboration: A tool addressing ethical issues for elderly patients near the end of life in intensive care units. *Journal of Gerontological Nursing,* September, 41–46.

Blackhall, L., Frank, G., Palmer, J., Murphy, S., Michel, V., & Azen, S. (1999). Ethnicity and attitudes toward withholding and withdrawing medical care. *Social Science and Medicine, 48,* 1979–1989.

Buscaglia, L. (1983). The *Fall of Freddie the Leaf.* Henry Holt and Company.

Cassell, C., & Foley, K. (1999). *Principles of care of patients at the end of life: An emerging consensus among the specialties of medicine.* New York: Millbank Memorial Fund.

Chamberlain, B. (2002). For those who practice pain management in the trenches. In C. Tollison, J. Satterwaite, and J. Tollison (Ed.), *Practical pain management (3rd ed.).* Philadelphia, PA: Lippincott & Wilkins.

Cheng, B. (1997). Cultural clash between providers of majority culture and patients of Chinese culture. *Journal of Long-Term Health Care, 16*(2), 39–43.

Corr, C. (1998). Death in modern society. In D. Doyle, G. Hanks, & N. MacDonald (Eds.), *Oxford textbook of palliative medicine* (2nd ed.). New York: Oxford University Press.

Crowther, C., & Edmunds, M. (2000). *Death and dying: Basic concepts for the clinician.* Washington, DC: American College of Nurse Practitioners National Clinical Symposium.

Dembner, A. (2004, September 14). Hospices widen care services. *Boston Globe,* B24.

Education on Palliative and End-of-Life Care (EPEC) Project. (1999). Retrieved August 13, 2001, from www.epec.net. Chicago: Author.

End-of-Life Nursing Education Consortium (ELNEC). (2003). Care Curriculum. American Association of College of Revising and City of Hope National Medical Center, Los Angeles, City.

Ersek, M., Kraybill, B., & Hansberry, J. (2000). Assessing the educational needs and concerns of nursing home staff regarding end-of-life care. *Journal of Gerontological Nursing,* October, 16–25.

Feudtner, C. (2000). *Dare we go gently. Journal of the American Medical Association, 284,* 1621–1622.

Field, M., & Cassel, C. (1997). *Approaching death: Improving care at the end of life.* Report of the Institute of Medicine Task Force. Washington, DC: National Academy Press.

Hallenbeck J. (2002). Fast facts and concepts #10: Tube feed or not tube feed? *Journal of Palliative Medicine, 5* (6), 909–910.

Hartford Institute for Geriatric Nursing. (1999). *Best nursing practices in care for older adults. Pain/palliation in older adults.* Retrieved September 12, 2004, from www.hartfordign.org.

Hegge, M., & Fischer, C. (2000). Grief responses of senior and elderly widows: Practice implications. *Journal of Gerontological Nursing, 26*(2) February, 35–43.

Hospice and Palliative Nurses Association (HPNA). (2003). *Value of professional nurse in end of life care. Position statement.* Retrieved November 1, 2004, from www.hpna.org.

Joint Commission on Accreditation of HealthCare Organizations. (2000). *Pain standards.* Retrieved August 23, 2002, from www.jcaho.org.

Kirkwood, N. (1993). *A hospital handbook on multiculturalism and religion.* Sydney, Australia: Millennium Books.

Knox, J. (2001). *Death and dying.* Philadelphia: Chelsea House.

Krakauer, E., Crenner, C., & Fox, K. (2002). Barriers to optimum end-of-life care for minority patients. *Journal of the American Geriatrics Society, 50,* 182–190.

Krohn, B. (1998). When death is near: Helping families cope. *Geriatric Nursing, 19,* 276–278.

Kübler-Ross, E. (1969). *On death and dying. What the dying have to teach doctors, nurses, clergy, and their own families.* New York: MacMillan.

Kyba, F. (1999). Improving care at the end of life: Barriers, challenges and resources. *Texas Nursing,* September, 6–13.

Labyak, M. (2001). Ten myths and facts about hospice care. Hospice care part I: A policymaker's primer. *State Initiatives in End-of-Life Care, 11,* Last Acts, 3.

Last Acts. (2002). *Means to a better end: A report on dying in America.* Retrieved April 14, 2003, from www.lastacts.org.

Lewis, L. (2002). Should patients with advanced dementia be tube fed? *Caring for the Ages,* July, Vol. 2, 17–18.

Lunney, J., Lynn, J., Fole, D., Lipson, S., & Guralnik, J. (2003). Patterns of functional decline at the end of life. *Journal of the American Medical Association, 289*(18), 2387–2392.

Lynn, J. (1997). Unexpected returns: Insights from SUPPORT. In S. Isaacs & J.R. Knickman (Eds.), *To improve health and health care: The Robert Wood Johnson anthology.* San Francisco: Jossey-Bass.

May, C. (2002). Do you have an advance directive? *Nursing Spectrum,* July 15, Vol. 7, 5.

McClaugherty, L. (2002). Chronic pain: We're undertreating the elderly. *Nursing Homes,* August 01, 79–86.

National Consensus Project (NCP) for Quality Palliative Care. (2004). *Clinical practice guidelines for quality palliative care.* Retrieved September 14, 2004, from www.nationalconsensusproject.org.

National Hospice and Palliative Care Organization. (2000). *Hospice fact sheet.* Alexandria, VA: Author. Retrieved September 14, 2002, from www.nhpco.org.

New York State. (2003). *Health care proxy. Information for consumers.* Retrieved November 9, 2004, from www.health.state.ny.us/nysdoh/hospital/healthcareproxy/instructions.htm.

North American Nursing Diagnosis Association. (2002). *Nursing diagnoses: Definitions and classification.* Philadelphia: Author.

Phillips, R. S., Wenger, N. S., Teno, J., Oye, R. K., Youngner, S., Califf, R., et al. (1996). Choices of seriously ill patients about cardiopulmonary resuscitation: Correlates and outcomes. *American Journal of Medicine, 100*(2), 128–137.

Quill, T. (2000). Perspectives on care at the close of life. Initiating end-of-life discussions with seriously ill patients: Addressing the "elephant in the room." *Journal of the American Medical Association, 284* (19), 2501–2507.

Robert Wood Johnson Foundation. (2000). *Pioneer programs in palliative care: Nine case studies.* New York: Milbank Memorial Fund.

Rosen, J. (1995, January 22). Rewriting the end: Elisabeth Kubler-Ross. *New York Times Magazine,* 22, 24–25.

Ross, D., & Alexander, C. (2001). Management of common symptoms in terminally ill patients: Part II. Constipation, delirium and dyspnea. *American Family Physician, 64*(5) September, 1–11.

Ross, H. (2000). *Islamic tradition at the end of life.* Unpublished manuscript.

Somogyi-Zalud, E., Likurrezos, A., Chichin, E., & Olson, E. (2001). Surrogate decision makers' attitudes towards tube feeding in the nursing home. *Archives of Gerontology and Geriatrics, 31,* 101–111.

Steinhauser, K. E., & Christakis, N. (2000). Factors considered important at the end of life by patients, family, physicians and other care providers. *Journal of the American Medical Association, 284*(19), 2476–2482.

SUPPORT Principal Investigators. (1995). A controlled trial to improve care for seriously ill hospitalized patients. The study to understand prognoses and preferences for outcomes and risks of treatment. *Journal of the American Medical Association, 274*(20), 1591–1598.

Tilden, V. (1998). *Dying in America: Ethics and end-of-life care.* Phoenix, AZ: Proceedings from the Communicating Nursing Research Conference and the Western Institute of Nursing Assembly.

von Gunten, C. (2002). Secondary and tertiary palliative care in U.S. hospitals. *Journal of the American Medical Association, 287,* 875–881.

von Gunten, E. (1999). *The education for physicians on end-of-life care curriculum.* Medical College of Wisconsin, Modules 1-10 Retrieved June, 12,1999, from www.EPERC. MCW.EDU.

Wilson, S., & Daley, B. (1999). Family perspectives on dying in long-term care settings. *Journal of Gerontological Nursing, 25*(11), November, 19–25.

World Health Organization. (1990). *Cancer pain relief and palliative care (Technical Report Series, 804).* Geneva, Switzerland: Author.

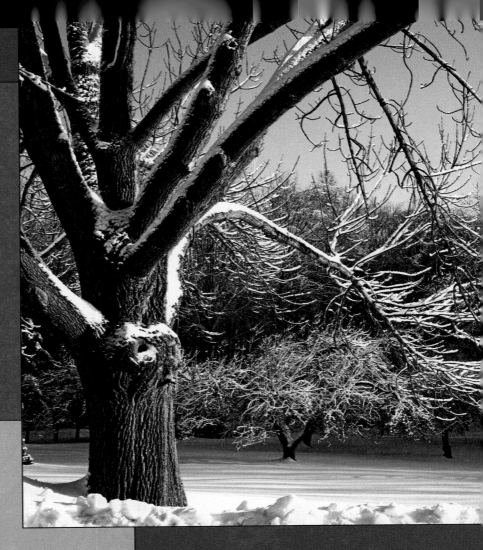

Physiological Basis of Practice

CHAPTER 12

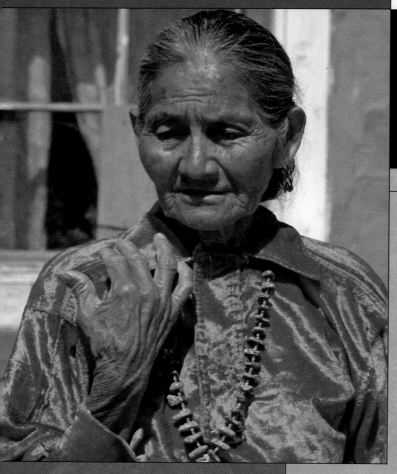

The Integument

Rita Olivieri, RN, EdD

CHAPTER OBJECTIVES

Upon completion of this chapter, the reader will be able to:

- **Describe normal skin changes associated with aging.**
- **Identify risk factors related to common skin illnesses of older persons.**
- **Delineate skin changes associated with benign and malignant skin changes.**
- **List nursing diagnoses related to common skin illnesses.**
- **Discuss the nursing responsibilities related to pharmacological and nonpharmacological treatment of common skin illnesses.**
- **Explain the nursing management principles related to the care of pressure ulcers.**

KEY TERMS

actinic keratosis 336
actinic keratotic lesions 336
autolytic debridement 355
cellulitis 335
chemical debridement 354
debridement 354
desquamation 329
extrinsic factors 341
friction 334
intrinsic factors 341
mechanical debridement 354
melanocytes 337
photoaging 336
pressure ulcer 335
sebum 330
senile purpura 334
sharp debridement 354
shearing forces 338

MediaLink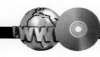

Additional resources for this chapter can be found on the Student CD-ROM accompanying this textbook and on the Companion Website at **www.prenhall.com/tabloski**. Click on Chapter 12 to select the activities for this chapter.

CD-ROM
- Animation/Video
    Pressure Ulcers
    Skin Cancer
- NCLEX Review
- Case Studies
- Tools

COMPANION WEBSITE
- Audio Glossary
- Additional NCLEX Review
- Case Study
- MediaLink Applications

The skin comprises between 15% and 20% of body weight. It has three layers, the epidermis, dermis, and subcutaneous layers. The epidermal accessory structures, or appendages, are downgrowths of the epidermal layer and include the hair, nails, and sweat glands. The skin, along with the accessory structures, is considered the integumentary system. The skin covers the entire body and protects it from external forces such as microorganisms, traumatic injury, and sun exposure. In addition, it prevents loss of body fluid, synthesizes vitamin D, regulates normal body temperature, and provides both touch and pressure neuroreception. The overall health of a person is often reflected by assessment of skin color, texture, warmth, general appearance, and overall grooming. Obvious changes in the skin and hair are an inevitable part of aging that lead to changes in a sense of self as well as how the individual is perceived by others. When these changes, such as graying of hair and wrinkling of the skin, are viewed as negative, considerable time and money may be spent on efforts to alter these outward appearances by using cosmetics and hair coloring. An important part of the nurse's role is to teach the older person techniques that will minimize and treat changes that are associated with aging and the skin's exposure to environmental hazards.

Usual Structure and Function of Skin Layers

The skin is the largest organ of the body and is formed in major layers. These layers include the epidermis, dermis, and hypodermis.

EPIDERMIS

The epidermis of the skin has up to five layers and is continually regenerating and shedding in a process called **desquamation.** The major cells of the epidermis, the keratinocytes, produce keratin, which provides the tough outer barrier of the skin. Langerhans' cells reside in the keratinocytes and provide immune protective function. Ultraviolet radiation may damage Langerhans' cells, decreasing their ability to protect the skin against cancer. At the junction of the epidermis and dermis are melanocytes. These produce melanin, which gives the skin its color and shields the body from the harmful effects of the sun. Skin tone results from the size and quantity of melanosomes (granules in the melanocyte) and the melanin activity rate. Persons with dark skin have larger melanosomes and more active melanin production than those with lighter skin. Skin also derives a reddish tone from the vascular bed that is located in the dermis (Corwin, 2000; Huether & McCance, 2000).

DERMIS

The dermis, the second layer of the skin, is made up of connective tissue and is rich in blood supply, lymph, and neurosensory receptors. The dermis provides nourishment and support for the epidermis, which does not have its own blood supply. This is the thickest skin layer and contains fibroblasts, mast cells, and lymphocytes. The white elastin fibers and yellow fibrous collagen produced by the fibroblasts provide strength to the skin and give it the ability to stretch during movement. Dermal ground substances retain water and play a role in skin turgor. Sensory nerve endings in the dermis provide responses to temperature, touch, pressure, and pain.

HYPODERMIS

The subcutaneous layer, or superficial fascia, is specialized connective tissue that lies beneath the dermis and attaches to the muscles below. This layer also contains blood vessels, lymphatic channels, hair follicles, and sweat glands that extend from the dermis as well as adipose or fat tissue. Fat tissue gives shape to the body and provides cushioning for the bones, protection for delicate internal organs, and insulation from extremes in temperature. Subcutaneous fat is most abundant on the lower back and buttocks and is absent on areas such as the eyelids and tibia. The amount of fat tissue is dependent on age, gender, and hereditary factors. This layer also contains blood vessels, lymphatic channels, hair follicles, and sweat glands that extend from the dermis.

Dermal Accessory Structures

Accessory structures of the skin include the hair, nails, and glands and together with the skin account for 20% of the body's weight. Each accessory structure has a unique purpose and function.

HAIR

Hair color, distribution, thickness, and texture vary greatly based on age, gender, and race as well as overall health. Hair is located on all skin surfaces except the soles of the feet and the palms of the hands. Each strand of hair grows independently in a cyclic fashion and can differ in its rate of growth depending on its location on the body. At any given time, about 10% of the hair on the scalp is in the resting phase. Hair develops from the mitotic activity of the hair bulb that is located in the dermal layer of the skin. As hair grows up the follicle, it becomes differentiated and is fully hardened by the time it reaches the skin surface. Hair growth occurs up the dermis at an angle. When the body temperature drops, the erector pili muscles contract and hair "stands up on end," creating "goose bumps." Hair color, like skin color, is related to the melanin production in the hair follicle (Corwin, 2000).

NAILS

Nails are rapidly dividing extensions of the keratin-producing epidermal layer of the skin. The crescent-shaped portion of the nail that is located at the proximal end of the nail plate is the nail matrix. In the nail matrix, specialized, nonkeratinized cells differentiate into keratinized cells, which form nail protein. Fingernail protein grows up the nail from the nail matrix at about .1 mm per day. Toenails grow at a slower rate.

GLANDS

Sebaceous glands are found on most skin areas with the exception of the palms of the hands and the soles of the feet. They are most abundant on the face, head, and chest. Sebaceous glands are usually associated with a hair follicle, forming a pilosebaceous unit. These glands secrete **sebum**, an oily substance that keeps hair supple and lubricates the skin. Sebum protects the skin from water loss and provides protection against infection.

Apocrine sweat glands are large glands that produce a milky substance that causes odor when bacteria that is present on the skin act upon it. These glands begin functioning after puberty and require a high level of sex hormone activity for functioning. They are found primarily in the axillary, perineum, and breast areolae.

Eccrine glands produce sweat, a dilute form of plasma. Sweat production from the eccrine glands is stimulated by exercise, heat (forehead, neck, chest), and psychic origins (palms of the hands, soles of the feet, axillae). Thus, they play an important role in regulating the heat and cooling of the body.

Usual Functions of the Skin

The skin is an amazing organ that protects the entire body from external environmental hazards. It contributes to the immune function, regulates temperature, and provides the vehicle for vitamin synthesis and sensory reception for the central nervous system.

REGULATION OF BODY FLUIDS AND TEMPERATURE

The skin contains epithelial cells that provide a barrier that prevents insensible loss of body fluids from the deeper layers of the skin and the internal organs. The epithelial cells also provide selective transport of nutrients and body wastes, and have a semi-regulated permeability to water. Damage to the skin, due to injuries such as burns, may result in life-threatening loss of this protective function.

The epidermis of the skin provides the vehicle for radiation, conduction, and convection of heat from the body. Blood vessels in the dermis help to regulate body temperature by dilating during warm temperatures and constricting during cold. The hypothalamus plays a role in maintaining an approximate core temperature of 37°C by regulating dermal blood flow to the extremities, as well as some facial areas. Body temperature in an older person is usually lower. During periods of intense exercise, or periods of increased external temperature, additional cooling mechanisms are needed. At these times, the eccrine glands produce large volumes of sweat that contribute greatly to the overall ability of the body to regulate temperature. The subcutaneous tissue provides insulation to retain body heat.

REGULATION OF THE IMMUNE FUNCTION

Intact skin is an important barrier to prevent infection from bacterial invasion and other microorganisms. Skin is not only a physical barrier, but also an important part of the body's immune response against various antigens. The cells that provide this specialized function are Langerhans' cells and keratinocytes in the epidermis, and lymphocytes in the dermis. These cells make it possible for a healthy skin surface to neutralize an attack against various antigenic substances. However, if the skin is damaged or diseased, it may be possible for an antigen to induce an immune response and cause inflammation or infection to occur (Huether & McCance, 2000).

PRODUCTION OF VITAMIN D

The epidermal layer of the skin provides the vehicle for the synthesis of vitamin D. A complex steroid called a sterol is present in the malpighian cells (7-dehydrocholesterol) and is activated by ultraviolet light to produce vitamin D. Vitamin D is important in the absorption of calcium and phosphorus from food.

SENSORY RECEPTION

General sensory receptors located in the skin provide the central nervous system with information about changes in the external environment. When stimulated, these specialized receptors detect touch, pressure, temperature, and pain. For example, Merkel disks in the epidermis detect light pressure, Meissner's corpuscles in the dermis detect light and discriminative touch as well as vibration, and Pacini's corpuscles in the subcutaneous tissue detect deep pressure. Figure 12-1■ illustrates these corpuscles and their distribution in the skin.

FIGURE ■ 12-1

Corpuscles and their
distribution in the skin.

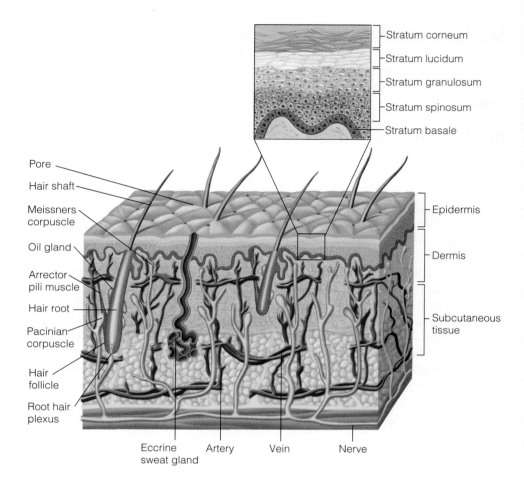

FIGURE ■ 12-1

Corpuscles and their
distribution in the skin.

- Stratum corneum
- Stratum lucidum
- Stratum granulosum
- Stratum spinosum
- Stratum basale

Pore
Hair shaft
Meissners corpuscle
Oil gland
Arrector pili muscle
Hair root
Pacinian corpuscle
Hair follicle
Root hair plexus

Epidermis
Dermis
Subcutaneous tissue

Eccrine sweat gland   Artery   Vein   Nerve

Normal Changes of Aging

Although changes occur in all of the body systems throughout life, skin and hair changes are the most visible and therefore greatly contribute to a person's self-perception and self-esteem. With normal aging, there is a decrease in the thickness and elasticity of the skin. These changes occur slowly, but by the seventh and eighth decade of life, they contribute to the appearance of wrinkled and sagging skin in the face, neck, and upper arms. The age-related changes in the skin's appearance correlate with changes in function. Exposure and damage by the sun, known as *actinic damage,* also affect the aging appearance of the skin. It is important for the older person to understand the normal changes, as well as environmentally induced damage, to decrease risk factors and minimize negative consequences. The decrease in melanocytes and a person's genetic makeup determine the graying pattern of hair. Figure 12-2■ illustrates normal changes of aging in the integumentary system.

EPIDERMIS

The epidermal cells of the older person contain less moisture. This contributes to a dry, rough skin appearance. After 50 years of age, epidermal mitosis slows by 30%, resulting in a longer healing time for the older person. This increased healing time also may be a contributing factor for infection. Rete ridges, which connect the dermis and epi-

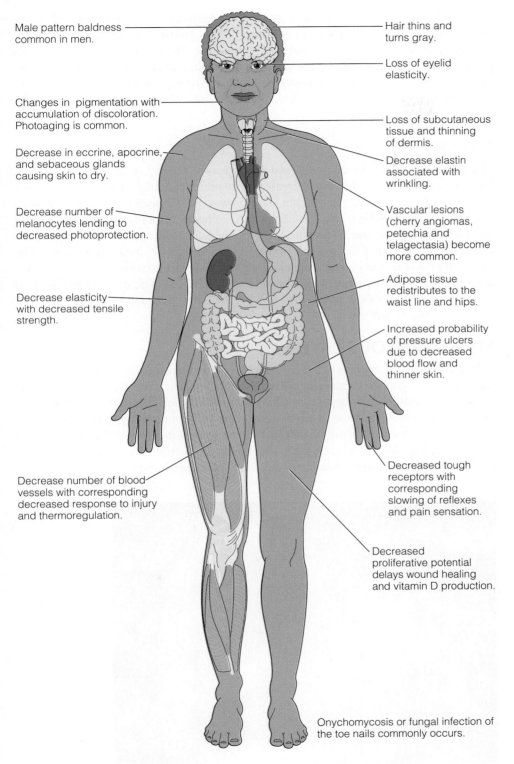

Male pattern baldness common in men.

Changes in pigmentation with accumulation of discoloration. Photoaging is common.

Decrease in eccrine, apocrine, and sebaceous glands causing skin to dry.

Decrease number of melanocytes lending to decreased photoprotection.

Decrease elasticity with decreased tensile strength.

Decrease number of blood vessels with corresponding decreased response to injury and thermoregulation.

Hair thins and turns gray.

Loss of eyelid elasticity.

Loss of subcutaneous tissue and thinning of dermis.

Decrease elastin associated with wrinkling.

Vascular lesions (cherry angiomas, petechia and telagectasia) become more common.

Adipose tissue redistributes to the waist line and hips.

Increased probability of pressure ulcers due to decreased blood flow and thinner skin.

Decreased tough receptors with corresponding slowing of reflexes and pain sensation.

Decreased proliferative potential delays wound healing and vitamin D production.

Onychomycosis or fungal infection of the toe nails commonly occurs.

FIGURE ■ **12-2**

Normal changes of aging in the integumentary system.

dermis, flatten, resulting in fewer contact areas between these two layers. This increases the risk for skin tears when seemingly slight **friction** occurs against the skin. Melanocytes decrease in number and activity with age. This contributes to a paler complexion and an increased risk for damage from ultraviolet radiation for the light-skinned older person. The remaining cells may not function normally, resulting in scattered pigmented areas such as nevi, age spots, or liver spots and an increase in the number and size of freckles.

DERMIS

The dermis decreases in thickness and functionality beginning in the third decade. Elastin decreases in quality but increases in quantity, resulting in the wrinkling and sagging of the skin. Collagen become less organized and causes a loss of turgor. Men have a thicker dermal layer than women, which explains the more rapidly apparent age-associated changes in the female facial appearance. The vascularity of the dermis decreases and contributes to a paler complexion in the light-skinned older person. The capillaries become thinner and more easily damaged, leading to bruised and discolored areas known as **senile purpura** as depicted in Figure 12-3■. There is a gradual decline in both touch and pressure sensations, causing the older person to be at risk for injury such as burns and pressure sores.

SUBCUTANEOUS LAYER

With increasing age, there is a gradual atrophy of subcutaneous tissue in some areas of the body, and a gradual increase in others. Subcutaneous tissue becomes thinner in the face, neck, hands, and lower legs, resulting in more visible veins in the exposed areas, and skin that is more prone to damage. Some other areas of the body have a gradual hypertrophy of subcutaneous tissue that leads to an overall increase in the proportion of body fat for the older person. Overall, with aging, fat distribution is more pronounced in the abdomen and thighs in women, and in the abdomen in men.

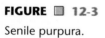

FIGURE ■ 12-3

Senile purpura.

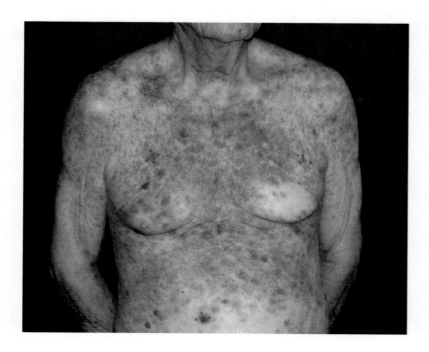

HAIR

The hair of the older person looks gray or white due to a decrease in the number of functioning melanocytes and the replacement of pigmented strands of hair with nonpigmented ones. The texture and thickness of the hair also changes, becoming coarse and thin. Hormones decline, resulting in gradual loss of hair in the pubic and axillary areas and the appearance of facial hair on women and hair in the ears and nose of men. By age 50, many older men have experienced a gradual loss of hair and often develop a symmetrical W-shaped balding pattern. Women have less pronounced hair loss than men. The actual age when graying and hair loss begins, as well as the pattern of baldness, is determined in part by a person's genetic makeup. However, many 50-year-olds have gray, or partly gray, scalp hairs.

NAILS

The nails of the older person become dull, and yellow or gray in color. Nail growth slows, which results in thicker nails that are likely to split. Longitudinal striations also appear due to damage at the nail matrix.

GLANDS

With aging, there is a decrease in the size, number, and function of both eccrine and apocrine glands. The decrease in eccrine or sweat glands results in a decrease in the older person's ability to regulate body temperature through perspiration and evaporation from the skin. As the ability to sweat decreases, the older person may be unable to control body temperature by the normal sweating mechanism, and therefore is at a high risk for heat exhaustion.

SEBACEOUS GLANDS

The sebaceous glands increase in size with age, but the amount of sebum produced is decreased. The decrease in sebum hastens the evaporation of water from the stratum corneum, which results in cracked, dry skin.

Common Illnesses of Older Persons

Some of the common illnesses of the older person include skin cancer, skin tears, **pressure ulcer**, delayed skin healing, **cellulitis**, and fingernail and toenail problems.

SKIN CANCER

Although a tan is often admired and the person with it is thought to look attractive and healthy, a tan is a protective response of the body to damage caused by the sun. Tanning is a sign of skin damage. The skin never "forgets" the damage done by exposure to ultraviolet radiation (UVR). In fact, several sunburns over the course of a lifetime can double the risk for developing melanoma later in life (Skin Cancer Foundation, 2001b). A tan may be attractive, but the cumulative effect of sun exposure throughout a lifetime leads to premature aging and increases the risk for skin cancer. UVR is responsible for approximately 90% of nonmelanoma skin cancers (Skin Cancer Foundation, 2001b).

The combination of normal age-related changes and UVR-related damage is a complex issue and not entirely understood. However UVR-related skin damage is thought to be distinct from the normal aging process. UVR may also accelerate the extrinsic and intrinsic skin changes of aging.

MediaLink Skin Cancer Video

There are two important types of UVR: UVA and UVB. Both have been implicated in skin cancer. UVA rays are responsible for deep skin penetration, cause premature aging, and may also decrease immune system function. One source estimates that up to 90% of skin changes attributed to aging are caused by sun exposure (Centers for Disease Control, 2002).

The older person who has spent a lot of time outdoors, either working or at leisure, may have long-term UVR damage known as **photoaging.** These changes occur on exposed areas such as the face, neck, arms, and hands and include freckling, loss of elasticity, damaged blood vessels, and a general coarse and weathered appearance. Continued damage may result in the development of a precancerous lesion, **actinic keratosis**, which can progress to skin cancer.

Skin cancer is the most common type of cancer in the United States (Greenlee, Murray, Boldem, & Wingo, 2000). As a person ages, the incidence of skin cancer increases, especially for those between 50 and 80 years of age. This is because older persons have had more time to be exposed to UVR, and the ability to repair damage caused by the sun has diminished. Both basal cell carcinoma and squamous cell carcinoma are more common in individuals over 55 years of age. Pigmented spots that bleed easily and are enlarging characterize these carcinomas.

Skin cancers that primarily result from sun exposure are basal cell carcinoma, squamous cell carcinoma, and malignant melanoma (Schober-Flores, 2001). The risks for skin cancer seem to be associated with the type of sun exposure. Intense, intermittent exposures, such as severe sunburns, are associated with both basal cell carcinoma and malignant melanoma. The risk for squamous cell carcinoma is strongly associated with chronic sun exposure but not with intermittent exposure (Centers for Disease Control, 2002).

ACTINIC KERATOSIS

The most common precancerous lesion is actinic keratosis, also known as solar keratosis and senile keratosis. **Actinic keratotic lesions** are more common in men than women. It is estimated that 1 in 1,000 will progress to skin cancer, usually squamous cell carcinoma, in a 1-year period. Erythematous actinic keratosis is the most common type and appears as a sore, rough, scaly, erythematous papule or plaque. Other types of actinic keratosis include hypertrophic and cutaneous horn. The most common sites for all types of actinic keratosis are sun-exposed areas such as the hands, face, nose, tips of the ears, and bald scalp (Leber, Perron, & Sinni-McKeehan, 1999).

Basal cell carcinoma is the most common form of skin cancer in Caucasians and accounts for about 80% of nonmelanoma skin cancers. Basal cell carcinoma can extend below the skin to the bone, but metastasis is rare. This cancer originates in the lowest layer of the epidermis and appears as small fleshy bumps (Figure 12-4■). Basal cell carcinoma can occur on any exposed skin surface but is frequently found on the head, neck, nose, and ears.

Squamous cell carcinoma is the second most common form of skin cancer in Caucasians and represents the remaining 20% of nonmelanoma skin cancers. It is the most common form of skin cancer in persons with dark skin. Squamous cell carcinoma originates in the higher levels of the epidermis. It appears as flesh colored to erythematous, indurated scaly plaques, papules, or nodules and may have ulceration or erosions in the center (Figure 12-5■). Metastasis can occur and is more common in lesions of the mucous membranes, such as the lips, and in individuals with a history of inflammatory

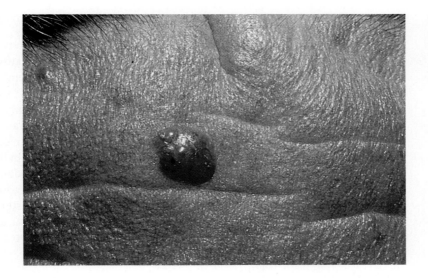

FIGURE ■ 12-4

Basal cell carcinoma.

disease, immune suppression, or exposure to chemicals and other hazardous substances (Schober-Flores, 2001).

Melanoma is the most serious of skin cancers. It is estimated that 53,000 persons were diagnosed with melanoma in 2001, accounting for 7,400 deaths. Melanoma is responsible for more than three quarters of all skin cancer deaths (American Cancer Society, 2002). About one half of melanomas occur in those over 50 years of age. Melanoma originates in the **melanocytes** and may grow from an existing mole or a new lesion. The moles or lesions may enlarge; become brown, black, or multicolored; develop nodules or plaques; and have a black, irregular outline that spreads. The lesions may crust or bleed and are usually greater than 6 mm in diameter. The most common type of melanoma, the superficial spreading type, accounts for 70% of the melanomas and is commonly found on the upper back on men and women and the lower legs of women. The risk factors for melanoma include a family or past history of melanoma, light skin and hair, a history of severe sunburns, or numerous atypical moles.

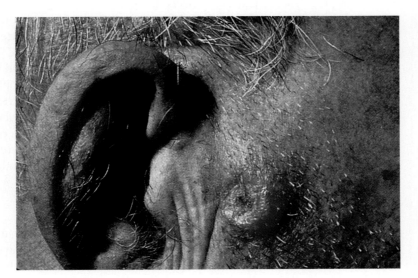

FIGURE ■ 12-5

Squamous cell carcinoma.

SKIN TEARS

A skin tear is a traumatic separation of the epidermis from the dermis, occurring primarily on the extremities of older persons. Skin tears can be caused by friction alone, or by a combination of **shearing forces** and friction. The nurse caring for a frail older person may remove an adhesive dressing from an intravenous insertion site, which may result in a skin tear on the thin vulnerable epidermis. These painful injuries can also occur with simple activities such as dressing, transferring, turning, or lifting. Independent older persons frequently sustain skin tears in the lower legs by bumping into chairs, beds, tables, or open dresser drawers in their home environment. Skin tears may be accompanied by ecchymosis and edema because of subcutaneous tissue atrophy. This is particularly true in those areas of the skin at risk such as the face, hands, shins, and feet. A three-category system, the Payne-Martin Classification for Skin Tears, can be used to assess, plan, and document outcomes of skin tear care. The categories, which are based on the amount of epidermal loss, are:

1. Skin tears without tissue loss.
2. Skin tears with moderate to large tissue loss.
3. Skin tears with complete tissue loss (Baranoski, 2001).

PRESSURE ULCERS IN THE OLDER PERSON

Pressure ulcers affect more than 1 million people each year. The majority of pressure ulcers occur on persons over 70 years of age. The costs associated with treatment of these millions of pressure ulcers is between $5 billion and $8.5 billion each year (Beckrich & Aronovitch, 1999). Based on a comprehensive review of the literature, the Agency for Health Care Policy and Research (AHCPR) published guidelines for all clinicians (AHCPR, 1992; Bergstrom et al., 1994). Van Rijswijk and Braden provided a review and update of the guidelines in 1999. The AHCPR guideline panel advises each agency to develop a team to monitor the quality of pressure ulcer prevention and care (Bergstrom et al., 1994). One of the first tasks of the team is to determine the scope of the pressure ulcer problem by measuring pressure ulcer incidence and prevalence. Incidence reflects the number of patients who develop a pressure ulcer while at a specific agency. Prevalence reflects the total number of patients with pressure ulcers on any given day at the agency. AHCPR reported that the incidence of pressure ulcers in hospital settings was from 2.7% to 29.5%. The prevalence rates were from 3.5% to 29.5% (Agency for Healthcare Research and Quality, 2003). Prevalence rates increase dramatically for high-risk groups of hospitalized patients. These include patients with quadriplegia, orthopedic patients with fractures, patients admitted to the critical care unit, and older patients admitted with a fracture of the neck of the femur. In all patient care environments, individuals more than 65 years old are considered at high risk for developing pressure ulcers. One source reports that over 66% of older people with hip fractures develop pressure ulcers (Boynton, Jaworski, & Paustian, 1999).

Definition and Stages of Pressure Ulcers

A pressure ulcer is defined as a lesion caused by unrelieved pressure that results in damage to underlying tissue. Pressure ulcer formation often occurs on the soft tissue over a bony prominence, although it can occur on any tissue that is exposed to external pressure for a length of time that is greater than capillary closing pressure.

The stages of pressure ulcers and the general guidelines for nursing management are presented in Table 12-1. The actual layers of the skin and depth of each stage are presented in Figure 12-6 ■.

The purpose of defining the specific stages of pressure ulcers is to have a standard for the documentation of clinical data in order to study the best practices and outcomes. Although the stages of a pressure ulcer describe a lesion that begins on the external surface of the skin and progresses inward, this is not always the case in clinical practice.

A review of the research literature by Nixon (2001) clarified the three different types of pressure ulcers and three different pathophysiological mechanisms that lead to pressure ulcers. The three types of pressure ulcers are:

1. A necrosis of the epidermis or dermis, which may or may not progress to a deep lesion.
2. A deep or malignant pressure ulcer where necrosis is observed initially in the subcutaneous tissue and tracks outward.
3. Full-thickness wounds of dry black eschar (Nixon, 2001).

The three types of pressure ulcers are thought to be distinct. The first, necrosis of the epidermis or dermis, may be caused by friction against the skin. An example might be if a sheet is pulled from under a patient, causing damage to the epidermis. The second type of pressure ulcer, malignant or deep pressure ulcers, occurs from an unrelieved

TABLE 12-1

Pressure Ulcer Stages and Management

Stage	Wound Cleaning/ Definition	Debridement	Change Dressing Choices	Frequency*
I	Nonblanchable erythema of intact skin		Transparent film; adherent hydrocolloid	q 3–7 days prn
II	Partial-thickness skin loss involving epidermis, dermis, or both	Normal saline or approved cleaner	Transparent film, hydrogel, hydrocolloid	q 3–7 days prn 3× week q 3–7days prn
III	Full-thickness skin loss involving damage or necrosis of subcutaneous tissue that may extend down to, but not through, underlying fascia	Normal saline or approved cleaner If necrotic tissue present, debridement must be done	1. Wet-to-dry saline dressings; or hydrogel, moistened gauze or calcium alginate 2. Cover with gauze, or foam wafer 3. Use least irritating taping method	q 4–6 h prn q 3–7 days prn q 12 h prn
IV	Full-thickness skin loss with extensive destruction, tissue necrosis, or damage to muscle, bone, or supporting structures	Same as stage III	Same as stage III	

*Change frequency depends on amount and type of drainage present. Read specific product instructions.
Source: AHCPR, 1994.

FIGURE ■ 12-6

Layers of the skin and depth of each ulcer.
I. Skin does not blanch but is intact.
II. Partial-thickness skin loss of the dermis and epidermis.
III. Full-thickness skin loss involving damage or necrosis of the subcutaneous tissue that may extend down to but not through the underlying fascia.
IV. Full-tissue skin loss with extensive destruction extending to muscle, bone, or supporting structures.

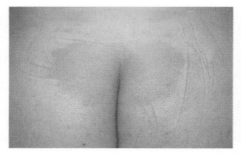

Stage I

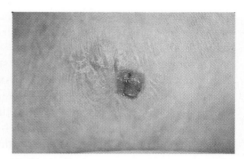

Stage II

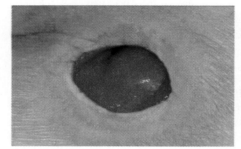

Stage III

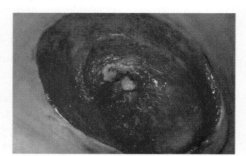

Stage IV

Source: Karen Lou Kennedy-Evans, RN, CS, FNP. Used with permission.

pressure over a long period of time. This type of ulcer begins deep in the subcutaneous tissue and tracks outward toward the dermis. Studies have shown that a significant number of pressure ulcers occur on patients undergoing surgical procedures lasting 3 hours or more. For example, hip fractures are largely a problem for older adults and have a 30% occurrence of pressure ulcers (Beckrich & Aronovitch, 1999). The third type of pressure ulcer, full-thickness wounds of dry black eschar, appear in areas that were previously normal, and occur due to chronic arterial narrowing and inadequate tissue perfusion. When a stage IV pressure ulcer occurs, it is not clear which tissue layer has the primary ischemic injury (Nixon, 2001).

Pathophysiological Mechanisms

Three mechanisms lead to tissue breakdown, although research in this area is limited because of the difficulty in replicating the clinical situation. The first mechanism is the occlusion of blood flow to the skin and the subsequent injury when the occlusion is removed and there is an abrupt reperfusion of the ischemic vascular bed. The second mechanism is caused by damage to the lining of the arterioles and smaller vessels due to the application of disruptive and shearing forces. This mechanism seems to be consistent with the most common body sites affected by pressure ulcers, the sacrum and trochanter. Sliding down in the bed from a sitting position causes disruptive shearing forces and results in damage to the underlying subcutaneous muscle or deep dermis in the sacral area. The trochanter site may be exposed to long periods of external pressure if the patient has not been moved or turned at appropriate times or is in the same position for a long time during surgery. The third cause of pressure ulcers is direct occlusion of the blood vessels by external pressure for a prolonged time period, resulting in cell death. The development of black eschar is usually seen in the lower limbs of patients where the skin is thin, and close to a bony prominence. These individuals usually have a history of arterial narrowing over a long period of time (Nixon, 2001).

Etiology of Pressure Ulcers

The general etiology of a pressure ulcer is the intensity and duration of pressure as well as the tolerance of the skin and its supporting structures to pressure. Changes in the skin and supporting structures due to the aging process are significant predictors for a pressure ulcer. In addition to normal age-related skin changes, older people have to cope with a myriad of both acute and chronic illnesses. Over 80% of people over 65 have one or more chronic diseases. Many patients over 75 have to cope with three of more chronic health problems (Boynton et al., 1999). Chronic health problems such as immobility, malnutrition, or declining mental status increase the risk for pressure ulcers. However, the particular variables that determine the actual development of a pressure ulcer will be unique to each person.

Tissue Tolerance: Extrinsic Factors. **Extrinsic factors** that affect the skin tolerance to pressure forces include shear, friction, moisture, and skin irritants. Pressure is the primary force that occludes blood flow and causes tissue damage, but shearing forces are also an important factor in the development of pressure ulcers. Shearing, the sliding of parallel surfaces against each other, occurs most commonly when the patient slides down in the bed. Shearing forces reduce the amount of pressure needed to occlude the blood vessels by up to 50%. Friction, which occurs with the lateral movement of pulling sheets or clothing from under a person's weight, may remove the stratum corneum, which could disrupt the epidermis and lead to a pressure ulcer. Various skin irritants, such as starch, soaps, and detergents, affect tissue tolerance by removing sebum, which normally protects the skin. The skin then may become dehydrated, decreasing its resistance to other irritants and bacteria.

Tissue Tolerance: Intrinsic Factors. **Intrinsic factors** that affect tissue tolerance and lead to skin breakdown include two major areas. The first is the structure and function of the skin and surrounding structures, and the second is the ability of the vascular system to provide circulation to the skin. Intrinsic factors that affect skin integrity include changes in collagen, advancing age, poor nutrition, and steroid administration. Factors that affect the ability of the vascular system to provide adequate perfusion to the skin include blood pressure, smoking, skin temperature, and vascular disease. Collagen seems to play an important role within the skin structure by protecting microcirculation and preventing damage from pressure. The total collagen content of the skin falls gradually after the age of 30, with a dramatic loss of collagen after 60 years of age. Nutritional factors associated with pressure ulcer development include decreased body weight, decreased serum albumin, and anemia (McLaren & Green, 2001).

WOUND HEALING

The process of wound healing is complex and continuous. It involves three major phases or stages:

1. Inflammation and destruction
2. Proliferation
3. Maturation

Inflammatory Phase

The inflammatory phase of healing in partial- and full-thickness wounds lasts about 5 days and is characterized by the classic symptoms of inflammation: redness, heat, pain, and edema or swelling. The damaged tissues release histamine and other chemicals, resulting in vasodilation. This enhances blood supply to the area, provides additional nutrients, and promotes tissue rebuilding. Neutrophils and macrophages control bacteria and remove debris from the wound. Macrophages also secrete growth factors, such as growth factor beta, that are essential for the initiation and control of wound repair.

Proliferation Phase

Proliferation, the second phase of healing, begins soon after injury and continues for up to 3 weeks. This phase is responsible for rebuilding the damaged tissue by three processes: epithelialization, granulation, and collagen synthesis. In a shallow or partial-thickness wound, viable hair follicles often provide the main source for epidermal regeneration. Epidermal cells migrate across the wound surface and cover and protect it from bacteria. This process of reepithelialization continues to cover the wound base in layers until the area has a normal epidermal thickness. For deeper wounds, healing takes much longer because hair follicles are lost and the wound margins provide the only source for epidermal cell regeneration.

In full-thickness wounds, granulation tissue is formed by new blood vessels and collagen strands. The support matrix of collagen provides strength to the new tissues. Oxygen, vitamin C, dietary amino acids, and trace elements are essential in this process. Granulation tissue becomes beefy red and grainy in appearance as the capillary bed builds. Wound healing usually fills in from the wound bottom so the depth decreases before the wound width is decreased (Stotts, 2001).

Maturation Phase

The last phase of healing for a full-thickness wound is maturation. This phase begins about 3 weeks after the injury and may last for up to 2 years. The process of collagen synthesis continues and the wound becomes thicker and more compact. Another part of the healing process, called contraction, results in a healed scar much smaller in size than the original wound. This process, initiated by myofibroblasts, is an important healing mechanism for wounds with tissue loss because it decreases the area to be healed. The wound is initially dark red in color and, over time, fades to a silver-white color. The scarred area never reaches the strength of the prewound tissue and is therefore more prone to reinjury than normal tissue.

Delayed Healing

The following are signs of delayed healing:

- Wound size is increasing.
- Exudate, slough, or eschar is present.
- Tunnels, fistula, or undermining has developed.
- Epithelial edge is not smooth and continuous and does not move toward wound.

A wound that does not heal within 6 weeks is considered a chronic wound. Common problems that often lead to chronic wounds are diabetes, peripheral vascular disease, and pressure ulcers. Normal aging and chronic disease factors that are often present in older persons will affect their ability to heal.

Some of the considerations related to delayed or impaired wound healing for the older person are (Boynton, Jaworski, & Paustian, 1999; Demling & DeSanti, 2001):

- Inadequate blood supply.
- Inadequate nutrition.

- Immunocompetence.
- Damage to the wound.

Adequate blood volume and cardiac output are the most important components of wound blood flow and oxygen delivery. Oxygen is needed for every phase of the healing process. Chronic cardiac disease, smoking, dehydration, hypovolemia, and the vascular complications of diabetes cause a decrease in blood supply to the tissues, which delays wound healing.

Wound healing cannot take place without large amounts of energy (glucose) and protein (amino acids) as well as other substances. Many older persons have protein-energy malnutrition, in which the intake of protein and energy is inadequate to meet the body's demand. In the malnourished person, the amino acids must come from muscle and other stores. The body can deal with this demand until there is a loss of 15% of lean body mass. After that, the supply of protein is inadequate to provide muscle replacement and wound healing, thus compromising the healing process.

Older persons have delayed immune function, which impairs the natural ability to fight infection. This delays the normal inflammatory response. Wounds cannot heal without the inflammatory process. Medications that further diminish the immune response include steroids and anti-inflammatory drugs. Weight loss due to an acute and chronic illness results in loss of body protein (lean body mass) and also compromises immune function.

The wound can be damaged by both too much and too little moisture. A dry wound surface impairs epithelial migration and leads to tissue injury and necrosis. The buildup of tissue exudates is toxic to new growth and leads to tissue hypoxia, which impairs healing. The older person may also be subject to wound maceration due to urine or fecal contamination, which will further damage the wound. Nursing interventions used to treat the pressure ulcers or chronic wounds can also cause damage. Topical antibiotics, cleansing solutions, and mechanical trauma during dressing changes may all contribute to damage to the wound bed.

CELLULITIS

Cellulitis is an acute bacterial infection of the skin and subcutaneous tissue that may cause an older person a great deal of pain and distress. Cellulitis, which occurs most frequently on the lower legs and face, is characterized by symptoms of inflammation, which include intense pain, heat, redness, and swelling. It may appear in a localized area as a complication of a wound infection, or it may involve an entire limb. In severe infections, fever may be present, as well as an increase in white blood cells and tender lymph nodes (lymphadenopathy). An elevated temperature, although a common sign of infection, may not be present in the older person. The organisms most commonly responsible for cellulitis are hemolytic streptococci (group G streptococci and *Streptococcus pyogenes*), and *Staphyloccus aureus* (Baddour, 2000). Older persons at risk for cellulitis include those with any break in the skin such as a leg ulceration or pressure ulcer. In addition, those with predisposing factors such as diabetes, obesity, a previous history of cellulitis, peripheral vascular disease, or tinea pedis are at risk (Baxter & McGregor, 2001; Dupuy et al., 1999; Koutkia et al., 1999). Many normal changes of aging increase the older person's risk for developing cellulitis. Changes in the thickness of the skin make the older person more susceptible to breaks in the skin. After the skin is broken, the older person is at higher risk for infection since wound healing is often delayed.

FINGERNAIL AND TOENAIL CONDITIONS

The distal phalanges are protected from injury and trauma by the nails. Changes in the nail plate occur with aging, and are also affected by trauma, systemic diseases such as diabetes and circulatory disorders, as well as dermatological conditions.

Onychomycosis, a fungal infection (i.e., *Trichophyton rubrum, T. mentragrophytes*) of the toenail, most commonly occurs on the big toe. The toenail appears thick, discolored, and protruding from the nail bed (Fielo, 2001). Older persons may complain of severe pain when their shoe presses on the deformed toe, often causing them to reduce their activity or wear open shoes and sandals. The older person should see a doctor for treatment to prevent the condition from spreading to the other parts of the foot.

Onychia is inflammation of the nail matrix; paronychia is inflammation of the matrix, plus the surrounding and deeper structures. This is a common condition in older adults and is caused by bacteria or fungus. Older persons who have been exposed to wet work such as dishwashing, cleaning, or fishing for many years are at high risk. Trauma caused by tight shoes may also be the source of the problem. This disorder is characterized by separation of the cuticle from the nail, which allows organisms to enter. The organisms may cause swelling, redness, and tenderness of the nail fold, accompanied by purulent drainage.

Onychogryphosis is a chronic hypertrophy of the nail plate characterized by a hooked or curved nail. Any pressure on the nail may cause severe pain. The deformed nail may cause pressure on an adjacent toe, leading to a dangerous pressure necrosis in a vulnerable older person. Diabetes and circulatory conditions are predisposing factors for these complications (Collett, 2000).

NURSING DIAGNOSES

Nursing diagnoses appropriate to the older person with problems of the skin may include any of the following (North American Nursing Diagnosis Association, 2002):

- *Impaired skin integrity related to lesions and inflammatory response*
- *Risk for impaired skin integrity related to physical immobility*
- *Risk for impaired skin integrity related to decreased skin turgor*
- *Risk for impaired skin integrity related to the effects of pressure, friction, or shear*
- *Risk for impaired tissue integrity related to decreased circulation*
- *Risk for infection related to pressure ulcer*
- *Pain related to destruction of tissue due to pressure and shear*

The two major nursing diagnoses related to integumentary problems are *risk for impaired tissue integrity,* and *impaired skin integrity.*

Impaired tissue integrity is defined as "a state in which an individual experiences, or is at risk for damage to the integumentary, corneal, or mucous membrane tissues of the body." Defining characteristics (major) that must be present include "disruptions of integumentary tissue or invasion of body structure (incision, dermal ulcer)" (Carpenito, 2002, p. 696). *Impaired skin integrity* is defined as "a state in which the individual experiences, or is at risk for damage to the epidermal and dermal tissue" (Carpenito, 2002, p. 705). The major defining characteristic that must be present is disruption of epidermal and dermal tissue. There is both overlap and possible confusion as to when to use these diagnoses. According to Carpenito (2002), *impaired tissue integrity* is the broad category under which more specific diagnoses fall. *Impaired skin integrity* should be used to describe pressure ulcers that have damaged the epidermal and dermal tissue only. *Impaired tissue integrity* would describe pressure ulcers that are deeper than the dermis (i.e., connective tissue, muscle).

The nursing diagnoses terminology for pressure ulcers can cause conceptual confusion because of the lack of specificity in the diagnosis as well as the etiologies. Franz (2001) has suggested the formulation of a nursing diagnosis that correctly identifies a pressure ulcer by giving it the label *pressure ulcer.* This label would correctly identify the problem and would be consistent with the terminology accepted by experts in skin and wound care. The signs and symptoms of pressure ulcer could address the patterns of partial-thickness pressure ulcer (which involves the epidermis and dermis) and full-thickness pressure ulcer (which involves damage to subcutaneous tissue and may extend to underlying tissue) (Franz, 2001).

LABORATORY AND TESTING VALUES

Total body photography, skin surface microscopy, machine vision, and skin biopsy are the current modalities that can be used to diagnose malignant melanoma.

Total Body Photography

A series of 24 slides are taken of high-risk patients and used during subsequent visits to identify changes in nevi (Oliviero, 2002). Skin surface microscopy uses a handheld instrument to provide a 10× illuminated review of the skin. This process is very time intensive to learn and requires training.

Machine Vision

This is a newly developed technology that provides a computerized analysis of a lesion and gives a quantitative score. The score reflects whether the lesion is benign or malignant.

Skin Biopsy With Histologic Examination

A skin biopsy is indicated in all skin lesions that are suspected of being neoplasms. A variety of techniques are available for the examination of the tissue, including immunofluorescence and electron microscopy. A biopsy is indicated for any lesion that has been present for longer than a month.

Wound Cultures to Determine Infection

Wound cultures and microscopic examination can identify infectious organisms. Wound cultures should be obtained by the aspiration method or a tissue biopsy. The swab method is not considered useful for obtaining a wound culture since it examines bacteria present on the wound surface, not in the wound bed itself. The tissue that is obtained must be healthy, viable tissue to ensure capturing the greatest number of microorganisms. If there is eschar or exudate visible, it must be removed so that the healthy tissue is accessible. The wound is then washed with saline and dried gently with sterile gauze.

The wound biopsy is considered the gold standard for culture (Robson, Mannari, Smith, & Payne, 1999). This is done by the removal of a small piece of tissue from the ulcer, which is then sent to the laboratory. The disadvantage of the wound biopsy, however, is that the removal of tissue from the ulcer will delay healing.

The aspirate method requires inserting a needle with a 10-cc syringe into the wound and aspirating fluid from the site while moving the needle around the wound base. All air must be removed from the syringe before injecting it into the container. The container must be labeled clearly with the location of the pressure ulcer (e.g., sacral area). The final results are available in 48 hours, but preliminary results can identify if an infection is present and whether it is gram negative or gram positive. This will allow antibiotic treatment to begin if indicated. Some of the common organisms found in wounds are *S. aureus,* group A streptococci, gram-negative bacilli, and fungi. Deep wounds may produce anaerobic bacteria such as clostridia or anaerobic streptococci (Corbett, 2000).

LABORATORY VALUES TO DETERMINE RISK FOR PRESSURE ULCER

Serum albumin and serum transferrin, as well as lymphocyte count, are useful values that will help to determine nutritional status. These values will be decreased in protein-energy malnutrition. They may also be affected by other illnesses.

Serum albumin indicates the level of protein stores. A serum albumin level below 3.5 g/dl is considered low, and below 2.5 g/dl is a serious depletion in protein.

Serum transferrin is considered a more accurate indicator of protein stores since it is more responsive to acute changes. A serum transferrin level below 200 mg/dl is considered low, and below 100 mg/dl is a serious depletion in protein.

A total lymphocyte count below 1,500 mm^3 indicates loss of energy to skin. A moderate decrease is 800 to 1,200/mm^3. The synthesis of lymphocytes is depressed when protein-energy malnutrition exists, which contributes to the decreased ability of the white blood cells to fight infection.

Pharmacology and Nursing Responsibilities

Pharmacological treatment of skin problems may include topical or systemic administration of medications. The following agents are used extensively in the clinical setting for management of dermatological problems in the older adult.

TOPICAL ANTIFUNGAL AGENTS

Antifungal agents such as itraconazole are used in the treatment of onychomycosis of the toenails and fingernails. The topical preparation is applied to the affected area and has few side effects. The suggested dosage for treatment of onychomycosis of the toenails is itraconazole 200 mg po daily for 12 weeks. Adverse effects include renal and hepatic damage.

TOPICAL ANTIBIOTICS

The use of topical antibiotics on local pressure ulcers has met with some debate. If the wound has foul-smelling exudate and is not healing after 2 to 4 weeks of optimal care, a short course of topical antibiotics should be instituted. Some other wounds without local signs may have a high level of bacteria and may also benefit from topical antibiotic therapy.

The topical antibiotics of choice for the nonhealing ulcer, or one with high bacterial levels (10^5/g of tissue), are silver sulfadiazine and triple antibiotic (combination of polymyxin B, neomycin, and bacitracin). These agents have a broad spectrum and have been found to be effective against gram-negative, gram-positive, and anaerobic organisms (NPSource, 2001). Topical antibiotics are indicated for short-term use and are reevaluated in 2 weeks. Patient teaching includes limiting the product to the number of applications and the condition prescribed. Overuse of topical antibiotics can lead to bacterial resistance.

SYSTEMIC ANTIBIOTICS

If a pressure ulcer shows signs of infection, such as cellulitis, osteomyelitis, or septicemia, appropriate systemic antibiotics should be instituted. Common offending organisms of bacteremia and sepsis include *S. aureus,* gram-negative rods, and *Bacteroides fragilis.* A blood culture will allow the causative organisms to be identified, and antibiotics can be directed at the offending organisms. These are very serious complications of pressure ulcers, and immediate medical attention is advised.

SELECTED ANTIMICROBIALS

Penicillinase-resistant penicillins (methicillin, nafcillin, oxacillin) are indicated against staphylococcal and beta-hemolytic streptococci infections of soft tissue. These drugs have a high degree of safety, but the dose should be adjusted for older persons with renal impairment to prevent nephrotoxicity.

AMINOGLYCOSIDES

Gentamicin, tobramycin, and streptomycin are rapidly bactericidal against staphylocci and gram-negative aerobic bacteria. The dose of these drugs should be reduced in the elderly person because of the risk of renal impairment. Risk of ototoxicity increases with age and is more likely in older persons with pre-existing hearing problems.

PRESCRIPTION CREAMS AND LOTIONS FOR DRY SKIN

Often corticosteroids are prescribed as topical treatment for dermatological problems in older people. These creams should be applied sparingly in thin layers to maximize therapeutic outcome and minimize the risk of side effects.

Hydrocortisone 1% or 2.5% is a low-potency topical corticosteroid, that can be applied for short-term treatment of inflamed dry skin. Long-term use may cause systemic absorption.

Drug Alert !

Older persons have a high rate of adverse reactions to corticosteroids and antihistamines, both of which are frequently prescribed for skin problems. Older persons should be reminded not to buy over-the-counter preparations of these drugs without specific instructions from their primary care provider. If these medications are prescribed, directions should be strictly followed and any unusual symptoms reported promptly.

Nonpharmacological Treatment of Skin Problems in Older Persons

Prevention and early treatment of skin problems in older people may also include nonpharmacological interventions and patient education. Identification and correction of factors that may contribute to pathological skin changes is a key nursing responsibility.

BOX 12-1 **ABCDs of Skin Cancer**

Asymmetrical. One half of the lesion is different from the other half.
Borders are ragged or irregular.
Color is varied within the same lesion.
Diameter is larger than 6 mm (and size is enlarging).

Source: Hwang, 1999. Used with permission.

SKIN CANCER AND PRECANCER CONDITIONS

The nurse's role in the nonpharmacological treatment of skin cancer focuses on giving the older person and family members the correct knowledge they need for the prevention and early diagnosis of this disease. Teaching the family and older person the correct methods for self-assessment, as well as practices for daily life, will empower them to focus on self-care and primary prevention.

Older persons should be taught the ABCDs of skin cancer, as listed in Box 12-1. If they have any skin changes, such as moles or pigmented lesions, the ABCDs should be noted.

Patients should also be taught the guidelines on protection from the sun, as listed in Box 12-2. The nurse should emphasize the importance of adhering to these guidelines and assist older persons in adapting the guidelines to their daily lives.

When assessing the skin of people of color, the nurse should become familiar with the characteristics of darker skin. Nurses and other healthcare professionals may find the assessment of darker skin to be more challenging because the traditional hallmarks of redness and color changes may be obscured by the darker skin tone. Box 12-3 illustrates guidelines for assessment of darker skin.

BOX 12-2 **Guidelines on Sun and Wearing Protective Clothing**

- Avoid the sun during midday (10 a.m. to 4 p.m.).
- Seek shade during midday (trees, umbrella, hats).
- Wear hats that protect the face:
  - Hats with at least a 3" brim
  - Legionnaire hats (baseball hat with ear and neck flaps)
- Wear protective clothing:
  - Fabrics with tighter weave transmit less UVR.
  - Darker colors transmit less UVR than lighter ones.
  - Wet or stretched fabrics transmit more radiation.
- Use a broad-spectrum sunscreen (UVA and UVB) with a sun protection factor of 15 or above.
- Use 1 to 2 oz of sunscreen and reapply after leaving the water, sweating, or drying off.

Source: Adapted from Centers for Disease Control and Prevention, 2002.

BOX
12-3

The Integument: Considerations for People of Color

- Some dark-skinned persons have bluish lips or gums.
- Black persons have freckle-like pigmentation of gums, buccal cavity, and borders of the tongue.
- A dark-skinned person may lose reddish tones if pallor is present.
- Cyanosis is difficult to assess in a dark-skinned person. The nurse should check soles and heels for color.
- Erythema is an area of inflammation on the skin. On a dark-skinned person, the skin assumes a purplish color when inflammation is present. To assess erythema in a dark-skinned person, the nurse should palpate for warmth and check for hardness and smoothness.
- Ecchymotic lesions are large bruises. Purple or dark color usually can be seen.
- To determine if an area of concern is erythema or ecchymosis, the nurse should use a glass slide and press gently over the area. If the color changes and becomes lighter, it is an erythema. If no change occurs, it is an ecchymotic area.
- Dermatosis papulosa nigra is a type of seborrheic keratoses that occurs only in Blacks. It is characterized by the appearance of many dark, small papules on the face.

Source: Gilchrist & Chiu, 2000.

NONPHARMACOLOGICAL TREATMENT OF SKIN CANCER

The treatment of skin cancers may include any of the following techniques and are appropriate interventions for older people.

Basal Cell Carcinoma and Squamous Cell Carcinoma

The diagnosis of basal cell carcinoma and squamous cell carcinoma must be confirmed by biopsy. Treatment options for basal cell carcinoma and squamous cell carcinoma depend on the size, depth, and location of the tumor. Electrodesiccation and curettage can be used for small tumors. Surgical excision has the highest cure and can be done on an outpatient basis. Mohs' surgery, a microscopically controlled surgical technique, is used for high-risk or large basal cell carcinoma, especially of the head and neck (Leber et al., 1999). Mohs' surgery helps to prevent tissue loss by sparing uninvolved tissue. Less common treatment includes cryosurgery and radiotherapy. Radiotherapy may be chosen for the older person who cannot tolerate surgery. Follow-up is anywhere from 3 to 12 months, and should include a complete skin check.

Malignant Melanoma

Excisional biopsy is done to confirm diagnosis, and prognosis depends on the vertical (depth) thickness of the lesion in millimeters. Treatment of melanoma is excision, with surgical margins dependent on tumor thickness. Adjuvant therapies may be offered depending on the stage of the tumor. Therapy for metastatic disease may include chemotherapy, chemoimmunotherapy, and regional radiation therapy (Leber et al., 1999). Advanced melanoma with metastasis is usually incurable, thus supportive care is offered. Focus should be on determining the wishes of the patient in relation to end-of-life care and pain management.

PREVENTION AND MANAGEMENT OF SKIN TEARS

Skin tears are common in the older person, with 1.5 million occurring each year. A preventive approach is therefore the key to decrease the risk for skin tears. Older persons, caregivers, and family members should be aware of the following preventive interventions:

- Do not use any pulling or sliding movements when assisting older persons with a change in their position.
- Protect the older person by padding any surfaces that come in contact with leg and arm movements such as side rails, wheelchair arm and leg supports, and table corners.
- Keep the environment free of obstacles and well lit.
- Keep skin moist with adequate fluids and skin moisturizing creams.
- Use paper tape and remove it cautiously, or substitute tape with gauze or stockinette.
- Encourage long sleeves and long pants to add a layer of protection over the skin.

The depth of the skin tear, and the agency protocol, will determine the management of skin tears. As yet, there is no evidence-based method for skin tear care. The recommended clinical care of a skin tear would include the following (Baranoski, 2001):

1. Clean with normal saline or other nontoxic cleaner.
2. Pat or air dry.
3. Gently place the torn skin in its approximate normal position.
4. Apply dressing (saline, foam, gels) and change per protocol or product requirements.
5. Document the assessment and intervention. Photograph if permitted.

NONPHARMACOLOGICAL TREATMENT OF PRESSURE ULCERS

The nonpharmacological treatment of pressure ulcers has evolved over the last two decades. Research that supports practice has provided nurses and other healthcare workers with evidence-based practice guidelines as well as a synthesis of current expert opinion. The AHCPR *Clinical Practice Guideline: Treating Pressure Ulcers* (Bergstrom et al., 1994) provides the clinical community with a synthesis of research and expert opinion of the treatment options for pressure ulcer and wound healing. It is a great resource for both nurses and physicians. Areas of nursing responsibility that will be addressed for pressure ulcers include risk assessment for pressure ulcers, prevention and modification of pressure ulcer risk factors, and treatment of pressure ulcers.

Risk Assessment for Pressure Ulcers

The nursing care of the older person should begin with an assessment of the risk for pressure ulcers. The Hartford Institute for Geriatric Nursing Best Nursing Practices in Care for Older Adults Curriculum Guide (2003) recommends the use of the Braden Scale for Predicting Pressure Sore Risk. The Hartford Institute recommends this scale be used for risk assessment in the following categories of older patients:

- All bed- or chair-bound patients, or those whose ability to reposition is impaired
- All at-risk patients on admission to healthcare facilities and regularly thereafter
- All older patients with decreased mental status, incontinence, and nutritional deficits

Accepted risk factors that form the basis of this scale generally include mobility, incontinence, nutrition, and mental status. Some of the variables used to develop this scale are expert derived and not based on accepted research evidence. See the Best Practices feature on the following page.

The Braden Scale (Braden & Bergstrom, 1994) is a widely used tool that assesses mobility, activity, sensory perception, skin moisture, friction, shear, and nutritional status. Each dimension is rated from 1 to 4 on a Likert type scale, and the total score range is from 6 to 23. A score of 16 or less indicates a pressure sore risk and a need for a prevention plan. The Braden scale has been subjected to several validation studies and is considered the most valid of the available risk assessment tools. Once a risk assessment is completed, and a deficit exists, the nursing care plan should reflect on-going prevention as well as complete documentation of the older person's progress.

BRADEN SCALE FOR PREDICTING PRESSURE SORE RISK

Patient's Name _____ Evaluator's Name _____ Date of Assessment

SENSORY PERCEPTION ability to respond meaningfully to pressure-related discomfort	1. Completely Limited Unresponsive (does not moan, flinch, or grasp) to painful stimuli, due to diminished level of consciousness or sedation. OR limited ability to feel pain over most of body	2. Very Limited Responds only to painful stimuli. Cannot communicate discomfort except by moaning or restlessness OR has a sensory impairment which limits the ability to feel pain or discomfort over ½ of body.	3. Slightly Limited Responds to verbal commands, but cannot always communicate discomfort or the need to be turned. OR has some sensory impairment which limits ability to feel pain or discomfort in 1 or 2 extremities.	4. No Impairment Responds to verbal commands. Has no sensory deficit which would limit ability to feel or voice pain or discomfort.				
MOISTURE degree to which skin is exposed to moisture	1. Constantly Moist Skin is kept moist almost constantly by perspiration, urine, etc. Dampness is detected every time patient is moved or turned.	2. Very Moist Skin is often, but not always moist. Linen must be changed at least once a shift.	3. Occasionally Moist: Skin is occasionally moist, requiring an extra linen change approximately once a day.	4. Rarely Moist Skin is usually dry, linen only requires changing at routine intervals.				
ACTIVITY degree of physical activity	1. Bedfast Confined to bed.	2. Chairfast Ability to walk severely limited or non-existent. Cannot bear own weight and/or must be assisted into chair or wheelchair.	3. Walks Occasionally Walks occasionally during day, but for very short distances, with or without assistance. Spends majority of each shift in bed or chair	4. Walks Frequently Walks outside room at least twice a day and inside room at least once every two hours during waking hours				
MOBILITY ability to change and control body position	1. Completely Immobile Does not make even slight changes in body or extremity position without assistance.	2. Very Limited Makes occasional slight changes in body or extremity position but unable to make frequent or significant changes independently.	3. Slightly Limited Makes frequent though slight changes in body or extremity position independently.	4. No Limitation Makes major and frequent changes in position without assistance.				
NUTRITION usual food intake pattern	1. Very Poor Never eats a complete meal. Rarely eats more than ⅓ of any food offered. Eats 2 servings or less of protein (meats or dairy products) per day. Takes fluids poorly. Does not take a liquid dietary supplement OR is NPO and/or maintained on clear liquids or IV's for more than 5 days.	2. Probably Inadequate Rarely eats a complete meal and generally eats only about ½ of any food offered. Protein intake includes only 3 servings of meat or dairy products per day. Occasionally will take a dietary supplement OR receives less than optimum amount of liquid diet or tube feeding	3. Adequate Eats over half of most meals. Eats a total of 4 servings of protein (meat, dairy products) per day. Occasionally will refuse a meal, but will usually take a supplement when offered OR is on a tube feeding or TPN regimen which probably meets most of nutritional needs.	4. Excellent Eats most of every meal. Never refuses a meal. Usually eats a total of 4 or more servings of meat and dairy products. Occasionally eats between meals. Does not require supplementation.				
FRICTION & SHEAR	1. Problem Requires moderate to maximum assistance in moving. Complete lifting without sliding against sheets is impossible. Frequently slides down in bed or chair, requiring frequent repositioning with maximum assistance. Spasticity, contractures, or agitation leads to almost constant friction.	2. Potential Problem Moves feebly or requires minimum assistance. During a move skin probably slides to some extent against sheets, chair, restraints, or other devices. Maintains relatively good position in chair or bed most of the time but occasionally slides down.	3. No Apparent Problem Moves in bed and in chair independently and has sufficient muscle strength to lift up completely during move. Maintains good position in bed or chair.					

Total Score

Prevention and Modification of Pressure Ulcer Risk Factors

Mobility and activity are important considerations in preventing and modifying risk factors as well as allowing healing to occur. Topics that will be discussed include position schedules, activities, and bed surface devices. All of these interventions will protect against external mechanical forces, including friction, shearing, and pressure. The older person who is at risk for a pressure ulcer should have a turning and activity schedule. Nurses and nurse assistants should consistently document their interventions in the flow sheet or progress notes. Mobility and activity considerations for preventing pressure ulcers include the following:

- Reposition q2h. Use a pull sheet to prevent shear and friction. If redness occurs, consider a 1½-hour turning schedule.
- Ensure proper positioning. Use pillows or wedges to prevent the skin from touching the bed on trochanter, heels, and ankles (Figure 12-7)▆. Do not use rings or donuts.
- Avoid sitting. The sitting position, either in bed or in the chair, should be limited to 2 hours. Time in the chair should be scheduled around meal times. The person in bed should not be left in the 90-degree position except during meals.
- Increase activity. Encourage older persons to change positions by making small body shifts. This will redistribute weight and increase perfusion. Range of motion exercises should be done every 8 hours, and the techniques should be taught to family and patients.
- Choose a mattress surface based on the assessment and diagnosis:
  - A low-air-loss bed or air-fluidized bed is indicated for any stage pressure sore, and for persons having grafts or surgery.
  - A water mattress is indicated for high-risk persons, and for stage I, II, and III pressure ulcers.
  - An alternating pressure mattress is indicated for high-risk persons and for stage I and II pressure ulcers.
  - A convoluted foam pad is indicated for short-term use (Bergstrom et al., 1994).

Practice Pearl

High-risk older persons should not be placed in a 90-degree side-lying position. This position places intense weight on the trochanter. Older persons at risk should be turned from supine to the right or left 30-degree oblique position. This position relieves pressure on the bony prominences of the trochanter and lateral malleolus.

Skin care practices for older persons include correct bathing procedure, prevention of injury, and dietary support. These skin care interventions are important to maintain healthy tissue as well as to improve the tissue tolerance to decrease further risk of injury. Adequate skin care should be considered a high priority for all patients at risk for pressure ulcers. Older persons and their families should be given educational materials and demonstrations when appropriate. Skin care considerations to prevent pressure ulcers in older persons at risk include the following:

- Keep the skin clean and dry.
- Lubricate the skin with a moisturizer. Massage the area around the reddened area or bony prominence. Do not massage any reddened area. Then apply a thin layer of a

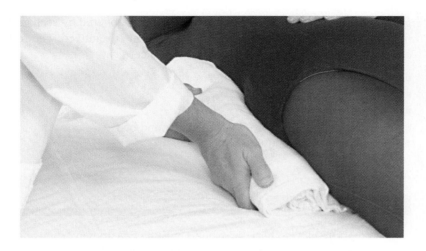

FIGURE ▪ 12-7

It is important to use pillows or wedges to prevent the skin from touching the bed on trochanter, heels, and ankles.

petroleum-based product, followed by a baby powder cornstarch product, to reduce friction and moisture.

- Evaluate and manage incontinence. A bowel and bladder management program should be in place. If soiling occurs, skin should be cleansed per routine. Underpads should be used that absorb moisture and present a quick drying surface to the skin. Plastic-lined bed pads should not be in contact with the person's skin. Use minimal pads and cover them with a sheet or pillowcase.

Practice Pearl

The area at risk for pressure sores should be washed gently with tepid water, with or without minimal soap. Soap removes natural oils from the skin, and cleaning the soap off may cause additional friction damage.

- Monitor nutrition. Determine factors that might cause inadequate nutrition. Obtain laboratory data. Provide additional canned supplements, vitamin C, and zinc to promote skin healing. Consider alternative methods such as total parenteral nutrition as needed (see Chapter 5 for further information). ⊂▭⊃

TREATMENT OF PRESSURE ULCERS

The AHCPR *Clinical Practice Guideline, Treating Pressure Ulcers* (Bergstrom et al., 1994) provides a review of research on all aspects of treating pressure ulcers. The first step in effective pressure ulcer care is to assess the wound. This assessment should include the history of the wound, the pressure ulcer size and depth, and any evidence or signs of tunneling, undermining, exudate, and infection. Once the wound is assessed and documented, an effective pressure ulcer care plan should be established. The specific treatment of pressure ulcers is determined by the ulcer stage. The AHCPR has adopted a four-stage criteria for the assessment of pressure ulcers (see pages 339-340), which is widely used in healthcare institutions in the United States.

The nursing care related to pressure ulcers is an important part of nursing practice. Therefore, many agencies have established protocols that offer specific nursing care guidelines for each stage of the ulcer. If an ulcer is covered by eschar, it is usually removed. An ulcer cannot be staged until the eschar is removed. The following are the components of the nursing care of a pressure ulcer:

- Assessing and staging the wound
- Debriding necrotic tissue
- Cleansing the wound
- Applying dressings to provide a moist wound bed
- Preventing and treating infection

Practice Pearl

For a pressure ulcer to heal, the wound must be free from infection and necrotic tissue. Moist, devitalized tissue supports the growth of bacteria, delaying the healing process. Necrotic tissue is avascular; therefore, treatment with systemic antibiotics is not effective.

Debriding of Necrotic Tissue

Debridement is the removal of devitalized necrotic (black) tissue or yellow slough tissue. Four methods are available for debridement: sharp, mechanical, enzymatic, and autolytic debridement.

Sharp debridement involves the use of a scalpel or other sharp instrument to remove necrotic tissue. It is the quickest form of debridement and is indicated when a dangerous sepsis or cellulitis is imminent. Large extensive ulcers, such as stage IV ulcers with thick adherent eschar, often require sharp surgical debridement in the operating room.

Mechanical debridement is the removal of stringy exudate by the use of wet-to-dry dressings, wound irrigations, and hydrotherapy. Wet-to-dry dressings are a common method of mechanical debridement. They are effective for wounds with a small-to-moderate amount of exudate and are usually changed every 4 to 6 hours. For a wet-to-dry dressing, gauze pads are moistened with saline and placed in the open wound, covering the necrotic tissue only. The wet dressing adheres to the dead tissue and is allowed to dry. When the dry dressing is removed, the dead, devitalized tissue is removed with it. The dry dressing should not be moistened before removal or the purpose of the wet-to-dry dressing is defeated. The wet dressing should not be in contact with any intact skin, or it will cause maceration. It is important to use a skin sealant to protect the ulcer border. Once the wound is clean and dry, wet-to-dry dressings are not appropriate. Instead, moist dressings are used to promote tissue healing.

Wound irrigations are done using gentle pressure, about 4 to 5 psi, to clean the wound and soften eschar. The nurse should use a 35-ml syringe with a 19-gauge angiocatheter to deliver the cleaning agent. A bulb syringe does not deliver adequate pressure for debridement.

Chemical debridement is the use of topical enzymatic agents to break down devitalized tissue. It can be used alone, after sharp debridement, or with mechanical debridement.

Autolytic debridement involves the use of a moisture retentive dressing to cover the wound and allow the enzymes in the wound bed to liquefy selective dead tissue.

Practice Pearl

The purpose of debridement is to remove dead, devitalized tissue from the wound bed to allow healing to progress. Therefore, debridement is discontinued once all the dead tissue is removed and the wound is clean (no necrotic tissue). Continuing debriding of any kind will cause damage to delicate new tissue.

Cleansing the Wound

The purpose of cleansing the wound is to remove bacteria, debris, and small amounts of devitalized tissue to allow optimal healing. Cleansing should not be confused with disinfection or antisepsis, both of which relate to the killing of microorganisms. Topical antiseptics such as povidone-iodine, acetic acid, hydrogen peroxide, and Dakin's solution should not be used on a wound because these products have been found to be toxic to the wound fibroblasts and macrophages (Ovington, 2001). The safest, most cost-effective and most common cleansing agent for wounds is isotonic saline (0.9%). Wound cleansing can be done by (1) pouring a saline solution over the wound, (2) applying saline-soaked gauzes to clean the debris, or (3) squeezing a saline-filled bulb syringe over the wound. For a wound that requires the removal of small areas of nonadherent devitalized tissue, irrigation may be needed. To irrigate for the purpose of cleansing, the nurse should use saline in a catheter tip syringe (60 cc) and apply gentle pressure (4 psi) (Thompson, 2000). Wounds with large adherent areas of necrotic tissue or yellow slough should be irrigated (debrided) with a higher pressure stream between 8 and 15 psi. Pressure should not exceed 15 psi, or tissue damage and edema could result (Krasner & Sibbald, 1999).

Dressings to Provide a Moist Wound Bed

To heal a pressure ulcer, a clean, moist environment must be maintained. A moist wound environment promotes cellular activity in all phases of wound healing, provides insulation, increases the rate of epithelial cell growth, and reduces pain. A dry wound environment has been found to result in further tissue death, or dry necrosis, beyond the cause of the wound (Ovington, 2001). Since scientific research demonstrated that a moist wound bed provided the best environment for wound healing, a thriving industry has emerged with hundreds of products developed to promote moist wound healing. Although many of these advanced products are appropriate, many common conventional dressing materials have the advantage of being readily available, effective, and less expensive. These products have been reviewed in the literature, and useful evaluations can be found elsewhere (Krasner & Sibbald, 1999; Moore, 2000).

The frequency of dressing change will be determined by the manufacturer's recommendations for the product selected and the type and amount of exudate and drainage.

The amount of wound moisture may change during the healing stages, so the wound may need added absorption during one period, and added moisture during another (Thompson, 2000).

Preventing and Treating Infection

One of the most complex and controversial aspects of wound care has been the use of antibiotics. The presence of an infection is determined by the microbial state of the wound. In order to apply clinical reasoning to the treatment of wound infection, it is important to understand and differentiate between the three microbial states of a wound.

Contamination is the presence of microorganisms on the wound. All open wounds are contaminated. The human body has various organisms living both on and in it. Thus, the skin is never sterile.

Colonization is the presence and proliferation of organisms (bacteria) in the wound but with no signs of local infection, thus no host response. Stage II, III, and IV pressure ulcers are generally considered to be colonized. Therefore, wound cleansing and debriding are instituted to prevent the development of infection.

Infection is the proliferation of bacteria in healthy cells that produces symptoms of local redness, pain, fever, and swelling. Examples of serious infections that can be complications of pressure ulcers are bacteremia, sepsis, osteomyelitis, and advancing cellulitis.

Use of Topical and Systemic Antibiotics

Urgent care is required for older persons with systemic signs of infection. This care includes obtaining wound cultures and blood cultures, and providing treatment with appropriate systemic antibiotics that will cover the offending organism. All of these conditions could cause delayed healing or further complications from tissue destruction, and may result in death.

Certain local conditions would warrant the use of topical antibiotics:

- A clean pressure ulcer that has not shown signs of healing over a 2-week period
- A pressure ulcer that has increased local discharge but shows no local signs of infection (See the section titled Pharmacology and Nursing Responsibilities for selected antibiotic information.)

Management of Cellulitis

Interventions for cellulitis focus on the immediate treatment of the acute infection and prevention of further complications such as abscess formation and tissue damage. The treatment includes appropriate antibiotics, prevention of further infection, immobilization and elevation of the affected limb, pain relief, and possibly anticoagulant therapy.

Appropriate antibiotics are the priority of treatment. They are usually given intravenously until the infection begins to resolve, and then they are changed to an oral route. Any existing wounds should be assessed, and a wound culture obtained if an infection is suspected. Bed rest should be maintained. If the cellulitis is on the lower extremities, the foot of the bed should be elevated to decrease swelling and allow the leg to be fully supported. The nurse should encourage active foot exercises and calf pumping to decrease pain and swelling and allow the older person to maintain normal function. Pain should be assessed with a 0 to 10 visual analog scale and medicated with appropriate analgesics. Sheets and blankets must not be allowed to rub against the area and cause friction and added pain.

NONPHARMACOLOGICAL TREATMENT OF FINGERNAIL AND TOENAIL CONDITIONS

Nonpharmacological treatment of fingernail and toenail problems focuses on the immediate treatment of the problem and prevention of further complications.

The treatment of onychomycosis will include relief of pain, patient education, and oral antifungal agents as appropriate. As a temporary measure, older persons should be advised to reduce the pressure on the toe by cutting a hole in their slipper or shoe. In addition, the podiatrist should be consulted periodically for reduction of the nail plate. Patient education includes frequent treatment to prevent the condition from spreading to the other parts of the foot. Oral antifungal agents may provide a cure (O'Dell, 1998).

The treatment of chronic paronychia will include keeping affected nails dry and perhaps antibiotics. The older person should be advised to keep the affected nails out of water and to keep the area protected. Drainage is sometimes needed. A physician or nurse practitioner should be consulted for appropriate antibiotic treatment.

The treatment of onychogryphosis will include a podiatry consultation and perhaps surgical intervention for refractory problems. The podiatrist should trim thickened toenails with an electric drill and burrs, or a carbon dioxide laser. Nails should be kept short. Proper foot care and hygiene are essential. If all conservative measures fail, the older person who is disabled by this disorder should consider surgery.

Nursing Management Principles

Nursing care and documentation of the older person with a skin problem should focus on careful assessment of the risk factors, provision of nursing interventions to minimize the risk of skin breakdown, documentation of care, and evaluation of the older patient's status.

NURSING PROCESS AND DOCUMENTATION

Nursing care of the older patient should focus on the prevention of pressure ulcers. This goal is difficult to achieve, but research has shown that a large majority of pressure ulcers can be prevented. For the older person who has a pressure ulcer, the nursing care plan should be a guide for nursing interventions. Ongoing nursing process and clinical reasoning should be reflected in each step. Documentation is necessary to ensure that the care plan is appropriate.

The wound is assessed initially, and an evaluation is done with each dressing change. If the nurse assesses that the wound has improved, documentation should reflect the actual changes that the nurse evaluated to make that decision. Wound healing is a process. As the wound changes and evolves, there may be a need to make changes in the dressing protocol. If the wound does not show signs of healing in 2 weeks, the treatment should be reevaluated.

KNOWLEDGE-BASED DECISION MAKING

In order to make knowledge-based decisions, the nurse should have access to all appropriate current knowledge regarding research on pressure ulcer care, pressure-relieving devices, and current products for topical treatment. Access to current literature will support decision making and provide information for families and other staff. Product information is helpful, but independent controlled trials of the product provide the needed unbiased results.

The following questions are useful when assessing wound care products:

1. What is the wound assessment? What is the stage, drainage, moisture, eschar?
2. What does the wound need? This will depend on the assessment and is ongoing. Does it need absorption, debridement, moisture?
3. What products are available in the setting? Many similarities exist between products, and all agencies will not have every product. It is important to understand what the product does.
4. What is the evaluation of the product? What materials are available? Is there a resource manual at the agency that will assist this process? If not, the nurse should begin the process.
5. What is practical? If the nurse is in the home or if a family member has to do the dressing, the process will have to be as simple as possible to ensure correct technique.

EVALUATION AND REVISION OF NURSING CARE PLAN

Critical evaluation of the care plan is the key to excellence in nursing practice. It is important to determine what practices were successful for the individual patient and what practices need to be modified. Careful, ongoing evaluation of nursing care is the key to a practice base that is constantly being changed to update skills and education that will benefit the older patient. The evaluation step of nursing process provides the opportunity to determine if the client goals were met. Possible outcome criteria for an older person with a pressure ulcer are the prevention of further tissue damage and the promotion of normal wound healing. The goals and outcome criteria are individualized for each older person. In the evaluation and revision of the care plan, the needs and opinions of the older person should always be considered. The nurse should evaluate if the goals were realistic for the older person's age and condition. If the older person was at home, were resources sufficient to make success possible? The evaluation of the family situation, resources available, and needs and desires of the older person will determine the revision of the care plan and the goals and outcome criteria that can be successful. Suggested patient-family teaching guidelines are included to assist the nurse in the process of educating patients and families.

Patient-Family Teaching Guidelines

PREVENTION OF SKIN CANCER

1. What can older persons do to decrease their risk of skin cancer?

- Remember that the sun penetrates through clouds, water, and shade throughout the year.
- Use the appropriate sunscreen protection, at least 15 SPF. It is never too late to protect yourself against further damage.
- Do a total body check, using a mirror if needed, and record any spots so that change can be noted.

RATIONALE:

Education is the key to decrease the older person's risk of skin cancer. On a cloudy day, 80% of the damaging UVR still penetrates to the skin. Sand and snow are equally risky, reflecting 85% to 95% of the sun's rays. It is important to know one's skin type and apply the

Patient-Family Teaching Guidelines

- Be aware that many drugs can cause increased photosensitivity and accelerate damage to the skin.
- Reapply sunscreen when needed. Be aware of ears and bald scalp areas when applying sunscreen. These areas are often the sites of skin cancer.

appropriate sunscreen so that burning is avoided. If actinic keratotic lesions have developed, avoidance of the sun may be sufficient therapy for the regression of mild cases. Self-examination is the key. Any precancerous lesions should be checked every 6 months.

Older persons often take multiple medications. All drug labels should be checked for photosensitivity precautions. Examples of common medications that can cause photosensitivity include Bactrim, tetracycline, and ibuprofen.

2. What causes dry skin (xerosis) in the older person?

Factors that are thought to contribute to dry skin include:

- Age-related changes in circulation (vascularity), sebum secretion, and decreased perspiration.
- Systemic variables such as vitamin A deficiency, hormones, and stress.
- Environmental factors such as smoking, sun damage, and low humidity.
- Personal practices such as excess bathing or the use of harsh bath products (Sheppard & Brenner, 2000).

RATIONALE:

The main source of skin hydration or moisture is provided from the underlying vasculature of the tissues. Sebum also helps to maintain hydration by adding a protective lipid layer to the skin that prevents loss of water through the epidermis. The changes of aging slowly decrease these features. The result is dry skin from a lack of moisture in the stratum corneum, resulting in less pliable epidermis. This decrease in pliability results in the rough texture and flaking of dry skin.

3. What treatment is most effective for dry skin?

Personal practices to improve or relieve dry skin include the following:

- Bathe once a day, using superfatted soaps such as Dove or Caress. Avoid any drying agents such as alcohol.
- Dry with a soft towel, including between the toes.
- Apply emollients liberally to the skin immediately after bathing, while skin is moist. Reapply frequently.
- Use white petroleum for an effective emollient for dry skin treatment. It is inexpensive and does not contain irritating additives such as perfumes.
- Keep humidity as high as possible, especially during the winter months.
- Wear soft, nonirritating clothing next to the skin.
- Prescription creams may also be useful (see Pharmacological Interventions).

RATIONALE:

Research findings indicate that dry skin increases with age and is more severe in winter. Excess bathing depletes the older person's skin of moisture and increases dryness. The use of superfatted soap for bathing helps to retain moisture in the older person's skin. The skin should not be rubbed with a towel; it will increase irritation. Applying emollients after bathing retains the moisture in the skin. It also helps to keep home temperature low and use a humidifier, especially in the winter.

Care Plan

A Patient With a Pressure Ulcer

Case Study

A registered nurse who works for a home health agency has been assigned to Mrs. Krebs, a 75-year-old patient with a chronic stage III ulcer on her heel that has not shown any progress in the last 3 months. The nurse notes that Mrs. Krebs has a smoking history of 40 pack years and has not followed her diet instruction. The supervisor of the home health agency has warned the nurse that if Mrs. Krebs does not improve, the insurance company will not continue to provide payment for the visits and treatment. Mrs. Krebs has refused to be admitted to the hospital for ulcer care and feels the nurses and physician do not understand her situation.

Applying the Nursing Process

ASSESSMENT

On the first visit, the nurse did a complete assessment and discussed the patient's history, which includes peripheral vascular disease and hypertension. Mrs. Krebs's physical examination showed blood pressure 140/82, pulse 76, respirations 20, and temperature 98°F. On examination of the heel ulcer, the nurse noted a 4 cm by 6 cm stage III ulcer with a minimal amount of serous drainage and no local signs of inflammation.

Mrs. Krebs is eating poorly, mostly freezer and canned foods with little protein and high sodium. She admits that she is smoking and not following her diet. She states, "I lost my husband 6 months ago and have not been able to take care of things. I tried to quit smoking but it only lasted 5 days. I have been smoking for 40 years and it is just too hard to stop. I'm doing the best I can."

DIAGNOSIS

The current nursing diagnoses for Mrs. Krebs include the following:

- *Impaired skin integrity,* stage III ulcer, related to prolonged pressure, inadequate nutrition, decreased vascular perfusion
- *Ineffective management of therapeutic regimen related to complex regimen,* limited resources and impaired adjustment as manifested by patient self-assessment of poor dietary intake, inability to rest and elevate foot, and smoking behavior
- *Risk for altered nutrition: less than body requirements* related to lack of physical and economic resources, and increased nutritional requirements related to ulcer

A Patient With a Pressure Ulcer

EXPECTED OUTCOMES

The expected outcomes for the plan specify that Mrs. Krebs will:

- Describe measures to protect and heal the tissue, including wound care.
- Report any additional symptoms such as pain, redness, numbness, tingling, or increased drainage.
- Demonstrate an understanding of nutritional needs, including the need for supplemental protein drink and vitamins.
- Collaborate with the nurse to develop a therapeutic plan that is congruent with her goals and present lifestyle.

PLANNING AND IMPLEMENTATION

The following nursing interventions may be appropriate for Mrs. Krebs:

- Establish a trusting relationship with Mrs. Krebs.
- Begin to explore what the patient's goals are in relation to her healthcare.
- Determine her daily habits and schedule and find some small measures that can be started for health improvement.
- Begin to determine ways to work with Mrs. Krebs's family to motivate her toward a healthy lifestyle (i.e., nutrition, smoking, foot care).
- Set priorities of care that Mrs. Krebs will agree to such as (1) ulcer improvement, (2) diet adjustments, and (3) smoking reductions.

EVALUATION

The nurse hopes to develop a long-term relationship with Mrs. Krebs and make an impact on her health and well-being. The nurse will consider the plan a success based on the following criteria:

- Mrs. Krebs will develop a trusting relationship and develop a plan with the nurse to improve her health.
- A family member will agree to assist Mrs. Krebs with her wound care and shopping issues.
- Mrs. Krebs will begin a smoking reduction effort.
- Mrs. Krebs will agree that if the ulcer is not healing in 4 weeks, she will seek inpatient treatment.

Ethical Dilemma

The primary ethical dilemma that evolves from this situation is the conflict between the moral obligation of the nurse to respect the autonomy of the patient and the principle of beneficence. The patient has a right to self-determination, independence, and freedom. It is important to allow patients to make their own decisions, even if the healthcare provider does not agree with them. However, the nurse has a responsibility to "do good" and "do no harm" based on the principles of beneficence and nonmaleficence. These ethical obligations are outlined in the American Nurses Association Code for Nurses. A second ethical dilemma is the conflict between the nurse's obligation to the patient and to the home health agency.

(continued)

A Patient With a Pressure Ulcer *(continued)*

The nurse hopes to work with Mrs. Krebs and the supervisor to set new goals and priorities and make progress toward them. The nurse understands that the patient has a right to make any final decisions.

Critical Thinking and the Nursing Process

1. What are the intrinsic and extrinsic factors that can cause skin problems in elderly adults? Make a list with two columns and see how many factors you can identify.
2. How important is nutrition to the dermatological health of your skin?
3. What type of dressings do you see used in your clinical rotations with older people? Are they consistent with current guidelines and recommendations?
4. What positioning techniques have you seen used in your clinical rotations?

- Evaluate your responses in Appendix B. ⊂▭

EXPLORE MediaLink

NCLEX review, case studies, and other interactive resources for this chapter can be found on the Companion Website at **www.prenhall.com/tabloski**. Click on Chapter 12 to select the activities for this chapter. For animations, video tutorials, more NCLEX review questions, and case studies, access the accompanying CD-ROM in this textbook.

Chapter Highlights

- The most common precancerous lesion is actinic keratosis, also known as solar keratosis and senile keratosis. Erythematous actinic keratosis is the most common type and appears as a sore, rough, scaly, erythematous papule or plaque. The most common sites for all types of actinic keratosis are sun-exposed areas such as the hands, face, nose, tips of the ears, and bald scalp.
- Basal cell carcinoma is the most common form of skin cancer in White people and accounts for about 80% of nonmelanoma skin cancers.
- Melanoma is the most serious of skin cancers. It is estimated that 53,000 persons were diagnosed with melanoma in 2001, accounting for 7,400 deaths.
- A wound that does not heal within 6 weeks is considered a chronic wound. Common problems of older persons that often lead to chronic wounds are diabetes, peripheral vascular disease, and pressure ulcers.
- The wound can be damaged by both too much and too little moisture. A dry wound surface impairs epithelial migration and leads to tissue injury and necrosis. The buildup of tissue exudates is toxic to new growth and leads to tissue hypoxia, which impairs healing.

- Wound cultures should be obtained by the aspiration method or a tissue biopsy. The swab method is not considered useful for obtaining a wound culture, since it examines bacteria present on the wound surface, not in the wound bed itself.

- Skin care practices for older persons include correct bathing procedure, prevention of injury, and dietary support. These skin care interventions are important to maintain healthy tissue as well as to improve the tissue tolerance to decrease further risk of injury.

- The nurse should encourage older persons to change or shift positions by making small body shifts. This will redistribute weight and increase perfusion. Range of motion exercises should be done every 8 hours and the techniques should be taught to family and patients.

- Topical antiseptics such as povidone-iodine, acetic acid, hydrogen peroxide, and Dakin's solution should not be used on a wound, since they have been found to cause damage.

- To heal a pressure ulcer, a clean, moist environment must be maintained. A moist wound environment promotes cellular activity in all phases of wound healing, provides insulation, increases the rate of epithelial cell growth, and reduces pain. A dry wound environment has been found to result in further tissue death.

- Colonization is the presence and proliferation of organisms (bacteria) in the wound but with no signs of local infection, thus no host response. Stage II, III, and IV pressure ulcers are generally considered to be colonized. Therefore, wound cleansing and debriding are instituted to prevent the development of infection.

- Infection is the proliferation of bacteria in healthy cells that produces symptoms of local redness, pain, fever, and swelling. Examples of serious infections that can be complications of pressure ulcers are bacteremia, sepsis, osteomyelitis, and advancing cellulitis.

References

Agency for Health Care Policy and Research (AHCPR). U.S. Department of Health and Human Services. Panel for the Prediction of Pressure Ulcers in Adults. (1992). *Pressure ulcers in adults: Prediction and prevention. Clinical Practice Guideline No. 3* (AHCPR Bulletin No. 920047). Rockville, MD: Author.

Agency for Healthcare Research and Quality. (2003). *Hospitals that had a lower rate of licensed nurses in the 1990s had higher rates of bedsores and pneumonia.* Retrieved November 12, 2004, from www.ahrq.gov.

American Cancer Society. (2002). *Cancer prevention and early detection—Cancer facts and figures 2002.* Atlanta, GA: Author.

Armstrong, D., & Bortz, P. (2001). An integrative review of pressure relief in surgical patients. *Association of Operating Room Nurses (AORN), 73*(3), 645–657.

Ayello, E. A. (2003). *Predicting pressure ulcer risk.* The Hartford Institute for Geriatric Nursing Division of Nursing, New York University. Retrieved www.hartfordign.org.

Baddour, L. (2000). Cellulitis syndromes: An update. *International Journal of Antimicrobial Agents, 14*(2), 113–116.

Baranoski, S. (2001). Skin tears: Guard against the enemy of frail skin. *Nursing Management, 32*(8), 25–31.

Baxter, H., & McGregor, F. (2001). Understanding and managing cellulitis. *Nursing Standard, 15*(44), 50–56.

Beckrich, K., & Aronovitch, S. A. (1999). Hospital-acquired pressure ulcers: A comparison of costs in medical vs surgical patients. *Nursing Economics, 17*(5), 263–271.

Beers, M., & Berkow, R. (Eds.). (2000). *The Merck manual of geriatrics.* Whitehouse Station Merck & Co.

Bergstrom, N., Allman, R., Alvarez, O., Bennett, M., Carlson, C., & Franz, R. (Eds.). (1994). *Treatment of pressure ulcers: Clinical Practice Guideline No.15 (AHCPR Publication No. 95-0652).* Rockville, MD: Agency for Health Care Policy and Research, Public Health Service, U.S. Department of Health and Human Services.

Boynton, P. R., Jaworski, D., & Paustian, C. (1999). Meeting the challenges of healing chronic wounds in older adults. *Nursing Clinics of North America, 34*(4), 921–932.

Braden, B., & Bergstrom, N. (1994). Predictive validity of the Braden scale for pressure sore risk in a nursing home population. *Research in Nursing and Health, 17,* 459–479.

Carpenito, L. J. (2002). *Nursing diagnosis: Application to clinical practice.* Philadelphia: Lippincott.

Centers for Disease Control and Prevention. (2002). Guidelines for school programs to prevent skin cancer. *Morbidity and Mortality Weekly Report, 51* (No.RR-4), 1–5.

Collett, B. (2000). Disorders of the foot. In M. Beers & R. Berkow (Eds.), *The Merck manual of geriatrics* (pp. 544–557). Whitehouse Station, Merck & Co.

Corbett, J.V. (2000). Laboratory tests and diagnostic procedures with nursing diagnoses. Upper Saddle River: Prentice Hall Health.

Corwin, E. (2000). *Handbook of pathophysiology* (2nd ed.). Philadelphia: Lippincott.

Demling, R., & DeSanti, L. (2001). Protein-energy malnutrition, and the non-healing cutaneous wound. *CME*. Retrieved 2003, from www.medscape.com/viewprogram/714?

Dupuy, A., et. al. (1999). Risk factors for erysipelas of the leg (cellulitis): Case control study. *British Medical Journal, 318*(7198), 1591–1594.

Fielo, S. (2001). Focus on feet. *Nursing Spectrum, 5*(12NE), 12–15.

Franz, R. (2001). Impaired skin integrity: Pressure ulcer. In M. Maas, K. Buckwalter, M. Hardy, T. Tripp-Reimer, M. Titler, & J. Specht (Eds.), *Nursing care of older adults: Diagnoses, outcomes & interventions* (pp. 117–136). St. Louis, MO: Mosby.

Gilchrist, B., & Chiu, N. (2000). Pressure sores. In M. Beers & R. Berkow (Eds.), *The Merck manual of geriatrics* (chap. 14, pp. 155–169): Merck & Co. Whitehouse Station.

Greenlee, R., Murray, T., Boldem, S., & Wingo, P. (2000). Cancer statistics. *CA: A Cancer Journal for Clinicians, 50,* 7–33.

Huether, S., & McCance, K. (2000). *Understanding pathophysiology.* St. Louis, MO: Mosby.

Hwang, M. (1999). Detecting skin cancer. *Journal of the American Medical Association, 281*(7), 676.

John A.Hartford Foundation Institute for Geriatric Nursing. (2003). *Best nursing practices in care for older adults: Incorporating essential geriatric content into baccalaureate and staff development education: A curriculum guide, 4e.* New York: New York University, The Steinhardt School of Education, Division of

Nursing, The John A. Hartford Foundation Institute for Geratric Nursing.

Koutkia, P. (1999). Cellulitis: Evaluation of possible predisposing factors in hospitalized patients. *Diagnostic Microbiology and Infectious Disease, 34*(4), 325–327.

Krasner, D., & Sibbald, G. (1999). Nursing management of chronic wounds. *Nursing Clinics of North America, 34*(4), 933–948.

Leber, K., Perron, V., & Sinni-McKeehan, B. (1999). Common skin cancers in the United States: A practical guide for diagnosis and treatment. *Nurse Practitioner Forum, 10*(2), 106–112.

Lyder, C., Preston, J., Grady, J., Scinto, J., Allman, R., & Bergstrom, N. (2001). Quality of care for hospitalized Medicare patients at risk for pressure ulcers. *Archives of Internal Medicine, 161*(12), 1549–1554.

Maklebust, J. (1999). Interrupting the pressure ulcer cycle. *Nursing Clinics of North America, 34*(4), 861–871.

McLaren, S., & Green, S. (2001). Nutritional factors in the etiology, development and healing of pressure ulcers. In M. J. Morison (Ed.), *The prevention and treatment of pressure ulcers* (pp. 195–215). New York: Mosby.

Moore, A. (2000). Market choices: Wound care products. *RN, 63*(1), 55–58.

Morison, M. J. (Ed.). (2001). *The prevention and treatment of pressure ulcers.* Edinburgh: Mosby.

Nixon, J. (2001). The pathophysiology and aetiology of pressure ulcers. In M. J. Morison (Ed.), *The prevention and treatment of pressure ulcers* (pp. 17–36). Edinburgh: Mosby.

North American Nursing Diagnosis Association. (2002). *Nursing diagnoses: Definitions and classification 2002–2003.* Philadelphia: Author.

NPSource. (2001, August). Treating secondarily infected wounds: Topical antibiotics or oral cephalosporin therapy? *NP Source, 1,* 1, 4.

O'Dell, M. (1998). Skin and wound infections: An overview. *American Family Physician, 57*(10), 2424–2432.

Oliviero, M. (2002). How to diagnose malignant melanoma. *Nurse Practitioner, 27*(2), 26–35.

Ovington, L. (2001). Wound management: Cleansing agents and dressings. In M. J. Morison (Ed.), *The prevention and treatment of pressure ulcers* (pp. 135–154). Edinburgh: Mosby.

Robson, M., Mannari, R., Smith, P., & Payne, W. (1999). Maintenance of wound bacterial balance. *American Journal of Surgery, 178*(5), 399–402.

Schober-Flores, C. (2001). The sun's damaging effects. *Dermatology Nursing, 13*(4), 279–286.

Sheppard, C. M., & Brenner, P. S. (2000). The effects of bathing and skin care products on skin quality and satisfaction with innovative product. *Journal of Gerontological Nursing, 26*(10), 36–45.

Skin Cancer Foundation. (2001a). About basal cell carcinoma, Retrieved March 5, 2005, from www.skincancer.org/basal/index/html.

Skin Cancer Foundation. (2001b). Skin: A concern for all ages. Retrieved March 5, 2005, from www.skincancer.org/older/indexphp.

Stotts, N. (2001). Assessing a patient with a pressure ulcer. In M. J. Morison (Ed.), *The prevention and treatment of pressure ulcers* (pp. 99–118). Edinburgh: Mosby.

Thompson, J. (2000). A practical guide to wound care. *RN, 63*(1), 48–57.

van Rijswijk, L., & Braden, B. J. (1999). Pressure ulcer patient and wound assessment: An AHCPR Clinical Practice Guideline update. *Journal of Ostomy and Wound Management, 45*(1), 26s–40s.

Vap, P., & Dunaye, T. (2000). Pressure ulcer risk assessment in long-term care nursing. *Journal of Gerontological Nursing, 26*(6), 37–45.

Whittington, K., Moore, R., Wilson, W., Patrick, M., & Briones, B. (1999). Managing pressure ulcers: A multisite CQI challenge. *Nursing Management, 30*(10), 27–30.

CHAPTER 13

The Mouth and Oral Cavity

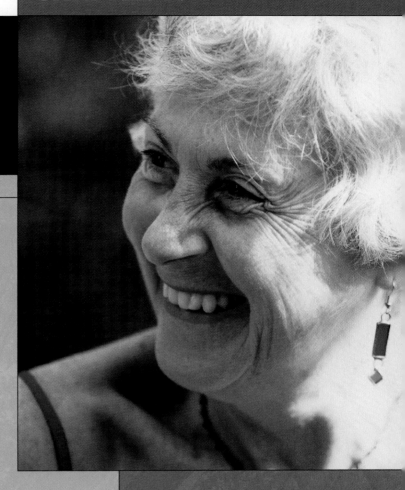

CHAPTER OBJECTIVES

Upon completion of this chapter, the reader will be able to:

- Explain normal changes of aging in the mouth and oral cavity.
- List common nursing diagnoses of older persons related to oral problems.
- Recognize nursing interventions that can be implemented to assist the aging patient with oral problems.
- Identify medications that may cause or aggravate oral problems.

KEY TERMS

angular cheilosis 370
caries 367
edentulous 367
gingivitis 372
glossitis 370
hypogeusia 366
leukoplakia 369
periodontal disease 367
stomatitis 374
xerostomia 368

MediaLink

Additional resources for this chapter can be found on the Student CD-ROM accompanying this textbook and on the Companion Website at **www.prenhall.com/tabloski**. Click on Chapter 13 to select the activities for this chapter.

CD-ROM
- Animation
  Caries
- NCLEX Review
- Case Studies
- Tools

COMPANION WEBSITE
- Audio Glossary
- Additional NCLEX Review
- Case Study
- MediaLink Applications

Oral assessment and care are important responsibilities of gerontological nurses caring for older adults. The mouth is the beginning of the digestive system and also serves as an airway for the respiratory system. The oral cavity consists of the lips, palate, cheeks, tongue, salivary glands, and teeth.

Normal Changes of Aging

With aging, there is thinning of the epithelium and tissue atrophy in the soft tissue of the oral cavity. The single most important factor relating to oral health in aging is maintaining good oral hygiene. In healthy aging with proper oral hygiene, the teeth and gums appear normal. However, with aging it becomes more difficult to maintain good oral hygiene because of multiple factors, including the number and condition of dental restorations, changing alignment between adjacent teeth due to recession of the gums, impaired visual acuity, possible loss of manual dexterity, restricted range of motion, and the effects of medications on oral health (Stark, 2001). Figure 13-1■ depicts the mouth and oral cavity.

Practice Pearl

Urge your older patients to brush with soft-bristled toothbrushes. Stiff bristles lack the flexibility needed to clean curved tooth surfaces and get into crevices between teeth (Stark, 2001).

The taste buds of the tongue decrease in number with a resulting **hypogeusia**, or loss of ability to taste. Salivary function also decreases over time and results in production of less saliva. The gums may recede, leaving teeth vulnerable to cavities below the gum line. The enamel on the surface of teeth may be worn away or abraded, leaving teeth open to staining, damage, and cavities. With tooth loss, malocclusion may result as remaining teeth become misaligned with use in chewing. With tooth loss and malocclu-

FIGURE ■ 13-1

Normal structures of the oral cavity. Over time, the epithelium becomes thinner and there is soft tissue atrophy.

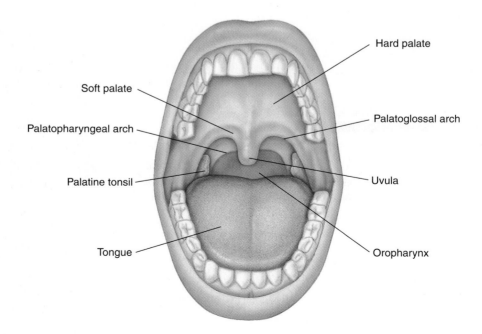

sion, the older person may avoid eating healthy foods high in fiber such as fruits and vegetables, causing further problems related to poor nutrition. Older patients with geriatric dental problems are urged to seek care from dentists with training and expertise in care of older persons and the restorative and preventive skills needed to adequately care for these patients. Dentists skilled in geriatric care have an important role to play in the diagnosis and treatment of oral cancer, soft tissue lesions, salivary gland dysfunction, and taste, smell, and swallowing disorders (Yellowitz, 2001).

Common Diseases of Aging Relating to the Mouth and Oral Cavity

Oral diseases and conditions are common to those older people who grew up without the benefit of community water fluoridation and other fluoride products. About 30% of adults 65 and older no longer have any natural teeth and are **edentulous** (without teeth) (Centers for Disease Control, 2001). Rates of toothlessness vary, with 48% of older Americans in West Virginia having no teeth compared to only 14% in Hawaii. Having missing teeth can affect nutrition because older persons with no teeth have difficulty chewing and swallowing foods with fiber and texture. Poor oral hygiene and ill-fitting dentures can further cause problems with an older person's self-esteem, speech, and facial appearance, and may be a source of halitosis. Even those with dentures and partial plates may choose softer foods and avoid fresh fruits and vegetables because artificial teeth are not as efficient as natural teeth in the chewing and biting process. **Periodontal disease** (gum disease) or dental **caries** (cavities) most often cause tooth loss. The severity of periodontal disease increases with age. About 23% of 65- to 74-year-olds have severe disease, measured by a 6-mm loss of attachment of the tooth to the adjacent gum (receding gum disease). Men are more likely than women to have more severe gum disease, and older people at the lowest socioeconomic level have the most severe periodontal disease (Centers for Disease Control, 2001). However, more older adults are retaining their teeth into advanced age as edentulism is reducing and is no longer considered a normal part of aging (Matear, 2000).

Older Americans with the poorest oral health are those who are economically disadvantaged, lack insurance, and are members of racial and ethnic minorities. Being disabled, homebound, or institutionalized also increases the risk of poor oral health. About 7% of older adults report having had tooth pain at least twice during the past 6 months. Older adults who belong to racial or ethnic minorities or who have a low level of education are more likely to report dental pain than older adults who are White or better educated (Centers for Disease Control, 2001).

Many Americans lose their dental insurance when they retire, and hence do not have access to regular dental care. The situation may be even worse for older women, who generally have lower incomes and may never have had dental insurance. Medicare, which provides health insurance for people over 65 and some people with disabilities, does not provide coverage for routine dental care. Medicaid, the jointly funded federal-state health insurance program for low-income people, funds dental care in some states, but reimbursement rates are so low that it is often difficult to locate a dentist who will accept Medicaid patients.

Oral and pharyngeal cancers, diagnosed in 30,000 Americans every year, result in about 8,000 deaths annually. These cancers, primarily diagnosed in older people, carry a poor prognosis. The 5-year survival rate for White Americans is 56% and for African Americans is only 34% (Centers for Disease Control, 2001).

MediaLink Dental Caries Animation

Most older Americans take prescription and over-the-counter medications that can decrease salivary flow and result in **xerostomia** or dry mouth. For example, antihistamines, diuretics, antipsychotics, and antidepressants can reduce salivary flow. Decreased salivation is associated with increased oral disease as saliva contains antimicrobial components and minerals that help rebuild tooth enamel attacked by decay-causing bacteria. This can be especially problematic for institutionalized elderly adults, who take an average of eight medications a day and often drink very little fluid.

Painful conditions that affect the facial nerves are more common among elderly adults and can be severely debilitating. These conditions can affect mood, sleep, and oral-motor functions such as chewing and swallowing. Further, neurological diseases such as Parkinson's disease, Alzheimer's disease, and stroke can affect oral sensory and motor functions, limiting the older person's ability for self-care (Centers for Disease Control, 2001).

BARRIERS TO MOUTH CARE

Although many older people regularly seek and receive dental care, older adults' use of dental services is the lowest of all adults (Walton, Miller, & Tordecilla, 2002). Frail or institutionalized older adults may not have the physical or financial resources to travel to the dentist and receive needed care. Less than one third of the older adult population visits their dentist annually and almost half have not seen a dentist in 5 years. Older people who are edentulous may erroneously think they no longer need dental services, and they are five times less likely to see a dentist than their peers who still have teeth. Further, many older persons think that tooth loss is a natural consequence of aging and that dental care is expensive, causes pain, and requires frequent and lengthy visits (Walton et al., 2002).

The oral healthcare needs of institutionalized older persons therefore fall to the gerontological nurse and nursing assistants. Many feel that these needs are not being met, and the way nurses provide mouth care has changed little in the last 50 years. Barriers to mouth care include lack of training and knowledge about the importance of oral hygiene, lack of perceived need for oral care, heavy workloads, and resistance by older persons with dementia (Matear, 2000). Further, some nurses find cleaning the mouth or handling dentures unacceptable and unpleasant. However, regular and meticulous mouth care decreases the presence of halitosis, difficult to clean dentures, and other unpleasant mouth conditions, making the process quicker and more pleasant for the older patient and the nurse providing the care.

A recent study of 442 institutionalized older persons in Edinburgh, Scotland, revealed that 65% of the persons wearing dentures had visible soft debris, calculus, and stains that would not wash off and 53% had denture-induced pathology requiring treatment of which the nursing staff was not aware. A study in Canada found that in a similar sample of older nursing home residents, more than 33% had mucosal lesions associated with ill-fitting dentures that had been fitted over 15 years ago; 50% had thick layers of plaque on their dentures; and 20% were using dentures with missing parts, fractures, and other structural defects. Fifty-five percent of subjects with teeth showed evidence of tooth decay and 11% had severe periodontal disease with loose teeth (Coleman, 2002). Studies done in the United States have produced similar findings.

NEGATIVE EFFECTS OF POOR ORAL CARE

Poor oral care can have serious adverse effects on the physical and psychosocial function and health of the older person. Consequences of poor oral care include the following:

- Social isolation and depression
- Systemic illness such as aspiration pneumonia and perhaps heart disease
- Periodontal disease, which can negatively affect glycemic control in persons with diabetes
- Malnutrition, vitamin deficiencies
- Pain, halitosis, tooth loss, dental caries, periodontal disease
- Denture stomatitis

(Coleman, 2002; Connell, McConnell, & Francis, 2002; Yoneyama et al., 2002)

RISK FACTORS FOR ORAL PROBLEMS

All older adults are at risk for oral problems. Normal changes of aging may predispose to the development and detection of these problems. Additionally, diseases commonly found in the older person such as diabetes mellitus can suppress neutrophil production, alter the structure of the lining of the blood vessels, and cause decreased circulation to the skin and mucous membranes. This results in poor healing of oral ulcerations and an increased potential for secondary infections, especially candidiasis (Walton, Miller, & Tordecilla, 2001). Table 13-1 lists risk factors for oral problems.

Practice Pearl

Virginia Henderson, a noted nurse theorist, stated over 40 years ago that the overall standard of nursing care can be judged by the state of the patient's mouth (Henderson, 1960). It remains true today.

Nursing Assessment of Oral Problems

Patients should be carefully questioned regarding their oral health history, including date of last dental examination, presence and function of dentures, missing or loose teeth, bleeding gums, dry mouth, presence of sores or lesions, medications, usual oral hygiene routine, altered sense of taste, chewing or swallowing difficulties, and presence of bad breath or halitosis.

A complete oral cavity assessment includes examination of the lips, teeth, interior of the buccal mucosa, anterior and base of the tongue, gums, soft and hard palate, and back of the throat. Careful notation of any cracks, lesions, ulcers, swelling, induration, gingival bleeding, hypertrophy, or dental caries should be made in the patient's record. **Leukoplakia**, or a white patchy coating on the surface of the oral mucosa, should be referred to a dentist or oral surgeon for further evaluation and biopsy.

Wearing gloves, the nurse should lift the tongue with a 4 × 4 inch dressing to examine the posterior surface. Extra light will be required to complete visualization. Observe any tremor, coating, or deviation of the tongue.

The lymph nodes of the head and neck should be carefully palpated and any tenderness or enlargement noted. The condition and number of natural teeth should also be noted. Loose or broken teeth should be referred for dental evaluation because the patient is at risk for losing and swallowing the tooth during a meal. Likewise, dentures should be examined for fit and condition. Cracks, poor fit, and missing or broken teeth should be noted.

TABLE 13-1

Risk Factors for Oral Problems

Risk Factor	Potential Cause of Oral Problem
Diseases	Cancer
	HIV/AIDS
	Sjögren's syndrome
	Diabetes mellitus
	Renal failure
	Endocrine disorders
	Dementia
	Psychiatric illness
	Viruses (e.g., herpes simplex, zoster, Coxsackie)
Vitamin deficiencies	
Glossitis	Niacin, folic acid, B_6, B_{12}
Glossodynia	B vitamins (riboflavin, niacin, folic acid, B_6, B_{12}, zinc and iron)
Stomatitis	Niacin, folic acid, B_{12}
Xerostomia	Vitamin A, vitamin B_{12}
Bleeding gums	Vitamin C, vitamin K
Angular cheilosis	B vitamins, iron
Medications	Antibiotics
	Antineoplastics
	Biological response modifiers
	Phenytoin
	Antihistamines
	Anticholinergics
	Reserpine and chlorpromazine
	Glucocorticoids (inhaled and oral)
Normal aging changes	Thinner enamel on teeth
	Stress lines and cracks in teeth
	Gingiva, periodontal ligament, and bone recede
	Mucosa becomes thinner and smoother, and loses elasticity
	Decreased salivary production
Functional problems	Institutionalization
	Caregiver stress/unavailability
	Transportation problems
	Cognitive impairment
	Mistrust of healthcare providers
	Poor vision/manual dexterity
Financial problems	Lack of dental insurance
	Unwillingness/inability to spend money on dental care
Confounding factors	Oxygen therapy
	Tachypnea/mouth breathing
	Oral or nasal suctioning
	Radiation therapy to head/neck
	Tobacco or alcohol use
	Ill-fitting dentures
	Medication toxicity
	Orthopedic replacements or organ transplants

Source: Hornick, 2002; Walton et al., 2001, 2002.

Common Oral Problems

Common problems of the mouth that occur with aging include xerostomia, oral candidiasis, oral pain, stomatitis, oral cancer, and gingival disease.

XEROSTOMIA

The most common oral problem occurring in the older adult is xerostomia and may affect as many as 30% of older people (Ship, Pillemer, & Baum, 2002; Walton et al., 2001). Dry mouth can result from mouth breathing, dehydration due to diuretic use, oxygen therapy, oral and systemic diseases, and head and neck radiation. The most common cause appears to be drug induced, with 80% of the most commonly prescribed drugs (about 400 medications) reported to cause xerostomia (Ship et al., 2002). The most common offenders are tri cyclic antidepressants, sedatives, tranquilizers, antihistamines, antihypertensives (alpha- and beta-blockers), diuretics, calcium channel blockers, ACE inhibitors, cytotoxic agents, antiparkinsonian agents, and antiseizure drugs (Ship et al., 2002). Chemotherapy drugs have also been associated with salivary disorders.

Oral symptoms associated with xerostomia include altered taste; difficulty eating, chewing, and swallowing (particularly dry foods); halitosis; chronic burning sensation in the mouth; and intolerance to spicy foods (Ship et al., 2002). Difficulty with swallowing leads to increased episodes of choking and aspiration pneumonia.

Sjögren's syndrome is a debilitating systemic autoimmune disorder associated with inflammation of epithelial tissue and xerostomia and occurs in association with other autoimmune disorders such as rheumatoid arthritis, systemic lupus erythematosus, scleroderma, polymyositis, and polyarteritis. Other components of the disorder include dry eyes, skin changes, and thyroid disease (Ship et al., 2002). Diagnosis is confirmed by the presence in the serum of autoantibodies to Ro (SS-A) or La (SS-B) antigen or both.

Nursing interventions to improve xerostomia include the following:

- Urging regular dental evaluation
- Low-sugar diet
- Mouth rinses
- Sugar-free chewing gum, hard candies, and mints
- Artificial saliva and mouth lubricants (Salivart, Xero-Lube)
- Bedside humidifiers
- Dietary modifications including avoidance of foods known to be difficult to chew or swallow and careful use of fluids while eating

ORAL CANDIDIASIS

Oral candidiasis is a frequent complication of dry mouth and is treated with oral antifungal agents. Persons who have diabetes and have high or elevated glucose levels are at risk for candidiasis (thrush) because the oral flora is altered and the organism *Candida albicans* is encouraged to overgrow. Additionally, persons with diabetes have an altered immune response including decreases in leukocyte activity, decreased phagocytosis, and decreased neutrophil resistance.

The usual treatment is rinsing with topical antifungal agents (nystatin) four times a day for 2 weeks. The nurse should carefully observe older patients to make sure they adequately "swish" the solution for about 2 minutes but do not swallow the solution. If an oral troche (a medicated lozenge to soothe the throat) is used, it must be held in the mouth and allowed to slowly dissolve. The troche contains sugar and should not be used with patients who have diabetes (Walton et al., 2002). Patients with dentures should remove their dentures before rinsing to ensure that the medication reaches all areas of the oral mucosa. One millimeter of nystatin oral suspension should be added to the water used to soak dentures at nighttime, and dentures should soak for at least 6 hours. If the older person is taking medications associated with xerostomia, the primary care provider should be consulted to see if these drugs might be discontinued. Careful denture cleaning and attention to mouth hygiene are essential.

A small soft toothbrush is considered the most effective mechanical method to control dental plaque. Teeth or gums should be brushed twice daily for about 3 to 4 minutes. Toothbrushes perform substantially better than foam swabs in the ability to remove plaque from the teeth and gingival margins and from the areas between teeth (Pearson & Hutton, 2002). Swabs are useful to cleanse and moisten oral mucosa and prevent damage to delicate tissue and may be effectively used when caring for the dying, but a moist toothbrush is more effective in reducing bacterial plaque and cleaning the oral cavity (Coleman, 2002).

> ### Practice Pearl
>
> Lemon and glycerine swabs are not only ineffective, but are in fact harmful and should not be used (Coleman, 2002).

Mouth rinses are available and can serve the purposes of cleansing, moisturizing, or killing germs. Nurses commonly use hydrogen peroxide and sodium bicarbonate although recent evidence suggests hydrogen peroxide harms the oral mucosa and causes negative subjective reaction in patients. Sodium bicarbonate dissolves mucous and oral debris but has an unpleasant taste and can burn oral mucosa if not diluted properly. Chlorhexidine (Peridex) is used widely to treat gingival and periodontal disease and other oral infections. It can improve oral hygiene in populations with special needs in whom mechanical plaque removal is difficult, such as those with Alzheimer's disease or those who do not possess the dexterity or strength for manual plaque removal.

ORAL PAIN

Oral pain is an advanced problem in a tooth or the gingival tissues. Although pain may resolve with time, an untreated problem can result in a tooth abscess or serious infection. When older patients complain of mouth pain, the gerontological nurse should carefully inspect the mouth, teeth, and tongue for signs of infection or abscess. Additional information includes checking the patient's temperature, pulse, and respiration to rule out acute infection. Patients with a dental abscess will often have swollen or enlarged lymph nodes under the ear or jaw. Clusters of vesicles of "punched out looking" ulcers on the lips and mucosa can indicate the presence of herpes simplex or zoster. Treatment with an antiviral topical ointment or suspension is indicated after referral and assessment by the primary care provider.

GINGIVITIS AND PERIODONTAL DISEASE

Inflammation of the gums associated with redness, swelling, and a tendency to bleed are the common presenting signs of gingivitis. **Gingivitis** is a precursor to chronic periodontitis. About 80% of older Americans have some sort of periodontal disease

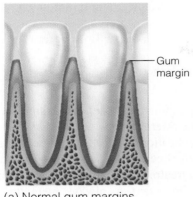

(a) Normal gum margins and teeth

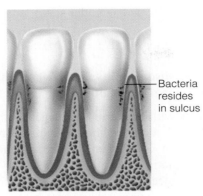

(b) Plaque formation and early gum erosion

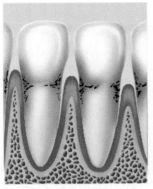

(c) Progressive gum erosion with early inflammatory response

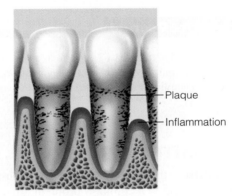

(d) Loss of alveolar bone with full gum erosion

FIGURE ◻ 13-2

Gingivitis and resulting gum erosion.

(Centers for Disease Control, 2001). Gingivitis results from bacterial colonization at the gum margin and in the sulcus between the margin and the tooth (Figure 13-2◻). When bacteria are not removed from the mouth, they form a sticky, colorless plaque on the teeth that will harden and form a sheltered area for colonies to flourish. The longer plaque and tartar remain on the teeth, the more harmful they become. These bacteria and their products have a direct inflammatory effect and also evoke an immunological response. This response can cause erosion of the gingival sulcus or pocket and resorption of alveolar bone around the tooth, leaving the tooth at risk for a cavity below the gum line. The gums will become red and swollen and bleed easily. Daily flossing and twice-daily brushing with fluoride toothpaste often helps reduce the symptoms of gingivitis. An oral hygienist is needed to remove plaque and tartar with special instruments.

Risk factors for gingivitis include:

- **Smoking.** Smoking cigarettes greatly increases the risk of periodontal disease and lowers the chances of success of dental treatments.
- **Diabetes.** Persons with diabetes are at higher risk of all forms of periodontal disease.
- **Medications.** Many drugs can reduce saliva production, and thus the protective effect of saliva on the teeth and gums is lost.
- **Poor nutrition.** A poor diet, especially one low in calcium, can lower resistance to gum disease. Eating and drinking foods and drinks high in sugars can damage teeth.

- **Stress.** Older people under stress have more difficulty fighting infection, including gingivitis.
- **Illness.** Diseases like HIV/AIDS and cancer can make fighting any infection more difficult.
- **Genetic susceptibility.** Although not directly inherited, gum disease seems more common in some families.

Patients with bright red or magenta-colored gums or those complaining of gum bleeding with toothbrushing or eating should be referred to the dentist or periodontist for evaluation. The dentist will recommend medications such as antimicrobial mouth rinses, antibiotic gels, and perhaps surgery with bone and tissue grafts to replace lost bone and protect the vitality of the teeth. These treatments are difficult and expensive; therefore, prevention and early intervention is important. As always, meticulous oral hygiene is necessary to prevent tooth loss and progression of the disease.

> ### Practice Pearl
>
> Urge all older patients to engage in self-care activities to prevent gum disease, including daily flossing, twice-daily brushing with fluoride toothpaste, twice-yearly dental cleaning and evaluation, eating a well-balanced diet, and avoiding tobacco products.

STOMATITIS

Stomatitis is the inflammation of the mouth that is frequently caused by chemotherapy agents and is a common problem among older patients undergoing cancer treatment. Approximately 40% of patients undergoing cancer treatment will experience this painful condition (Walton et al., 2001). Anticancer drugs cause cell destruction throughout the body, and the cells of the mouth can become damaged leading to erosion, ulceration, inflammation, and secondary infections. Eating and drinking can be painful, and nutritional problems may occur as a result of stomatitis.

Treatments include meticulous oral hygiene, frequent use of a mild saline mouthwash, and avoiding extremes of hot, cold, or very spicy food and liquids. In extreme cases, a swish-and-spit solution of kaolin and pectin, diphenhydramine hydrochloride, and lidocaine may provide relief before mealtime.

ORAL CANCER

Benign and malignant tumors can occur in the mouth and pharynx. Like other cancers, malignant tumors of the mouth and pharynx can metastasize and invade other parts of the body, making early diagnosis crucial. Oral cancer that metastasizes will usually travel via the lymph nodes in the neck. Squamous cell carcinoma is the most frequent cancer of the oral cavity and occurs most often in older persons. The 5-year survival rate for treated oral cancer is about 50%, with mortality the highest for cancers of the tongue and lowest for cancers of the lips (National Cancer Institute, 2002).

Oral cancer usually occurs in people over the age of 45 but can develop at any age. Symptoms of oral cancer include the following:

- A sore on the lip or mouth that does not heal
- A lump on the lip or in the mouth
- A white or red patch on the gum, tongue, or buccal mucosa

- Unusual bleeding, pain, or numbness in the mouth
- A feeling that something is always caught in the throat
- Difficulty or pain with chewing or swallowing
- Swelling of the jaw that changes the fit and comfort of dentures
- Changes in the voice
- Pain in the ear

(National Cancer Institute, 2002)

Patients with these symptoms should seek treatment from their dentist or primary care provider for further assessment and diagnosis. Currently, diagnosis of oral cancer involves checking histopathology of suspicious cells after biopsy and x-ray techniques like computerized axial tomography scans or magnetic resonance imaging. Treatment involves surgery, radiation therapy, and chemotherapy. A team approach is needed when treating older patients with oral cancer. Key team members usually include an oral surgeon, the gerontological nurse, a medical oncologist, a plastic surgeon, a dietitian, a social worker, and a speech therapist.

Rehabilitation is an important follow-up to treatment for patients with oral cancer. Regular follow-up appointments are needed to check the healing process and monitor for signs of returning cancer. Patients with weight loss should work closely with the dietitian. Most physicians advise patients to stop using tobacco and alcohol to reduce the risk of developing a new cancer (National Cancer Institute, 2002).

Risk factors for the development of oral cancer include:

- **Tobacco use.** Smoking cigarettes, pipes, and cigars accounts for 90% of oral cancers. Cigar, pipe, and chewing tobacco users have the same risk as cigarette smokers.
- **Chronic and heavy alcohol use.** The risks are even greater for older people who smoke and use alcohol.
- **Sun exposure to the lips.** Wearing a brimmed hat and lip balm with sunscreen reduce the risk. Pipe smokers are especially prone to lip cancer.
- **History of leukoplakia.** Older people with white patches in the mouth should be closely monitored.
- **Erythroplakia.** People in their 60s and 70s may develop red or magenta patches in the mouth.

Black men have the highest rates of oral cancer, followed by White men. Black men tend to be younger at age of diagnosis (peaks at 65 to 69 and at 75 to 79 years) than White men (peaks at 80 to 84). This may reflect underlying genetic predisposition and smoking habits. Figure 13-3■ illustrates oral cancer incidence and death rates by race and sex.

See the Best Practice feature on page 377 for the Geriatric Oral Health Assessment Index (GOHAI).

NURSING STRATEGIES FOR PROVIDING ORAL CARE TO PATIENTS WITH COGNITIVE IMPAIRMENTS

Many older nursing home residents with cognitive impairments will resist or refuse the nursing staff's attempts to provide mouth care. Some will refuse to open their mouths, resist inserting or removing dentures, try to bite the caregiver or clamp down on the toothbrush, or refuse to swish or swallow mouth rinses. These problems can discourage the nurses and the nursing assistants that are providing mouth care. Nursing research is clearly needed in this area to identify appropriate and effective nursing interventions. Some strategies that may be used and adapted in the nursing home

Oral cancer incidence and death rates among persons 65 years of age and older by sex and race, 1993-1997, (rate per 100,000 persons)

Incidence Rate

	Total	Male	Female
All races	44	68	27
White	45	69	28
Black	40	65	21

Death Rate

	Total	Male	Female
All races	14	21	9
White	14	20	9
Black	17	30	9

Source: Centers for Disease Control, 2001.

setting when providing mouth care for difficult residents with a cognitive impairment include:

- **Task breakdown.** Time is taken to slowly break down the task into small steps. For instance, "Now I will place some toothpaste on the toothbrush. Does this look like enough to you?" The resident should be involved in each step of the process.
- **Distraction.** Playing music or looking at family pictures may provide some distraction while the caregiver carries out oral care.
- **Hand over hand.** The caregiver places a hand over the resident's hand and guides the activity.
- **Chaining.** The caregiver starts the activity and then asks the resident to complete it. For instance, the nurse may move the toothbrush back and forth a few times and then say, "Now you do it, Mrs. Jones. I may not be doing it exactly how you like it."
- **Protection.** Nurses should never insert their fingers into the mouth of a resident who bites or resists care. Human bites can be painful and infection prone. In extreme circumstances, several tongue blades may be taped together and inserted into the resident's open mouth, providing some small measure of protection should the resident decide to clamp down.

(Modified from Chalmers, 2000)

As always, timing is key to approaching residents with cognitive impairments. Choose the time of day when the resident is most calm and accepting of care. Should the resident vehemently refuse oral care, it is best to walk away and reapproach the resident at a later time. It is seldom effective to try to force the resident to open the mouth and accept oral care. Even if successful care is achieved during the forced event, the next time oral care is offered, the resident will probably violently refuse again and experience a great deal of distress as a result.

Sometimes the presence of a family member can be reassuring and calming to the resident. A staff member who seems to have a good rapport with the resident should take responsibility for the provision of oral care. Effective and ineffective nursing interventions should be carefully noted in the nursing care plan so that a consistent approach can be used and the resident will come to associate oral care with the pleasant feeling of having a clean mouth.

The Hartford Institute for Geriatric Nursing Try This assessment series recommends the Geriatric Oral Health Assessment Index (GOHAI) for use in the clinical setting (Atchison, 1997). The GOHAI has been tested and used extensively primarily in the community and acute care setting; however, it is appropriate for the long-term care facility as well. This is a 12-item scale. A score of 57 to 60 is considered a high score, 51 to 56 a medium score, and below 50 a low score. Individuals with a high score or troublesome symptoms should be referred for a dental examination and follow-up (Hartford Institute for Geriatric Nursing, 1999).

The Geriatric Oral Health Assessment Index

Indicate, in the past three months, how often you feel the way described in each of the following statements. Circle one answer for each.

	1	2	3	4	5
1. How often did you limit the kind or amounts of food you eat because of problems with your teeth or dentures?	Always	Often	Sometimes	Seldom	Never
2. How often did you have trouble biting or chewing any kinds of food such as firm meat or apples?	Always	Often	Sometimes	Seldom	Never
3. How often were you able to swallow comfortably?*	Always	Often	Sometimes	Seldom	Never
4. How often have your teeth or dentures prevented you from speaking the way you wanted?	Always	Often	Sometimes	Seldom	Never
5. How often were you able to eat anything without feeling discomfort?*	Always	Often	Sometimes	Seldom	Never
6. How often did you limit contacts with people because of the condition of your teeth or dentures?	Always	Often	Sometimes	Seldom	Never
7. How often were you pleased or happy with the looks of your teeth and gums or dentures?*	Always	Often	Sometimes	Seldom	Never
8. How often did you use medication to relieve pain or discomfort from around your mouth?	Always	Often	Sometimes	Seldom	Never
9. How often were you worried or concerned about the problems with your teeth, gums, or dentures?	Always	Often	Sometimes	Seldom	Never
10. How often did you feel nervous or self-conscious because of problems with your teeth, gums, or dentures?	Always	Often	Sometimes	Seldom	Never
11. How often did you feel uncomfortable eating in front of people because of problems with your teeth or dentures?	Always	Often	Sometimes	Seldom	Never
12. How often were your teeth or gums sensitive to hot, cold, or sweets?	Always	Often	Sometimes	Seldom	Never

Total Score: _____

*Items 3, 5, 7 are reverse scored with a "1" for never and a "5" for always. All other items are a "1" for always.

Adapted from Atchison, K. A. (1997). The Geriatric Oral Health Assessment Index. In Slade, G. D. (Ed.), Measuring Oral Health and Quality of Life. Chapel Hill: University of North Carolina, Dental Ecology 1997. Kurlowicz., L. *Try This: Best Practices in Care for Older Adults* (2002). New York: New York University, The Steinhardt School of Education, Division of Nursing, The John A. Hartford Foundation Institute for Geriatric Nursing.

Nursing Diagnoses

The nursing diagnoses of *impaired dentition* and *impaired oral mucous membrane* may be used for older patients with mouth problems. The presence of acute and chronic pain and nutrition problems would also be noted. The presence of infection, communication difficulties, and self-esteem problems should also be indicated.

The patient-family teaching guidelines in the following feature will assist the nurse to instruct older persons about problems relating to the mouth and oral cavity.

Patient-Family Teaching Guidelines

EDUCATION GUIDE TO ORAL HEALTH

Being older does not necessarily mean wearing dentures and being toothless. Older patients should be urged to take these steps to protect their oral health and preserve their teeth.

1. What can I do to protect my teeth now that I am older?

Suggestions for good oral health include:

- Drink fluoridated water and use fluoridated toothpaste; fluoride provides protection against dental decay at all ages.

- Practice good oral hygiene. Brush teeth carefully twice a day and floss daily to reduce dental plaque and prevent periodontal disease. Use an egg timer to ensure that brushing is carried out for at least 3 minutes.

- Get professional oral healthcare, even if you have no natural teeth. Professional care helps to maintain the overall health of the teeth and mouth, and provides for early detection of precancerous or cancerous lesions. For patients with teeth, see the dentist and dental hygienist twice a year for evaluation, cleaning, and scaling. For the patient without teeth, see the dentist yearly for an oral cancer check.

RATIONALE:

Good oral self-care and professional care are needed to maintain oral health. Ongoing yearly or twice-yearly appointments augment self-care practices.

2. Are there substances I should avoid in my daily habits?

- Avoid tobacco. In addition to the general health risks of tobacco use, smokers have 7 times the risk of developing periodontal disease compared to nonsmokers. Tobacco used in any form—cigarettes, cigars, pipes, and smokeless (chewing) tobacco—increases the risk for periodontal disease, oral and throat cancers, and oral fungal infections.

- Limit alcohol. Excessive alcohol consumption is a risk factor for oral and throat cancers. Alcohol and tobacco use together greatly increase the risk.

- Get dental care before, after, and during cancer treatment with chemotherapy and radiation. Careful attention is needed to treat and prevent damage that can destroy teeth and oral tissues.

RATIONALE:

Many older patients and their families are unaware of how important oral health is to their overall health and function. Those without teeth or with dentures may feel that they need not worry about mouth care. By reinforcing these guidelines, older patients' oral health and general health can be improved (Centers for Disease Control, 2001).

Caregivers should attend to the daily oral hygiene of older people who cannot care for themselves. This includes older people with cognitive impairments and physical frailty. It is important to note effective techniques and provide a consistent approach.

Care Plan

A Patient With a Problem of the Mouth/Oral Cavity

Case Study

Mr. Graham is a 72-year-old African American man who is admitted to a rehabilitation facility for recovery after falling and breaking his right hip. He is now 3 days post-operative after an open reduction with internal fixation with replacement of his hip with a prosthesis. He is awake and alert, but the nurse notices that he looks slightly de-hydrated and emaciated. His height is 66 inches and his weight is 120 lb. He reports that his appetite has been poor for the last few months and he has lost some weight. Mr. Graham wears dentures but they seem to move about in his mouth a lot, and he is con-stantly covering his mouth with his hand. The nurse is concerned that if he does not im-prove his nutritional intake, his wound might not heal properly and he is at risk for infection.

Applying the Nursing Process

ASSESSMENT

The nurse should assess the dietary history including meal preferences, eating habits, use of tobacco and alcohol, and list of current medications. Also, the gerontological nurse should carefully assess Mr. Graham's mouth to determine his state of oral health, assess skin turgor, and check postural blood pressures. As he has fallen and fractured a hip, he is at risk for future falls. With dehydra-tion, he may exhibit postural hypotension and become dizzy when arising from a chair.

He seems to have loose-fitting dentures, which is common after a person has weight loss. Weight loss of about 10 lb can mean that dentures need to be refit-ted to provide the tight fit needed for chewing food. He may have ulcerations from ill-fitting dentures, causing pain and discomfort when he ingests food and fluids.

DIAGNOSIS

Appropriate nursing diagnoses for Mr. Graham include the following:

- *Nutrition imbalanced: less than body requirements,* as evidenced by his weight loss
- *Risk for injury,* as evidenced by his recent fall and hip fracture
- *Impaired dentition,* as evidenced by his toothlessness and ill-fitting dentures
- *Impaired oral mucous membrane,* if evidence exists of gum or mucous mem-brane ulceration or erosion

(continued)

A Patient With a Problem of the Mouth/Oral Cavity (*continued*)

EXPECTED OUTCOMES

The expected outcomes for the plan specify that Mr. Graham will:

- Describe dietary preferences and eat at least 50% of each meal.
- Report any oral symptoms such as pain, redness, swelling, or taste disturbances.
- Demonstrate an understanding of nutritional needs, including the need for supplemental protein drink and vitamins.
- Collaborate with the nurse to develop a therapeutic plan that is congruent with his goals and present lifestyle situation.

PLANNING AND IMPLEMENTATION

The nurse may wish to observe Mr. Graham at mealtime to ascertain his oral intake, chewing ability, and food preferences. Careful documentation regarding the kinds of food and amount of food consumed at each meal is needed. Additionally, family members should be encouraged to bring in favorite foods to stimulate appetite. Pain, if present, should be monitored and treated so that Mr. Graham is not in pain during mealtimes. Should his dentures need adjustment, temporarily lining them with a gel pad may improve his eating ability. A referral to a dentist will ultimately be needed for a permanent adjustment and realignment for a proper fit. Any ulcers or abrasions to the gums and oral mucosa should be carefully cleaned and monitored to prevent infection and aid healing.

EVALUATION

The nurse will evaluate the success of the care plan based on the following:

- Mr. Graham will develop a trusting relationship and work with the nursing staff to improve his nutritional intake.
- He will maintain a stable weight or begin to gain weight slowly over time.
- He will show evidence of recovery from his surgery, including skin and bone healing on x-ray.
- Mr. Graham will report his dentures fit well and he can chew and swallow without difficulty.

Ethical Dilemma

Mr. Graham states, "I'm hooked on cigarettes. I've smoked a pack a day since I was 15 years old. If I don't have a cigarette I'll crawl out of my skin, and my daughter won't bring me any. Can you get some for me?"

The nurse knows that quitting cigarette smoking "cold turkey" can be very difficult, especially for a patient who has a long smoking history. However, the nurse also knows that continued smoking will probably further suppress appetite, delay the healing of any ulcerations in the mouth, and increase the risk for many cancers, including oral cancer. The nurse may wish to consult with the patient, family, and primary care provider regarding the use of a nicotine patch or other nicotine substitute. Additionally, some medications (buspirone) can ease nicotine withdrawal. It would be unethical to ignore the patient's request entirely and equally unethical to procure cigarettes for him. By involv-

A Patient With a Problem of the Mouth/Oral Cavity

ing Mr. Graham, his family, and the primary care provider, his tobacco addiction can be considered and hopefully addressed.

Critical Thinking and the Nursing Process

1. How would you feel receiving mouth care from another person? Ask a close friend to brush your teeth, and then brush your friend's teeth. What feelings are elicited? Does your mouth feel fresh and clean afterwards? What suggestions for improvement do you have for your friend?

2. Imagine you are caring for a patient who has smoked cigarettes for many years and now has oral cancer. Are you likely to "blame the patient" for getting the disease because he or she continued to smoke and knew the risks?

3. Your nursing home patient has significant periodontal disease, loose teeth, and many dental caries. He is in pain or discomfort most of the day. The director of nursing cannot locate a dentist who will come to the nursing home, and it is difficult to get the patient to the dentist's office because he has had a stroke and is paralyzed on the right side and is wheelchair-bound. Describe your feelings.

4. You observe a nurse's aid approach a nursing home resident with dementia and say brusquely, "Open your mouth." The resident refuses and the aid walks away, telling you later that the resident refused oral care. What would be an appropriate response?

■ Evaluate your responses in Appendix B.

EXPLORE MediaLink

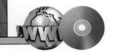

NCLEX review, case studies, and other interactive resources for this chapter can be found on the Companion Website at **www.prenhall.com/tabloski**. Click on Chapter 13 to select the activities for this chapter. For animations, video tutorials, more NCLEX review questions, and case studies, access the accompanying CD-ROM in this textbook.

Chapter Highlights

■ Mouth care and maintenance of oral health is well within the role of the gerontological nurse.

■ Normal changes of aging, common diseases affecting older people, and many treatments and medications can negatively affect the teeth and oral cavity.

■ There is convincing evidence that oral problems are associated with weight loss, malnutrition, infection, social isolation, depression, and mortality.

■ Institutionalized elderly adults, especially those with cognitive impairments, are completely dependent upon nursing staff for oral care and maintenance.

■ Conscientious assessment and adherence to promoting oral hygiene and instituting preventive care can improve the quality of life for older patients.

References

Atchison, K. (1997). The general oral health assessment index (the geriatric oral health assessment index). In G. D. Slade (Ed.), *Measuring oral health and quality of life.* Chapel Hill: University of North Carolina, Dental Ecology.

Centers for Disease Control. (2001). *Oral health for older Americans.* Retrieved November 12, 2004, from www.cdc.gov.

Chalmers, J. (2000). Behavior management and communication strategies for dental professionals when caring for patients with dementia. *Special Care Dentistry, 20,* 147–154.

Coleman, P. (2002). Improving oral health care for the frail elderly: A review of widespread problems and best practices. *Geriatric Nursing, 23*(4), 189–198.

Connell, B., McConnell, E., & Francis, T. (2002). Tailoring the environment of oral health care to the needs and abilities of nursing home residents with dementia. *Alzheimer's Care Quarterly, 3*(1), 19–25.

Hartford Institute for Geriatric Nursing. (1999). *Best practices in nursing care to older adults.* New York: New York University.

Henderson, V. (1960). *Basic principles of nursing care.* Geneva, Switzerland: International Council for Nursing.

Hornick, B. (2002). Diet and nutrition implications for oral health. *Journal of Dental Hygiene, 76*(1), 67–82.

Kurlowicz., L. *Try this: Best practices in care for older adults (2002).* New York: New York University, The Steinhardt School of Education, Division of Nursing, The John A. Hartford Foundation Institute for Geriatric Nursing.

Matear, D. (2000). How should we deliver and assess oral health education in seniors' institutions? *Journal of the Gerontological Nursing Association, Perspectives, 24*(2), 15–21.

National Cancer Institute. (2002). *What you need to know about oral cancer.* Retrieved November 12, 2004, from www.cancer.gov.

Pearson, L., & Hutton, J. (2002). A controlled trial to compare the ability of foam swabs and toothbrushes to remove dental plaque. *Journal of Advanced Nursing, 39*(5), 480–489.

Ship, J., Pillemer, S., & Baum, B. (2002). Xerostomia and the geriatric patient. *Journal of the American Geriatrics Society, 50,* 535–543.

Stark, A. (2001). Oral health. In M. Mezey (Ed.), *The encyclopedia of elder care.* New York: Springer.

Walton, J., Miller, J., & Tordecilla, L. (2001). Elder oral assessment and care. *MEDSURG Nursing, 10*(1), 37–44.

Walton, J., Miller, J., & Tordecilla, L. (2002). Elder oral assessment and care. *ORL—Head and Neck Nursing, 20*(2), 12–19.

Yellowitz, J. (2001). Geriatric dentistry. In M. Mezey (Ed.), *The encyclopedia of elder care.* New York: Springer.

Yoneyama, T., Yshoda, M., Ohrui, T., Mukaiyama, H., Okamoto, H., Hoshiba, K., et al. (2002). Oral care reduces pneumonia in older patients in nursing homes. *Journal of the American Geriatrics Society, 50,* 430–433.

CHAPTER 14

Sensation: Hearing, Vision, Taste, Touch, and Smell

Bridgette Maclaughlin Warnat, MS, RNBC
Patricia Tabloski, PhD, GNP

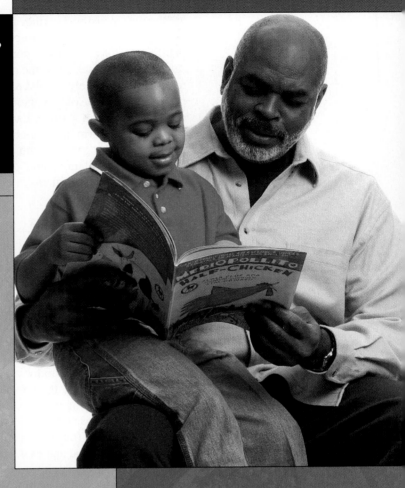

CHAPTER OBJECTIVES

Upon completion of this chapter, the reader will be able to:

- Explain normal changes of aging on the five senses—vision, hearing, taste, smell, and touch.
- List common nursing diagnoses of older persons related to sensory problems.
- Recognize nursing interventions that can be implemented to assist the aging patient with sensory changes.
- Identify medications that may cause or aggravate sensory dysfunction.

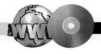

MediaLink

Additional resources for this chapter can be found on the Student CD-ROM accompanying this textbook and on the Companion Website at **www.prenhall.com/tabloski**. Click on Chapter 14 to select the activities for this chapter.

CD-ROM
- Animation/Video
    Allergic Rhinitis
    Audiology
    Cataracts
    Conjunctivitis
    Ear and Eye A&P
- NCLEX Review

- Case Studies
- Tools

COMPANION WEBSITE
- Audio Glossary
- Additional NCLEX Review
- Case Study
- MediaLink Applications

KEY TERMS

accommodation 387
age-related macular
  degeneration (ARMD) 384
cataracts 384
cerumen 398
conductive hearing loss 400
diabetic retinopathy 384
glaucoma 384
hyposmia 410
presbycusis 402
presbyopia 387
sensorineural hearing loss 402
tinnitus 405
xerostomia 408

Changes in vision, hearing, smell, taste, and touch occur naturally throughout the aging process. However, impairments in sensory functioning can greatly alter the capabilities of older adults to complete everyday activities, affecting quality of life and safety. Intact senses allow the older person to accurately perceive the environment and remain appropriately involved with other people, places, and objects. Safety is compromised when the older person cannot see fall hazards on the floor, cannot smell a natural gas leak from a stove, cannot recognize the taste of spoiled milk, cannot hear a signaling fire alarm, and cannot feel a pebble in the shoe that could lead to a blister or foot ulcer. Older persons with sensory dysfunction may suffer functional impairment, injury, social isolation, and depression. This chapter will discuss normal sensory changes, common problems, management, treatment, and nursing interventions.

Vision

Normal age-related changes in vision occur gradually; however, over time these changes can limit the functional ability of the older adult. Approximately 1.8 million community-dwelling older people report some difficulty with basic activities such as bathing, dressing, and walking around the house, in part because they are visually impaired. Unfortunately, visual impairment increases with age. Visual impairment is defined as visual acuity of 20/40 or worse while wearing corrective lenses, and legal blindness or severe visual impairment is 20/200 or more as measured by a Snellen wall chart at 20 feet.

The prevalence of blindness also increases with age, reaching its peak at about the age of 85. Fortunately, the prevalence of blindness in both eyes in the United States is low, about 1% among persons 70 to 74 years of age and 2.4% in persons 85 and older (Centers for Disease Control, 2002). Visual impairment and blindness in the older person is the result of four main causes: **cataracts, age-related macular degeneration (ARMD), glaucoma,** and **diabetic retinopathy.**

Visual impairment can lead to a loss of independence, social isolation, depression, and a decreased quality of life. Visual impairment increases the risk of falls and fractures, making it more likely that an older person will be admitted to a hospital or nursing home, be disabled, or die prematurely (Centers for Disease Control, 2002). It is important for the nurse to understand normal versus abnormal changes and how to assist the older adult to improve safety and well-being.

The gerontological nurse should urge all older patients to schedule routine eye examinations with an ophthalmologist to maintain and protect vision. The healthy older adult should schedule a complete eye examination every other year. During this examination, visual acuity should be evaluated, pupils should be dilated with examination of the retina, and intraocular pressure should be tested. Older persons with diabetes should have this complete visual evaluation yearly (Reuben et al., 2002).

When assessing the vision of an older person, the nurse should first observe the patient's appearance. Older patients with stains on their clothing, older women with too much or poorly applied makeup, or patients with multiple bumps and bruises may be exhibiting signs of visual impairment. Older patients should be questioned regarding adequacy of vision, recent changes in vision, visual problems, and the date of their last complete visual examination. The gerontological nurse should inspect the eyes for any abnormalities, including movement of the eyelids, abnormal discharge, excessive tearing, abnormally colored sclera, and abnormal or absent pupillary response. A Snellen chart (Figure 14-1 ■) can be used to measure visual acuity, or the patient can be asked to read from a magazine or newspaper with various print sizes. Visual field testing can

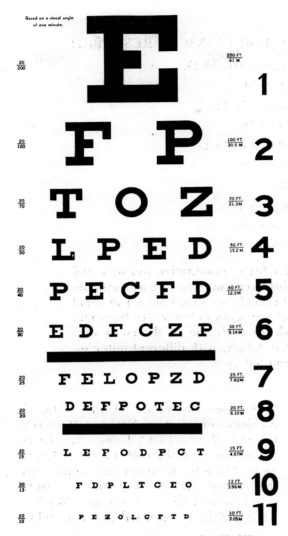

Source: National Eye Institute, National Institutes of Health, 2004.

FIGURE ▨ 14-1

The Snellen chart, used to measure visual acuity.

detect blind spots or loss of peripheral vision. Ask the patient to follow your fingers as they move from point to point without changing the head position to check extraocular movements. The older person with glasses should wear them during the vision assessment.

In addition to annual or biennial examinations, the gerontological nurse should urge all older persons who complain of a visual problem to seek a visual evaluation if they experience any of the following problems:

- Red eye
- Excessive tearing or discharge
- Headache or feeling of eyestrain when reading or doing close work
- Foreign body sensation in the eye
- New-onset double vision or rapid deterioration of visual acuity
- New-onset haziness, flashing lights, or moving spots
- Loss of central or peripheral vision
- Trauma or eye injury

The majority of older people wear some kind of glasses or contact lenses to correct their vision. Ninety-two percent of persons over 70 wear glasses. An additional 18% also use a magnifying glass for reading or close work. Even with glasses, many older people report trouble seeing. Fourteen percent of persons age 70 to 74 report difficulties seeing even with correction, and 32% of those over 85 offer this complaint.

Although visual aids and suggestions offered by low-vision clinics can assist an older person with visual impairment, fewer than 2% of persons over the age of 70 use these services. Telescopic lenses, books in braille, computer scanners and readers, tinted glasses to reduce glare, large-print books and magazines, guide dogs, and canes are often rejected because of the stigma attached to them. As many of these items can be very expensive and are not covered by Medicare, the older person should request the opportunity to try them at home for a few days to see if the visual aid offers improvement of vision and function. Most states offer assistance to persons who are legally blind. Older persons who are registered with the Commission for the Blind can borrow books on tape with a tape player, telephones with large numbers, and high-intensity lighting, without cost, if they can furnish a letter from a physician noting that they are legally blind.

Independence may be limited and freedom restricted when visual impairments interfere with the ability to drive, read, and write. Older adults are forced to rely on friends and family to drive them to the grocery store, assist with paying bills, take medications, and do things they were previously able to do on their own. Lack of transportation or the desire not to burden family and friends may leave them socially isolated, with the inability to get places. Leaving home may induce anxiety and fear related to visual difficulties, ultimately leading to voluntary isolation and depression.

NORMAL AGE-RELATED CHANGES

External changes of the eye related to age include graying and thinning of the eyebrows and eyelashes. Wrinkling of the skin surrounding the eyes occurs as a result of subcutaneous tissue atrophy. The eyes may appear sunken as orbital fat decreases and the eyelids sag (geronurseonline.org, 2005). Figure 14-2 ■ illustrates the aging eye.

Table 14-1 describes commonly occurring age-related changes in the eye.

A decrease in endothelial cells on the cornea reduces ocular sensitivity and pain, which may delay awareness for treatment of injuries and infections. Arcus senilis,

FIGURE ■ 14-2

Normal changes of aging in the eye include a thinning of skin surrounding the eye.

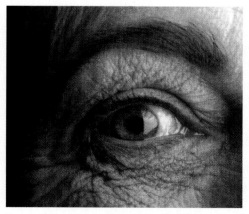

Source: National Eye Institute, National Institutes of Health, 2004.

TABLE 14-1

Age-Related Changes in the Eye and Nursing Implications

Age-Related Changes	Implications
Thinning of skin surrounding the eye	Cosmetic implications only.
Decrease in musculature in eyelids	Ophthalmologic evaluation and correction.
Ectropion—the bottom lid sags outward and is no longer in contact with the eye.	
Entropion—the lid turns inward, bringing the eyelashes in contact with the eyeball and causing irritation and abrasion to the cornea.	
Arcus senilis (corneal calcium deposits)	Cosmetic implications only (rare correlation with systemic hyperlipoproteinemia).
Musculature in the iris	Results in smaller pupil size. Use extra light, gradual change from light to dark, avoid glare.
Visual acuity	Decreased reading and color discrimination ability. Wear corrective lenses and use extra light.
Atrophy of lacrimal glands	Results in dry eyes. Saline drops can bring relief.
Intraocular pressure	Regular ophthalmologic evaluation can detect glaucoma and prevent visual loss.

grayish yellow rings around the peripheral cornea, develop due to lipid deposits; however, this condition is unrelated to hypercholesterolemia or lipid abnormalities except in rare cases.

The lenses thicken and harden with age and appear yellowish and opaque. Thickening of the lenses can cause light to scatter, and opaqueness of the lenses will interfere with color discrimination. This greatly increases the risk for falls and dangerous night driving. Lens thickness also reduces the space for aqueous humor to drain and increases the risk for glaucoma. Hardening impedes **accommodation**, the ability of the lens to change shape and focus images clearly. This loss of pliability in the lens contributes to **presbyopia** or the decrease in near vision, which generally occurs around the age of 40. Visual acuity tends to diminish gradually after 50 years of age and then more rapidly after the age of 70.

Pupils continue to react to light by dilating and constricting; however, this process occurs more slowly with increased age. Accommodation, or the ability to focus on objects at varying distances, declines with age. The greatest declines in accommodation occur between 45 and 55 years of age, making this more a problem of middle-aged adults than older adults. There is usually no change in accommodation after 60 years of age (Burke, 2002). A delay in pupillary reaction makes it difficult for older adults to adapt to light changes, putting them at greater risk for falls. Overall pupil diameter is also decreased, which reduces the amount of light reaching the retina, and more light is required to see clearly (Burke, 2002). The iris loses color and eyes appear gray or light blue.

Light sensitivity, or the ability to adapt to varying degrees of light, declines with age. With increased age, there is a need for increased light (Burke, 2002). Three functions are associated with light sensitivity:

1. **Brightness contrast.** This is the ability to discriminate between objects in varying degrees of light. Starting at about age 50, more light is needed to see dimly lit objects or objects in shadows on a sunny day.

2. **Dark adaptation.** This is the ability to see objects upon entering a dimly lit room after entering from daylight. An older person will not see objects at first, but with time, outlines will become more discernible.
3. **Recovery from glare.** Glare is excessive light reflected back into the eye. Glare will obliterate normal vision for a period of time (for example, after a flash picture is taken). With age, recovery from glare takes more time.

NURSING IMPLICATIONS RELATED TO CARING FOR PATIENTS WITH VISION PROBLEMS

Understanding the normal changes in vision that occur with age enables the nurse to share appropriate interventions to help the patient adjust and regain confidence. Signs that an older adult may be having difficulty with vision include squinting or tilting the head to see; changes in ability to drive, read, watch television, or write; holding objects closer to the face; difficulty with color discrimination and walking up or down stairs; and hesitation in reaching for objects or not being able to find something (American Society on Aging, 2003).

The gerontological nurse can recommend environmental modifications to assist an older person with visual impairment to maintain independence. The Home Safety Inventory (Box 14-1) will assist the gerontological nurse to identify safety problems in the home. Recommendations include the following:

- Provide adequate lighting in high-traffic areas.
- Recommend motion sensors to turn on lights when an older person walks into a room.
- Look for areas where lighting is inconsistent. Dark or shadowy areas can obscure objects.
- Use proper lampshades to prevent glare.
- Use contrast when painting so that the older person can easily discriminate between walls, floors, and other structural elements of the environment.
- Avoid reflective floors.
- When designing signs, use bright colors such as red, orange, and yellow. Avoid soft blues, grays, and light greens because the contrast between colors will be poor.
- Use supplementary lamps near work and reading areas.
- Use red-colored tape or paint on the edges of stairs and in entryways to provide warning and signal the need to step up or down.
- Avoid complicated rug patterns that may overwhelm the eye and obscure steps and ledges.

Safety is a major concern with vision changes in the older adult. Since pupillary reaction slows with age, it takes an older adult more time to become acclimated to changes in light intensity. Nurses should instruct patients on the importance of walking slowly when entering a room with brighter or dimmer light.

The leading cause of accidental death in persons over the age of 65 is a motor vehicle accident; in those older than 75, it is the second leading cause after falls (Li & Smith, 2003). Therefore, it is very important for elderly adults to have their vision and driving ability screened regularly. In the United States, driving is sometimes seen as a right, and many older people are hesitant to relinquish their driver's licenses because they fear loss of independence.

Many older adults restrict their driving to short distances only during the daytime in an effort to compensate for visual impairment. As a result of recent publicity given to

		BOX 14-1
Home Safety Inventory—Older Person		

Safety Consideration	Yes	No
1. Lighting adequate on stairs?	[ ]	[ ]
2. Stair rails present and in good repair?	[ ]	[ ]
3. Nonskid surfaces on stairs?	[ ]	[ ]
4. Throw rugs present safety hazard?	[ ]	[ ]
5. Crowded living area presents safety hazard?	[ ]	[ ]
6. Tub rails installed?	[ ]	[ ]
7. Tub has nonslip surface?	[ ]	[ ]
8. Space heaters present safety hazard?	[ ]	[ ]
9. Adequate provision made for refrigeration of food?	[ ]	[ ]
10. Medications kept in appropriately labeled containers with readable print?	[ ]	[ ]
11. Toxic substances have labels with readable print and are stored well away from food?	[ ]	[ ]
12. Home is adequately ventilated and heated?	[ ]	[ ]
13. Neighborhood is safe?	[ ]	[ ]
14. Fire and police notified of older person in home?	[ ]	[ ]

Source: Clark, M. J. C. (2002). *Community health nursing: Caring for populations* (4th ed.). Upper Saddle River, NJ: Prentice Hall.

older drivers who were involved in fatal pedestrian accidents, many states are struggling to develop systems that would detect older drivers with cognitive and visual impairments on a more timely and accurate basis. Although most states require periodic vision testing for all drivers regardless of age, few require road tests that would simulate actual conditions that an older person may encounter when driving. Such conditions may include driving in the rain and using windshield wipers, encountering oncoming vehicles with headlights on, and driving in bright sunlight with various reflections and solar glare. The debate will continue; however, young male drivers have the highest accident rates of any age group. Safe driving habits, including avoiding drugs or alcohol, wearing seat belts, obeying the speed limit, and limiting driving in poor weather conditions, are recommended for all drivers regardless of age. Families with concern over an older person's driving safety are urged to observe firsthand the older person's performance behind the wheel. AARP offers an 8-hour safe driving course in which older people are taught the effects of aging on driving. There is a nominal charge for the course, and it is taught throughout the United States. Visit the AARP website to find the location of driver safety courses.

If the older person is deemed unsafe, the Department of Motor Vehicles should be notified so the older person will be called in for a road test. If the road test is failed, the older person's license will be revoked.

MediaLink ● AARP and Driver Safety Courses

Drug Alert !

It is important to be aware of the potential for visual disturbance as a side effect of the following drugs:

- **Hydroxychloroquine (Plaquenil).** retinopathy, blurred vision, and difficulty focusing
- **Tamoxifen (Nolvadex).** decreased visual acuity and blurred vision
- **Thioridazine (Mellaril).** blurred vision, impaired night vision, and color discrimination problems
- **Levodopa.** blurred vision
- **Propranolol.** dry eyes, visual disturbances

Source: Wilson, Shannon, & Stang, 2002.

VISUAL PROBLEMS

Age-related macular degeneration (ARMD) is a degenerative disorder of the macula, which affects both central vision (scotoma) and visual acuity. The macula is situated in the posterior region of the retina, surrounding the fovea, and is dense with photoreceptor cells (cones and rods) (Wood, 2000).

There are two types of ARMD: a dry and wet form. The dry form, or atrophic form, occurs as a result of atrophy, retinal pigment degeneration, and drusen accumulations. Drusen are deposits of cellular debris and appear as yellow spots on ophthalmic examination. Visual loss as a result of this type of ARMD is generally slow in progression, and accounts for only 10% to 20% of severe vision loss. In the wet form, also known as neovascular exudate ARMD, blood or serum leaks from newly formed blood vessels beneath the retina. This seepage of fluid ultimately leads to scar formation and visual problems. Although less prevalent than the dry form, the wet form of ARMD is responsible for the majority of severe vision loss (Lee & Beaver, 2003).

Patients with ARMD often require more light for reading. They often experience blurry vision, central scotomas (blind spots within the visual field), and metamorphopsia in which images are distorted to look smaller (micropsia) or larger (macropsia) than they actually are.

Another symptom typical of wet ARMD is that straight lines appear crooked or wavy. The Amsler grid was developed as a screening tool to assess for ARMD; patients with this condition experience visual distortions of the lines and central scotomas. A sample grid and the appearance of the grid to a patient with normal vision and ARMD are depicted in Figure 14-3■.

Central vision is mainly affected by this disorder, and peripheral vision remains intact (Rosenthal, 2001). A person with macular degeneration will experience a dark spot in the center of the field of vision and must learn to rely upon and interpret peripheral vision in order to function. A person with ARMD might experience vision as depicted in Figure 14-4■.

Risk factors for ARMD include the following:

- Age above 50
- Cigarette smoking
- Family history of ARMD
- Increased exposure to ultraviolet light
- Caucasian race and light-colored eyes

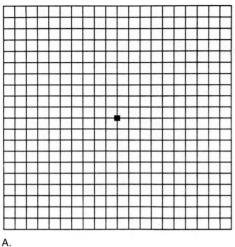

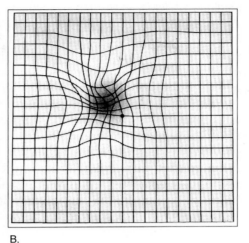

A.   B.

Source: National Eye Institute, National Institutes of Health, 2004.

FIGURE ■ 14-3

A. Amsler grid as it appears to a person with normal vision.
B. Amsler grid as it appears to a person with macular degeneration.

- Hypertension or cardiovascular disease
- Lack of dietary intake of antioxidants and zinc

(Fine, Berger, Maguire, & Ho 2000; Uphold & Graham, 2003)

Treatment and prevention of ARMD with steroid injections, plasmapheresis, and radiation therapy is still under investigation. Currently, there are no treatments for the dry form of ARMD; however, the wet form may benefit from laser treatments to stop neovascularization. Laser therapy may result in secondary vision loss due to collateral damage; however, use of photosensitive dye may decrease damage to the normal retina. Surgery may be another option for some patients, but benefits have been limited (Weston, Aliabadi, & White, 2000).

Due to the severity of vision loss as a result of ARMD nurses can play an important role in patient education. According to the American Academy of Ophthalmology (2003), people over the age of 65 should be examined every 1 to 2 years. Routine ophthalmic examinations are important to detect early signs of this disease. Nurses should encourage preventive measures such as wearing ultraviolet protective lenses in the sun,

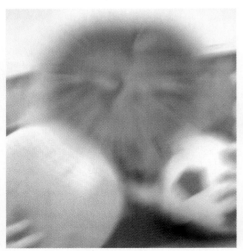

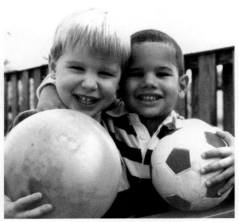

A.   B.

Source: National Eye Institute, National Institutes of Health, 2004.

FIGURE ■ 14-4

A. Simulation of vision with macular degeneration.
B. Normal vision.

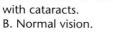
smoking cessation, and exercising routinely. In addition, a healthy diet consisting of fruits and vegetables may be helpful not only to increase consumption of antioxidants, but also to reduce the risk of cardiovascular disease (Elfervig, 1998). The role of vitamins is being studied, and current recommendations for those with ARMD include zinc oxide 80 mg, cupric oxide 2 mg, beta-carotene 15 mg, vitamin C 500 mg, and vitamin E 400 IU taken in divided doses twice a day to slow the risk of progression (Reuben et al., 2002).

Cataracts are opacities or yellowing of the lenses. Lenses are normally clear structures through which light passes to reach the retina. Cataracts cloud the lens, decrease the amount of light able to reach the retina, and inhibit vision. Development is slow and painless, and may be unilateral or bilateral. Cataracts are the leading cause of blindness in the world. More than 50% of adults over the age of 65 years have visual problems as a result of cataracts (Solomon & Donnenfeld, 2003). Ultraviolet light exposure may be a contributing factor to cataract formation.

There are four classifications of cataracts based on their location on the lens: nuclear cataracts (central aspect of lens), cortical cataracts (cortex of the lens), posterior subcapsular (posterior or back of the lens), and mixed cataracts. The most prevalent type of cataracts requiring surgery in older adults is a nuclear cataract (Solomon & Donnenfeld, 2003).

Patients with cataracts may experience blurry vision, glare, halos around objects, double vision, lack of color contrast or faded colors, and poor night vision. They may need more light or illumination when reading, and repeated alterations of their corrective lens prescriptions (Solomon & Donnenfeld, 2003). Figure 14-5■ provides depictions of normal vision and vision of a person with cataracts.

Risk factors for the development of cataracts include the following:

- Increased age
- Smoking and alcohol
- Diabetes, hyperlipidemia
- Trauma to the eye
- Exposure to the sun and UVB rays
- Corticosteroid medications

Surgical removal of the affected lens is generally the treatment of choice because there are no medications to treat this problem (Lee & Beaver, 2003). Corrective lenses

FIGURE ■ 14-5

A. Simulation of vision with cataracts.
B. Normal vision.

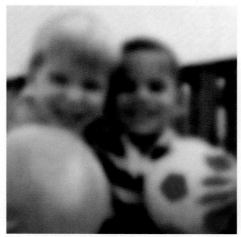
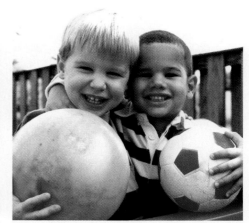

A.   B.

that filter out glare may be effective in managing symptoms in the early phases, but do not stop progression of vision loss. Surgical recommendations are made when vision problems interfere with daily activities such as reading and driving. Cataract surgery is recommended in the following circumstances:

- Visual acuity is 20/50 or less with symptoms of loss of functional ability.
- Visual acuity is 20/40 or better with disabling glare or frequent exposure to low light situations, diplopia, disparity between eyes, or occupational need.
- Cataract removal will treat another lens-induced disease such as glaucoma.
- Cataract exists with other diseases of the retina, such as diabetic retinopathy, requiring unrestricted monitoring.

(National Guideline Clearinghouse, 2001)

The outpatient surgical procedure involves removal of the affected lens and insertion of an artificial lens or intraocular lens. Cataract surgery is generally a nonemergency procedure. Newer surgical procedures with laser photolysis and sonic phacoemulsification have shown to be valuable in making smaller surgical incisions (Solomon & Donnenfeld, 2003). Cataract surgery is contraindicated when the patient wishes to avoid surgery, glasses or visual aids provide satisfactory vision, the patient's lifestyle is not compromised, or the patient has been diagnosed with medical problems that make surgery a high-risk procedure.

Patient education and support are two important aspects of care that nurses can provide for older adults with cataracts. Cataracts may prevent people from driving and completing their normal daily activities, which can ultimately lead to a loss of independence, feelings of hopelessness, and depression. It is important for patients to understand what cataracts are, their symptoms, and treatment options. For patients who undergo surgery, postsurgical education includes reinforcement not to lift any heavy objects, strain at stool, or bend at the waist. Complications of cataract surgery include infection, wound dehiscence, hemorrhage, severe pain, and uncontrolled elevated intraocular pressure (IOP). Patients with cognitive impairments such as Alzheimer's disease must be carefully supervised for at least 24 hours after surgery to ensure that they do not remove the protective eye patch and do not rub the eye. When surgery is needed in both eyes, one eye is done first and the second procedure is scheduled a month or so later to allow healing and recovery. Adequate home care and support is needed to prevent complications.

Preventive measures should also be implemented into teaching such as wearing hats and sunglasses when in the sun, smoking cessation, eating a low-fat diet, and avoiding ocular injury. In addition, the nurse can provide patients with information regarding support groups and other resources that offer psychological and emotional support.

Glaucoma is associated with optic nerve damage due to an increase in IOP, which can ultimately lead to vision loss. Glaucoma accounts for about 10% of all blindness in the United States. When the IOP is greater than 21 mmHg, the optic nerve has the potential for atrophy and vision loss.

Aqueous humor or fluid within the eye serves as nourishment for surrounding tissues. Normally, this fluid is produced in the anterior chamber and drains outward via the trabecular meshwork, maintaining an average or normal IOP of 15 mmHg (normal range is 10 to 20 mmHg). If the outflow of aqueous fluid is obstructed, aqueous humor accumulates, increasing the pressure within the eye and damaging the optic nerve. The two types of glaucoma are open-angle glaucoma and angle-closure glaucoma (Weston et al., 2000).

Open-angle glaucoma occurs when the flow of aqueous humor through the trabecular meshwork is slowed and eventually builds up. If the IOP remains elevated, vision may

FIGURE ☐ 14-6

A. Simulated glaucoma vision.
B. Normal vision.

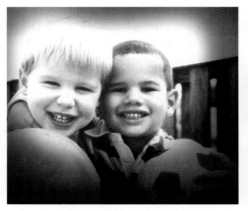
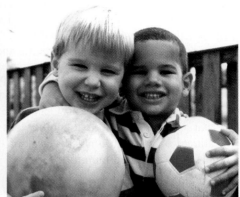

A.   B.

Source: National Eye Institute, National Institutes of Health, 2004.

be lost due to damage of the retinal nerve fiber layer. Vision loss is painless and gradual with midperipheral visual field loss being the classic symptom (Lee & Beaver, 2003). Simulated vision loss from the effects of glaucoma is pictured in Figure 14-6☐.

Another form of open-angle glaucoma is termed *normal-tension* glaucoma, where the IOP remains within the normal range, but damage to the optic nerve and visual changes still occur. In this circumstance, it is believed that damage to the nerve occurs as a result of ischemia or inadequate blood flow. Damage due to open-angle glaucoma can be visualized in ophthalmic examination by enlargement of the optic cup in relation to the optic disc, nicking of the neuroretinal rim, and small hemorrhages near the optic disc (Weston et al., 2000).

In angle-closure glaucoma, which is not as common, the angle of the iris obstructs drainage of the aqueous humor through the trabecular meshwork. It may occur suddenly as a result of infection or trauma; symptoms include unilateral headache, visual blurring, nausea, vomiting, and photophobia. Acute-closure glaucoma is an ophthalmic emergency requiring immediate attention by an ophthalmologist to preserve vision (Weston et al., 2000).

Risk factors for glaucoma include the following:

- Increased intraocular pressure
- Older than 60 years of age
- Family history of glaucoma
- Personal history of myopia, diabetes, hypertension, migraines
- African American ancestry

(Whitaker, Whitaker, & Dill, 1998)

Patients do not generally report symptoms of glaucoma until advanced stages of the disease, so monitoring of IOP during routine ophthalmic examinations for patients with any of the above risk factors is essential. The American Academy of Ophthalmology (2003) recommends that patients over the age of 65 be examined and screened for glaucoma at least every 1 to 2 years. A complete examination includes the patient's visual acuity with corrective lenses, visual field test to assess peripheral vision, measurement of the IOP noting the time of day as pressures may vary throughout the day, slit lamp inspection of the iris to assess whether the anterior angle is open or closed, and a complete dilated examination to inspect the optic nerve and retina (Whitaker et al., 1998). The image in Figure 14-7☐ illustrates an older patient undergoing IOP testing.

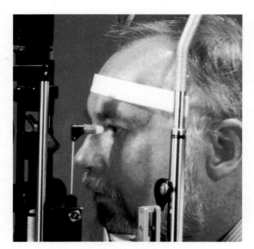

Source: National Eye Institute, National Institutes of Health, 2004.

FIGURE ■ 14-7

Intraocular pressure testing.

Management of glaucoma involves lowering the IOP to stop damage to the optic nerve and prevent further vision loss. Therapy involves medications (oral or topical) to decrease IOP, and/or laser surgery to increase the flow of aqueous humor, by creating a new drainage exit (Weston et al., 2000). Follow-up care with the ophthalmologist is essential to monitor the adequacy of treatment and to ensure that the IOP remains below 20 mmHg. Open-angle glaucoma is usually managed with one or several of the following medications: beta-blockers, miotics, alpha-adrenergic agonists, prostaglandin analogues, and carbonic anhydrase inhibitors. Beta-blockers remain the first-line therapy for glaucoma because they decrease the rate of intraocular fluid production (Weston et al., 2000).

Potential adverse effects of ophthalmic solutions include the following:

- **Beta-blockers (Betagan, Timoptic, Ocupress)** (*bottles with blue or yellow caps*). Bradycardia, congestive heart failure, syncope, bronchospasm, depression, confusion, sexual dysfunction.
- **Adrenergics (Lopidine, Alphagan, Epinal)** (*bottles with purple caps*). Palpitation, hypertension, tremor, sweating.
- **Miotics/cholinesterase inhibitors (pilocarpine, Humorsol)** (*bottles with green caps*). Bronchospasm, salivation, nausea, vomiting, diarrhea, abdominal pain, lacrimation.
- **Carbonic anhydrase inhibitors (Trusopt, Azopt)** (*bottles with orange caps*). Fatigue, renal failure, hypokalemia, diarrhea, depression, exacerbation of chronic obstructive pulmonary disease.
- **Prostaglandin analogues (Xalatan, Lumigan).** Changes in eye color and periorbital tissues, itching.

(Epocrates.com, 2003; Reuben et al., 2002)

When administering eyedrops it is important for the nurse to first wash his or her hands, ask the patient to tip the head backward and look upward, then slightly pull the lower lid down to make a small pouch. The nurse should try not to drop the medication directly onto the eye but rather into the eyelid pouch to prevent a violent blink reflex and excessive tearing. It is important not to contaminate the dropper by touching it to the eye, and to wait several minutes before administering an additional dose of the same medication or a second medication to allow time for complete absorption and prevent additional medication from simply running out of the eye. The nurse should provide the patient with a facial tissue to blot any medication or tears that may run down the cheek, and when finished, wash the hands carefully again.

If medications are unable to decrease IOP or are contraindicated, then surgery may be an option. Acute angle-closure glaucoma is initially treated with medication (both oral and topical) to decrease IOP, but surgery is usually indicated to improve aqueous fluid drainage (Lee & Beaver, 2003). A small opening is made at the base of the iris (iridotomy) to allow the IOP to equalize on either side and prevent the iris from obstructing the outflow channel. Iridotomy with a laser can be performed in the outpatient setting.

Diabetic retinopathy is a microvascular disease of the eye occurring in both type 1 and type 2 diabetes. Damage to the ocular microvascular system impairs the transportation of oxygen and nutrients to the eye (McCance & Huether, 2001).

There are two forms of diabetic retinopathy—nonproliferative and proliferative. In the nonproliferative form, the endothelium layers of blood vessels within the eye become damaged and microaneurysms develop. These microaneurysms may leak and the surrounding area may become edematous. If swelling occurs near the macula (macular edema), vision is impaired. Proliferative diabetic retinopathy is a more advanced stage and is a result of retinal ischemia due to damaged blood vessels. To increase the blood and nutrient supply to the retina, new blood vessels develop in a process known as neovascularization. The new blood vessels are fragile and tend to leak red blood cells, which can obscure vision depending on the location and degree of hemorrhage. The new blood vessels may also attach themselves to various areas such as the optic disc, retina, vitreous body, and iris. Tension exertion on the retinal surface and vitreous body increases the risk for retinal detachment or further damage to the surrounding blood vessels and hemorrhage. If neovascularization occurs on the iris (rubeosis iridis), drainage of the aqueous humor may be impaired, placing the patient at risk for neovascular glaucoma (Lee & Beaver, 2003).

Prevention of diabetic retinopathy is dependent on tight glycemic control in addition to managing hypertension and hyperlipidemia. Goals of treatment for patients with diabetes include maintaining an average preprandial blood glucose of 80 to 120 mg/dl, an average bedtime capillary blood glucose of 100 to 140 mg/dl, and a Hemoglobin (HbA$_{1c}$) of less than 7. (Refer to Chapter 19 for additional details on care of the patient with diabetes. ⊂⊃) Patients should be referred for ophthalmic examination after diagnosis of diabetes, and recommendations for follow-up will be made at that time (Lee & Beaver, 2003). Patients with diabetic retinopathy experience gradual vision loss with generalized blurring and areas of focal vision loss. Figure 14-8■ is a simulation of vision for a person with diabetic retinopathy.

Treatment involves laser therapy for both types of retinopathy. Laser therapy can repair leaking microaneurysms, reducing the amount of ocular edema. Neovascularization may also be halted through the use of laser therapy, decreasing the risk of retinal detachment, hemorrhage, and neovascular glaucoma. Secondary visual impairment including peripheral and central vision loss may result from laser therapy if the retina or fovea is damaged (Lee & Beaver, 2003).

Nurses can play a major role in educating patients about diabetes mellitus and the importance of glycemic control to prevent retinopathy. Proper nutrition, including a low-carbohydrate and low-cholesterol diet, is imperative to keep blood glucose levels down and decrease the risk of cardiovascular disease and hypertension. Exercise helps to lower glucose levels, burns extra calories for weight management, and reduces insulin resistance in persons with type 2 diabetes. The nurse should educate patients on how to check serum sugar levels, when and how to administer medications (insulin or oral hypoglycemic medications), and signs and symptoms of hypoglycemia and hyperglycemia.

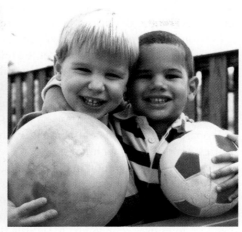

A.   B.

Source: National Eye Institute, National Institutes of Health, 2004.

FIGURE ▢ 14-8
A. Simulated diabetic retinopathy vision.
B. Normal vision.

NURSING DIAGNOSES ASSOCIATED WITH VISUAL IMPAIRMENT

Nursing diagnoses associated with visual impairment are diverse and depend upon the older person's ability to compensate for visual problems. The gerontological nurse should consider the older patient's functional ability and not just the results of visual acuity testing using the Snellen chart. The nurse should assess the older person's ability to perform activities of daily living, including the ability to read medication labels, to drive or take public transportation, to ambulate safely in familiar and strange environments, to shop and pay for food and personal items, to prepare food while maintaining a safe and hygienic environment, and to engage in recreational and leisure activities.

The nursing diagnosis *sensory/perceptual alterations visual* encompasses a variety of nursing goals and interventions including communication, safety, mobility, self-care activities, and mood assessment.

> **Practice Pearl**
>
> If an older person reports visual problems while wearing glasses, check to see that the glasses are clean and free from scratches. Dirty, scratched lenses can reflect light and distort vision.

Hearing

Auditory problems and hearing loss can severely impact quality of life. Hearing loss can interfere with communication, enjoying certain forms of entertainment such as music and television, safety, and ultimately independence.

Hearing impairments make communication difficult and are often frustrating for both the patient and family. It is difficult for older adults to understand conversations with background noise, and difficulties become apparent at restaurants, stores, and social gatherings. The inability to participate in dialogue with family and friends may result in the lack of desire to attend functions, feelings of social isolation, and depression. The need to repeat oneself or miscommunication can lead to stressful interactions. Sound distortion may impair the ability to listen to music, hear favorite television shows, or enjoy other forms of entertainment including movies, plays, or concerts. Turning up the volume of the television or radio to a level that one can hear may be unpleasant for others in the room. Hearing impairments also may endanger individuals living alone, due to the inability to hear a smoke detector or security alarm. Crossing the street and driving a car are dangerous if one is unable to hear oncoming traffic, horns, and sirens. As a result of these challenges, independence may be jeopardized because healthcare providers, family, or friends may want to limit activities normally done alone.

Hearing loss is common in older adults. Over 30% of persons age 65 to 74 and 50% over 75 have some degree of hearing loss (Demers, 2001). Older men of all ages are more likely to be hearing impaired than older women; White men and women are more likely than African American men and women to report hearing problems. Complete deafness in both ears accounts for a little over 20% of all hearing impairments in older people. About 3 million people in the United States wear hearing aids in one or both ears (Centers for Disease Control, 2002).

Hearing loss related to normal aging is the most common cause, but other risk factors include the following:

- Long-term exposure to excessive noise
- Impacted **cerumen** (earwax)
- Ototoxic medications
- Tumors
- Diseases that affect sensorineural hearing
- Smoking
- History of middle ear infection
- Chemical exposure (e.g., long duration of exposure to trichloroethylene)

Because of the trend toward an aging population in the United States, the number of people with hearing problems will increase significantly as will the demand for hearing-related services and hearing corrective devices.

AGE-RELATED CHANGES

The external appearance of the ear changes with age as the auricle tends to wrinkle and sag. Cerumen or earwax produced by the ceruminous glands is a normal finding. In the older adult, cerumen tends to be drier and harder and tends to accumulate in the ear canal due to decreased activity of the apocrine glands. Hearing may become impaired if cerumen accumulates to impact the canal. Dryness of the canal can also cause pruritus, and the epithelial lining of the ear canal may be easily irritated and injured if anything is inserted into the ear, increasing the risk of infection (Hazzard, Blass, Ettinger, Halter, & Ouslander 1999).

Changes in the inner ear involve atrophy of the organ of Corti and cochlear neurons, loss of the sensory hair cells, and degeneration of the stria vascularis (Danner & Harris, 2003). Aging produces gradual bilateral hearing loss in many individuals starting as early as age 20 to 30 but appearing more commonly in the 50s and 60s. About one third of all hearing impairments are at least partially attributable to damage from exposure to loud sounds. Sounds that are sufficiently loud to damage sensitive inner ear structures can produce hearing loss that is not reversible. Very loud sounds of short duration, such as an explosion or gunfire, can cause immediate, severe, and permanent loss of hearing. Virtually all of the structures of the ear can be damaged, in particular the organ of Corti, the delicate sensory structure of the auditory portion of the inner ear (cochlea), which may be torn apart. Figure 14-9 ▢ illustrates the anatomical structure of the ear.

Moderate exposure to loud noise may initially cause temporary hearing loss termed *temporary threshold shift (TTS).* Many people have experienced TTS after being in a loud environment like a rock concert or sports event. However, TTS can become permanent with continued and longer duration exposure to less intense but still loud sounds that erode hearing ability. This danger became apparent several years ago, and legislation was passed to protect workers from hearing loss from loud noise in the workplace. Sound levels of less than 75 dB(A) are unlikely to cause permanent hearing loss, whereas sound levels about 85 dB(A) with exposures of 8 hours per day will produce permanent hearing loss after many years (National Institutes of Health, 1990; U.S. Department of Labor, 2004). Some older adults have worked in industrial factories or occupations where loud noises were routinely encountered. The Occupational Safety and Health Administration (OSHA) now regulates the amount of noise workers can be routinely exposed to and mandates the use of ear protection in noisy environments such as airports and factories where noisy equipment is operated; however, many older persons worked their entire lives in factories that would now be considered unsafe by OSHA standards. Additionally, many veterans who served in active duty during wartime have suffered hearing loss from the firing of heavy artillery.

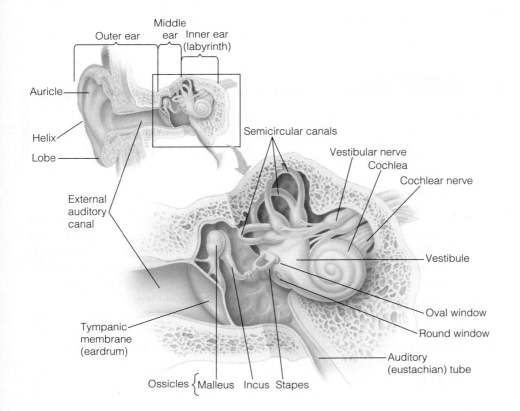

FIGURE ▢ 14-9

Structure of the ear.

TYPES OF HEARING LOSS

A thorough history and physical examination is important to help determine the cause of the hearing loss. It may be conductive, due to the external aspect of the ear, or sensorineural from inner ear problems.

Conductive hearing loss is related to a problem in the external or middle ear – canal, tympanic membrane, bones in the outer and middle ear, or the ossicles (Marcincuk & Roland, 2002). Sound is unable to be transmitted to the inner ear, creating reception and amplification problems. This type of hearing loss may be a result of an external ear infection (otitis externa), impacted cerumen, middle ear infection (otitis media), benign tumors or carcinoma, perforation of the tympanic membrane, foreign bodies, or otosclerosis (a disease affecting the mobility of the middle ear bones) (Marcincuk & Roland, 2002).

Cerumen impaction is one of the most common and reversible causes of conductive hearing loss in elderly adults. Nearly 35% of community-residing older adults have cerumen impaction in one or both ears, and the rate of impaction in the institutionalized elderly is thought to be much higher. As described earlier, cerumen becomes harder and drier with age, and may occlude the ear canal. Recommended aural hygiene involves gentle cleansing of the auricles (outside of the ears) during the bath or shower. The use of cotton-tipped applicators to cleanse the ear canal is not recommended because the applicator may push the cerumen deeper into the canal and thus increase the risk of impaction, as well as traumatize the canal wall and tympanic membrane (Moore, Voytas, Kowalski, & Maddens, 2002).

An occlusion of cerumen can greatly affect hearing, as sound is unable to reach the inner ear (Marcincuk & Roland, 2002). Examination of the ear canal for cerumen impaction is recommended as part of routine preventive healthcare screening for older adults. The person with cerumen impaction may complain of a feeling of fullness or itching in the ear canal. In addition to hearing loss, cerumen may also cause tinnitus, ear pain, or vertigo.

Practice Pearl

Contraindications for cerumen removal include perforated tympanic membrane, ear trauma, tumors, and cholesteatoma. Use extreme caution in patients with diabetes due to the increased risk for infection.

Two common methods for removal of cerumen from the ear canal are:

- **Curette.** A small instrument with a scoop on the end is inserted into the ear canal while the helix is lifted posteriorly and laterally. The tip of the curette is placed over the top of the impacted cerumen and pulled forward. It is helpful to use both hands and wear a headlamp to provide bright light to visualize the canal as much as possible. The advantage of this method is that no water is needed and therefore there is a lower risk of infection. The disadvantage is that the procedure requires a greater degree of skill, and the risk of injury to the tympanic membrane or ear canal is greater.
- **Lavage or irrigation.** Some nurses like to soften the cerumen for up to 3 days before attempting irrigation with mineral oil or Debrox eardrops up to three times daily. Irrigation is the simpler and more straightforward approach to cerumen removal. However, because it is a blind procedure, the risk exists that water and infectious agents could be pushed through a perforated tympanic membrane into the middle ear space.

Practice Pearl

Contraindications to ear lavage or irrigation include history of ear surgery and history of otitis externa (swimmer's ear). It is safer to make a referral to an ear, nose, and throat specialist.

To irrigate, the following equipment is needed: a clean bulb syringe, a clean container of warm water or saline solution, an emesis basin, an otoscope, and lots of towels.

The tip of a bulb irrigation syringe is placed into the external canal (Figure 14-10■). Water should be warmed to 37°C. The nurse can make sure the water is not too hot by testing it on the inside of a wrist. If it feels uncomfortably warm, more cool water is added to avoid burning the patient. Some patients can assist by holding an emesis basin below the ear to catch the water. A plastic cape can be used to protect the patient's clothing. Place gentle pressure on the syringe and angle the water stream posteriorly to wash the impacted cerumen away from the tympanic membrane. It is important to avoid getting air into the syringe as it will sound deafening to the patient and will terrify a patient with a cognitive impairment. Pulling the helix of the ear upward and outward will straighten the ear canal. Use the otoscope to check progress and stop the irrigation when you can visualize the tympanic membrane. If the patient experiences discomfort, the nurse should stop. Large pieces of cerumen will be apparent in the emesis basin. Following irrigation, swab and dry the canal carefully to reduce the risk of infection. Some nurses use a water jet dental device, but this is risky because the water pressure cannot be controlled and damage to the tympanic membrane may occur.

Because of the risk of tympanic membrane perforation or damage to the lining of the ear canal, the curette method should be performed only by an advanced practice nurse, physician, or gerontological nurse with specialized training and experience. Neither the curette nor irrigation method should be attempted if a perforated tympanic membrane is present or suspected.

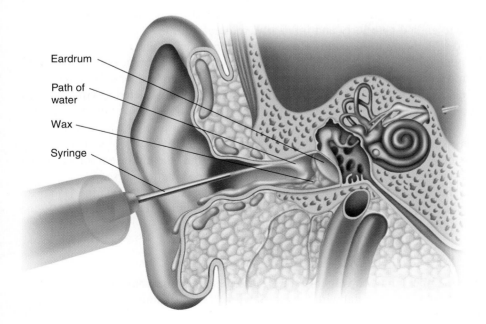

Eardrum

Path of water

Wax

Syringe

FIGURE ■ 14-10

The tip of a bulb irrigation syringe is placed into the external canal.

> **Practice Pearl**
>
> Use only sterilized equipment to avoid spreading bacteria and possibly infection from one patient to another during ear irrigation for cerumen impaction.

Sensorineural hearing loss is a manifestation of problems within the inner ear. Sound is transmitted to the inner ear, but problems with the cochlea and auditory nerve (eighth cranial nerve) create sound distortion. Causes of this type of hearing loss include **presbycusis** (loss of hearing due to age-related changes in the inner ear), damage due to excessive noise exposure, Meniere's disease, tumors, and infections (Danner & Harris, 2003).

Presbycusis affects approximately 75% of people over the age of 60 (Jackler, 2003). Loss of hair cells in the cochlea (sensory loss) and degradation of neurons (neural loss), which occur as part of the normal aging process, result in this form of sensorineural hearing loss (Sandor, 2000). The incidence is greater in men than women and believed to be related to noise-induced hearing loss. Presbycusis occurs gradually and is usually bilateral, impairing the ability to hear high-pitched tones (Jackler, 2003). There are currently no interventions to slow the progression of presbycusis; however, it rarely causes severe hearing loss or deafness (Jackler, 2003).

The American Speech-Language-Hearing Association recommends that asymptomatic adults should be screened every 10 years until the age of 50, and every 3 years thereafter with an audiometric battery test (Jackler, 2003). Many patients do not report symptoms of hearing loss, and studies have shown 8- to 20-year time lapses from when patients recognize the problem to the time they report it (Sandor, 2000).

Evaluation of hearing loss is dependent on a thorough history and physical examination. Inspect the auricle for lumps, lesions, and deformities. Examine the ear canal with an otoscope. It is important to select a speculum for the otoscope that is the appropriate size for the patient. Hold the otoscope in your dominant hand and place the ulnar surface on the patient's occiput to stabilize the instrument and prevent damage to the ear canal should the patient suddenly move his or her head. Most adult ear canals are angled anteriorly and inferiorly, so gently pulling the pinna upward and outward with the opposite hand helps to straighten the canal and allows a better look at the tympanic membrane. Enter the ear canal slowly (only about ½ inch) to prevent discomfort to the patient and inspect the canal for cerumen, redness, foreign bodies, swelling, or discharge. If the tympanic membrane is not obstructed it will appear as a smooth, pearly gray object at the end of the ear canal. Some older adults have jagged white scars across the tympanic membrane as a result of ruptured eardrums from infections when they were children before the widespread use of antibiotics. Carefully document all findings. A red bulging membrane is a sign of a middle ear infection and requires immediate referral to a physician or advanced practice nurse.

The Hartford Institute recommends the screening version of the Hearing Handicap Inventory for the Elderly (HHIE-S) for assessing hearing loss in older adults. See the Best Practice feature on the following page.

ASSESSING HEARING LOSS

Family members may be valuable sources because they may have noticed communication problems or social withdrawal (Sandor, 2000). Examination of the ear may reveal an external infection or impaction that can be treated appropriately to resolve

The Hartford Institute for Geriatric Nursing Try This assessment series (2002) recommends stresses the importance of good communication with an older adult. Questioning the patient about hearing problems involves inquiring about communication difficulties in person or over the phone, in conversation with more than one person, and with others when a high level of background noise is present. The Hartford Institute recommends the use of the screening version of the Hearing Handicap Inventory for the Elderly (HHIE-S). This instrument is a 5-minute, 10-item questionnaire developed to assess how the individual perceives the social and emotional effects of hearing loss. Persons who perceive their hearing loss to be a problem are more likely to have further testing and accept the need for a hearing aid. The higher the HHIE-S score, the greater the handicapping effect of a hearing impairment. Audiologic referral is recommended for individuals scoring 10 or higher on this inventory (Demers, 2001).

Hearing Handicap Inventory for the Elderly — Screening Questionnaire

Instructions: Check one answer for each question. Do not skip a question if you avoid a situation because of a hearing problem. If you use a hearing aid, please answer according to the way you hear without the aid.

1. Does a hearing problem cause you to feel embarrassed when you meet new people?
2. Does a hearing problem cause you to feel frustrated when talking to members of your family?
3. Do you have difficulty hearing when someone speaks in a whisper?
4. Do you feel handicapped by a hearing problem?
5. Does a hearing problem cause you difficulty when visiting friends, relatives, or neighbors?
6. Does a hearing problem cause you to attend religious services less often than you would like?
7. Does a hearing problem cause you to have arguments with family members?
8. Does a hearing problem cause you difficulty when listening to TV or radio?
9. Do you feel that any difficulty with your hearing limits or hampers your personal or social life?
10. Does a hearing problem cause you difficulty when in a restaurant with relatives or friends?

Scoring: No = 0; Sometimes = 2; Yes = 4 Interpretation of Total Scores: 0–8 = no handicap; 10–24 = mild to moderate handicap; 26–40 = severe handicap. Ventry, I., Weinstein, B. 1983; Identification of elderly people with hearing problems. *ASHA. 25:*37-42. Reproduced by permission of the author and the American Speech and Hearing Association, © 1983.
Adapted from *Try This Best Practices in Care for Older Adults.* (2002). New York: New York University, The Steinhardt School of Education, Division of Nursing, The John A. Hartford Foundation Institute for Geriatric Nursing.

the hearing loss. If the problem is not that obvious, a tuning fork may be helpful in distinguishing conductive versus sensorineural loss; however, it is not appropriate for bilateral hearing loss (Jackler, 2003). The Weber test involves placement of a tuning fork on top of the patient's head. If the sound is heard from the vibrating fork equally in both ears, hearing is normal. If the sound is lateralized or perceived louder in one ear, this may indicate unilateral conductive hearing loss in that ear. With sensorineural loss, sound will be heard in the unaffected ear. The Rinne test involves placing the tuning fork on the mastoid bone to assess bone conduction. The patient is asked to tell the examiner when he or she can no longer hear the sound, and the tuning fork is then placed next to the ear to measure air conduction. Normally air conduction should be longer than bone conduction, so the patient should be able to hear the tuning fork after it is moved alongside the patient's ear. A patient with conductive hearing loss will perceive the bone conduction to be longer and will not hear the tuning fork through the air, as there is an external ear problem (Bates, 2003).

Patients whose hearing does not resolve after treatment of an ear infection, removal of cerumen, or discontinuation of ototoxic medications; patients with sudden unexplained hearing loss; and those with abnormal unilateral Rinne or Weber tests should be referred to an audiologist (Bogardus, Yueh, & Shekelle, 2003).

HEARING AIDS

Hearing aids amplify sounds and deliver them directly into the ear. Improvements have made them smaller and more discreet. Gerontological nurses should be aware of the cleaning, inserting, and troubleshooting involved with hearing aids. The first priority is to identify patients wearing hearing aids on admission to the hospital or nursing home and make an appropriate notation on each patient's nursing care plan. It is helpful to note the type, model number, and serial number of the hearing aid in case it should become lost. The working condition of the hearing aid is then assessed. Assessment parameters include:

- **Integrity of the ear mold.** Are there cracks or rough areas? Is there a good fit?
- **Battery.** Use a battery tester if one is available. Are the contacts clean? Is the battery inserted correctly with + on battery matched to + in compartment?
- **Dials.** Are they clean? Easily rotated? Does the patient report variation of volume when the volume dial is moved?
- **Switches.** Do they easily turn on and off? Is there excessive static or feedback?
- **Tubing for behind the ear aids.** Are there cracks? Is there good connection to the earpiece?

(Modified from Palumbo, 2000)

All nursing personnel, including nursing assistants, should know how to care for hearing aids. Professional nurses can serve as role models, educators, and instructors for nursing assistants who are unfamiliar with the care of these expensive items. It is also critical to reinforce that patients who wear hearing aids should have them inserted during morning care so that they can effectively communicate throughout the day. Some older people have been labeled as cognitively impaired because they respond inappropriately to questions, while in reality they are hearing impaired. Even the patient diagnosed with Alzheimer's disease will become more withdrawn, increasingly socially isolated, and more disoriented without the benefit of a hearing aid.

Each evening at bedtime, the hearing aid should be removed and cleansed with warm water or saline and a cotton pad. Harsh soaps or alcohol should not be used, as they will degrade the plastic. Any cerumen should be carefully removed from the earpiece while still soft. The battery should be disengaged from the contacts and the hearing aid stored securely in its case in a safe place. Many nursing home residents and their caregivers routinely misplace hearing aids, eyeglasses, and dentures when they are placed on meal trays or get mixed into bedding and laundry. Frequent inventory and labeling will assist the staff to keep track of these expensive and difficult-to-replace items.

Hearing aids are appropriate for most persons with a hearing impairment. In order to be fitted with the device most appropriate for the individual patient's hearing loss, it is recommended that an independent audiologist be visited for testing and evaluation. Audiologists who do not sell hearing aids have a wider variety of devices to choose from and will not feel pressured to recommend the type of aid sold by their employer. Older hearing aids amplified all noise at the same level, and some older people were not able to tolerate them because of the amplification of loud background noise. Newer aids enhance selected frequencies where the patient exhibits hearing loss and thus are more acceptable to many patients. Amplification in both ears (binaural) achieves the best understanding of speech. Unilateral amplification may be appropriate for those with hearing loss only in one ear, those who cannot afford two aids, or those who may be challenged by the care of two hearing aids.

The U.S. Food and Drug Administration (FDA) has approved implantable hearing devices (cochlear implants) for older adults with moderate-to-severe sensorineural hearing loss. The device must be implanted into the skull behind the ear. This procedure requires a hospital stay and the administration of anesthesia. After the implantation, significant training is needed with a speech pathologist to recognize and interpret the new electronic sounds produced by the implant. A small battery pack is worn around the waist with a cable that attaches to the implant behind the ear. The device allows many people who were previously unable to do so to speak on the telephone, thus improving safety and quality of life.

ASSISTIVE LISTENING DEVICES

Older persons with hearing impairments may also use assistive listening devices. Many theaters are equipped with these devices that amplify the performers' voices by the use of small microphones and then transmit them to headphones or earpieces that are worn in the ear. Wireless transmission using infrared technology is useful for persons with central auditory processing disorders (Reuben et al., 2002). A telecommunications device for the deaf (TDD) is an assistive device that allows telephone conversation for a deaf person via a keyboard that transmits signals over the telephone wires to another person with a TDD receiver. Special TDD operators can assist with emergency calls when the older person must call someone without a TDD receiver. The use of computers and e-mail has greatly assisted many deaf people to communicate with the hearing world.

COMMON HEARING PROBLEMS IN OLDER PERSONS

Tinnitus (ringing in the ears) can occur with or without hearing loss and is associated with increased age. Tinnitus is classified into two categories: objective and subjective. Patients with *objective* tinnitus hear pulsatile sounds caused by turbulent blood flow within the ear; clicking or low-pitched buzzing is indicative of spastic muscles within the ear or spontaneous vibrations of the hair cells. *Subjective* tinnitus is the perception of sound when there is no actual sound stimulus. Causes of this type of tinnitus are medications, infections, neurological conditions, and disorders related to hearing loss (Lockwood, Salvi, & Burkard, 2002).

A thorough history including a complete description of the sound is extremely important to assist in determining the cause. The underlying condition that may be causing the tinnitus must first be addressed (for example, stopping a medication suspected as the source of the tinnitus or treating the infection). Patients with pulsatile tinnitus need a complete workup because they may have hypertension, anemia, or hyperthyroidism (Lockwood et al., 2002).

No drugs have yet been approved by the FDA to treat tinnitus specifically; however, benzodiazepines and tricyclic antidepressants have been shown to be effective (Danner & Harris, 2003). Approved therapies include tinnitus retraining therapy, relaxation, biofeedback, and masking devices to cover up the sounds (Lockwood et al., 2002).

Although many feel the urge to shout when they are communicating with older people, in many cases shouting is not helpful. Box 14-2 provides tips for communicating with older persons who have hearing impairments.

Drug Alert !

If a patient on one or more of the following drugs reports a change in hearing, be suspicious of a drug side effect:

- Aminoglycoside antibiotics (gentamicin)—ototoxic
- Antineoplastics (cisplatin)—ototoxic
- Loop diuretics (furosemide)—ototoxic
- Baclofen—tinnitus
- Propranolol (Inderal)—tinnitus and hearing loss

Source: Epocrates.com, 2003; Jackler, 2003; Wilson et al., 2002.

NURSING DIAGNOSES ASSOCIATED WITH HEARING IMPAIRMENT

Nursing diagnoses associated with older patients with hearing impairment are diverse and depend upon the ability to compensate for hearing problems. The gerontological nurse should consider the older patient's functional ability and not just the results of audiology testing. The nurse should assess the older person's ability to perform activities of daily living, including the ability to communicate, to drive or take public transportation, to hear alarms and doorbells, and to engage in leisure and recreational activities.

BOX 14-2   Nursing Interventions to Use When Speaking With a Hearing Impaired Individual

- Eliminate extraneous noise in the room. For example, turn the television or radio down or off.
- Stand 2 to 3 feet from the patient.
- Have the patient's attention before speaking. Touch lightly on the arm or shoulder if needed.
- Try to lower the pitch of your voice.
- Pause at the end of each phrase or sentence.
- If the patient has a hearing aid, provide assistance with the device, plus glasses if needed.
- Assess the illumination in the room and make sure that the patient can see you. Face the patient at all times during the conversation.
- The patient may read lips, so it is important not to cover your mouth or chew gum. Do not speak into the chart or converse with someone over your shoulder. The patient will misinterpret your message.
- Speak slowly and clearly in a normal tone of voice—do not shout.
- If the patient does not understand your message, rephrase it rather than repeating the same words.
- Gestures, if appropriate, may help.
- Use written communication if the patient is able to see and read.
- Ask the patient for an oral or written response to determine if the communication was successful.

Source: McConnell, 2002; Reuben et al., 2002.

The nursing diagnosis *sensory/perceptual alterations: hearing* encompasses a variety of nursing goals and interventions including communication, safety, self-care activities, mood, and leisure activities.

Taste

The sense of taste allows full appreciation of the flavor and palatability of food and serves as an early warning system against toxins and spoiled food products. Physiologically, taste triggers normal digestion by stimulating gastrointestinal secretions (Bromley, 2000). Taste deficits can result in weight loss, malnutrition, impaired immunity, and worsening of medical illness. Older people sometimes use excessive sugar or salt to compensate for a diminished sense of taste.

A diminished sense of taste, hypogeusia, is a normal sensory change usually occurring after the age of 70. The exact pathophysiology behind age-related gustatory changes remains unclear. However, studies have shown that both taste discrimination and sensitivity significantly change with age. Taste thresholds for protein, salt, and sweeteners are on average 2.5 to 5 times higher in the older person than in the young (Schiffman, 1997). The sense of taste is mediated by taste buds located on the dorsal surface of the tongue, in the lateral folds on the side of the tongue, on the epiglottis, on the larynx, and even on the first third of the esophagus. Many nerves are responsible for transmitting taste information to the brain, including cranial nerves VII, IX, and X. Taste buds are continually bathed in secretions from the salivary glands, and excessive dryness can distort taste sensation.

Additional factors that may influence alterations in taste include oral condition, olfactory function, medications, diseases, surgical interventions, and environmental exposure (McCague, 1999). Medical conditions that affect the sense of taste are listed in Table 14-2.

TABLE 14-2

Medical Conditions Affecting Taste

System	Condition
Central Nervous System	Head trauma
	Multiple sclerosis
Endocrine	Cushing syndrome
	Hypothyroidism
	Diabetes mellitus
Systemic	Cancer
	Chronic renal failure
	Burns
	Nutritional deficiencies (zinc, niacin)
	Liver disease (cirrhosis)
	HIV/AIDS
Other	Hypertension
	Psychiatric disorders
	Laryngectomy
	Acute infections
	Mouth and gum diseases
	Radiation to head/neck
	Candidiasis
	Gingivitis
	Epilepsy

Source: Bromley, 2000; Schiffman, 1997.

Gustatory function may be impaired by poor dentition or improperly fitting dentures that inhibit the ability to chew food properly for flavor release. Dentures covering the soft palate obstruct food from reaching the palate and decrease taste perception. Oral infections can release acidic substances, which alter taste. Impaired salivary glands produce less saliva, decreasing the ability for food to dissolve and release flavor (Hazzard et al., 1999). Olfactory dysfunction (discussed later in this chapter) can also greatly impair taste sensation because smell stimulates taste and enhances flavor.

Medications can alter taste sensation by affecting peripheral receptors and chemosensory pathways (Schiffman, 1997). Drugs known to alter taste are listed in Table 14-3.

NURSING ASSESSMENT OF THE OLDER PATIENT WITH TASTE DISTURBANCES

A thorough assessment of the head and neck should be performed to rule out obvious deformity, injury, infection, or obstruction. Mucous membranes should be assessed for dryness, ulceration, or presence of candidiasis. If older patients are noted to have severe gum disease or dental caries, referral to a dentist or oral surgeon is indicated. If the patient wears dentures, they should be removed in order to thoroughly inspect the gums. It is also helpful to question the patient regarding past dietary habits, most enjoyable foods, use of salt and sugar, and preferred beverage at mealtime.

There are no pharmacological treatments to improve taste; however, seasonings and additives to enhance flavor and aroma may amplify taste. Encouraging patients to alternate and eat the different foods on their plate rather than sticking to one food may decrease sensory exhaustion. An intervention used in nursing homes to stimulate gustatory sensation is brewing coffee at mealtimes (Schiffman, 1997).

Hypogeusia can lead to malnutrition because a decreased ability to sense flavor in foods can lead to lack of motivation and enjoyment in preparing and consuming a well-balanced diet. The inability to distinguish between salt and sugar can have grave implications for patients with hypertension or diabetes who may not realize that they are consuming too much (Schiffman, 1997).

Xerostomia, or dry mouth, occurs with salivary gland dysfunction. In the absence of disease and medication effects, salivary function in the older adult generally remains normal. Conditions that may induce xerostomia include systemic diseases (diabetes, HIV, Alzheimer's disease), radiation, medications (anticholinergic drugs), and Sjögren's syndrome. The leading cause of dry mouth in the geriatric population is a result of medication. Xerostomia has been described as a side effect of 80% of the most commonly prescribed medications (Ship, Pillemer, & Baum, 2002).

Implications of dry mouth include altered taste, difficulty swallowing (dysphagia), periodontal disease (dental caries, gingivitis, oral lesions), speech difficulties, dry lips, halitosis, and sleeping problems (Ship et al., 2002). Decreased ability to chew and swallow places those affected at risk for malnutrition and aspiration pneumonia. Dry lips and oral mucosa increases the incidence of infection and dental caries as the dry tissues are more easily injured. In addition, dentures can irritate dry oral mucosa. Speech and eating difficulties may be embarrassing and discourage individuals from wanting to socialize, ostracizing themselves from loved ones (Ship et al., 2002).

Management of xerostomia involves good oral care, regular dental examinations, and a diet low in sugar. See Chapter 13. ⏤ Sugar-free candies, mints, and chewing gum may help stimulate salivary secretions. Over-the-counter artificial saliva, oral lubricants, and drinking fluids with meals may help relieve symptoms and dysphagia. Using a humidifier adds moisture to the air and can help with xerostomia that may

TABLE 14-3

Drugs Affecting Taste

Class	Drug
Antibiotics	Ampicillin
	Azithromycin
	Ciprofloxacin
	Clarithromycin
	Griseofulvin
	Metronidazole
	Ofloxacin
	Tetracycline
Anticonvulsants	Carbamazepine
	Phenytoin
Antidepressants	Amitriptyline
	Desipramine
	Doxepin
	Imipramine
	Nortriptyline
Antineoplastics	Cisplatin
	Doxorubicin
	Methotrexate
	Vincristine
Lipid-Lowering Agents	Fluvastatin
	Lovastatin
	Pravastatin
Sympathomimetics	Amphetamines
Miscellaneous	Etidronate
	Iron supplements
	Vitamin D
Antihistamines/Decongestants	Loratadine
	Pseudoephedrine
	Chlorpheniramine
Cardiac/Antihypertensives	Captopril
	Diltiazem
	Enalapril
	Nifedipine
	Nitrogylcerin
	Propranolol
	Spironolactone
Anti-inflammatory Agents	Colchicine
	Dexamethasone
	Hydrocortisone
Antiparkinsonian Agent	Levodopa
Muscle Relaxants	Baclofen
	Dantrolene

Source: Bromley, 2000; Schiffman, 1997.

interfere with sleep. Pilocarpine (Salagen) and cevimeline (Evoxac) are both secretagogues approved by the FDA to relieve symptoms associated with xerostomia (Ship et al., 2002).

Since a large percentage of medications have xerostomia as a side effect, a careful assessment of all medications should be completed to determine if substitutions are possible. Other strategies that may be tried to decrease symptoms include prescribing an anticholinergic medication to be taken during the day instead of at night when salivary secretion normally diminishes, or dividing a larger medication dose from once a day to twice a day to decrease symptoms associated with the larger dose (Ship et al., 2002).

Nurses can assist patients with xerostomia by suggesting these interventions to help relieve symptoms. Understanding which prescriptions cause xerostomia can facilitate discussions with the patient's healthcare provider about a possible medication review.

NURSING DIAGNOSES ASSOCIATED WITH TASTE IMPAIRMENT

Nursing diagnoses associated with older patients with taste impairment include *sensory/perceptual alterations: gustatory.* Additional diagnoses may include *intake less than necessary for caloric requirements.* Nursing interventions may include appetite enhancement strategies such as adding flavors, checking dentures for fit and cleanliness, inspecting the mouth for ulcers or gingivitis, carefully reviewing medications and identifying any possible offenders known to affect taste, encouraging fluids, maintaining bowel records, and assessing the palatability of the food. The gerontological nurse working with the institutionalized older person should also survey the dining area with a critical eye and try to ensure that older patients have a pleasant environment in which to eat and are seated with others of their own functional and cognitive levels. Pleasant background music, appetizing smells, clean table settings, and a small bunch of flowers can greatly improve sociability and enjoyment of the mealtime experience.

> ### Practice Pearl
>
> Gerontological nurses working in long-term care facilities are encouraged to routinely sample the food. Eat with your patients once a week or so and you may have additional insights into how to improve the meal service.

Smell

Olfactory dysfunction is more common than taste dysfunction. The three most common causes of loss of smell are nasal and sinus disease, upper respiratory infection, and head trauma (Bromley, 2000). Normal age-related changes influencing olfactory function are attributed to injury of the olfactory mucosa and reduction in both the number of sensory cells and neurotransmitters. Structural alterations of the upper airway, olfactory tract and bulb, hippocampus, amygdaloid complex, and hypothalamus have also been observed within elderly adults as contributing factors for diminished sense of smell, or **hyposmia** (Schiffman, 1997). Smell thresholds for common odors are frequently 11 times higher for older people than in the young (Schiffman, 1997).

Research has shown that olfactory sensory impairment is prevalent in older adults, with incidence being greater in men than in women (Murphy, Schubert, Cruickshanks,

Klein, Klein, & Nondahl, 2002). Although hyposmia may be due to age-related changes, it might also be the result of olfactory nerve damage (cranial nerve I), as this nerve is the sole innervation for smell (Broihier, 2000). Upper respiratory infections (cold, flu, or bronchitis), head trauma, inflammatory conditions (sinusitis or allergic rhinitis), and neurodegenerative diseases (Alzheimer's and Parkinson's disease) are the four major causes of olfactory damage (Murphy et al., 2002). Other forms of damage may occur as a result of chemotherapy, radiation, and medications (Broihier, 2000). Current or past use of cocaine or tobacco has also been associated with sense of smell (Bromley, 2000).

Similar to taste disturbances, poor dentition can inhibit olfactory perception if food is not chewed properly because most flavors are perceived retronasally. Dentures covering the soft palate can also block aroma from reaching these receptors (McCague, 1999).

Chemosensory impairment can be dangerous because an inability to smell smoke or gas odors increases the potential for fire and explosions. Older adults may also become ill if they lack the ability to smell spoiled food products. Malnourishment is another major implication of hyposmia. Normally, adults experience a decline in metabolic rate with age and consume fewer nutrients. Impaired olfactory function affects appetite, as odor cannot simulate it. Diminished flavor perception makes food less appealing and enjoyable. Loss of sensation can also affect the older adult emotionally and psychologically because the sense of smell triggers memories and pleasurable experiences such as smelling fragrant flowers.

Certain medications have also been known to affect sense of smell. These are listed in Box 14-3.

NURSING ASSESSMENT OF THE OLDER PATIENT WITH DISTURBANCES OF SMELL

One reason decreased sense of smell fails to be detected is that it is not adequately tested. Most physical examination records state "cranial nerves II–XII intact," completely omitting cranial nerve I. The gerontological nurse can examine the mucous membranes of the

---

BOX 14-3

Medications That Affect Sense of Smell

- Anesthetics, local
- Antihypertensives
- Antibiotics
- Opiates
- Antidepressants
- Sympathomimetics
- Cocaine hydrochloride
- Diltiazem, nifedipine
- Streptomycin, tyrothricin
- Codeine, hydromorphone, morphine
- Amitriptyline
- Amphetamines

Other
- Head/neck radiation
- Antiallergy medications
- Environmental exposure to toxins
- Chemicals and pesticides
- Overuse of antihistamine nasal spray

Source: Schiffman, 1997.

nares using an otoscope and speculum. The mucous membranes of the nares should be free from polyps, slightly red in color, and without ulceration or copious exudates. The nurse can then ask the patient to occlude one side of the nose, close the eyes, and identify a familiar smell such as vanilla, coffee, or an alcohol swab. This maneuver is repeated on the opposite side using a different odor. Using familiar odors enhances the validity of the test. Commercially prepared scratch-and-sniff tests are available in some smell assessment clinics. These tests contain over 40 odorants and provide more complete information regarding deficits in smell. Patients with obvious deficits in smell should be referred to their primary care provider, an otolaryngologist, and a neurologist of a specialized smell or taste center, usually housed in a large medical center.

NURSING DIAGNOSIS

Nursing diagnoses associated with older patients with hyposmia include *sensory/perceptual alterations: olfactory.* Additional assessment should focus on patient safety and nutrition. Patient education for hyposmia involves safety precautions such as dating and labeling all foods, placing natural gas detectors in the home if the patient has gas heat or stove, placing smoke detectors in strategic locations, and establishing schedules for personal hygiene and house cleaning. Urge the removal of kitchen waste every evening to prevent a garbage smell from permeating the house, which may be offensive to visitors and go undetected by the older person with hyposmia.

Physical Sensation

As people age, tactile sensation diminishes, in addition to the ability to detect temperature extremes (Watson, 2000). Touch is the tactile sense that is perceived by nerve endings and transmits signals to the brain for interpretation. Touch orients a person to the environment and allows the exchange of information and sensation. Psychological benefits to touch include the ability to be soothed, comforted, held, and loved. Some cultures rely heavily on touching others during routine communication and find it difficult to refrain from touching others when they are unable to use their hands. Touch also can be protective by stimulating movement or withdrawal from hot, sharp, or unpleasant stimuli.

Much research has been done to document the importance of touch early in life. Infants in incubators who are not touched will stop eating and fail to thrive. The same may be true for older people, especially those with cognitive or sensory impairments. Institutionalized older persons deprived of caring touch and nurturing physical contact experience a diminishing quality of life, a lessening of their desire to relate to others, and a weakening of what may already be a fragile relationship with physical reality (Nelson, 2001).

Loss of physical sensation may be harmful for older adults because it increases their risk for injury. Inability to feel the heat of bath or shower water may lead to harmful burns. Injuries or infections may go unnoticed in the lower extremities, delaying needed treatment. Certain medical diagnoses such as diabetes mellitus are associated with peripheral neuropathies that can further decrease touch sensation.

Sedating medications can decrease touch sensation by clouding the sensorium and inducing lethargy. Patients taking opioids require additional supervision and monitoring to ensure that foot ulcers or other injuries do not occur without apparent notice.

Research in nursing homes has indicated that back rubs, hand and foot massages, and touch therapy sessions can greatly decrease dementia-associated problems such as restlessness, wandering, agitation, and withdrawal (Nelson, 2001). Gerontological nurses will want to be well versed in nonpharmacological techniques to improve the quality of life for older persons with dementia. The use of caring touch and massage offers promise as a nursing intervention.

NURSING ASSESSMENT OF THE OLDER PERSON WITH TACTILE IMPAIRMENT

Touch is usually assessed using a wisp of cotton. Patients are asked to close their eyes and nod or say "yes" when they are touched on the face, upper back, and extremities. A cotton swab can also be used with the wooden end pressed lightly against the skin for a sensation of "sharp" and the cotton end for the sensation of "dull." Patients should first be instructed by the nurse with their eyes open so that the sensation can be adequately interpreted. Small test tubes can also be filled with warm (not hot) and cold water and the tubes pressed to various points on the body for identification with the eyes closed. The patient's ability to discriminate between one and two points can also be assessed using the wooden ends of a cotton swab. Deficits in touch may be referred for further evaluation to the patient's primary care provider or a neurologist.

NURSING DIAGNOSES ASSOCIATED WITH TACTILE IMPAIRMENT

Nursing diagnoses associated with older patients with tactile impairment are diverse and depend upon the older person's ability to compensate for tactile problems. Using the diagnosis of *sensory/perceptual alterations: tactile,* the gerontological nurse should assess safety and preventive measures.

For patients with impaired sense of touch, nursing interventions could focus on continuous monitoring of the intactness of the skin, assessment of safety risks, and the development of a safety plan with instructions to minimize injury. Water heaters should be turned down to 110°F to prevent scalding. Protective padding of upper and lower extremities can prevent bruising and protect skin integrity. Older patients with diabetes mellitus should place a mirror on the wall close to the floor, remove their shoes, and examine the bottom of their feet daily for blisters, redness, or ulcerations. The use of a good strong light will ease the process and compensate for visual impairment.

Practice Pearl

Advise all older persons to use heating pads on the low setting only. Serious burns can result from use of the higher settings.

Teaching Guidelines for Patient and Family With Sensory Impairments

Gerontological nurses require skills and knowledge related to teaching patients and families about the key concepts of gerontology and gerontological nursing. The patient-family teaching guidelines in the following feature will assist the nurse to assume the role of teacher and coach. Educating patients and families is critical so that nurses can interpret scientific data and individualize the nursing care plan.

Patient-Family Teaching Guidelines

FREQUENTLY ASKED QUESTIONS ABOUT SENSORY CHANGES

1. How can I protect my eyes as I get older?

With aging, vision problems become more common. Some are serious and some are easily treated. The best way to protect your eyes is to:

- Have regular eye examinations every 1 to 2 years.
- Find out if you are at high risk for vision loss (diagnosis of diabetes, family history of eye disease, hypertension).
- Wear sunglasses and a wide brim hat. This will protect your eyes from the sun and prevent cataracts.
- See an eye professional at once if you have loss or dimness of eyesight, eye pain, double vision, swelling, or redness of the eyes.

RATIONALE:

Regular eye examinations and early detection can reduce the risk of vision loss.

2. What are some common eye complaints experienced by older people?

Some common complaints include:

- *Floaters.* These are tiny spots that float across your eyes. They are usually normal but if you see floaters with spots or flashes, call your eye care professional right away.
- *Tearing.* This can result from light sensitivity or dry eye as your body tries to compensate by producing excess tears.
- *Eyelid problems.* Pain, itching, tearing, drooping, or irritation can be corrected with eyedrops or minor surgery.
- *Conjunctivitis.* Also called pink eye, this condition results from allergies or infection. It is easily treated with eyedrops.
- *Presbyopia.* This is the loss of ability to see close objects or small print. Reading glasses can usually correct the problem.

RATIONALE:

Education regarding common complaints can help the older person to evaluate vision changes and decide when to call the eye care professional for more serious problems.

3. What can I do to function better if I have low vision?

Low-vision adaptations can help you to carry out your normal routines. See a low-vision expert for help choosing the right product because they are not all covered by insurance and can be expensive. Most clinics will let you try out some devices to improve your function at home for a week or so before you make the decision to buy them. Simple things you can do at home include:

- Write with bold felt-tip markers.
- Put colored tape on the edge of steps to prevent falls.
- Use contrast whenever possible, like light furniture on dark floors, red dishes on a light-colored table, and so on.
- Use motion lights that turn on by themselves when you walk into a room and timers that turn on lights at dusk.

RATIONALE:

Less than perfect vision does not mean that older persons cannot function. The nurse can help them to come up with creative solutions to maximize independence.

Patient-Family Teaching Guidelines

- Use telephones, clocks, and watches with large numbers.
- Have several pairs of magnifying glasses around the house so that you can set the microwave, adjust the TV, and read the mail easily.
- Use appropriate assistive devices and environmental interventions to improve safety, functional ability, and quality of life.

4. I think I am getting a little hard of hearing. Is this common at my age?

Yes, about one third of Americans over 60 have hearing problems. It is important to get testing and find out the severity of your problem. See your doctor if:

- You cannot hear on the phone.
- It is hard to keep up with a conversation when several people are talking.
- You need to turn the TV up so loud others complain.
- You have trouble hearing women and children talking.

RATIONALE:

Older people sometimes gradually adjust to hearing loss and do not recognize they have a problem. Pointing out specific behaviors will help them assess their own situation.

5. What causes hearing loss?

Many things such as earwax, noise exposure over a long period of time, viral or bacterial infections, heredity, certain medications, and other factors cause hearing loss. The only way to know is to see a doctor for examination and testing.

RATIONALE:

Some causes of hearing loss are reversible, and treatment can improve the quality of a person's life. Further testing is always indicated.

6. How can I help myself to overcome my hearing loss?

Some tips include:

- Look at people's faces when they speak.
- Ask people to speak slowly and clearly.
- Read facial expressions like grins or frowns.
- Be patient and ask people to repeat if you do not hear the first time.
- Use a hearing aid if you need it.

RATIONALE:

Some commonsense tips can help an older person to function more effectively.

7. I have a decreased sense of touch and smell. What should I be concerned about?

The main issue is safety. Our sense of touch and smell alert us to dangers in the environment like smoke from a fire or spoiled food in the refrigerator. It is a good idea to see an ear, nose, and throat doctor for further testing if you have problems with smell, and an internist or neurologist for problems with touch. Some of these problems can be treated and your safety improved.

RATIONALE:

Special safety and home modifications are needed for older people with problems of touch and smell. Older patients should be urged to seek testing, to correct the problem if appropriate, and to institute a plan of safety. It is essential to have intact and functioning smoke detectors in the home and natural gas detectors if the patient has gas heat or a gas stove.

Care Plan

Case Study

Mrs. Owen is a 78-year-old woman who has just been admitted to the hospital's rehabilitation unit. She is recovering from an open reduction with internal fixation of her right hip. She broke her hip 5 days ago at home when she fell getting up to go to the bathroom in the middle of the night. The circumstances of the fall were not documented because she lives alone, but Mrs. Owen states, "I got my feet all tangled up in an electrical cord I was using to run the fan because it was so hot in my room. I just didn't see it." Mrs. Owen has a daughter who lives in a nearby town. The daughter states she is unaware of any other falls her mother may have had, but has noticed numerous bumps and bruises on her mother's arms and legs within the last few months. Mrs. Owen denies this, saying, "Oh, I bruise easily. I always have. It's worse since I'm taking an aspirin every day." Additional medications include atenolol for hypertension, imipramine for depression, and pilocarpine eyedrops for glaucoma.

Mrs. Owen has a regular primary care provider, but has not seen her eye doctor for several years. She states, "Oh, he never does a thing for me. He only tests the pressure in my eyes and says OK, you're good."

Applying the Nursing Process

ASSESSMENT

Mrs. Owen has suffered a fall with resultant serious injury. Falls in the older person can result from a number of factors, so a complete health assessment is needed. However, the nurse should carefully check postural blood pressures because the patient is taking atenolol and imipramine, both of which can contribute to postural hypotension, dizziness, and falls. Additional information that Mrs. Owen uses pilocarpine for glaucoma but has not been vigilant in following up with her eye care provider or monitoring her intraocular pressures should raise a red flag. This patient needs a complete nursing assessment including functional abilities, mental status and mood testing, nutritional assessment, and safety evaluation.

DIAGNOSES

Appropriate nursing diagnoses for Mrs. Owen might include the following:

- *Sensory/perceptual alterations/visual* as evidenced by her fall at night and possibly because of damage secondary to poorly controlled IOP as the result of glaucoma
- *Risk for falls* related to decreased vision and environmental hazards, multiple medications that can affect blood pressure and cause postural hypotension, and

A Patient With Visual Impairment

decreased safety awareness as evidenced by placing an electrical appliance with a cord in a walkway

- *Altered health maintenance behaviors* as evidenced by failure to seek ongoing care and evaluation regarding her glaucoma

EXPECTED OUTCOMES

The expected outcomes for the plan of care specify that Mrs. Owen will:

- Become aware of the need to follow up with her eye care provider to monitor her IOP.
- Utilize risk reduction measures to decrease fall hazards in her home.
- Develop a more trusting and open relationship with her daughter regarding her health status.
- Agree to establish a therapeutic relationship with the nurse and develop a mutually acceptable plan to work toward these outcomes.

PLANNING AND IMPLEMENTATION

The following nursing interventions may be appropriate for Mrs. Owen:

- Urge family to conduct a safety assessment of Mrs. Owen's home environment so that she will not suffer additional falls or injury after discharge from the hospital.
- Educate Mrs. Owen regarding the importance of seeing her ophthalmologist to have her IOP monitored to avoid further visual impairment as the result of poorly managed glaucoma. Encourage Mrs. Owen to arrange an appointment within one month of discharge from the hospital.
- Assess the support system and services needed for Mrs. Owen when she completes her rehabilitation and is discharged to home. Meals-on-wheels, visiting nurse services, physical therapy, shopping, and transportation services can be supplied as needed.
- Begin to explore Mrs. Owen's problem-solving and coping strategies that she has used to solve problems in the past. Mrs. Owen should be aware of the risk of injury and the need to modify her environment for safety.

EVALUATION

The nurse hopes to work with Mrs. Owen over time to increase her functional status, decrease her fall risk, and monitor the management of her chronic illnesses. The nurse will consider the plan a success based on the following criteria:

- Mrs. Owen will return to her home or the least restrictive institutional environment that is acceptable to her, her daughter, and her healthcare providers.
- A family meeting will be held to discuss Mrs. Owen's overall health.
- She will begin to identify fall hazards in her home and make a plan to minimize risk from falls.

Ethical Dilemma

Change the previous scenario slightly to reflect that Mrs. Owen's fall was caused by her dog Muffin, a toy poodle who constantly runs under her feet. Mrs. Owen states,

(continued)

A Patient With Visual Impairment *(continued)*

"I don't care if I did fall on Muffin. I can't imagine life without him. I'll never give him up." How should the nurse respond?

Obviously, Mrs. Owen cares deeply for her dog. Pets improve the quality of life of their owners by providing unconditional love and companionship. However, older people with impaired vision may have difficulty ambulating around a quickly moving dog. Assuming Mrs. Owen is cognitively intact, has good judgment (appropriate assessment required), and can adequately care for Muffin and herself, she has the right to keep her pet.

Should the pet be removed against her will, she would probably suffer from depression and grief, both of which can be detrimental to the function and quality of life of an older person. However, there may be interventions appropriate to improving the situation. For instance:

■ Asking a neighbor to walk the dog vigorously once or twice a day to provide a release of energy and perhaps calm Muffin. If a high school student lives nearby, a small payment would ensure the daily walk and provide socialization for Mrs. Owen.
■ Asking Mrs. Owen to use a cane when ambulating. If Muffin should run under her feet, she could use the cane to steady herself.
■ Placing a bell on Muffin's collar so that Mrs. Owen can be alerted when he runs into the room, and changing Muffin's collar to a bright red or orange color to improve Mrs. Owen's ability to see him.
■ Using motion sensors to turn on lights at night so that when Mrs. Owen has to get up to go to the bathroom, her way will be well lighted.

Mrs. Owen and all involved with her care and support should be aware of the risks and benefits involved with keeping a pet and the chance of another fall. Careful monitoring and ongoing assessment will be needed.

Critical Thinking and the Nursing Process

1. What strategies can the gerontological nurse use when asking an older person to make environmental changes in the home to improve safety?
2. How can nurses become more proactive and improve the environment for safety in the nursing home and hospital settings?
3. Many older people refuse the use of assistive devices like canes and hearing aids because of vanity. What strategies can gerontological nurses use to increase acceptance of assistive devices?
4. How can the mealtime environment be improved in the facilities where you have had clinical rotations?
5. Wear knit gloves for a few hours at home and try to describe the experience of being unable to directly touch and experience your environment.
6. Examine your own habits in your clinical experiences relating to touch. Do you routinely touch older patients? How do you respond when they touch you? Practice touching others in a caring manner, especially if they are vision and hearing impaired. The insights gained will be invaluable.

■ Evaluate your responses in Appendix B.

EXPLORE MediaLink

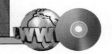

NCLEX review, case studies, and other interactive resources for this chapter can be found on the Companion Website at **www.prenhall.com/tabloski**. Click on Chapter 14 to select the activities for this chapter. For animations, video tutorials, more NCLEX review questions, and case studies, access the accompanying CD-ROM in this textbook.

Chapter Highlights

- Sensory impairments occur commonly in older people as a result of normal changes of aging, the side effects of medications, pathology in certain illnesses, and exposure to environmental insults and chemicals.

- Visual changes involve decreased night vision, color discrimination, and lens accommodation, inhibiting near vision.

- Hearing loss may result from previous occupational exposure to loud noises for prolonged periods of time.

- Taste, smell, and touch perception gradually decrease over time, but large losses may be the result of comorbid diseases and toxic side effects of medication.

- Older persons with one or more sensory impairments are at risk for injury, weight loss, falls, malnutrition, and social isolation. Careful assessment of the duration, extent, and degree of impact on the functional ability of the older person with a sensory impairment is within the role of the gerontological nurse.

- The nurse can urge older people to seek medical evaluation and advice on assistive devices that can improve function, safety, and quality of life.

- Modifications in the older person's environment can be made to improve safety and function.

References

Agency for Health Care Policy and Research. (1993). *Management of cataract in adults. Clinical Practice Guideline No. 4. (AHCPR Publication No. 93–0543).* Rockville, MD: U.S. Department of Health and Human Services.

American Academy of Ophthalmology. (2003). *Take care of your family's eyes at every stage of life.* Retrieved July 10, 2003, from www.aao.org/aao/news/release/091702.cfm.

American Society on Aging. (2003). *Technologies for independence.* Retrieved July 1, 2003, from www.asaging.org/ameritech/V003b_signs_of_vision_loss.html.

Bates, B. (2003). *Health assessment and guide to history taking.* Philadelphia: Lippincott, Williams & Wilkins.

Bogardus, S.T., Yueh, B., & Shekelle, P. (2003). Screening and management of adult hearing loss in primary care. *Journal of the American Medical Association, 289*(15), 1986–1990.

Broihier, K. (2000). Taste and smell: Tactics to triumph over declining senses as you age. *Environmental Nutrition, 23*(2), 1.

Bromley, S. (2000). Smell and taste disorders: A primary care approach. *American Family Physician, 61,* 427–436, 438.

Burke, T. (2002). *A grey area: Colour specification in dementia-specific accommodation.* Retrieved December 10, 2002, from www.dementia.com.au/papers/TimBurkeFINALVERSION.htm.

Centers for Disease Control. (2002). *Trends in vision and hearing among older Americans.* Retrieved March 24, 2003, from www.cdc.gov.

Danner, C. J., & Harris, J. P. (2003). Hearing loss and the aging ear. *Geriatrics and Aging, 6*(5), 40–43.

Demers, K. (2001). *Hearing screening. Try this: Best practices in nursing to care for older adults,* Hartford Institute for Geriatric Nursing, 12.

Elfervig, L. S. (1998). Age-related macular degeneration. *Nurse Practitioner Forum, 9*(1), 4–6.

Epocrates.com. (2003). *Prescription medication information program.* Retrieved March 14, 2003, from www.Epocrates.com.

Fine, S. L., Berger, J.W., Maguire, M. G., & Ho, A. C. (2000). Age-related macular degeneration. *New England Journal of Medicine, 342*(7), 483–492.

Geronurseonline.org. (2005). Normal aging changes. Want to know more. Received March 4, 2005, from www.gewnekseonLine.org.

Hartford Institute for Geriatric Nursing. (1999). *Best nursing practices in care of older adults.* New York: New York University.

Hazzard, W. R., Blass, J. P., Ettinger, W. H., Halter, J. B., & Ouslander, J.G. (1999). *Principles of geriatric medicine and gerontology.* New York: McGraw-Hill.

Jackler, R. K. (2003). A 73-year-old man with hearing loss. *Journal of the American Medical Association, 289*(12), 1557–1565.

Lee, A. G., & Beaver, H. A. (2003). Visual loss in the elderly — Part 1: Chronic visual loss: What to recognize and when to refer. *Clinical Geriatrics, 11*(6), 46–53.

Li, I., & Smith, R. V. (2003). Driving and the elderly. *Clinical Geriatrics, 11*(5), 40–46.

Lockwood, A. H., Salvi, R. J., & Burkard, R. F. (2002). Tinnitus. *New England Journal of Medicine, 347*(12), 904–910.

Marcincuk, M. C., & Roland, P. S. (2002). Geriatric hearing loss: Understanding the causes and providing appropriate treatment. *Geriatrics, 57*(4), 44.

McCague, P. A. (1999). Taste and smell losses in normal aging and disease. *Journal of Dental Hygiene, 73*(2), 105.

McCance, K., & Huether, S. (2001). *Pathophysiology: The biologic basis of disease in adults and children.* New York: Mosby.

McConnell, E. A. (2002). How to converse with a hearing-impaired patient. *Nursing 2002, 32*(8), 20.

Moore, A., Voytas, J., Kowalski, D., & Maddens, N. (2002). Cerumen, hearing and cognition in the elderly. *Journal of the American Medical Directors Association, 3*(3), 136–139.

Murphy, C., Schubert, C. R., Cruickshanks, K. J., Klein, E., Klein, R., & Nondahl, D. M. (2002). Prevalence of olfactory impairment in older adults. *Journal of the American Medical Association, 288*(18), 2307–2312.

National Eye Institute, National Institutes of Health. (2004). *Eye photos.* Retrieved November 7, 2004, from www.nei.nih.gov.

National Guideline Clearinghouse. (2001). *Cataract in the adult eye.* Retrieved August 14, 2003, from www.guideline.gov.

National Institutes of Health. (1990). *Noise and hearing loss. Consensus Statement, 8*(1). Rockville, MD: U.S. Department of Health and Human Services.

National Institute on Aging. (2004). *Age page. Aging and your eyes.* Retrieved April 23, 2003, from www.nia.nih.gov.

Nelson, D. (2001). The power of touch in facility care. *Massage & Bodywork, 16*(1), 12–18.

Palumbo, M. V. (2000). Increasing awareness of the hearing impaired. Hearing Access 2000. *Journal of Gerontological Nursing, 16* (9), 26–30.

Reuben, D., Herr, K., Pacala, J., Potter, J., Pollock, B., & Semla, T. (2002). *Geriatrics at your fingertips.* Malden, MA: Blackwell.

Rosenthal, B. P. (2001). Screening and treatment of age-related and pathologic vision changes. *Geriatrics, 56*(12), 27–32.

Sandor, N. (2000). Is your elderly patient hard of hearing? *Geriatrics and Aging, 3*(8), 6–11.

Schiffman, S. S. (1997). Taste and smell losses in normal aging and disease. *Journal of the American Medical Association, 278*(16), 1357–1362.

Ship, J.A., Pillemer, S. R., & Baum, B. J. (2002). Xerostomia and the geriatric patient. *Journal of the American Geriatrics Society, 50*(3), 535–543.

Solomon, R., & Donnenfeld, E. D. (2003). Recent advances and future frontiers in treating age-related cataracts. *Journal of the American Medical Association, 290*(2), 248–251.

Try This Best Practices in Care for Older Adults. (2002) New York: New York University, The Steinhardt School of Education, Division of Nursing, The John A. Hartford Foundation Institute for Geriatric Nursing.

Uphold, C. R., & Graham, M. V. (2003). *Clinical guidelines in adult health* (3rd ed.). Gainesville, FL: Barmarre Books.

U.S. Department of Labor. Occupational Safety and Health Administration. (2004). *Occupational noise exposure, 1910–95.* Retrieved December 15, 2004, from www.osha.gov.

Ventry, I., Weinstein, B. (1983); Identification of elderly people with hearing problems. *ASHA. 25:*37–42. Reproduced by permission of the author and the American Speech and Hearing Association, © 1983.

Watson, R. (2000). Assessing neurological functioning in older people. *Elderly Care, 12*(4), 25–27.

Weston, B. C., Aliabadi, Z., & White, G. L. (2000). Glaucoma — Review for the vigilant clinician. *Clinician Reviews, 10*(8), 58–74.

Whitaker, R., Whitaker, V. B., & Dill, C. (1998). Glaucoma: What the nurse practitioner should know. *Nurse Practitioner Forum, 9*(1), 7–12.

Wilson, B. A., Shannon, M. T., & Stang, C. L. (2002). *AgingEye Times.* Retrieved October 15, 2003, from www.agingeye.net/ visionbasics/eye&meds.php.

Wood, A. J. (2000). Age-related macular degeneration. *New England Journal of Medicine, 342*(7), 483–492.

CHAPTER 15

The Cardiovascular System

Susan K. Chase, EdD, RN

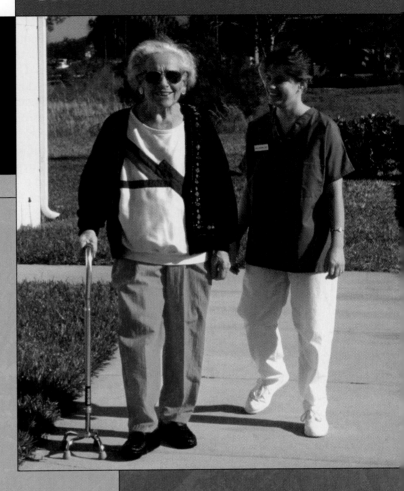

CHAPTER OBJECTIVES

Upon completion of this chapter, the reader will be able to:

- Describe changes in the cardiovascular system that occur with aging.

- List focus areas of assessment for cardiovascular patients.

- Relate physiological concepts to the diagnosis and management of common cardiovascular conditions, including hypertension, angina, congestive heart failure, and peripheral vascular disease.

- List nursing diagnoses commonly occurring in the cardiovascular patient.

- Describe specific nursing interventions used with cardiovascular patients.

- Outline an education plan for cardiovascular patients.

KEY TERMS

adrenergic receptors 424
cardiac output 423
diastole 422
refractory period 424
stroke volume 423
systole 422

MediaLink

Additional resources for this chapter can be found on the Student CD-ROM accompanying this textbook and on the Companion Website at **www.prenhall.com/tabloski**. Click on Chapter 15 to select the activities for this chapter.

CD-ROM
- Animation/Video
  Cardiac A & P
  Cardiac Drugs
  Coronary Artery Disease
- NCLEX Review
- Case Studies

- Tools

COMPANION WEBSITE
- Audio Glossary
- Additional NCLEX Review
- Case Study
- MediaLink Applications

The cardiovascular system pumps blood to all parts of the body for the purpose of delivering oxygen and nutrients and removing metabolic waste products. Because its purpose is to supply all parts of the body, the functioning of the system affects functioning of all other systems. Cardiovascular conditions are the chief cause of death in the United States and other developed countries. In recent years, advanced technology has prolonged the lives of many people with cardiovascular diseases, but this has resulted in increased numbers of people living with the chronic effects of cardiovascular disease. Any nurse working with older persons will encounter cardiovascular disorders. By understanding key principles of physiology, the nurse can understand how new treatment modalities work to reduce symptoms and improve function and quality of life. Nurses need to be able to assess cardiovascular problems, provide effective nursing interventions, and explain conditions and treatments to older patients and their families. Helping older people learn to manage their chronic conditions is very rewarding for the nurse. By better managing their chronic cardiovascular problems, patients have the opportunity to enjoy improved quality of life. Recent studies have led to new treatments and knowledge about diet and exercise that can make a difference in function and quality of life. Working with older persons to improve their ability to manage their cardiovascular health is a rewarding aspect of gerontological nursing.

This chapter reviews the changes related to aging, the pattern of specific cardiovascular conditions, and the medical and nursing interventions used to support older patients who have these conditions. As with all healthcare delivered to older persons, it is important to consider changed response patterns due to age, to preserve function and quality of life, and to maintain patient dignity and choice. Changes in cardiovascular function are a feature of every life stage, but this chapter will focus on changes for the young-old (65 to 74), the old (75 to 85), and the old-old (86 and older). This last age group is the fastest growing segment of the U.S. population.

Structure and Function

The heart is a four-chambered organ slightly left of the sternum. The two upper chambers of the heart are the atria. The two lower chambers of the heart are the ventricles. The ventricles generate power to pump blood through the body systems to which they are connected. The left side of the heart generates greater power to overcome the systemic resistance of the blood vessels of the body. The system of chambers and valves allows for one-way flow of blood from the general circulation, through the right side of the heart, to the lungs where blood gases are exchanged to allow for the release of carbon dioxide and the absorption of oxygen. The blood returns to the left side of the heart and then to the general circulation where oxygen is delivered to tissue and carbon dioxide and other wastes are removed. The cardiac cycle is the sequence and timing of contraction and relaxation in the heart. It is determined by the electrical system of the heart. Figure 15-1 ■ illustrates the structure of the heart and the valves.

The inferior and superior venae cavae return blood from the circulation to the right atrium. Pressures in this chamber are relatively low which allows for easy return of blood from the peripheral circulation. When the tricuspid valve opens, pressures in the resting right ventricle are lower than in the right atrium and blood flows across the tricuspid valve into the right ventricle. The resting phase of the ventricle is called **diastole.** Atrial contraction forces even more blood into the filling right ventricle. With ventricular contraction, also called **systole**, pressure rises in the ventricle and the tricuspid valve is forced closed, preventing blood from flowing back into the right atrium.

FIGURE ▢ **15-1**

The structure of the heart and the valves.

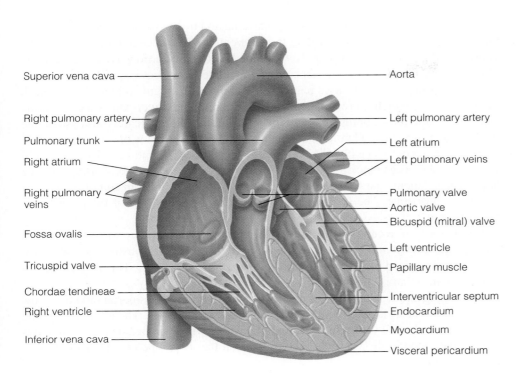

Superior vena cava

Right pulmonary artery

Pulmonary trunk

Right atrium

Right pulmonary veins

Fossa ovalis

Tricuspid valve

Chordae tendineae

Right ventricle

Inferior vena cava

Aorta

Left pulmonary artery

Left atrium

Left pulmonary veins

Pulmonary valve

Aortic valve

Bicuspid (mitral) valve

Left ventricle

Papillary muscle

Interventricular septum

Endocardium

Myocardium

Visceral pericardium

As the pressure rises, the pulmonic valve is opened, forcing blood from the high-pressure right ventricle into the lower pressure pulmonary artery.

The pulmonary artery leads blood into branching vessels of the lungs. During ventricular diastole, the pulmonic valve closes, preventing blood from returning from the pulmonic artery to the right ventricle. Eventually in the lung capillaries, gas exchange takes place. The pulmonary veins return the oxygenated blood from the lungs to the left atrium. On the left side of the heart, the sequence of events is similar and simultaneous with the right-sided events. The opening of the mitral valve allows blood to flow into the relaxed left ventricle. Atrial contraction forces even more blood into the filling left ventricle. When the left ventricle contracts, the mitral valve is forced closed. The aortic valve opens to allow blood to be pumped into the aorta from which it distributes to the entire systemic circulation. When the left ventricle relaxes, the aortic valve closes, preventing blood from flowing back into the left ventricle. The pressures generated on the left side of the heart are greater than the pressure generated on the right side of the heart. This greater pressure is necessary to ensure the adequate flow of blood to and from all systems in the body. Over time and especially when there is increased resistance such as encountered with peripheral vascular disease, this can put stress on the structures of the valves that are associated with the left ventricle, specifically the aortic and mitral valves. The valves can become leaky and damaged, resulting in regurgitation of blood back into the atrium and left ventricular hypertrophy or increased muscle mass to the left ventricle. This can decrease the valuable space needed for blood in the left ventricle.

The amount of blood pumped from the left ventricle with each beat is the **stroke volume.** The amount pumped per minute is the **cardiac output.** This value is reflective of overall functioning of the heart. It can be calculated using the following formula:

$$\text{cardiac output} = \text{heart rate} \times \text{stroke volume}$$

The cardiac output is affected by the heart rate and by the venous blood returned to the heart. The amount of blood filling the left ventricle is reflected in the preload. The afterload reflects the resistance to flow of blood across the aortic valve or through the blood vessels. Cardiac function can be partly regulated by affecting preload, afterload, and contractility. The body uses neurochemical means to regulate these factors such as epinephrine, which increases heart rate, and norepinephrine, which increases the force of contraction. Among the many functions of the autonomic nervous system, the regulation of pressure and volume in the cardiovascular system is of vital importance. Sympathetic receptors can be divided into alpha and beta receptors. A large group of cardiovascular drugs block the alpha and beta receptors, reducing the workload on the heart. The balancing parasympathetic nervous system has neurotransmitters that cause decreased heart rate. The vagus nerve is one of the major nerves of the parasympathetic system.

Stimulation of receptors of the sympathetic nervous system, sometimes called **adrenergic receptors**, causes increased blood pressure, vasoconstriction, increased heart rate, decreased blood flow to the kidneys, and other effects. This is the fight-or-flight response that is elicited in times of stress.

With aging and the diagnosis of cardiovascular disease, it is important to know how efficiently the heart is able to pump blood throughout the body. The amount of blood pumped from the left ventricle at the end of diastole with each beat is not the full volume of the blood in the ventricle. The proportion that is pumped is the ejection fraction. Its formula is:

$$\text{ejection fraction} = \text{stroke volume/end diastolic volume of left ventricle}$$

The efficiency of the ventricle's ability to pump is reflected in this volume. The ejection fraction can be affected by the strength of the contraction of the ventricles, the amount of blood contained in the ventricles, the ability of the valves to prevent regurgitation, and the amount of peripheral vascular resistance. The higher the ejection fraction, the more efficiently the heart is able to provide adequate circulation to the body systems.

CONDUCTION SYSTEM

The mechanical events related to heart function are regulated and coordinated by a series of complex electrical events. All cells of the heart are capable of generating and responding to electrical stimulation. The cells of the myocardium are connected in a mesh that allows the transmission of electrical impulses that regulate heartbeat and stimulate coordinated muscle contractions.

When an action potential is generated or transmitted to a cardiac muscle cell, it initiates a chain of events that result in contraction of the muscle. Returning the cell membrane to its resting state requires energy and time. The period before a cell is at its resting state is called the **refractory period.** Disease states can change the length of the refractory period. A cell that receives and responds to an impulse during the refractory period may initiate an irregularity of heart rhythm called an arrhythmia.

The normal rhythm of cardiac contraction is initiated by the sinoatrial (SA) node in the right atrium. The cells of this region generate action potential at the fastest rate of all the cells of the heart; therefore, they initiate a new impulse and maintain the ongoing heartbeat. This impulse travels across the atria in a coordinated wave and results in atrial contraction.

A band of nonconductive tissue separates the atria from the ventricles. The slight delay in atrial and ventricular contraction allows for efficient filling of the chambers of the heart and a coordinated heartbeat. This fibrous tissue is where the valves are attached. Only one section of the band that separates the atria from the ventricles allows conduction of impulses. It is called the atrioventricular (AV) node. The impulse through the AV node is delayed somewhat and then is allowed to transmit the action potential wave through the bundle of His and bundle branches, which allow for fast conduction. The bundle branches branch and allow for essential simultaneous activation of the thick ventricular walls. When activated, the ventricles contract at the same time. After the refractory period, the SA node generates a new action potential and the sequence repeats itself.

ELECTROCARDIOGRAM

The electrocardiogram (ECG) can offer valuable information about the cardiac function and electrical regulation of the heart. The ideal ECG deflections represent depolarization and repolarization of cardiac muscle tissue in a regular pattern and rhythm. The waves of interest include the P, QRS, and T waves. The P wave represents atrial depolarization. The PR interval represents delay in conduction at the AV node. The QRS complex represents ventricular depolarization. The T wave represents ventricular repolarization. A diagram of a normal ECG is illustrated in Figure 15-2■.

THE CIRCULATORY SYSTEM

Blood vessels that circulate blood throughout the body include arteries and their smaller branches called arterioles, capillaries, the smallest diameter and thinnest vessels; and veins, which include the smaller venules. Arteries carry blood away from the heart. In the pulmonary circuit, this blood is unoxygenated and is on the way to capillaries in the lungs where gases can be exchanged and the blood is oxygenated. The walls of arteries have several layers of smooth muscle that allow for some local control of diameter and pressure in the system. With contraction of the smooth muscle, the

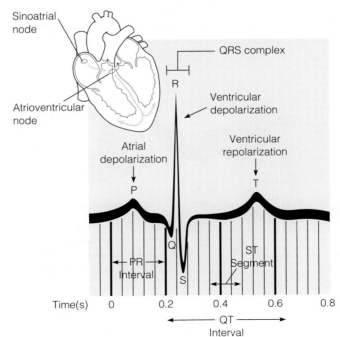

FIGURE ■ **15-2**

Normal electrocardiogram.

artery becomes smaller, allowing less space for circulating blood and resulting in increased systemic pressure.

The inside layer of the artery is called the tunica intima, including the endothelium, and the basal membrane. The next layer out is the tunica media, which has collagen and fibrous tissue including smooth muscles. The outer layer is called the tunica adventitia, which is composed of connective tissue. The capillaries have an endothelial layer and a basal lamina. The spacing between the cells of the endothelium varies from one part of the body to another. Serum of the blood, the fluid portion, and the smaller dissolved substances are filtered though the spaces between endothelial cells of the capillaries. Most of the filtered fluid is returned to the bloodstream in the veins, which have lower pressure than the arteries or capillaries.

The veins have a larger diameter than arteries. Because they carry blood under decreased pressure, they have thinner walls. The veins of the legs have valves that assist in returning blood from the lower extremities to the heart. As the muscles of the legs contract, they squeeze the blood upward, facilitating the return of venous blood to the heart. Valves prevent the blood from flowing back due to the pull of gravity. Figure 15-3☐ illustrates the capillary network between the arterial and venous blood vessels.

REGULATION OF BLOOD FLOW

Blood flow in any area of the body is under several types of control. Local control allows for more or less flow of blood due to local conditions—for example, as a result of trauma or inflammation. The endothelial lining of the arteries and veins is metabolically active and capable of the release of nitric oxide, which causes vasodilation or relaxation. Extreme cold in the extremities may shunt blood away from the extremities to vital organs like the heart and brain to prevent loss of essential body heat. This can result in frostbite to fingers and toes. Areas of the circulation that are metabolically active will receive more circulation than areas that are at rest. Increased blood flow can be initiated by acidosis. Metabolic activity causes the production of acids as a byproduct, so acidosis causes a relaxation of local sphincters and allows more blood to an area. For instance, circulation to the large muscles of the legs will increase during stren-

FIGURE ☐ 15-3

The capillary network between arterial and venous blood.

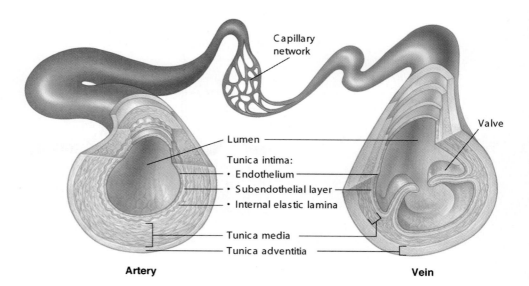

Capillary network

Lumen

Tunica intima:
• Endothelium
• Subendothelial layer
• Internal elastic lamina

Tunica media

Tunica adventitia

Valve

Artery

Vein

uous activity such as jogging or stair climbing. When the area rests, acidosis decreases and the circulation also decreases. This allows the body to conserve energy and to perfuse those areas that are in greatest need.

The lymphatic system is a separate pathway that collects excess tissue fluid and returns it to the circulatory system. The lymphatic system is a pumpless system and consists of lymphatic vessels and lymph nodes. A series of valves ensures one-way flow of excess interstitial fluid toward the heart. Usually, the lymphatic system drains interstitial fluid (lymph) through a system of nodes where immune system cells screen and protect the body from infection. When the capillary outflow exceeds venous reabsorption, some fluid remains in the interstitium or extracellular space. This fluid must be returned to the blood system to ensure ongoing efficient cardiovascular function. If too much fluid leaves the capillaries because of excessive arterial pressure, or if the pressure in the venous system is too great and the interstitial fluid cannot reenter the venous circulation, then extra interstitial fluid collects and is termed *edema*. This edema often collects in the lower extremities as the result of gravity.

CARDIAC CIRCULATION

The heart is supplied with blood by the coronary circulation. The function of the heart muscle depends on adequate circulation to provide oxygenated blood and prevent pain caused by myocardial ischemia or angina. The two coronary arteries arise from the aorta just above the aortic valve. The left coronary artery branches to become the left anterior descending and the circumflex artery. The right coronary artery supplies the right side of the heart. The coronary arteries travel on the outside of the heart, and the branches penetrate to the deeper layers of muscle. Increased cardiac workload such as increases in rate in response to activity and movement requires increased blood flow through the coronary arteries. Atherosclerotic changes in the coronary arteries and the plaque accumulation of coronary artery disease can result in myocardial ischemia, myocardial infarction, and sudden death.

The heart is surrounded by the pericardium, a double-walled sac filled with a small amount of fluid. This fluid decreases friction and allows for smooth movement of the muscle within the sac when it contracts and relaxes. Increased fluid in the pericardium is called *cardiac tamponade* and can result in cardiac compression and death.

Normal Changes With Aging

It is often difficult to distinguish between disease processes and natural consequences of aging. A decrease in cardiovascular reserve or a decrease in cardiac output may be the result of deconditioning or disease and not the result of natural aging processes as was once thought. A wide range of changes can occur with aging, and differences in cardiovascular functioning exist from one person to another. The very old person with a good family history and healthy lifestyle can enjoy much greater cardiac function than a middle-aged person with a family history of cardiovascular problems or a history of smoking. It is important to remember the concept of compensation in cardiovascular function. Changes may occur with aging, such as decreased renal functioning. This causes a change in other systems in order to try to improve functioning. Sometimes these compensatory changes cause problems of their own. For example, kidneys that are poorly perfused due to decreased cardiac output produce renin that eventually increases blood pressure and sodium retention. These gradual compensatory changes are initially benign but can lead to decreased cardiac and renal function and fluid overload. See Figure 15-4■ for normal changes of aging in the cardiovascular system.

FIGURE ▢ 15-4

Normal changes of aging in the cardiovascular system.

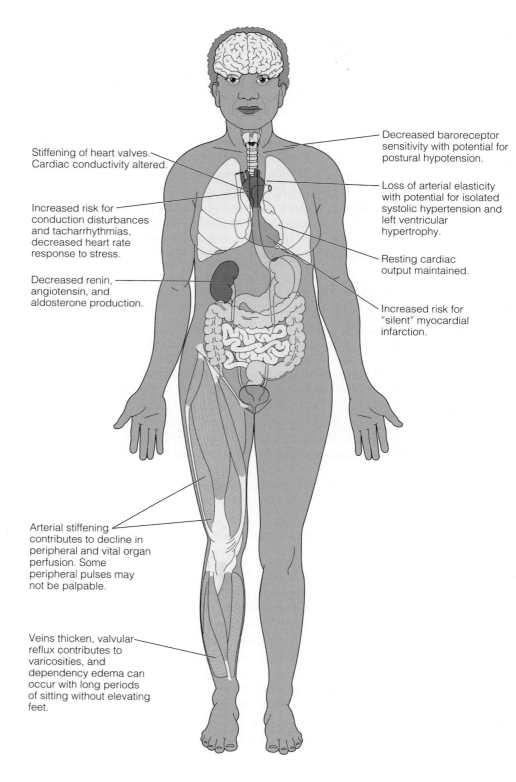

Stiffening of heart valves. Cardiac conductivity altered.

Increased risk for conduction disturbances and tacharrhythmias, decreased heart rate response to stress.

Decreased renin, angiotensin, and aldosterone production.

Arterial stiffening contributes to decline in peripheral and vital organ perfusion. Some peripheral pulses may not be palpable.

Veins thicken, valvular reflux contributes to varicosities, and dependency edema can occur with long periods of sitting without elevating feet.

Decreased baroreceptor sensitivity with potential for postural hypotension.

Loss of arterial elasticity with potential for isolated systolic hypertension and left ventricular hypertrophy.

Resting cardiac output maintained.

Increased risk for "silent" myocardial infarction.

How an individual person ages is determined by genetic factors as well as by physical and social environments. Aging changes are gradual and may not be noticed by the individual or by members of the family. Different body systems age at different rates. One person might have orthopedic problems but relatively few cardiovascular problems. Many cardiovascular functions involve neurological or endocrine systems. These interrelated processes are vulnerable to aging in that a change in one system can affect functioning in many others. Furthermore, physical or emotional stress can cause greater response and require longer time for recovery. Taking a trip or getting the flu can cause much greater stress and negative changes for a frail older person. Another feature of aging is the atypical presentation of disease in an older person. For example, a middle-aged person experiencing a myocardial infarction will most likely complain of the typical substernal chest pain with radiation down the left arm. However, the older person may complain of heartburn, nausea and vomiting, or excessive fatigue. Nurses must be alert to possible problems and must include a wide range of diagnostic possibilities in a given situation. Mental status changes, agitation, and falls may be the first sign of cardiac problems in the older person. Mental status changes should never be assumed to be the result of dementia. Sudden changes in cognitive ability should be assessed completely and aggressively (Craven, 2000).

Practice Pearl

Many older women will complain of vague symptoms when having a myocardial infarction, including fatigue, sleep disturbances, and epigastric pain. Be sure to refer older patients with these complaints for medical evaluation.

Specific changes in the cardiovascular system with aging include myocardial hypertrophy, an increase in the size of muscle cells of the myocardium. This will change the function of the left ventricular wall and the ventricular septum. The left ventricular wall is 25% thicker for the average 80-year-old as compared with the average 30-year-old. Inside individual cardiac cells, lipofuscin and amyloid desposits accumulate and the structure of the myocardium shows increased collagen and connective tissue (McCance & Huether, 2001). Heart valves become stiff with aging as the result of fibrosis and calcification. In addition, changes in the valve rings can contribute to stenosis or incompetence. These changes then have an effect on the heart muscle and chamber sizes (Reuben et al., 2004).

Resting heart rate is relatively unchanged with normal aging. In the absence of disease, cardiac output is not much changed. However, there is a slight decline in cardiac output after age 20. The average man with a cardiac output of 5.0 L/min at age 20 will likely have a cardiac output of 3.5 L/min at age 75. This cardiac output is sufficient to maintain normal adult functioning. The ability of the heart to increase its rate in response to stress has been demonstrated (Craven, 2000).

Practice Pearl

The older heart cannot respond to stressful stimuli as well as the younger heart. Caution your sedentary older patients not to engage in stressful activities like vigorous shoveling of snow or heavy yard work without engaging in a gradual exercise program.

Electrical activity of the heart is affected in aging with a decrease in the number of normal pacemaker cells in the sinus node. By age 75, only 10% of original pacemaker cells are still functional, but under normal circumstances this number can still support cardiac function. Similarly, the number of cells in the AV node and in the left bundle branch is lower for the older person. Similar changes have been demonstrated that show a decrease in cells in the bundle of His at age 40 and a decrease in right bundle branch cells by age 50. Other studies show an increase in fat and collagen in these regions. Fibrosis of the AV node can lead to AV block with no other cardiac pathology. The AV node refractory period is also increased with aging. The electrocardiogram shows no specific changes with age, although some lengthening of the PR, QRS, and QT interval has been described. The stress of illness can precipitate conduction difficulties for the older person (Craven, 2000).

Practice Pearl

New-onset atrial fibrillation and other arrythmias may signal the onset of serious underlying illness such as hyperthyroidism, electrolyte disturbances, or myocardial infarction. All older patients with complaints of "skipped beats" or "fluttering in the chest" should be referred for medical evaluation.

The vascular system undergoes a range of changes with aging. The layers of the vascular system change with a thickening of the intimal and medial layers. For arteries, the endothelial layer becomes irregular with more connective tissue. Lipid deposits and calcification occur. Calcification can extend to the medial layer with increased collagen deposits. These changes can all lead to decreased elasticity or "hardening" of the arterial walls. Blood pressure elevation frequently occurs with aging, although it is not considered a normal variant. Isolated systolic hypertension (systolic >140 mmHg) is frequently seen in the older person. Normally, the arterial wall diameter is controlled by a balance of systems including the autonomic nervous system and beta-adrenergic stimulation. With aging, decreased responsiveness to beta-adrenergic stimulation is noted (Craven, 2000).

Practice Pearl

If left uncontrolled, high systolic pressure can lead to stroke, myocardial infarction, congestive heart failure, kidney damage, blindness, or other conditions. Although it cannot be cured once it has developed, isolated systolic hypertension (ISH) can be controlled.

Pulmonary changes that occur with aging can affect cardiovascular function. Decreased chest wall compliance is the result of decreased elasticity of lung tissue and stiffness of thoracic and spinal joints. An increase in anteroposterior diameter is seen with aging. This can lead to higher residual volumes. Airway closure in dependent lung areas can occur at higher volumes. This removes portions of the lung from exchange functions. A combination of early airway closure, decreased diffusing capacity, increased lung volumes, and changes in alveolar structure can lead to lower arterial oxygen tension (PaO_2). Because carbon dioxide is diffused more readily, no change in $PaCO_2$ is noted with aging. Elevated $PaCO_2$ would indicate pathology. Ciliary function is decreased with age. This fact along with decreased immune function makes the older person more susceptible to pneumonia or other infections (Craven, 2000).

Renal function declines with age, and the kidneys decrease in size and weight. By the ninth decade, the weight of the kidney is 25% less than the weight of the young adult kidney. Functional decline is also the result of decreased renal blood flow and decreased glomerular filtration. By age 80, the glomerular filtration rate is reduced 30% to 50% as compared with that of the 30-year-old. Because of a concomitant decrease in muscle mass, serum creatinine levels are not elevated. However, the clearance rate for creatinine and other chemicals, including many medications, is reduced. This results in a longer half-life for drugs administered to the older person. With aging, decreased levels of renin and aldosterone are found in the plasma. This leads to an increased sensitivity to dietary sodium consumption. Decreased ability to clear sodium from the blood can lead to body water overload. This increased preload can tax the myocardium. Additionally, antidiuretic hormone is less able to be suppressed when serum osmolality is low. This results in further retention of body water. A decreased ability to concentrate urine can result in dehydration. In general, older persons are less able to adapt to fluid volume changes (Craven, 2000).

In summary, aging brings change to the cardiovascular system. Older people should not expect to become debilitated from aging alone. Complaints of fatigue, decreased activity, sleep disturbance, or pain are not normal and should be investigated. The older person has a decreased capacity to adapt to stress to the cardiovascular system and may need medical or nursing interventions.

Common Illnesses With Older Persons

In the United States, it is difficult to determine the actual prevalence of cardiovascular disorders because there is no national database that tracks such things. Some recent surveys have failed to include patients over 80 years of age or patients who live in nursing homes (Centers for Disease Control, 2004). Heart disease is the number one cause of death for older people in the United States. Figure 15-5 illustrates the most common causes of death in the United States in 1999.

Cardiovascular disease develops slowly and can take years to develop. Some common conditions such as hypertension or hyperlipidemia are risk factors for developing more serious conditions at any stage in life, and these conditions require ongoing assessment and treatment at any age.

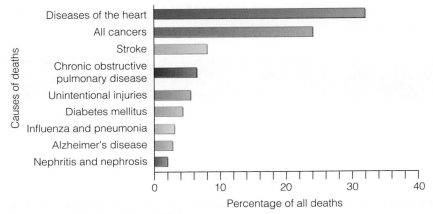

Source: Centers for Disease Control, 2004.

FIGURE 15-5

Most common causes of death in the United States, 1999.

HYPERTENSION

Hypertension is a major risk factor for other cardiovascular conditions, although it does not usually produce symptoms of its own. Since the 1960s, the death rates due to cardiovascular conditions in industrialized nations have decreased, largely due to better control of hypertension with medications. An estimated 43 million Americans (24% of adults) have hypertension, with even more having blood pressures higher than optimal. In a recent study, only 69% of people with elevated blood pressure were aware of their condition (National Heart, Lung, and Blood Institute, 2004). This represents a major risk for the development of cardiovascular conditions in these individuals. The nurse should use the term *high blood pressure* with patients and family members since the term *hypertension* can be mistakenly associated with anxiety or tension. Patients sometimes mistakenly take blood pressure medication only when they feel tense. This fails to control blood pressure (Cunningham, 2000a).

Drug Alert !

Instruct your older patients to take blood pressure medication regularly as prescribed. It is important to keep constant drug levels for effective blood pressure control.

The definition and cutoff readings for diagnosis hypertension are revised as new research is evaluated. The Joint National Committee of the National High Blood Pressure Education Program (JNC) has defined hypertension in stages with recommendations for treatment at each stage. Its most recent version was published in 2003 and is referred to as *JNC 7* (Joint National Committee on Prevention, Detection, Evaluation, and Treatment of High Blood Pressure, 2003) (see Table 15-1). When the systolic and diastolic of a particular reading fall in different categories, the higher category should be identified. Isolated systolic hypertension is common in the older person. It is defined as systolic blood pressure greater than 140 mmHg.

Highlights from the *JNC 7* report include the following:

- In persons older than 50 years, systolic blood pressure greater than 140 mmHg is a much more important cardiovascular disease (CVD) risk factor than diastolic blood pressure.
- The risk of CVD beginning at 115/75 mmHg doubles with each increment of 20/10 mmHg; individuals who are normotensive at age 55 have a 90% lifetime risk for developing hypertension.

TABLE 15-1

Classification of Blood Pressure

Category	Systolic Pressure (mmHg)	Diastolic Pressure (mmHg)
Optimal	<120	<80
Prehypertension	120–139	80–89
Hypertension		
Stage 1	140–159	90–99
Stage 2	≥ 160	≥ 100

Source: Adapted from Joint National Committee, 2003.

- Individuals with a systolic blood pressure of 120 to 139 mmHg or a diastolic blood pressure of 80 to 89 mmHg should be considered as prehypertensive and require health-promoting lifestyle modifications to prevent CVD.
- Thiazide-type diuretics should be used in drug treatment for most patients with uncomplicated hypertension, either alone or combined with drugs from other classes. Certain high-risk conditions are compelling indications for the initial use of other antihypertensive drug classes (angiotensin-converting enzyme inhibitors, angiotensin receptor blockers, beta-blockers, calcium channel blockers).
- Most patients with hypertension will require two or more antihypertensive medications to achieve goal blood pressure (<140/90 mmHg, or <130/80 mmHg for patients with diabetes or chronic kidney disease).
- If blood pressure is more than 20/10 mmHg above goal blood pressure, consideration should be given to initiating therapy with two agents, one of which usually should be a thiazide-type diuretic.
- The most effective therapy prescribed by the most careful clinician will control hypertension only if patients are motivated. Motivation improves when patients have positive experiences with, and trust in, the clinician.
- Empathy builds trust and is a potent motivator (Joint National Committee, 2003).

Practice Pearl

Older patients with chronic kidney disease or diabetes should be more aggressively treated because of additional risk. Their blood pressure goal is below 130/80 mmHg.

Blood pressure readings increase with age with a higher incidence in men than in women up to age 70, after which the incidence in women is higher. Furthermore, non-Hispanic Black men and women at almost every age group have higher blood pressures than other racial cohorts (National Heart, Lung, and Blood Institute, 2004). Since publication of the Framingham Heart Study, it has been known that blood pressure increases with increased body weight (National Heart, Lung, and Blood Institute, 2004). High blood pressure in genetically related individuals has also been shown to be a risk factor for hypertension (Hunt & Williams, 1999). In the United States, the southern states have been designated the "stroke belt" because of the high incidence of cardiovascular conditions. It is not known if the cause of this higher incidence is genetic or environmental. This part of the country has high rates of obesity, high rates of eating high-sodium and fried food, and lower rates of physical exercise as compared with other areas (Hall, 1999).

The physiological changes associated with hypertension involve an increase in cardiac output or an increase in systemic vascular resistance or both. Baroreceptors in the body constantly assess blood pressure and control blood pressure with a neurohormonal feedback system. Some associated factors include renal regulation of vascular volume. Low-pressure baroreceptors also have an effect on vascular volume. Over long periods of time, high blood pressure results in increased systemic vascular resistance and a decreased cardiac output and stroke volume (Cunningham, 2000a).

Practice Pearl

Because changes of aging cause the baroreceptors to be less efficient, it is essential to check postural blood pressures in older patients to prevent postural hypotension and falls.

The underlying causes of hypertension are not known in most cases. In a small number of cases, specific causes can be determined. In general, several mechanisms may be involved, including (1) autonomic nervous system dysfunction with an exaggerated response to autonomic triggers; (2) genetic differences in renal sodium reabsorption, which may be particularly prevalent among non-Hispanic blacks; (3) dysfunction of the renin-angiotensin aldosterone system, which results in increased body water; (4) impaired endovascular responsiveness; and (5) insulin resistance, noted because hypertension and diabetes frequently occur together. Primary hypertension is diagnosed when no specific cause is known. Secondary hypertension is diagnosed in 5% to 10% of cases with specific causes such as renal artery stenosis or adrenal dysfunction (Cunningham, 2000a).

Untreated hypertension results in several physical changes in the body. The medial layer of artery walls hypertrophies in early stages of hypertension. This results in a narrowing of the lumen of the vessel. Eventually, the endothelium becomes unable to support vasodilation. Hypertension accelerates the rate at which atherosclerosis develops in the aorta and large vessels (Cunningham, 2000a). Arteriosclerosis occurs when lesions are concentric and dilated. These arteries become stiff as elastin is lost and collagen increases (O'Rourke, 1999). The heart develops left ventricular hypertrophy and an increased risk for coronary artery disease. In long-term hypertension the renal afferent arterioles fail to protect the glomerular membrane, resulting in increased filtration pressure. Dissolved proteins, which normally do not cross the glomerular membrane, can be forced across and lost in the urine as proteinuria. Vascular changes in the retina are visible on ophthalmoscopic examination and appear as hemorrhages, exudates, cotton-wool patches, and changes in vascular wall thickness. Arterial-venous nicking results when a thickened artery wall crosses a vein and causes an indentation. Blood vessels to the brain change in long-term hypertension, resulting in narrowing of the internal lumen. Stroke rates are increased in patients with hypertension. Stroke is the number one cause of disability and the number three cause of death in the United States (Cunningham, 2000a).

Assessment of the patient with hypertension includes accurate blood pressure monitoring. The nurse should record pressures in both upper extremities and in the positions of lying, sitting, and standing. Diagnosing hypertension requires multiple readings on multiple occasions. Blood pressure can vary widely by time of day and with activity level. Some people react to the stress of having their blood pressure examined in an office setting by having higher readings than when tested in other settings. This is called *white coat hypertension.* Patients should be taught to monitor their own blood pressure at home, to record the readings, and to bring both the readings record and their equipment to the office to check the validity of their equipment and technique. Assessment should also include looking for evidence of target organ damage with ophthalmic examination and urinalysis for proteinuria. For blood pressure that develops suddenly or is refractory to treatment, secondary hypertension should be considered.

Management of hypertension begins with setting blood pressure goals and teaching lifestyle modification. For patients with multiple risk factors such as diabetes and previous MI, lower targets are set than for those with fewer risk factors. The target is 120/80. Lifestyle change is always attempted at every stage of hypertension. Weight loss of even 10 lb will reduce blood pressure to a certain extent. Even without weight loss, increasing the consumption of fruits, vegetables, and whole grains will lower blood pressure. The Dietary Approaches to Stop Hypertension (DASH) diet was tested in a clinical study and found to be effective in significantly lowering blood pressure in older patients with hypertension (National Heart, Lung, and Blood Institute, 2004). Beginning an exercise program, stopping smoking, and reducing alcohol intake are also effective measures to lower blood pressure (Cunningham, 2000a).

Medication management in the older person can be complicated because there are many choices of medications that are considered appropriate options. In addition, the older person may have coexisting conditions that will affect medication selection. For patients with liver or renal disease, different medications may be required. All medications have side effects, and choosing medications with minimal effects for the particular person is important. The major classes of drugs used in hypertension are listed in Table 15-2.

The nurse's role in caring for older patients with hypertension is to screen for high blood pressure in a variety of community settings and to promote healthy lifestyles through low-fat and low-sodium diets, exercise, smoking cessation, and controlled alcohol consumption. Another important role is to teach older patients who are diagnosed with hypertension about the importance of staying on medications even though they do not feel any different, or perhaps feel worse because of side effects. Monitoring the effect of medication and determining barriers to healthy living are important in supporting the patient in self-management.

HYPOTENSION

Low blood pressure, or hypotension, can occur in the older person. It is a frequent side effect of many cardiovascular conditions and many medications. Blood pressure varies widely during the day. As a person ages, the ability to autoregulate blood pressure can decrease. Normally, if there is a transient decrease in cardiac output, the sympathetic nervous system causes an increase in heart rate to maintain cardiac output. With aging, the responsiveness declines. Additionally, decreased muscle tone in the lower extremities can contribute to postural or orthostatic hypotension, which is a rapid decline in blood pressure when the older person rises to a standing or sitting position from a lying position. Diagnosis of orthostatic hypertension can be made by having the patient maintain a supine position for at least 5 minutes. The nurse should check the blood pressure while the patient is supine, and 1 and 3 minutes after sitting or standing. If the pressure drops as much as 20 mmHg systolic or 10 mmHg diastolic, postural hypotension exists (Stone & Wyman, 1999).

Medications that can cause postural hypotension include alpha-adrenergic blockers, centrally acting antihypertensive agents, psychotropic drugs and tranquilizers, high-dose antibiotics, and nonsteroidal anti-inflammatory drugs (NSAIDs). Patients who experience hypotension can be taught to rise slowly from a lying or sitting position, to use a cane or walker if unsteady, and to drink water, unless restricted, to maintain blood volume (Reuben et al., 2004).

Drug Alert !

Persons taking alpha-blockers like doxazosin mesylate or prazosin HCl should be taught to rise slowly to prevent a drop in blood pressure.

HYPERLIPIDEMIA

The body produces a range of lipid-based chemicals that are useful in cell membrane structure and that form the basis of other chemicals such as steroid hormones. Lipid chemicals circulating the body come from either dietary sources or from the production of liver cells. Lipids can be classified into several categories, including high-density

TABLE 15-2

Medications Used for the Management of Hypertension

Medication Group	Sample Drugs	Reason to Choose	Side Effects/ Precautions
Diuretics	Hydrochlorothiazide (HydroDIURIL) Furosemide (Lasix) Bumetanide (Bumex) Spironolactone (Aldactone) Triamterene (Dyrenium)	Good first-line agent, inexpensive, useful with heart failure	Can increase cholesterol and glucose, uric acid, decrease potassium hyperkalemia
Adrenergic inhibitors Beta-blockers	Acebutolol (Sectral) Atenolol (Tenormin) Betaxolol (Kerlone) Metoprolol (Lopressor, Toprol-XL) Nadolol (Corgard) Penbutolol sulfate (Levatol) Propranolol HCl (Inderal) Timolol HCl (Blocadren)	Coexisting coronary artery disease, angina, arrhythmias, post–myocardial infarction	Asthma exacerbation, bradycardia, reduced peripheral circulation, fatigue, decreased exercise tolerance
Adrenergic inhibitors Alpha-blockers	Doxazosin mesylate (Cardura) Prazosin HCl (Minipress) Terazosin HCl (Hytrin)	Dyslipidemia, benign prostatic hypertrophy	Postural hypotension, bronchospasm
Adrenergic inhibitors Combined alpha- and beta-blockers	Carvedilol (Coreg)	Heart failure	Postural hypotension
Adrenergic inhibitors Centrally acting inhibitors	Clonidine HCl (Catapres) Guanfacine HCl (Tenex) Methyldopa (Aldomet)		Sedation, dry mouth bradycardia
ACE inhibitors	Benazepril HCl (Lotensin) Captopril (Capoten) Enalapril maleate (Vasotec) Fosinopril Na (Monopril) Lisinopril (Prinivil, Zestril) Moexipril (Univasc) Quinapril HCl (Accupril) Ramipril (Altace) Trandolapril (Mavik)	Diabetes mellitus, heart failure, renal insufficiency	Dry cough angioedema, hyperkalemia
Angiotensin receptor blockers	Losartan K (Cozaar) Valsartan (Diovan) Irbesartan (Avapro)	Heart failure	Angioedema, hyperkalemia
Calcium channel blockers Nonhydropyridines Dihydropyridines	Diltiazem HCl (Cardizem SR) Verapamil (Isoptin, Calan, Verelan, Covera) Amlodipine besylate (Norvasc) Felodipine (Plendil) Isradipine (DynaCirc) Nicardipine (Cardene SR) Nifedipine (Procardia XL, Adalat CC) Nisoldipine (Sular)	Angina Atrial tachycardia Isolated systolic hypertension	Slows conduction, decreased cardiac output Ankle edema, flushing, headache
Vasodilators	Hydralazine HCl (Apresoline) Minoxidil (Loniten)		Headache, tachycardia, fluid retention

Source: Data from Cunningham, 2000a, pp. 796, 798–799.

Note: Information pertinent to full group presented first. Specific information on line right of drug name.

Risk Category	LDL Goal (mg/dl)	LDL to Consider Therapy (mg/dl)
Coronary heart disease or high-risk equivalents	< 100	≥ 130 (100–129 drug optional)
Two or more risk factors	< 130	130–190
Zero or one risk factor	< 160	≥ 190 (160–189 drug optional)

TABLE 15-3

Categories of Risk and LDL Cholesterol Goals

Source: Data from Expert Panel on Detection, Evaluation and Treatment of High Blood Cholesterol in Adults, 2001.

lipoprotein (HDL), low-density lipoprotein (LDL), and triglycerides. High-fat diets and certain hereditary patterns can result in elevated serum lipids. Elevated cholesterol has been shown to be a risk factor for the development of cardiovascular disorders. LDLs have been shown to be the type of lipid associated with increased risk for mortality or morbidity. HDLs have been shown to have a beneficial effect on overall vascular health, probably because they help to mobilize cholesterol from the blood vessels and carry it back to the liver for processing.

The Adult Treatment Panel (ATP III) has recently made recommendations for evaluating and managing elevated cholesterol. The new approach considers the individual's risk factor profile in recommending how aggressive to be in lowering cholesterol levels. The Heart Protection Study (HPS) has also shown that controlling LDL with simvastatin assists in the prevention of coronary heart disease. Risk factors include having other known atherosclerosis such as peripheral arterial disease or abdominal aortic aneurysm, or the presence of diabetes mellitus (Braun & Davidson, 2003). Table 15-3 shows the new recommendations, which include starting medications for people with no evidence of coronary heart disease but with positive risk factors.

The HMG-CoA reductase inhibitors (also known as statins) have been shown to be the most powerful and best tolerated group of drugs in lowering LDL. The greatest benefit is achieved for the patients most at risk for developing coronary heart disease. These include people with multiple risk factors for cardiovascular disorders. Research has also shown that reducing LDL with medications reduces coronary events for older persons and for women of all ages. Some have argued that older persons may not benefit from drug therapy to improve lipid profiles because mortality is approaching and the time for prevention of adverse outcomes is shortened. Others have shown that reducing cardiac events decreases morbidity and disability. In addition to lowering LDL cholesterol, statins have such protective effects as being anti-inflammatory and antithrombotic. They also protect intravascular plaque stability.

It is anticipated that many more patients will be placed on statins in the future, and nurses need to be able to teach patients about their medications. In general, statins are well tolerated, but a small minority of patients experience liver inflammation with elevated liver enzymes or muscle pain and weakness with myopathies.

Drug Alert !

Patients taking statins should be taught to report muscle aches and symptoms to their healthcare provider.

TABLE 15-4

Drugs Used in the Treatment of Hyperlipidemia

Medication Group	Sample Drugs	Reasons to Use	Side Effects/Precautions
HMG-CoA reductase inhibitors	Lovastatin (Mevacor) Pravastatin (Pravachol) Simvastatin (Zocor) Fluvastatin (Lescol XL) Atorvastatin (Lipitor)	Reduce LDL	Gastrointestinal distress, elevation of liver enzymes, myopathies
Bile acid sequestrants	Cholestyramine (Questran) Colestipol (Colestid) Colesevelam (WelChol)	Reduce LDL Reduce triglycerides	Constipation, bloating, decreased fat-soluble vitamin absorption
Fibrates	Gemfibrozil (Lopid) Fenofibrate (Tricor)	Reduce triglycerides	Gastrointestinal distress, abdominal pain
Nicotinic acid	Niacin (Niaspan)	Reduce LDL Elevate HDL Reduce triglycerides	Skin flushing, pruritus, gastrointestinal distress

Source: Data from Fair & Berra, 2000, p. 830.

Other medications useful in reducing serum cholesterol are most often used to augment the effect of the statins. These have adverse effects that make them less tolerable for many patients, so nurses need to explain their benefits and strategize on minimizing unpleasant effects. The first group of drugs also used for cholesterol control is the bile acid sequestrants. They attach to bile in the gut and prevent its return to the liver. Gastrointestinal bloating or constipation are the chief side effects. Secondly, fibrates can be useful in reducing elevated triglycerides. Nausea and abdominal pain are the main side effects. Finally, nicotinic acid is useful in lowering LDL and triglycerides as well as increasing HDL. The major side effect from nicotinic acid is skin flushing (Fair & Berra, 2000). Starting with low doses and gradually increasing can minimize this effect (Stein, 2002). Table 15-4 lists medications used for the management of hyperlipidemia.

CHEST PAIN

Chest pain can occur for a variety of reasons, but the nurse should always consider the possibility of heart-related problems. When the myocardium is deprived of sufficient blood supply and thereby oxygen, ischemia occurs. Ischemia causes pain and loss of function. Chronic ischemic pain is referred to as angina. In addition to coronary artery disease, aortic stenosis and pericarditis are cardiovascular causes of chest pain. Gastrointestinal problems such as heartburn, acid reflux, and ulcers can also cause chest pain. Musculoskeletal causes of chest pain are chondritis. Pulmonary problems such as pulmonary embolus, pneumonia, and pleural effusion are other causes. Herpes zoster (shingles) can cause pain in the skin of the chest. The evaluation of chest pain should be part of a full nursing assessment, which is discussed later in the chapter. The absence of chest pain does *not* indicate the absence of cardiovascular disease. For the older person and for women, myocardial infarction can occur with no chest pain. Patients who describe sudden breathlessness or activity intolerance or a feeling of impending doom should be evaluated as aggressively as those who describe chest pain.

Practice Pearl

The absence of chest pain in the older person does not indicate an absence of ischemic heart disease. Older persons can present with fatigue, weakness, shortness of breath, and gastrointestinal complaints.

ANGINA

The gradual process of atherosclerosis results in narrowing of the arteries that supply blood to the heart muscle. The incidence of atherosclerosis increases with age. There are two kinds of ischemic heart disease. *Supply ischemia* results from a decreased blood flow to the myocardium, and *demand ischemia* results from increased demand for oxygen related to such conditions as a fast heart rate or thick heart muscle. An inadequate supply of oxygen and nutrients leads to a decrease in adenosine triphosphate production because of a shift to anaerobic metabolism. Anaerobic metabolism is less efficient and produces waste products such as pyruvate and lactate. The acidic condition as well as the loss of adenosine triphosphate results in decreased sodium potassium pump activity and can eventually lead to cell death. Intracellular calcium ion concentration also increases. The accumulation of waste products leads to the release of inflammatory mediators and the activation of white blood cells. Cardiac cells that are stressed can initiate arrhythmias and are less effective in contracting. Ischemia is a reversible condition and can be improved with lifestyle, medication, or surgical management (Cunningham, 2000b).

Patients with stable angina report chest pain that is relieved with rest. It is precipitated by activities that increase the workload on the heart. Angina is frequently managed with sublingual nitroglycerin, which causes vasodilation and increases blood flow to the heart. Patients who need multiple doses of nitrates every day can be placed on long-term nitrate therapy. Many older people do not experience typical chest pain but have anginal equivalent symptoms such as fatigue or weakness, arm or jaw pain, palpitations, sweating, or dizziness. Symptoms that are not relieved with rest or medication can indicate progression of the angina or myocardial infarction. This requires immediate medical intervention. Unstable angina occurs when angina is not relieved with rest or medication. It indicates a progression of the coronary artery disease.

Prinzmetal's angina or atypical angina is less common and is characterized by chest pain experienced at rest. The pain is not relieved with nitroglycerin, but does not usually progress to myocardial infarction. It is thought to be caused by transient coronary artery constriction.

The development of coronary heart disease is related to identifiable risk factors, some of which are modifiable. By working on risk factors, patients will decrease their chance of developing heart disease. Even if they have developed heart disease, they can improve their quality of life by following a healthy lifestyle.

Nurses can help older patients with angina by supporting lifestyle change and by teaching proper medication usage. Many patients are reluctant to use medications, particularly when prescribed "as needed." The nurse can present scenarios and ask patients what they would do if they have sudden weakness or if they take the medication and it does not help.

MYOCARDIAL INFARCTION

Ischemic heart disease is the major cause of death in the United States. It is caused by clot development within the coronary arteries, which causes a blockage in blood flow to the areas normally served by the particular artery. The blockage in blood flow results in myocardial cell death or myocardial infarction (MI). Ischemia is reversible, but cell death is not. Once the myocardial cell has died, it cannot be resuscitated and the loss of the cell's contraction will decrease the function of the heart itself. Damage to the heart muscle is determined by the size and location of the area of injury and infarct. Left ventricle anterior wall infarcts occur because of a blockage of the left anterior descending coronary artery. Infarcts of the anterior wall result in reduced cardiac output and electrical conduction blockages because the left anterior descending artery also supplies the intraventricular septum. Another type of MI is classified as inferior or posterior. The right coronary artery supplies these areas for most patients. The sinus node and atria are perfused by this artery, and arrhythmias or blocked conduction can occur in these areas. Parasympathetic signs such as nausea, vomiting, or other gastrointestinal complaints are often seen with this type of MI. Lateral wall MIs occur with occlusion of the circumflex branch of the left main coronary artery. This artery also supplies the AV node and ventricular papillary muscles, so dysfunction in these areas can be seen with this type of MI. The right ventricle can also experience an MI (Del Bene & Vaughan, 2000).

The diagnosis of MIs involves good history and physical assessment as well as laboratory and electrocardiographic analysis. An MI is an event with several stages, and interpreting these findings requires consideration of the stage of the MI. A history of chest pain may be the major presenting complaint, but in many patients, particularly older women, pain may not be experienced. Accompanying symptoms include nausea or vomiting, weakness, shortness of breath, diaphoresis, confusion, or syncope. The physical examination is often unremarkable (Del Bene & Vaughan, 2000).

Electrocardiographic changes associated with MI include ST segment elevation in the leads associated with the area of the infarct. New bundle branch blocks can be seen with widened QRS complexes. The presence of a Q wave (a 1-mm negative deflection before the QRS complex) indicates infarcted tissue. Q waves persist after recovery from MI, so one cannot assume that a Q wave represents a new or recent event (Del Bene & Vaughan, 2000).

Laboratory findings consistent with MI include creatine kinase (CK) and the specific enzyme found in heart muscle (CK-MB) elevation 4 to 6 hours after tissue necrosis. Troponin levels rise 6 to 8 hours after infarct. Lactate dehydrogenase is elevated later with a peak at 36 hours after infarct. This is important to remember because patients frequently fail to report significant events when they occur and only mention the problem later or after they feel bad for a day or two (Del Bene & Vaughan, 2000).

Other examinations performed in evaluating the patient with suspected MI might include hemodynamic monitoring if heart failure is suspected, and echocardiography to determine wall motion, estimated cardiac output, and valve function.

Immediate complications of MI include arrhythmia and blockages of electrical conduction, heart failure with possible pulmonary edema, and extension of an infarct. Long-term complications from MI include ventricular aneurysms, which are a weakened area of the ventricle wall that has paradoxical motion during systole. Another long-term complication is pericarditis, an inflammation of the pericardial space resulting in pain. Patients are sometimes concerned that they are having another heart attack when they develop the pain of pericarditis. Treatment with anti-inflammatory medications is indicated for this complication.

New medications that can dissolve clots in evolution can prevent permanent loss of myocardial cells if they are used within the first several hours of the myocardial event. These clot-busting drugs have many precautions because they dissolve all clots in the body and can result in sudden and excessive bleeding. However, they are considered worth the risk and to be lifesavers in certain older persons. Patients with risk factors for

MI should be taught to report any change in symptom pattern promptly so that they can receive appropriate therapy. Many cardiologists advise older patients with symptoms of heart attack to chew one aspirin while waiting for the ambulance to arrive.

Some patients benefit from coronary angioplasty procedures, which can be done when unstable angina develops or at the time of MI. This procedure is relatively non-invasive. By threading a balloon-tipped catheter into the coronary artery, the blockage of the artery can be opened. Stents or mechanical supports to keep the artery open can be placed during angioplasty.

If an MI does occur, patients are usually admitted to the hospital for monitoring of hemodynamic status and for arrhythmias. Patients will receive oxygen therapy, pain control, and antiarrhythmic drugs as needed. The nurse's role is to monitor for changes in the patient's condition and treat complications from MI using protocols or to refer to the cardiologist for treatment. The nurse can do much to reduce stress on the myocardium by providing a safe, quiet environment, which reduces endogenous catecholamine release. After the initial insult is survived, a cardiac rehabilitation program can be designed to offer gradual, supervised increase in activity and to support other healthy lifestyle changes.

Many medications that are important during the evolving MI event and following recovery are useful in other cardiovascular conditions. Beta-blockers are useful during and after MI to reduce the workload of the heart. Patients given beta-blockers have a reduced rate of death and of reinfarction following MI. Beta-blockers have negative effects on patients with asthma and can reduce the cardiac output, which causes symptoms of heart failure. Calcium channel blockers can be substituted for patients who cannot tolerate beta-blockers, although the research basis for using calcium channel blockers is not as well established as for beta-blockers. Calcium channel blockers also reduce workload on the heart and can cause bradycardia. ACE inhibitors can reduce afterload and improve endothelial function. Aspirin or warfarin (Coumadin) therapy can help to prevent new clots from forming.

Drug Alert !

Patients at risk for falling may not be appropriate for Coumadin therapy. Anticoagulated patients who fall can sustain life-threatening bleeds.

VALVULAR HEART DISEASE

Because of age-related changes and the long-term effect of conditions such as hypertension, stress on the cardiac valves can result in structural and functional changes. Two categories of disorders affect heart valve function. Stenosis can occur in all heart valves and results in reduced flow across the valve with a resultant increased pressure required in the chamber from which the blood is being pumped. For example, aortic stenosis results in higher than normal pressure in the left ventricle as well as reduced cardiac output. The second type of disorder is incompetence, regurgitation, or insufficiency. In this case, the valve fails to close properly, which allows blood to flow backwards when pressure in a chamber rises. For example, mitral regurgitation results in blood flow from the left ventricle to the left atrium. This stretches the left atrium and also reduces forward pumping of the blood from the left ventricle. Valve disorders can arise in the leaflets themselves, in the fibrous tissue ring to which the leaflets are attached, or in papillary muscles that hold valve leaflets in place. Most valve disease in the older person involves the valves that control flow for the left ventricle, the highest pressure chamber, and the aortic and mitral valves (LeDoux, 2000).

In years past, the long-term effects of rheumatic heart disease led to many heart valve problems including mitral stenosis, aortic stenosis, and tricuspid stenosis. Because of the widespread use of antibiotics, the incidence of rheumatic heart disease is decreasing.

The most common valve disorder in the older person is aortic stenosis. It usually involves changes in the valve leaflets, but can also be caused by abnormal tissue in the cardiac septum or aorta. For older persons who develop aortic stenosis, the major cause is calcified degenerative stenosis. Risk factors include hyperlipidemia, diabetes, and hypertension. As the condition progresses, patients tolerate a decrease in cardiac output and an increase in left ventricular hypertrophy quite well. Eventually a critical loss of valve area can lead to symptoms. If the patient develops congestive heart failure, the condition can deteriorate rapidly. Angina can be experienced because blood has difficulty perfusing a thickened myocardium. Syncope can occur because of reduced blood flow to the brain. Orthostatic changes in blood pressure can also reflect a low cardiac output. Increased ventricular and atrial arrhythmias can also occur.

The diagnosis of aortic stenosis is begun during the history and physical examination. Progressive shortness of breath should indicate that aortic stenosis is a possible diagnosis. On physical examination, the murmur of aortic stenosis can be detected as a systolic ejection murmur heard most prominently in the second intercostal space. As the condition progresses, the murmur may decrease as less blood is being pumped forward. Jugular venous pressure is normal unless heart failure has developed. The echocardiogram is a good way to evaluate all heart valve function. This test allows the visualization of the valves as they open and close. Using this test, one can determine valve area, cardiac output, and any regurgitant flow. The size of cardiac chambers and movements of the heart muscle can also be tracked. If coronary heart disease is suspected, cardiac catheterization may be performed. This allows direct measurement of chamber pressures and cardiac output (LeDoux, 2000).

Definitive therapy for aortic stenosis requires mechanical or surgical intervention. During cardiac catheterization, a balloon device can be used to open the tight valve leaflets. This procedure is less invasive than open-heart surgery but offers less direct control of valve opening. This procedure can improve function but does not correct the underlying problem. Aortic valve replacement is required for true correction of aortic stenosis. However, surgical mortality is higher in the older person, and only 50% of older patients with heart failure from aortic stenosis will survive 2 years (LeDoux, 2000).

Nursing considerations in the care of patients with aortic stenosis are to maintain an index of suspicion with patients who have signs of congestive heart failure, particularly without MI. Nurses should explain the progression of the condition to patients and answer their questions. Monitoring the progression of the disease is important because many patients minimize their symptoms. Caring for patients undergoing cardiac surgery is beyond the scope of this book, but principles of cardiac rehabilitation can be followed during the recovery period.

CONGESTIVE HEART FAILURE

Heart failure is a growing problem as baby boomers age and as more people survive such damaging events as MI. It is estimated that 4.79 million Americans have heart failure, with more than 500,000 new cases each year (Centers for Disease Control, 2004). One third of all hospital admissions are caused by heart failure, costing the healthcare system $27.9 billion annually (American Heart Association, 2005). Heart failure is equally divided between men and women. Since the 1950s, the incidence of heart failure for men has remained unchanged, but the incidence for women has declined between 31% and 49%. The mortality rates for both men and women are declining by about 12% every 10 years. Men tend to develop heart failure following MI. Women tend to develop heart failure as a result of long-standing hypertension. Treatment for both hypertension and heart failure is improving through the use of new drugs and technology. However, long-term prognosis is not good. The 5-year survival rate for patients with systolic dysfunction is 50% (Levy et al., 2002). In addition to being a threat to life, heart failure causes symptoms that have a negative impact on quality of life for the older person.

The loss of contractility of the myocardium results in the inability of the heart to produce a sufficient cardiac output to meet the needs of the body. The muscles do not receive enough blood supply to respond to increased demand, and the person experiences activity intolerance. Heart failure is the number one cause of hospital admissions as patients experience recurring bouts with fluid retention. The body responds to decreased cardiac output using several compensatory mechanisms. One of these compensatory mechanisms is mediated by the sympathetic nervous system and results in increased heart rates and increased vascular resistance. Another compensatory mechanism is mediated by the kidneys, which respond by reproducing renin, which in turn leads to the formation of angiotensin I. This is transformed by enzymes to angiotensin II, a potent vasoconstrictor, elevating both blood pressure and vascular resistance. This increases afterload and further reduces cardiac output. Angiotensin II also promotes the release of aldosterone, which results in sodium and water retention. This further taxes the failing heart. Increased blood volume results in edema of the extremities and can cause pulmonary edema. Another compensatory mechanism involves dilation of the ventricles, a situation that can take advantage of the Frank-Starling response under normal circumstances. In the Frank-Starling response, the stretched myocardial fibers are able to contract with increased force, resulting in increased cardiac output. If fibers become overstretched, however, the force of contraction is decreased, further exacerbating the heart failure.

Heart failure was once thought to be due entirely to pump failure and was diagnosed with an ejection fraction less than 40%. Systolic dysfunction can be the result of loss of functional myocardium due to muscle death in MI or from generalized cardiosuppression as found in alcoholic cardiomyopathy. Recent research has described another facet of heart failure due to diastolic dysfunction. During diastole, the ventricle cannot relax and open enough to allow returning blood to fill it. This is called noncompliance and can be due to a thickened muscle or septal wall (Caboral & Mitchell, 2003).

The most common risk factors for heart failure include coronary artery disease and hypertension. The high prevalence of these conditions makes many people susceptible to heart failure. Other risk factors include family history, cardiotoxic drugs (some cancer chemotherapy drugs), smoking, obesity, alcohol abuse, and diabetes mellitus. Reducing modifiable risk factors is important at all stages of heart failure, and the nurse can do much to support patients in making lifestyle changes.

Clinical manifestations of heart failure can be divided into those that are the result of left-sided heart failure and are evidenced by pulmonary symptoms, and those that are the result of right-sided heart failure and are evidenced by systemic signs. Most heart failure symptoms include breathlessness or dyspnea. This can take the form of orthopnea, which is an inability to breathe comfortably while lying flat. Paroxysmal nocturnal dyspnea occurs when edema fluid, which has been collecting in the legs and feet, moves into the circulation when the patient lies down. This extra fluid produces pulmonary edema experienced as dyspnea at night. Crackles detected on lung auscultation are a sign of left-sided heart failure. Physical signs of right-sided heart failure include edema in the extremities, dilated neck veins, and congested liver.

Laboratory and diagnostic tests used to evaluate heart failure include electrocardiogram, which may reveal ST-T wave changes indicating myocardial ischemia, atrial fibrillation, or Q waves from previous MIs. Echocardiograms can reveal chamber size and valve function and can provide an estimated stroke volume, ejection fraction, and cardiac output. Blood tests include the complete blood count to evaluate anemia, which can aggravate heart failure; tests for elevated serum creatinine, which may indicate renal insufficiency; and thyroid function tests. Hyper- or hypothyroid conditions can aggravate heart failure (Laurent-Bopp, 2000).

Ways of classifying heart failure patients to guide therapy have been proposed by the New York Heart Association. A more recent classification system has been proposed by the American College of Cardiology and the American Heart Association to focus on prevention as well as on treatment (Hunt et al., 2001). Table 15-5 summarizes both sets of classification systems for heart failure patients. The newer guidelines emphasize the progressive nature of heart failure and guide the gradual increase in therapies as the disease advances.

Heart failure patients have a high incidence of sleep disorders. This is a synergistic relationship. Heart failure symptoms disturb sleep, and sleep disturbances cause physiological changes that can exacerbate heart failure. After a complete sleep history, patients may benefit from treatment with low-dose nocturnal oxygen therapy for identified central sleep apnea or Cheynes-Stokes respirations. Obstructive sleep apnea can be treated with continuous positive airway pressure (Parker & Dunbar, 2002).

Patients with stage B heart failure benefit from taking ACE inhibitors for several reasons. Healthy endothelial function is supported. That means local areas are less reactive to vasoconstricting factors and fewer structural changes occur. ACE inhibitors prevent the release of aldosterone, thereby allowing sodium to be lost in the urine, maintaining a normal sodium balance. ACE inhibitors decrease the blood pressure, decreasing afterload. They also support healthy renal function for patients with diabetes. The troublesome side effect of dry hacking cough occurs in 10% of patients. These patients may be placed on angiotensin receptor blockers, although the research is not as clear on the long-term helpfulness.

Beta-blockers are helpful in treating heart failure patients by decreasing the workload on the heart. Some (e.g., carvedilol) have been shown to promote healthy remodeling of heart muscle with long-term therapy. Other medications frequently used with heart failure include diuretics. Most Stage C patients will require furosemide (Lasix) therapy to keep body water from increasing. Digoxin was once thought to be a major drug used in heart failure therapy. Research has shown that only patients with systolic dysfunction benefit from digoxin therapy; with its narrow therapeutic index, close monitoring is required to detect toxic levels. Women who were randomly assigned digoxin therapy had higher death rates from all causes than women in the placebo control group. The effects of digoxin differ between men and women (Rathore, Wang, & Krumholz, 2002). Hydralazine and nitrates are vasodilators that can be helpful in stage C patients. Nitrates are useful for patients who also have angina.

Patients need to weigh themselves daily to monitor body water. If their weight increases by 2 lb in a day, they should call their provider to report the change as this may be the first sign of fluid retention. Waiting to report it until the next appointment could result in an episode of pulmonary edema. Guided exercise is useful for all patients with heart failure except those with an acute exacerbation. Exercise can contribute to better

TABLE 15-5

Functional and Therapeutic Classification Systems

New York Heart Association Functional Classification (1964)	American College of Cardiology/American Heart Association Task Force (2002)	Recommendations
	Stage A: Asymptomatic and no evidence of structural problems but high risk for developing heart failure.	• Manage: -Hypertension. -Lipid disorders. -Diabetes mellitus. • Teach: -Smoking cessation. -Exercise promotion. -Moderate EtOH. • ACE inhibitor if indicated.
Class I: Evidence of cardiac disease but no limitation in physical activity.	Stage B: Evidence of structural disease but no symptoms of heart failure.	• All stage A therapies. • ACE inhibitor unless contraindicated. • Beta-blocker unless contraindicated.
Class II: Evidence of cardiac disease with slight limitation in physical activity. Comfortable at rest. Ordinary activity results in fatigue, palpitations, dyspnea, or angina.	Stage C: Evidence of structural disease with current or prior symptoms of heart failure.	• All stage A and B therapies. • Sodium-restricted diet. • Diuretics, digoxin. • Avoid antiarrhythmic agents, most calcium channel blockers, NSAIDs. • Consider aldosterone antagonists, angiotensin receptor blockers, hydralazine, and nitrates.
Class III: Evidence of cardiac disease with marked activity limitation, comfortable at rest. Less than ordinary activity causes symptoms.		
Class IV: Evidence of cardiac disease, symptomatic at rest, any activity causes discomfort.	Stage D: Heart failure refractory to stage C treatment outlined above, requiring specialized interventions.	• All therapies as above. • Mechanical assist devices, biventricular pacemakers, left ventricular assist device. • Continuous inotropic IV therapy. • Hospice care.

Source: Adapted from Caboral & Mitchell, 2003, p. 16.

activity tolerance. The chronic nature of heart failure treatment makes it an ideal condition for nurses to manage and support in heart failure clinics. Being able to detect subtle changes in patient function through home visits or phone calls can alert the team that treatment changes are required to prevent hospitalization (Caboral & Mitchell, 2003).

Practice Pearl

The guidelines for obtaining daily weights include same scale, same clothing, and same time of day. Daily weights can vary by many factors. Adopting these rules will minimize the risk of error.

ARRHYTHMIAS AND CONDUCTION DISORDERS

Arrhythmias and conduction disorders are frequently seen in the older person. They can affect function and quality of life and may require medical management. The nurse can assist patients by explaining complicated medical problems, supporting self-care, and monitoring the effects of therapy.

Atrial fibrillation is the most common sustained arrhythmia and is characterized by rapid and disorganized atrial activity. The ECG shows no P wave. The incidence of atrial fibrillation increases with age. Common causes include hypertension, valvular stenosis that causes stretching of the atria, and ischemic heart disease. Thyroid disorders can also precipitate atrial fibrillation.

The random arrival of impulses to the AV node results in an irregular heart rate. When the atrial fibrillation first begins, the ventricular response can be as high as 160 beats per minute. Atrial fibrillation that is of long-standing duration often slows to a rate in the normal range (60 to 100 beats per minute). Some loss of cardiac output occurs with new-onset atrial fibrillation because of fast rate and short ventricular filling times. A loss of the atrial contraction to fill the ventricles can also decrease the cardiac output.

Atrial fibrillation is not a life-threatening arrhythmia, but it can cause morbidity and mortality increases. One complication of atrial fibrillation is embolic cerebrovascular accidents. This is the result of the failure of the atria to fully empty with an organized atrial contraction. Clots that form in the blood and stagnate in the atria can break loose and follow the circulation to any part of the body. The incidence of stroke is five times baseline for people with atrial fibrillation. Anticoagulant therapy is indicated for any patient with atrial fibrillation for more than 24 hours.

Short-term anticoagulation is usually begun with heparin. The blood test that determines the level of anticoagulant activity is the activated partial thromboplastin time. Heparin is given either intravenously or subcutaneously. For long-term therapy, warfarin (Coumadin) is usually prescribed. It can take several days for Coumadin levels to reach a steady state, and patients are usually maintained on heparin until this occurs. The laboratory test that assesses the blood-thinning effects of Coumadin is the international normalized ratio (INR), formerly called the protime.

Drug Alert !

Patients taking Coumadin need to be taught that green leafy vegetables contain vitamin K, which is an antidote to warfarin. Patients should limit or maintain an even intake of green vegetables to prevent fluctuation in warfarin levels.

Overall treatment goals for atrial fibrillation are to correct hemodynamic instability, control ventricular rate, and restore sinus rhythm if possible. Several medication groups are frequently used for atrial fibrillation. Conversion to sinus rhythm can be achieved by using antiarrhythmic drugs. Ventricular response can be slowed with beta-blockers, calcium channel blockers (particularly verapamil) and with digoxin.

If drug therapy is not successful, electrophysiologic studies can be performed to determine whether one particular area of the atria is initiating the irregular rhythm. If an area is located, it can be ablated using radio frequency waves. This can prevent the recurrence of new atrial fibrillation.

Conduction disturbances can occur with age as well. These are blocks in the transmission of electrical impulses. First-degree heart block is blockage of the impulse at the AV node, resulting in prolonged PR interval. First-degree block can progress so that no atrial impulses are transmitted and only the underlying ventricular rate (30 beats per minute) maintains circulation. This is called complete heart block. Heart blocks that result in decreased cardiac output will need to be treated with an internal pacemaker insertion. Patients usually tolerate this procedure well. The nurse will need to monitor functioning of the pacemaker by checking pulse rates and looking for pacemaker activity on the ECG.

PERIPHERAL VASCULAR DISEASE

Over time, disorders can develop in the arterial system, the venous system, or both. Because the etiology of arterial and venous disease is different, the disorders will be described separately.

Arterial Disease

Arterial disease is usually the result of atherosclerosis, which is a diffuse process causing changes in many places in the arterial system. Occlusion of specific vessels causes loss of function and symptoms of pain in the areas perfused by the artery. Intermittent claudication is the experience of burning pain in legs or buttocks during exercise, which is relieved by rest. Pain felt in the calf indicates superficial femoral artery blockage. Thigh pain indicates external iliac artery disease, and buttock pain indicates aortic disease. Pain occurs at rest as the disease progresses. Patients will frequently allow the affected leg to dangle over the edge of the bed to relieve the rest pain. Without therapy the disease progresses to cause tissue necrosis and gangrene. This usually occurs in the toes of the affected leg.

A good history can indicate the extent and location of the blockage, but arteriograms need to be performed to determine the extent of the blockage. To evaluate circulation of the leg, the ankle brachial index (ABI)—equal to the systolic pressure of the ankle divided by the systolic pressure of the brachial artery—is useful. In the normal extremity, the ABI is close to 1.0. Decreased arterial flow to the leg is indicated by values less than 1.0. Intermittent claudication is often seen with ABIs of .5 to .7. Rest pain, arterial ulcers, or gangrene can occur with ABIs of .3 or less (Fahey, 1999).

New classes of drugs can improve peripheral circulation. Antithrombotic agents, prostaglandins, and calcium channel blockers are frequently prescribed. Surgical bypass of the occluded artery is often required to preserve circulation to the leg and prevent amputation. Meticulous care of surgical sites and ischemic extremities can preserve tissue, prevent infection, and preserve function (Fahey & McCarthy, 1999).

Vascular rehabilitation programs can improve function and quality of life for patients with arterial occlusive disease. Programs are appropriate for patients who are not in crisis or who are being discharged from revascularization procedures. After a full assessment of risk factors and capacity of exercise, a gradual increase in physical exercise is planned. Patients need support and teaching from the nurse to maintain motivation for lifestyle change (Ekers & Hirsch, 1999).

Venous Disease

Several risk factors predispose the development of venous insufficiency. The most common site is the veins of the leg. Thrombophlebitis sometimes results in damage to the valves of the deep veins. Obesity and occupations that require prolonged standing or sitting can also lead to venous insufficiency. When the valves of the veins are incompetent, higher than normal pressures develop in the veins. This pressure is transmitted to the capillaries of the lower extremities. Over time, a thickening of the tissues around the ankles develops along with a brownish discoloration due to red blood cells that are pressed outside the capillaries. As the cells break down, hemosiderin (a breakdown product of hemoglobin) deposits collect. Eventually, chronic venous insufficiency can lead to nonhealing ulcers. The chronic ulcers caused by venous insufficiency tend to develop over the medial malleolus, the ankle area. The ulcers are different from arterial ulcers in that they are wide and have irregular borders.

Treatment for chronic venous insufficiency often involves wearing external compression hose every day. Because venous insufficiency can co-occur with arterial insufficiency, the ankle brachial index should be measured before external compression is begun. Nonhealing ulcers can be effectively treated with multilayer compression bandages such as the Unna's boot. Occasionally, skin grafts must be performed. Even after ulcers heal, patients need to be instructed that the underlying cause has not been removed and that external compression hose must continue to be worn to prevent recurrence of the ulcers (Fahey, 1999).

NURSING MANAGEMENT PRINCIPLES

The nurse is in an ideal situation to intervene with older persons with cardiac problems. Nursing interventions for promotion of cardiac health should be grounded in an understanding of the relationship between lifestyle modification, judicious use of medications, and ongoing assessment of the older person's cardiac status.

Nursing Assessment

Nursing assessment of cardiovascular function for the older person follows the same principles as health assessment in general. The history is the most important part of the assessment. Taking a history from an older person requires a balance between encouraging the person to share any concerns along with the ability to focus data gathering on the particularly important factors. Older persons may have many physical complaints and a long list of illnesses, surgical procedures, and medications that must be sorted out in building a picture of the health status. Nurses collect information to support medical diagnoses as well as nursing diagnoses to establish treatment and monitoring plans for their patients.

Assessments need to be appropriate to the situation. In an emergency, a focused assessment will streamline care planning, whereas in a long-term or community setting, more extensive assessments can be performed. Comprehensive histories include demographic information, chief complaint, history of the present illness, past history, a review of systems, family history, social history, and a functional health pattern assessment. When working in a tertiary setting where many providers have access to the patient, the nurse may not need to initiate the medical history. In this setting, the nurse can verify data collected by others and focus on the functional assessment. In the community setting, however, the nurse will need to conduct the entire history and physical to obtain information necessary to plan and monitor care.

The nurse should collect vital demographic information including the patient's date of birth. The source of history other than the patient should be noted. For the older person, a family member or caretaker frequently becomes an important source of information. Sometimes a decrease in function is more obvious to an outside observer than to the patient.

The nurse should carefully note the chief complaint in the patient's own words. The chief complaint is defined as the main reason the person has sought attention by the healthcare provider. The nurse should use quotation marks if possible to record the words of the patient. This minimizes the chance for misinterpretation. Many patients come to a clinic for screening or follow-up and will have no specific complaint. In these cases, the nurse would note the reason for the follow-up or any prompt to the screening. For patients with multiple complaints, a numbered problem list can help to focus assessment and treatment planning. Many patients who come for care unrelated to cardiovascular problems will have a cardiovascular history. For example, the patient who is admitted for a joint replacement may have a history of coronary artery disease and will require monitoring and assistance with rehabilitation.

Next the nurse should assess the history of the present illness, again using the patient's own words to describe the present health problem. Asking specific questions will help to fill in missing pieces of information. A full description of the symptom will include when and how it began, exactly where it is experienced, how long it has been noticed, associated symptoms, anything that makes it better or worse, and the characteristics of pain. Pain and fatigue can be assessed using numeric scales, although these may be harder for the older person to quantify. The thermometer scale might be more easily understood for some patients. The nurse should pay attention to how serious the patients feel their problems are. Patients frequently know if their problem is serious or life threatening. Laboratory test results can be included in this section for documentation purposes. Tests of interest for cardiac patients include clotting studies, serum electrolytes, and specific indicators such as CK-MB and troponin levels. More indirectly important might be thyroid studies. See Table 15-6 for a list of frequently used cardiovascular laboratory studies.

The next step is to assess the older person's past health history. This section includes health problems other than the present illness; it includes hospital admissions and surgical procedures. The current medication list is a clue to medical problems. The patient may forget to report thyroid disease, but listing Synthroid prompts the nurse to clarify thyroid status. The medication list should include prescription and over-the-counter medications as well as vitamins and supplements. Allergies should be noted in this section. Another way to uncover history of cardiac disease is to ask if cardiac catheterization, stress tests, or other cardiac studies have been conducted. Many patients with serious conditions such as congestive heart failure may never have been told the level of their problem, or may not understand what the diagnostic label means. The nurse must go below the surface to determine the real picture of the patient's medical history.

Assessing family history is important to identify risk factors for cardiovascular disorders. For the older person, asking age and cause of death of parents and health status of siblings and children can offer evidence on genetic risk factors. Such conditions as coronary events, cerebrovascular accidents, peripheral vascular disease, aneurysms, diabetes, alcoholism, and depression all have family patterns of incidence and can affect cardiovascular status.

Next the nurse assesses the older person's personal or social history. This area contains much information that the nurse will need to plan appropriate care. Different healthcare systems will organize this information in different ways. In some systems, a nursing functional health pattern assessment can form the basis of this material and offers broad categories of interest to the nurse. Other settings are structured according to the medical care system. This information can be referred to as current living situation, resources, and supports. The nurse must use the framework that allows essential information to be gathered and report it in this section. Functional health pattern assessments will gather information in 11 pattern areas. The pattern areas are not rigid categories; information from several can be combined and used as evidence to support problem identification (Gordon, 1994). Table 15-7 lists functional health pattern areas and pertinent data that might affect cardiovascular status.

Finally, the nurse conducts a complete review of systems. For older patients with cardiovascular problems, the nurse should focus on the presence or absence of chest pain, shortness of breath, syncope, palpitations, edema, nocturnal dyspnea, nocturia, pain in the extremities, cough, and fatigue. It is important to ask if the patient has been less active than previously or seems more easily fatigued. The function of other body systems may

TABLE 15-6

Laboratory Testing Values

Test	Normal Range	Significance
Hematologic Studies		
Red blood cell count	Men $4.6–6.2 \times 10^6$	Anemia if too low or diluted, polycythemia if too high
	Women $4.2–5.4 \times 10^6$	
Hematocrit	40–50% men	Anemia if too low or diluted
	38–47% women	Polycythemia if too high or dehydrated
Hemoglobin	13.5–18.0 g/100 mg/dl	Reflects oxygen-carrying capacity of blood
	12.0–16.0 g/100 mg/dl	
Coagulation Studies		
Platelet count	250,000–500,000 /mm³	Thrombocytopenia if too low, can decrease clotting ability
Prothrombin time (PT)	12–15 sec	Prolonged with Coumadin, reflects slower clotting
Partial thromboplastin time (PTT)	60–70 sec	Prolonged with heparin, reflects slower clotting
Activated partial thromboplastin time	35–45 sec	Prolonged with heparin, reflects slower clotting
Fibrinogen level	160–300 mg/dl	Reflects clotting factor in serum
Serum chemistries		Can interfere with normal electrical impulse conduction
Electrolytes		
Sodium (Na)	135–145 mEq/L	
Potassium (K)	3.3–4.9 mEq/L	
Chloride (Cl)	97–110 mEq/L	
Carbon dioxide	22–31 mEq/L	
Creatinine	0.9–1.4 mg/dl men	Elevation reflects renal insufficiency
	0.8–1.3 mg/dl women	
Glucose (fasting)	65–110 mg/dl	Elevation reflects diabetes mellitus
Urea nitrogen (BUN)	8–26 mg/dl	Elevation reflects renal insufficiency or dehydration
Uric acid	4.0–8.5 mg/dl men	Elevation can precipitate gout
	2.8–7.5 mg/dl women	
Serum Enzymes		
Creatine Kinase-MM	95–100%	Skeletal muscle fraction
Creatine Kinase-MB	0–5%	Elevation reflects cardiac muscle damage: peaks day 2, gone day 4
Creatine Kinase-BB	0%	Brain fraction
LDH-1	Varies with test system	Reflects muscle damage; elevated in MI: peaks day 4, gone day 12
Myocardial Proteins		
Troponin I	0–2 ng/mL	Elevation reflects cardiac damage
Troponin T	0–3.1 ng/mL	Elevated in muscle damage and renal failure
Myoglobin	10–75 ng/mL	Elevation reflects general muscle damage
Cholesterol		
Total blood cholesterol	<200 mg/dl	Desirable
	200–239 mg/dl	Borderline high
	≥ 240 mg/dl	High
LDL cholesterol	<130 mg/dl	Desirable
	130–159 mg/dl	Borderline high
	≥160 mg/dl	High
HDL cholesterol	≥ 35 mg/dl	Desirable
Apoprotein A	120 mg/dl	Elevation reflects increased risk of atherosclerosis
Apoprotein B	134 mg/dl	
C reactive protein	0–2 mg/dl	Elevation reflects increased risk of coronary disease

Source: Adapted from Woods, Froelicher, & Motzer, 2000, p. 238.

TABLE 15-7

Functional Health Patterns and Cardiovascular Data

Pattern Area	Cardiovascular Data
Health perception/health management	Do you see yourself as healthy? What do you do to stay healthy? Do you understand what each of your medications is for? Do you have any difficulty getting or taking medications? Do you smoke? Did you ever smoke? How much and for how long? How much alcohol do you drink in a week? If you have a problem, do you call your healthcare provider or do you wait until your next appointment?
Nutrition/metabolic	Have you gained or lost weight in the past (2 months to few days)? What did you eat yesterday? Are you able to shop for food that is healthy? Do you weigh yourself daily?
Elimination	What is your pattern of urination? How often do you waken at night to urinate? How often do you have a bowel movement?
Activity/exercise	How far can you walk before you get short of breath? How many flights of stairs can you climb? When was the last time you climbed that many? What is your typical day like? Do you shop for yourself? Do you need help dressing, bathing, toileting, eating, keeping house, or cooking?
Sleep/rest	Do you sleep through the night? Do you feel refreshed? Do you need pillows to sleep comfortably? Does your partner say that you snore?
Cognitive/perceptual	Do you have limitations in hearing or seeing? Do you need hearing aids or glasses? Have you noticed a change in your memory? How do you like to receive new information?
Self-perception/self-concept	How would you describe yourself? Are you comfortable with your own life?
Role/relationship	Who do you live with? How many people do you see in a day or week? Where do you see people? Do you have one or two good friends you can count on?
Sexuality/reproductive	Are you sexually active? Do you have any concerns about sexuality?
Coping/stress tolerance	What do you do to cope with stresses in your life? Do you feel stressed or worried right now?
Value/belief	What gives your life meaning? Are religious practices important to you? Are there any things about your values that your healthcare providers need to know?

point to cardiovascular disorders as well. Peripheral neuropathy may suggest diabetes, which has implications for cardiovascular risk factors. Pulmonary problems may be the result of smoking, which can also cause cardiovascular problems. The patient may not understand that shortness of breath may have a cardiovascular cause. Indigestion may be a misinterpreted angina symptom. Many cardiac drugs cause constipation, which may be noted on the review of systems. Peripheral edema can indicate fluid retention.

Functional classification of patients with cardiovascular conditions allows for monitoring progress and for planning appropriate support. Table 15-5 lists two classification systems that nurses may encounter in use in the practice environment.

Pharmacology and Nursing Implications

Many patients have more than one disease and require multiple medications to control cardiovascular conditions. This can lead to a common problem in the older person known as polypharmacy. Many older persons have multiple physicians or other providers. The cardiologist may be prescribing medications without knowing what medications the rheumatologist is prescribing. The nurse and the pharmacist are often the only providers to see the full range of medications a patient is taking.

Medications can be both a support and a stress. Because medications cause changes in body systems, the older person takes time to adjust to changes. The general rule of starting with low doses and increasing them slowly is a good practice. The nurse should be alert to side or toxic effects even when the older person is taking medications in the normal adult dosage range.

Nonpharmacological Treatments

One of the most useful methods to help patients adjust to cardiovascular problems is the concept of rehabilitation. Cardiac rehabilitation can be used for patients with angina, recent MI, heart failure, recent revascularization, or other risk factors for heart disease. Most rehabilitation programs include information on exercise and are available while patients exercise in case arrhythmias develop. They also include information on diet and stress management. Topics such as sexuality can also be addressed in a rehabilitation setting. Having a cardiac diagnosis can cause fear of death or progression of disease. The support of rehabilitation programs can encourage patients to engage in healthy lifestyle patterns.

Nursing Diagnoses

Many cardiovascular conditions require long-term management. Many patients will describe *fatigue* or *activity intolerance,* which are both nursing diagnoses. The nursing diagnosis *ineffective management of therapeutic regimen* is important for patients with heart failure or angina, and for those with risk factors who do not yet have overt disease. For patients with heart failure, *deceased cardiac output* and *fluid volume overload* can direct nursing interventions. For patients with orthopnea or paroxysmal nocturnal dyspnea, *sleep pattern disturbance* may be identified (North American Nursing Diagnosis Association, 2002).

Nursing Interventions

Specific nursing interventions are useful in a variety of cardiovascular conditions. *Risk factor reduction* can be done in a variety of settings from home to hospital to long-term care. Patients can be encouraged to maintain a normal weight, to stop smoking, to moderate alcohol intake, and to exercise. The creativity of nursing is to reach each patient as an individual. Patients who love baseball can be motivated by being in their own "spring training." Feeling well enough to travel to see grandchildren can be a strong motivator for lifestyle change.

Activity and exercise support is an intervention that provides for supervised increase in activity. Patients should be monitored for changes in vital signs and sudden fatigue. Along with exercise, planning is important for rest.

Diet therapy will involve teaching and may also involve consultation with dietitians. It is best to start with the patient's preferred diet and suggest small changes that are acceptable to the patient.

Smoking cessation is important for cardiovascular patients, and it can be used to prevent cardiovascular problems. Research has shown that healthcare providers often fail to ask patients about their smoking and fail to offer support in stopping smoking. One useful method is to ask patients to record each cigarette daily for a week. Then they select the one time that they think they can comfortably avoid cigarettes and do so for another week. Gradually, the patient is smoking less, which makes stopping more likely. Medication can also assist in smoking cessation.

Medication management is important because so many medications are useful in treating cardiovascular concerns. Older persons need to be able to open their medication bottles. They need to remember to take medications and need to know when they should report side effects.

Caregiver support is important in any chronic condition. Family members need to understand medications and their effect and they need to know what signs or symptoms should be reported to the nurse or doctor. Adult day health programs can offer respite for the caregiver and support for the patient.

Advance directives should be discussed with the patient and family members. Does the patient want aggressive treatment for the condition and understand the burdens of that treatment? Has the patient discussed treatment preferences with a healthcare proxy or with the physician? These are topics best addressed during a stable time. Crisis is a bad time to begin these discussions. The nurse can assist patients in clarifying their values and wishes and can support them in preparing written advance directives.

Community resources are important in chronic conditions. The American Heart Association has many programs that support healthy living. Many senior centers have cardiovascular programs available. The nurse can become familiar with resources in the community and can refer patients appropriately.

The patient-family teaching guidelines in the following feature will assist the nurse to assume the role of teacher and coach. Educating patients and families is critical so that nurses can interpret scientific data and individualize the nursing care plan.

Patient-Family Teaching Guidelines

HIGH BLOOD PRESSURE OR HYPERTENSION

The following are guidelines that the nurse may find useful when instructing older persons and their families about hypertension.

1. What is high blood pressure?

High blood pressure is a condition of higher than normal pressures inside the blood vessels. It can cause:

- Changes in the thickness of the blood vessels.
- Increased risk of heart attack and stroke.
- Damage to kidneys.

RATIONALE:

Long-term hypertension increases the endothelium of the blood vessels, increases atherosclerosis, and damages renal arteries.

2. What causes high blood pressure?

The cause of most high blood pressure is frequently not known, but is most likely an imbalance in:

- the body's ability to control body water.
- the body's ability to control sodium levels.
- neuroendocrine controls of blood pressure.

RATIONALE:

Primary hypertension has no direct cause.

(continued)

Patient-Family Teaching Guidelines, *cont.*

3. What can a person do to decrease blood pressure to a healthy level?

It is important to make healthy choices such as the following:

- Maintaining a normal body weight
- Decreasing intake of high-fat and high-sodium foods
- Exercising regularly
- Stopping smoking
- Limiting alcohol intake
- Taking prescribed medications
- Having blood pressure checked regularly

RATIONALE:

All these lifestyle changes will decrease blood pressure. Even losing 10 lbs can significantly lower blood pressure.

4. What is heart failure?

Heart failure happens when the heart is not able to pump enough blood to the body to allow a person to do the things he or she wants or needs to do. People who have heart failure often experience these symptoms:

- Fatigue
- Shortness of breath
- Inability to be comfortable lying flat in bed
- Shortness of breath at night
- Needing to use the bathroom frequently at night
- Swollen ankles

Heart failure patients frequently need to be hospitalized to balance fluid in their body and ease their breathing.

RATIONALE:

Fatigue is caused by inadequate pumping ability of the heart. Shortness of breath and ankle swelling are caused by fluid retention that happens when kidneys do not receive the amount of blood flow that they need. At night, fluid that has collected in the legs is moved into the full circulation, and fluid backs into the lungs.

5. What causes heart failure?

Heart failure is caused by damage to the heart muscle. This can occur from heart attacks (myocardial infarctions) or from long-standing high blood pressure. In some cases, heart valve problems can lead to heart failure. Either the heart cannot pump as well as it should or the workload that the heart is pumping against is increased.

RATIONALE:

Once a heart attack occurs, heart muscle dies and cannot contribute to the pumping function of the heart. Long-standing high blood pressure can cause enlarged heart muscle that prevents blood from entering the heart.

6. What can a person do to live with heart failure?

Heart failure patients can improve the quality of their life and reduce hospitalizations by:

- Taking medications as prescribed. If there is any trouble with the medications, either in obtaining them or from side effects, the doctor or nurse should be told.
- Avoiding high-sodium and salty foods.
- Balancing activity and rest.
- Weighing themselves daily to determine if they are holding fluid.
- Reporting any change in how they feel to a doctor or nurse.

RATIONALE:

Medications can assist the body in balancing fluid and sodium. Medications can decrease the workload on the heart. Some patients cannot afford all the medications that they have been prescribed. They should notify their doctor rather than decrease their medication. Salty food causes the body to hold sodium and water, which increases the workload on the heart.

Care Plan

A Patient With Heart Failure

Case Study

Mrs. Lockhart lives in senior housing in the small town where she has lived her entire life. She is an 87-year-old widow who was recently hospitalized for exacerbation of her congestive heart failure. She has had two other such admissions already this year. She has a son and daughter-in-law who live about an hour away.

Applying the Nursing Process

ASSESSMENT

When the home care nurse comes to Mrs. Lockhart's apartment the morning after her discharge from the hospital, her vital signs include heart rate of 82, irregular, and blood pressure 138/80. Her lung sounds are clear and she has a mild systolic ejection murmur. Her laboratory values on discharge were normal. She says her medications have not been delivered by the pharmacy yet, but the list from the discharge sheet includes Lasix 20 mg daily, enalapril maleate 5 mg daily, digoxin 0.125 mg, and Feldene 10 mg twice daily. She seems evasive when questioned about her medications. When asked, she states, "I'm not sure I can afford all these new medications. I hate to ask my son for help." The nurse notes that her kitchen cabinets contain mostly canned and prepared foods such as soup, macaroni and cheese, and beef stew. The nurse asks about where she obtains food, and she says that her son brings things once a week. She has difficulty walking in a store because of her arthritis. When asked, she says that she does not own a bathroom scale.

DIAGNOSIS

The current nursing diagnoses for Mrs. Lockhart include the following:

- *Ineffective management of therapeutic regimen* due to insufficient resources and knowledge
- *High risk for fluid volume excess* due to limited food choices and insufficient knowledge
- *Activity intolerance* due to pain and deconditioning

EXPECTED OUTCOMES

The expected outcomes for Mrs. Lockhart include that she will:

- Weigh herself daily and record the readings in a chart that she will take to the doctor's appointment.

(continued)

A Patient With Heart Failure (continued)

- Obtain fresh food twice a week from a delivery service, including fruits, vegetables, and whole grains that are low in sodium.
- Have an organized system for taking medications.
- Gradually increase her activity through participation in senior center activities.
- Discuss more openly with her son what she needs to stay independent.
- Discuss with her doctor the cost of her medications.

PLANNING AND IMPLEMENTATION

The following nursing interventions would be appropriate for Mrs. Lockhart:

- Establish a relationship of trust with the patient.
- Plan a family meeting to discuss obtaining food, bathroom scale, and medications.
- Plan medication and weight sheet to record medications and daily weight.
- Consult with physicians to coordinate medications that are economical.

EVALUATION

The nurse can evaluate the patient plan by reviewing daily weight recording and assessing Mrs. Lockhart's heart, lungs, and peripheral edema. The evaluation of the plan will be reduced rate of hospitalization and improved functional level and quality of life for Mrs. Lockhart.

Ethical Dilemma

The ethical dilemma in this case balances Mrs. Lockhart's wish for autonomy and not being dependent upon her son and the principle of beneficence, which motivates care providers to do what is best for the patient. The key to bridging this gap is to help Mrs. Lockhart see that her independence is ultimately supported by accepting some level of care.

Critical Thinking and the Nursing Process

1. Why is cardiac rehabilitation indicated following angioplasty or revascularization with coronary artery bypass grafting?
2. How is knowing and following up a cardiovascular patient over time important to the caring process?
3. How do you respond when a patient says, "I don't want to run a marathon. Why should I go to rehab?"
4. What supports are necessary to assist older persons who live alone to maintain their independence when they are diagnosed with heart failure?
5. Suppose you are designing an intergenerational program in an inner-city community center. What health issues would benefit both older and younger people?

- Evaluate your responses in Appendix B. ⊂⊃

EXPLORE MediaLink

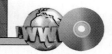

NCLEX review, case studies, and other interactive resources for this chapter can be found on the Companion Website at **www.prenhall.com/tabloski.** Click on Chapter 15 to select the activities for this chapter. For animations, video tutorials, more NCLEX review questions, and case studies, access the accompanying CD-ROM in this textbook.

Chapter Highlights

- Caring for cardiovascular patients is complicated but can be very rewarding. Nearly all older persons have some cardiovascular condition or risk factor. Managing cardiovascular conditions well can add quality of life and years to life.

- Most cardiovascular conditions are chronic and require long-term support.

- Assessment skills are important in monitoring cardiovascular conditions.

- Lifestyle factors such as normalizing body weight; choosing foods that include fruits, vegetables, and whole grains; and getting enough exercise can improve quality of life and reduce the risk of further disease.

- Blood pressure should be controlled with lifestyle and with medications to prevent stroke and heart attack.

- Isolated systolic hypertension is frequently seen in older persons, particularly women, and contributes to high rates of stroke.

- African American patients have higher rates of hypertension and may benefit from sodium restriction.

- Heart failure has a poor prognosis, requires frequent expensive hospitalizations, and interferes with quality of life.

- Patient teaching is best conducted in short sessions over time.

- Older persons frequently experience ischemia with symptoms other than chest pain. These include shortness of breath, fatigue, jaw or arm pain, and gastrointestinal distress.

References

American Heart Association. (2005). *Heart disease and stroke statistics. 2005 update.* Dallas, TX: American Heart Association.

Braun, L. T., & Davidson, M. H. (2003). Cholesterol-lowering drugs bring benefits to high-risk populations even when LDL is normal. *Journal of Cardiovascular Nursing, 18*(1), 44–49.

Caboral, M., & Mitchell, J. (2003). New guidelines for heart failure focus on prevention. *Nurse Practitioner, 28*(1), 13, 16, 22–23.

Centers for Disease Control. (2004). *Chronic disease overview.* Retrieved October 15, 2004, from www.cdc.gov/nccdphp/overview.htm.

Craven, R. F. (2000). Physiologic adaptation with aging. In S. L. Woods, E. S. S. Froelicher,

& S. A. Motzer (Eds.), *Cardiac nursing* (4th ed., pp. 180–185). Philadelphia: Lippincott.

Cunningham, S. (2000a). High blood pressure. In S. L. Woods, E. S. S. Froelicher, & S. A. Motzer (Eds.), *Cardiac nursing* (4th ed., pp. 777–817). Philadelphia: Lippincott.

Cunningham, S. (2000b). Pathophysiology of myocardial ischemia and infarction. In

S. L. Woods, E. S. S. Froelicher, & S. A. Motzer (Eds.), *Cardiac nursing* (4th ed., pp. 495–505). Philadelphia: Lippincott.

Del Bene, S., & Vaughan, A. (2000). Diagnosis and management of myocardial infarction. In S. L. Woods, E.S.S. Froelicher, & S. A. Motzer (Eds.), *Cardiac nursing* (4th ed., pp. 513–540). Philadelphia: Lippincott.

Ekers, M. A., & Hirsch, A. T. (1999). Vascular medicine and vascular rehabilitation. In V. A. Fahey, *Vascular nursing* (3rd ed., pp. 188–211). Philadelphia: Saunders.

Expert Panel on Detection, Evaluation and Treatment of High Blood Cholesterol in Adults (Adult Treatment Panel III). (2001). Executive summary of the third report of the National Cholesterol Education Program (NCEP). *Journal of the American Medical Association, 285,* 2486–2497.

Fahey, V. A. (1999). *Vascular nursing* (3rd ed.). Philadelphia: W. B. Saunders.

Fahey, V. A., & McCarthy, W. J. (1999). Arterial reconstruction of the lower extremity. In V. A. Fahey, *Vascular nursing* (3rd ed., pp. 233–269). Philadelphia: W. B. Saunders.

Fair, J. M., & Berra, K. A. (2000). Lipid management and coronary heart disease. In S. L. Woods, E. S. S. Froelicher, & S. A. Motzer (Eds.), *Cardiac nursing* (4th ed., pp. 819–834). Philadelphia: Lippincott.

Gordon, M. (1994). *Nursing diagnosis: Process and application* (3rd ed.). St. Louis, MO: Mosby.

Hall, W. D. (1999). Geographic patterns of hypertension in the United States. In J. L. Izzo, Jr., & H. R. Black (Eds.), *Hypertension primer* (pp. 226–228). Philadelphia: Lippincott, Williams & Wilkins.

Hunt, S. A., Baker, D. W., Chin, M. W., Cinquegrani, M. P., Feldman, A. M., Francis, G.S., et al. (2001). ACC/AHA guidelines for the evaluation and management of chronic heart failure in the adult: Executive summary. *Journal of the American College of Cardiology, 38,* 2101–2113.

Hunt, S. C., & Williams, R. R. (1999). Genetics and family history of hypertension. In J. L. Izzo, Jr., & H. R. Black (Eds.), *Hypertension primer* (pp. 218–221). Philadelphia: Lippincott, Williams & Wilkins.

Joint National Committee on Prevention, Detection, Evaluation, and Treatment of High Blood Pressure & National High Blood Pressure Education Program Coordinating Committee. (2003). *The seventh report of the Joint National Committee on Prevention, Detection, Evaluation, and Treatment of High Blood Pressure.* Retrieved November 9, 2004, from www.nhlbi.nih.gov/guidelines/hypertension.

Laurent-Bopp, D. (2000). Heart failure. In S. L. Woods, E. S. S. Froelicher, & S. A. Motzer (Eds.), *Cardiac nursing* (4th ed., pp. 560–579). Philadelphia: Lippincott.

LeDoux, D. (2000). Acquired valvular heart disease. In S. L. Woods, E. S. S. Froelicher, & S. A. Motzer (Eds.), *Cardiac nursing* (4th ed., pp. 699–717). Philadelphia: Lippincott.

Levy, D., Kenchaiah, S., Larson, M. G., Benjamin, E. J., Kupka, M. J., Ho, K. K. L., et al. (2002). Long-term trends in the incidence of and survival with heart failure. *New England Journal of Medicine, 347,* 1397–1402.

McCance, K., & Huether, S. (2001). *Pathophysiology: The biologic basis for disease in adults and children.* St. Louis, MO: Mosby.

National Heart, Lung, and Blood Institute. (2004). *Your guide to lowering blood pressure: The DASH diet.* Retrieved November 9, 2004, from www.nhlbi.nih.gov.

North American Nursing Diagnosis Association. (2002). *Nursing diagnoses: Definitions and classification 2001–2002.* Philadelphia: Author.

O'Rourke, M. F. (1999). Arterial stiffness and hypertension. In J. L. Izzo, Jr., & H. R. Black (Eds.), *Hypertension primer* (pp. 160–162). Philadelphia: Lippincott, Williams & Wilkins.

Parker, K. P., & Dunbar, S. B. (2002). Sleep and heart failure. *Journal of Cardiovascular Nursing, 17*(1), 30–41.

Rathore, S. S., Wang, Y., & Krumholz, H. M. (2002). Sex-based differences in the effect of digoxin for the treatment of heart failure. *New England Journal of Medicine, 347,* 1403–1411.

Reuben, D., Herr, K., Pacala, J., Pollock, B., Potter, J., & Semla, T. (2004). *Geriatrics at your fingertips.* Malden, MA: American Geriatrics Society, Blackwell.

Stein, E. A. (2002). Management of dyslipidemia in the high-risk patient. *American Heart Journal, 144*(6), S43–S50.

Stone, J. T., & Wyman, J. F. (1999). Falls. In J. T. Stone, J. F. Wyman, & S. A. Salisbury (Eds.), *Clinical gerontological nursing: A guide to advanced practice* (2nd ed., pp. 341–366). Philadelphia: W. B. Saunders.

Stone, J. T., Wyman, J. F., & Salisbury, S. A. (Eds.). (1999). *Clinical gerontological nursing: A guide to advanced practice* (2nd ed.). Philadelphia: W. B. Saunders.

Woods, S. L., Froelicher, E. S. S., & Motzer, S. A. U. (2000). *Cardiac nursing* (4th ed.). Philadelphia: Lippincott.

CHAPTER 16

The Respiratory System

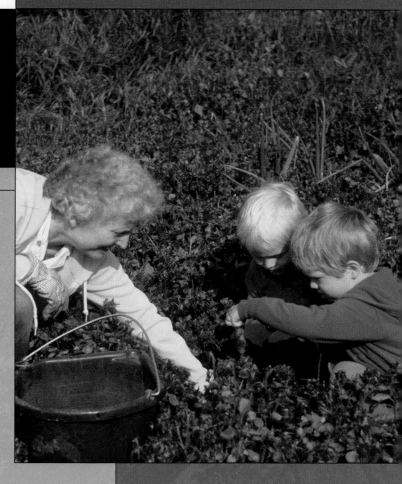

CHAPTER OBJECTIVES

Upon completion of this chapter, the reader will be able to:

- Identify normal changes of aging of the respiratory system.
- Describe appropriate health promotion and disease prevention guidelines relating to the respiratory system.
- Discuss the nurse's role in caring for older persons with respiratory problems.
- Describe common diseases of the respiratory system.
- Identify the nursing assessment process and formulation of nursing diagnoses relating to the respiratory system.

KEY TERMS

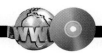

MediaLink

Additional resources for this chapter can be found on the Student CD-ROM accompanying this textbook and on the Companion Website at **www.prenhall.com/tabloski**. Click on Chapter 16 to select the activities for this chapter.

CD-ROM
- Animations/Videos
  Asthma
  Nebulizer Treatments
  Respiratory System A & P
  Using a Metered-Dose Inhaler
  Using a Nasal Cannula
- NCLEX Review

- Case Studies
- Tools

COMPANION WEBSITE
- Audio Glossary
- Additional NCLEX Review
- Case Study
- MediaLink Applications

During a normal day, the average person takes 25,000 breaths and inhales more than 10,000 L of air. The air inhaled is composed mainly of oxygen and nitrogen, but there are also small amounts of other gases, contaminants such as bacteria and viruses, and environmental pollutants such as tobacco smoke and automobile exhaust.

Most air pollution is simply irritating, but some pollution can lead to permanent injury or death. The lungs have a series of built-in barriers and defenses to protect function and life; however, with aging and disease, damage to the lungs can occur. Over time, the lungs will become damaged by smoking, occupational exposure, the effects of air pollution, and chronic infection and inflammation. These processes will degrade the lung's defenses, and the result is chronic respiratory problems or various lung diseases.

Anatomy and Physiology

The respiratory system is composed of the lungs, the airways leading to the lungs, the blood vessels serving the lungs, and the chest wall. The right lung has three lobes (upper, middle, and lower). To leave space for the heart, the left lung has two lobes (upper and lower). The lobes consist of segments and lobules. They are shaped like cones and textured like a fine-grained sponge that can be inflated with air. The lungs occupy the thoracic cage and stretch from the trachea to below the heart. About 10% of the lung is solid tissue, and the remainder is composed of air and blood (National Heart, Lung, and Blood Institute, [NHLBI], 2002).

The lung is delicate enough to allow the exchange of oxygen and carbon dioxide, yet strong and resilient enough to maintain its shape. Two support systems, the airways for ventilation and the circulatory system for perfusion, are coordinated by special muscles and nerves. This coordinated system enables the lung to perform its primary function of rapidly exchanging oxygen from inhaled air with the carbon dioxide in the blood.

Air enters the body through the nose or mouth, and travels down the throat and trachea into the chest through a pair of tubes called **bronchi**. The bronchi divide and subdivide into successive generations of narrower and shorter tubes of unequal length and diameter. The final destination for inhaled air is the network of about 3 million air sacs, called **alveoli**, located at the ends of the air passages.

The first branching of the trachea divides toward the left and right lung. The two lungs fill most of the chest cavity. The **mediastinum** is the space between the lungs that contains the heart, the esophagus, the trachea, lymph nodes, and large blood vessels. The chest wall with its muscle and skeletal structure supports the lungs. Through the process of expanding and contracting, it allows movement of air in and out of the lungs during ventilation. The chest wall is lined with a membrane called the pleura that adheres to the surface of the lungs. Normally, a small amount of fluid is present in the pleural space between the pleural lining of the chest wall and the pleural attachment to the lungs. Typically, the pleural space contains only a small amount of fluid and is free of any gas, blood, or other matter. This fluid provides lubrication and permits free and easy movement of the chest wall and lung expansion during respiration. Figure 16-1 ■ illustrates the normal anatomy of the lungs and airways.

Blood vessels, bronchi, and nerves come together at the entrance to the lung called the *hilum.* Bronchopulmonary lymph nodes, important for the drainage of the lungs, are located here. The nervous system of the lungs extends from the hilum to almost all of the lungs' anatomical areas.

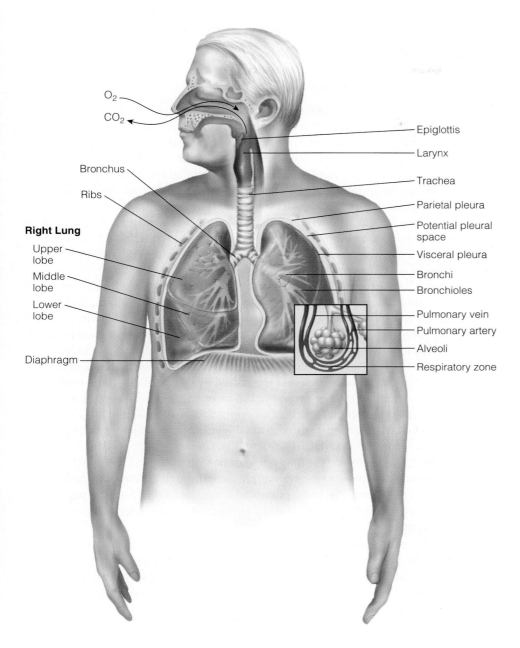

FIGURE ■ 16-1

Normal anatomy of the lungs and airways.

O_2

CO_2

Epiglottis

Larynx

Bronchus

Trachea

Ribs

Parietal pleura

Right Lung

Potential pleural space

Upper lobe

Visceral pleura

Middle lobe

Bronchi

Bronchioles

Lower lobe

Pulmonary vein

Pulmonary artery

Diaphragm

Alveoli

Respiratory zone

The first 16 subdivisions of the bronchi ending in terminal **bronchioles** are called the conducting airways. Terminal bronchioles are the smallest airways without alveoli. They further divide into respiratory bronchioles, ending in alveolar ducts. Respiratory bronchioles have occasional alveoli budding from their walls, and alveolar ducts are completely lined with alveoli. The last seven branches of the bronchioles where gas exchange occurs are called the *respiratory zone*. The terminal respiratory unit of the lung from the respiratory bronchiole to the alveolus is called the *acinus*.

The lungs have two major functions: one is respiratory and the other is nonrespiratory. Respiratory functions include gas exchange or the transfer of oxygen from the air into the blood and the removal of carbon dioxide from the blood.

Respiration or breathing is accomplished via three mechanisms:

1. Movement of the muscles in the chest wall
2. Elastic recoil in the lungs and chest
3. Airway resistance that encourages the flow of air into the lungs

Normally, breathing is an automatic process that most people take for granted. However, if one of the three conditions is compromised, breathing can become labored, consume a tremendous amount of energy, and cause a great deal of anxiety and stress. Gas exchange between inhaled air and blood takes place in the alveoli. Blood is delivered to the alveoli via a fine network of pulmonary capillaries where it is spread into a thin film. The barrier separating the air and the blood is extremely thin, 50 times thinner than a sheet of tissue paper. A large surface area ($80 m^2$, or about the size of a tennis court) is available for gas exchange within the lungs. While at rest, it takes about a minute for the total blood volume of the body (about 5 L) to pass through the lungs. It takes a red cell a fraction of a second to pass through the capillary network. Gas exchange is almost instantaneous during this period (NHLBI, 2002).

Movement of the air into the lungs is controlled by the respiratory muscles of the thorax. These muscles, part of the apparatus responsible for ventilation, include the diaphragm (the muscle that separates the chest from the abdominal cavity) and the muscles that move the ribs. When respiratory muscles contract, the chest enlarges and air rushes in for inhalation, causing lung expansion. During exhalation, the lungs recoil, forcing air out, returning the lungs to their original size. The performance of the respiratory apparatus is coordinated and monitored by specific nerve sites called respiratory centers, located in the brain and in the carotid arteries. The respiratory centers respond to changes in blood levels of oxygen, carbon dioxide, and blood pH. The body works to maintain homeostasis or normal levels of these chemicals by altering rate and depth of respiration (NHLBI, 2002)

Once the oxygen has entered the lungs, it must be distributed to the rest of the body. The oxygen in the lungs passes via alveolar pressure through the capillary beds to enter the circulatory system. The heart pumps to continuously perfuse the pulmonary circulation. When ventilation and perfusion are consistent, the arterial blood is saturated with oxygen.

The nonrespiratory functions of the lungs are mechanical, biochemical, and physiological. The lungs provide the first line of defense against airborne irritants and bacterial, viral, and other infectious agents by entrapping and **lysing** foreign invaders. The lungs also remove volatile and toxic substances generated from metabolism occurring in the body and exhale them with carbon dioxide. Sensitive sensors in the lungs control the flow of water, ions, and large proteins across its various cellular structures. With the liver and kidneys, the lungs remove and control various products of the body's metabolic reactions. Finally, the lungs manufacture a variety of essential hormones and other chemicals that direct and carry out biochemical reactions (NHLBI, 2002).

Normal Changes of Aging

The aging process is accompanied by physiological changes to the respiratory system. Differentiating the normal changes of aging from disease-related changes can be difficult. The effects of chronic exposure to tobacco smoke, air pollution, and environmental toxins can further complicate the process of differentiation.

The following changes occur in lung structure and function with normal aging:

- Stiffening of elastin and the collagen connective tissue supporting the lungs
- Altered alveolar shape resulting in increased alveolar diameter
- Decreased alveolar surface area available for gas exchange
- Increased chest wall stiffness

The functional implications of these changes are a decreased elastic recoil of the lung that produces increased residual volume (the amount of air remaining in the lungs at the end of exhalation), decreased vital capacity (the amount of air that moves in and out with inspiration and expiration), and premature airway closure in dependent portions of the lungs. With early airway closure, the mismatch of ventilation and perfusion increases and arterial oxygen tension decreases. Another factor that can contribute to the decrease in arterial oxygen tension is a decrease in pulmonary diffusion, apparently as a result of the decreased area available for gas exchange. However, the precise mechanisms for the decrease in diffusing capacity with age are still unclear (NHLBI, 1997). With aging, the amount of oxygen carried by the blood is likely to be lower, and gas exchange will occur more slowly and less efficiently. Figure 16-2 ■ illustrates the normal changes of aging in the respiratory system.

CHANGES IN CARDIOVASCULAR FUNCTION

Changes in cardiovascular function that can affect the pulmonary system include the following:

- Increased stiffness of the heart and blood vessels, rendering these vessels less compliant to increased blood flow demands
- Diastolic dysfunction due to impaired diastolic filling
- Systolic dysfunction due to increased left ventricular afterload
- Decreased cardiac output with rest and with exercise

Although not a normal change of aging, congestive heart failure is frequent among elderly adults, occurring six times as often in the seventh decade of life than in the fifth. In 75% of older patients with congestive heart failure, hypertension or coronary artery disease is the underlying cause (NHLBI, 2002).

CHANGES IN IMMUNE FUNCTION

The following changes that occur in immune function with normal aging can affect pulmonary function:

- A decrease in the nature and quantity of antibodies produced
- A decrease in effectiveness of the protective cilia of the respiratory tract in removing debris from the airways, allowing more foreign bodies to travel to the lungs
- Decreased production of antibodies after immunization
- Use of medications that can suppress immune function

Decreased levels of total serum IgE, reduced T lymphocyte function, and less efficient phagocytosis result in decreased cell-mediated immune function. For older people, the overall decline in immune function results in increased susceptibility to tuberculosis, pneumonia, and influenza. Even after immunization, older people mount a less efficient immune response, and immunity is reduced and of shorter duration (NHLBI, 2002). Use of glucocorticoid and antineoplastic medications can suppress immune response and further place an older person at risk for acquiring a respiratory bacterial or viral infection.

FIGURE ◻ 16-2

Normal changes of aging in the respiratory system.

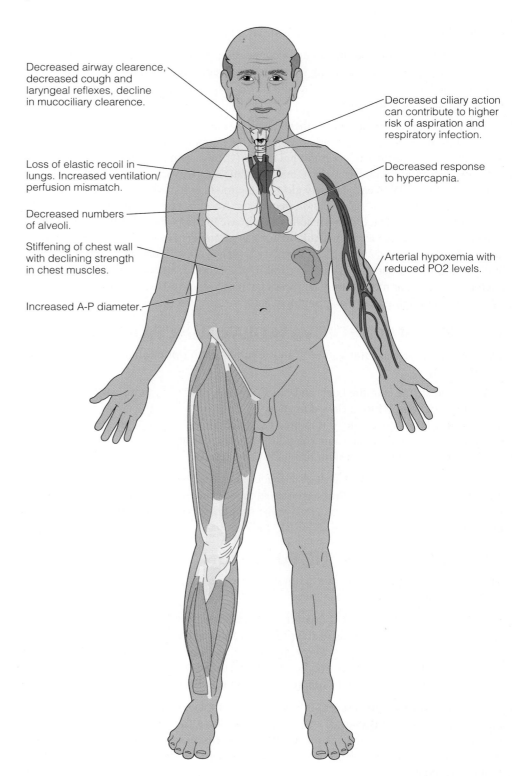

Decreased airway clearence, decreased cough and laryngeal reflexes, decline in mucociliary clearence.

Decreased ciliary action can contribute to higher risk of aspiration and respiratory infection.

Loss of elastic recoil in lungs. Increased ventilation/perfusion mismatch.

Decreased response to hypercapnia.

Decreased numbers of alveoli.

Stiffening of chest wall with declining strength in chest muscles.

Arterial hypoxemia with reduced PO2 levels.

Increased A-P diameter.

CHANGES IN NEUROLOGIC, NEUROMUSCULAR, AND SENSORY FUNCTIONS

Aging results in neuron loss in the brain and central nervous system, which increases reaction time, decreases the ability to respond to multiple complex stimuli, and may impair the ability to adapt and interact with the environment. Changes that can affect pulmonary function include the following:

- Loss of muscle tone, exacerbated by deconditioning and sedentary lifestyle
- Increased thoracic rigidity and osteoporotic changes to the spine (kyphosis)
- Use of medications that can cause fatigue, depression of the cough reflex, insomnia, dehydration, and bronchospasm
- Diagnosis of neurologic disease or impairment (dementia, Parkinson's disease, stroke or cerebrovascular accident)
- Increased anteroposterior diameter of the thorax, causing a "barrel chest" appearance

Older people with decreased muscle tone and osteoporosis of the spine are less able to accomplish complete chest expansion and as a result are more likely to have decreased tidal volumes. Inability to completely fill the lungs with air can lead to atelectasis (areas of the lung that become incapable of expansion and gas exchange) over time, further decreasing respiratory efficiency. Sedating and opioid medications, diuretics, anxiolytics, cough suppressants, and beta-blockers can also decrease neuromuscular function. They make oral secretions thicker, suppress the cough reflex (which may lead to aspiration pneumonia), increase hours of sleep within a 24-hour period, decrease time for drinking fluids and socialization, and trigger bronchospasm and trapping of secretions, further inhibiting gas exchange (NHLBI, 2002).

Respiratory Diseases Common in Older People

Age-related changes in the lungs, years of exposure to air pollutants and cigarette smoke, and presence of comorbidities may predispose the older person to respiratory diseases and pulmonary dysfunction. The following diseases are commonly diagnosed pulmonary diseases in the older person.

ASTHMA

Asthma is a respiratory disease characterized by usually reversible airflow obstruction, airway inflammation, increased mucous secretion, and increased airway responsiveness (contraction of airway smooth muscles) to a variety of stimuli. Asthma can present as a newly diagnosed disease or as a chronic disease that the older person has lived with for many years. In older patients, complete reversibility of airflow problems becomes more difficult, especially in those patients with severe and persistent problems, because of the irreversible damage done to the airways by years of inflammatory changes. Over time, plugging of the bronchioles occurs along with scarring and narrowing of the airways. Normal changes of aging in the lung may interact with asthma-related pathophysiology to further produce irreversible airflow obstruction (NHLBI, 2002a). Figure 16-3 ■ illustrates a comparison of a normal airway and a scarred and inflamed airway typically found in an older patient with asthma, bronchitis, or emphysema.

With asthma, inflamed airways are characterized as "twitchy" and overreact to common irritants like viruses, cigarette smoke, cold air, and allergens. These triggers can activate an inflammatory response including mobilization of mast cells, eosinophils,

FIGURE ■ 16-3

Note the differences between the normal bronchiole and the asthmatic bronchiole.

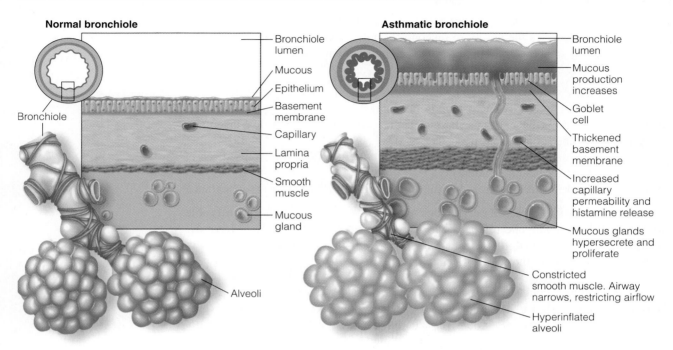

Normal bronchiole

- Bronchiole lumen
- Mucous
- Epithelium
- Basement membrane
- Capillary
- Lamina propria
- Smooth muscle
- Mucous gland
- Bronchiole
- Alveoli

Asthmatic bronchiole

- Bronchiole lumen
- Mucous production increases
- Goblet cell
- Thickened basement membrane
- Increased capillary permeability and histamine release
- Mucous glands hypersecrete and proliferate
- Constricted smooth muscle. Airway narrows, restricting airflow
- Hyperinflated alveoli

macrophages, and T lymphocytes. With these inflammatory changes, airway smooth muscle contracts, swells, and produces excessive mucous secretions. With this airway narrowing and inflammation, it becomes difficult for the older person to breathe. The common symptoms of an asthma attack include the following:

- Coughing
- Wheezing
- Shortness of breath
- Chest tightness

(Nurses Asthma Education Partnership Project, 2003)

Figure 16-4 ■ illustrates the relationship between airway inflammation, hyperresponsiveness, airway obstruction, and asthma symptoms.

Mortality from asthma in older adults is reportedly increasing, but it is difficult to define the cause of death in many older people with lung diseases. Asthma is thought to occur in about 1 in 1,000 older people (NHLBI, 2002). Hospital admission rates are 40% to 70% higher in African Americans than in Caucasians, and the admission rates for women are approximately 20% to 40% higher than for men in both races. Although African Americans represent only 12% of the U.S. population, close to 26% of asthma deaths occur in this group. In 2001, an estimated 3 million African Americans had asthma. The asthma prevalence rate among African Americans was more than 23% higher than for Caucasians (American Lung Association, 2003).

At any age, the diagnosis of asthma is based on the clinical history, physical examination, and laboratory studies. When asthma is diagnosed in an older person, other lung and cardiovascular diseases must be eliminated. It is sometimes difficult to distinguish between exacerbations of chronic bronchitis, **chronic obstructive pulmonary disease**

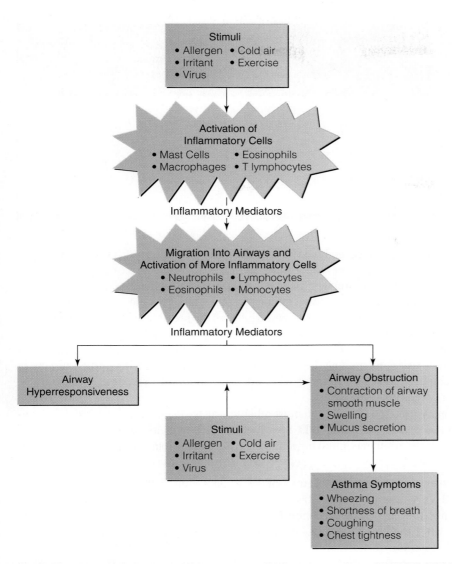

Relationships between airway inflammation, airway hyperresponsiveness, airway obstruction, and asthma symptoms.

(COPD), and asthma, especially in current and former smokers (NHLBI, 2002). Additionally, many older people with congestive heart failure will present with signs and symptoms that mimic those of asthma. Table 16-1 presents some of the signs and symptoms of common lung diseases.

Practice Pearl
Nocturnal dyspnea occurring with asthma is most likely to take place between 4 a.m. and 6 a.m., whereas nocturnal dyspnea occurring with congestive heart failure typically occurs 1 to 2 hours after retiring. The nurse should try to pinpoint the exact time that breathing difficulties occur.

Diagnostic Studies

The physician will most likely examine the results of pulmonary function tests, chest radiography, electrocardiography, and a complete blood count with differential to confirm the diagnosis of asthma in the older person. The electrocardiogram will help identify the

TABLE 16-1

Signs and Symptoms
of Common Lung
Diseases

Symptom	Asthma	Chronic Bronchitis	Chronic Obstructive Pulmonary Disease	Congestive Heart Failure
Wheezing	+	+	+	+
Chest tightness	+			
Chronic cough with sputum	+	+		+/−
Nocturnal dyspnea	+			+
Smoking history		+	++	+/−

presence of cardiac disease and the risk associated with certain medications that may be used to treat the older patient with asthma and cardiac disease (e.g., theophylline). The chest x-ray in the older person with asthma is usually negative, but the presence of lesions may indicate acute infection, lung tumor, or other abnormalities. Additionally, cardiomegaly and pulmonary congestion would indicate the presence of underlying heart disease. Hyperinflation of the lungs would indicate **emphysema**. The presence of a large number of eosinophils in the blood may indicate an allergic component as a predictor of asthma, but these numbers may be low in some older patients taking corticosteroids or chemotherapeutic agents or in those with a decreased immune response because of the presence of other illnesses.

Pulmonary function tests are the most reliable way to diagnose asthma and differentiate it from other illnesses like COPD. Spirometry is used to measure the volume of air expired in 1 second from maximum inspiration (FEV_1) and the total amount of air expired as rapidly as possible (forced vital capacity, FVC). The diagnosis of asthma is confirmed by:

- Demonstrated airflow obstruction of FEV_1 less than 80% of predicted and an FEV_1/FVC ratio of less than 70%.
- Evidence that airflow obstruction is reversible (greater than 12% and 200 ml in FEV_1, after the administration of a bronchodilator or over time after a course of corticosteroids).
- Peak expiratory flow (PEF) measurements indicating the maximum flow (expressed in liters per second) that can be generated during a forced expiratory maneuver with fully inflated lungs as measured using a peak flow meter. PEF measurements before and after bronchodilator administration may be useful in confirming the asthma diagnosis. A pattern of greater than 20% variation in PEF from late afternoon to arising the next morning confirms the presence of variable airflow obstructions, often indicative of asthma.

(American Thoracic Society, 2002).

Spirometry testing in the older adult can pose practical problems that must be addressed to obtain accurate results. Increasing rigidity of the chest wall, anxiety, weakness or paresthesia in the upper extremities, cognitive impairment, and poor eye-hand coordination can be factors leading to poor results. The gerontological nurse along with the pulmonologist, allergist, and respiratory therapist may be called upon to assist the older patient with spirometry testing. Accurate and reproducible spirometry techniques will provide the necessary information to reach an accurate diagnosis.

Once diagnostic testing is completed, asthma is classified as to severity so that the appropriate treatment and monitoring may be initiated. Table 16-2 presents the four

TABLE 16-2

Classification of Asthma Severity: Clinical Features Before Treatment

	Days With Symptoms	Nights With Symptoms	PEF or FEV$_1$[*]	PEF Variability
Step 4 Severe Persistent	Continual	Frequent	≤ 60%	> 30%
Step 3 Moderate Persistent	Daily	≥ 5/month	> 60%–<80%	> 30%
Step 2 Mild Persistent	3–6/week	3–4/month	≥ 80%	20–30%
Step 1 Mild Intermittent	≤ 2/week	≤ 2/month	≥ 80%	< 20%

[*] Percent predicted values for forced expiratory volume in 1 second (FEV$_1$) and percent of personal best for peak expiratory flow (PEF) (relevant for children 6 years old or older who can use these devices).

Notes:

• Patients should be assigned to the most severe step in which *any* feature occurs. Clinical features for individual patients may overlap across steps.

• An individual's classification may change over time.

• Patients at any level of severity of chronic asthma can have mild, moderate, or severe exacerbations of asthma. Some patients with intermittent asthma experience severe and life-threatening exacerbations separated by long periods of normal lung function and no symptoms.

• Patients with two or more asthma exacerbations per week (i.e., progressively worsening symptoms that may last hours or days) tend to have moderate-to-severe persistent asthma.

Source: NHLBI, 2002.

categories of asthma severity before treatment based on duration of symptoms, presence and severity of nocturnal symptoms, and results of spirometry testing.

Based upon the classification of severity, medications are prescribed using the following goals of therapy for asthma control:

- Minimal or no chronic symptoms day or night
- Minimal or no exacerbations
- No limitations on functional ability and ability to perform activities of daily living
- Maintenance of normal or nearly normal pulmonary function
- Minimal use of "rescue" short-acting inhaled beta$_2$-agonist (less than once daily or one canister per month)
- Minimal or no adverse effects from medication

(Nurses Asthma Education Partnership Project, 2003)

Medications required to maintain long-term control are prescribed according to the level of severity of asthma using the four-step classification system. It is recommended that the treatment protocol be reviewed on a regular basis, about every 6 months, to review the medication technique, to monitor for adherence and environmental control, and to step up or down a level according to progression and manifestation of symptoms and PEF variability. Increased use of short-acting beta$_2$-agonists on a daily basis or more than three to four times in one day would indicate the need to seek physician advice and possibly step up to the next level to achieve better control. Referral to an asthma specialist for consultation or comanagement with the primary care provider is recommended if there is difficulty maintaining control or if the older patient requires step 3 or step 4 care. Table 16-3 indicates preferred daily medications by asthma classification.

TABLE 16-3

Stepwise Approach for Managing Asthma in Adults and Children Older Than 5 Years of Age: Treatment

Classify Severity: Clinical Features Before Treatment or Adequate Control

	Symptoms/Day Symptoms/Night	PEF or FEV, PEF Variability	Daily Medications
Step 4 Severe Persistent	Continual Frequent	≤ 60% > 30%	• **Preferred treatment:** — High-dose inhaled corticosteroids AND — Long-acting inhaled beta$_2$-agonists AND, if needed, — Corticosteroid tablets or syrup long term (2 mg/kg/day, generally do not exceed 60 mg per day). (Make repeat attempts to reduce systemic corticosteroids and maintain control with high-dose inhaled corticosteroids.)
Step 3 Moderate Persistent	Daily > 1 night/week	> 60% − < 80% > 30%	• **Preferred treatment:** — Low-to-medium dose inhaled corticosteroids and long-acting inhaled beta$_2$-agonists. • Alternative treatment (listed alphabetically): — Increase inhaled corticosteroids within medium-dose range OR — Low-to-medium dose inhaled corticosteroids and either leukotriene modifier or theophylline. If needed (particularly in patients with recurring severe exacerbations): • **Preferred treatment:** — Increase inhaled corticosteroids within medium-dose range and add long-acting inhaled beta$_2$-agonists. • Alternative treatment: — Increase inhaled corticosteroids within medium-dose range and add either leukotriene modifier or theophylline.
Step 2 Mild Persistent	> 2/week but < 1x/day > 2 nights/month	≥ 80% 20–30%	• **Preferred treatment:** — Low-dose inhaled corticosteroids. • Alternative treatment (listed alphabetically): cromolyn, leukotriene modifier, nedocromil, OR sustained release theophylline to serum concentration of 5–15 mcg/mL.

The medications used to treat asthma in the older person do not differ significantly from those used with younger people. However, the risk of adverse effects and the potential for drug interactions are greater because of the use of additional medications to treat coexisting conditions.

Corticosteroid therapy is the most effective anti-inflammatory treatment for asthma. Used of inhaled corticosteroids has reduced the morbidity and mortality associated

TABLE 16-3

Stepwise Approach for Managing Asthma in Adults and Children Older Than 5 Years of Age: Treatment

Classify Severity: Clinical Features Before Treatment or Adequate Control			
	Symptoms/Day **Symptoms/Night**	**PEF or FEV,** **PEF Variability**	**Daily Medications**
Step 1 **Mild Intermittent**	≤ 2 days/week ≤ 2 nights/month	≥ 80% < 20%	• No daily medication needed. • Severe exacerbations may occur, separated by long periods of normal lung function and no symptoms. A course of systemic corticosteroids is recommended.
Quick Relief **All Patients**	• Short-acting bronchodilator: 2–4 puffs short-acting inhaled beta$_2$-agonists as needed for symptoms. • Intensity of treatment will depend on severity of exacerbation; up to 3 treatments at 20-minute intervals or a single nebulizer treatment as needed. Course of systemic corticosteroids may be needed. • Use of short-acting beta$_2$-agonists > 2 times a week in intermittent asthma (daily, or increasing use in persistent asthma) may indicate the need to initiate (increase) long-term control therapy.		

↓ Step down

Review treatment every 1 to 6 months; a gradual stepwise reduction in treatment may be possible.

↑ Step up

If control is not maintained, consider step up. First, review patient medication technique, adherence, and environmental control.

Note

• The stepwise approach is meant to assist, not replace, the clinical decision making required to meet individual patient needs.

• Classify severity: assign patient to most severe step in which any feature occurs (PEF is % of personal best; FEV$_1$ is % predicted).

• Gain control as quickly as possible (consider a short course of systemic corticosteroids); then step down to the least medication necessary to maintain control.

• Provide education on self-management and controlling environmental factors that make asthma worse (e.g., allergens and irritants).

• Refer to an asthma specialist if there are difficulties controlling asthma or if step 4 care is required. Referral may be considered if step 3 care is required.

Goals of Therapy: Asthma Control

• Minimal or no chronic symptoms day or night
• Minimal or no exacerbations
• No limitations on activities; no school/work missed

• Maintain (near) normal pulmonary function
• Minimal use of short-acting inhaled beta$_2$-agonist (< 1x per day, < 1 canister/month)
• Minimal or no adverse effects from medications

Source: Nurses: Partners in Asthma Care, 1998.

with asthma exacerbations (NHLBI, 2002b). Adverse effects of inhaled corticosteroids include electrolyte and fluid imbalances in older patients with cardiac or renal disease, the possibility of hypokalemia when the patient is taking a thiazide diuretic, worsening of hypertension, and elevated blood sugar and blood urea nitrogen (BUN) readings in patients with diabetes. Additionally, oral corticosteroids can negatively affect cognitive function, accelerate osteoporosis, increase intraocular pressure, and aggravate peptic and gastric ulcers (NHLBI, 2002b). As with all drugs, the benefits of inhaled corticosteroids must be weighed against the risks. Inhaled corticosteroids are important to facilitate control of asthma in older adults and to avoid the adverse effects of systemic corticosteroids and asthma exacerbations. Although safer than systemic therapy, long-term inhaled corticosteroid use in relatively high doses (>1.6 mg/day) can cause dose-dependent adverse effects similar to those seen with oral doses (NHLBI, 2002b).

Cromolyn sodium does not appear to be as effective in the older person as it is in children, but this may be related to the presence of additional lung pathology in the older person with asthma. Leukotriene antagonists interfere with the synthesis or action of leukotrienes that can cause bronchospasm, and their use may decrease the need for inhaled steroids in some older people.

Inhaled beta$_2$-agonists are short-acting medications that are effective bronchodilators for all asthma patients. Both long- and short-acting beta$_2$-agonists are available. Only short-acting beta$_2$-agonists (Proventil, Ventolin) should be used for rescue from sudden onset of wheezing, tightness in the chest, or shortness of breath. Long-acting bronchodilators have a duration of action exceeding 12 hours and may reduce asthma symptoms and the frequency of exacerbations. However, long-acting beta$_2$-agonists (Serevent) are not to be used as rescue medications because of their delayed onset and longer duration of action. Side effects from long-acting beta$_2$-agonist therapy include the following:

- Increased consumption of myocardial oxygen (can induce angina in some older patients)
- Electrocardiographic changes, including ventricular arrythmias
- Hypokalemia
- Increased blood pressure
- Tremor
- Hypoxemia

(NHLBI, 2002b)

Practice Pearl

Patients who require the use of rescue inhalers should obtain prescriptions for extra canisters and keep several inhalers in strategic places in the home. It also helps to label them with bright red tape so they can be easily seen if needed quickly.

Methylxanthine (theophylline) is a bronchodilator that may be useful in the treatment of asthma in the older person but is associated with the following adverse effects:

- Supraventricular tachycardia
- Exercise-induced angina and ST-segment depression
- Toxicity due to metabolic changes in older people

If used, careful monitoring is needed to keep the serum concentrations between 8 and 12 µg/ml.

Ipratropium bromide is a synthetic atropine-like compound that is sometimes used to treat asthma in the older person. Ipratropium has a lower incidence of tremor and arrhythmia and is associated with the relatively mild side effects of dry mouth and pharyngeal irritation. Older patients on this medication should be carefully monitored for symptoms of xerostomia. Table 16-4 lists common asthma medications and potential adverse effects.

Some older patients with asthma may prefer nebulizer rather than metered-dose inhaler delivery because of the moisturizing effect and decreased need for hand-diaphragm coordination. Nebulizer treatments are an effective way to administer

TABLE 16-4

Asthma Medications and Potential Adverse Effects

Class of Therapeutic Agent	Drug	Potential Adverse Clinical Effects
Anti-inflammatory	Oral corticosteroids	↑ Blood pressure, edema, congestive heart failure due to Na^+ retention
		Hypokalemia, alkalosis, and resulting arrhythmias due to K^+ and H^+ excretion
		Worsening diabetes mellitus, cataracts, polyuria with dehydration due to elevated blood glucose
		Thinning of the skin, reduced muscle mass with myopathy, osteoporosis, ↑ blood urea nitrogen without change in renal blood flow due to protein catabolism
		Hypoadrenalism due to decreased ACTH
		Cataracts
		Altered cognitive function, depression
		Joint effusions and articular pain with corticosteroid withdrawal
		Osteoporosis due to decreased calcium absorption
		Glaucoma due to decreased absorption of aqueous humor
		Aggravation of existing peptic ulcer disease
	Inhaled corticosteroids	Cough; dysphonia, loss of taste, laryngomalacia, oral candidiasis
	(High doses, e.g., > 1.6 mg/day)	Effects on ACTH secretion with hypoadrenalism may be related to the effects on calcium absorption with acceleration of osteoporosis
		Development of cataracts
	Cromolyn sodium	No significant adverse effect known
	Nedocromil	No significant adverse effect known
Bronchodilator	Short-acting beta$_2$-agonists	Myocardial ischemia due to ↑ myocardial oxygen consumption and mild increase in hypoxemia
		Complex ventricular arrhythmia due to ↑ myocardial irritability
		Cardiac arrhythmias and muscle weakness related to hypokalemia
		Hypotension or hypertension
		Tremor
		With excessive use, ↓ bronchodilator effect and ↑ airway hyperresponsiveness related to downregulation of beta receptors
	Long-acting beta$_2$-agonists	Same as for short-acting beta$_2$-agonists
	Theophylline	Cardiac arrhythmias, effect is related to ↑ catecholamine release and is additive with beta$_2$-agonists
		Nausea and vomiting from gastric irritation, gastroesophageal reflux
		Insomnia, seizures related to central nervous system stimulant
		Cardiac arrhythmia due to inotropic and chronotropic effects
		Serum levels increased by heart failure, liver disease, beta-blocker therapy, selected H_2 blocker therapy, quinolone therapy, macrolide therapy, ketoconazole therapy
	Ipratropium bromide	Mucosal dryness

Source: Nurses: Partners in Asthma Care, 1998.

inhaled medications to those with cognitive impairments. Regardless of whether the older patient is using a metered-dose inhaler or nebulizer, proper instruction is needed to administer the medication and care for the equipment. Those choosing a metered-dose inhaler should use a spacer that will allow the medication to be inhaled at a slower rate and be less likely to stimulate a cough reflex. See Figure 16-5 ☐ for the proper use of a metered-dose inhaler, spacer, and nebulizer.

Practice Pearl

Several medications now come prepared as dry powder inhalers and contain no propellant. Patients should activate the dispenser, place their lips around the mouthpiece, and inhale quickly. The dry powder is inhaled into the upper airway when done properly.

Older patients using inhaled steroids should rinse their mouths with warm water and expectorate after medication administration. This will prevent the overgrowth of candidiasis or thrush, prevent gum disease, and deter tooth decay. The nurse should report the presence of painful white lesions in the mouth to the physician for treatment.

FIGURE ☐ 16-5

Instructions for proper use of a metered-dose inhaler, spacer, and nebulizer.

SPACERS: MAKING INHALED MEDICINES EASIER TO TAKE

Unless you use your inhaler the right way, much of the medicine may end up on your tongue, on the back of your throat, or in the air. Use of a spacer or holding chamber can help prevent this problem.

A spacer or holding chamber is a device that attaches to a metered-dose inhaler. It holds the medicine in its chamber long enough for you to inhale it in one or two slow deep breaths.

The spacer makes it easier to use the medicines the right way. It helps you not cough when using an inhaler. A spacer will also help prevent you from getting a yeast infection in your mouth (thrush) when taking inhaled steroid medicines.

There are many models of spacers or holding chambers that you can purchase through your pharmacist or a medical supply company. Ask your doctor about the different models.

HOW TO USE A SPACER

1. Attach the inhaler to the spacer or holding chamber as explained by your doctor or by using the directions that come with the product.

2. Shake well.

3. Press the button on the inhaler. This will put one puff of the medicine in the holding chamber.

4. Place the mouthpiece of the spacer in your mouth and inhale slowly. (A face mask may be helpful for a young child.)

5. Hold your breath for a few seconds and then exhale. Repeat steps 4 and 5.

6. If your doctor has prescribed two puffs, wait between puffs for the amount of time he or she has directed and repeat steps 2 through 5.

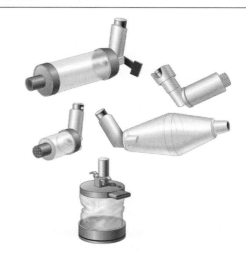

There are a variety of spacers.

FIGURE ■ 16-5 *(continued)*

YOUR METERED-DOSE INHALER: HOW TO USE IT

Using a metered-dose inhaler is a good way to take asthma medicines. There are few side effects because the medicine goes right to the lungs and not to other parts of the body. It takes only 5 to 10 minutes for inhaled beta$_2$-agonists to have an effect compared to the liquid or pill form, which can take 15 minutes to 1 hour. Inhalers can be used by all asthma patients age 5 and older. A spacer or holding chamber attached to the inhaler can help make taking the medicine easier.

The inhaler must be cleaned often to prevent buildup that will clog it or reduce how well it works.

- ■ The guidelines that follow will help you use the inhaler the correct way.
- ■ Ask your doctor or nurse to show you how to use the inhaler.

USING THE INHALER

1. Remove the cap and hold the inhaler upright.
2. Shake the inhaler.
3. Tilt your head back slightly and breathe out.
4. Use the inhaler in any one of these ways. (A and B are the best ways. B is recommended for young children, older adults, and those taking inhaled steroids. C is okay if you are having trouble with A or B.)
   A. Open mouth with inhaler 1 to 2 inches away.
   B. Use spacer (refer to previous section).
   C. Put inhaler in mouth and seal lips around the mouthpiece.

5. Press down on the inhaler to release the medicine as you start to breathe in slowly.
6. Breathe in *slowly* for 3 to 5 seconds.
7. *Hold* your breath for 10 seconds to allow the medicine to reach deeply into your lungs.
8. Repeat puffs as prescribed. Waiting 1 minute between puffs may permit the second puff to go deeper into the lungs.

Note: Dry powder capsules are used differently. To use a dry powder inhaler, close your mouth tightly around the mouthpiece and inhale very fast.

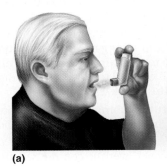 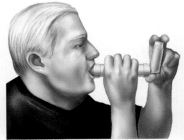 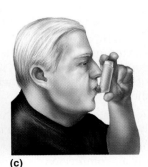

(a)   (b)   (c)

CLEANING

1. Once a day clean the inhaler and cap by rinsing it in warm running water. Let it dry before you use it again. Have another inhaler to use while it is drying. Do not put the canister holding cromolyn or nedocromil in water.
2. Twice a week wash the L-shaped plastic mouthpiece with mild dishwashing soap and warm water. Rinse and dry well before putting the canister back inside the mouthpiece.

CHECKING HOW LONG A CANISTER WILL LAST

1. Check the canister label to see how many "puffs" it contains.
2. Figure out how many puffs you will take per day (e.g., 2 puffs, 4 times a day = 8 puffs a day). Divide this number into the number of puffs contained in the canister. That tells you how long the canister should last.

Example:
Canister contains 200 puffs.
You take 2 puffs, 4 times a day, which equals 8 puffs/day.
$200 \div 8 = 25$. The canister will last 25 days.

(continued)

FIGURE ■ 16-5 *(continued)*

HOW TO USE AND CARE FOR YOUR NEBULIZER

A nebulizer is a device driven by a compressed air machine. It allows you to take asthma medicine in the form of a mist (wet aerosol). It consists of a cup, a mouthpiece attached to a T-shaped part or a mask, and thin, plastic tubing to connect to the compressed air machine. It is used mostly by three types of patients:

- Children under age 5.
- Patients who have problems using metered-dose inhalers.
- Patients with severe asthma.

A nebulizer helps to make sure you get the right amount of medicine.

Routinely cleaning the nebulizer is important because an unclean nebulizer may cause an infection. A good cleaning routine keeps the nebulizer from clogging up and helps it last longer. (See instructions with nebulizer.)

Directions for using the compressed air machine may vary (check the machine's directions), but generally the tubing has to be put into the outlet of the machine before it is turned on.

HOW TO USE A NEBULIZER

1a. If your machine is premixed, measure the correct amount of medicine using a clean dropper and put it into the cup. Go to step 2.

1b. If your medicine is not premixed, measure the correct amount of saline—using a clean dropper—and put it into the cup. Then measure the correct amount of medicine using a *different* clean dropper and put it into the cup with the saline. (Do NOT mix the droppers; use one for saline and another for the medicine.) Put an "S" for saline on one dropper with nail polish.

2. Fasten the mouthpiece to the T-shaped part and then fasten this unit to the cup OR fasten the mask to the cup. For a child over the age of 2, use a mouthpiece unit because it will deliver more medicine than a mask.

3. Put the mouthpiece in your mouth. Seal your lips tightly around it OR place the mask on your face.

4. Turn on the air compressor machine.

5. Take slow, deep breaths in through the mouth.

6. Hold each breath 1 to 2 seconds before breathing out.

7. Continue until the medicine is gone from the cup (approximately 10 minutes).

8. Store the medicine as directed after each use.

CLEANING THE NEBULIZER

Don't forget: Cleaning and getting rid of germs prevent infection. Cleaning keeps the nebulizer from clogging up and helps it last longer.

Cleaning Needed After Each Use

1. Remove the mask or the mouthpiece and T-shaped part from the cup. Remove the tubing and set it aside. The tubing should not be washed or rinsed. The outside should be wiped down. Rinse the mask or mouthpiece and T-shaped part—as well as the eyedropper or syringe—in warm running water for 30 seconds. Use distilled or sterile water for rinsing, if possible.

2. Shake off excess water. Air dry on a clean cloth or paper towel.

3. Put the mask or the mouthpiece and T-shaped part, cup, and tubing back together and connect the device to the compressed air machine. Run the machine for 10 to 20 seconds to dry the inside of the nebulizer.

4. Disconnect the tubing from the compressed air machine. Store the nebulizer in a ziplock plastic bag.

5. Place the cover over the compressed air machine.

Cleaning Needed Once Every Day

1. Remove the mask or the mouthpiece and T-shaped part from the cup. Remove the tubing and set it aside. The tubing should not be washed or rinsed.

2. Wash the mask or the mouthpiece and T-shaped part—as well as the eyedropper or syringe—with a mild dishwashing soap and warm water.

3. Rinse under a strong stream of water for 30 seconds. Use distilled (or sterile) water if possible.

FIGURE ■ 16-5 *(continued)*

4. Shake off excess water. Air dry on a clean cloth or paper towel.

5. Put the mask or the mouthpiece and T-shaped part, cup, and tubing back together and connect the device to the compressed air machine. Run the machine for 10 to 20 seconds to dry the inside of the nebulizer.

6. Disconnect the tubing from the compressed air machine. Store the nebulizer in a ziplock plastic bag.

7. Place a cover over the compressed air machine.

Cleaning Needed Once or Twice a Week

1. Remove the mask or the mouthpiece and T-shaped part from the cup. Remove the tubing and set it aside. The tubing should not be washed or rinsed. Wash the mask or the mouthpiece and T-shaped part—as well as the eyedropper or syringe—with a mild dishwashing soap and warm water.

2. Rinse under a strong stream of water for 30 seconds.

3. Soak for 30 minutes in a solution that is one part distilled white vinegar and two parts distilled

water. Throw out the vinegar water solution after use; do not reuse it.

4. Rinse the nebulizer parts and the eyedropper or syringe under warm running water for 1 minute. Use distilled or sterile water, if possible.

5. Shake off excess water. Air dry on a clean cloth or paper towel.

6. Put the mask or the mouthpiece and T-shaped part, cup, and tubing back together and connect the device to the compressed air machine. Run the machine for 10 to 20 seconds to dry the inside of the nebulizer thoroughly.

7. Disconnect the tubing from the compressed air machine. Store the nebulizer in a ziplock plastic bag.

8. Clean the surface of the compressed air machine with a well-wrung, soapy cloth or sponge. You could never use an alcohol or disinfectant wipe. NEVER PUT THE COMPRESSED AIR MACHINE IN WATER.

9. Place a cover over the compressed air machine.

Source: *Nurses: Partners in Asthma Care,* National Asthma Education and Prevention Program, National Heart, Lung, and Blood Institute, NIH Publication No. 95-3308, 1995.

Certain medications should be avoided when treating patients with asthma because adverse reactions can exacerbate asthmatic problems. These drugs include:

- **Beta-blockers.** Commonly used to treat hypertension in older people, beta-blockers (propranolol) can induce bronchospasm. Even ophthalmologic solutions like timolol should be avoided if possible. Hypoxemia can result from bronchospasm and lead to serious consequences.
- **Nonsteroidal anti-inflammatory drugs (NSAIDs).** Sudden, potentially life-threatening bronchospasm has been associated with NSAID and aspirin use in older patients.
- **Diuretics.** Hypokalemia can develop for patients taking thiazide (non–potassium sparing) diuretics. Hypokalemia can be associated with cardiac arrythmias, especially for those taking digitalis.
- **Antihistamines.** The QT interval can be prolonged in older patients taking beta$_2$-agonists or diuretics. The sedative effect of some antihistamines is also of concern.
- **Angiotensin-converting enzyme (ACE) inhibitors.** Widely used as antihypertensives, ACE inhibitors can produce cough in some patients. This may exacerbate

TABLE 16-5

Medications With Increased Potential for Adverse Effects in the Elderly Patient with Asthma

Medication	Comorbid Condition(s) for Which Drug Is Prescribed	Adverse Effect	Comment
Beta-adrenergic blocking agent	Hypertension Heart disease Tremor Glaucoma	Worsening asthma • bronchospasm • decreased response to bronchodilator Decreased response to epinephrine in anaphylaxis	Avoid where possible; when must be used, use a highly beta-selective drug
Nonsteroidal anti-inflammatory drugs	Arthritis Musculoskeletal diseases	Worsening asthma • bronchospasm	Not all older adults with asthma have intolerance of NSAIDs, but are best avoided if possible
Non-potassium-sparing diuretics	Hypertension Congestive heart failure	Worsening cardiac function/dysrhythmias due to hypokalemia	Additive effect with antiasthma medications that also produce potassium loss (steroids, beta-agonist); elderly also more likely to be receiving drugs (e.g., digitalis) where hypokalemia is of increased concern
Certain nonsedating antihistamines (terfenadine and astemizole)	Allergic rhinitis	Worsening cardiac function/ventricular arrythmias due to prolonged QT_C interval	
Cholinergic agents	Urinary retention Glaucoma	Bronchospasm Bronchorrhea	Also note that some over-the-counter asthma medications contain ephedrine, which could aggravate urinary retention, glaucoma
ACE inhibitors	Heart failure Hypertension	Increased incidence of cough	

Source: Nurses: Partners in Asthma Care, 1998.

asthma symptoms, causing asthma medications to be increased or diagnostic category moved a step upward.

■ **Antidepressants.** Corticosteroids can worsen underlying depression in the older person and interact with monoamine oxidase (MAO) inhibitors and tricyclic antidepressants.

Table 16-5 lists nonasthma medications with increased potential for adverse effects in older patients with asthma. The gerontological nurse should carefully review the therapeutic effects and side effects, and monitor for interactions with other medications. Beta-adrenergic blocking agents can trigger acute bronchospasm and hypoxemia, even when administered as ophthalmologic solutions (timolol) and should be avoided if possible.

After the physician has classified the severity of the asthma and prescribed a treatment plan, it is crucial that the patient be instructed in the use of a peak flow meter. The peak flow meter measures how well air moves in and out of the lungs and will alert older patients to narrowing of the airways hours before the onset of asthma symptoms. By taking medications before the onset of symptoms, the asthma attack may be lessened in severity or stopped completely. Further, the peak flow meter can alert the patient and the physician by:

- Illustrating the response of various conditions like exercise, exposure to cold weather, and psychological stress.
- Monitoring the effect of medications.
- Indicating when medication changes are needed.
- Indicating that emergency care is needed.

The peak flow meter should be used:

- Every day for the first 2 weeks after diagnosis or with change in treatment.
- Mornings after awakening and between noon and 2 P.M.
- Before and after taking beta$_2$-agonists to document effect.
- When symptoms occur such as wheezing or tightness in the chest.
- When the patient feels he or she is coming down with a cold or respiratory infection.

Patients should keep a peak flow diary and carefully record readings. At the time of asthma diagnosis, the physician will inform patients of their "personal best" or highest peak flow number achieved over a 2-week period when asthma is under good control. Good control indicates a feeling of respiratory well-being for the patient and absence of asthma symptoms. Peak flow readings can be classified into three categories:

1. Green zone (80% to 100% of personal best) indicating *good control.* No asthma symptoms are present and medication should be taken as usual.
2. Yellow zone (50% to 79% of personal best) indicating *caution.* An asthma attack may be starting and the patient may not be under control. Medication changes may be needed.
3. Red zone (below 50% of personal best) indicating *danger.* The patient should take a short-acting beta$_2$-agonist immediately and notify the physician.

Figure 16-6 ▪ includes instructions for the proper use of a peak flow meter, a sample peak flow diary, and a sample asthma management plan. The gerontological nurse can greatly improve the asthma management plan by teaching the older patient and family members about the peak flow meter and diary so that asthma attacks can be minimized or avoided. Having a written plan and instructions to refer to can improve medication adherence and reduce confusion should the older patient become short of breath or start to wheeze.

Older patients with asthma should be instructed that because of their sensitive airways, they may need to avoid allergens and triggers to asthma attacks. Many times, older patients will undergo allergy testing or report anecdotal evidence that being

FIGURE ☐ 16-6

Instructions for using a peak flow meter.

How to Use Your Peak Flow Meter

A peak flow meter is a device that measures how well air moves out of your lungs. During an asthma episode the airways of the lungs begin to narrow slowly. The peak flow meter will tell you if there is narrowing in the airways days—even hours—before you have any symptoms of asthma.

By taking your medicine(s) early (before symptoms), you may be able to stop the episode quickly and avoid a severe episode of asthma. Peak flow meters are used to check your asthma the way that blood pressure cuffs are used to check high blood pressure.

The peak flow meter can also be used to help you and your doctor.

- Learn what makes your asthma worse.
- Decide if your medicine plan is working well.
- Decide when to add or stop medicine.
- Decide when to seek emergency care.

A peak flow meter is most helpful for patients who must take asthma medicine daily. Patients age 5 and older are able to use a peak flow meter. Ask your doctor or nurse to show you how to use a peak flow meter.

How to Use Your Peak Flow Meter

- Do the following five steps with your peak flow meter:
  1. Put the indicator at the bottom of the numbered scale.
  2. Stand up.
  3. Take a deep breath.
  4. Place the meter in your mouth and close your lips around the mouthpiece. Do not put your tongue inside the hole.
  5. Blow out as hard and fast as you can.
- Write down the number you get.
- Repeat steps 1 through 5 two more times and write down the numbers you get.
- Write down in "My Asthma Symptoms and Peak Flow Diary" the highest of the three numbers achieved.

Find Your Personal Best Peak Flow Number

Your personal best peak flow number is the highest peak flow number you can achieve over a 2-week period when your asthma is under good control. Good control is when you feel good and do not have any asthma symptoms.

Each patient's asthma is different, and your best peak flow may be higher or lower than the peak flow of someone of your same height, weight, and sex. This means that it is important for you to find your own personal best peak flow number. Your medicine plan needs to be based on your own personal best peak flow number.

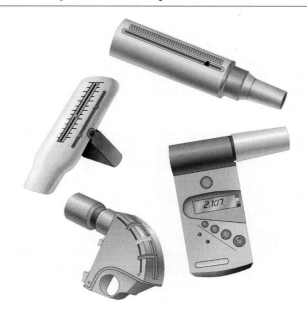

There are a variety of peak flow meters.

To find out your personal best peak flow number, take peak flow readings:

- Every day for 2 weeks.
- Mornings and early afternoons or evenings (when you wake up and between 12:00 and 2:00 P.M.).
- Before and after taking inhaled beta$_2$-agonist (*if* you take this medicine).
- As instructed by your doctor.

Write down these readings in your peak flow diary.

FIGURE ☐ **16-6** *(continued)*

The Peak Flow Zone System

Once you know your personal best peak flow number, your doctor will give you the numbers that tell you what to do. The peak flow numbers are put into zones that are set up like a traffic light. This will help you know what to do when your peak flow number changes. For example:

Green Zone (80% to 100% of your personal best number) signals *good control*. No asthma symptoms are present. You may take your medicines as usual.

Yellow Zone (50% to 79% of your personal best number) signals *caution*. You may be having an episode of asthma that requires an increase in your medicine. Or your overall asthma may not be under control, and the doctor may need to change your medicine plan.

Red Zone (below 50% of your personal best number) signals *danger!* You must take a short-acting inhaled beta$_2$-agonist right away and call your doctor immediately if your peak flow number does not return to the Yellow or Green Zone and stay in that zone.

Record your personal best peak flow number and peak flow zones at the top of "My Asthma Symptoms and Peak Flow Diary."

Use the Diary to Keep Track of Your Peak Flow

Write down your peak flow number on the diary every day, or as instructed by your doctor.

Actions to Take When Peak Flow Numbers Change

■ PEFR goes more than 20% below your personal best (PEFR is in the Yellow Zone).

ACTION: Take an inhaled short-acting bronchodilator as prescribed by your doctor.

■ PEFR changes 20% or more between the morning and early afternoon or evening (measure your PEFR before taking medicine).

or

■ PEFR increases 20% or more when measured before and after taking an inhaled short-acting bronchodilator.

ACTION: Talk to your doctor about adding more medicine to control your asthma better (for example, an anti-inflammatory medication).

(continued)

around certain things can trigger an asthma attack. The common offenders are the following:

- House-dust mites
- Animals
- Cockroaches
- Tobacco smoke
- Wood smoke
- Strong odors and sprays
- Colds and infections
- Exercise
- Weather
- Pollens
- Molds

Figure 16-7 ☐ indicates tips for persons who are allergic or bothered by any of these items. Additional items and strategies may be recommended by the pulmonologist or allergist caring for the older patient.

FIGURE ■ **16-6** *(continued)*

My Asthma Symptoms and Peak Flow Diary

_____ My predicted peak flow   _____ My personal best peak flow

_____ My Green (Good Control) Zone	_____ My Yellow (Caution) Zone	_____ My Red (Danger) Zone
80–100% of personal best	50–79% of personal best	below 50% of personal best

Date:	a.m.	p.m.	a.m.	p.m.	a.m.	p.m.	a.m.	p.m.	a.m.	p.m.	a.m.	p.m.	a.m.	p.m.
Peak Flow Reading														
No Asthma Symptoms														
Mild Asthma Symptoms														
Moderate Asthma Symptoms														
Serious Asthma Symptoms														
Medicine Used to Stop Symptoms														
Urgent Visit to the Doctor														

Directions:

1. Take your peak flow reading every morning (a.m.) when you wake up and every afternoon or evening (p.m.). Try to take your peak flow readings at the same time each day. If you take an inhaled beta$_2$-agonist medicine, take your peak flow reading **before** taking that medicine. Write down the highest reading of three tries in the box that says peak flow reading.

2. Look at the box at the top of this sheet to see whether your number is in the Green, Yellow, or Red Zone.

3. In the space below the date and time, put an "X" in the box that matches the symptoms you have when you record your peak flow reading; see description of symptom categories below.

4. Look at your Asthma Management Plan for what to do when your number is in one of the zones or when you have asthma symptoms.

5. Put an "X" in the box inside "medicine used to stop symptoms" if you took **extra** asthma medicine to stop your symptoms.

6. If you made any visit to your doctor's office, emergency department, or hospital for treatment of an asthma episode, put an "X" in the box marked "urgent visit to the doctor." Tell your doctor if you went to the emergency department or hospital.

No symptoms	= No symptoms (wheeze, cough, chest tightness, or shortness of breath) even with normal physical activity.
Mild symptoms	= Symptoms during physical activity, but not at rest. It does not keep you from sleeping or being active.
Moderate symptoms	= Symptoms while at rest; symptoms may keep you from sleeping or being active.
Severe symptoms	= Severe symptoms at rest (wheeze may be absent); symptoms cause problems walking or talking; muscles in neck or between ribs are pulled in when breathing.

FIGURE ◼ **16-6** (continued)

Date: _____   Personal Best PEFR _____

Asthma Management Plan for _____

Green Zone = Good control

Green Zone: _____ to _____ Peak Flow Rate (80–100% of personal best; no symptoms)

To keep your asthma under control: Stay away from things that make your asthma worse (such as animals, smoke, etc.; talk to your doctor about these things). **Take your medicine(s).**

Name of Medicine	How Much to Take	How Often/ When to Take It

Yellow Zone = Caution

Yellow Zone: _____ to _____ Peak Flow Rate (50–79% of personal best)

Take medicine listed below to get your asthma back under control.

Symptoms: Coughing, wheezing, shortness of breath, tightness in the chest, or other symptoms of an asthma episode. Symptoms may be mild.

Early signs your asthma is getting worse: _____

Take your Yellow Zone medication when these early signs occur.

Name of Medicine	How Much to Take	How Often/ When to Take It

- ◼ Peak flow rate or symptoms not better in _____ minutes after taking the medicine listed above? Call the doctor.
- ◼ Keep taking your Green Zone medicine(s). Keep staying away from things that make your asthma worse.

(continued)

FIGURE ■ **16-6** *(continued)*

Red Zone = Danger!

Red Zone: Below _____ Peak Flow Rate (below 50% of personal best)

Take the medicine listed below. Then call your doctor.

Symptoms: Coughing, very short of breath, trouble walking and talking, tightness in the chest, other symptoms.

Name of Medicine	How Much to Take	How Often/ When to Take It

- Call your doctor or emergency room NOW, say this is an emergency, and ask what you should do next.
- Go to the doctor or hospital **right away** or call an ambulance without delay if:
  —You are struggling to breathe or your lips or fingernails turn a little blue or grey.
  —Your peak flow remains in the Red Zone level 20 minutes after taking your medicine.
- Keep taking your Green Zone medicine(s).

Doctor: _____

Office Phone: _____

Phone Number After Office Hours: _____

Emergency Room: _____

Notes

Source: *Nurses: Partners in Asthma Care,* National Asthma Education and Prevention Program. National Heart, Lung, and Blood Institute, NIH Publication No. 95-3308, 1995.

FIGURE ■ 16-7

Guidelines for patients with asthma.

How to Stay Away From Things That Make Your Asthma Worse

Because you have asthma, your airways are very sensitive. They may react to things that can cause asthma attacks or episodes. Staying away from such things will help you keep your asthma from getting worse.

■ Ask your doctor to help you find out what makes your asthma worse. Discuss the ways to stay away from these things. The tips listed below will help you.

■ Ask your doctor for help in deciding which actions will help the most to reduce your asthma symptoms. Carry out these actions first. Discuss the results of your efforts with your doctor.

Tips for Those Allergic to or Bothered by Any Item Listed Below

House-Dust Mites

The following actions should help you control house-dust mites:

■ Encase your mattress and box spring in an airtight cover.

■ Either encase your pillow or wash it in hot water once a week every week.

■ Wash your bed covers, clothes, and stuffed toys once a week in hot water (130°F).

The following actions will also help you control dust mites—but they are not essential:

■ Reduce indoor humidity to less than 50%. Use a dehumidifier if needed.

■ Remove carpets from your bedroom.

■ Do not sleep or lie on upholstered furniture. Replace with vinyl, leather, or wood furniture.

■ Remove carpets that are laid on concrete.

■ Stay out of a room while it is being vacuumed.

■ If you must vacuum, one or more of the following things can be done to reduce the amount of dust you breathe in: (1) Use a dust mask. (2) Use a central vacuum cleaner with the collecting bag outside the home. (3) Use double-wall vacuum cleaner bags and exhaust-port HEPA (high-efficiency particulate air) filters.

Animals

Some people are allergic to the dried flakes of skin, saliva, or urine from warm-blooded pets. Warm-blooded pets include ALL dogs, cats, birds, and rodents. The length of a pet's hair does not matter. Here are some tips for those allergic to animals:

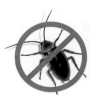

■ Remove the animal from the home or school classroom.

■ Choose a pet without fur or feathers (such as a fish or a snake).

■ If you must have a warm-blooded pet, keep the pet out of your bedroom at all times. Keeping the pet outside of your home is even better.

■ If there is forced air-heating in the home with a pet, close the air ducts in your bedroom.

■ Wash the pet weekly in warm water.

■ Do not visit homes that have pets. If you must visit such places, take asthma medicine (cromolyn is often preferred) before going.

■ Do not buy or use products made with feathers. Use pillows and comforters stuffed with synthetic fibers like polyester. Also do not use pillows, bedding, and furniture stuffed with kapok (silky fibers from the seed pods of the silk-cotton tree).

■ Use a vacuum cleaner fitted with a HEPA filter.

■ Wash hands and change clothes as soon as you can after being in contact with pets.

Cockroaches (Some people are allergic to the droppings of roaches.)

■ Use insect sprays; but have someone else spray when you are outside of the home. Air out the home for a few hours after spraying. Roach traps may also help.

■ All homes in multiple-family dwellings (apartments, condominiums, and housing projects) must be treated to get rid of roaches.

Tobacco Smoke

■ Do not smoke.

■ Do not allow smoking in your home. Have household members smoke outside.

■ Encourage family members to quit smoking. Ask your doctor or nurse for help on how to quit.

■ Choose no-smoking areas in restaurants, hotels, and other public buildings.

(continued)

FIGURE ■ 16-7 *(continued)*

Wood Smoke

- Do not use a wood-burning stove to heat your home.
- Do not use kerosene heaters.

Strong Odors and Sprays

- Do not stay in your home when it is being painted. Use latex rather than oil-based paint.
- Try to stay away from perfume; talcum powder, hair spray, and products like these.
- Use household cleaning products that do not have strong smells or scents.
- Reduce strong cooking odors (especially frying) by using an exhaust fan and opening windows.

Colds and Infections

- Talk to your doctor about flu shots.
- Stay away from people with colds or the flu.
- Do not take over-the-counter cold remedies, such as antihistamines and cough syrup, unless you speak to your doctor first.

Exercise

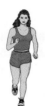

- Make a plan with your doctor that allows you to exercise without symptoms. For example, take inhaled beta$_2$-agonist or cromolyn less than 30 minutes before exercising.
- Do not exercise during the afternoon when air pollution levels are highest.

- Warm up before doing exercise and cool down afterward.

Weather

- Wear a scarf over your mouth and nose in cold weather. Or pull a turtleneck or scarf over your nose on windy or cold days.
- Dress warmly in the winter or on windy days.

Pollens

During times of high pollen counts:

- Stay indoors during the midday and afternoon when pollen counts are highest.
- Keep windows closed in cars and homes. Use air conditioning if you can.
- Pets should either stay outdoors or indoors. Pets should not be allowed to go in and out of the home. This prevents your pet from bringing pollen inside.
- Do not mow the grass. But if you must mow, wear a pollen filter mask.

Mold (Outdoor)

- Avoid sources of molds (wet leaves, garden debris, stacked wood).
- Avoid standing water or areas of poor drainage.

REMEMBER: Making these changes will help keep asthma episodes from starting. These actions can also reduce your need for asthma medicines.

Notes

_____

_____

_____

_____

_____

_____

_____

_____

_____

_____

Source: *Nurses: Partners in Asthma Care,* National Asthma Education and Prevention Program. National Heart, Lung, and Blood Institute, NIH Publication No. 95-3308, 1995.

Nursing Assessment

The gerontological nurse will have the opportunity to work with older patients with asthma over time and get to know them as individuals. It is recommended that each visit follow a three-part process. These three parts can occur more than once in any given session:

1. Assess the older patient's needs, expectations, and progress.
2. Introduce or review an action the older patient should take.
3. Obtain an agreement to take specific actions and schedule a follow-up visit to discuss the patient's progress.

Box 16-1 provides the organizing framework with specific suggestions for the nurse caring for patients with asthma (Nurses: Partners in Asthma Care, 1998).

Physical assessment of the older patient with asthma should include observation of the overall shape and movement of the thorax during respiration. The nurse should auscultate the lungs beginning at the apices of one lung and comparing that sound to the same area of the other lung. Usually auscultation proceeds from posterior to anterior and from the apex downward to the eighth rib. It is important to note the presence of crackles, wheezes, rhonchi, or pleural rub. Wheezing is a sign that air is having difficulty passing through airways narrowed by edema, spasm, or mucus. If wheezing is present, the nurse should note whether it occurs on inspiration or expiration and also note the use of accessory muscles during respiration. Chest excursion is measured by placing the thumbs beside the spine and noting their movement during deep inspiration. Tactile and vocal fremitus, vibrations felt on the surface of the chest, may be slightly decreased in the patient with asthma.

Nursing Diagnoses

Nursing diagnoses associated with the older person with asthma may include *activity intolerance* for those persons with exercise-induced asthma, *ineffective airway clearance* for those with chronic cough with mucus production, *ineffective breathing patterns* for those with tachypnea and wheezing with poorly controlled asthma, *altered tissue perfusion: respiratory* for those with hypoxemia, and *ineffective management of therapeutic regimen, individual* for those who are unable or unwilling to monitor the peak flow recordings and adjust medications to prevent asthma attacks and exacerbations. The nurse should seek advice from the social worker if older patients do not have medication coverage and are having difficulty purchasing the more expensive asthma medications.

CHRONIC OBSTRUCTIVE PULMONARY DISEASE

Chronic obstructive pulmonary disease is a term used for two closely related diseases of the respiratory system: chronic bronchitis and emphysema. Chronic bronchitis is defined as cough and sputum production present on most days for a minimum of 3 months for at least 2 successive years or for 6 months during 1 year. In chronic bronchitis, there may be narrowing of the large and small airways, making it more difficult to move air in and out of the lungs. An estimated 12.1 million Americans have chronic bronchitis. In emphysema, there is permanent destruction of the alveoli, the tiny elastic air sacs of the lung, because of irreversible destruction of elastin, a protein in the lung that is important for maintaining the strength of the alveolar walls. The loss of elastin also causes collapse or narrowing of the smallest air passages, called bronchioles, which in turn

Assessing and Meeting Needs: Examples of Patient Education for Each Clinic Visit

The way you organize and conduct your visits with patients will have a dramatic effect on their following your directions, their satisfaction with their care, and their management of their asthma. Specific examples of patient education for the first and subsequent visits are described in detail. The following three-part patient education process is used to organize every visit. These "parts" can recur more than once within a single session (e.g., assess progress and agree on next steps for two or more actions).

I. Assess needs, expectations, and progress.

II. Introduce/review an action patient needs to take.
   - Review the *benefits* of doing the action.
   - Identify concerns and *barriers,* and problem solve.
   - *Teach the action*—describe action, show action, have patient do the action, give feedback.
   - Devise ways to *help the patient remember* when to take the action.

III. Obtain an agreement with the patient to take specific action(s), and say you will discuss his or her progress at the next visit.

First Visit: Patient Assessment and Expectations

I. a. Introduce yourself and agree on expectations for the visit.
   - Explain what will happen during the visit.
   - Ask if the patient has concerns that he or she wants to have addressed at this visit.
   - Tell the patients when their concerns will be addressed during the visit. Ask if the plans for this visit are likely to meet the patient's needs.

   b. Determine if patients are at high risk for an asthma-related death or life-threatening episode. Patients at high risk should receive greater attention and vigilance. The following are risk factors for asthma-related death:
   - Age: 17–24, >55 years old.
   - African American, especially those 15 to 44 years of age.
   - Previous life-threatening acute asthma episode.
   - Hospital admission for asthma in the past year.
   - Inadequate general medical management.
   - Psychological and psychosocial problems (e.g., depression, alcohol abuse, recent family death and disruption, recent unemployment, schizophrenia, extreme anxiety).

   c. Assess resources and family support with simple questions requiring only "yes" and "no" answers (discuss periodically after the first visit).
   - **Insurance.** "Are your doctor's visits and medications covered by private insurance, Medicare, or Medicaid?" "Do you think you may need financial assistance?"
   - **Family opinions.** "Does your family understand your problems with asthma?" "Are they helpful and supportive of your getting proper treatment?" Discuss responses if there is time.
   - **Companion at visits.** "Would you like to bring a family member to your next appointment so he or she can learn about your asthma and its treatment?"

   d. Ask about *consequences* of asthma.
   - "How does asthma affect your life?" Identify the consequences of asthma that they would like to prevent. Discuss how likely it is that problems will continue if they do *not* take the appropriate action.

e. Ask about expected *benefits* of treatment.
   - "What do you expect the treatment will help you to do?" Review the goals of asthma management and tell the patient that these can be achieved by the patient and healthcare team working together. Present the benefits that would be *lost* by *not* taking the steps needed to control asthma (e.g., lose control of asthma).

f. Identify patient *concerns*/issues.
   - "What concerns do you have about your asthma and its treatment?"

II. Teach patients how and when to use their metered-dose inhaler(s).

III. Explain and agree on the demands of treatment.
   - Explain *generally* what the course of treatment will be, that treatment will be ongoing and long term, and how often they will need to come to the office. Tell them you will be helping them to achieve and maintain control of their asthma. Ask if this is acceptable to them.
   - Ask patient to agree to take specific actions (e.g., taking medicine) discussed in this visit.

Routine Visits: Assessment, Instruction, Review, and Agreement

I. a. Agree on expectations for the visit.
   - Explain what will happen during the visit.
   - Ask if the patient has concerns that he or she wants to have addressed at this visit.
   - Tell the patients when their concerns will be addressed during the visit. Ask if the plans for this visit are likely to meet the patient's needs.

   b. **Assess achievement of the goals of asthma management.** (Simple questions requiring only "yes" and "no" answers can be quickly asked.)
   - **Symptoms.** "Do you have any of the following symptoms during the day or night since your last visit or in the last month—coughing, wheezing, chest tightness, shortness of breath?"
     - If yes, ask when, where, how often, and during what activity they occurred.
   - **Exercise.** "Do you have symptoms during or after exercising or after exertion?" "Do activities such as running, climbing stairs, cleaning house, or laughing cause any symptoms in you?" "How many times a week do you usually exercise?"
   - **Routine interrupted.** "Has your asthma kept you from going to school, working, or doing other routine activities?"
   - **Emergency/additional care.** "Have you gone to an emergency department, hospital, or walk-in clinic for your asthma since the last visit?"
   - **Side effects.** "What side effects have you had from your medicines?" "Do you feel shaky or nervous?" "Are you having a bad taste, cough, or upset stomach?" "Are you having trouble working?" "Do you have any other problems with medicines?"

   c. **Assess activities in the components of asthma management.**
   - Objective measures—peak flow monitoring
     - Ask what time the patient checks his or her peak flow rate each day.
     - Review the pattern of the patient's daily peak flow rate.
     - Have patient demonstrate peak flow meter technique.
   - Environmental control
     - **Problems.** "What seems to make your asthma worse?"

(continued)

BOX
16-1
Assessing and Meeting Needs: Examples of Patient Education for Each Clinic Visit, *continued*

- **Actions.** "What have you done (or will you do) to stay away from things that make your asthma worse?"
- Pharmacotherapy
  - **Medications taken now.** "How much and how often do you take _____ medication?" If inhaled, "What is the name and color of the inhaler?"
  - **Treatment of symptoms.** "What do you do when you begin noticing symptoms?" "What medication do you take?" Review asthma management plan.
  - What other medications do you take for your asthma?
  - **Access to medicines.** "Do you have any problems getting your medicine at any time (e.g., at school or work)?"
  - **Effectiveness of medications.** "Do the medicines seem to be working for you?" (Clarify/reinforce benefits.)
  - **Concerns or questions.** "Do you have any concerns or questions about your medicine?"
  - **Demonstration by patient** of his or her inhaler/spacer and/or nebulizer technique.
  d. **Review an activity patients agreed to do at last visit (follow-up visits only).**
  - **Review activities/praise.** "What were you able to do regarding _____ [specific action]?" Praise some aspect of the patient's effort.
  - **Define problems/barriers.** "Did you have trouble with any actions that we discussed at the last visit?" "What seemed to be the problem?"
    - Unclear what action was
    - Benefits not achieved/believed
    - Lacked skills/confidence
    - Forgot
    - Barriers present—time, circumstances, other people, finances, etc.
  - **Problem solve with patient.** Discuss how to resolve the problem with the patient. For example, if patients forget, help them find ways to remind themselves. If they lack skills and confidence, reinforce previous teaching if needed, reduce the number and complexity of management activities if possible.
  - **Be positive.** Suggest that patients learn from and then forget about any mistakes they may have made. Encourage them to keep trying. They will succeed with time.
  - **Reinforce benefits.** "How helpful was _____ [a specific asthma management activity]?" For example, "What effects do you think the inhaled steroids had?" Remind patients that it can take a few weeks before they no-

limits airflow out of the lung. The estimated number of persons with emphysema in the United States is over 2 million (NHLBI, 2002a).

In the general population, emphysema usually develops in older people with a long smoking history; however, there is a form of emphysema that tends to run in families. People with familial emphysema have a hereditary deficiency of a blood component, alpha$_1$-proteinase inhibitor, also called alpha$_1$-antitrypsin. It is estimated that only 1% to 3% of all cases of emphysema are due to this deficiency (NHLBI, 2002a).

In many older patients, chronic bronchitis and emphysema occur together, although one may present more symptoms than the other. Most patients with these diseases have a long history of heavy cigarette smoking. More than 13.5 million Americans are thought to have COPD. It is the fifth-leading cause of death in the United States, and the

tice benefits from inhaled steroids. Reinforce benefits mentioned and address any problems.

- **Agree upon patient's plans to act.** Ask the patient to agree to take the specific action and say you will discuss his or her experience with him or her at the next visit.

II. **Introduce a new activity using the process below (as needed).**
- **Propose an action.** Tell the patient what action he or she needs to learn next (e.g., peak flow rate monitoring). "I would like to talk to you about this action today. Is that OK?"
- **Present benefits.** Present the key benefits to the patient. Ask, "How do you think this could be helpful to you given your experience with asthma?"
- **Teach.** Use the four R's to guide teaching: Reach agreement, rehearse, repeat, reinforce.
- **Address barriers.** "What do you think might keep you from doing this asthma management activity?" "What might make it difficult?" "How can these problems/difficulties be reduced?"
- **Make specific plans.** "During the next month, what do you plan to do regarding _____ [specific action] (e.g., taking peak flow rate every morning when I brush my teeth and record the rate on my peak flow diary at that time)?" Or simply ask, "How likely are you to do _____ [specific action], _____[frequency], over the next month?"
- **Devise reminders.** Discuss how patients can remind themselves to take the agreed-upon actions.

Closing for All Visits

Assess satisfaction. "Were your concerns and questions during this visit addressed satisfactorily?" Other satisfaction questions include: "How did your visit with Dr. _____ go?" "Is there anything that was said that you weren't sure you understood?" "How could we make your visit more helpful to you in the future?" Provide feedback to the rest of the health professionals and make appropriate notations in the patient record.

Review/confirm agreements. Obtain or confirm the patient's commitment and plans to take each recommended action.

Express interest in future progress. ALWAYS tell patients you will talk to them about their agreed-upon actions at their next visit. Convey interest in their progress and do not make this sound like you are checking up on them.

Source: Nurses: Partners in Asthma Care, 1998.

death rate has been steadily increasing. Although COPD is still more common in men than in women, the greatest increases in the COPD death rate have occurred in women, especially African Americans. In 2000, 23.2% of African Americans smoked; more than 45,000 African Americans die from smoking-related diseases annually. Although African Americans smoke fewer cigarettes per day than Whites, on average, they tend to smoke brands with higher nicotine levels (American Lung Association, 2003).

The symptoms of COPD tend to emerge in the middle years of life, and many persons with COPD become disabled with constant shortness of breath. COPD causes 18 million office visits per year and over 2 million hospital days. COPD costs about $9 billion annually in healthcare and another $10 billion in lost productivity. It is a disease with high individual and societal costs.

Pathophysiology

When COPD develops, the walls of the small airways and alveoli lose their elasticity and thicken, closing off some of the smaller air passages and narrowing larger ones. The lungs contain 300 million alveoli whose ultrathin walls form the gas exchange surface. Enmeshed in the wall of each of these air sacs is a network of tiny capillaries that bring blood to the gas exchange surface. Air can enter the alveoli during inspiration; but on expiration, the air becomes trapped because of collapsing airways. Stale air cannot leave the lungs, and this residual volume adversely affects gas exchange. Over time, pathological changes occur with COPD. Blood flow and airflow to the walls of the alveoli become uneven and mismatched. In some alveoli, blood flow exceeds airflow; in others, the opposite occurs. The end result is that blood is poorly oxygenated and tissue perfusion is less efficient.

Pushing air through the narrow air passageways becomes harder with time, and the respiratory muscles become fatigued. Carbon dioxide cannot be adequately removed from the blood and may accumulate to critical levels, resulting in respiratory acidosis and ultimately respiratory failure.

The ability to efficiently move air into and out of the lungs declines gradually with age, but in most cases lung function remains adequate in nonsmokers, those free from occupational and household exposure to airborne contaminants and secondhand smoke, and those living in geographical areas with relatively clean air. It is never too late to quit smoking because lung function declines much more rapidly in smokers. If smoking stops before serious lung damage occurs, the rate at which lung function declines returns to nearly normal. However, some lung damage cannot be reversed, and over time it is unlikely that lung function will return to normal (NHLBI, 2002). Figure 16-8 ▢ illustrates the relationship between smoking and lung function.

COPD also strains the heart, especially the right ventricle that is responsible for pumping blood into the lungs. As COPD progresses, the amount of oxygen in the blood decreases, causing blood vessels in the lungs to further constrict. As a result, more force is required to circulate blood throughout the lungs. The right ventricle enlarges and thickens, which can result in abnormal rhythms called *cor pulmonale*. Older patients with cor pulmonale suffer from fatigue, rhythm disturbances, and palpitations, and are at risk for heart failure should additional strain be placed on the heart such as acquiring a respiratory illness.

FIGURE ▢ 16-8

Age-related change in the lung function and effect of smoking and smoking cessation.

Source: NHLBI: National Heart, Lung, and Blood Institute, 2002a. *The Lungs in Health and Disease.*

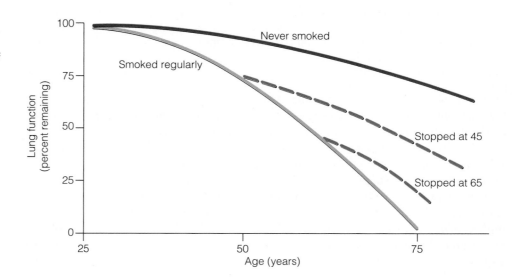

As COPD progresses, the body tries to boost the amount of oxygen carried in the blood by making extra red blood cells. This condition is *secondary polycythemia* and results in a larger than normal number of red cells in the general circulation. Although these cells are helpful to carry extra oxygen, they clog up small blood vessels and thicken the blood. This results in the formation of a bluish color in the skin, lips, and nail beds called *cyanosis*. Eventually, clubbing of the fingers will become apparent. Too little oxygen can also affect the brain, resulting in headache, irritability, impaired cognition, and sleep problems.

Symptoms

The earliest presenting symptom of COPD is early morning cough with the production of clear sputum. The sputum will turn to yellow or green should the older person develop a respiratory infection. Periods of wheezing may occur during or after colds. Shortness of breath on exertion develops later and becomes more pronounced with severe episodes of **dyspnea** occurring during even modest activity like walking or making a bed.

The typical progression of COPD is as follows:

- Usually no symptoms occur for the first 10 years after beginning smoking.
- At about 10 years after beginning smoking, chronic cough with clear sputum develops.
- At about the age of 40 or 50, dyspnea begins to occur.
- At about age 50, increased susceptibility to colds occurs with longer recovery time needed.

Survival of patients with COPD is closely related to the level of their lung function when they are diagnosed and the rate at which they lose their lung function. Mouth breathing, puffing, use of accessory muscles of breathing, and inability to finish a sentence without catching one's breath are signs of dyspnea from air hunger (McGann & Fitzgerald, 2001). Patients with severe lung damage sleep in a semisitting position because they are unable to breathe when they lie flat. Dyspnea is the most common reason for emergency department visits and has been associated with an increased risk of hospitalization in older patients with COPD (McGann & Fitzgerald, 2001). Overall, the median survival is about 10 years for patients with COPD who have lost approximately two thirds of their normally expected lung function at diagnosis (American Lung Association, 2003).

Practice Pearl

Older patients with COPD often have calluses on their elbows as a result of leaning over tables to stretch out their torsos so that more air can enter and exit during respiration.

Diagnosis

At present, it is impossible to diagnose COPD before irreversible lung damage occurs. Spirometry is the preferred diagnostic method for testing pulmonary function. The three volume measures most relevant to COPD are:

1. **Forced vital capacity.** The maximum volume of air that can be forcibly expelled after inhaling as deeply as possible.
2. **Residual volume.** The amount of air remaining in the lungs after forced vital capacity is measured.
3. **Total lung capacity.** Combination of the forced vital capacity and residual volume.

Although most of the measured lung volumes change with COPD, residual volume usually increases dramatically. This increase is the result of the weakened airways collapsing before all of the normally expired air can leave the lungs. The increased residual volume makes breathing more difficult because the trapped air occupies a large area and impedes the influx of fresh air.

The FEV_1 (forced expiratory volume in 1 second) also provides valuable information as COPD results in narrowed air passages. When FEV_1 is used as an indicator of lung function, the average rate of decline in patients with COPD is two to three times the normal rate of loss of 20 to 30 mm per year. As COPD progresses, less air can be expelled in 1 second. A greater than expected fall in FEV_1 is the most sensitive test for COPD progression and a fairly good predictor of early disability and death (NHLBI, 2002).

As the primary function of the lung is to remove carbon dioxide from the blood and add oxygen, another indicator of pulmonary function is the measurement of blood oxygen and carbon dioxide levels. As COPD progresses, the amount of oxygen in the blood decreases and the amount of carbon dioxide rises. Blood oxygen can be measured by obtaining arterial blood gas levels (the gold standard, but often difficult to obtain in older persons) or by using pulse oximetry (more convenient but less reliable). PaO_2 and $PaCO_2$ are measures of arterial oxygen and carbon dioxide. Pulse oximetry is reported in percentage of oxygen in capillary blood. Under normal conditions, the hemoglobin in arterial blood is 97.4% saturated with oxygen while the patient is breathing room air. This level of oxygen saturation is decreased with progressive pulmonary disease.

In most cases, it is necessary to monitor the results of a series of spirometry tests to determine the rate of disease progress or improvement. Measurement of FEV_1 and FEV_1/FVC ratio should be a routine part of the physical examination of every patient with COPD. The ratio is normally 75% to 85%, depending on the patient's age (NHLBI, 2002). The ratio is reduced in COPD.

Treatment

Although there is no cure for COPD, treatment can reduce disabling symptoms. Because cigarette smoking is the most significant cause, quitting smoking can most always prevent COPD progression. The goals of treatment are to reduce disability, prevent acute exacerbations, reduce hospitalization, and avoid premature mortality.

Home oxygen therapy has been shown to increase the survival rate of patients with advanced COPD who have hypoxemia, low blood oxygen levels. This treatment can improve a patient's exercise tolerance and ability to perform on cognitive and physical tests, reflecting improvement in the function of the brain and increased muscle coordination. Oxygen also improves cardiac function and prevents the development of cor pulmonale. Continuous oxygen therapy is recommended for patients with low oxygen levels at rest, during exercise, and while sleeping (NHLBI, 2002a). Many oxygen sources are available for home use including compressed gaseous oxygen or liquid oxygen devices that concentrate oxygen from room air. The patient's insurance may reimburse some of the expense of continuous oxygen therapy (can be hundreds of dollars a month) once hypoxemia is verified and documented. It is imperative that the older patient not smoke anywhere near oxygen or oxygen equipment because of the danger of explosion.

Medications used to treat patients with COPD are similar to those used to treat patients with asthma and include:

■ Bronchodilators to help open narrowed airways to improve airflow and gas exchange. The *sympathomimetics* (isoproterenol, metaproterenol, terbutaline, albuterol), the *parasympathomimetics* (atropine, ipratropium bromide), and *methylxanthines* (theophylline and its derivatives) all can be inhaled or taken by mouth.

- Corticosteroids to lessen inflammation of the airway. Inhaled steroids include beclomethasone, dexamethasone, triamcinolone, and flunisolide. By decreasing inflammation and swelling, more air can pass through the narrowed airways. Additionally, less inflammation usually means less mucus production.
- Antibiotics (tetracycline, ampicillin, erythromycin, and trimethoprim-sulfamethoxazole combinations) to fight infections. Antibiotics are usually prescribed at the first sign of infection or when sputum color changes from clear to yellow or green. The goal is to prevent the development of pneumonia and serious illness requiring hospitalization.
- Expectorants to loosen mucus and clear the airways.
- Other drugs to treat associated symptoms. Diuretics for heart failure, analgesics for pain, cough suppressants for cough, and anxiolytics for anxiety and restlessness.

Additional Treatment Options

Bullectomy or lung reduction surgery has shown some limited success in selected patients. Portions of the lung that are nonfunctional and filled with stagnant air are removed to make room for the more healthy parts of the lung to expand. However, this is major surgery and many patients with COPD are poor surgical risks and prone to life-threatening surgical complications. Lung transplantation has also been used with some COPD patients. The 1-year survival in patients with transplanted lungs is over 70%.

Pulmonary rehabilitation is useful in patients with COPD. The goals are to improve overall physical stamina and compensate for the conditions that cause dyspnea and limit functional ability. General exercise training increases performance, improves sense of well-being, and strengthens muscles. Administration of oxygen and nutritional supplements when needed can improve exercise tolerance. Intermittent mechanical ventilatory support relieves dyspnea and rests respiratory muscles in selected patients. **Continuous positive airway pressure** is used as an adjunct to weaning from mechanical ventilation to minimize dyspnea during exercise (see Figure 8-8 on page 233). The positive pressure keeps the narrowed airways from collapsing and trapping air. Relaxation techniques may also reduce the perception of ventilatory effort and dyspnea. Breathing exercises and techniques such as pursed lip breathing can improve functional status.

Clearing the air passages of mucus can be difficult in patients with end-stage COPD. **Intermittent positive pressure breathing (IPPB)** may be prescribed for frail and debilitated patients for short-term ventilatory support and delivery of aerosol medications. The IPPB treatment can clear secretions and stimulate a cough reflex. Additional methods that may help to loosen and remove troublesome secretions include:

- **Postural drainage.** The patient lies with the head and chest over the side of the bed. Gravity forces secretions at the bottom of the lungs upward and stimulates a cough reflex. Postural drainage is more effective following inhalation of a bronchodilator.
- **Chest percussion.** Lightly clapping the chest and back helps to loosen secretions.
- **Controlled coughing.** The patient can be taught to cough while contracting the diaphragm to maximize the cough response.
- **Tracheal suctioning.** This method may be needed during the end-of-life phase for frail older patients who are unable to clear their own secretions.

Smoking Cessation

The most important thing a patient with COPD can do is to quit smoking. Older patients and their families may think that if lung damage has occurred, it is too late and therefore not worth the effort. The gerontological nurse can function as educator and change agent for the older smoker.

The NHLBI has developed a smoking IQ test for older smokers. It can be a good way to open a discussion regarding smoking cessation with older patients who smoke and their families. The nurse should ask the older patient to complete the test and then discuss the correct answers. Box 16-2 lists the questions, scoring, and rationale for each response.

The nurse should investigate community resources and availability of smoking cessation support groups. Many hospitals and community agencies offer programs stressing behavior modification techniques. In addition, nicotine patches and gum with supportive counseling can be effective for some older people. If nicotine replacement transdermal patches are used, they should be applied to clean, nonhairy skin on the upper arm or torso daily. Sites should be rotated to prevent skin irritation. Nicoderm comes in three strengths (21 mg, 14 mg, and 7 mg). It is recommended that older patients begin with the 14-mg strength to prevent possible cardiovascular side effects. After 2 to 4 weeks, the dose should be reduced to 7 mg for 2 to 4 weeks and then discontinued. For older patients reporting sleep difficulties, the patch should be removed one hour before bedtime and reapplied first thing in the morning. Patients who smoke while wearing the patch are at risk for cardiovascular problems, including heart attack, and should be clearly informed of this risk. If they decide to start smoking during treatment with the patch, they should remove the patch and wait a minimum of 2 hours before having a cigarette (overnight is better).

For patients choosing Nicorette gum, it is recommended that 9 to 12 pieces be used daily. The nurse should instruct patients to chew one piece at a time when they get the urge to smoke. After chewing the gum a few times to soften it, it should be held in the buccal cavity for at least one-half hour to release all the medication.

The physician can also prescribe bupropion (Zyban) for 7 to 12 weeks to ease tobacco cravings during the cessation process. Bupropion is contraindicated in persons with seizure disorder. When it is combined with nicotine replacement, the quit rate doubles to 30% at 12 months (Reuben et al., 2002).

Practice Pearl

Cessation of smoking is the best way to slow the progression of COPD. Nurses should be persistent in educating and urging older patients to quit. The smoking addiction is difficult to beat. Many older people try to quit several times before they are ultimately successful. It is important for nurses not to smoke. Nurses who smoke lose credibility with their patients and put themselves at risk for developing this debilitating disease.

Additional suggestions for patients with COPD include the following:

- Avoid exposure to dust and fumes. Ensure good ventilation when working with solvents, chemicals, and paints. Wear a mask when doing woodwork or sanding furniture. Avoid woodstoves and smoky fires, perfumes, and other indoor pollutants.
- Avoid air pollution, including secondhand smoke. Do not exercise when air pollution or smog levels are high.
- Refrain from close contact with people who have colds or the flu. Be sure to receive a yearly flu shot and pneumococcal vaccine at age 65.
- Avoid excessive heat, cold, and high altitudes. A commercial aircraft maintains a cabin pressure equivalent to an elevation of 5,000 to 10,000 feet. This can result in hypoxemia for some patients with COPD. Supplemental oxygen may be needed and can be arranged in advance of the flight.
- Drink lots of fluids. Being hydrated can keep sputum loose and secretions easier to clear.

| **Check Your Smoking I.Q.** | **BOX 16-2** |

An Important Quiz for Older Smokers

If you or someone you know is an older smoker, you may think that there is no point in quitting now. Think again. By quitting smoking now, you will feel more in control and have fewer coughs and colds. However, with every cigarette you smoke, you increase your chances of having a heart attack, a stroke, or cancer. Need to think about this more? Take this older smokers' I.Q. quiz. Just answer "true" or "false" to each statement below.

True or False

1. ○ True ○ False If you have smoked for most of your life, it's not worth stopping now.
2. ○ True ○ False Older smokers who try to quit are more likely to stay off cigarettes.
3. ○ True ○ False Smokers get tired and short of breath more easily than nonsmokers the same age.
4. ○ True ○ False Smoking is a major risk factor for heart attack and stroke among adults 60 years of age and older.
5. ○ True ○ False Quitting smoking can help those who have already had a heart attack.
6. ○ True ○ False Most older smokers don't want to stop smoking.
7. ○ True ○ False An older smoker is likely to smoke more cigarettes than a younger smoker.
8. ○ True ○ False Someone who has smoked for 30 to 40 years probably won't be able to quit smoking.
9. ○ True ○ False Very few older adults smoke cigarettes.
10. ○ True ○ False Lifelong smokers are more likely to die of diseases like emphysema and bronchitis than nonsmokers.

Test Results

1. If you have smoked for most of your life, it's not worth stopping now.

   False. You have every reason to quit now and quit for good—even if you've been smoking for years. Stopping smoking will help you live longer and feel better. You will reduce your risk of heart attack, stroke, and cancer; improve blood flow and lung function; and help stop diseases like emphysema and bronchitis from getting worse.

2. Older smokers who try to quit are more likely to stay off cigarettes.

   True. Once they quit, older smokers are far more likely than younger smokers to stay away from cigarettes. Older smokers know more about both the short- and long-term health benefits of quitting.

3. Smokers get tired and short of breath more easily than nonsmokers the same age.

   True. Smokers, especially those over 50 years old, are much more likely to get tired, feel short of breath, and cough more often. These symptoms can signal the start of bronchitis or emphysema, both of which are suffered more often by older smokers. Stopping smoking will help reduce these symptoms.

(continued)

BOX 16-2 **Check Your Smoking I.Q.,** *continued*

---

4. Smoking is a major risk factor for heart attack and stroke among adults 60 years of age and older.

   True. Smoking is a major risk factor for four of the five leading causes of death including heart disease, stroke, cancer, and lung diseases like emphysema and bronchitis. For adults 60 and over, smoking is a major risk factor for six of the top 14 causes of death. Older male smokers are nearly twice as likely to die from stroke as older men who do not smoke. The odds are nearly as high for older female smokers. Cigarette smokers of any age have a 70% greater heart disease death rate than do nonsmokers.

5. Quitting smoking can help those who have already had a heart attack.

   True. The good news is that stopping smoking does help people who have suffered a heart attack. In fact, their chances of having another attack are smaller. In some cases, ex-smokers can cut their risk of another heart attack by half or more.

6. Most older smokers don't want to stop smoking.

   False. Most smokers would prefer to quit. In fact, in a recent study, 65% of older smokers said that they would like to stop. What keeps them from quitting? They are afraid of being irritable, nervous, and tense. Others are concerned about cravings for cigarettes. Most don't want to gain weight. Many think it's too late to quit—that quitting after so many years of smoking will not help. But this is not true.

7. An older smoker is likely to smoke more cigarettes than a younger smoker.

   True. Older smokers usually smoke more cigarettes than younger people. Plus, older smokers are more likely to smoke high nicotine brands.

8. Someone who has smoked for 30 to 40 years probably won't be able to quit smoking.

   False. You may be surprised to learn that older smokers are actually more likely to succeed at quitting smoking. This is more true if they're already experiencing long-term smoking-related symptoms like shortness of breath, coughing, or chest pain. Older smokers who stop want to avoid further health problems, take control of their life, get rid of the smell of cigarettes, and save money.

9. Very few older adults smoke cigarettes.

   False. One out of five adults aged 50 or older smokes cigarettes. This is more than 11 million smokers, a fourth of the country's 43 million smokers! About 25% of the general U.S. population still smokes.

10. Lifelong smokers are more likely to die of diseases like emphysema and bronchitis than nonsmokers.

    True. Smoking greatly increases the risk of dying from diseases like emphysema and bronchitis. In fact, over 80% of all deaths from these two diseases are directly due to smoking. The risk of dying from lung cancer is also a lot higher for smokers than nonsmokers: 22 times higher for males, 12 times higher for females.

- Maintain good lifestyle habits. Good nutrition, exercise, weight control, and moderation in alcohol consumption can add years and function to the life of a patient with COPD.
- Have spirometry done routinely and get to know the numbers.

Nursing Assessment and Nursing Diagnosis

The gerontological nurse will have the opportunity to work with older patients with COPD over time and get to know them as individuals. Guidelines for care of the patient with COPD are similar to those developed for patients with asthma. It is recommended that each visit include:

- Assessment of the older patient's needs, expectations, and progress.
- Introduction or review of actions the older patient should take.
- Obtaining an agreement to take specific actions and scheduling a follow-up visit to discuss the patient's progress.
- Careful review of the patient's progress toward smoking cessation or continued abstinence from smoking.

Physical assessment of the older patient with COPD should include observation of the overall shape and movement of the thorax during respiration. The lungs should be auscultated beginning at the apices of one lung and comparing that sound to the same area of the other lung. Usually auscultation proceeds from posterior to anterior and from the apex downward to the eighth rib, noting the presence of crackles, wheezes, rhonchi, or pleural rub. Wheezing is a sign that air is having difficulty passing through airways narrowed by edema, spasm, or mucus. If wheezing is present, the nurse should note whether it occurs on inspiration or expiration. The nurse notes the use of accessory muscles during respiration, measures chest excursion by placing the thumbs beside the spine and noting their movement during deep inspiration, and notes the presence or absence of lung sounds in the base of each lung. Absence of lung sounds indicates air trapping and lack of air movement. Tactile and vocal fremitus, vibrations felt on the surface of the chest, may be slightly decreased in the patient with COPD.

Nursing diagnoses associated with the older person with COPD may include *activity intolerance* for those persons with fatigue and air hunger, *ineffective airway clearance* for those with chronic cough with mucus production, *ineffective breathing patterns* for those with tachypnea and wheezing with advanced COPD, *altered tissue perfusion: respiratory* for those with hypoxemia, and *ineffective management of therapeutic regimen, individual* for those who are unable or unwilling to refrain from cigarette smoking and to adjust medications to prevent exacerbations. The nurse should seek advice from the social worker if older patients do not have medication coverage and are having difficulty purchasing the more expensive medications.

TUBERCULOSIS

Tuberculosis (TB) infects about one third of the world's population, approximately 2 billion people. It is the worldwide leading killer of young adults. *Mycobacterium tuberculosis* is spread through the air and usually infects the lungs, although other organs are sometimes involved. Most persons infected with *M. tuberculosis* harbor the bacterium without symptoms but may develop active disease. Each year, 8 million people worldwide develop active TB and 3 million die (National Institute of Allergy and Infectious Diseases, 2002).

In the United States, TB has reemerged as a serious public health problem. The number of active cases has been decreasing, mainly due to improved public health control measures. The disease burden is greatest in developing countries where 95% of the cases occur. However, those in the U.S. who develop TB are often poor, lack acccess to adequate health care, and often have low cure rates because they have been infected by drug-resistant strains (Sandoz Biochemicals, 2005). In addition to those with active TB, an estimated 10 million to 15 million people in the United States are infected without displaying symptoms and are considered to have latent TB. About 10% of these persons will develop TB at some time in their lives.

Minorities are disproportionately affected by TB. Fifty-four percent of active cases in 1999 were among African Americans and Hispanics, with an additional 20% found in Asians. In 2001, the total number of new TB cases among non-Hispanic African Americans was 4,796. Although African Americans represent 12% of the American population, they account for 30% of the TB cases. African Americans are eight times more likely to contract active TB than are Whites (American Lung Association, 2003).

The number of new cases of TB dropped rapidly in the 1940s and 1950s when the first effective antibiotic therapies and treatments were introduced. In 1985, the decline ended and the number of active cases in the United States began to rise. Several factors were behind this resurgence:

- The HIV/AIDS epidemic. People diagnosed with HIV are vulnerable to manifesting active TB when they are exposed to *M. tuberculosis.*
- Increased numbers of foreign-born persons entering the United States from parts of the world where TB is indigenous such as Africa, Asia, and Latin America. TB cases among these people account for nearly half of the U.S. total number of cases.
- Increased poverty, injection drug use, and homelessness. Transmission is rampant in crowded shelters and prisons where people weakened by poor nutrition, drug addiction, and alcoholism are exposed to *M. tuberculosis.*
- Failure of patients to take medications as directed, increasing resistant strains of *M. tuberculosis.*
- Increased numbers of residents in long-term care facilities such as nursing homes. Many older people in nursing homes are frail and have weakened immune systems. If exposed to *M. tuberculosis,* they can rapidly develop active TB (National Institute of Allergy and Infectious Diseases, 2002).

TB in older people can be the reactivation of old disease or a new infection due to exposure to an infected individual. Risk factors for developing or reactivating TB include the following:

- Living in an institution
- Diabetes mellitus
- Use of immunosuppressive drugs like corticosteroids or anticancer medications
- Malignancy
- Malnutrition
- Renal failure

(Reuben et al., 2002)

Transmission

TB is primarily an airborne disease that is spread by droplets when an infected person coughs, sneezes, speaks, sings, or laughs. Only people with active disease are contagious. It usually takes repeated exposure to someone with active TB before a person becomes infected. On average, most people would have a 50% chance of becoming infected if they spent 8 hours a day for 6 months or 24 hours a day for 2 months working or living with someone with active TB. The odds of contracting the disease are increased if the person exposed has any of the above risk factors. However, people with TB who have been treated with appropriate drugs for at least 2 weeks are no longer contagious and are incapable of spreading the disease (National Institute of Allergy and Infectious Diseases, 2002). Adequate ventilation is the most important measure to prevent transmission.

Diagnosis

About 2 to 8 weeks after infection with *M. tuberculosis,* a person's immune system responds by walling off infected cells. From then on the body maintains a standoff with the infection, sometimes for years. Most people undergo complete healing of their initial infection, and the bacteria eventually die off. A positive TB skin test and old scars on a chest x-ray may provide the only evidence of past infection. If, however, resistance is low because of aging, infection, malnutrition, or other reason, the bacteria may break out of hiding and cause active TB (National Institute of Allergy and Infectious Diseases, 2002).

The risk of developing active TB is greatest in the first year after infection, but it can occur at any time. Early symptoms include weight loss, night sweats, and loss of appetite. One in three patients with TB will die within weeks to months if the disease is not treated. For the rest, the disease either goes into remission or becomes chronic with debilitating cough, chest pain, and bloody sputum.

The hallmarks of TB diagnosis are the skin test and the chest x-ray. People who should be skin tested include:

- Those known to have spent time with someone with active TB.
- Those with HIV or malignancy.
- Those who think they may have the disease.
- Those from parts of the world where TB is common (Latin America, the Caribbean, Africa, Asia, eastern Europe, and Russia).
- Those who use intravenous drugs and alcohol to excess.
- Those living in institutions where TB is common (homeless shelters, migrant farm camps, prison, nursing homes).

The purified protein derivative (PPD) skin test involves the injection of 5 TU (Bioequivalent) per dose (0.1 mL) under the skin in the forearm. It should not be given subcutaneously, but rather subdermally. It should barely raise a wheal. If an area of induration results (raised, reddened area) around 72 hours after the PPD has been injected, it should be measured and recorded. Figure 16-9 ▪ illustrates how to correctly measure the tuberculin skin test. Guidelines for considering the PPD positive are found in Table 16-6.

When PPD testing in an older adult, the two-step approach is recommended. If the initial PPD is negative, testing is repeated after waiting 1 to 2 weeks. The second PPD provides a more accurate reading because the older person's immune system may be sluggish and not adequately react to the first exposure. It is unclear how the PPD results should be interpreted for those who have received the BCG, the antituberculosis vaccine. The BCG vaccine is not used in the United States but many people coming from other parts of the world have received it in the past. A general rule is to interpret the PPD results in patients who have received BCG using the same criteria as nonvaccinated

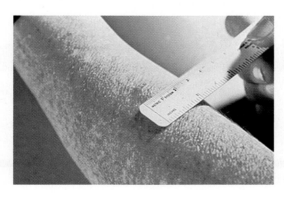

FIGURE ▪ **16-9**

The tuberculin skin test. Read the tuberculin skin test 48–72 hours after injection. Measure only induration, and record reaction in millimeters.

Source: Centers for Disease Control, 2003.

TABLE 16-6	Population	Area of Induration
Interpretation of Tuberculin Skin Testing by Risk	Low risk, healthy adult	15 mm
	Employees of hospitals, nursing homes, prisons, etc.	10 mm
	Recent immigrants (<5 years) from high-risk countries	
	Intravenous drug users	
	Persons with diabetes, chronic renal failure, leukemia, lymphoma, cancer, or weight loss of unexplained origin	
	Recent contact with TB patients	5 mm
	Fibrotic changes on chest x-ray	
	HIV-positive or on corticosteroids	

Source: Centers for Disease Control, 2003; National Institute of Allergy and Infectious Diseases, 2002; Reuben et al., 2002.

patients. Others do not recommend PPD testing in persons who have received BCG because the results will most likely be positive and large areas of induration can result. These patients should be closely followed up with symptom checklists and chest x-rays if they are in high-risk categories. Patients with a positive test are referred to physicians for further testing including a chest x-ray and sputum analysis to check for acid-fast bacillus.

Treatment

Successful treatment of TB depends on close cooperation between the patient and healthcare workers. Usually several antibiotics are prescribed and given for between 6 and 12 months. Patients must take their medication at the same time every day to prevent resistance.

Treatment of active TB involves the medications listed in Table 16-7.

With appropriate antibiotic treatment, TB can be cured in more than 90% of patients. Serious side effects of isoniazid include loss of appetite, nausea, vomiting, jaundice, fever for more than 3 days, abdominal pain, and tingling in the fingers and toes (Centers for Disease Control, 2003). Patients taking isoniazid are urged not to drink alcoholic beverages, including wine, beer, and liquor.

When the antibiotic treatment is interrupted because of unpleasant side effects or financial reasons, the TB bacteria may become resistant and be more difficult to eradicate when treatment is started again. Multidrug-resistant TB resists eradication with more than one drug. Treatment of multidrug-resistant TB requires the use of special drugs that have more serious side effects. However, even with this enhanced treatment, between 40% and 60% of patients with multidrug-resistant TB will die, a rate similar to untreated TB patients with nonresistant organisms (National Institute of Allergy and Infectious Diseases, 2002).

TABLE 16-7	Drug	Dose/Duration
Medications Used to Treat Tuberculosis	Isoniazid (INH)	5 mg/kg/day (max 300 mg/day) for 6–9 months
	Rifampin plus	10 mg/kg/day (max 600 mg/day)
	Pyrazinamide	15–20 mg/kg/day (max 2 g/day) for 2 months
	Rifampin	10 mg/kg/day (max 600 mg/day) for 4 months

Source: Reuben et al., 2002.

Prevention

TB is largely a preventable disease. In the United States, once persons infected with *M. tuberculosis* are identified they are treated with isoniazid to prevent active disease. This drug can cause hepatitis in a small percentage of patients and is especially a risk for those over 35. Liver function tests should be routinely monitored in the older patient to prevent liver complications.

Hospitals and clinics should take special precautions and isolate patients with active TB. Special filters and ultraviolet light can sterilize the air. Patients with TB should be in special rooms with controlled ventilation and reverse airflow. Healthcare workers should be tested with PPD every year.

Approximately 10 million people worldwide are infected with *M. tuberculosis* and HIV at the same time. The primary cause of death in these patients is TB, not AIDS. In the United States, it is estimated that about 20% of persons who have TB also have HIV. TB can be prevented and cured, even in people with HIV. Patients should be referred to clinics where physicians and nurses have experience in the treatment of HIV-positive patients.

LUNG CANCER

Deaths from lung cancer were virtually unknown in the United States until 1900, but the death rate has steadily increased since then. Lung cancer is responsible for almost one third of all cancer deaths in this country. The incidence of lung cancer may have reached its peak in men, but it is continuing to rise in women. More than 90% of patients with lung cancer are, or have been, cigarette smokers. Quitting cigarette smoking reduces the incidence of lung cancer, but the level of risk reaches that of a nonsmoker only after the person has remained a nonsmoker for 10 to 15 years (NHLBI, 2002).

Lung cancer and smoking are significant health problems for African Americans. In 2000, 23.2% of African Americans smoked. More than 45,000 African Americans die from smoking-related diseases annually. If current patterns continue, an estimated 1.6 million African Americans who are now under the age of 18 will become regular smokers and many will develop health problems in the future. The incidence rate (newly diagnosed cases) of lung cancer for African American men is more than 45% higher than that of White men. The mortality rate in African American men is almost 34% higher than that of White men. Women of both races have similar rates (American Lung Association, 2003). Cigarette smoking and exposure to environmental or occupational toxins (air pollution, asbestos, or lead exposure) may have a synergistic effect and speed the production of lung cancer.

Lung cancer deaths are more common in the young-old than in the old-old. Deaths from lung cancer appear at 35 to 44 years of age, and a sharp increase occurs between the ages of 45 and 55 years. The incidence continues to increase through the ages of 65 to 74 years, after which it levels off and decreases among the very old (McCance & Huether, 2002).

Types of Lung Cancer

At least 12 different types of tumors are included under the broad heading of lung cancer. Cancers of the cells that line the major bronchi or their primary branches are called squamous cell carcinomas. This type of cancer metastasizes mostly to other sites within the thorax. Adenocarcinomas are cancers of the glandular cells that line the respiratory tract. They most often start at the outer edges of the lungs and spread to the brain, the other lung, the liver, and bones. Large cell carcinomas usually begin in the outermost parts of the lung. By the time of diagnosis, they are often large, bulky tumors. Small cell carcinomas, also called "oat cell" cancers, usually begin in the bronchi. Small cell carcinomas metastasize widely to the mediastinum, liver, bones, bone marrow, central nervous system, and pancreas (NHLBI, 2002). Growth rate and metastasis rate vary by tumor type. Squamous cell carcinoma grows slowly and metastasizes late, and small cell carcinoma grows rapidly and metastasizes early.

Symptoms

The symptoms of lung cancer are vague and mimic the symptoms of other pulmonary illness, making diagnosis difficult. Chronic cough, **hemoptysis** (coughing up of blood or production of bloody sputum), chest pain, shortness of breath, fatigue, weight loss, and frequent lung infections such as pneumonia and bronchitis that do not resolve with antibiotic treatment could all be warning signs to refer the older person to the primary care provider for further testing. The chest x-ray is usually the first examination the physician will order. Suspicious masses seen on the chest x-ray may signal the need for a computerized axial tomography (CAT) scan or a magnetic resonance imaging (MRI) scan. Both the CAT scan and MRI can provide additional information about soft tissue masses. Further tests may include pulmonary function tests; bronchoscopy with the collection of lung tissue, cells, or fluids for analysis under the microscope; and biochemical and cellular studies of respiratory fluids removed from the lungs by lavage. Other important tests may include measures of arterial blood gas tensions (Pao_2 and $Paco_2$) (NHLBI, 2002).

Older patients with lung cancer may undergo surgical removal of the tumor or the lung if they are good surgical candidates and are not diagnosed with comorbid conditions. Chemotherapy, ionizing radiation to the thorax, and palliative care are less aggressive approaches used for older patients with comorbid conditions. Only 14% of White and 11% of African American patients live 5 years or longer after the diagnosis of lung cancer. Survival rates have improved only slightly over the last 10 years (American Lung Association, 2003).

RESPIRATORY INFECTIONS

Infections are a major cause of respiratory illness. They can be caused by bacteria or virus and can infect the lung, the nose, sinuses, and upper airways. Respiratory infections can also complicate other chronic illnesses and lung disease. Because of the decreased function in the immune system, older people with lung infections may not cough, exhibit an elevated temperature, or show other classic signs of respiratory infection. They may instead become lethargic, exhibit loss of cognitive or physical function, or simply stop eating and drinking. The gerontological nurse must be cognizant of the atypical presentation of respiratory infection in the older person.

Most respiratory tract infections such as the common cold, pharyngitis, and laryngitis affect only the upper airway and require no treatment. These infections, although uncomfortable, are probably viral in nature and will not respond to antibiotics. Supportive care such as rest, cough medication to suppress nighttime cough, throat lozenges, and humidifiers can ease symptoms and improve comfort.

Sinusitis is inflammation of the mucosal lining of the paranasal sinuses that can lead to mucous stasis, obstruction, and subsequent infection. Sinusitis should not be confused with rhinitis, a condition characterized by inflammation of the mucous membranes of the nose, usually accompanied by nasal discharge. Rhinitis can occur in conjunction with an upper respiratory infection or may be allergic in origin.

Sinusitis can also be caused by allergens, air pollution, and irritants such as the use of inhaled recreational drugs. Normally the sinuses will drain up to 2 pints of mucus daily and are self-cleaning through the use of cilia that propel mucus outward to the nose. When bacterial infection occurs, this drainage can be impeded by mucosal swelling induced by the inflammatory response. Sinusitis can also be induced by dental abscess, irritation of nasogastric tubes, and immune deficiency syndromes.

Acute sinusitis may be diagnosed by the presence of dull pain over the maxillary sinuses that is worsened by bending over. Congestion, green nasal discharge, periorbital edema, and fever may also be present. Acute sinusitis often follows an upper respiratory infection. Chronic sinusitis with symptoms lasting longer than 3 months is usually related to allergies. Usually, radiological examinations are not necessary and the symptoms can confirm the diagnosis. Transillumination of the sinuses with a flashlight is seldom effective to confirm the diagnosis of sinusitis in an older person and is difficult to perform in many clinical settings.

Treatment of sinusitis usually involves nasal decongestants (phenylephrine 0.25%), one or two sprays every 4 hours in each nostril for up to 5 days; saline spray to lubricate and moisten the nares; and acetaminophen for discomfort. Humidified air may provide some relief. For acute sinusitis, some clinicians advocate treatment with antimicrobials such as Augmentin 500 mg every 12 hours for 2 weeks. As the sinuses are poorly perfused, longer treatment may be necessary to ensure that all areas of infection receive adequate concentrations of antibiotics and that the responsible bacteria are truly eradicated.

The use of antibiotics to treat upper respiratory infections and simple pharyngitis is not recommended because it encourages antibiotic resistance. Most upper respiratory infections will resolve spontaneously within 7 to 10 days. However, infections of the lower respiratory tract such as bronchitis and pneumonia are more serious in the older person and require aggressive evaluation and treatment.

Infections of the lower respiratory tract are the sixth leading cause of death in the United States and the fourth leading cause of death in Americans 80 years of age and older (Karnath, Agyeman, & Lai, 2003). Pneumonia, or inflammation of the lungs, is the most common type of infectious disease of the lung. Infectious pneumonias are usually identified by naming the cause of the infection or the pattern of infection in the lung (e.g., lobar pneumonia). Mortality rates from pneumonia have not decreased significantly since the 1950s. Among patients with community-acquired pneumonia, mortality approaches 20%. Mortality from nosocomial pneumonia, an infection acquired while institutionalized in a hospital or nursing home, can approach 30% and reflects both the underlying frailty of the older person and the predominance of virulent pathogens present in institutional settings.

The following risk factors are thought to increase susceptibility to respiratory infection in the older lung and to affect the outcome of pneumonia:

- History of nosocomial pneumonia within the last 6 months to 1 year
- Diagnosed lung disease (COPD)
- Recent hospitalization
- Nursing home residence
- Smoking
- Alcoholism
- Neurologic disease (dementia, cerebrovascular accident)
- Immunosuppression (corticosteroid use, malignancy)
- Use of oxygen therapy
- Severe protein-calorie malnutrition
- Heart failure

- Antibiotic therapy during the previous month
- Eating dependency
- Enteral feeding by nasogastric tube

(Reichmuth & Meyer, 2003; Rothan-Tondeur et al., 2003)

Aspiration is a major risk factor for the development of pneumonia and stroke, dementia, and dysphagia. Gastric tube placements are major risk factors for aspiration. Sedative and narcotic use is associated with decreased levels of consciousness, lethargy, and nighttime aspiration. Viral infections, in particular influenza A, are a risk factor for secondary bacterial pneumonia (Reichmuth & Meyer, 2003).

Pathogens

Bacterial pathogens are the most frequent cause of pneumonia. *Streptococcus pneumoniae* remains the most prevalent bacterial pathogen and is estimated to account for approximately 50% of all infections. In addition, *Haemophilus influenzae, Staphylococcus aureus,* and Enterobacteriaceae cause more pneumonia in the older person than in the young. Atypical agents such as *Legionella* make up a smaller portion of pneumonias in elderly patients than in younger patients, and pneumonia caused by *Mycoplasma pneumoniae* is rare after the age of 55. *H. influenzae* and *Moraxella catarrhalis* bronchial infections are commonly associated with lower tract infections in patients with COPD (Reichmuth & Meyer, 2003). Influenza is four times more common in persons over 70 years of age than in younger adults. In most years, persons over 65 account for about 90% of influenza-associated deaths in the United States. Epidemics, sometimes associated with high mortality, are a problem in institutional settings. Virus can be spread by airborne droplets, caregivers, and exposure to contaminated respiratory equipment.

Inflammatory Response

The inflammatory response of the lung in pneumonia varies depending on the type of infection and might include:

- **Lobar consolidation.** Solidification of the lung as air spaces are filled with fluid and cellular debris.
- **Interstitial inflammation.** Inflammatory changes and scarring, along with alveolar wall injury.
- **Necrosis.** Death and decay of lung tissue. Dead and dying cells accumulate in the lungs and impede air exchange.
- **Cavitation.** Hollow spaces walled off by scar tissue.
- **Abscess.** Formation of pus.
- **Granuloma formation.** Production of tumorlike masses of different kinds of cells due to a chronic inflammatory response.

(NHLBI, 2002a)

Symptoms of Pneumonia

The classic symptoms of pneumonia are cough, fever, and sputum production. Fever may be absent because many older people have a lower basal temperature and will not exhibit a fever response in the face of infection. Bacterial pneumonias are commonly preceded by a viruslike prodrome of headache, myalgia, and lethargy. Other symptoms may include abrupt onset of shaking chills (rigors). Nonbacterial pneumonia may be accompanied by substernal chest pain and dyspnea. However, the gerontological nurse must be alert for subtle changes in behavior and baseline physical signs. New-onset tachycardia and tachypnea are important clues to illness with both viral and bacterial pneumonia. Changes in function, appetite, continence, and other subtle symptoms may be the first signs of the onset of illness.

Nursing Assessment of Pneumonia

When the gerontological nurse suspects pneumonia, health assessment should include checking vital signs, inspecting the thorax, and auscultating the lungs. The skin should be examined for cyanosis. Crackles that do not clear with coughing may be suggestive of pneumonia. Signs of consolidation (bronchial breath sounds, dullness to percussion, and egophony) are common findings with late-stage pneumonia.

The primary care provider will probably request a chest x-ray; however, it may be negative in early stages of the disease. Physical findings will probably precede the appearance of an infiltrate by about 24 hours. After resolution of the pneumonia, the chest x-ray will not appear normal for about 6 weeks. Sputum for analysis is difficult to obtain from an older person as it requires a vigorous cough reflex. Many sputum samples sent for analysis contain mostly saliva or secretions from the upper airways that may reveal "carriage" or "colonization" (the bacteria an older person has living in the upper airway). These organisms may be completely different from the pathogens in the lungs responsible for the pneumonia. Pulse oximetry of arterial blood gases provides valuable information about the patient's status. Hypoxemia is associated with poor outcome. Older patients with severe hypoxemia should be referred to the acute care setting for immediate evaluation. A blood chemistry analysis may reveal marked leukocytosis, indicating white blood cells are being produced to try to fight off the infection.

Hospitalization for pneumonia should be considered when:

- Comorbidities are present (lung disease, alcoholism, malnutrition, congestive heart failure).
- Respiratory rate exceeds 30 breaths per minute.
- Hemoptysis is present.
- Diastolic blood pressure is less than 60 mmHg or systolic blood pressure is less than 90 mmHg.
- Temperature exceeds 38.3°C or 101°F.
- PaO_2 is less than 60 mmHg on room air.
- Chest x-ray shows more than one lobe involvement, presence of a cavity, or presence of a pleural effusion.
- There is evidence of sepsis.
- Patient is unable to take oral fluids.

(American Thoracic Society, 2002).

Treatment of Pneumonia

In the 1940s, widespread use of penicillin helped reduce mortality from *S. pneumoniae* infections. In the 1960s, resistance to penicillin by some organisms began to be reported, with patients dying despite treatment. Resistance was not considered a major problem until the early 1990s. Studies indicate that about 25% of isolates of *S. pneumoniae* are now resistant to penicillin (Karnath et al., 2003). The emergence of drug-resistant pneumococci and the development of new antimicrobials have changed the empirical treatment of pneumonia. Newer fluoroquinolones with activity against *S. pneumoniae* offer alternatives in the treatment of drug-resistant *S. pneumoniae* infection. New macrolides such as azithromycin and clarithromycin may be preferable to erythromycin because of better gastrointestinal tolerance (Epocrates, 2003).

The treatment recommendations for older outpatients with community-acquired pneumonia are an oral macrolide (erythromycin, azithromycin, or clarithromycin) or an oral beta-lactam (cefuroxime, amoxicillin, or amoxicillin-clavulanate). Patients allergic to a macrolide or a beta-lactam may take a fluoroquinolone (Reuben et al., 2002). For critically ill hospitalized older patients, an intravenous third-generation cephalosporin in combination with a macrolide is recommended.

Additional supportive treatments include chest percussion to clear secretions, inhaled beta-adrenergic agonists to dilate constricted airways, oxygen if needed, and rehydration. Although treatment of pneumonia is the same for all patients regardless of age, the older person requires more careful monitoring. Agents with nephrotoxic potential, like the aminoglycosides, should be used with caution. Hypersensitivity reactions are more frequent in older patients, and risk of antibiotic-associated diarrhea or colitis is common with ampicillin or clindamycin. Drug interactions may also occur between antibiotics and other therapeutic agents commonly used in older persons such as warfarin. Intravenous fluids should be administered slowly in patients with congestive heart failure to prevent overhydration and pulmonary edema.

Prevention

The current 23-valent pneumococcal vaccine was developed in 1983. Although there are over 80 serotypes of pneumococci that can cause pneumonia, the 23 most common serotypes are covered in the vaccine. The vaccine is approved by the U.S. Food and Drug Administration, and Medicare covers the cost of administration.

Vaccination is recommended for all persons 65 years of age and older and all adults with immunosuppression or chronic illnesses. It is estimated that only about 25% of older patients with risk factors have received the pneumococcal immunization. The vaccine is approximately 80% effective with decreasing effectiveness over time. Revaccination every 6 years is recommended for persons with renal failure, those who have had splenectomies, those with underlying malignancy, and patients with HIV/AIDS. When an older person's immunization status is unknown, the pneumococcal vaccine should be administered (Morbidity and Mortality Weekly Report, 2003). Revaccination has minimal side effects, with the most common being a localized reaction at the injection site.

The influenza vaccine should also be received yearly in persons who are at risk for pneumonia. The pneumococcal and influenza vaccines may be administered at the same time. The influenza vaccine alone is associated with a 52% reduction in hospitalizations for pneumonia, and the pneumococcal vaccine alone is associated with a 25% reduction in hospitalization for pneumonia. When both vaccines are given, the reduction in hospitalizations for pneumonia is 63% (American Thoracic Society, 2004).

Practice Pearl

When an older person has been hospitalized for pneumonia and discharge planning is under way, remind the physician to order the pneumococcal vaccine before the patient leaves the hospital. An older person who has had one pneumonia is at high risk for acquiring another.

Nursing Diagnoses

The following nursing diagnoses may be appropriate for nursing care plans of older patients with pneumonia: *risk for infection,* based on advanced age or immunosuppression; *altered health maintenance,* based on poor nutrition, tobacco or alcohol use; *noncompliance,* based on inability or unwillingness to take medications as prescribed; *ineffective airway clearance,* based on altered cough reflex and excessive secretions; *risk for aspiration,* based on diagnosis with neurologic disease such as cerebrovascular accident or dementia; and *ineffective tissue perfusion,* based upon the presence of hypoxia.

Patient-Teaching Guidelines for the Older Patient With Lung Disease

Older patients with pneumonia should be urged to rest and restrict activities to allow themselves time to heal and completely recover. Many will begin to recover after 5 to 7 days of antibiotic therapy. Additional patient education points include the following:

- Stop smoking (permanently if possible, mandatory during acute treatment).
- Take 10 deep breaths an hour to aerate lungs and loosen secretions.
- Drink plenty of fluids to keep secretions moist.
- Take antibiotics as prescribed and finish all medication.
- Report any adverse reactions immediately such as diarrhea, gastrointestinal irritation, rash or hives, and difficulty breathing.
- Avoid contact with others who are ill, infants, and frail older persons.
- Avoid coughing in public and practice good hand washing.
- Receive the pneumococcal vaccine as soon as possible after recovery and get a flu shot yearly to minimize the risk of further infection.

ACUTE BRONCHITIS

Acute bronchitis is an acute inflammation of the bronchi. It is usually a self-limiting viral illness. The signs and symptoms are similar to those of pneumonia and include productive cough, chills, lethargy, and low-grade fever. Chest x-ray will be negative, showing no active disease or infiltrates. Chest pain may be produced by muscle strain from prolonged and excessive coughing. Treatment consists of rest, humidification of the air, use of cough suppressants, and acetaminophen for aches.

Persons with COPD will usually be treated for bronchitis with antibiotics because their bronchitis may easily progress to pneumonia. This condition is sometimes called acute exacerbation of chronic bronchitis. Some physicians instruct their COPD patients to phone immediately upon noticing a change in sputum color from clear to white or green.

PULMONARY EMBOLISM

Pulmonary embolism is an occlusion of a portion of the pulmonary vascular bed by an embolus consisting of a thrombus, an air bubble, or a fragment of tissue or lipids. The highly branched network of blood vessels in the lung aerates the blood as it flows through the lungs. When the blockage occurs, gas exchange can no longer take place in this section of the lung. The result is shortness of breath, heart failure, or death. Pulmonary emboli in older persons most often originate from deep vein thrombosis in the calf.

Pulmonary emboli are the third leading cause of death in the United States and account for about 100,000 deaths per year (American Lung Association, 2003). Depending on the size of the embolism, various degrees of hypoxemia can occur. A large occlusion in a major artery will cause severe results such as pain from infarcted lung tissue, decreased cardiac output, hypotension, and death. Smaller emboli may be chronic or recurrent in nature and result in vasoconstriction, pulmonary edema, and atelectasis. If the embolus does not cause infarction, the clot will usually dissolve and the lung will return to normal. If an infarction does occur, scarring will develop and lung function may be permanently lost.

Risk factors for formation of pulmonary embolus include clotting disorders, immobility, dehydration, recent surgery, atherosclerotic changes in the circulatory system, atrial fibrillation, and obesity. As many as 65% of patients with lower extremity trauma or surgery will develop deep vein thrombosis (American Thoracic Society, 2004).

Symptoms

Typical symptoms of pulmonary embolus include tachypnea, dyspnea, chest pain, hypoxia, decreased cardiac output, systemic hypotension, and possible shock.

Nursing Assessment

Patients with leg swelling, duskiness, and a positive Homans' sign (calf pain on dorsiflexion of the foot) are at risk for pulmory embolus. In persons with suspected deep vein thrombosis, the calf of the affected leg should be carefully measured and the size noted and compared to the other leg. Asymmetry of more than 1 cm increases the likelihood of deep vein thrombosis from 27% to 56% in an at-risk individual (McCance & Huether, 2002). Positive ultrasound studies of the leg warrant the initiation of anticoagulation therapy for prevention of pulmonary embolus (Reuben et al., 2002).

Hypoxemia and hyperventilation are suggestive of the diagnosis of pulmonary embolus. A perfusion scan, in which lungs are scanned after injection of a radioactive dye into the venous circulation, can indicate obstruction of pulmonary circulation.

Treatment

Treatment consists of intravenous administration of heparin and other anticoagulant therapy. For large, life-threatening pulmonary obstructions, a fibrinolytic agent such as streptokinase is sometimes used; however, streptokinase cannot be administered within 7 to 10 days after surgery (Reuben et al., 2002). Warfarin therapy may be continued for 3 to 6 months after discharge to prevent the formation of another pulmonary embolus.

The gerontological nurse can play a vital role in the prevention of pulmonary embolus by identifying persons at risk and reducing risk factors. Appropriate interventions include minimizing venous stasis by leg elevation, urging passive and active range of motion exercises in the immobile older person, encouraging early postoperative ambulation, and placing elastic compression stockings and pneumatic calf compression boots on the postoperative patient. Low-dose anticoagulation therapy with heparin is sometimes beneficial to prevent clots in postoperative patients until they become mobile. Prevention is key because less anticoagulant is needed to prevent a clot than to dissolve one already formed.

Nursing Diagnoses

Nursing diagnoses for older patients with pulmonary embolism may include (North American Nursing Diagnosis Association, 2004) *ineffective breathing patterns* when inspiration and/or expiration does not provide adequate ventilation, *risk for suffocation* (in life-threatening situations, anxiety, fear) *activity intolerance* related to hypoxia, *death anxiety,* and *acute pain.* Dyspnea or air hunger as a result of pulmonary embolism will usually result in extreme anxiety and requires emergency treatment.

SEVERE ACUTE RESPIRATORY SYNDROME (SARS)

Within the recent past, an international outbreak of a virus suspected to be a mutated form of the Coronavirus has occurred. About 26 countries have been affected, with the most severe problems occurring in the Far East and parts of Canada. At this time, there is no definite cure for SARS, but treatment with antivirals and supportive care including oxygen administration and mechanical ventilation has been effective for some SARS patients.

The primary symptoms of SARS are lethargy, muscle aches, dry cough, difficulty breathing, and persistent fever over 38°C or 100.4°F (Centers for Disease Control,

2003). Older people with these symptoms who have traveled to a high-risk country, or have been exposed to someone who has, should seek medical attention immediately.

Preventive measures include wearing a face mask when in public areas of high-risk countries, strict isolation of infected persons, and careful hand washing. The virus is hardy and has been shown to survive on various surfaces for 24 hours. The mortality rate from SARS is highest in persons over 50. Intensive efforts to find an accurate diagnostic test and effective treatment or cure are under way at the time of this writing.

Patient-Family Teaching Guidelines

Gerontological nurses require skills and knowledge related to teaching patients and families about the key concepts of gerontology and gerontological nursing. The patient-family teaching guidelines in the following feature will assist the nurse to assume the role of teacher and coach. Educating patients and families is critical so that nurses can interpret scientific data and individualize the nursing care plan.

Patient-Family Teaching Guidelines

LUNG DISEASE

The following are guidelines that the nurse may find useful when instructing older persons and their families about lung disease.

1. How can I prevent lung disease?

Because respiratory problems are so often caused or aggravated by environmental exposure to toxins and pollutants, try to avoid these substances if at all possible. Some points to consider are:

- Do not smoke cigarettes or other tobacco products.

- Do not visit or work in areas where dangerous substances or irritants are in the air (oven cleaner, glues, spray paints, etc.).

- Do not go outside or exercise when smog is present or air pollution warnings are in effect.

- Try to avoid contact with ill people and places where illness rates are high.

RATIONALE:

The prevention of respiratory disease is easier and safer than the treatment and cure. Stress prevention principles whenever appropriate.

2. If I already have lung disease, is there anything I can do to stop it?

Yes. If you smoke, stop immediately! Also carry out all the suggestions listed in question 1. If you are prescribed medication by your doctor, take it exactly as directed. Report any worsening of your condition or new symptoms to your doctor. Have your disease monitored with spirometry testing as often as recommended by your doctor and get to know your numbers.

RATIONALE:

Chronic lung disease requires careful ongoing monitoring to prevent crises and exacerbations. Careful ongoing assessment is needed.

3. Is there anything else I should do to make the most of living with lung disease?

Yes. Exercise to keep your muscles fit and strong, eat a healthy diet, control your weight, get a flu shot every fall, get the pneumonia shot at age 65 and then every 6 years afterward, and visit the dentist regularly. Good oral hygiene can decrease respiratory infections and keep you healthy.

RATIONALE:

Improvement and maintenance of general good health will improve function and quality of life for an older person with respiratory disease. Education regarding health maintenance is always appropriate.

Care Plan

Case Study

Mr. Lehman is admitted to the nursing home with the diagnoses of moderate dementia, COPD, and frequent falls. He is 84 years old. He no longer smokes, although he has a 50-year smoking history. He has an involved and loving son who lives nearby and a daughter in California who has not seen her father for several years. He has specified no advance directives.

About 1 week after admission, Mr. Lehman begins to exhibit symptoms of dyspnea on exertion. He had been walking approximately 50 feet to the dining room without difficulty and now finds he has to rest after walking about 20 feet. When questioned, Mr. Lehman states, "I just seem to run out of air when I walk." He has no fever, chills, chest pain, or lower extremity edema. His pulse is 96 and his respiratory rate is 26 at rest.

Applying the Nursing Process

ASSESSMENT

The gerontological nurse faces a dilemma because there is not a lot of baseline information regarding Mr. Lehman. However, even with only 1 week of observation and experience, it seems clear that he is having a change from his baseline level of function. The nurse should think broadly and perform a head-to-toe nursing assessment to get further information. Vital signs should be carefully assessed because he presents with tachypnea and tachycardia at rest. Obtaining pulse oximetry at rest and on exertion may yield valuable information. Should hypoxemia be noted, activity should be restricted and oxygen provided to prevent cardiac complications.

Even though Mr. Lehman has a diagnosis of dementia, he should be carefully questioned about any symptoms of chest pain, difficulty breathing at other times, or presence of sore throat or cough that could indicate onset of new illness. It is useful to quantify dypsnea if possible. Sudden and unexpected onset of dyspnea can be associated with pulmonary embolus, pneumonia, or exacerbation of chronic bronchitis. Nocturnal dyspnea may be associated with congestive heart failure. Mr. Lehman should be weighed and his baseline weight compared with the current weight. A change of over 2 or 3 lbs may indicate congestive heart failure with the retention of excessive fluid. Just because he does not have a fever, the gerontological nurse cannot be assured he is not developing a respiratory infection. The medical record should be reviewed to see whether Mr. Lehman received the pneumococcal vaccine within the last 6 years and the flu shot within the last year.

A Patient With Lung Disease

Another possibility is that Mr. Lehman may have an undisclosed swallowing disorder and have aspirated a foreign body that is partially occluding his bronchus. A careful review of his eating habits and preferences will assist the nurse in this area.

DIAGNOSIS

The nursing diagnosis for Mr. Lehman would be:

- *Activity intolerance related to hypoxia.*

EXPECTED OUTCOMES

The expected outcomes for the plan of care specify that Mr. Lehman will:

- Return to baseline function with appropriate treatment and monitoring of his chronic lung disease and hypoxia.
- Maintain or return to normal body weight with adequate nutritional intake.
- Agree to establish a therapeutic relationship with the nurse and develop a mutually acceptable plan to work toward these outcomes.
- Identify wishes toward treatment and establish advance directives as appropriate to patient and family preferences.

PLANNING AND IMPLEMENTATION

The nurse should contact Mr. Lehman's primary care provider and report the change in condition and the information gathered in the nursing assessment. As Mr. Lehman has no advance directives and has a diagnosis of moderate dementia, the family should also be contacted. They may be able to provide valuable information regarding his past medical history, including any previous episodes of dyspnea.

Mr. Lehman and his family should also discuss and communicate to the healthcare team regarding the way they would like him to be treated. For instance, they may want him to be sent to the hospital for aggressive assessment and care, they may wish diagnosis and treatment to occur in the nursing home, or they may prefer palliative care be delivered with emphasis on symptom control and patient comfort. This information is crucial and will form the basis for future healthcare decisions.

EVALUATION

The nurse hopes to work with Mr. Lehman and will consider the plan a success based on the following criteria:

- Mr. Lehman will exhibit normal pulse and respiratory rates and oxygen saturation readings at rest and on exertion.
- A family meeting will be held to discuss his overall health, values, and advance directives.
- Mr. Lehman will maintain or work toward normal body weight, functional status, and satisfactory quality of life.
- He will receive appropriate immunizations (pneumonia and yearly flu vaccines) to prevent exacerbation of chronic lung disease.

(continued)

A Patient With Lung Disease *(continued)*

Ethical Dilemma

When Mr. Lehman is questioned about naming a healthcare proxy or someone to make decisions for him if he should become unable, he states, "Yes, I'd like to name my daughter in California. I love my son but I don't trust him to make the right decisions for me." The nurse reports this to the physician and the appropriate papers are signed.

The next day, the physician brings this up in discussion with Mr. Lehman and his son. His son seems offended and states, "Well you know he is ill and sometimes his mind wanders. I think I should be the one to make all healthcare decisions for my dad."

The issue here is the conflict between Mr. Lehman's autonomy (the right to determine his healthcare proxy) and beneficence (what is in his best interest). Clearly, further information and involvement of the healthcare team are needed. On the surface, it seems to make more sense for Mr. Lehman's son to be the healthcare proxy. He lives locally, is involved in his father's care, visits daily, and keeps track of his progress and health status. However, just because the daughter lives in California and seems less involved does not negate Mr. Lehman's desire to name her as proxy if he has the capacity to make an informed decision.

The nursing code of ethics supports the patient's right to self-determination and believes that nurses will and must play a primary role in implementing this right. The nurse should identify and mobilize mechanisms in place within the facility to resolve this conflict. Hopefully, the nursing home has an interdisciplinary ethics team with nursing representation to address and resolve this dispute.

Critical Thinking and the Nursing Process

1. What nursing interventions can you identify to help older persons to quit smoking?
2. What advice would you give to a teenager who is just starting to smoke cigarettes?
3. Describe your feelings regarding older people who are reliant on the use of portable oxygen and a nasal cannula to function adequately.

■ Evaluate your responses in Appendix B.

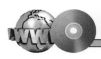

EXPLORE MediaLink

NCLEX review, case studies, and other interactive resources for this chapter can be found on the Companion Website at **www.prenhall.com/tabloski**. Click on Chapter 16 to select the activities for this chapter. For animations, video tutorials, more NCLEX review questions, and case studies, access the accompanying CD-ROM in this textbook.

Chapter Highlights

- The two major functions of the respiratory system are related to respiration and metabolic function.

- Normal changes of aging, exposure to environmental toxins and pollution, and concomitant illness can affect the structure and function of the respiratory system.

- Because many problems related to respiratory function are a direct result of years of cigarette smoking, the gerontological nurse can function as an educator and change agent to assist the older patient to quit smoking. African Americans are disproportionately affected by smoking-related respiratory illness.

- Tuberculosis is a serious problem that can affect older people by reactivation of an old infection or the acquisition of new-onset disease after exposure to others with the disease.

- Immunosuppression, chronic illness, and living in a long-term care facility are risk factors for developing tuberculosis. Purified protein derivative testing in the older person should involve the two-step approach with another vaccine administered 1 week after the first one with negative results.

- Respiratory infections like pneumonia and influenza can cause death and disability for the older person, especially in the presence of diagnosed neurologic disease and immunosuppression. Because of the decreased immune response, it may be difficult to diagnose pneumonia in the older person.

- The gerontological nurse should suspect pneumonia when the older person exhibits changes in behavior, appetite, continence, or function. Tachypnea and tachycardia may be early warning signs of pneumonia.

- Antibiotic therapy and supportive treatment are necessary to treat pneumonia in the older person. Prevention using the pneumococcal and influenza vaccine is recommended.

- Pulmonary embolism is a potentially life-threatening blockage of the blood vessels in the lungs and accounts for about 100,000 deaths per year. Preventive measures include minimizing venous stasis through early postoperative ambulation and calf compression. Low-dose anticoagulation may be needed for immobile older persons.

- SARS is a serious respiratory illness. At the present time it is difficult to diagnose and cure. Travel to high-risk countries should be curtailed or delayed if outbreaks are known to be occurring.

References

American Lung Association. (2003). *American Lung Association fact sheet: African Americans and lung disease.* Retrieved November 14, 2003, from www.lungusa.org.

American Thoracic Society. (2002). *Diagnosis and care of patients with COPD.* Retrieved September 17, 2002, from www.thoracic.org.

American Thoracic Society. (2004). *Statement on cardiopulmonary exercise testing.* Retrieved November 9, 2004, from www.thoracic.org.

Centers for Disease Control. (2003). *Questions and answers about TB.* www.cdc.gov.

Epocrates. (2003). Retrieved September 14, 2003, from Drug Program www.epocrates.

Karnath, B., Agyeman, A., & Lai, A. (2003). Pneumococcal pneumonia: Update on therapy in the era of antibiotic resistance. *Consultant, 43*(3), 321–326.

McCance, K., & Huether, S. (2002). *Pathophysiology: The biologic basis for disease in adults and children.* St. Louis, MO: Mosby.

McGann, E., & Fitzgerald, C. (2001). Dyspnea. In M. Mezey (Ed.), *The encyclopedia of elder care.* New York: Springer.

Morbidity and Mortality Weekly Report. (1997). *Advisory committee on immunization practices.* Retrieved September 14, 2003, from www.cdc.gov/mmwr.

Morbidity and Mortality Weekly Report. (2003). *Influenza and pneumococcal vaccination coverage among persons > 65 years and persons 18–64 years with diabetes and asthma.* (Vol. 53: No. 43). Retrieved December 15, 2004, from Center for Disease Control www.cdc.gov/mmwr/pdf/wk/mm5343.pdf.

NANDA. (2004). Nursing Diagnoses: Definitions and Classifications. NANDA International: Philadelphia.

National Heart, Lung, and Blood Institute (NHLBI). (2002a). *The lungs in health and disease.* National Institutes of Health, U.S. Department of Health and Human Services, No. 97–3279.

National Heart, Lung, and Blood Institute (NHLBI). (2002b). *Considerations for diagnosing and managing asthma in the elderly.* National Asthma Education and Prevention Program, National Institutes of Health, No. 96-3662.

National Institute of Allergy and Infectious Diseases. (2002). *Tuberculosis.* National Institutes of Health, U.S. Department of Health and Human Services. Retrieved November 12, 2003, from www.niaid.nih.gov.

Nurses Asthma Education Partnership Project. (2003). Nurses: Partners in Asthma Care. National Heart, Lung, and Blood Institute, National Institutes of Health. Retrieved November 12, 2003, from www.nhlbi.nih.gov.

Nurses: Partners in Asthma Care. (1995). National Asthma Education and Prevention Program, National Heart, Lung, and Blood Institute, NIH Publication No. 95-3308.

Nurses: Partners in Asthma Care. (1998). *Guidelines for the diagnosis and management of asthma.* National Institutes of Health. Retrieved December 12, 2003, from www.nhlbi.nih.gov.

Nursing Diagnoses: Definitions and Classification. NANDA International: Philadelphia.

Reichmuth, K., & Meyer, K. (2003). Management of community-acquired pneumonia in the elderly. *Annals of Long-Term Care, 11*(7), 27–31.

Reuben, D., Herr, K., Pacala, J., Potter, J., Pollock, B., & Semla, T. (2002). *Geriatrics at your fingertips.* Malden, MA: American Geriatrics Society, Blackwell.

Rothan-Tondeur, M., Meaume, S., Gizard, L., Weill-Engerer, S., Lancien, E., Abdelmalak, S., et al. (2003). Risk factors for nosocomial pneumonia in a geriatric hospital: A control-case one-center study. *Journal of the American Geriatrics Society, 51,* 997–1001.

Sandoz Biochemicals (2005). TB facts and figures. Retrieved June 23, 2005, from www.sandoz.com.

CHAPTER 17

The Genitourinary and Renal Systems

Tamara L. Zurakowski, PHD, CRNP, APRN, BC

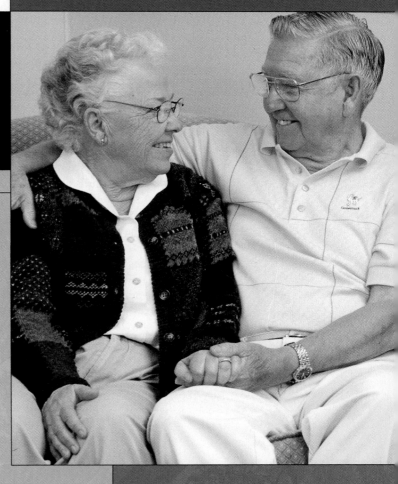

CHAPTER OBJECTIVES

Upon completion of this chapter, the reader will be able to:

- Describe the normal changes of aging in the physiology of the genitourinary and renal systems.

- Differentiate among normal and disease-related changes in genitourinary and renal function in the older adult.

- Identify the impact of changes in urinary function on the quality of life of older persons.

- Define appropriate nursing interventions for improving the effect of genitourinary status on quality of life of older adults.

- Recognize one's own biases related to sexuality and aging.

- Discuss the effect of the social and physical environment on genitourinary concerns in elderly adults.

MediaLink

Additional resources for this chapter can be found on the Student CD-ROM accompanying this textbook and on the Companion Website at **www.prenhall.com/tabloski**. Click on Chapter 17 to select the activities for this chapter.

CD-ROM
- Animations/Videos
    Breast Cancer
    Erectile Dysfunction
    Genitourinary/Renal A&P
    Kidney Stones
    Renal Failure
- NCLEX Review

- Case Studies
- Tools

COMPANION WEBSITE
- Audio Glossary
- Additional NCLEX Review
- Case Study
- MediaLink Applications

KEY TERMS

atrophic vaginitis 534
bladder training 531
detrusor muscles 521
dyspareunia 541
erectile dysfunction 524
functional incontinence 529
intimacy 539
nocturia 533
overflow incontinence 529
pelvic floor exercises (Kegel exercises) 532
renal failure 525
sexuality 518
sexually transmitted diseases 536

Discussing matters relating to **sexuality**, the reproductive organs, and elimination of body waste is considered to be socially taboo and may be deeply embarrassing to the older adult. Most individuals have been independent in toileting since toddlerhood, and may be reluctant to admit having difficulty in this most private matter. Today's elderly adults grew up in an era when sexuality was not discussed, and they have carried this sensibility into advanced age. It is unlikely that they discussed sex with their own parents; therefore, they may have very little information about what to expect as they age. In addition, many people accept as "normal" such genitourinary phenomena as incontinence, impotence, and dyspareunia.

Nurses may also find it embarrassing or uncomfortable to discuss sexuality or urination, and may hold unconscious biases about aged individuals. Some may consider elderly adults to be asexual, neither desiring nor needing an active sex life. Others may consider incontinence to be a minor annoyance and may overlook the effects it has on the quality of life of an older individual. It is important to be aware of one's belief system and to identify possible biases. Sensitivity to the emotions of both client *and* nurse is crucial if the nurse is to intervene effectively to promote or restore the health of persons with concerns related to the genitourinary tract.

Compassionate and skillful nursing care for older adults requires scientific knowledge, self-awareness, and strong communication skills. The North American Nursing Diagnosis Association (2001) has identified 14 nursing diagnoses related to *urinary elimination* or *sexuality patterns,* and they are as pertinent to older adults as they are to younger people.

Normal Changes of Aging

It is difficult to differentiate normal aging of the genitourinary system from that related to common pathologies found in older people. It is prudent, therefore, to keep an open mind when discussing age-related changes.

The genitourinary system includes the organs of urinary elimination (kidneys, ureters, bladder, and urethra) and reproduction in both men (penis, testis, epididymis, vas deferens, seminal vesicles, and prostate) and women (ovaries, fallopian tubes, uterus, cervix, vagina, and vulva). Hormones, such as testosterone, luteinizing hormone–releasing hormone (LHRH), luteinizing hormone (LH), follicle-stimulating hormone (FSH), estrogens, progesterone, and antidiuretic hormone (ADH), are responsible for regulation of the system (McCance & Huether, 2001). The urinary system removes wastes from the body and participates in the regulation of fluid and electrolyte balance, blood pressure, and red blood cell production. The genital system provides for the conception and birth of children, and is integral to expressions of intimacy and self-concept. Figure 17-1 ■ illustrates the normal changes of aging in the male and female genitourinary system.

AGE-RELATED CHANGES IN THE KIDNEY

The kidney in a 90-year-old person weighs 20% to 30% less than that of a 30-year-old, with a concomitant decrease in size and loss of 30% to 40% of the glomeruli (Beck, 1999). Sclerosis may be found in as many as 40% of the remaining glomeruli, and fibrous changes in the interstitial tissues may be found in older persons without kidney

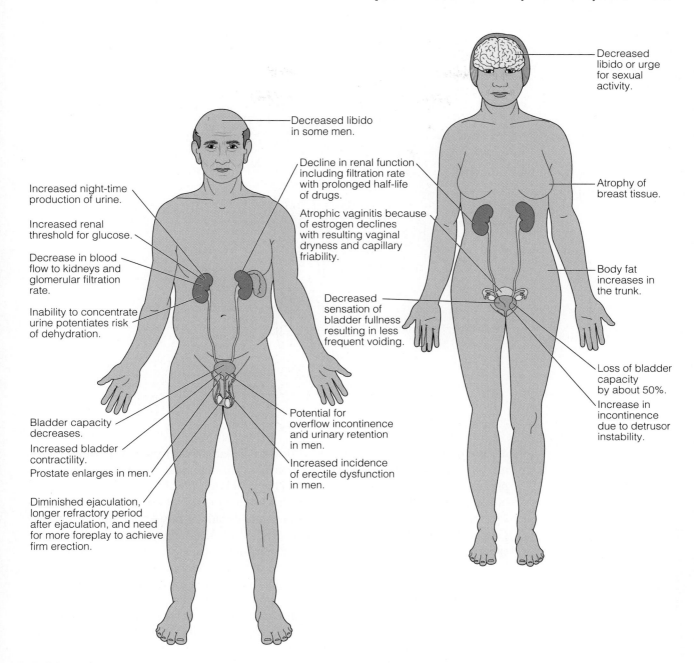

Decreased libido
in some men.

Decline in renal function
including filtration rate
with prolonged half-life
of drugs.

Atrophic vaginitis because
of estrogen declines
with resulting vaginal
dryness and capillary
friability.

Increased night-time
production of urine.

Increased renal
threshold for glucose.

Decrease in blood
flow to kidneys and
glomerular filtration
rate.

Inability to concentrate
urine potentiates risk
of dehydration.

Decreased
sensation of
bladder fullness
resulting in less
frequent voiding.

Bladder capacity
decreases.

Increased bladder
contractility.

Prostate enlarges in men.

Diminished ejaculation,
longer refractory period
after ejaculation, and need
for more foreplay to achieve
firm erection.

Potential for
overflow incontinence
and urinary retention
in men.

Increased incidence
of erectile dysfunction
in men.

Decreased
libido or urge
for sexual
activity.

Atrophy of
breast tissue.

Body fat
increases in
the trunk.

Loss of bladder
capacity
by about 50%.

Increase in
incontinence
due to detrusor
instability.

FIGURE ◻ 17-1

Normal changes of aging in the genitourinary system.

FIGURE ◼ **17-2**

Anatomy of a nephron.

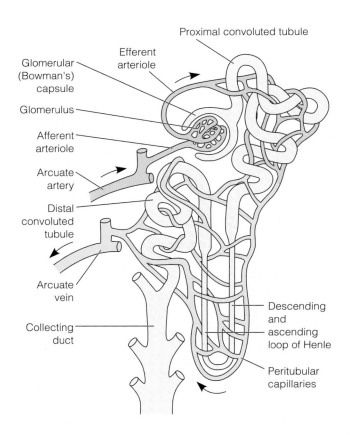

Proximal convoluted tubule

Efferent arteriole

Glomerular (Bowman's) capsule

Glomerulus

Afferent arteriole

Arcuate artery

Distal convoluted tubule

Arcuate vein

Collecting duct

Descending and ascending loop of Henle

Peritubular capillaries

disease (Sands & Vega, 1999). Blood flow to the kidney decreases as a result of atrophy in the supplying blood vessels, particularly in the renal cortex. In addition, the proximal tubules decrease in number and length. Figure 17-2 ◼ illustrates the anatomy of a nephron. Although these changes start around the age of 40, they do not become significant until an individual reaches the ninth decade of life. At that time, decreased glomerular filtration rate, renal blood flow, maximal urinary concentration, and response to sodium loss are marked. The older adult will usually demonstrate a lower creatinine clearance than a young adult. The older person will typically excrete lower levels of glucose, acid, and potassium, and the specific gravity of the urine will be lower (less concentrated). The serum creatinine level, however, may increase to as much as 1.9 mg/dl without negative consequences, and the blood urea nitrogen (BUN) may rise to 69 mg/dl (Kennedy-Malone, Fletcher, & Plank, 2000). The older kidney, in contrast to the kidneys in younger adults, excretes more fluid and electrolytes at night than in the daytime. More urine is formed at night, potentially interrupting sleep patterns. In addition, because older adults excrete lower levels of glucose in the urine, testing for glycosuria is not an accurate method of monitoring blood glucose levels.

Drug Alert

Because of renal excretion changes, be particularly vigilant for signs of toxicity when older patients are taking antibiotics, digoxin, diuretics, beta-blockers, statin lipid-lowering agents, ACE inhibitors, and oral antidiabetic agents (Schwartz, 1999).

The ability to respond to a fluid overload by increasing urine production is also decreased in the older adult. One of the consequences of these changes is an impairment in the excretion of drugs and their metabolites, making older adults extremely susceptible to drug overdoses and other adverse medication effects, even within a normal dose range (McCance & Huether, 2001). Another consequence is an increased probability of hyperkalemia, particularly when potassium sparing diuretics, ACE inhibitors, nonsteroidal anti-inflammatory drugs (NSAIDs), and beta-blockers are used (Beck, 1999). The changed ability to concentrate urine makes the elderly adult more susceptible to dehydration, a problem that is further complicated by a deficit in the thirst response; therefore, the elderly person will not feel thirsty even when significantly dehydrated (Beck, 1999).

BLADDER AND URETHRAL CHANGES WITH AGING

Changes in the bladder and urethra also occur with aging. The bladder becomes more fibrous, with subsequent decreased capacity and increased postvoiding residuals (Bravo, 2000). Figure 17-3 ■ illustrates the structure of the bladder and supporting detrusor muscles. Autonomic innervation of the bladder decreases with age, affecting not only contraction of the detrusor muscle, but also the external sphincter. The **detrusor muscles**, three layers of muscle that cover the bladder, become less contractile but also somewhat unstable. This means the older adult is subject to both inability to completely empty the bladder and involuntary contractions of the bladder (McCance & Huether, 2001). There is age-related weakening of the voluntary pelvic floor muscles that are important to controlling the release of urine from the urethra. These changes make older adults more likely to have difficulty delaying urination and predispose them to urinary incontinence and urinary tract infection. Even though there are anatomical and physiological changes that make incontinence more probable with increased age, urinary incontinence is *not* a normal part of aging.

The urethral changes in women are mostly related to the loss of estrogen following menopause (Bravo, 2000). The external sphincter muscle becomes thinner and less able to resist the pressure of urine from the bladder. In men, there is no muscle thinning, but the enlargement of the prostate may constrict the urethra (Saxon & Etten, 2002).

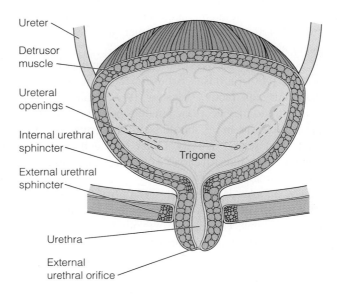

Ureter

Detrusor muscle

Ureteral openings

Internal urethral sphincter

External urethral sphincter

Trigone

Urethra

External urethral orifice

FIGURE ■ **17-3**

The structure of the bladder and supporting detrusor muscles.

Practice Pearl

Due to estrogen-mediated changes in the perineal area of postmenopausal women, the urinary meatus may be difficult to visualize. When attempting urinary catheterization, you may wish to consider placing the older woman in a side-lying position, and visualize the perineum by lifting the buttock. If you are right-handed, assist the woman to lie on her left side, with her back towards you. If you are left-handed, assist the woman to her right side. By lifting the buttock, you should be able to visualize the urinary meatus on or near the anterior vaginal wall.

ANTIDIURETIC HORMONE AND THE AGING PROCESS

Older adults tend to have higher basal levels of ADH than younger adults, and the pituitary responds more vigorously to osmotic stimuli by secreting more ADH than in younger people (Gruenewald & Matsumoto, 1999). ADH release in relation to hypotension and hypovolemia, however, is blunted in elderly adults. The aging kidney is less responsive to circulating ADH, producing urine that is poorly concentrated and rich in sodium. This puts the older adult at increased risk of hyponatremia, which can be magnified with the use of diuretics.

MALE REPRODUCTIVE SYSTEM AND ADVANCED AGE

The weight of the testis does not decrease in old age, although the testes become less firm. Approximately half of all men continue to produce viable sperm up to the age of 90 years (McCance & Huether, 2001). The number of seminiferous tubules that contain sperm decreases dramatically with age, but the adage "it only takes one" seems to apply here.

The testes gradually produce less testosterone, starting at approximately age 50 (Tan, 1999). Concomitantly, FSH and LH levels increase, probably in response to a decrease in circulating testosterone. The secondary sex characteristics supported by testosterone, such as muscle mass and body and facial hair growth, tend to diminish.

The older man will notice several age-related changes in his sexual response and performance, but it is important for both the client and nurse to know that sexual response and performance should be present in the older adult. For both men and women, the major age-related change in sexual response is timing. It takes longer to become sexually aroused, longer to complete intercourse, and longer before sexual arousal can occur again (Butler & Lewis, 2003).

The decreased levels of testosterone in the older man change the vascular responses that are part of arousal. Arousal occurs more in response to direct penile stimulation than to psychic factors (Masters, 1986; Schiavi & Rehman, 1995). In general, the older man's libido may decrease but does not disappear. If an older man reports a loss in sexual interest, the nurse should be as concerned as when a younger man reports a loss of interest in sexual activity. Older men achieve an erection that is less firm than in younger men, but still capable of penetration. Ejaculation may take longer to occur, and the older man may have difficulty anticipating or delaying ejaculation.

The orgasm of older men differs from that of younger men in that there are fewer contractions of the urethra, the amount of seminal fluid decreases, and the force of ejaculation lessens. The nipples may not engorge to firm erections, and the rectal sphincter contractions that accompany climax are less frequent. After orgasm, the erection is rapidly lost. The refractory period (time to next erection) is lengthened to several hours, or in some cases, as long as 24 hours (McCance & Huether, 2001).

FEMALE REPRODUCTIVE SYSTEM AND ADVANCED AGE

The most obvious change in the female reproductive tract as a woman ages is the cessation of menstruation, although the hormonal changes that bring on menopause are also responsible for a number of changes in the older woman's body. Menopause is the complete cessation of menstruation secondary to the lack of ovarian function. Perimenopause, however, may begin as early as 38 years of age or as late as 53 years (Duffy, 1998) and may last up to 8 years before menopause. During perimenopause, FSH levels increase, although LH remains constant, and estrogen levels vary widely (Merry & Holehan, 1994). Follicles mature irregularly, and ovulation may occur sporadically. Since most of the estrogen is produced by the corpus luteum after ovulation, the fluctuating estrogen levels may be explained by the irregularity of ovulation. Once menopause has occurred, FSH and LH stabilize at levels much higher than in younger women. Estrogen levels fall off dramatically and remain at very low levels for the rest of the woman's life.

Estrogen affects many other target organs, in particular the mucous membranes of the genitourinary tract. The decreased levels of estrogen cause the vaginal tissues to thin and become less elastic, and the vagina to shorten (Duffy, 1998). There is less vaginal lubrication, potentially making intercourse more painful. The uterus shrinks; the cervix, urethra, and trigone of the bladder also atrophy (McCance & Huether, 2001). When these changes are compounded by the alterations in the bladder and urethra, the older woman is at increased risk for urinary incontinence and infection.

Just as the decrease of testosterone in the man causes changes in secondary sex characteristics, so does the decrease of estrogen cause similar changes in older women. Pubic and axillary hair may become more sparse. As women also produce small amounts of testosterone, loss of libido in an older woman may be related to a decrease in testosterone (Duffy, 1998). Breast tissue grows in response to estrogen. As estrogen levels taper off, the breasts become less firm and somewhat pendulous. The glandular tissue in the breast is gradually replaced by fat, and the ligaments supporting the breast (Cooper's ligaments) no longer maintain the lobular shape of the breast. The ducts near the areola become less elastic and may be palpated as firm stringlike structures (Bickley & Szilagyi, 2003). Cystic changes, however, are not normal and should be promptly evaluated (Mansel & Harland, 1998). The mons and vulva also lose fullness, and the clitoris may become smaller (Duffy, 1998). The level of circulating androgens in the woman, no longer opposed by estrogen, may cause coarsening of the skin and an increase in facial hair.

Older women also experience changes in their sexual responses. It takes longer for the older woman to become sexually aroused and produce vaginal lubrication. The labia and uterus do not fully elevate, making penetration slightly more difficult (Monga, Monga, Tan, & Grabois, 1999). The clitoris remains an important part of orgasm, but may become irritated more easily because the clitoral hood is less protective than in younger women (Duffy, 1998). During orgasm, the uterus will contract less frequently, but the contractions remain vigorous, and orgasm is as intense as in younger women. Box 17-1 summarizes the normal changes of aging related to the genitourinary tract for men and women.

GAY AND LESBIAN OLDER ADULTS

Older adults whose sexual orientation is homosexual experience the same physical changes as do their heterosexual peers. Older gays and lesbians, however, are affected by many social factors that may exacerbate those physical changes. For example, most gay and lesbian people who are now older adults have experienced blatant hostility for their sexual orientation (Pope, 1997). They may be even more hesitant than other older adults to discuss sexuality for fear of prejudice or rejection.

BOX 17-1 **Major Age-Related Genitourinary Changes**

Kidney

↓ Weight, glomeruli, glomerular filtration rate
↓ Concentration of urine
↑ Serum creatinine, blood urea nitrogen
↑ Nighttime formation of urine
↓ Drug excretion
↑ Basal level of antidiuretic hormone

Bladder and Urethra

↓ Autonomic innervation
↓ Capacity
↓ Detrusor contractility
↑ Postvoid residual

Male Reproductive Tract

↓ Sperm production
↓ Testosterone
↑ Time to arousal, ejaculation, refractory period
↓ Firmness of erection, force of ejaculation

Female Reproductive Tract

Menopause
↓ Estrogen levels
↓ Thickness, elasticity, and lubrication of vaginal tissues
↓ Glandular tissue in breasts
↑ Time to arousal

In addition, older gays and lesbians may be rejecting of their own sexual orientation. They may have never "come out" to themselves or significant others, leaving them in a state of identity confusion. Older lesbians, as a group, are less sexually active than their male counterparts, but still seek intimacy with others. An insensitive or judgmental nurse may easily compromise the sexual health of this group of older adults.

Common Genitourinary Concerns in Older Adults

The popular press has brought **erectile dysfunction** into common discourse, but there are other genitourinary diseases and problems that are also important to older adults. Some, such as malignancies, require effective collaboration among health professionals. The nurse, however, may be the primary healthcare provider for such concerns as urinary incontinence and unsatisfactory sexual activity.

ACUTE AND CHRONIC RENAL FAILURE

Age-related changes in the kidney, particularly the decrease in glomeruli and glomerular filtration rate, make the older adult particularly vulnerable to renal disease (Bailey & Sands, 2003). **Renal failure**, the inability to remove nitrogenous waste from the body and to regulate fluid and electrolytes, may arise from problems in blood flow to the kidney (prerenal), injury to the glomeruli or tubules (renal), or out-flow obstruction (postrenal). The failure may be acute, with a sudden onset; or chronic, in which irreversible damage accumulates, usually over time. Renal failure in the elderly adult can be difficult to diagnose and treat, in part because of the pres-entation of symptoms, and in part because of the delicate balance of kidney function in old age.

Acute renal failure is found in approximately one fifth of older adults (Bailey & Sands, 2003) and may comprise up to 10% of all older adults admitted to acute care settings (Jassal, Fillit, & Oreopoulos, 1998). Prerenal causes are common in older adults and lead to poor perfusion of the kidney (Table 17-1). Renal causes may be sec-ondary to chronic diseases such as hypertension and diabetes mellitus. The most preva-lent postrenal cause is prostatic hypertrophy.

Renal failure has different presentations in older and younger adults. In younger adults, marked oliguria is the most dramatic symptom of acute renal failure, but the older adult may not display this symptom. Postural hypotension is a common finding in prerenal acute renal failure (Bailey & Sands, 2003), and the nurse is in a position to monitor. BUN and serum creatinine levels increase, and dependent edema may be pres-ent (see Table 17-2). Ultrasound may demonstrate changes in the size of the kidney, or presence of calculi, in renal and postrenal causes. The complex nature of renal failure in older adults makes an interdisciplinary approach critical. The nurse, nephrologist, and nutritionist are essential members of the care team. A nephrology consult is impor-tant in limiting kidney damage and decreasing mortality (Bailey & Sands, 2003). Nu-tritional support is also important, but weight loss of up to 1 lb per day is expected in the older adult with acute renal failure. Any attempt to prevent the weight loss may overtax multiple systems and lead to cardiac failure. For example, the use of nutritional supplements that are high in calories may be contraindicated in the older adult with acute renal failure. Allowing weight loss to occur during this acute phase may better

TABLE 17-1

Causes of Renal Failure in Older Adults

Prerenal Causes	Renal Causes	Postrenal Causes
Dehydration	Acute glomerulonephritis	Benign prostatic hyperplasia
Shock	Aminoglycoside antibiotics	Prostate cancer
Vomiting and diarrhea	Sepsis	Bladder cancer
Surgery	Acute pyelonephritis	Calculi
Cardiac failure	Aneurysms	Fecal impaction
Diuretics	Cholesterol embolus	Urethral strictures
NSAIDs	Allergic response to radiocontrast media	Gynecological cancers
ACE inhibitors		
Hypotension	Diabetic nephropathy	

Source: Beers & Berkow, 2000; Jassal et al., 1998; Sands & Vega, 1999.

TABLE 17-2

Comparisons of Signs and Symptoms of Renal Failure in Older Adults

	Acute Renal Failure	Chronic Renal Failure
Onset	Sudden onset	Gradual onset
Blood pressure	Postural hypotension	Hypertension
Electrolytes	Increased BUN and serum creatinine	Increased serum phosphate, calcium
		Decreased serum calcium
		Metabolic acidosis
Edema	Dependent edema	Generalized edema
Well-being	Fatigue and drowsiness	Fatigue and drowsiness
Urine output	Possible decreased urine output	Nonspecific changes
Gastrointestinal symptoms	Nausea and vomiting	Nausea and vomiting
	Rapid weight loss	Anorexia
		Weight loss
Other symptoms	Flank pain	Decreased glomerular filtration rate
		Anemia
		Pruritus
		Altered mental status

Source: Beers & Berkow, 2000; Jassal et al., 1998; Sands & Vega, 1999.

protect the long-term health of the older adult. Dehydration in the older adult is a causative factor in acute renal failure; therefore, fluid restrictions should be modest (Jassal et al., 1998).

Chronic renal failure is caused by irreversible damage to the kidney and is much more common in older adults than in younger adults (Beers & Berkow, 2000). Diabetes mellitus, benign prostatic hyperplasia, hypertension, and long-term use of NSAIDs all contribute to the higher prevalence of chronic renal failure in older adults. The symptoms and signs are similar to those exhibited by younger persons, and include decreased glomerular filtration rate, hyperphosphatemia, hypocalcemia, hyperkalemia, metabolic acidosis, hypertension, and anemia. The assessment of chronic renal failure in the older adult is made more difficult by the age-related decrease in glomerular filtration rate and the low correlation between serum creatinine and glomerular filtration rate (Jassal et al., 1998). As the disease progresses, the older adult may experience pruritus, general lack of well-being, generalized edema, altered cognition, anorexia, nausea, and weight loss. As with acute renal failure, prompt consultation by a nephrologist is critical to improving the older adult's quality of life and long-term survival (Bailey & Sands, 2003).

The treatments for chronic renal failure should be modified for the older adult. The restrictions on fluid intake and dietary protein should be less stringent, since most older adults have already decreased their protein and sodium intakes (Jassal et al., 1998). Constipation, a concern for many older adults, may exacerbate the hyperkalemia that accompanies chronic renal failure. Nursing and medical management for regularity are important contributions to the treatment plan. Thinning and dry skin is a common concern for all older adults, and the pruritus of chronic renal failure can present a real challenge. Careful skin care by the nurse, including moisturizing the skin, will be much appreciated by the older patient.

The definitive treatment for chronic renal failure is renal replacement therapy, either through dialysis or through renal transplant (Bailey & Sands, 2003). Older adults in the United States are underrepresented among those receiving any type of dialysis or transplant (U.S. Renal Data System, 2002); however, they are more likely than younger adults to receive in-center hemodialysis, if they are receiving renal replacement therapy at all. This trend is consistent with Binstock's (1999) concerns that de facto age-based rationing of expensive healthcare services is being practiced. The nurse must be a strong advocate to ensure that older adults with chronic renal failure are well informed about treatment options and are not discriminated against in care decisions.

URINARY TRACT INFECTION

Changes in the urinary tract of older adults make them more susceptible to urinary tract infections. A **urinary tract infection (UTI)** is the presence of bacteria in the urethra, bladder, or kidney, although the majority of UTIs in older adults are asymptomatic (Nicolle, 2003). Some authors term this condition *asymptomatic UTI,* whereas others apply the term *UTI* only to those older adults with symptoms, and use *bacteriuria* to define the presence of bacteria in the urine with no concomitant symptoms (Nicolle, 2003). (In the following discussion, *UTI* will indicate bacteriuria, symptomatic or not. If indicated, the phrase *asymptomatic UTI* will be used.) Eleven percent of all women experience UTIs annually (National Institute of Diabetes and Digestive and Kidney Diseases, 2001), and that number may double in older women (Krogh & Bruskewitz, 1998). Older men have about one third the rate of UTIs of older women (McCue, 1999). Older adults who have indwelling catheters have a nearly universal rate of asymptomatic UTI, and the rate of symptomatic UTI is much higher than in persons without indwelling catheters (McCue, 1999). UTIs in catheterized older adults tend to be polymicrobial and difficult to eradicate. Before using an indwelling catheter, the potential benefits to the older adult must be carefully weighed against the serious risks posed.

Older adults do not present the same symptoms of UTI as do younger adults. Particularly in a long-term care setting, a change in behavior may be the only indicator of a UTI (McCue, 1999). The symptoms usually seen in younger adults with UTIs—urgency and frequency—are common age-related changes in the older adult and therefore lack diagnostic usefulness. If, however, an older adult has not previously experienced **urinary urgency**, the shortened period of time between the urge to void and actual urination, or **urinary frequency**, more than seven voids per 24-hour period, these symptoms should be thoroughly investigated.

Practice Pearl

It is important to remember the principle of nonmaleficence (do no harm). Although it may seem inappropriate not to treat bacteriuria, if the older patient is not troubled with symptoms, offering an antibiotic will not improve the outcome and may cause harm.

Asymptomatic UTI does not require treatment. In fact, treatment does not improve the morbidity or mortality in affected older persons (Krogh & Bruskewitz, 1998; McCue, 1999; Nicolle, 2003; Steers, 1999). Routine urinalysis for older adults without symptoms is neither appropriate nor cost-effective. In the presence of symptoms, however, treatment decisions should be based on urine culture and sensitivity test. UTI in an older person with an indwelling catheter is considered to be complicated and may include a variety of microorganisms, such as *Escherichia coli, Proteus mirabilis, Klebsiella pneumoniae, Citrobacter* spp., *Providencia* spp., and *Pseudomonas aeruginosa* (Nicolle, 2003). Even in older adults without indwelling catheters, a wide variety of organisms may be found in the urine. The only way to accurately identify the causative organism, and thus treat the infection effectively, is to obtain a urine culture (McCue, 1999). If an older adult is able to follow directions and cooperate with the nurse, obtaining a clean-catch urine specimen is done according to standard procedure. A clean, newly applied condom catheter and collection bag can be used with an older man who cannot participate in specimen collection. Immediately prior to applying the condom catheter, the nurse should thoroughly clean and dry the glans of the penis (Nicolle, 2003). Many experts recommend straight catheterization for collecting an uncontaminated specimen from older women who are unable to cooperate. However, Brazier and Palmer (1995) empirically demonstrated that two other methods also provide an uncontaminated sample. External collection pouches are effective if the labia are properly cleaned and separated. The other method requires an in-toilet collection pan with a sterile bowl placed inside. The nurse assists the older woman to the toilet, separates and cleans the labia with disposable moist towelettes, and then maintains the separation of the labia until the patient voids. The specimen may then be poured from the sterile bowl into a sterile specimen container, and the older woman is assisted to wipe and re-dress herself. Once the microorganisms are identified, an appropriate antibiotic is prescribed. The duration of therapy will depend, in part, on the virulence of the identified pathogen. Sex is also a consideration in treatment choices, because men require longer periods of treatment than women. The longer urethra in men makes it less likely that bacteria can ascend into the bladder. When bacteria do reach the older man's bladder, the infection is considered to be complicated and requires a longer course of treatment.

URINARY INCONTINENCE

Urinary incontinence (UI), the involuntary loss of urine, affects over 13 million adults and costs older adults approximately $19.5 billion per year (Hu et al., 2004). Approximately one third of noninstitutionalized older women experience UI (Ouslander, 2000), and nearly one fifth of community-dwelling older men report UI (Assad, 2000). These figures rise to nearly 50% for older men and women in long-term care settings (Assad, 2000; Ouslander, 2000). Nurses are in a key position to decrease those staggering numbers.

> **Practice Pearl**
>
> Some older persons will not mention incontinence because they consider it embarrassing or just a normal part of aging. It is important to explicitly ask about involuntary loss of urine.

UI may be classified by the cause of the involuntary loss (Table 17-3). **Stress incontinence** is defined as the involuntary loss of urine when the intra-abdominal pressure is increased, such as during coughing or laughing. Either the pelvic floor muscles or the internal urethral sphincter is not strong enough to counter the pressure on the bladder, and urine is released. **Urge incontinence** occurs when the detrusor muscles contract forcefully and unexpectedly, and the internal sphincter is unable to

TABLE 17-3

Types of Urinary Incontinence

Type	Etiology	Examples	Group Most Affected
Stress	Weakened external sphincter/pelvic floor, increased intra-abdominal pressure	Urine loss during sneezing, laughing, exercise	Women under age 60 Men after prostate surgery
Urge	Detrusor instability, internal sphincter weakness	Overactive bladder	Older adults of both sexes, older men somewhat more affected
Overflow	Bladder muscles overextended and have poor tone, overflow of retained urine	Enlarged prostate causes obstruction of the urethra, urine backs up in bladder; diabetic nephropathy affects the contractility of the detrusor muscles	Persons with diabetes mellitus Men with enlarged prostates Persons taking calcium channel blockers, anticholinergics, and adrenergics
Functional	Physical or psychological factors impair ability to get to the toilet	An older adult unable to transfer from wheelchair to toilet is unable to obtain needed assistance	Frail elderly adults Nursing home residents Persons with dementias

Source: Assad, 2000; Hartford Institute for Geriatric Nursing, 2001; Malone-Lee, 1998; Ouslander, 2000.

retain urine in the bladder. **Overflow incontinence** is sometimes known as mechanical incontinence because a blockage of the urethra may be the cause of the bladder overfilling and stretching the bladder muscles beyond the point of contractility. Overflow may also occur if the muscles are unable to contract properly because of lack of innervation, as in spinal cord injury or in diabetes mellitus. Finally, **functional incontinence** is defined as incontinence related to causes external to the urinary apparatus, such that the older adult is unable to get to a toilet to void. For example, a person who is restrained may be aware of the need to void and can control the release of urine (up to a point), but is not assisted to the toilet in a timely manner. Older persons with dementia may experience functional incontinence because they are unable to find the toilet.

Practice Pearl

New-onset urinary incontinence is always a nursing priority.

The nurse is in an ideal position to collect data to assist in diagnosing and treating UI. Assessment should include the six areas of health history related to UI, mental status evaluation, functional evaluation, environmental assessment, social supports, bladder records, and physical examination (Jarvis, 2004). Health history questions related to UI should include (Kennedy-Malone et al., 2000; Lekan-Rutledge & Colling, 2003; Ouslander, 2000):

- Is there a concurrent medical condition, such as UTI, cerebrovascular accident (CVA), or diabetes mellitus that may be affecting continence status?
- Has UI occurred before, and under what conditions?

- What is the pattern of UI? The nurse should ask questions that will help categorize the type of UI (see Table 17-3).
- What medications are currently being used?
- What amount, type, and timing of fluid intake are present? It is important to assess fluids that may irritate the bladder or increase urine production such as caffeine-containing coffee or tea, carbonated beverages, alcohol, citrus juices, and diet drinks containing aspartame (Bottomley, 2000).
- How does the UI affect the older person's quality of life?

In addition to these health history questions, a mental status examination (see Chapter 8) and functional assessment (see Chapter 7) must be completed to evaluate the effect these areas might have on continence. ⚊⚊ A careful assessment of the environment should include locating the toilet and any obstacles to its use (long distance from where the older adult is, lack of grab bars, poor lighting, lack of room to maneuver, and interior decorating that "disguises" the toilet room) (Lekan-Rutledge & Colling, 2003). The clothing that an older adult wears is also part of the environment and should be evaluated to see if it is impairing continence. For example, can the older person easily remove clothing to use the toilet? The presence of significant others is an important part of the social support that is available to the older adult. The ability and willingness of the significant others to assist in toileting should be assessed. Paid assistants, such as certified nurse aids, are also part of this social support evaluation.

New-onset urinary incontinence should be aggressively investigated by the gerontological nurse. The earlier the cause is identified, the sooner nursing interventions can be instituted to correct the problem and improve the patient's situation. The following Best Practices feature represents a standard for health professionals to use in assessing and treating new-onset urinary incontinence.

Bladder records or diaries are a critical tool in evaluating and managing UI. A wide variety of diaries are available, including the example in Figure 17-4 ■. This diary is available on the World Wide Web and may be downloaded for the nurse or older patient (Agency for Health Care Policy and Research, 1996).

The nurse should perform a physical assessment, focusing on areas that may contribute to incontinence. These include an abdominal examination, particularly looking for distended bowel or bladder; rectal examination, evaluating for impacted stool; and genital examination, observing for skin condition and presence of organ prolapse (Kane, Ouslander, & Abrass, 2004).

Once transient conditions contributing to UI have been identified and treated, and a diagnosis of type of UI has been made, a treatment plan may be implemented. A certified wound, ostomy, and continence nurse (CWOCN) is a valuable asset to both nurse and client. The CWOCN is educationally prepared to treat clients with wound, ostomy, or continence concerns, and must pass a rigorous written examination (Wound, Ostomy and Continence Nursing Certification Board, 2003). They are expert nurses, able to treat patients directly or to offer consultation to nurses who will then implement a plan of care.

Treatments for UI are categorized into five groups: lifestyle modification, scheduled voiding regimens, pelvic floor muscle strengthening, anti-incontinence devices, and supportive interventions (Wyman, 2003). Medications form a sixth category. A combination of interventions from several categories is usually referred to as a toileting program (Lekan-Rutledge & Colling, 2003). The older adult must be a partner in choosing the interventions (Palmer, 2000) (Table 17-4).

Several of these interventions merit further discussion, as the nurse may be responsible for a major portion of the actual implementation. Timed voiding has been demon-

FIGURE ◼ 17-4

Sample bladder record.

NAME:					
DATE:					
INSTRUCTIONS: Place a check in the appropriate column next to the time you urinated in the toilet or when an incontinence episode occurred. Note the reason for the incontinence and describe your liquid intake (for example, coffee, water) and estimate the amount (for example, 1 cup).					
Time interval	Urinated in toilet	Had a small incontinence episode	Had a large incontinence episode	Reason for incontinence episode	Type/amount of liquid intake
6–8 A.M.					
8–10 A.M.					
10–noon					
Noon–2 P.M.					
2–4 P.M.					
4–6 P.M.					
6–8 P.M.					
8–10 P.M.					
10–midnight					
Overnight					
No. of pads used today:			No. of episodes:		
Comments:					

strated to be effective for older women with stress incontinence and for some older men after prostatectomy (Wyman, 2003). It requires consistency among caregivers, or an older adult who is independent in toileting (Meadows, 2000). A schedule is established for toileting, usually every 2 hours, but as long as 3 hours may be acceptable. The older adult is assisted (if needed) to the toilet and encouraged to relax the pelvic floor muscles and attempt to urinate. Because of the importance of adequate sleep (see Chapter 8 ⬤▭), the nurse and older adult should carefully consider if the schedule will continue throughout the night. **Bladder training** is similar to timed voiding, but the intervals between trips to the toilet are gradually lengthened, training the bladder to hold slightly increased amounts of urine. Prompted voiding also uses some of the techniques of timed voiding,

The Hartford Institute for Geriatric Nursing (1999) recommends the use of the mnemonic **DIAPPERS** for identifying the cause of new-onset urinary incontinence:

- **D**elirium
- **I**nfection (urinary or systemic)
- **A**trophic urethritis/vaginitis (irritation, inflammation)
- **P**harmaceuticals (diuretics, psychotropics)
- **P**sychological (depression, agitation)
- **E**ndocrine (diabetes mellitus)
- **R**estricted mobility/restraints (gait disorders, CVA, environmental obstacles)
- **S**tool impaction

Source: Resnick & Yalla, 1985; Reuben et al., 2004.

but rather than assisting the older adult to the toilet every 2 hours, the nurse reminds the older adult every 2 hours to go to the toilet.

Practice Pearl

An older adult who is taking diuretics should be helped to identify the onset and peak action of the diuretic, and then aided in developing a toileting schedule to maximize continence.

Pelvic floor exercises, or **Kegel exercises**, are another UI intervention frequently employed by nurses. The technique works well for urge and stress incontinence. It requires that the older adult be motivated to perform the exercises and be cognitively intact enough to learn them (Wyman, 2003). The older adult is instructed to tighten the muscles of the perineum, without also tensing the muscles of the abdomen, thigh, or buttock (Assad, 2000). Imagining the perineum as an elevator that goes from floors one through five may help. The "fifth floor" represents a very intense tightening and may produce muscle fatigue, particularly if the contraction is held for more than 10 seconds (Meadows, 2000). Suggest quick trips only to the fifth floor! A recommended pattern is 15 repetitions of rapid contractions, one to three sets, daily (Assad, 2000).

Several medications are available to assist the person with stress or urge UI. Urge UI medications are generally anticholinergic and inappropriate for persons with narrow-angle glaucoma or urinary retention, or antiadrenergics that may potentiate other antihypertensives (Smith & Ouslander, 2000). Stress incontinence in women may be treated with estrogen applications, and in both men and women with pseudoephedrine, which is contraindicated in people with hypertension (Smith & Ouslander, 2000). Medications should be used as an adjunct to other therapies. Research by Ouslander, Maloney, Grasela, Rogers, and Walawander (2001) demonstrated that the addition of tolterodine (Detrol) to a behavioral UI therapy in nursing home residents was helpful in maintaining continence.

Many older adults who experience UI use disposable incontinence pads or protective undergarments. Although these may be helpful in managing the social consequences of

TABLE 17-4

Examples of Treatments for Urinary Incontinence

Lifestyle Modifications	Scheduled Voiding Regimens	Pelvic Floor Muscle Strengthening	Anti-Incontinence Devices	Supportive Interventions
Smoking cessation	Timed voiding	Kegel exercises	Pessaries	Elevated toilet seats
Weight reduction	Prompted voiding	Biofeedback	Condom catheter	Gait training
Bowel management	Bladder training	Electrical stimulation	External clamps or urethral plugs	Modified clothing
Caffeine reduction				Absorbent pads or undergarments
Appropriate fluid intake				

Source: Bottomley, 2000; Meadows, 2000; Wyman, 2003.

UI, they are neither a cure nor without adverse effects. Excellent skin care remains a nursing priority because urine can be very damaging to the skin. That damage can be exacerbated by anything that decreases airflow to the affected area. Pads or undergarments must be changed frequently and after every episode of incontinence. They should be disposed of in ways that minimize environmental impact, especially the patient's immediate sur-

> **Practice Pearl**
>
> It is essential to be considerate of a patient's dignity and self-esteem. The term *diapers* is demeaning to many. The nurse should use the product name (Depends, for example), or *products* or *protective undergarments,* which could be abbreviated *PUGs.*

roundings. Used incontinence products can have an unpleasant odor, and care should be taken to keep the older adult's room or home aesthetically pleasing.

BENIGN PROSTATIC HYPERPLASIA

Benign prostatic hyperplasia (BPH) affects 50% of men between the ages of 51 and 60 years, and 90% of men over age 80 (National Institute of Diabetes and Digestive and Kidney Diseases, 2001). BPH is classified in three ways. Microscopic BPH is diagnosable only by histologic changes. Macroscopic BPH is characterized by palpable enlargement of the gland during rectal examination (Chow, 2001). Clinical BPH refers to observable symptoms related to BPH (Chow, 2001). The growth of the prostate is influenced by androgens and occurs mostly in the transitional zone that surrounds the urethra (Letran & Brawer, 1999). BPH affects older men without regard to race, tobacco use, level of sexual activity, or vasectomy (Chow, 2001).

The symptoms of BPH are sometimes referred to as "nuisances," although they can have a profound effect on daily living. They include difficulty starting a stream of urine, weak stream, straining to urinate, longer time needed to urinate, and a feeling of incomplete bladder emptying (Letran & Brawer, 1999). As the prostate continues to grow, urinary retention may occur. Symptoms of bladder irritation secondary to the enlarged prostate include urinary urgency, frequency, and **nocturia**. Some men experience urge incontinence as a result of BPH.

> **Drug Alert** ❗
>
> Urinary retention in men with BPH can be precipitated by several classes of medications, including those with anticholinergic properties and over-the-counter medications for the common cold.

Treatment for BPH includes managing urge incontinence (discussed earlier) and decreasing the other urinary symptoms. Alpha-adrenergic blocking medications such as tamsulosin and doxazosin mesylate may be prescribed. Saw palmetto is an over-the-counter herbal preparation that appears to be effective in improving BPH symptoms and has relatively few side effects (Chow, 2001). As with any herbal preparation, saw palmetto is not regulated by any organized group. Problems of inconsistent packaging, mixing, and bioavailability should be considered. When urinary retention becomes refractory to other treatments, or renal insufficiency due to bladder outlet obstruction develops, surgical intervention may be recommended (Letran & Brawer, 1999).

The most commonly performed surgery for BPH is transurethral resection of the prostate, although rates of this surgery have decreased since a peak in 1987 (Bubolz, Wasson, Lu-Yao, & Barry, 2001). The percentage of men over 80 years of age who undergo this surgery has increased, and their postsurgical mortality has decreased (Bubolz et al., 2001). Older men who have the surgery are at risk for erectile dysfunction, retrograde ejaculation, hemorrhage, and infection, although most have dramatic improvement in their presurgery symptoms (Chow, 2001; Letran & Brawer, 1999).

MENOPAUSE-RELATED CONCERNS

Although menopause is an age-related process, not pathology, some women have troublesome health experiences after the cessation of menses. These include decreased vaginal lubrication, **atrophic vaginitis** (thinning and atrophy of the vaginal epithelium usually resulting from diminished estrogen levels), more frequent UTIs, UI, cognitive changes, vasomotor instability (hot flashes), sleep disturbances, osteoporosis, and increased cardiovascular disease (Welner, 1999). Hoerger et al. (1999) have estimated that annual medical costs for postmenopausal health problems are $186 billion, with the majority spent on cardiovascular disease. Menopause is an emotionally laden subject with many cultural implications. Different societies view aging women differently, and the older woman may internalize some of these views. Women may experience negative changes in their body image, or a feeling that they are no longer sexually viable people (Daniluk, 1998). Some women may celebrate menopause; others attach no significance to it.

The mediating factor in postmenopausal health concerns appears to be estrogen. Until recently, estrogen or hormone replacement therapy (HRT) was commonplace to relieve the problematic effects of menopause. In 2001, however, the American Heart Association strongly advised healthcare providers to stop prescribing HRT to postmenopausal women for cardioprotection ("AHA Cautions," 2001). The recommendation was based on a number of clinical research trials that demonstrated that HRT was not cardioprotective and could be deleterious to women with concomitant cardiovascular disease (Manson et al., 2003). In this large clinical investigation, women on HRT had demonstrated higher rates of myocardial infarction, stroke, breast cancer, pulmonary embolism, and deep vein thrombosis. In 2003, the U.S. Food and Drug Administration went even further, requiring explicit labeling of HRT products to caution potential users of a number of serious risks related to use ("FDA Orders Estrogen Safety Warnings," 2003). Current recommendations are that HRT be used only for the relief of vasomotor symptoms related to menopause, for women at high risk of osteoporosis, and for prevention of colorectal cancer (Nelson, Humphrey, Nygren, Teutsch, & Allan, 2002). The potential for harm from HRT should be thoroughly discussed with the older woman before she initiates the therapy.

Older women may be anxious about using estrogen-containing preparations, even if their vasomotor symptoms are severe. The hot flashes of menopause range from mild feelings of being overly warm to intense feelings of uncomfortable heat over the upper body (Noblett & Ostergard, 1999). Some women find that dressing in layers allows them to remove and replace clothing as the hot flashes come and go. If the hot flashes occur frequently, the older woman should discuss her concerns with her primary care provider. Soy products and black cohosh have been shown to relieve hot flashes without serious side effects and may be acceptable to older women (Morelli & Naquin, 2002).

Atrophic vaginitis may result in urogenital infection, ulceration, and uncomfortable sexual intercourse. The treatment of choice is topical estrogen as a cream that is applied to the affected tissues (Messinger-Rapport & Thacker, 2001). Topical creams have not demonstrated the link to adverse effects that systemic HRT has (Strandberg, Ylikorkala, & Tikkanen, 2003).

GENITOURINARY MALIGNANCIES

Older adults are more susceptible to a number of cancers than are younger adults. These include cancer of the bladder, breast, prostate, uterus, ovary, and kidney (Ries et al., 2002). The early symptoms of renal cancer are fairly vague, including anemia, weight loss, fever, hypertension, and hypercalcemia. More specific and obvious signs, such as microhematuria, flank pain, and a mass on the affected kidney, occur at a much more advanced stage of the disease (Beers & Berkow, 2000). Microscopic examination of the urine is an important screening mechanism. Surgical removal of the kidney is the only recommended course of action, as neither radiation nor chemotherapy is effective.

Cancer of the Urinary Bladder

Bladder cancer is one of the more common malignancies that affect older adults. Older men are almost four times more likely to develop bladder cancer than are older women, and approximately one in every 42 men between the ages of 60 and 79 will develop it (American Cancer Society, 2002). White, non-Hispanic men are particularly susceptible to the disease, although African American men have a higher mortality rate, probably reflecting the quality of healthcare available to both groups (Etzioni, Berry, Legler, & Shaw, 2002). Common risk factors include cigarette smoking and occupational exposure to certain chemicals known as arylamines.

Some symptoms of bladder cancer are similar to those of other urinary tract diseases: microhematuria, urinary frequency, urgency, and dysuria (Beers & Berkow, 2000). Pyuria, the presence of pus in the urine, may also be a symptom of bladder cancer. There are no recommended screening tests for bladder cancer, although hematuria testing and urinary cytology testing have been evaluated for this purpose (National Cancer Institute, 2003). These tests carry a high frequency of false positives, making them too nonspecific for screening. Any patient who presents with the previously listed symptoms, however, should be carefully evaluated. In the absence of UTI, an older adult with either gross or microhematuria should be referred for cystoscopy. In many cases, this procedure can be carried out in a physician's office.

The treatments for bladder cancer are dependent on the anatomical structures involved, the degree of invasiveness, and recurrent status (Beers & Berkow, 2000). Available treatments range from depositing chemotherapeutic agents into the bladder to removal of the bladder and surrounding organs. If the bladder is removed, a reservoir for urine will be created. A loop of intestine may be used to create the reservoir. The ureters are attached to the loop, and a stoma on the abdomen is created. The older adult then wears an external collection device over the stoma. Newer interventions include a reservoir that is capable of storing urine and is catheterized intermittently. These surgeries present challenges to the older adult's body image, and the nurse must work with the patient to address these challenges. Specific concerns include the psychomotor skills of managing the urinary reservoir, ongoing fear of cancer, and "the bag" (Beitz & Zuzelo, 2003).

Prostate Cancer

Prostate cancer is even more common in older men than bladder cancer, and will affect one of every eight men over the age of 60 (American Cancer Society, 2002). African American men are more likely to develop prostate cancer, as are men with a family history and those with diets high in animal fats (Balducci, Pow-Sang, Friedland, & Diaz, 1997; Cozen & Liu, 2000). Furthermore, higher levels of sexual activity have been demonstrated to correlate with an increased risk of prostate cancer (Cozen & Liu, 2000). This relationship probably reflects the role of androgens in both prostate cancer and sexual activity. No reliable links among **sexually transmitted diseases** (diseases contracted through sexual intercourse or intimate sexual contact) and prostate cancer have been found.

The most commonly used screening tests for prostate cancer are digital rectal examination (DRE) combined with prostate-specific antigen (PSA) testing (Gambert, 2001). A normal PSA level is below 4 ng/ml. Values over 10 ng/ml are strongly indicative of prostate cancer, while values between 4 ng/ml and 10 ng/ml are difficult to interpret. During the DRE, the practitioner is able to palpate the prostate, feeling for nodules suspicious for cancer. If either of these screens demonstrates abnormalities, a transrectal ultrasound is usually recommended. There is diversity of opinion on which populations of men should be screened, and with which tests, given that older men (those over 75 years) with a negative DRE rarely die from prostate cancer. Some experts recommend that DRE and PSA be done annually on all men over age 50. Others recommend DRE alone for men over age 75 and DRE with PSA for men between ages 50 and 75 (Gambert, 2001). The U.S. Preventive Services Task Force (2003) has stated that the evidence on the value of DRE and PSA in decreasing mortality is insufficient to recommend for or against this screening. Older men are probably wise to rely on the advice of their primary care provider.

Once prostate cancer is diagnosed, the older man has a variety of treatment options. No one option appears to have significant benefits over the others (Letran & Brawer, 1999). If the cancer is localized, there are three options. *Radical prostatectomy* involves removing the prostate through a perineal or retropubic incision. *Radiation ther-*

apy may be applied externally or through implants in the prostate. *Surveillance* is watchful waiting. If the cancer is more advanced, external radiation or hormonal treatment may be recommended (Balducci et al., 1997). The older patient should be offered a thorough discussion of all options with a urologist.

Rates of other genitourinary cancers in older men are low. Testicular cancer is predominantly a disease of young men, and cancer of the penis is rare in all age groups (Ries et al., 2002).

Gynecological Malignancies

Ovarian, uterine, and breast cancer are more prevalent in older women than in younger women (Ries et al., 2002). Cervical cancer, although more prevalent in young and midlife women, remains a concern. Vulvar cancer, signaled by a palpable nodule on the labia and pruritus, is not common in any age group (Brown & Cooper, 1998).

Seventy-five percent of ovarian cancer is diagnosed in women over the age of 55 (Ries et al., 2002). It is associated with a poor prognosis, particularly in older women (Termrungruanglert et al., 1997). The symptoms are vague, including diffuse abdominal discomfort and gastrointestinal distress (Beers & Berkow, 2000). The vagueness of the symptoms may account, in part, for the poor prognosis because women are rarely diagnosable when the tumor is confined to the ovary. More obvious symptoms, such as ascites or a palpable mass, are not frequently present until lymph nodes are involved or metastases are found.

Although there are no screening tests *per se* for ovarian cancer, there is a blood test for a tumor marker that is both sensitive and specific (Brown & Cooper, 1998). However, the CA-125 is not recommended as a screening tool because there is little conclusive evidence that it would decrease the mortality from ovarian cancer (National Cancer Institute, 2003). Similarly, transvaginal ultrasonography to detect ovarian cancer has not demonstrated a benefit in terms of decreased mortality.

Treatment options for the older woman with ovarian cancer include surgery to remove the uterus, ovaries, fallopian tubes, and omentum (Balducci et al., 1997). Chemotherapeutic agents may also be used, but recurrent disease is common (Brown & Cooper, 1998).

Cancer of the body of the uterus or endometrium is the most common gynecological cancer in older women (Ries et al., 2002). Risk factors include celibacy, late menopause, obesity, hypertension, and diabetes mellitus (Brown & Cooper, 1998). HRT, particularly estrogen, has also been implicated in the development of endometrial cancer (Nelson et al., 2002). The most common symptom is uterine bleeding after menopause, which occurs early in the disease, making early diagnosis and treatment possible. Any older woman who reports postmenopausal uterine bleeding should be assumed to have endometrial cancer until proved otherwise (Balducci et al., 1997). The diagnosis is usually made by endometrial biopsy, and treatment includes hysterectomy, oophorectomy, and salpingectomy. Chemotherapy after surgery is common. Prognosis is much better if the treatment is begun earlier in the course of the disease.

Cervical cancer in the older woman is primarily a concern because of the confusion around screening for the disease, the Papanicolaou (Pap) smear. The disease itself is more prevalent in younger women. The risk factors of cervical cancer include infection with human papillomavirus, early onset of sexual activity, history of abnormal Pap smears, HIV-positive status, and many sexual partners (Brown &

Cooper, 1998; National Cancer Institute, 2003). Current recommendations are that women who are over age 65, who have had a regular history of normal Pap smears, and who are not at high risk because of other factors (as previously noted) should *not* receive routine Pap smears (U.S. Preventive Services Task Force, 2003). Older women who have had a total hysterectomy (cervix removed) for nonmalignant reasons do not need to be screened with Pap smears (Table 17-5).

Breast cancer affects nearly 1 in every 14 women over age 60 (American Cancer Society, 2002). Risk factors include advanced age, family history of breast cancer, early menarche and late menopause, estrogen replacement therapy, none or late pregnancy, regular alcohol use, abdominal obesity, exposure to radiation, and personal history of benign breast disease (Kimmick & Muss, 1997). Three specific screening tests are available for breast cancer: mammography, clinical breast examination, and breast self-examination.

Strong evidence exists that yearly mammography for all women over the age of 40 decreases mortality from breast cancer and should be encouraged (U.S. Preventive Services Task Force, 2003). There is less consensus about the value of examinations done by a healthcare provider and those performed by the older woman herself. The American Cancer Society (2002) continues to recommend these practices, whereas the U.S. Preventive Services Task Force (2003) does not. As clinical breast examinations can easily be integrated into other health visits, it is wise for the healthcare provider to continue to perform them when possible. Teaching an older woman breast self-examination, however, may be socially unacceptable to her. Women who do not examine their breasts on a regular basis cannot enjoy the same preventive value as women who perform this examination regularly.

The treatment for breast cancer depends on the stage of the tumor when detected. Small, contained tumors may be treated with modified radical mastectomy, or lumpectomy with radiation (Kimmick & Muss, 1997). The presence of comorbidities in older women makes treatment choices more challenging because some conditions, such as cardiovascular disease, may militate against extensive reconstructive surgery (Munster & Hudis, 1999). The use of tamoxifen after surgery appears to increase survival from breast cancer for older women with metastases to the lymph nodes. However, the nurse must carefully monitor the older woman on tamoxifen, as these women develop higher serum concentrations of tamoxifen per dose than do younger women (Munster & Hudis, 1999). Age alone should not be the determining

TABLE 17-5

Pap Smear Recommendations for Women 65 Years and Older

Risk Factor → Uterine Status↓	History of Abnormal Pap Smears	HIV-Positive	Human Papillomavirus Positive	Hysterectomy for Previous Cancer	History of Regular, Normal Pap Smears
With intact cervix	Screen	Screen	Screen	Screen	Do not screen
Without intact cervix	Screen	Do not screen	Do not screen	Screen	Do not screen

Source: U.S. Preventive Services Task Force, 2003.

Note: If "screen" appears under any risk factor for a particular older woman, she should be advised to have an annual Pap smear.

factor in treatment options offered to the older woman. The nurse can be a powerful advocate for the older woman, ensuring that she receives adequate information and access to all treatment options.

Sex and the Senior Citizen

Older adults continue to need **intimacy**, chosen emotional interconnectedness between two people that includes mutual caring and responsibility, although there may be fewer opportunities and strong social sanctions against this. Intimacy entails five important aspects: commitment, affective intimacy, cognitive intimacy, physical intimacy, and mutuality (Blieszner & de Vries, 2001). Close friendships, sexual relationships, strong ties to family members, and beloved pets can all contribute to meeting the older adult's need for intimacy but are not always available. Nursing care may include touching intimate areas of an older person's body, but in a detached and clinical fashion. This may leave the older adult feeling bereft. Awareness on the part of the nurse can be an asset to older adults and their quest for intimacy.

Practice Pearl

The same things that stop you having sex with age are exactly the same as those that stop you riding a bicycle (bad health, thinking it looks silly, no bicycle).

Attributed to Alex Comfort (1974)

The age-related changes in sexual response in both men and women do not preclude a satisfying sex life. Because arousal takes longer in both sexes, foreplay is even more important than in younger adults. Hugging, kissing, and caressing are sexual activities that both men and women enjoy. They can be preludes to sexual intercourse or satisfying activities in themselves (Johnson, 1996). The older adults Johnson studied were generally open-minded and knowledgeable about sexual matters, but health status was a barrier to sexual expression.

Chronic pain and osteoarthritis are two common problems that have deleterious effects on sexual activity and older adults. Arthritis in the hip joint presents the greatest challenge to satisfying sexual activity (Butler & Lewis, 2003), but it can be ameliorated by changes in coital position, use of heat applications, and timing during the day when joints are less painful. The "spoon" position, in which partners lie on their sides with the woman in front, allows for penile penetration of the vagina without undue strain to either partner (Monga et al., 1999). Warm baths can also help relieve pain and can be incorporated as foreplay.

Many older adults who suffer from cardiovascular disease are concerned about the safety of sex. In general, if an older adult can climb two flights of stairs or walk at a rate of 2 miles per hour without chest pain or shortness of breath, he or she should have no cardiac problems during sexual intercourse (Butler & Lewis, 2003). Consideration should be given to the partner with the less stable vital signs, particularly blood pressure, and that person should not be positioned on top. Sexual intercourse with one partner in a chair, and the other directly in front of the chair, is another variation that may help some older couples (Monga et al., 1999). Figure 17-5■ illustrates these positions.

MediaLink

Erectile Dysfunction Video

FIGURE ■ **17-5**

Coital positions for older adults with cardiovascular disease.

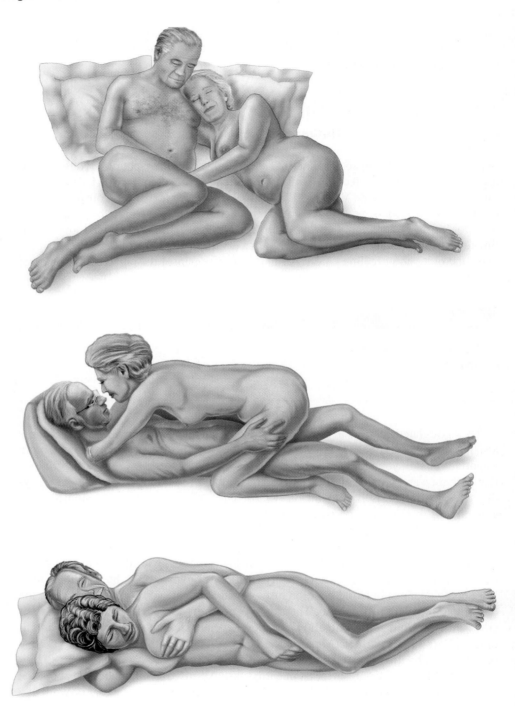

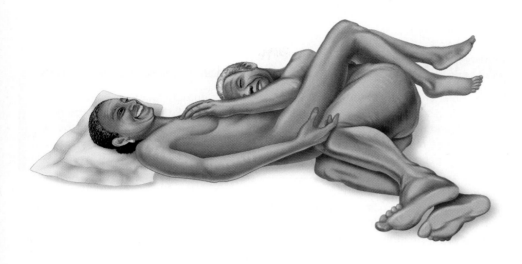

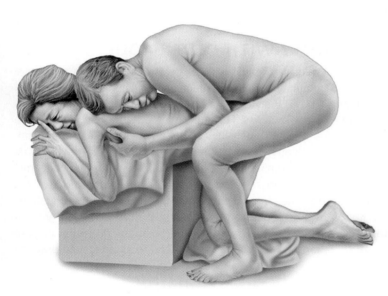

Drug Alert !

A wide range of medications can have negative effects on sexual expression, including many antipsychotics, tricyclic antidepressants, monoamine oxidase inhibitors, diuretics, beta-blockers, ACE inhibitors, and clonidine ("Focus on Effects," 2000).

Dyspareunia, painful intercourse for the older woman, may be related to decreased vaginal lubrication as well as lack of elevation of the labia during sexual arousal (Monga et al., 1999). Penetration is difficult as the vaginal opening may be partially obscured by the labia, and the lack of lubrication further inhibits entrance of the penis. The older couple might be advised to use a vaginal lubricant as part of their sexual activity and to have the woman use her hand to guide her partner's penis into the vagina.

> **Practice Pearl**
>
> The nurse should be prepared for nervous giggles or outright laughter when discussing sexuality with an older adult. Many people think that older adults do not and should not have sexual needs or desires. It is important to assure patients that a wide range of feelings about sexuality are appropriate for seniors, just as they are for younger people.

Diabetes mellitus can have negative effects on the sexual expression of both men and women. It is correlated with erectile dysfunction in the man and even greater reduction of lubrication in the woman (Monga et al., 1999). Alternative expressions of sexuality, such as body caressing, manipulation of the partner's genitals with the hand, or mutual masturbation, may be suggested.

DISCUSSING SEXUALITY WITH OLDER ADULTS

The **PLISSIT** model of intervention for sexual concerns was developed over 30 years ago, but is still a valid method for nurses to use with older adults (Annon, 1974; Hartford Institute for Geriatric Nursing, 2001). **P** stands for permission, in which the nurse validates the older adult's desire for sexual activity. The nurse may start the conversation with a neutral phrase such as, "Many people think older adults aren't interested in sex any more, but that's not true. I wonder if you have questions that I might answer for you." The permission phase is concerned with normalizing the older adult's feelings and concerns.

LI is limited information, and the nurse offers specific, factual information pertinent to the older patient. For example, an older man may appreciate knowing that although his erection is not as firm as it once was, he can still satisfy himself and his partner. **SS** stands for specific suggestions, such as coital positions or timing of pain medication. **IT** is intensive therapy, which requires a referral to an advanced practice nurse or other expert.

SEXUALITY IN LONG-TERM CARE

Meeting the intimacy needs of older adults in long-term care settings can be a challenge to the nurse. A poignant description of the negative view nurses hold of sexuality and older adults in institutions was written by Nay (1992), who concluded, "It is not possible to provide care that aims at maximizing potential, independence, and control, while denying or ridiculing a 'core' aspect of identity. It is not enough to care for the body; recognition of the whole person, including sexuality, must be reflected in nursing care" (p. 314). That being said, there are both legal and ethical concerns when it comes to sexual activity among residents of long-term care facilities.

Nursing homes have a lack of privacy for residents, and safety is a concern when there are no beds large enough to accommodate two people and sexual activity. Pushing two beds together is not a safe option, unless they are securely fastened together. The attitudes of staff and adult children, however, may be the biggest hurdle sexually active elders have to face (Lichtenberg, 1997; Nay, 1992). Adult children may collude with staff members to keep their parent away from a romantic interest.

If one or both of the older adults involved in physical intimacy is cognitively impaired, both legal and ethical responsibilities arise. The nurse must intervene to ensure that both parties are making an informed decision to participate in sexual activity, or at least that there is no exploitation involved (Lichtenberg, 1997). A person with dementia who is unable to make an informed decision should be protected from exploitation. There is no generally accepted standard for when a person with cognitive changes is no longer able to give informed consent, and the nurse will have to assess each situation. Many individuals may have concerns related to physical intimacy between nursing home residents, including the adult children of the involved residents, the unit staff, governmental agencies, and the administrative team of the nursing home.

Some older adults with dementias will engage in sexual activity that is inappropriate, for example, masturbation in public. One nursing intervention is to redirect the older adult to a private area or provide distraction (Monga et al., 1999). It is important to consider the motive that may be driving the sexual behavior and attempt to meet those needs (Duffy, 1998). For example, fondling the genitals may be an indication that the older person needs to urinate. At no time should a punitive approach be taken.

ERECTILE DYSFUNCTION

Impotence, or erectile dysfunction (ED), affects as many as two thirds of all men over 70 (Jensen & Burnett, 2002). It is defined as the inability to achieve or maintain an erection sufficient for sexual satisfaction (Carbone & Seftel, 2002). ED may be caused by vasculogenic, neurologic, hormonal, or psychogenic factors. Vasculogenic ED may be caused by poor arterial blood flow into the penis or poor return of blood through the veins. Hypertension, diabetes mellitus, dyslipidemia, and smoking may all cause arterial damage significant enough to lead to ED.

There are no universally recommended diagnostics for ED. Treatment is dependent on etiology, so some laboratory studies and specific physical examinations may be conducted. Thyroid-stimulating hormone and serum testosterone may give important information, as may imaging studies (Stern, 1997). A review of the medications an older man takes is critical, as many drugs have ED as a side effect. A neurologic examination and assessment for depression may also be performed (Carbone & Seftel, 2002).

A variety of treatments are available for ED, including oral medication, self-administered injections into the penis, vacuum erection devices, and surgical implants (Carbone & Seftel, 2002). The nurse may act as an advocate to ensure the older man is offered all appropriate treatment options.

SEXUALLY TRANSMITTED DISEASES

Sexually active older adults are at risk for the same sexually transmitted diseases that affect younger adults. They should be offered the same education about safer sex, including the use of condoms. The death rate from AIDS in persons over 65 years of age was 2.4 per 100,000 in 1997, a small but significant number (National Center for Health Statistics, 1999). Gonorrhea and syphilis are also found in the older population, with Black and Hispanic older adults having higher incidence rates than their White counterparts (National Center for Health Statistics, 1999). This may be a reflection of greater acceptance of sexuality among older persons in these populations. Questions related to symptoms of sexually transmitted diseases should be included in the review of systems and nursing assessment of an older adult.

Patient-Family Teaching Guidelines

INSTRUCTING OLDER PERSONS ABOUT URINARY TRACT INFECTIONS

The following are guidelines that the nurse may find useful when instructing older persons and their families about urinary tract infections.

1. What is a urinary tract infection?

A urinary tract infection is the result of the growth of bacteria (germs) in the kidney or bladder, or in the tubes that connect them. It might also be called a bladder infection, cystitis, or UTI.

RATIONALE:

The older patient may not understand that several different words and diagnoses can specify the same or similar conditions. The nurse should include the terms UTI, cystitis, and bladder infection when educating older patients.

2. Who gets urinary tract infections?

Women who have been through menopause are likely to get urinary tract infections.
Men with prostate problems are also likely to get urinary tract infections.
Men or women who have a urinary catheter may also get them.

RATIONALE:

UTIs are much less common in men than women because of underlying anatomical differences between the sexes. Men who present with symptoms of UTI and who have not been catheterized should seek advice from a urologist as they may have an undiagnosed prostate problem.

3. What are the symptoms?

Common symptoms of UTI may include:

- Burning or itching during urination.

- Feeling of urgency and need to urinate frequently.

- Involuntary loss of urine or urinary incontinence.

- Back pain, fatigue, nausea, and dull pain or ache in the lower abdomen.

- Sometimes confusion, especially in those who already have memory problems.

RATIONALE:

The symptoms of UTI may be vague and nonspecific. It is important to describe the wide variety of symptoms that may signal UTI in the older person.

4. How does the healthcare provider know a patient has a urinary tract infection?

A simple urine test may show white blood cells and the bacteria causing the infection. The healthcare provider will test your urine as a result of your complaints and symptoms. One test can be done quickly in the office or clinic, and the other test (culture and sensitivity) must be sent to the laboratory and takes about 3 days to obtain the final results. If you are very uncomfortable and having severe urinary symptoms, your healthcare provider will probably treat you right away with an antibiotic while awaiting the final test results.

RATIONALE:

Educating older patients and their families about the assessment and treatment process for UTIs will empower patients and facilitate positive outcomes.

5. What is the treatment for urinary tract infections?

If you are found to have a UTI with troubling symptoms and bacteria, white blood cells, or blood in your urine, you will probably be given an antibiotic by your healthcare provider. It is very important to take *all* the medicine, even if you start to feel better before it is all gone. Drink at least 8 large glasses of water per day.

RATIONALE:

The symptoms of UTI may resolve within the first few days of treatment, but to prevent reinfection the entire 5- to 7-day course of antibiotics should be taken as ordered by the healthcare provider.

Patient-Family Teaching Guidelines

6. How do I prevent another infection?

Many older people are prone to frequent UTIs. You can help prevent recurrent infections by taking the following steps:

- Make sure you keep drinking at least 8 large glasses of water per day.

- Drink a few glasses of cranberry juice if you feel the symptoms of UTI starting to bother you.

- Wear all-cotton underwear, and put on a clean set every day.

- Go to the toilet as soon as you need to urinate—do not wait.

- Wipe from the front to the back after you use the toilet.

- Make sure to pass a few drops of urine after you have sexual intercourse.

RATIONALE:

These self-care measures can prevent recurrent UTI and are part of a regimen of good urinary health practices.

Care Plan

A Patient With a Genitourinary Problem

Case Study

Mr. and Mrs. Brown are 92 and 89 years of age, respectively. They live in their own apartment, with the occasional services of a housekeeper and a visiting nurse. Their adult children and grandchildren live within easy commuting distance. Mr. Brown has osteoarthritis, most significantly in his spine, hands, hips, and knees. He has hypertension that is controlled with hydrochlorothiazide, 25 mg, po, qd; and lisinopril, 20 mg, po, qd. He takes acetaminophen, 1,000 mg, po, tid for his osteoarthritis, and it is moderately effective in controlling his pain. Mrs. Brown had a CVA 3 months ago. She has no motor deficits, and her speech is intact. Since the CVA, Mrs. Brown has had marked disinhibition, but no other health problems. She does not take routine medications, but has a prescription for Ambien, 10 mg, po, hs, prn.

At the completion of a home visit, Mr. Brown follows the visiting nurse to the front door of the apartment and asks for a word in private. He appears quite anxious, looks over his shoulder frequently at Mrs. Brown, lowers his voice, and says, "Nurse, I've got a problem. I think my wife is oversexed."

(continued)

A Patient With a Genitourinary Problem *(continued)*

Applying the Nursing Process

ASSESSMENT

Upon calm, deliberative questioning from the nurse, Mr. Brown reveals that shortly after her CVA, Mrs. Brown began to initiate sexual activity with Mr. Brown every night, sometimes several times a night. Her preferred sexual activity is intercourse. She becomes quite angry when Mr. Brown cannot achieve an erection and has frequently accused him of "fooling around with other women," although Mr. Brown vehemently denies this. Mr. Brown's feelings are hurt by Mrs. Brown's accusations. In addition, sexual intercourse makes his arthritic joints very painful, and he is not getting enough sleep due to nightly intercourse. Mr. Brown loves his wife very much and is concerned about "not satisfying her" as well as "living with a pervert." Mr. Brown tried to discuss this matter with his wife's physician, who told Mr. Brown that he had "never heard of anything as abnormal as an 89-year-old woman wanting sex." Mr. Brown has become increasingly desperate and admits to sometimes giving Mrs. Brown two Ambien tablets "just to keep her from attacking me in the middle of the night." He finishes his tale by poignantly saying, "Fifty years ago she always had a headache, now I'm getting a headache!"

DIAGNOSIS

The current nursing diagnoses for the Brown family include:

- *Deficient knowledge of human sexuality*
- *Chronic pain related to* Mr. Brown's osteoarthritis
- *Ineffective sexuality patterns*
- *Disturbed sleep pattern*
- *Disturbed thought processes related to* Mrs. Brown's CVA
- *Hopelessness related to* Mr. Brown's perception of his marital and caregiving roles
- *Interrupted family processes*

EXPECTED OUTCOMES

The expected outcomes for the plan of care specify that the Browns will:

- Achieve a mutually satisfying pattern of sexual activity.
- Develop accurate and sufficient knowledge of human sexuality.
- Manage Mr. Brown's pain to increase activity tolerance and quality of life.
- Establish productive communication patterns within their marriage.
- Experience adequate rest.
- Identify options and choices in selected situations.
- Agree to establish a therapeutic relationship with the nurse to facilitate these outcomes.

A Patient With a Genitourinary Problem

PLANNING AND IMPLEMENTATION

The following nursing interventions may be appropriate for Mr. and Mrs. Brown:

- Establish a therapeutic relationship.
- Provide sources of accurate, appropriate information related to sexuality and older adults.
  - Include information about sexual activities other than intercourse.
  - Include information about positions for sexual intercourse that may be less painful for Mr. Brown.
- Involve Mr. and Mrs. Brown in discussions about their individual concerns and desires for intimacy.
- Assess their sleep and activity patterns.
  - Look for lack of synchronization, e.g., does one partner nap from 2 p.m. to 4 p.m., and the other from 1 p.m. to 3 p.m.?
  - Consider the need for additional help with household chores, giving Mr. Brown more rest time.
  - Evaluate the need for occasional respite services for Mrs. Brown, allowing Mr. Brown to have personal time.
- Encourage Mr. Brown to share his concerns with the nurse or other health professional.
- Approach Mr. and Mrs. Brown in an open, nonjudgmental manner.
- Explore Mr. Brown's need for additional support in caring for Mrs. Brown.
- Explore Mrs. Brown's need for increased meaningful activity.

EVALUATION

The nurse will consider the plan a success based on the following outcomes:

- Mr. and Mrs. Brown will verbalize satisfying and fulfilling sexual activity.
- Mr. Brown will report that he is able to maintain a satisfactory level of physical activity without pain.
- Mr. and Mrs. Brown will demonstrate open and effective communication about their needs and feelings to each other.

Ethical Dilemma

An ethical dilemma exists when two equally compelling ethical principles are in conflict. The ethical dilemma in this situation is the conflict between beneficence for Mrs. Brown and nonmaleficence for Mr. Brown. Beneficence is the moral duty to do good, and nonmaleficence is the imperative to do no harm. The nurse has to work toward optimal outcomes for both family members, but their needs appear to be in opposition to each other. For example, Mr. Brown needs adequate sleep, but giving extra sleeping medication to Mrs. Brown may be dangerous. Similarly, Mrs. Brown needs to have her sexual needs met, but Mr. Brown needs to be pain-free.

(continued)

A Patient With a Genitourinary Problem *(continued)*

Critical Thinking and the Nursing Process

1. Are you comfortable talking with your older patients about sexuality?
2. What are some responses nurses can provide to those who say that older adults interested in sex are abnormal or "dirty old men or women"?
3. What resources do you have in your clinical setting for referral of older people with sexual problems if they need further assistance?
4. What environmental modifications might enhance sexual activity and satisfaction for older adults?

- Evaluate your responses in Appendix B.

EXPLORE MediaLink

NCLEX review, case studies, and other interactive resources for this chapter can be found on the Companion Website at **http://www.prenhall.com/tabloski**. Click on Chapter 17 to select the activities for this chapter. For animations, video tutorials, more NCLEX review questions, and case studies, access the accompanying CD-ROM in this textbook.

Chapter Highlights

- There are many age-related changes in the genitourinary systems of older men and women.
- Sexuality continues to be a human need throughout the life span.
- Understanding the changes in renal, urinary, and reproductive functions will help the nurse provide safe, effective nursing care that is holistic in nature.
- The kidney becomes less efficient in old age, producing urine that is less concentrated and making the older person more susceptible to fluid and electrolyte disorders.
- Urinary incontinence is not a normal part of aging, but age-related changes make the older adult more vulnerable to it. Urinary incontinence should always be carefully evaluated, and an individualized treatment plan developed.
- Both older men and older women have age-related changes in sexual function, but are fully able to have satisfying sexual experiences.
- Renal failure and genitourinary cancers become more common with increasing age.
- Nursing care for genitourinary concerns requires self-awareness on the part of the nurse and sensitivity to the dignity of the older adult.

References

Agency for Health Care Policy and Research. (1996). *Urinary incontinence in adults: Acute and chronic management* (AHCPR Publication No. 96-0682). Retrieved November 18, 2002, from www.ahcpr.gov/clinic/cpgarchv.htm.

AHA cautions against using HRT to prevent CVD. (2001). *Geriatrics, 56*(9), 15–16.

American Cancer Society. (2002). *Cancer facts and figures, 2002.* Retrieved August 2, 2003, from www.cancer.org/docroot/STT.

Annon, J. (1974). *The behavioral treatment of sexual problems: Volume I, Brief therapy.* Honolulu, HI: Enabling Systems.

Assad, L. A. D. (2000). Urinary incontinence in older men. *Topics in Geriatric Rehabilitation, 16*(1), 33–53.

Bailey, J. L., & Sands, J. M. (2003). Renal disease. In W. R. Hazzard, J. P. Blass, J. B. Halter, J. G. Ouslander, & M. E. Tinetti (Eds.), *Principles of geriatric medicine and gerontology* (5th ed., pp. 551–568). New York: McGraw-Hill.

Balducci, L., Pow-Sang, J., Friedland, J., & Diaz, J. I. (1997). Prostate cancer. *Clinics in Geriatric Medicine, 13*(2), 283–306.

Beck, L. H. (1999). Aging changes in renal function. In W. R. Hazzard, J. P. Blass, W. H. Ettinger, J. B. Halter, & J. G. Ouslander (Eds.), *Principles of geriatric medicine and gerontology* (4th ed., pp. 767–776). New York: McGraw-Hill.

Beers, M. H., & Berkow, R. (2000). *The Merck manual of geriatrics* (3rd ed.). Whitehouse Station, NJ: Merck Research Laboratories.

Beitz, J. M., & Zuzelo, P. R. (2003). The lived experience of having a neobladder. *Western Journal of Nursing Research, 25,* 294–316.

Bickley, L. S., & Szilagyi, P. G. (2003). *Bates' guide to physical examination and history taking* (8th ed.). Philadelphia: Lippincott Williams & Wilkins.

Binstock, R. H. (1999). Older persons and health care costs. In R. N. Butler, L. K. Grossman, & M. R. Oberlink (Eds.), *Life in an older America* (pp. 75–96). New York: Century Foundation Press.

Blieszner, R., & deVries, B. (2001). Perspectives on intimacy. *Generations, 25*(2), 7–8.

Bottomley, J. M. (2000). Complementary nutrition in treating urinary incontinence. *Topics in Geriatric Rehabilitation, 16,* 61–77.

Bravo, C. V. (2000). Aging of the urogenital system. *Reviews in Clinical Gerontology, 10,* 315–324.

Brazier, A. M., & Palmer, M. H. (1995). Collecting clean-catch urine in the nursing home: Obtaining the uncontaminated specimen. *Geriatric Nursing, 16,* 217–224.

Brown, A. D. G., & Cooper, T. K. (1998). Gynecologic orders in the elderly—sexuality and aging. In R. Tallis, H. Fillit, & J. C. Brocklehurst (Eds.), *Brocklehurst's textbook of geriatric medicine and gerontology* (5th ed, pp. 987–997). Edinburgh Scotland: Churchill Livingstone.

Bubolz, T., Wasson, J. H., Lu-Yao, G., & Barry, M. (2001). Treatments for prostate cancer in older men, 1984–1997. *Urology, 58* (6), 977–982.

Butler, R. N., & Lewis, M. I. (2003). Sexuality and aging. In W. R. Hazzard, J. P. Blass, J. B. Halter, J. G. Ouslander, & M. E. Tinetti (Eds.), *Principles of geriatric medicine and gerontology* (5th ed., pp. 1277–1282). New York: McGraw-Hill.

Carbone, D. J., & Seftel, A. D. (2002). Erectile dysfunction: Diagnosis and treatment in older men. *Geriatrics, 57*(9), 18–24.

Chow, R. D. (2001). Benign prostatic hyperplasia: Patient evaluation and relief of obstructive symptoms. *Geriatrics, 56*(3), 33–38.

Comfort, A. (Ed.). (1974). *The joy of sex: A cordon bleu guide to lovemaking.* New York: Fireside Books.

Cozen, W., & Liu, L. (2000). Risk factors for prostate cancer. In P. K. Mills (Ed.), *Prostate cancer in California* (pp. 30–35). Berkeley, CA: Public Health Institute.

Daniluk, J. C. (1998). *Women's sexuality across the life span: Challenging myths, creating meanings.* New York: Guilford Press.

Duffy, L. M. (1998). Lovers, loners, and lifers: Sexuality and the older adult. *Geriatrics, 53* (Suppl. 1), S66–S69.

Etzioni, R., Berry, K., Legler, J. M., & Shaw, P. (2002). PSA testing in black and white men: An analysis of Medicare claims from 1991–1998. *Urology, 59,* 251–255.

FDA orders estrogen safety warnings: Agency offers guidance for HRT use. (2003). *Journal of the American Medical Association, 289,* 537–538.

Focus on effects of commonly used drugs on sexual function. (2000). *Focus on Geriatric Care and Rehabilitation, 13*(10), 12.

Folstein, M., Folstein, S., & McHugh, P. (1975). Mini Mental State: A practical method for grading the cognitive state of patients for the clinician. *Journal of Psychiatric Research, 12,* 189–194.

Gambert, S. R. (2001). Prostate cancer: When to offer screening in the primary care setting. *Geriatrics, 56,* 22–31.

Ganong, W. F. (2001). *Review of medical physiology* (20th ed.). New York: Lange Medical Books.

Gruenewald, D. A., & Matsumoto, A. M. (1999). Aging of the endocrine system. In W. R. Hazzard, J. P. Blass, W. H. Ettinger, J. B. Halter, & J. G. Ouslander (Eds.), *Principles of geriatric medicine and gerontology* (4th ed., pp. 949–965). New York: McGraw-Hill.

Hartford Institute for Geriatric Nursing. (1999). *Best nursing practices in care of older adults.* New York: New York University.

Hartford Institute for Geriatric Nursing. (2001). *Incorporating essential gerontologic content into baccalaureate nursing education and staff development* (3rd ed.). New York: Author.

Hoerger, T. J., Downs, K. E., Lakshmanan, M. C., Lindrooth, R. C., Plouffe, L., Jr., Wendling, B., et al. (1999). Healthcare use among U.S. women aged 45 and older: Total costs and costs for selected postmenopausal health risks. *Journal of Women's Health and Gender-Based Medicine, 8,* 1077–1089.

Hu, T. W., Wagner, T. H., Bentkover, J. D., Leblanc, K., Zhou, S. Z., & Hunt, T. (2004). Costs of urinary incontinence and overactive bladder in the United States: A comparative study. *Urology, 63* (3), 461–465.

Jarvis, C. (2004). *Physical examination and health assessment* (4th ed.). Philadelphia: Saunders.

Jassal, V., Fillit, H., & Oreopoulos, D. G. (1998). Diseases of the aging kidney. In R. Tallis, H. Fillit, & J. C. Brocklehurst (Eds.), *Brocklehurst's textbook of geriatric medicine and gerontology* (5th ed., pp. 949–971). Edinburgh: Churchill Livingstone.

Jensen, P. K., & Burnett, J. K. (2002). Erectile dysfunction: Primary care treatment is appropriate and essential. *Advance for Nurse Practitioners, 10*(4), 45–52.

Johnson, B. K. (1996). Older adults and sexuality: A multidimensional perspective. *Journal of Gerontological Nursing, 22*(2), 6–15.

Kane, R. L., Ouslander, J. G., & Abrass, I. B. (2004). *Essentials of clinical geriatrics* (5th ed.). New York: McGraw-Hill.

Kennedy-Malone, L., Fletcher, K. R., & Plank, L. M. (2000). *Management guidelines for gerontological nurse practitioners.* Philadelphia: F. A. Davis.

Kimmick, G., & Muss, H. B. (1997). Breast cancer in older women. *Clinics in Geriatric Medicine, 13*(2), 265–282.

Krogh, R. H., & Bruskewitz, R. C. (1998). Disorders of the lower genitourinary tract. *Clinical Geriatrics, 6*(13), 19–25.

Lekan-Rutledge, D., & Colling, J. (2003). Urinary incontinence in the frail elderly. *American Journal of Nursing, 103*(Suppl. 3), 36–46.

Letran, J. L., & Brawer, M. K. (1999). Disorders of the prostate. In W. R. Hazzard, J. P. Blass, W. H. Ettinger, J. B. Halter, & J. G. Ouslander (Eds.), *Principles of geriatric medicine and gerontology* (4th ed., pp. 809–821). New York: McGraw-Hill.

Lichtenberg, P. A. (1997). Clinical perspectives on sexual issues in nursing homes. *Topics in Geriatric Rehabilitation, 12*(4), 1–10.

Malone-Lee, J. (1998). Urinary incontinence. In R. Tallis, H. Fillit, & J. C. Brocklehurst (Eds.), *Brocklehurst's textbook of geriatric medicine and gerontology* (5th ed., pp. 1343–1357). Edinburgh: Churchill Livingstone.

Mansel, R. E., & Harland, R. N. L. (1998). Carcinoma of the breast. In R. Tallis, H. Fillit, & J. C. Brocklehurst (Eds.), *Brocklehurst's textbook of geriatric medicine and gerontology* (5th ed., pp. 999–1002). Edinburgh: Churchill Livingstone.

Manson, J. E., Hsia, J., Johnson, K. C., Rossouw, J. E., Assaf, A. R., Lasser, N. L., et al. (2003). Estrogen plus progesterone and the risk of coronary heart disease. *New England Journal of Medicine, 349,* 523–534.

Masters, W. H. (1986). Sex and aging: Expectations and reality. *Hospital Practice, 21*(8), 177.

McCance, K., & Huether, S. (2001). *Pathophysiology: The biologic basis of disease in adults and children.* St. Louis, MO: Mosby.

McCue, J. D. (1999). Treatment of urinary tract infections in long-term care facilities: Advice, guidelines, and algorithms. *Clinical Geriatrics, 7*(8), 11–17.

Meadows, E. (2000). Physical therapy for older adults with urinary incontinence. *Topics in Geriatric Rehabilitation, 16,* 22–32.

Merry, B. J., & Holehan, A. M. (1994). Aging of the female reproductive system: The menopause. In P. S. Timiras (Ed.), *Physiological basis of aging and geriatrics,* (2nd ed., pp. 147–170). Boca Raton: CRC Press.

Messinger-Rapport, B. J., & Thacker, H. L. (2001). Prevention for the older woman: A practical guide to hormone replacement therapy and urogynecologic health. *Geriatrics, 56*(9), 32–42.

Miller, C. A. (1995). Medications can cause or treat urinary incontinence. *Geriatric Nursing, 16,* 253–254.

Monga, T. N., Monga, U., Tan, G., & Grabois, M. (1999). Coital positions and sexual functioning in patients with chronic pain. *Sexuality and Disability, 17,* 287–297.

Morelli, V., & Naquin, C. (2002). Alternative therapies for traditional disease states: Menopause. *American Family Physician, 66,* 129–134.

Munster, P. N., & Hudis, C. A. (1999). Systemic therapy for breast cancer in the elderly. *Clinical Geriatrics, 7*(7), 70–80.

National Cancer Institute. (2003). *Physician data query.* Bethesda, MD: Author. Retrieved 11/14/2003 from www.cancer.gov/cancerinfo/pdq.

National Center for Health Statistics. (1999). *Health, United States, 1999 with health and aging chartbook.* Hyattsville, MD: Author.

National Institute of Diabetes and Digestive and Kidney Diseases. (2001). *Kidney and urologic diseases statistics for the United States* (NIH Publication No. 02-3895). Washington, DC: U.S. Department of Health and Human Services.

Nay, R. (1992). Sexuality and aged women in nursing homes. *Geriatric Nursing, 13*(6), 312–314.

Nelson, H. D., Humphrey, L. L., Nygren, P., Teutsch, S. M., & Allan, J. D. (2002). Postmenopausal hormone replacement therapy: Scientific review. *Journal of the American Medical Association, 288,* 872–881.

Nicolle, L. E. (2003). Urinary tract infections in the elderly. In W. R. Hazzard, J. P. Blass, J. B. Halter, J. G. Ouslander, & M. E. Tinetti (Eds.), *Principles of geriatric medicine and gerontology* (5th ed., 1107–1116). New York: McGraw-Hill.

Noblett, K. L., & Ostergard, D. R. (1999). Gynecologic disorders. In W. R. Hazzard, J. P. Blass, W. H. Ettinger, J. B. Halter, & J. G. Ouslander (Eds.), *Principles of geriatric medicine and gerontology* (4th ed., 797–807). New York: McGraw-Hill.

North American Nursing Diagnosis Association. (2001). *Nursing diagnoses: Definitions and classification.* Philadelphia: Author.

Ouslander, J. G. (2000). Urinary incontinence. In D. Osterweil, K. Brummel-Smith, & J. C. Beck (Eds.), *Comprehensive geriatric assessment* (pp. 555–572). New York: McGraw-Hill.

Ouslander, J. G., Maloney, C., Grasela, T. H., Rogers, L., & Walawander, C. A. (2001). Implementation of a nursing home urinary incontinence management program with and without tolterodine. *Journal of the American Medical Directors Association, 2,* 207–214.

Palmer, M. H. (2000). Interdisciplinary approaches to the treatment of urinary incontinence in older adults. *Topics in Geriatric Rehabilitation, 16,* 1–9.

Pope, M. (1997). Sexual issues for older lesbians and gays. *Topics in Geriatric Rehabilitation, 12*(4), 53–60.

Resnick, N. M. (1984). Urinary incontinence in the elderly. *Medical Grand Rounds, 3,* 281–290.

Resnick, N., & Yalla, S. (1985). Current concepts: Management of urinary incontinence in the elderly. *New England Journal of Medicine, 313,* 800–805.

Reuben, D., Herr, K., Pacala, J., Pollick, B., Potter, J., & Semla, T. (2004). *Geriatrics at your fingertips.* Malden, MA: American Geriatrics Society, Blackwell.

Ries, L. A. G., Eisner, M. P., Kosary, C. L., Hankey, B. F., Miller, B. A., Clegg, L., &

Edwards, B. K. (Eds.). (2002). *SEER cancer statistics review, 1973–1999.* Bethesda, MD: National Cancer Institute. Retrieved September 19, 2003, from http://seer.cancer.gov/csr/1973_1999/.

Sands, J. M., & Vega, S. R. (1999). Renal disease. In W. R. Hazzard, J. P. Blass, J. B. Halter, J. G. Ouslander, & M. E. Tinetti (Eds.), Principles of geriatric medicine and gerontology (4th ed., pp. 777–796). New York: McGraw-Hill.

Saxon, S. V., & Etten, M. J. (2002). *Physical changes and aging: A guide for the helping professions* (4th ed.). New York: Tiresias Press.

Schiavi, R. C., & Rehman, J. (1995). Sexuality and aging. *Urological Clinics of North America, 22,* 711–726.

Schwartz, J. B. (1999). Clinical pharmacology. In W. R. Hazzard, J. P. Blass, W. H. Ettinger, J. B. Halter, & J. G. Ouslander (Eds.), *Principles of geriatric medicine and gerontology* (4th ed., pp. 303–331). New York: McGraw-Hill.

Smith, D. A., & Ouslander, J. G. (2000). Pharmacologic management of urinary incontinence in older adults. *Topics in Geriatrics Rehabilitation, 16,* 54–60.

Strandberg, T. E., Ylikorkala, O., & Tikkanen, M. J. (2003). Differing effects of oral and transdermal hormone replacement therapy on cardiovascular risk factors in healthy postmenopausal women. *American Journal of Cardiology, 92*(2), 212–214.

Steers, W. D. (1999). Meeting the urologic needs of the aging population. *Clinical Geriatrics, 7*(5), 62–64, 73.

Stern, M. F. (1997). Erectile dysfunction in older men. *Topics in Geriatric Rehabilitation, 12*(4), 40–52.

Tan, R. S. (1999). Managing the andropause in aging men. *Clinical Geriatrics, 7*(8), 63–69.

Termrungruanglert, W., Kudelka, A., Edwards, C. L., Declos, L., Verschragen, C. F., & Kavanagh, J. J. (1997). Gynecologic cancer in the elderly. *Clinics in Geriatric Medicine, 13*(2), 363–379.

U.S. Preventive Services Task Force. (2003). *Guide to clinical preventive services, 3rd edition: Periodic updates.* Rockville, MD: Agency for Health Care Research and Quality. Retrieved November 14, 2003, from www.ahcpr.gov/clinic/uspstf/uspsprca.htm.

U.S. Renal Data System. (2002). *USRDS 2002 annual data report: Atlas of end-stage renal disease in the United States.* Bethesda, MD: National Institutes of Health, National Institute of Diabetes and Digestive and Kidney Diseases.

Welner, S. L. (1999). Menopausal issues. *Sexuality and Disability, 17*(3), 259–267.

Wound, Ostomy and Continence Nursing Certification Board. (2003). Retrieved April 9, 2003, from www.wocncb.org.

Wyman, J. F. (2003). Treatment of urinary incontinence in men and older women. *American Journal of Nursing, 103* (Suppl. 3), 26–35.

CHAPTER 18

The Musculoskeletal System

Rita Olivieri, RN, EdD

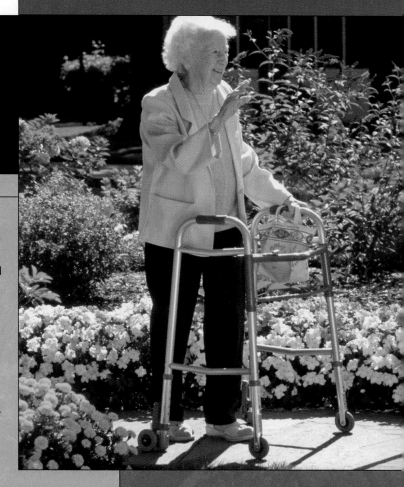

CHAPTER OBJECTIVES

Upon completion of this chapter, the reader will be able to:

- Explain normal changes in the musculoskeletal system associated with aging.
- Identify risk factors for the older person related to common musculoskeletal problems.
- List nursing diagnoses of older persons related to common musculoskeletal problems.
- Discuss the pharmacological management and nursing responsibilities related to the older person with common musculoskeletal problems, including osteoporosis, osteomalacia, Paget's disease, osteoarthritis, rheumatoid arthritis, gout, pseudogout, and hip fractures.
- Discuss the nonpharmacological management of the older person with common musculoskeletal problems, including osteoporosis, osteomalacia, Paget's disease, osteoarthritis, rheumatoid arthritis, gout, pseudogout, and hip fractures.
- Explain the nursing management principles related to the nursing care of older patients with arthritis.

 ## MediaLink

Additional resources for this chapter can be found on the Student CD-ROM accompanying this textbook and on the Companion Website at **www.prenhall.com/tabloski**. Click on Chapter 18 to select the activities for this chapter.

CD-ROM
- Animations/Videos
  Arthritis
  Bone Healing
  Bradykinesia
  Musculoskeletal System A&P
  Osteoporosis
- NCLEX Review

- Case Studies
- Tools

COMPANION WEBSITE
- Audio Glossary
- Additional NCLEX Review
- Case Study
- MediaLink Applications

KEY TERMS

The Normal Musculoskeletal System and Joints

The musculoskeletal system consists of the body's skeleton, muscles, ligaments, bursae, and joints. The skeleton provides form and support for the body. Bones provide protection for delicate body parts and are an important source of minerals as well as blood cells. The skeletal muscles provide movement of various body parts. All components of the system work together to produce the normal movement and actions that allow individuals to function independently in daily life.

Normal changes of aging often bring about complaints of musculoskeletal pain and various joint limitations, and aging appears to predispose an individual to the development of diseases such as osteoporosis and arthritis. The older person often suffers from these and other musculoskeletal chronic conditions that limit mobility and impair the ability to perform self-care activities such as bathing, dressing, and cooking. Impaired self-care abilities may result in the loss of independence. When the loss of mobility and self-care ability is permanent, it may result in a dependence on others for assistance in carrying out these activities of daily living. The older person may be forced to give up an independent lifestyle and become increasingly dependent on others for assistance.

SKELETAL SYSTEM: STRUCTURE AND FUNCTION

The adult body has 206 bones, which are divided into two major categories: the axial skeleton and the appendicular skeleton. Bones are also classified by shape, such as long bones (e.g., upper and lower extremities), short bones (e.g., tarsals, carpals), flat bones (e.g., ribs, cranium), and irregular bones (ear, vertebrae). The term *long* refers to the fact that the bone is longer than it is wide. For example, the bones of the fingers are considered long bones even though they are small. The two types of bones in the body are **compact (cortical) bone** and **spongy (cancellous) bone**. Both types of bone tissue have the same elements but are organized differently. Compact bone is solid and strong. At a microscopic level, compact bones are organized into structural units called haversian systems. These consist of concentric layers of crystallized matrix surrounding a central canal that contains blood vessels and nerves. Spongy bone is less complex and lacks the haversian systems. A typical long bone structure has a hard compact diaphysis, or shaft, fused with the spongy epiphysis at each end. The outer covering of the bone, the periosteum, is made up of fibrous connective tissue and is rich with blood vessels and nerves (McCance & Mourad, 2000).

Bones are composed of three types of cells and a bony matrix. The three types of cells are osteoblasts, osteocytes, and osteoclasts. Osteoblasts are bone-forming cells that lay down new bone. Osteocytes are mature bone cells that maintain bone. Osteoclasts are bone cells that reabsorb bone during repair and growth. The matrix consists of organic and inorganic substances. The organic substances, protein and fibers (especially collagen), are secreted by the osteoblasts and give tensile strength to the bone. The inorganic components of the matrix, calcium salts, account for the hardness that allows bone to resist compression. Bone salts allow the bones to persist long after death and have provided a great source of information about humans' ancestors (Corwin, 2000).

Bone appears to be lifeless and seems to lack the dynamics of other organ systems such as the heart and lungs. In fact, bone tissue is very active with as much as 0.5 g of calcium entering or leaving the human body per day. The functions of the skeletal system include hematopoiesis, bone remodeling and repair, and homeostasis. Bone is the site for hematopoietic tissues, which manufacture blood cells. In adults, the most active site of hematopoiesis is the red marrow cavities found within the cancellous bone spaces of the skull, vertebrae, ribs, sternum, and shoulder (Manolagas, 2003). Throughout life, new bone is continually deposited and reabsorbed in response to hormonal, dietary, and mechanical stimuli. Together, these processes are called *bone remodeling,* which is one of the major mechanisms for maintaining calcium balance in the body. The skeleton gradually undergoes replacement of old bone, and is completely regenerated every 10 years (Corwin, 2000; Manolagas, 2003).

JOINTS: STRUCTURE AND FUNCTION

Joints, the area where two bones are attached, provide stability and mobility to the skeleton. A joint may be (1) freely movable, called a diarthrodial joint; (2) immobile, a synarthrosis joint; or (3) only slightly movable, an amphiarthrosis joint. Diarthrodial joints are the most complex, and allow various positions depending upon the type of joint. The two ends of the bone are not directly connected but come together in a fibrous joint (articular) capsule that provides support. The joint capsule has two layers, an outer layer and a delicate inner layer called the synovial membrane. The synovial fluid, secreted by the synovial membrane, fills the joint cavity and provides lubrication and nourishment. Synovial joints have articulating surfaces covered by hyaline cartilage and a closed sac filled with fluid. The function of hyaline cartilage is to reduce friction in the joint and redistribute the forces of weight bearing. Bursae function as cushions in areas of potential friction. One example is the prepatellar bursa of the knee, which lies between the patella and the skin. It helps muscles and tendons glide smoothly over bone. Synovial joints include hinge, ball and socket, and pivot joints. Figure 18-1 ▪ illustrates the structure of a synovial joint.

Synarthrodial or fibrous joints are immovable and are found between the bones of the cranium, the bones of the lower arm (radius and ulna), and the bones of the lower leg (tibia and fibula). The amphiarthroses joints allow only slight movement. They are cartilaginous by construction and are found in the rib cage, vertebrae, and pubic bone.

Ligaments are fibrous connections between two bones that provide the joint with stability during movement. Ligaments both allow and limit joint motion. Commonly injured ligaments are the medial, collateral, anterior, and posterior cruciate ligaments of the knee. Tendons are collagen fibers that attach muscle to bone. These specialized

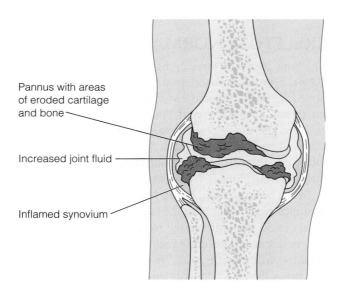

FIGURE ▪ **18-1**

Structure of a synovial joint.

Pannus with areas of eroded cartilage and bone

Increased joint fluid

Inflamed synovium

tissues are surrounded by synovial-like tissue. Ligaments and tendons protect the limbs from various sudden movements or changes in speed.

MUSCLES: STRUCTURE AND FUNCTION

Skeletal muscles are the largest organs of the body and account for 50% of lean body mass in a healthy young person (Manolagas, 2003). The more than 600 muscles in the body vary in size and shape. Their length ranges from 2 to 60 cm, and each muscle's shape is related to function. The muscle consists of a three-layer framework composed of connective tissue covered by fascia. The fascia provides support and protection for the muscle, connects muscle to bony prominences, and is the structure that houses the blood, lymph, and nerve supply.

The motor unit is the functional unit of the neuromuscular system. A motor unit consists of muscle fibers innervated by a single motor nerve, its axon, and an anterior horn cell. When the motor unit receives an electrical impulse, it contracts as a whole. The number of motor units per muscle varies greatly. Isotonic contractions, such as those that allow the person to pick up an object, produce movement. Isometric contractions do not produce actual movement, but increase the tension within the muscle. Muscle contraction occurs on the molecular level and leads to the actual observed muscle movement. A contraction occurs when an electrical charge moves along a nerve and across the neuromuscular junction to the muscles. Neurotransmitters, such as acetylcholine, permit neurologic impulses to be transmitted to the muscle. Nerve fibers may supply more than 100 individual skeletal muscle cells.

The number of muscle cells in the body does not change after birth. However, the size of the muscle cell will be determined by the work of the muscle. When the work of the muscle is demanding, the muscle will increase in diameter (hypertrophy). With lack of use, the muscle will shrink (atrophy).

Normal Changes of Aging

Significant alterations in human structure, function, biochemistry, and genetic patterns are responsible for the changes in the muscles, tendons, bones, and joints of the older person. These changes contribute to the appearance of aging in many older persons such as decreased height, stooped shoulders, and rigid movements. Figure 18-2 ■ illustrates the normal changes of aging and the musculoskeletal system.

SKELETON: NORMAL CHANGES OF AGING

The bone loss of normal aging has been described in two distinct phases (Manolagas, 2003). Type I, or menopausal bone loss, and type II, senescent bone loss. Menopausal bone loss is a rapid phase of bone loss that affects women in the first 5 to 10 years after menopause. Senescent bone loss is a slower phase that affects both sexes after midlife. These two phases are distinct in their clinical features, but in women there is eventual overlap, which leads to increased difficulty in differentiating the two phases. Other conditions may also contribute to skeletal deterioration in the older person and may alter the clinical symptoms.

In the older person, bones become stiff, weaker, and more brittle. Changes in appearance are evident after the fifth decade, and changes in height are the most obvious. At about 50 years of age the long bones of the arms and legs appear disproportionate in size due to the shrinking stature. An average loss of height is 1 to 2 cm every two decades, from about 20 to 70 years of age. This change in height is due to various processes that result in shortening of the vertebral column. Thinning of the vertebral

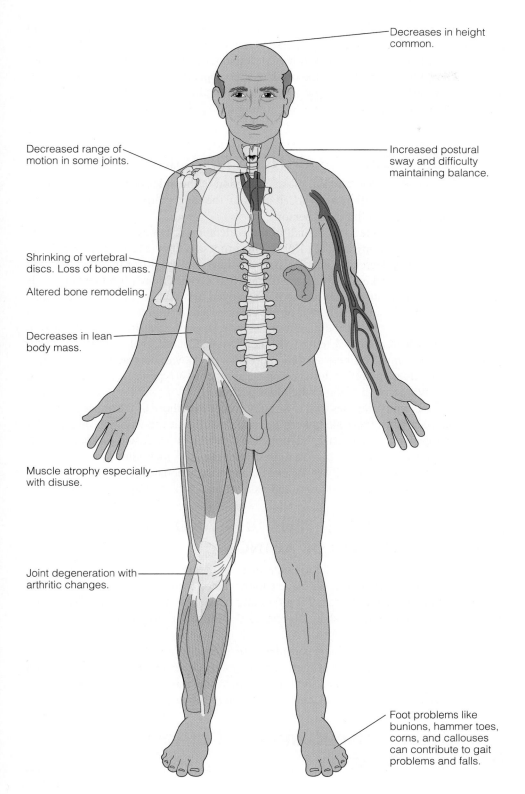

Decreases in height common.

Decreased range of motion in some joints.

Increased postural sway and difficulty maintaining balance.

Shrinking of vertebral discs. Loss of bone mass.

Altered bone remodeling.

Decreases in lean body mass.

Muscle atrophy especially with disuse.

Joint degeneration with arthritic changes.

Foot problems like bunions, hammer toes, corns, and callouses can contribute to gait problems and falls.

FIGURE ■ 18-2

Normal changes of aging in the musculoskeletal system.

disks occurs more commonly in midlife; in later years, there is a decrease in the height of individual vertebrae. As the older person enters the eighth and ninth decades, there is a more rapid decrease in vertebral height due to osteoporotic collapse of the vertebrae. The result is a shortening of the trunk and the appearance of long extremities. Additional postural changes are kyphosis and a backward tilt of the head to make eye contact. The result is a forward bent, or "jutting out" posture, with the hips and knees assuming a flex position.

MUSCLES: NORMAL CHANGES OF AGING

There is a great deal of variation in muscle function in the older person. Muscle function remains trainable well into advanced age, and the regenerative function of muscle tissue remains normal in the older person.

By age 75, most people lose one half of the skeletal muscle mass they had at the age of 30 (Metter, Lynch, Conwit, et al., 1999). This process is known as **sarcopenia**. Muscle tone and tension decreases steadily after the third decade. Some muscles decrease in size, resulting in weakness. The shape of muscles becomes more prominent and feels more distinct. Maximum muscle strength is achieved between 20 and 35 years of age. Muscle strength declines slowly, but by 50 years of age a decline in stamina is often noticed. By 80 years of age, the maximum muscle strength that the individual had in the mid-20s has decreased 65% to 85% (Metter, Lynch, Conwit, et al., 1999). The faster contracting type 2 muscle fibers atrophy more than the slower contracting type 1 muscles. Type 1 fibers maintain posture and perform repetitive-type exercise; for the most part, they maintain this function in the older person.

The lower extremity muscles tend to atrophy earlier than those of the upper extremity. Routine daily activities most likely keep the upper extremities functioning on a regular basis. By comparison, walking may be limited to a small living area and for short periods of time. Despite age-related change in muscle strength, the older adult can usually perform functional activities of daily living and demonstrate adequate muscle function when climbing stairs, walking a straight line, and rising from a sitting or squatting position.

JOINTS, LIGAMENTS, TENDONS, AND CARTILAGE: NORMAL CHANGES OF AGING

Hyaline cartilage, which lines the joints, erodes and tears with advancing age, allowing bones to be in direct contact with one another. Knee cartilage is subjected to a great deal of wear and tear, and the result is a thinning of about 0.25 mm per year. Thinning, damaged cartilage and diminished lubricating fluid result in discomfort and slowness of joint movement.

Ligaments, tendons, and joint capsules lose elasticity and become less flexible. There is a decrease in the range of motion of the joints due to changes in ligaments and muscles. Nonarticular cartilage, such as the ears and nose, grows throughout life, which may cause the nose to look large in relation to the face.

Common Musculoskeletal Illnesses of Older Persons

Osteoporosis, osteomalacia, and Paget's disease are metabolic bone diseases. Osteoarthritis, rheumatoid arthritis, gout, and pseudogout are joint diseases (arthropathies). The two major categories of arthropathies are inflammatory and noninflammatory joint diseases. Noninflammatory joint diseases (osteoarthritis) are distinguished from inflammatory joint diseases (rheumatoid arthritis, gout, and pseudogout) by the (1) lack of synovial inflammation, (2) absence of systemic manifestations, and (3) normal synovial fluid (McCance & Mourad, 2000).

OSTEOPOROSIS

Osteoporosis is the most common metabolic disease, affecting 50% of women during their lifetime. Current estimates suggest that 20 million women and 8 million men in the United States have osteoporosis. Of those estimated 20 million women, only 19% are receiving adequate care (Lie, 2000). Major risk factors for osteoporosis are increased age, female sex, White or Asian race, positive family history of osteoporosis, and thin body habitus. Additional risk factors include low calcium intake, prolonged immobility, excessive alcohol intake, cigarette smoking, and the long-term use of corticosteroids, anticonvulsants, or thyroid hormones.

Pathophysiology

Osteoporosis is characterized by low bone mass and deterioration of bone tissue leading to compromised bone strength that increases the risk for fractures. The bone strength reflects the integration of bone density and quality. Bone density is defined as grams of mineral per area or volume. Bone quality is explained as the architecture, turnover, and damage accumulation and mineralization (NIH Consensus Development Panel, 2000). At present, bone strength cannot be directly measured. Bone mineral density (BMD) is a replacement measure that accounts for 70% of the bone strength.

Bone loss in the older person is considered normal when bone mineral density is within 1 standard deviation (SD) of the young adult mean. Bone density between 1 and 2.5 SD below the young adult mean is termed osteopenic. Osteoporosis is defined as bone density 2.5 SD below the young adult mean. The three factors most likely to contribute to decreased bone mass in the older person are (1) failure to reach peak bone mass in early adulthood, (2) increased bone resorption, and (3) decreased bone formation.

Osteopenia and osteoporosis result in high mortality and morbidity. Estimated health costs are over $14 billion annually. Reduced BMD is highly predictive of spinal and hip fractures in women and men. In the United States, the number of osteoporotic fractures is 1.3 million annually (Lie, 2000). The greatest majority are fractures of the vertebrae, with about 500,000 individuals suffering from this injury each year. Hip and wrist fractures make up about one fifth of the total. One in five patients die within 1 year of a hip fracture, and only one third regain their prefracture mobility and independence level (NIH Consensus Development Panel, 2000). Figure 18-3■ illustrates normal and osteoporotic bone structure.

Classification of Osteoporosis

Primary osteoporosis is divided into type I, menopausal bone loss; and type II, senescent bone loss. Secondary osteoporosis, which is less common in elderly adults, may be caused by hyperparathyroidism, malignancy, immobilization, gastrointestinal disease, renal disease, or drugs that cause bone loss. Specific causes of secondary osteoporosis that commonly affect elderly adults are vitamin D deficiencies and the use of glucocorticoid drugs.

Menopausal Bone Loss

Before menopause, sex hormones (estrogen in women and testosterone in men) protect the body from bone loss. After menopause in women (or after castration in men), an overproduction of interleukin-6 results in an increased loss of bone mass of up to 10-fold. The

FIGURE ▢ 18-3

Normal bone compared to
osteoporotic bone.
A. Normal bone.
B. Osteopenia.
C. Osteoporosis.

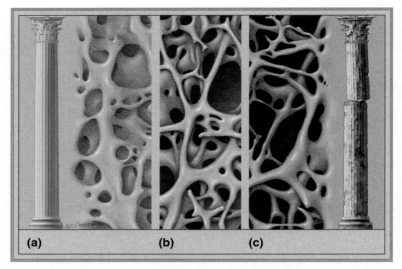

(a)   (b)   (c)

Source: Reprinted with permission from the National Osteoporosis Foundation (2003), Washington, DC 20037.
Physicians Guide to Osteoporosis. All rights reserved.

loss of bone matrix (resorption) occurs more rapidly than bone growth (deposition), resulting in the loss of bone density or osteoporosis. By age 70, susceptible women have
lost an average of 50% of their peripheral cortical bone mass from the shafts of the long
bones. Vertebral and Colles' fractures are the result of menopausal bone loss.

Senescent Bone Loss

In senescent bone loss, there is a decrease in the actual amount of bone formed during
remodeling. This occurs in both sexes and is due to the aging process. Osteoblast formation, bone mineral density, and the rate of bone formation continuously decrease,
leading to a decrease in bone wall thickness—especially in trabecular (cancellous)
bone. Trabecular bone mass is found in the vertebrae, pelvis, and shafts of long bones.
Vertebral and hip fractures may be the results of senescent bone loss.

Trajectory of Bone Loss for Women

In most cases, women in their third decade have lower peak bone mass than men. Women
generally have thinner bones, so they have less in the "bone bank." Women who have
children may lose additional bone mass with lactation. In the fifth decade during perimenopause, rapid withdrawal from the bone bank leaves the woman's bones even more
depleted. The longer life span for women further extends the risk for osteoporosis (see
Box 18-1 for gender differences in bone loss). Signs and symptoms of osteoporosis are
usually absent. Osteoporosis is a silent disease; the first sign is often a fracture.

OSTEOMALACIA

Osteomalacia is a metabolic disease in which there is inadequate mineralization of
newly formed bone matrix, usually resulting from vitamin D deficiency. Rickets,
which is similar to osteomalacia, occurs in the growing bones of children. Although osteomalacia and rickets are not common in the United States, they are endemic in Asia.
In the United States, these diseases are seen in elderly people, premature infants, people who adhere to strict macrobiotic vegetarian diets, and women who have had multiple pregnancies and have breast-fed their children.

<table>
<tr><td>

Gender Differences in Bone Loss

</td><td>

**BOX
18-1**

</td></tr>
</table>

It is generally accepted that women have a greater risk of decreased bone density and possible osteoporosis. Several factors contribute to this risk:

1. Factors during the adolescent years:
   a. Women accumulate less bone mass than men and have smaller, narrower bones with thinner cortices.
   b. Men have more bone mass growth and have bigger and stronger bones.
2. Factors related to loss of sex hormones:
   a. Abrupt loss of estrogen after menopause causes rapid loss in bone.
   b. Men have a slower decline of testosterone. Although bone mass is lost, it is at a slower rate.
3. Factors related to reproduction:
   a. Women may also lose bone mass during the reproductive years, especially with prolonged lactation.
4. Factors related to longevity:
   a. Women live longer than men and thus have an increased risk for senescent bone loss.

Data from Lie, 2000; Raisz, 2003.

Pathophysiological Mechanisms

The most common causes of osteomalacia are vitamin D deficiency, abnormal metabolism of vitamin D, and phosphate depletion. In osteomalacia, the volume of bone remains normal, but new bone replacement consists of soft osteoid rather than rigid bone. Osteoid continues to be produced, in excess of mineralization, and results in deformities of the long bones, spine, pelvis, and skull. Osteomalacia may be due to primary vitamin D deficiency from a lack of exposure to ultraviolet radiation of the sun, or to poor dietary intake. In the United States, primary vitamin D deficiency is rare because synthetic vitamin D is added to dairy and bread products. However, older persons are at risk for osteomalacia because of the inability to get outdoors, limited dietary intake of milk, as well as aging skin that is less able to produce vitamin D. In addition, many other pathological conditions in the older person may result in osteomalacia.

Clinical Manifestations

Osteomalacia causes varying degrees of bone pain and tenderness, which may be generalized or localized to the hips, pelvis, legs, ribs, or vertebrae. Bones are fragile, and fractures occur with minor injuries, making it difficult to differentiate from osteoporosis. Vertebral collapse is common, resulting in changes in posture and height. Deformities (gibbus deformity, leg bowing) occur occasionally in the severely affected older person. In severe osteomalacia, muscle weakness and easy fatigability may cause an unsteady gait. The muscle weakness is caused by lack of vitamin D to the muscle cells, as well as low calcium and phosphorus levels (Corwin, 2000).

Vitamin D Metabolism

Vitamin D is actually a group of vitamins that are essential for the metabolism of calcium and phosphorus. Each step in the process of vitamin D metabolism must be accomplished for the active form of the vitamin to be produced. Interference with any step may result in the insufficient bone mineralization that leads to osteomalacia.

The following are steps in the process of vitamin D metabolism and some of the pathological conditions that may cause a deficit at each step (Ignatavicius & Workman, 2002; Raisz, 2003):

Step 1. Normal process.
Vitamin D_3 (cholecalciferol) is manufactured by skin (from sun or certain food). *Vitamin D deficit occurs if there is* inadequate intake or inadequate exposure to sun or impairment of absorption in small bowel (postgastrectomy, small bowel resection, or Crohn's disease).

Step 2. Normal process.
Vitamin D_3 (cholecalciferol) is then carried to the liver and partly converted to calcidiol (25-hydroxy D_3). *Vitamin D deficit occurs if there is* severe liver disease and if certain drugs are taken, such as phenytoin, barbiturates, or carbamazepine.

Step 3. Normal process.
Calcidiol (25-hydroxy D_3) is then carried to the kidney and converted to calcitriol (1, 25-dihydroxy D_3). The amount produced is regulated by parathyroid hormone and plasma phosphate levels. *Vitamin D deficit occurs if there is* severe renal disease.

Step 4. Normal process.
Calcitriol (1, 25-dihydroxy D_3) is the active hormonal form that stimulates intestinal absorption of calcium and phosphorus, resulting in mineralization of the bone.

Practice Pearl

Muslim women often cover their entire body when out in public. This may prevent them from obtaining adequate vitamin D through exposure to sunlight and may increase the risk of osteomalacia.

PAGET'S DISEASE

Paget's disease, or **osteitis deformans**, is a chronic, localized bone disorder of unknown etiology in which normal bone is removed and replaced with abnormal bone. Paget's lesions may involve one or more locations of the skeleton, but are most common in the pelvis (68%), vertebrae (49%), skull (44%), and femur (55%) in both men and women, usually over 70 years of age (Corwin, 2000; Lewis, Tesh, & Lyles, 1999). Following osteoporosis, it is the second most common bone remodeling disease, affecting between 1 million and 3 million Americans. Paget's disease may be asymptomatic, the diagnosis made by abnormal x-ray findings for an unrelated problem.

Pathophysiology

Paget's disease begins with the accelerated activity of abnormally large osteoclasts, which resorb bone at specific sites. The resulting bone formation is too rapid, leading to new bone structure that is inferior to normal bone. The pagetic bone is less compact, more vascular, and especially prone to structural deformities, weakness, and pathological fractures. Although the etiology of Paget's disease is unknown, viral particles, genetics, and hereditary factors have all been implicated.

Clinical Manifestations

The clinical manifestations of Paget's disease are determined by the affected bone sites. Bone pain, the most frequently reported symptom, may be described as deep and aching, and may be accompanied by muscle spasms. Pain may occur at the site of the pagetic lesion, or at the osteoarthritic joints (hips and knees) that result from the disease. Pain, as well as the inherent mechanical deformities of the long bones, may result in bowing of the femur or tibia. Mobility impairments, gait changes, and stress fractures are also common lower extremity complications. Bony growths in the spine may cause kyphosis, cord compression, and paralysis.

When Paget's disease affects the skull, it may cause enlargement and disfigurement of the cranium, resulting in complications of the central nervous system such as mental deterioration and dementia. The older person may also experience headaches, tinnitus, and vertigo. Thickened bony growths on the interior of the skull may impinge cranial nerves, causing hearing loss and visual changes. Jaw deformities may result in dental problems such as malocclusion. The clinical manifestations of the disease may significantly affect the quality of life of older people.

JOINT DISORDERS: NONINFLAMMATORY AND INFLAMMATORY CATEGORIES

There are many joint diseases (arthropathies). The two major categories are inflammatory joint disease and noninflammatory joint disease. As mentioned previously, noninflammatory joint diseases (osteoarthritis) are distinguished from inflammatory joint diseases (rheumatoid arthritis, gout, and pseudogout) by the (1) lack of synovial inflammation, (2) absence of systemic manifestations, and (3) normal synovial fluid (McCance & Mourad, 2000).

Noninflammatory Joint Disease: Osteoarthritis

Osteoarthritis is the most common form of arthritis in the United States. Osteoarthritis (OA) affects more than 50% of people over the age of 65 and is the leading cause of disability for this age group (Agency for Healthcare Research and Quality, 2002). OA is a chronic disease that is a daily presence in the lives of over 20 million older adults. Women are affected more than men. The severity of the disease may vary greatly from being an insignificant problem to causing a major life disruption. Nodal disease at middle age is frequently associated with the development of knee OA in the 60s and 70s (Lozada & Altman, 2001). Osteoarthritis is a significant predictor of whether older persons will be functionally limited in their self-care abilities. Recent studies have determined that aging alone does not cause this disease. Associated factors include obesity, overuse of a joint, trauma, and a cold climate.

Primary or idiopathic osteoarthritis has no single, clear cause. It is likely a group of similar disorders that involve various complex biomedical, biochemical, and cellular processes. The typical changes can occur in several joints but have various causes. Secondary arthritis has an underlying condition such as trauma, bone disease, or inflammatory joint disease.

Pathophysiology. Osteoarthritis is characterized by the progressive erosion of the joint articular cartilage with the formation of new bone in the joint space (Figure 18-4 ■). The picture illustrates the hands of an older person diagnosed with osteoarthritis. The joints most commonly involved in OA are joints of the hands, the weight-bearing joints of the knee and hip, and the central joints of the cervical and lumbar spine.

FIGURE ■ 18-4

Osteoarthritis of the hands.

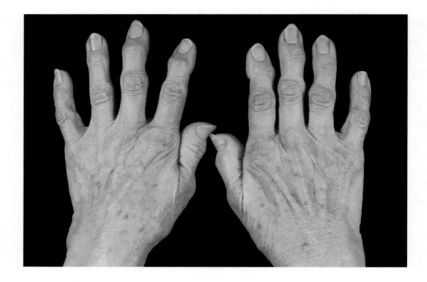

The normal joint cartilage covers the joint and bone ends and provides a cushioning structure to reduce the mechanical force of the joint. In OA, the cartilage thins and erodes. The underlying bone (subchondral bone) is no longer protected, particularly in areas of increased stress. Without the cartilage performing as a buffer, the subchondral bone becomes irritated, which leads to degeneration of the joint. As cartilage deteriorates, subchondral bone cells hypertrophy and eventually cause bony spurs (osteophytes). These bony spurs grow and enlarge, and often change the contour of the joint. Small pieces may break off (joint mice) and irritate the synovial membrane, causing a joint effusion and further limitation of movement.

Clinical Manifestations. By age 40, about 90% of all people have x-ray evidence of primary osteoarthritis in their weight-bearing joints. However, only 40% of people with severe OA (as determined by x-ray) have pain (Lozada & Altman, 2001). Generalized or systemic symptoms, such as fever and malaise, are not characteristic of OA. The most common symptoms are early morning stiffness and joint pain. Morning stiffness in the joints usually resolves in about 30 minutes. Pain usually occurs during activity and is relieved by rest. As the disease progresses, the pain may be present at rest and interrupt sleep patterns. The source of pain is often not known, but needs to be identified to provide treatment.

> **Practice Pearl**
>
> The damaged articular cartilage, the distinct feature of OA, is not the direct source of the pain because cartilage lacks nerve endings. Rather, the articular cartilage and surrounding structures cause pain indirectly. Examples of etiologies of pain include stretching of the joint capsule, muscle spasm in the surrounding area, and the release of inflammatory cells into the synovial fluid (Lozada & Altman, 2001).

Joint involvement is usually asymmetrical at first, and patients may complain of the bony appearance of their joints (see Table 18-1 for specific joints and characteristics). Pain is not usually associated with inflammatory symptoms (as with rheumatoid arthri-

TABLE 18-1

Osteoarthritis: Specific Sites, Joints, and Characteristics

Site	Joint	Features
Hand Women mainly in their 40s	Distal interphalangeal joint Proximal interphalangeal joint First carpometacarpal joint (thumb base)	Distal joint more common (flexion and lateral deviation have genetic component). Bony enlargement, malalignment (chronic). Can result in erosion, deformity, ankylosis.
Knee Women more than men in their 50s, 60s, and 70s	Medial, lateral, and patellofemoral compartment	Most often affected weight-bearing joint. Strong association with obesity. Crepitus on range of motion (chronic periarticular muscle atrophy). Limited range of motion (chronic). Bowed leg deformity—varus.
Spine	Lumbar area (facet joints) Cervical spondylosis	Pain referred to thigh—may mimic sciatic. Stiffness—muscle spasm. Spinal stenosis (chronic or severe).
Hip Men and women equally in their 40s, 50s, and 60s		Pain mainly at front of groin. Also at lateral thigh, buttocks, and radiating to knee. Characteristic limp (antalgic gait). Decreased range of motion, especially on internal rotation. Extremely disabling.
Foot	Big toe	

tis). Joints affected may have crepitus (a grating sound on movement), deficits in range of motion, and muscle weakness. Osteoarthritis of the hands may show new bone growth with the appearance of Heberden's nodes (distal interphalangeal joint) and Bouchard's nodes (proximal interphalangeal joint). Pain can be elicited on both active and passive motion. The joint damage, chronic pain, and muscle weakness of OA result in impaired balance and decreased activity.

Inflammatory Joint Disease

The three most common inflammatory joint diseases affecting the older person are rheumatoid arthritis, gout, and pseudogout. Redness, tenderness, and severe swelling around the circumference of the joints characterize inflammatory disease. Unlike osteoarthritis, inflammatory diseases are responsive to pharmacological intervention, which can improve the quality of life for the older person.

Rheumatoid Arthritis. **Rheumatoid arthritis (RA)** is the most prevalent inflammatory arthritis of any age group. It is quite common in elderly adults, and the incidence increases up to age 80. Women are affected more than men by a 3 to 1 ratio and tend to have more severe articular disease symptoms. The course of the disease varies greatly. For some patients, it may be a mild remitting disease; for others, it brings severe disability, joint deformity, and even premature death (Gornisiewicz & Moreland, 2001).

Pathophysiology. Rheumatoid arthritis is a chronic syndrome, characterized by symmetrical inflammation of the peripheral joints, with pain, swelling, significant morning stiffness, as well as general symptoms of fatigue and malaise. The cause of RA is unknown. RA is most likely due to a variety of unknown environmental factors (infectious agents, chemical exposures) that trigger an autoimmune response to an unidentified antigen. Genetic predisposition is a major factor in both the susceptibility and the severity of RA (Gornisiewicz & Moreland, 2001; Workman, 2000).

In RA, the long-term intense exposure to the offending antigen (unknown virus or bacteria) causes normal antibodies (IgG and IgM) to convert to autoantibodies. These transformed antibodies (rheumatoid factors) can then perpetuate the inflammatory response indefinitely. Rheumatoid factors are commonly (not always) present in the synovial fluid and blood of the person with RA. The initial pathological changes appear in the synovial tissue and result in mild cell proliferation. Over time, complex immune and inflammatory processes form a neoplasm-like mass in the synovium, known as a *pannus* (Browning, 2001).

The pannus is made up of granulation tissue. It erodes joint, soft tissue, cartilage, and bone, and may cause the development of bone spurs and osteophytes. The end result of pannus formation is the development of scar tissue that shortens tendons and joints, resulting in subluxation and contractures (loss of joint space, or juxta-articular bone erosion). The pannus formation causes the joint damage and is the focus of treatment for RA.

Clinical Manifestations. The course of RA may be slow and insidious, or it may present with an acute process affecting several joints (polyarticular). RA causes tenderness and limitation of movement. The older person may experience the first symptoms of RA after the age of 65. This is known as *de novo* development of RA. Clinical manifestations include disabling morning stiffness and marked pain in the joints, chiefly in the upper extremities. The morning stiffness of RA lasts more than an hour and may also occur after a period of rest. On assessment, the joints will have severe redness, swelling, and warmth of the soft tissue. These symptoms cause severe pain on movement, limitation of movement, and a disrupted sleep pattern. In the early stage of the disease, the older person may have symptoms that are severely disabling, but deformities are not present.

Rheumatoid arthritis commonly occurs in joints of the hands (proximal interphalangeal, metacarpophalangeal, wrist), elbows, shoulders, knees, ankle, and feet (metatarsophalangeal). Less frequently, joints of the shoulder, hip, and sternoclavicular are involved (Gornisiewicz & Moreland, 2001). Although RA is characterized by joint symptoms, it is a systemic inflammatory disease. Most patients with RA experience nonspecific systemic symptoms such as fatigue, malaise, weight loss, and fever, which often occur several weeks or months before the typical joint symptoms. Figure 18-5■ illustrates the hands of an older person diagnosed with rheumatoid arthritis.

Practice Pearl

The stiffness of RA is caused by the inflammatory process in the synovium that mechanically prevents the joint movement. The timing of the stiffness—lasting an hour—is especially characteristic of RA, and differentiates it from OA (stiffness due to OA lasts only a few minutes).

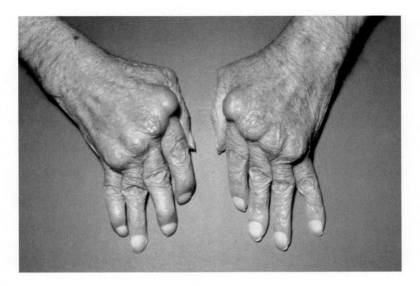

The hands of an older person diagnosed with rheumatoid arthritis.

The second category of RA in older persons occurs in those who have been diagnosed with the disease before 65 years of age. Over time, rheumatoid arthritis becomes a symmetrical additive disease of the joints. The physical stresses and inflammatory changes of the disease result in the characteristic joint deformities (see Table 18-2). Within 2 years of the establishment of the disease, more than 10% of RA patients will develop deformities of the hands. After 10 years, most RA patients will experience these changes. As described previously, these deformities are caused by the development of a pannus (long-term, severe proliferation of the synovial intimal layer).

Subcutaneous nodules also occur with advanced disease in more than one fourth of RA patients. They are located on pressure areas such as the elbows or sacrum, and are not attached to bone or underlying skin. Many older people who have had the disease for many years have multiple deformities due to progressive disease involvement. They may also have had various forms of drug treatment. In addition, these patients may have undergone one or more joint replacement surgeries.

Systemic and Nonarticular Manifestations.   In addition to joint symptoms, patients with severe and advanced RA have systemic and nonjoint manifestations of the disease. Although the disease is more common in women, these extra-articular manifestations are more common in men, especially pleural involvement, vasculitis, and

TABLE 18-2

Deformities of Chronic Advanced Rheumatoid Arthritis

Site	Deformity	Description
Hands	Swan neck deformity	Flexion of the distal interphalangeal and metacarpophalangeal joints, hyperextension of the proximal interphalangeal joint
	Boutonniere deformity	Avulsion of extensor hood of the proximal interphalangeal joint
	Ulnar deformity	Ulnar deviation of the fingers at the metacarpophalangeal joint
Feet	Hallux valgus	Displaced toes, angulation laterally

pericarditis. It is often difficult to determine if these conditions are from RA itself, or from the side effects of the drug used for treatment of the disease.

Systemic manifestations of RA include the following:

- Cutaneous manifestations: rheumatoid nodules, Sjögren's syndrome
- Ocular manifestations: episcleritis and scleritis
- Pulmonary involvement: pleurisy with effusion
- Cardiac: pericarditis and myocarditis
- Renal involvement
- Felty's syndrome (neutropenia and splenomegaly)
- Vasculitis

Multiple deformities of advanced RA are often present. These deformities are described in Table 18-2.

Gout. Gouty arthritis is the most common form of inflammatory joint disease in men over 25 years of age (Meiner, 2001). The peak onset of gout in men is between 40 and 50 years of age. Gout in women usually occurs after menopause. In general, estimates range from 2.6 to 8.4 per 1,000 adults, with the prevalence increasing with age. For persons between 65 and 74 years of age, the prevalence increases significantly to 16 per 1,000 for the older woman, and 24 per 1,000 for the older man (Sturrock, 2000). Gout is thought to be both misdiagnosed and underdiagnosed.

Pathophysiology. The pathophysiology of gout is closely linked to purine metabolism and kidney function. Uric acid is a by-product of purine, both ingested or synthesized from ingested foods. Patients with gout have a genetic abnormality of purine metabolism that results in either an overproduction or an underexcretion of uric acid. For example, some patients with gout have an abnormally high rate of purine synthesis as well as an excess production of uric acid. For these patients, reducing intake of purine foods does not affect the level of uric acid production.

Serum urate levels greater than 7 mg/dl are associated with an increased risk of gout, the risk increasing as the duration and level of urate increases (Kase & Ostrov, 2001). Hyperuricemia is due to an underexcretion or overproduction of urate, or both. In most cases of gout, underexcretion of urate is considered the most common metabolic abnormality (Meiner, 2001; Sturrock, 2000). The main predisposing factors for gout include family history, high purine diet, and obesity. Although genetics play a major role, drugs such as alcohol and acetylsalicylic acid (ASA) also result in low urate renal clearance. This may be a considerable problem for the older person who is frequently taking these drugs and may have decreased renal function, thus increasing the risk for hyperuricemia.

Clinical Manifestations. **Gout** results from the deposit of urate crystals in a peripheral joint where it initiates pain, inflammation, and destruction. Acute pain, warmth, and swelling in the metatarsophalangeal joint of the big toe are typically the first signs of gouty arthritis. A mild attack may last just a few hours, while a severe attack may last several weeks. Over time, the attacks continue and may affect other joints, including the knee, wrist, ankle, elbow, joints of the hand or feet, or bursa. General malaise, fever, and chills accompany these painful joint symptoms. Pain and tenderness are often so severe that the older person cannot tolerate the weight of a sheet or blanket, or even move the affected joint (Ettinger, 2003a). The diffuse periarticular erythema that is often present with an attack of gout may be mistaken for cellulitis. The white blood cell count (WBC) and erythrocyte sedimentation rate (ESR) may be elevated as well. The definitive finding for a diagnosis of gout is urate crystals in the synovial fluid.

Practice Pearl

Although hyperuricemia is a common feature of gout, it is not obligatory. Serum urate concentrations may be normal during an acute attack. Conversely, idiopathic hyperuricemia occurs more often than clinical gout (Sturrock, 2000).

Chronic gout, also known as tophaceous gout, can begin as early as 3 years or as late as 40 years after the initial acute attack (McCance & Mourad, 2000). The person with chronic gout will have persistent complaints of aching joints, soreness, and morning stiffness, most commonly in the hands and feet. Urate crystal deposits (tophi) occur in cartilage, synovial membranes, tendons, and soft tissue. The development of tophi is directly related to the duration and severity of hyperuricemia (Ettinger, 2003a; Kase & Ostrov, 2001). These white subcutaneous nodules, or tophi, vary in size and appear as irregular lumps or swellings of the joints. Tophi continue to grow and may eventually lead to severe limitation of movement and markedly deformed hands and feet.

Practice Pearl

In the older person, acute attacks of gout are less common. Instead, gout presents insidiously with symptoms of chronic arthritis and associated subcutaneous tophi deposits on the toes, fingers, and elbows. It is often misdiagnosed as rheumatoid arthritis (Sturrock, 2000).

Pseudogout. Pseudogout, or calcium pyrophosphate deposition disease, is a form of arthritis. It is caused by the formation of calcium pyrophosphate-dihydrate crystals in large joints. Pseudogout was so named because of the painfully similar goutlike nature of the acute attacks of joint pain that characterize the disease (see the earlier section on gout). This disease occurs in people 60 years of age or older, and women are affected more often than men. The knee is the most common joint affected for most people. Other joints that may be affected include the shoulder, hip, and elbow (Kerr, 2003).

Over time, pseudogout results in calcification of hyaline and fibrous cartilage (chondrocalcinosis). It may affect several joints at the same time and result in painful asymmetrical inflammatory polyarthritis. The mechanism of this disease is not fully understood. The tendency to develop pseudogout and chondrocalcinosis seems to run in families, although the exact genetic link is not clear. In some cases, the disease is associated with a history of hypothyroidism, hyperparathyroidism, and acromegaly.

Tendinitis and Bursitis. Tendinitis and bursitis are two of the most common and least understood causes of musculoskeletal pain. Many older persons who complain of acute pain in a joint area have soft tissue injuries and not the more serious, debilitating articular diseases. Both of these conditions are usually caused by repetitive injury due to age, sports, or occupational injuries (Reginato & Reginato, 2001). Bursitis is an irritation of subcutaneous tissue and inflammation of the underlying bursae. Bursitis also develops at pressure points such as the site of bunions. Acute bursitis is characterized by a deep aching pain on movement of any structure adjacent to the bursae. Tendinitis refers to inflammation of the tendon sheath (tenosynovitis). The course of soft tissue rheumatism, such as tendinitis and bursitis, is benign and responds to therapeutic regimens. The pain, however, is significant and will often temporarily decrease mobility.

Falls and the Older Person

Falls are a major health problem for the older person, with serious implications for medical as well as financial outcomes. Most falls occur in the home during normal routines. In the United States, falls are the leading cause of accidental death, and the seventh leading cause of death, in persons over 65 years of age (Hwang, Glass, & Moher, 1999b). The rate of death due to falls rises with increasing age. The statistics related to falls point out the seriousness of this problem and the need for ongoing prevention as part of the overall care of the older person. The National Center for Injury Prevention and Control (NCIPC, 2003) publishes a variety of statistics on this important topic. Information regarding falls and hip fractures in the older person includes the following:

- The cost of falls was over $20 billion in 1994. The cost is projected to be over $34 billion in 2020 (NCIPC, 2003).
- Each year, more than a third of people over 65 sustain a serious fall (Hausdorff, Rios, & Edelber, 2001).
- In 1999, about 10,000 people over 65 died from fall-related injuries (NCIPC, 2003).
- More than 60% of people who die from falls are 75 years of age or older (Murphy, 2000).
- Among older adults, the majority of fractures are caused by falls.
- Osteoporotic fractures of the hip, spine, and forearm are the most common fall-related injuries.
- As a person ages, he or she is more likely to sustain a hip fracture. A person 85 or older is 10 times more likely to sustain a hip fracture than a 65-year-old.
- Of all fall-related fractures, hip fractures cause the greatest number of deaths. They also result in enormous quality of life changes and numerous health problems due to immobility (Hall, Goldswain, & Criddle, 2000).
- After sustaining a hip fracture, about one quarter of older people remain in an institution for at least a year. Many are never able to return to their homes (NCIPC, 2003).

Prevention of falls in the clinical setting is one of the key goals of gerontological nursing practice. The goals are to recognize older persons at risk for falling; to identify and correct fall risk factors; to improve balance, gait, mobility, and functional independence using a structured interdisciplinary approach; to reduce or eliminate environmental factors that contribute to fall risk; and to evaluate outcomes with revision of the plan as needed. The Hartford Institute for Geriatric Nursing recommends using the Fall Assessment Tool when evaluating fall risk in the older adult; see pages 570–572.

HIP FRACTURE

Hip fractures are a serious problem for the older person, occurring in about 340,000 people annually. In 1999 in the United States, hip fractures resulted in approximately 338,000 hospital admissions (Popovic, 1999). One in three women and one in six men who reach age 90 will sustain a hip fracture. Hip fractures include those in the upper third of the femur, and may be intracapsular or extracapsular. Intracapsular fractures are those located within the joint capsule and are further categorized as femoral neck and subcapital fractures. Extracapsular fractures include intertrochanteric (in the trochanter) and subtrochanteric (below the trochanter).

Intracapsular fractures frequently impair the blood to the femoral head. A displaced femoral neck fracture can completely disrupt the blood supply to the femoral head, which may result in avascular necrosis and nonunion of the fracture. Extracapsular fractures cause acute blood loss from the vascular cancellous bone surfaces, but rarely cause avascular necrosis (Gerhart, 2003).

Most fractures in older persons result from low-energy trauma, and often occur in the home. Older persons with displaced fractures usually have a history of a fall and are unable to bear weight. Assessment findings usually reveal the older person lying with the injured leg shortened and externally rotated. The force of gravity and pull of the leg muscles cause this classic position. The extreme pain of the fracture prevents any movement, and the older person often cannot even crawl to reach a phone.

Selected Nursing Diagnoses for Common Musculoskeletal Illnesses of Older Persons

The following nursing diagnoses can be applied to many of the common musculoskeletal illnesses of older persons:

- *Impaired physical mobility* related to stiffness, pain, joint contractures, and decreased muscle strength
- *Acute pain* related to progression of inflammation
- *Chronic pain* related to joint abnormalities
- *Fatigue* related to pain and systemic inflammation
- *Body image disturbance* related to chronic illness, joint deformities, impaired mobility
- *Ineffective coping* related to personal vulnerability in a situational crisis

The most common nursing diagnosis for the older person with musculoskeletal problems is *impaired physical mobility,* which is defined as "the state in which an individual experiences a limitation of ability for independent physical movement" (Carpenito, 2002, p. 588). The major defining characteristics include the inability to purposefully move within the physical environment, and limited range of motion (Carpenito, 2002). Minor defining characteristics are decreased muscle strength, less control, inability to sit unsupported, and impaired coordination. For a diagnosis to be accurate, the North American Nursing Diagnosis Association suggests the patient should have most of the major or critical defining characteristics. Examples of related factors for impaired mobility include decreased strength and endurance, external devices such as casts, and acute or chronic pain (Carpenito, 2002).

Older people who have chronic musculoskeletal illnesses, such as arthritis, will experience both acute and chronic pain. They often accept pain as part of the aging process. As a result, pain is neither recognized nor well managed for this age group. Older people should be encouraged to express all their symptoms, including pain, so that they can be managed. Pain is defined as "a state in which an individual experiences and reports the presence of severe discomfort or an uncomfortable sensation" (Carpenito, 2002, p. 185). Chronic pain is defined as pain that is persistent for more than a 6-month period. The major defining characteristic of pain is the patient's report of pain. A rating scale of 0 to 10 should be used to identify the current pain level and to determine the goal for an acceptable pain level. Objective assessments of pain are variable and cannot be used in place of self-report. Some of the related factors for pain include actual or potential tissue damage, muscle spasm, and inflammation.

The Hartford Institute for Geriatric Nursing Best Nursing Practices in Care for Older Adults Curriculum Guide (2003) recommends that the nurse consider the following risk factors when assessing fall risk in the older person. These factors, taken from Best Nursing Practices, include:

- Cognitive impairment (dementia, impaired judgment, impulsive behavior)
- Medications (benzodiazepines, psychotropics, opioids)
- Impaired mobility, gait, or balance (cerebrovascular accident, osteoarthritis, peripheral neuropathies)
- Fall history (the occurrence of at least one previous fall)
- Acute or chronic illness
- Environmental factors (wet floor, loose and dangling wires, improper footwear, improper lighting, clutter, etc.)
- Sensory deficits (impaired vision, hearing)
- Alcohol use (ataxia)
- Postural hypotension (may be iatrogenic related to pharmacological treatment of hypertension)
- Depression (inattention to environment)
- Use of assistive devices (improper use and maintenance of canes, walkers, raised toilet seats)
- Frailty or deconditioning (loss of endurance and lean muscle mass)

The nurse is urged to develop a restraint-free attitude regarding falls in the older adult. The professional responsibility is to assess the older person and develop an individualized nursing care plan to minimize risk for falls and injury. Just because an older person has fallen does not mean that he or she should be restrained (Hartford Institute for Geriatric Nursing, 2003).

A falls prevention program is essential to the provision of holistic care for older adults. Since normal and pathological changes, which are common in aging, contribute to falls, assessment of the risk factors for falls is necessary. Recommendations for fall prevention are abundant throughout the literature, and many tools exist to identify individuals at highest risk for injurious falls. The Fall Assessment Tool presented here includes patient and environmental factors that contribute to falls. Additional environmental risks may be present depending on the physical setting. To administer the tool, the nurse circles the score that corresponds with the risk factor listed on the left-hand side of the instrument. The tool should be administered on admission to a long-term care facility or the first time an older patient is seen in an outpatient clinic. The assessment should be done again at specified intervals (yearly) and when warranted by changes in health status such as after an acute care hospitalization, the addition of a new medical diagnosis, or a significant change in the patient's condition. Scores of 15 and higher indicate high risk, and preventive fall measures should be implemented.

Instructions: Circle the score that corresponds with the risk factor listed on the left-handside of the instrument. The tool should be administered on admission to the facility or agency and again at specified intervals and when warranted by changes in health status.

FALL ASSESSMENT TOOL

Client Factors	Date	Initial Score	Date	Reassessed Score
History of falls		15		15
Confusion		5		5
Age (over 65)		5		5
Impaired judgment		5		5
Sensory deficit		5		5
Unable to ambulate independently		5		5
Decreased level of cooperation		5		5

FALL ASSESSMENT TOOL

Client Factors	Date	Initial Score	Date	Reassessed Score
Increased anxiety/emotional liability		5		5
Incontinence/urgency		5		5
Cardiovascular/respiratory disease affecting perfusion and oxygenation		5		5
Medications affecting blood pressure or level of consciousness		5		5
Postural hypotension with dizziness		5		5
Environmental Factors				
First week on unit [facility, services, etc.]		5		5
Attached equipment (e.g., IV pole, chest tubes, appliances, oxygen, tubing, etc.)		5		5

Total points: _____
Implement fall precautions for a total score of 15 or greater.

Source: Key Aspects of Elder Care: Managing falls, incontinence, and cognitive impairment. Funk, S. G., Tornquist, E. M., Champagne, M. T., & Wiese. R. A. (Eds.), *A Fall Prevention Program for the Acute Care Setting.* Hollinger, L., Patterson, R. Copyright (1992). New York. NY: Springer Publishing Company, Inc. Used by Permission.

Older nursing home residents at risk for falls should have an appropriate safety plan, including resident and environmental interventions to prevent falls and serious injuries. The following table illustrates appropriate interventions to prevent falls in long-term care facilities and delineates the roles and responsibilities of the members of the interdisciplinary team in fall prevention activities.

Resident & Environmental Interventions to Prevent Falls

These interventions show the multidisciplinary, facility-wide effort that comprises an effective falls-prevention program.

Resident-oriented Interventions

Medical Department
- Risk assessment and identification—e.g., joint and balance testing, muscle strength testing
- Medication evaluation
- Medical intervention for acute and chronic conditions

Nursing Department
- Risk-factor screening
- Care planning for risk factors
- Transfer and gait training
- Muscle-strengthening exercises
- Provide ambulation aids
- Provide proper footwear
- Provide pressure-graded stockings
- Investigate falls and suggest preventive measures

Occupational Therapy Department
- Provide chairs with arms, proper height
- Toilet pillows to raise seats
- Cervical collars

Environmental Modifications

Administration
- Provide facility philosophy, policy, and direction

Maintenance Department
- Paint edges of stairs in bright colors to help with depth-perception problems
- Install and maintain hand rails at proper height
- Install adequate, glare-free day-and-night lighting
- Use nonglare paint on walls
- Highlight night switches
- Install and maintain grab bars on toilets and tubs
- Install high toilet seats

Housekeeping Department
- Maintain nonskid, dry floors
- Position furniture in nonobstructing patterns
- Avoid placing obstacles while cleaning
- Provide proper clothing

(continued)

Therapeutic Recreation Department
- Exercise classes
- Motivation therapy
- Sensory stimulation

Social Service Department
- Provide psychosocial intervention with residents and families

Optometry/Ophthalmology Departments
- Vision screening
- Provision of glasses/lenses
- Eyecare, cataract extraction

Audiology/ENT Departments
- Audiological screening
- Provision of hearing aids

Podiatry Department
- Foot and nail care

Nursing Department
- Maintain proper staffing
- Maintain proper supervision (particularly at peak activity/accident time and shift changes)

Physical Therapy Department
- Provide proper shoes
- Provide and monitor ambulation devices

Occupational Therapy Department
- Provide advice on procurement of all seating equipment
- Provide and monitor all seating equipment

In-Service Department
- Provide transfer and ambulation training to prevent accidents that may occur during transfer
- Assure staff that no disciplinary action will be taken if an accident occurs while policies and procedures are properly followed
- Encourage staff to report accidents in a timely manner to ensure proper care

Medical Director/Nursing Director
- Monitor all accidents to identify possible hazards and formulate corrective action

Source: John A. Hartford Foundation Institute for Geriatric Nursing. (2003). *Best nursing practices in care for older adults: Incorporating essential geriatric content into baccalaureate and staff development education: A curriculum guide, 4e.* New York: New York University, The Steinhardt School of Education, Division of Nursing, The John A. Hartford Foundation Institute for Geriatric Nursing.

SELECTED DIAGNOSTIC TESTS AND VALUES FOR MUSCULOSKELETAL PROBLEMS

Some of the laboratory and radiological tests that can assist in the diagnosis and evaluation of musculoskeletal problems in the older adult include the following:

- Bone mineral density test
- Bone and joint radiography and computerized tomography
- Magnetic resonance imaging
- Bone and joint scanning

Bone Mineral Density Test

Dual energy x-ray absorptiometry (DEXA) is a common method to measure bone mineral density. DEXA of the proximal femur predicts hip fracture risk best and is the gold standard for fracture prediction. Other sites tested include spine, wrist, or total body. Bone mineral density is measured by having the patient lie on a table. An arm of the machine passes over the body part that is being tested. There is no contact of the machine with the patient, and radiation exposure is minimal. The test is considered expensive. The results are expressed in standard deviations, and compare the patient's results with the young adult mean. Results can also be compared with a norm group of the same age.

For instance, a BMD of 1 SD below the mean (-1 SD) indicates osteopenia. A BMD of 2.5 SD below the mean (-2.5 SD) indicates severe osteoporosis, according to the World Health Organization.

There are many pitfalls in the current densitometry systems (Raisz, 2003):

1. Elderly adults often have bone changes due to arthritis or disk disease in the lumbar spine, which complicates the measurement of BMD.
2. The cutoffs to determine diagnosis (-1SD, etc.) are arbitrary and must be considered in light of other factors.
3. The site of the measurement changes the relative risk. A 1 SD below the mean of the young adult (measured in the femoral neck) increases the relative risk for hip fracture 2.7 times. If the BMD is measured at other body sites, the risk is considered to be increased between 1.5 and 2 times.
   a. BMD results vary with technique and the position of the patient.
   b. Current criteria are based on postmenopausal White women and do not reflect sexual or cultural diversity (Raisz, 2003).

Bone and Joint Radiography

The routine x-ray is the basic imaging technique for diagnosis and staging of all rheumatic diseases, and for diagnosing fractures. X-rays detect musculoskeletal structure, integrity, texture, or density problems. X-rays also allow evaluation of disease progression and treatment efficacy. The routine x-ray is not sensitive enough to diagnosis BMD because change is not detected until 30% of bone mass is lost.

Computerized Tomography and Magnetic Resonance Imaging

Computerized tomography (CT) produces computer reconstruction that allows detection of images in a small area of tissue. This allows more detailed and precise diagnosis. CT scan is obtained with an x-ray machine that rotates 180 degrees around the patient's body or head (Corbett, 2000). Inflammation and degeneration that are not visible on a routine x-ray can be seen and diagnosed on a CT scan. CT also shows occult fractures and articular damage that are difficult to image on x-ray.

Magnetic resonance imaging (MRI) uses a large magnet and radio waves to produce an energy field that can be transferred to a visual image. It produces a more detailed image than CT without the use of radiation or a contrast medium. These factors give MRI advantages over CT.

However, MRI is more expensive than CT (by at least one third) and requires special facilities. MRI cannot show calcification or bone mineralization, and images of bone structure are not as useful as x-ray or CT. During an MRI, the patient hears noises that range from soft to thunderous. Earplugs may be used if desired. MRI can detect soft tissue changes such as synovitis, edema, and bone bruises that occur in traumatic injuries.

Bone Scan

A bone scan detects skeletal trauma and disease by determining the degree to which the matrix of the bone "takes up" a bone-seeking radioactive isotope. A bone scan may reveal the reason for an elevated alkaline phosphatase (ALP). It may help to diagnose a stress fracture in the elderly person who continues to experience pain after a skeletal x-ray has negative findings (Corbett, 2000).

Blood Serum Tests

Several blood tests are important in diagnosing and treating musculoskeletal disorders. They are as follows:

- Electrolytes: calcium level
- Serum uric acid (SUA)

- Joint tests: rheumatoid factor (RF)
- Acute-phase reactants: C-reactive protein
- Bone and muscle enzymes: ALP
- (CRP) and ESR

  Electrolytes: serum calcium and phosphorus decreased in the older person
  Serum calcium (normal range for older adult 8.8 to 10.2 mg/dl)
  Phosphorus (normal range for person older than 60 = 2.3 to 3.7 mg/dl)

Serum calcium and phosphorus or phosphate have an inverse relationship in a normal healthy state. Calcium is increased in Paget's disease, bone fractures, and immobility; it is decreased in osteoporosis and osteomalacia. Phosphorus is increased in bone fractures in the healing state and decreased in osteomalacia.

Serum Uric Acid

The value of SUA levels in the diagnosis of acute gout is not conclusive. A diagnosis of gout is not established unless SUA is found in tissue or synovial fluid. In general, the higher the level of SUA, the more likely the person is to have an attack of gout.

> **Practice Pearl**
>
> There are several limitations in the application of SUA levels. Elevated levels of SUA may occur in people who do not develop gout, and levels can be normal at the time of an acute attack. However, once the diagnosis of gout is made, the SUA levels can be helpful in monitoring medication levels.

Rheumatoid Factor

Rheumatoid factor is an antibody (IgM, IgG) that binds to the Fc fragment of immunoglobulin G. In the early stages of the disease, the RF is negative. However, 70% to 80% of patients with RA will become RF positive. A high RF (positive RF high titers > = 1:320) is a predictor of an increase in the severity of symptoms such as greater disability and extra-articular disease. RF is also elevated in patients with liver disease, lung disease, and other conditions. Rheumatoid factor is not diagnostic for RA, but it can confirm the diagnosis. RF does not change rapidly, so once the titer is high, the test is not repeated.

Acute-Phase Reactants: C-Reactive Protein and Erythrocyte Sedimentation Rate

Acute-phase reactants are proteins that increase serum concentration in response to acute and chronic inflammation. CRP and ESR are common acute-phase reactants. ESR is the most common measurement of acute-phase proteins in rheumatic disease. Sedimentation of red cells is directly related to the acute-phase proteins. This test can be done in the office in 1 hour. CRP is used for determining if an inflammatory process is present, such as a bacterial infection or rheumatic disease. CRP increases and goes back to normal quicker than ESR.

Alkaline phosphatase is an enzyme associated with bone activity. Normal values for men are 45 to 115 U/L, and for women 30 to 100 U/L. Values tend to increase after the age of 50. ALP studies identify increases in osteoblastic activity and inflammatory conditions. A person with Paget's disease will have a pronounced elevation of ALP (> 5×normal). Two isoenzymes—ALP_1 (liver origin) and ALP_2 (bone origin)—will help to determine if the source of the elevation is bone disease.

Synovial Fluid Analysis

Synovial fluid analysis involves evaluation of fluids drawn from a joint with a sterile needle. Synovial fluid is normally a viscous, straw-colored substance that is found in small amounts in a normal joint to provide lubrication and prevent friction during joint movement. The fluid is initially analyzed for color and clarity. Additional routine analysis may include evaluation of white blood cells, red blood cells, neutrophils, protein, glucose crystals, tests for rheumatoid factor (RA), uric acid for gout, and bacteria to establish the presence of infection. Abnormal joint fluid may look cloudy or abnormally thick.

For many diseases that have joint swelling, the aspiration and examination of synovial fluid is an important test to aid in the diagnosis. Based on visual inspection of the synovial fluid, it is classified into 4 groups (I=clear, II=transluscent, III =opaque, IV= bloody), and the appearance, volume, and cellular contents are analyzed (Wener, 2001). These four groups are on a continuum. Group I fluids are noninflammatory, have a low WBC (< 1,000/µl.), and are associated with osteoarthritis. Group II fluids are inflammatory, have a moderate WBC (2,000 to 20,000 /µl) and are associated with diseases such as rheumatoid arthritis. Group III fluids are purulent, have a high WBC (over 100,000/µl), and are infectious. Group IV fluids contain bloody fluid from a traumatic event.

Synovial fluid in groups II to IV should be cultured to determine if an infection is present in the joint. In addition, synovial fluids can be examined for monosodium urate crystals (gout) and calcium pyrophosphate-dihydrate crystals. Monosodium urate crystals are considered to be mandatory for establishing the diagnosis of gout and acute arthritis. Monosodium urate crystals are rod or needle shaped and can be seen with light microscope.

COMMON DIAGNOSTIC FINDINGS FOR MUSCULOSKELETAL ILLNESSES

A variety of tests (urine, blood, synovial fluid) and procedures may be done to diagnose and monitor the treatment of any musculoskeletal problem. Some of the common diagnostic findings are presented in Table 18-3.

Pharmacology and Nursing Responsibilities

The physiological changes of aging and resulting altered drug metabolism frequently cause serious side effects as well as drug toxicities. The older person often has more than one clinical problem and may be taking over-the-counter drugs as well. A complete history and physical as well as baseline tests should be done to determine baseline function. It is important to determine all the medications and doses the older person takes. Medication should be added to the regimen in the most safe and effective manner. Drug dosage should be based on age and renal function. Blood work should be routinely monitored for signs of toxicity. Nonsteroidal anti-inflammatory drugs (NSAIDs) are of particular concern because of their serious renal and gastric side effects. These medications are taken frequently by the older person, sometimes in inappropriate doses.

PHARMACOLOGY AND NURSING RESPONSIBILITIES FOR OSTEOPOROSIS

Bisphosphonates, selective estrogen receptor modulators (SERMs), and calcitonin are antiresorptive drugs prescribed for the treatment and prevention of osteoporosis in both

TABLE 18-3

Common Diagnostic Findings for Musculoskeletal Illnesses

Condition	Diagnostic Findings
Osteoporosis	• Decrease in bone mineral density (DEXA).
	• A bone mineral density of −1 SD below the mean (−1 SD) = osteopenia. Bone mineral density of −2.5 SD below the mean (−2.5 SD) = severe osteoporosis (Corbett, 2000; NIH Consensus Development Panel, 2000).
Osteomalacia	• Serum alkaline phosphatase (ALP) elevated.
	• X-ray studies are similar to osteoporosis. However, the classic finding of Looser's lines due to stress fractures or pseudofractures that have not healed would confirm the diagnosis.
Paget's Disease	• ALP elevated.
	• Serum calcium levels (Ca) low or normal.
	• X-rays, bone scan, or CT scans will indicate areas of increased bone resorption.
	• Depending on the stage of the disease, the bone mass may be enlarged and deformities may be present.
	• A bone biopsy may be done to confirm findings.
Osteoarthritis	• The x-ray will show joint space narrowing, spur formation, and bony sclerosis.
	• Conventional x-rays do not show cartilage changes and therefore are not helpful for early OA. X-ray pathology may be present without corresponding clinical symptoms.
	• Synovial fluid—group I.
	• White blood cell count (WBC) and erythrocyte sedimentation rate (ESR) normal.
Rheumatoid Arthritis	• The x-ray will show symmetrical disease, soft tissue swelling, and loss of articular cartilage. In late disease, joint space narrowing and joint osteoporosis.
	• Synovial fluid—group II.
	• WBC and ESR elevated in 80% of cases.
	• Positive C-reactive protein during acute phase.
	• Rheumatoid factor (RF) elevated in 50% of cases.
	• High RF (> = 1:320) is more specific to RA.
Gout	• Definitive finding is urate crystals in the synovial fluid of an affected joint.
	• WBC elevated.
	• ESR elevated.
	• Serum urate elevated (nonspecific).
Pseudogout	• Definitive finding is calcium pyrophosphates-dihydrate crystals in the synovial fluid of an affected joint.
	• WBC elevated.
	• ESR elevated.
	• Serum uric acid elevated.
Fractures	• X-ray will show fracture, trauma, and so on.
	• Hematocrit test determines blood loss from fractures.
	• ALP can be measured to show fracture healing.

men and women. Antiresorptive therapy preserves or increases bone density, and decreases the rate of bone resorption.

Bisphosphonates—alendronate (Fosamax) and risedronate (Actonel)—are potent drugs that inhibit osteoclastic activity and have decreased the incidence of vertebral and nonvertebral fractures by 40% to 50% in postmenopausal women (National Osteoporosis Foundation, 2002). Both of these drugs have been approved for the prevention of postmenopausal osteoporosis in women and for the treatment of osteoporosis in men and postmenopausal women (see Box 18-2 for drug dosages). Many people who take these drugs experience adverse gastrointestinal symptoms, such as esophageal irritation, heartburn, and difficulty swallowing. Refer to a pharmacology text for complete information (Wilson, Shannon, & Stang, 2003). Calcium should not be taken at the same time as bisphosphonates since this will interfere with the absorption of the drug.

Drug Alert ❗

The nurse is responsible for teaching the older person the specific instructions for taking Fosamax and Actonel. The older person must (1) take either drug on an empty stomach, first thing in the morning with 8 oz of water; (2) remain upright for 30 minutes; and (3) not eat or drink anything else for 30 minutes.

SERMs have been developed to provide the benefits of estrogens without the disadvantages. Raloxifene has been approved by the U.S. Food and Drug Administration (FDA) for the prevention and treatment of osteoporosis in postmenopausal women. SERMs are less effective antiresorptive drugs than bisphosphonates, but do reduce bone loss and decrease fracture risk (National Osteoporosis Foundation, 2002; Wilson et al., 2003).

Calcitonin is generally considered to be a safe but less effective treatment for osteoporosis. It has been found to decrease spinal fractures by up to 35%. It may be given intranasally or subcutaneously. It is approved for women who are at least 5 years postmenopausal (National Osteoporosis Foundation, 2002). Common pharmacological interventions for the prevention and treatment of osteoporosis are summarized in Box 18-2.

For many years, hormone replacement therapy (HRT) has been taken by postmenopausal women to reduce the risk of fractures and treat the symptoms of menopause. Many women believed that they gained extra benefits such as a reduction of cardiac events, cognitive changes, and mortality. However, many of those assumptions have been challenged. In 2000, the FDA withdrew its approval of estrogen replacement for the treatment of osteoporosis. More recent research results continue to

---

Common Pharmacological Interventions for Prevention and Treatment of Osteoporosis	**BOX 18-2**

Bisphosphonates
Alendronate (Fosamax)
    Osteoporosis prevention: 5 mg daily or 35 mg weekly po
    Osteoporosis treatment: 10 mg daily or 70 mg weekly po
SERMs
Raloxifene (Evista)
    Prevention: 60 mg daily po
Calcitonin (Miacalcin)
    Treatment: Intranasally. One spray daily delivers 200 IU.

Source: National Osteoporosis Foundation, 2002; U.S. Food and Drug Administration, 2003.

raise concerns. Several additional reports from a long-term study conducted by the Women's Health Initiative and funded by the National Institutes of Health have greatly increased the concerns of women taking these drugs. Recent results from this study have demonstrated that postmenopausal women taking estrogen plus progesterone have an increased risk of heart attack, stroke, breast cancer, and blood clots (FDA, 2003).

These new data have prompted the FDA to require pharmaceutical companies to share this new risk information with the healthcare providers and women. The FDA believes that this new information should be disseminated with the prescribing information that is given to physicians, and with the leaflet that is given to the patients, for all estrogen and estrogen plus progesterone products (FDA, 2003). Patients should be advised to discuss all drug options with their primary care provider.

> **Drug Alert** ❗
>
> In 2003, the results from the Women's Health Initiative demonstrated that postmenopausal women taking estrogen plus progesterone have an increased risk of heart attack, stroke, breast cancer, and blood clots (FDA, 2003). All nurses should keep current regarding these changes in risk factors (by visiting the FDA Website) so that they can discuss these options with their patients.

PHARMACOLOGY AND NURSING RESPONSIBILITIES FOR PAGET'S DISEASE

The many deformities, symptoms, and joint changes that occur in advanced Paget's disease are frequently irreversible. The FDA-approved treatment for Paget's disease includes two types of drugs: bisphosphonates and calcitonin (Paget Foundation, 2003). The goal of this treatment is to relieve bone pain and prevent progression of the deformities of this disease. The therapies of choice are the most potent bisphosphonates: Actonel, Fosamax, and Aredia. Common dosage examples include the following:

- Alendronate (Fosamax) given 40 mg daily for 6 months may produce a prolonged remission.
- Calcitonin (Miacalcin) by injection 50 to 100 units daily or 3 times a week for 6 months. Repeat course can be given after a short rest period (Paget Foundation, 2003).

Refer to the Paget Foundation Website for information and additional references on the treatment of Paget's disease. For some older persons, mild bone pain can be managed with ASA or NSAIDs. Adequate pain relief should be encouraged.

PHARMACOLOGY AND NURSING RESPONSIBILITIES FOR OSTEOMALACIA

The goal of the pharmacological treatment of osteomalacia is to remineralize the bone. The treatment of osteomalacia will depend on the cause. Vitamin D replacement is given in doses of 50,000 to 100,000 U/day for 1 to 2 weeks and followed by a daily dose of 400 to 800 U/day. The older person should be monitored for serum and urine calcium levels. Other forms of vitamin D such as calcidiol and calcitriol are given for the specific cause of vitamin D deficiency. All older persons with osteomalacia need to have adequate calcium intake (1,000 to 1,500 mg/day).

PHARMACOLOGY AND NURSING RESPONSIBILITIES FOR OSTEOARTHRITIS

At present, there is no therapy that will slow or halt the progression of OA (Lozada & Altman, 2001). Current therapy is directed at relief of pain and minimizing functional disability. Agents for pain relief for OA include topical agents, systemic oral agents, adjuvant agents, and intra-articular agents.

Capsaicin is a topical analgesic agent that is available as a nonprescription drug. It has been shown to be of value for OA (Lozada & Altman, 2001). Capsaicin is believed to prevent the reaccumulation of substance P (a neurotransmitter) in peripheral sensory neurons. It is applied 2 to 4 times daily to the affected area, and may cause heat or burning. It has been found to be most effective for the hands and knees (Ettinger, 2003a). Pain relief may require 4 to 6 weeks of applications (Wilson et al., 2003). Acetaminophen (Tylenol) is one of the safest drugs available and, according to the American College of Rheumatology guidelines, should be the first-line pharmacological therapy for OA (Miller, 2001). Acetaminophen can be given up to 4 g/day with minimal toxicity. Higher doses may cause liver damage. This drug has a ceiling effect, which means that increasing the dose does not increase the analgesic benefit. Acetaminophen can be used alone or as an adjunct to NSAIDs.

NSAIDs are a large group of drugs that are the most common treatment for pain and inflammation of OA. Pain of OA is intermittent; therefore, medications can be too. With most traditional NSAIDs, analgesia can be obtained at smaller doses than anti-inflammatory effects. COX-2 inhibitors, a new category of anti-inflammatory drugs, are considered safer for the gastrointestinal tract but have other side effects such as renal impairment (see Chapter 9 on pain for further information ▭).

Intra-articular corticosteroids may be of value when synovial inflammation is present. Synovial effusion is removed prior to injections. Injection should be limited to 4 per year in any one joint. Few published trials support their benefit in OA (Lozada & Altman, 2001).

The substance intra-articular hyaluronic acid for OA of the knee is a normal component of the joint involved in lubrication and nutrition. In general, hyaluronan derivatives have been found to decrease pain for longer periods than other intra-articular therapies. Intra-articular hyaluronic acid is administered in a series of 3 to 5 injections in the knee, on a weekly basis. It has been approved for use of OA of the knee, and studies on other joints are under way. There is conflicting evidence of the efficacy of hyaluronan derivatives (Lozada & Altman, 2001).

PHARMACOLOGY AND NURSING RESPONSIBILITIES FOR RHEUMATOID ARTHRITIS

Pharmacological therapies for RA include prednisone, NSAIDs, and disease-modifying antirheumatic drugs (DMARDs).

Corticosteroids such as prednisone are potent anti-inflammatory drugs used in the treatment of rheumatic diseases such as RA. They decrease inflammation rapidly and improve fatigue, pain, and joint swelling. The usual dose required for suppression of synovitis in the older person is low (2.5 to 7.5 mg per day) so toxicity is minimal. Low doses of prednisone take up to 10 years to produce osteoporosis, making it a good alternative for elderly adults who cannot tolerate other drugs. The long-term adverse effects of steroids (osteoporosis, cataracts, hypertension, and increased risk of infection) must be discussed with the patient and weighed against the functional and therapeutic benefits (Ettinger, 2003b). Some experts feel that the risk-benefit ratio for low-dose prednisone is a positive one (Kerr, 2003).

NSAIDs are another common drug category used for RA. However, the high doses required to relieve the inflammation in the elderly patient often cause toxic side effects such as gastrointestinal bleeding, gastrointestinal perforation, and renal failure. The COX-2 inhibitors are considered safer for the gastrointestinal tract, but have other damaging side effects such as renal impairment. Drugs in the category include Celebrex and Vioxx. Vioxx was withdrawn from the market in 2004 because of studies showing an increased incidence of myocardial infarction related to its use in older people. Users of Celebrex are urged to take the lowest dose possible, use the drug for only short periods of time, and investigate the use of alternative drugs.

Practice Pearl

Treatment of acute RA that offers quick relief and return of function is particularly important for the older person to prevent immobility and loss of independence. The complications of immobility, such as pressure ulcers, occur more often in the older person. When these complications develop, return to the previous level of health, function, and independence is unlikely.

DISEASE-MODIFYING ANTIRHEUMATIC DRUGS

For the older person who has been on low-dose steroids for several months, and whose symptoms have not subsided, the next pharmacological treatment offered may be the DMARDs (see Box 18-3). These drugs may offer some pain relief, but the older person may not show improvement for weeks or months. However, most of these agents have been shown to slow the rate of joint erosion and dysfunction (Browning, 2001; Gornisiewicz & Moreland, 2001). Several studies have shown a benefit to the patient when the drug is offered early in the disease process (Anderson, Wells, Verhoeven, & Felson, 2000). The disease symptoms may return when treatment ends.

DMARDs include broad-spectrum immunosuppressive agents as well as newer biological agents. All of these drugs suppress lymphocyte destruction of the synovial membrane, and each has specific toxic effects that must be monitored. The typical first choice is often methotrexate (Browning, 2001). The long-term safety of the newer biological agents has not been proven. In addition, these agents require parenteral administration and have many contraindications for use such as a history of cancer or chronic infections that are often present in older people (Kerr, 2003).

BOX 18-3 **Examples of Disease-Modifying Antirheumatic Drugs (DMARDs)**

Immunosuppressive Agents

Methotrexate
Antimalarial (hydroxychloroquine)
Sulfasalazine
Gold compounds (aurothioglucose)
Cytotoxic agents (azathioprine, cyclophosphamide, and cyclosporine)

Source: Gornisiewicz & Moreland, 2001; Kerr, 2003.

Suggested Pharmacological Options for an Acute Gout Attack

BOX 18-4

The drugs are given in the following situations:

1. NSAIDs for 2 to 7 days (should resolve the symptoms). If underlying pathology of renal, cardiac, or hepatic disease exists, NSAIDs are contraindicated.
2. If it is within 48 hours of the acute attack, colchicine can be given (normal renal function must be present). A dose of colchicine 0.6 mg given hourly to a 6-dose maximum will provide relief.
3. If symptoms are monoarticular, and the older person cannot tolerate other treatments, a long-acting steroid is injected (depomethylprednisolone) into the affected joint.
4. If the attack involves several joints, a course of oral steroids with a loading dose of 30 mg daily, with a tapering of the dose over 2 weeks, is indicated (Kerr, 2003).

PHARMACOLOGY AND NURSING RESPONSIBILITIES FOR ACUTE GOUT AND CHRONIC GOUT

Pharmacological options for the treatment of acute gout include NSAIDs, oral colchicine loading, intra-articular steroid injections, and systemic steroids (Kerr, 2003). Prompt treatment in the older person is indicated to improve symptoms and ensure a better quality of life. The pharmacological options for the treatment of pseudogout include NSAIDs or a short course of oral corticosteroids (see Box 18-4). If a large joint is involved, intra-articular corticosteroids may be effective.

Treatment for chronic gout includes colchicine, allopurinol, probenecid, and sulfinpyrazone (see Box 18-5). Colchicine (0.5 mg), an NSAID, is used to decrease inflammation. Colchicine may be given long term to reduce repeated attacks of gout. The maximum dose should be lowered for elderly patients. It is used less often today because of its liver, renal, and bone marrow toxicity (Miller, 2001). If serum urate levels remain high and colchicine is not effective, other agents may be indicated.

Drugs such as probenecid, sulfinpyrazone, and allopurinol prevent long-term complications by lowering serum uric acid blood level (see Box 18-5 for dose ranges). Probenecid and sulfinpyrazone are uricosuric agents that work by increasing the excretion of uric acid. Allopurinol is a uric acid synthesis inhibitor, which means it lowers formation of uric acid. It is more versatile than uricosurics because it may be given at all levels of renal function. The goal of therapy with these agents is to decrease serum urate levels to 6.5 mg/dl or less (Ettinger, 2003a; Miller, 2001).

Dose Ranges for Chronic Gout Medications

BOX 18-5

Probenecid (500 to 2,000 mg/day)
Sulfinpyrazone (100 to 800 mg/day)
Allopurinol (100 mg daily bid up to 600 mg/day if needed)

PHARMACOLOGICAL TREATMENT OF BURSITIS

The treatment of bursitis will depend on the cause of the problem. If infection is present (usually gram-positive staphylococcus or streptococcus, group A), antibiotics can be given orally. If microcrystalline disease and infection are absent, aspiration of fluid and injection of the bursal sac with corticosteroid is usually successful. For milder cases, resting the joint during acute phases of pain, physical therapy, use of braces or splints, and oral use of NSAIDs are also effective.

Nonpharmacological Treatment of Musculoskeletal Problems

Lifestyle changes such as increase in exercise, weight loss, and eating a healthy diet are important for all elderly adults. They are especially indicated for those with musculoskeletal problems to prevent disuse caused by immobility. Older persons should see their primary care provider, nurse, or other health professional for instructions or limitations related to fitness before beginning or changing normal routines. See specifics on exercise and rest later in the chapter.

NONPHARMACOLOGICAL TREATMENT OF OSTEOPOROSIS

Nonpharmacological treatment of osteoporosis for the older person focuses on assessment of risk factors and education to promote positive behaviors related to healthy bones. Nonmodifiable risk factors for osteoporosis are increased age, female sex, White or Asian race, positive family history of osteoporosis, thin body habitus, and the long-term use of corticosteroids, anticonvulsants, or thyroid hormones. Modifiable risk factors include low calcium intake, prolonged immobility, excessive alcohol intake, and cigarette smoking. Prevention programs should be aimed at older persons with risk factors and those with osteoporosis as determined by bone density of 2 SD below the young adult mean. However, all older people will benefit from positive lifestyle changes for osteoporosis such as diet, exercise, and other risk modifications.

ASSESSMENT AND PREVENTION OF RISK FACTORS FOR OSTEOPOROSIS

The National Osteoporosis Foundation recommendations include the following:

1. All women should be educated on the risk factors for osteoporosis. One-half of all White women will experience an osteoporotic fracture during their lifetime.
2. Any woman who has had a fracture should have a BMD test to determine osteoporosis diagnosis.
3. Any woman under 65 who has any risk factors for osteoporosis should have a BMD test, and all women over 65 should have a BMD test (National Osteoporosis Foundation, 2002).

Preventive activities are also important for older men. Many risk factors (with the exception of estrogen) are the same for men. Most men have bigger bones than women so they have increased protection. The following lifestyle modification activities to prevent or treat osteoporosis may be suggested by the gerontological nurse:

- **Promote a diet with adequate calcium and vitamin D.** Calcium intake tends to decrease in older people, sometimes due to lactose intolerance. In addition, decreased absorption of calcium from the gastrointestinal tract and changes in vitamin D metabolism contribute to the decrease in calcium absorption of the older person. All older persons should obtain an adequate intake of dietary calcium and vitamin D. Calcium supplements may slow the rate of bone loss. Calcium intake of at least 1,500 mg/day is recommended. Calcium citrate has better absorption than calcium carbonate and requires fewer pills. Patients should be instructed to take calcium with food to minimize side effects and enhance absorption. Vitamin D is necessary for calcium absorption into the bloodstream. The vitamin D requirement is 400 to 800 IU/day. Elderly adults, in whom vitamin D absorption may be reduced, should take 800 U of vitamin D daily. Many supplement options are available (AACE, 2001).
- **Encourage weight-bearing exercise.** The older person should participate in weight-bearing exercises to improve muscle strength, mobility, and agility, and to reduce the risks of falls (AACE, 2001). Regular resistance and high-impact exercises are likely the most beneficial types of physical activity. Weight-bearing exercises such as dancing, walking, and stair climbing may slow bone loss that occurs in the elderly because of disuse. Exercises should be done for 30 minutes, three times a week.
- **Reduce or eliminate smoking.** Cigarette smokers tend to be thinner and experience more fractures (AACE, 2001). Smoking depletes the body of ascorbic acid and exposes it to toxins that damage bone and interfere with calcium absorption. Tobacco use is associated with decreased bone mass and an increased risk of hip fracture in men and women.
- **Reduce or eliminate consumption of beverages containing alcohol, caffeine, and phosphorus.** Alcohol abuse is responsible for decreased bone mass and increased fractures. In addition, older persons with chronic alcoholism frequently use aluminum-containing antacids to treat gastrointestinal symptoms, which leads to calcium loss. The combination of alcohol and aluminum-containing antacids contributes to osteoporosis development.

The older adult can reduce the risk of fractures and falls by implementing the personal and home safety guidelines as listed in Box 18-9.

NONPHARMACOLOGICAL TREATMENT OF OSTEOMALACIA

Nonpharmacological treatments of osteomalacia that may be suggested to the older patient include:

- **Space activities to conserve energy.** By spacing tasks, the older person can partake in more activities, such as self-care, work-related, social, or recreational pursuits.
- **Monitor safety measures for the home.** Safety devices such as grab bars and ambulatory aids such as canes should be used to prevent falls and fractures. The fatigue experienced by the patient makes safety and protection an added concern to prevent falls and trauma.
- **Evaluate home hazards.** The risk of falls and fractures makes home safety important. Common home hazards such as scatter rugs, poor lighting, and furniture placement should be evaluated and proper steps taken to ensure safety.

NONPHARMACOLOGICAL TREATMENT OF PAGET'S DISEASE

Suggestions for nonpharmacological treatment of Paget's disease include:

- **Evaluate diet.** There is no relationship between diet and Paget's disease. In general, older people should be instructed to take adequate amounts of calcium and vitamin D and receive adequate sunshine. Older persons with Paget's disease should discuss the use of calcium and vitamin D if they have a history of kidney stones (see the instructions given earlier for osteoporosis).
- **Increase exercise.** Prevention of fractures is very important for Paget's disease. The older person should avoid undue stress on affected bones and take proper measures to avoid falls. Exercise is important to maintain joint mobility and overall skeletal health. Weight gain should also be avoided.

Healthy People 2010 and Living With Arthritis

An important part of treatment of the older person who has a chronic disease such as arthritis is learning how to live with the disease and attain the best quality of life. The *Healthy People 2010* Website contains the nation's goals and objectives for improved health for the years 2000 to 2010. One objective for arthritis patients states: "Increase the proportion of persons with arthritis who have had effective, evidence based arthritis education as an integral part of the management of their condition" (U.S. Department of Health and Human Services, 2000). Many arthritis self-help programs have been offered in the United States in the last decade. Strategies such as self-help groups, online courses, telephone support, and one-to-one instruction have been found to be effective. Patient benefits include decreased pain, increased arthritis knowledge, and an increase in the frequency of exercise. An additional benefit is reduced physician visits, which results in costs savings for both RA and OA patients (Boutaugh & Brady, 2001). Technology-supported arthritis programs also show promise for the future.

NONPHARMACOLOGICAL TREATMENT OF OSTEOARTHRITIS

For the older person with OA, early treatment can significantly affect outcomes and improve the overall quality of life. Older patients should also be offered a variety of cognitive-behavioral modalities (relaxation, imagery) to help them cope with the adjustment to chronic illness. (See Chapter 9 for cognitive-behavioral methods of pain management. ⊂▭⊃) The nonpharmacological strategies are applicable to most types of arthritis. Each strategy must be individualized to the older person's needs. Nonpharmacological treatment of OA includes:

- Education about the disease.
- Weight reduction to decrease stress on joints.
- Exercise to relieve pain and stiffness (and many other benefits).
- General and specific rest as needed to control symptoms.
- The use of canes, crutches, and walkers to protect joints.
- The use of assistive technology to help with functional ability.
- Surgical intervention for joint replacement (hips and knees).

PREVENTION AND TREATMENT OF OSTEOARTHRITIS

Older persons living with osteoarthritis may need to consider the following factors to prevent progression of their disease and to treat debilitating symptoms. Weight loss may be indicated for those who are overweight or obese, regular exercise may enhance joint health, and rest may ease pain and relieve fatigue for painful joints.

Weight Loss

The most important risk factor for OA that can be modified is obesity. Reducing weight can improve quality of life and reduce healthcare costs associated with OA. Karlson et al. (2003) studied 568 participants from the ongoing Nurses Health Study who received a hip replacement to treat OA. The researchers examined the following risk factors for hip replacement: body mass index (estimates body fat), use of hormone replacement therapy after menopause, age, alcohol consumption, physical inactivity, and cigarette smoking. Of all the risk factors, body mass index and age were associated with needing hip replacement. There was double the risk for a hip replacement for those with a high body mass index compared to participants with a low body mass index. The risk from obesity seems to begin early in life and to be established by age 18. This is one of the first long-term prospective studies to show an association between a modifiable risk factor and OA.

Practice Pearl

To prevent OA, the obese elderly person should lose weight. An obese person is five times more likely to have OA of the knees and twice as likely to have OA of the hips.

Exercise to Relieve Pain and Stiffness

Many older persons with OA (and other joint diseases) believe that exercise will cause a flare-up of their arthritis and lead to more pain. As a result, many are afraid to partake in activities that they previously enjoyed. Contrary to that misconception, exercise is an important part of treatment for the older person with arthritis. In fact, joints are dependent upon the surrounding muscles for strength, joint protection, and weight bearing. If the muscles are not used, atrophy may result and lead to weakness, falls, and mobility limitations (see exercise guidelines in Box 18-6).

Rest as Needed to Control Symptoms

Rest is also an important part of an overall plan for the older person with arthritis. Teaching the older person about rest must include both general rest and rest for the specific joints involved. General rest includes adequate sleep at night and rest periods to ensure overall health and to prevent the excessive fatigue that often occurs with inflammatory conditions. Rest should be done at specific times with proper positioning and should be limited to prevent disuse that occurs with prolonged immobility. Frequent short rest periods are better than long ones to prevent stiffness.

Practice Pearl

The correct balance between rest and exercise is extremely important for the patient with musculoskeletal problems such as OA and RA. Exercises such as swimming, stationary bicycling, and walking can be safely done with symptomatic (subacute or chronic) joints and not cause further aggravation of symptoms (Minor & Westby, 2001; Resnick, 2001).

BOX 18-6 **Exercise Guidelines for Older Persons With Arthritis**

1. Stretching of all muscle groups (prevent overstretching) 10 minutes daily.
2. Active range of motion daily for all joints.
3. Isometric exercises. Keep intensity low. Extremely forceful muscle contractions can cause intra-articular pressure and promote damage.
4. Isotonic exercises. Move the joint in an arc. Start gently and progress to weights. Attempts should be made to do full range of motion.
5. Resistive exercises twice a week. Increase weights gradually.
6. Aerobic exercises (aquatic, walking) are usually well tolerated by older adults with mild to moderate lower extremity OA. For some older persons with moderate to severe OA, walking as aerobic exercise may not be well tolerated. Alternative exercises such as swimming, biking, and water walking can be offered. Aerobics and strength training improve strength, exercise capacity, gait, functional performance, and balance (Resnick, 2001).

Specific rest relates to rest of joints that are painful or inflamed. This would include inflammatory arthritis (RA and gout) and osteoarthritis. This type of rest gives affected joints time to recover and prevents additional pain and injury, while maintaining overall physical activity and preserving function.

The older person should rest an acutely painful or inflamed joint by limiting particular activities and using assistive devices. It is important not to overstretch damaged tissues. During inflammation, tensile strength of the tissue is reduced by up to 50%; thus, overstretching and tearing can more easily occur (Minor & Westby, 2001). However, daily range of motion exercises of the remaining joints should continue because strong muscles support the damaged joint. It is important to rest painful joints to prevent overuse, provide support, and maintain function (see Box 18-7). Resting the joint should result in decreased pain, swelling, and fatigue.

Additional nonpharmacological strategies to enhance comfort for those with musculoskeletal problems such as OA and RA include:

- **Apply heat to painful joints.** Applying heat to a painful joint will decrease pain and improve flexibility. Hot packs can be applied for about 20 minutes to elevate skin temperature and then should be removed. Patients sometimes find hot showers and tub baths to be soothing. Moist heat is more effective than dry heat because it penetrates deeper (Robbins, Burckhardt, Hannan, & Dehoratius, 2001).
- **Use cold applications to reduce pain and swelling.** Cold is applied to the skin with ice packs or cold packs, usually for 10 to 30 minutes depending on the intensity of the cold source and depth of the tissue (Hayes, 2001). Mild cold is used for swelling, deeper cold for pain. Care should be taken not to frost the skin.
- **Use canes, crutches, and walkers to protect joints.** These devices are important for joint rest and safety, especially during times of acute joint pain and inflammation. The nurse should teach the patient the correct use of the device or consult with a physical therapist or occupational therapist for patient follow-up.
- **Use assistive technology.** Assistive devices are items that are used to maintain, increase, or improve function. They may be bought commercially or custom-made

---

**BOX
18-7**

Specific Methods to Rest a Painful Joint

These methods can be used during painful periods or when a joint is inflamed.

Modify activities to control joint loading:

- Avoid stairs and climbing if knees or hip joints are painful.
- Reduce time standing.
- Alternate weight bearing and non–weight bearing.
- Choose low-impact activities (swimming).
- Avoid carrying loads more than 10% of body weight.

Provide biomechanical support to reduce motion:

- Shoe modification to reduce metatarsal extension.
- Functional splints (usually of wrists, fingers, and thumbs).
- Resting splints for nighttime use.

Provide rest for joint repetitive movement:

- Keyboarding, sewing, playing musical instruments, and sitting are examples of repetitive movements.
- A regular schedule of rest breaks from these activities should be implemented.

Source: Minor & Westby, 2001.

---

for the patient. It may be as simple as a kitchen grip, an enlarged pen, a specialized motor scooter, or a dressing aid such as a sock holder. Assistive devices are available for general daily living, home management, school, and work activities. Compliance with their use increases if the patient has been adequately taught. Specific guidelines are available for environmental accessibility. The Job Accommodation Network (a service of the U.S. Department of Labor Office of Disability Employment) is a helpful resource for working with a patient in need of modification of environment.

NONPHARMACOLOGICAL TREATMENT FOR RHEUMATOID ARTHRITIS

The older person with RA generally has been living with the disease for many years. It is necessary that the patient and close family members understand the disease, symptoms that it may cause, and special care it may require (see the following Teaching Guidelines for Patient and Family for Rheumatoid Arthritis). General nonpharmacological treatment for RA is focused on reducing joint stress, maintaining joint function, promoting independence, and managing fatigue. Strength training can reverse muscle wasting. If a joint is inflamed, or if there is an exacerbation of the disease, high levels of activity are discouraged. Range of motion of the joints, however, should be maintained to prevent contractures and muscle atrophy. In general, rest can reduce joint stress. Once the acute inflammation subsides, muscle strengthening should continue to prevent atrophy around inflamed joints.

For the older person with RA, fatigue is a common problem. The chronic inflammatory response, muscle atrophy, disrupted sleep patterns, and pain all play a role in causing fatigue. Long rest periods should be scheduled in the morning and afternoon. Total body rest is important to prevent the development of fatigue. Splinting, canes, and walking aids are also useful to protect joints and reduce stress. Special devices are available for the home such as grab bars, cups, and utensils.

TEACHING GUIDELINES FOR RHEUMATOID ARTHRITIS

Education to prevent inappropriate treatment includes:

- Contacting the local Arthritis Foundation for materials and references.
- Visiting government Websites for accurate and up-to-date information.
- Talking to healthcare providers regarding advertisements for RA treatments.

Exercise and positioning to prevent contractures, muscle weakness, and atrophy include:

- Doing full range of motion daily.
- Participating in an exercise program.
- Staying active.
- Avoiding positions of deformity.

Steps to reduce joint stress during times of inflammation include:

- Resting the painful joint.
- Losing weight.
- Splinting specific joints (fingers, hands, wrist, etc.).
- Using larger stronger joints when possible.

Rest periods to prevent fatigue should include:

- Planned rest periods in morning and afternoon.
- Whole body rest to reduce inflammatory response.

Functional limitations can be minimized by:

- Using assistive devices to enhance self-care abilities.
- Modifying the environment to ensure social activities.
- Finding tools that allow leisure activities.

Box 18-8 summarizes nonpharmacological interventions useful for older patients diagnosed with gout and pseudogout.

Nonpharmacological treatment for bursitis includes moving the affected area as much as possible to the point of pain. Limited movements of the shoulder area could cause long-term problems with range of motion such as "frozen shoulder." Exercises should be reinforced with the older person to prevent disuse.

NONPHARMACOLOGICAL TREATMENT TO PREVENT FALLS AND FALL-RELATED INJURIES

Approximately 30% of older adults not in hospitals or care facilities fall each year. Because many older people lose bone density as they grow older, the risk of fractures from falls is a major concern. Falls and fall-induced injuries are increasing at a tremendous rate (Hwang et al., 1999a, 1999b). Vigorous prevention measures are needed to control

BOX 18-8

Nonpharmacological Treatment for Gout and Pseudogout

- Rest the joint during acute gout attack.
- Increase fluid intake to 3 L/day to promote renal function and prevent stones.
- Apply cold to relieve pain.
- Avoid heat application (if inflammation present).
- Avoid foods high in purine (shellfish and organ meats).
- Avoid alcoholic beverages.
- Prevent obesity to reduce urate production (for gout only).

the increasing numbers of injuries to the aging population (see Box 18-9, Fall Prevention Advice for Older Persons). Changes in vision, balance, or judgment; cardiovascular problems; medications; urinary incontinence; and other physical conditions can all contribute to an increased risk of falling (Brown et al., 2000). Many of the so-called safety measures that have been used in the past such as restraints and side rails have not been found to be effective and may even cause injury (Capezuti, 2002). Assessment of functional mobility, such as gait, balance, and position changes, provides valuable clues regarding a person's risk for future falls.

Practice Pearl

A simple assessment of routine mobility tasks can provide clinical information to determine fall risk. The older person is observed while doing the following activities: (1) getting up from a chair, (2) turning while walking, (3) raising the foot completely off the floor, and (4) sitting down. Difficulty with any of these activities often points to an increased risk for falls. The nurse should develop an individualized plan to increase muscle strength and prevent falls.

Difficulty with any one of the activities points to an increased risk for falls. The more difficulties that the older person has, the greater the risk for falls. Many functional and performance assessment tools are available that will provide quantitative data (a score) on an older person's limitation in mobility and risk for falls (Alexander, 2003; Patrick, Leber, Scrim, Gendron, & Eisener-Parche, 1999; Tinetti, 2003). Many exercise options are available to help the older person to regain and maintain muscle strength and improve general fitness (Bernick & Bretholz, 1999).

The older person should also be taught how to get up from a fall and how to get help. One method would be to turn over on the stomach and crawl to the phone. Another would be to scoot on the bottom or side to reach a phone, or the person may be able to crawl to a stairway and climb up until able to stand. If the injury does not allow movement, the person should cover up with anything handy and try to stay warm. The older person should have an emergency plan such as a bell or a phone near the floor (versus a wall phone). Daily calls to the elderly person to check on his or her safety will also give a feeling of reassurance.

BOX 18-9   Fall Prevention Advice for Older Persons

General Advice

- Have vision and hearing checked regularly.
- Talk to your doctor or nurse about side effects of medications.
- Wear rubber-soled shoes that fit well and support your feet.
- Avoid walking on icy sidewalks.
- Avoid slippery floor surfaces.
- Wear nonslip shoes at all times.
- Keep temperature at a comfortable level (Hwang et al., 1999a, 1999b).

Home Safety Advice

- Clean house and remove clutter.
- Keep lighting adequate and switches easy to reach.
- Have handrails installed where needed.
- Remove scatter rugs and mats.
- Ensure that bathtub and bathroom areas have nonskid mats.
- Secure all electrical cords

(Hwang et al., 1999a, 1999c).

TREATMENT OF HIP FRACTURES

Trained emergency staff should take the older person with a hip fracture to a hospital that offers 24-hour surgical care. Fractures must be immobilized immediately to prevent further damage. Surgery is the treatment of choice and should be performed as soon as possible. Older people will benefit from the increased mobility and pain relief that is experienced after surgery. The type of injury, the overall condition of the person, and any pre-existing orthopedic conditions will determine the type of surgical procedure. In general, the more invasive the surgical procedure, the more risk involved for the older person. For some older people with acute or chronic disease, the risk of surgery may be too great, and medical management may be the preferred course. For example, a person with severe osteoporosis who has been bedridden may not benefit from surgical interventions. The following are examples of fracture type and common surgical procedures:

1. **Nondisplaced subcapital and femoral neck fractures.** Surgical procedure is internal fixation with multiple pins.
2. **Displaced fractures of subcapital and femoral neck.** Surgical procedure includes open reduction internal fixation (ORIF), with any of the following: intermedullary rod, pins, prosthesis, or a fixed sliding plate such as a compression screw.
   a. ORIF is the surgical preference for active elderly adults who are able to use crutches with partial weight bearing.
   b. Moore's prosthesis (hemiarthroscopy, replacement of the femoral head with a smooth metal sphere) is preferred for the less active older person. Allows full weight bearing and return to active function. Figure 18-6 illustrates the repair of a hip fracture using Moore's prosthesis.
   c. Total hip replacement is done only when severe arthritis is present.

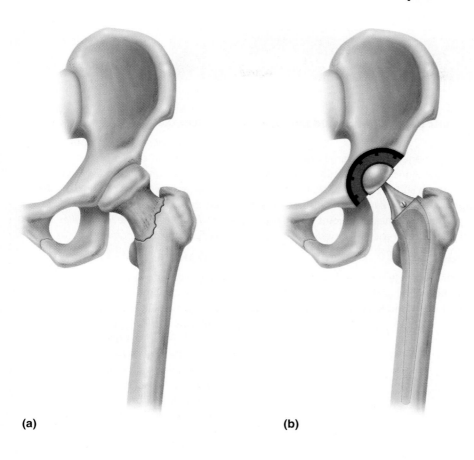

FIGURE ☐ **18-6**

A hip fracture and repair
with Moore's prosthesis in
an older person.

(a)   **(b)**

Figure 18-6 ☐ illustrates a hip fracture and repair with Moore's prosthesis in an older person.

Total joint replacement or arthroplasty involves removing the damaged part of the joint and replacing it with a prosthetic device made of metal or polyethylene. Joint replacements are indicated when pain, decreased range of motion, and increased disability interfere with daily function. The most common reason for a joint replacement is osteoarthritis, but other conditions such as RA, avascular necrosis, injury, and bone tumors may also require joint replacement.

The goals of joint replacement surgery are to decrease pain and increase joint function. In a total hip replacement, surgeons replace the head of the femur (the ball) and the acetabulum (the socket) with new parts that allow a natural gliding motion of the joint. The surgeon may use a cemented or uncemented prosthetic device. In the uncemented device, the person's own bone grows in the pores and holds the device in place. Cemented procedures were developed about 40 years ago, and have proven effective to reduce pain and increase function. They are used more frequently than cementless ones for people over 75 years and for people with osteoporosis (National Institute of Arthritis and Musculoskeletal Disease, 2001).

Nursing care of the older person with total hip replacement or internal fixation of the hip includes assessment and prevention for common complications, including dislocation of the device, avascular necrosis, infection, and delayed healing. General nursing care for the postoperative patient would depend on the specific surgical procedure.

Patient-Family Teaching Guidelines

MOBILITY PROBLEMS

1. I have osteoarthritis and chronic pain. What should I do to control my pain?

The pain of osteoarthritis should be managed with a variety of modalities. Pain initially occurs with increased activity and may be relieved by rest. As time goes on, the pain may take longer to subside and occur at rest as well. It is important that pain be managed effectively early in the disease in order to prevent inactivity that leads to muscle weakness and joint instability. Try Tylenol, topical rubs, hot and cold packs, and regular moderate exercise.

RATIONALE:

Pain levels should be adequately controlled so the older person can move about and stay active. If pain increases and limits activity, the older person may get discouraged and decide not to partake in activities because of fear of pain.

2. Why is it important to exercise?

In order to maintain or regain an active lifestyle you need to maintain muscle strength, coordination, balance, flexibility, and endurance. Exercise can do all of that for you plus benefit your heart and keep off excess weight that can further stress your joints.

RATIONALE:

Many older people have very little exercise beyond the minimum required to carry out normal routines. The stereotype of the frail elderly person quickly becomes a reality as the older person faces the challenges of the aging process. The older person should begin with a low-impact exercise and increase it gradually. Walking, dancing, and swimming are all examples of aerobic activities. Warm-up and cool-down should be included. There are numerous ways to take part in exercise, including local programs at the YMCA, local senior citizens groups, and walking groups at the mall. Each older person should determine the type of exercise he or she prefers and will continue to do.

3. What exercise can I do to keep myself moving?

Key exercises and activities that will help you to maintain functional performance include walking, pool or water aerobics, yoga or stretching exercises, dancing, golfing, fishing, or anything that is enjoyable and gets you moving.

RATIONALE:

The quadriceps muscle groups are needed when rising from a chair, stair climbing, and walking. Weakness of these muscles may prevent older persons from maintaining independence in many functional activities and cause them to be homebound or need assistance with activities of daily living. It is vital for the older person to maintain these activities on a regular basis as part of an exercise program.

Patient-Family Teaching Guidelines

4. What are some precautions I should take when I exercise?

Dress appropriately, wear proper footwear, and check with your doctor if you have chest pain, irregular heartbeat, shortness of breath, hernia, foot or ankle sores that do not heal, hot or red joints with pain, and certain eye conditions like bleeding in the retina or detached retina. If you have any of these conditions, it does not mean you cannot exercise, but modifications and precautions might be needed. See an expert who can help you get going.

5. How do I know if exercise is helping me?

Begin by seeing how far you can walk in 5 minutes. (Use a watch and record your distance in feet or blocks.) Then time yourself as you walk up a flight of stairs (at least 10 steps). After 1 month of exercising, repeat these tests and compare your times. If you are on the right track, it should be taking less time. Keep a diary and bring it with you the next time you come to the clinic.

RATIONALE:

Older people with chronic conditions should begin an exercise regimen slowly and seek advice from professionals familiar with their special needs, including cardiologists, physical therapists, sports medicine practitioners, and fitness instructors.

RATIONALE:

The nurse can discuss the patient's pain and activity diary and determine if the goals were achieved. If the patient is in the home, or the primary care setting, the nurse can evaluate the older person's functional abilities and focus on areas of concern such as hips and knees. If the older person met the goal, the nurse and patient can determine if the exercise goal can be increased to include a longer time period or increase in intensity of activities. Praise is given for achievement.

If the goal has not been met, the nurse and patient need to evaluate the data and revise the care plan to reflect the abilities of the older person. Compassion and understanding are important so that the older person does not get discouraged. If the patient is having an episode of acute joint pain, range of motion should continue on all noninvolved joints. Stiffness, muscle weakness, and atrophy can occur quickly if the person becomes immobile. Prescribed pain medication, as well as nonpharmacological pain management techniques, should be implemented to allow the patient to remain as active as possible during the acute pain.

Care Plan

A Patient With a Hip Fracture

Case Study

Mrs. Jerome is a patient in the orthopedic department of a large hospital. She is an 82-year-old widow who has lived alone for the last 5 years since her husband died. Her daughter found her on the floor of her home where she had fallen. Mrs. Jerome was admitted to the emergency department, where x-rays revealed a hip fracture due to severe osteoporosis. She is 4 days postoperative after an ORIF of the left femur. She is stable surgically and has been medicated for pain with Percocet 1 tablet. The night nurse reports that Mrs. Jerome has been crying at times during the night. When the nurse tried to talk to her, she said she was fine.

Applying the Nursing Process

ASSESSMENT

The registered nurse completes the nursing assessment and discusses Mrs. Jerome's history, which includes hypertension, high cholesterol, and asthma. The physical examination shows blood pressure 160/90, pulse 88, respirations 28, and temperature 98°F. The nurse notes a large hip dressing which is dry and intact. The patient has pain of 3 on a 0 to 10 scale. Mrs. Jerome states that she "has been living in her home alone and managing normal daily activities until this terrible thing happened." She enjoys cooking for herself, her daughter, and other family members when they visit. Her daughter, Rose, does her errands and takes her to the doctor. Mrs. Jerome does not go out alone. She gave up smoking many years ago and keeps to her diet to lower her cholesterol. She is on medications for asthma and hypertension. Mrs. Jerome starts to cry when she talks about her sister who recently passed away. She states, "My sister went to a nursing home after a fall and was never able to return to her own home again." Her daughter, Rose, has spoken with the nurse and doctor and does not feel that her mother would be safe living alone at home anymore. Rose is very upset about the situation. However, she does not wish to talk to her mother about this at the present time.

DIAGNOSIS

The current nursing diagnoses for Mrs. Jerome include the following:

- *Impaired physical mobility* related to tissue trauma secondary to fracture
- *Anxiety* related to anticipated postoperative dependence and living situation
- *Pain* related to surgical trauma
- *Risk for trauma: falls* related to weakness, *fatigue* related to surgery

A Patient With a Hip Fracture

EXPECTED OUTCOMES

Expected outcomes for the plan specify that Mrs. Jerome will:

- Demonstrate knowledge related to self-care after surgical procedure for a fractured hip.
- Verbalize fears to help cope with change due to injury and hospitalization.
- Report pain as tolerable (such as less than 3 on a 0 to 10 scale).
- Collaborate with the nurse and healthcare team to reach the goal of returning home with functional independence.

PLANNING AND IMPLEMENTATION

The following nursing interventions may be appropriate for Mrs. Jerome:

- Allow patient to complete self-care as much as possible to gain confidence in her abilities.
- Begin to explore the patient's problem-solving strategies to determine how she has resolved past changes or problems.
- Assess support systems that are available for the patient after hospitalization.
- Identify a plan to reduce the risk of falls in the future.
- Reinforce all exercises, ambulation, and transfer techniques that will achieve maximum physical mobility within restrictions of the surgery.

EVALUATION

The nurse hopes to resolve this patient situation. The nurse will consider the plan a success based on the following:

- Mrs. Jerome will learn the major concepts of self-care after hip fracture.
- She will report minimal pain and will have adequate pain control.
- Mrs. Jerome will progress in her muscle strength and maintain functional ability as much as possible to prevent disuse.
- She and her daughter will discuss the short-term and long-term options and develop a plan based on Mrs. Jerome's progress and her overall health.

Ethical Dilemma

The primary ethical dilemma in this situation is the conflict between the moral obligation of the nurse to be honest with the patient (veracity) and the daughter's wish for the nurse not to disclose to the patient that she does not believe her mother should return home. The patient is interested in doing all she has to do to get better and return home. Her daughter has been visiting and giving encouragement to her mother but has not been honest about her true feelings about the discharge plan.

The nurse has an obligation to be honest with the patient. The nurse also has an obligation to do good, based on the principle of beneficence, and to respect the patient's autonomy. The patient has the right to make decisions for herself and should be part of the discussions that are about her future.

(continued)

A Patient With a Hip Fracture *(continued)*

The nurse plans to ask the daughter to speak openly with her mother. The nurse also plans to set up a meeting with the entire healthcare team so that the daughter can appreciate the true potential and progress that Mrs. Jerome can make. The risks and benefits of Mrs. Jerome returning to her own home will also be discussed. The nurse hopes to help the daughter and mother make the decision together. The patient has the right to make the decision, but the daughter's help will be needed to support the patient in the home as she has been doing for the past 5 years.

Critical Thinking and the Nursing Process

1. What factors should the nurse consider when caring for older patients with osteoporosis?
2. What safety measures should the nurse and the older patient plan for the home environment to prevent falls?
3. What type of exercise program are you comfortable suggesting to your older patients with mobility problems?

■ Evaluate your responses in Appendix B.

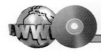

EXPLORE MediaLink

NCLEX review, case studies, and other interactive resources for this chapter can be found on the Companion Website at **www.prenhall.com/tabloski**. Click on Chapter 18 to select the activities for this chapter. For animations, video tutorials, more NCLEX review questions, and case studies, access the accompanying CD-ROM in this textbook.

Chapter Highlights

■ The older person loses 1 to 2 cm of height every two decades from about 20 to 70 years of age.

■ By age 75, older persons lose about one half of the skeletal muscle mass they had at 30 years of age.

■ The older person can usually perform the functional activities of daily living and demonstrate adequate muscle function.

■ There is a decrease in range of motion of joints due to loss of elasticity in ligaments, tendons, and joint capsules.

■ Diagnostic tests for musculoskeletal problems include bone mineral density, synovial fluid analysis, x-rays, CT, MRI, and blood tests including calcium level, rheumatoid factor, C-reactive protein, erythrocyte sedimentation rate, and serum uric acid.

- Osteoporosis is characterized by low bone mass and deterioration of bone tissue leading to a decrease in bone strength that increases the risk for fractures.

- The major risk factors for osteoporosis are increased age, female sex, White or Asian race, thin body, and positive family history of the disease.

- Treatment for osteoporosis includes increasing calcium in the diet, and drug therapy with antiresorptive agents such as Fosamax.

- Osteomalacia is a metabolic disorder caused by vitamin D deficiency that results in deformities of long bones. Muscle weakness and severe pain in the hip may cause gait problems.

- Paget's disease is a chronic disease of unknown etiology. It causes pain, physical deformity, motor impairments, and mental status changes that significantly affect the older person's quality of life.

- Gout is a metabolic disease caused by urate crystal deposits in joints, leading to local pain and inflammation in the joints. It primarily affects joints in the feet, often the big toe.

- Osteoarthritis is a chronic degenerative joint disease of the weight-bearing joints that is characterized by thinning and eroding of cartilage. Systemic symptoms such as fever are not present. Obesity is a major modifiable risk factor. Acetaminophen is often used to relieve the pain.

- Rheumatoid arthritis is a chronic syndrome that is characterized by symmetrical inflammation of peripheral joints. It causes pain, swelling, and morning stiffness lasting up to an hour. RA may cause chronic deformities and systemic nonjoint symptoms including renal, lung, and vascular involvement. Anti-inflammatory treatment should be started early to prevent deformities.

- Education is the key to success in adapting to chronic diseases. A program of exercise and rest is an important part of preventing and reversing many of the disabilities that accompany joint diseases.

References

AACE Osteoporosis Guidelines. (2001). *Endocrinology Practice, 7*(4), 300–306.

Agency for Healthcare Research and Quality. (2002). Managing osteoarthritis: Helping the elderly maintain function and mobility. *Research in Action,* Issue 3. Retrieved July 19, 2002, from www.ahrq.gov.

Alexander, N. (2003). Falls. In M. Beers & R. Berkow (Eds.), *The Merck manual of geriatrics* (Chap. 20). Whitehouse Station, NJ: Merck Research Laboratories.

Andersson, I. (2001). Case studies of food shopping, cooking and eating habits in older women with Parkinson's disease. *Journal of Advanced Nursing, 35*(1), 69–78.

Anderson, J., Wells, G., Verhoeven, A., & Felson, D. (2000). Factors predicting response to treatment in rheumatoid arthritis: The

importance of disease duration. *Arthritis and Rheumatism, 43*(1), 22–29.

Beers, M., & Berkow, R. (Eds.). (2003). *The Merck manual of geriatrics* (3rd ed.). Whitehouse Station, NJ: Merck Research Laboratories.

Berg, W., & Blasi, E. (2000). Stepping performance during obstacle clearance in women: Age differences and the association with lower extremity strength in older women. *Journal of the American Geriatrics Society, 48*(11), 1414–1423.

Bernick, L., & Bretholz, I. (1999). Safe mobility program: A comprehensive falls prevention program for a multilevel geriatric setting. *Journal of the Gerontological Nursing Association, 23*(3), 4–11.

Boutaugh, M., & Brady, T. (2001). Patient education for arthritis self-management. In

L. Robbins, C. Burckhardt, & R. Dehoratius (Eds.), *Clinical care in the rheumatic diseases* (pp. 155–161). Atlanta, GA: Association of Rheumatology Health Professionals.

Brown, J., Vittinghoff, E., Wyman, J., Stone, K., Nevitt, M., Ensrud, K., et al. (2000). Urinary incontinence: Does it increase risk for falls and fractures. *Journal of the American Geriatrics Society, 48*(7), 721–725.

Browning, M. (2001). Rheumatoid arthritis: A primary care approach. *Journal of the American Academy of Nurse Practitioners, 13*(9), 399–408.

Burman, K. (2001). Graves' disease in women. *Women's Health in Primary Care, 4*(4), 306–317.

Capezuti, E. (2002). Side rail use and bed-related fall outcomes among nursing home residents. *Journal of the American Geriatrics Society, 50*(1), 90–96.

Capezuti, E., Talerico, K., Cochran, I., Becker, H., Strumpf, N., & Evans, L. (1999). Individualized interventions to prevent bed-related falls and reduce siderails use. *Journal of Gerontological Nursing, 25*(11), 26–34.

Carpenito, L. J. (2002). *Nursing diagnosis: Application to clinical practice.* Philadelphia: Lippincott.

Choa, D., Espeland, M., Farmer, D., Register, T., Lenchik, L., Applegate, W., et al. (2000). Effect of voluntary weight loss on bone mineral density in older overweight women. *Journal of the American Geriatrics Society, 48*(7), 753–759.

Corbett, J. (2000). *Laboratory tests and diagnostic procedures with nursing diagnoses.* Upper Saddle River, NJ: Prentice Hall Health.

Corwin, E. (2000). *Handbook of pathophysiology* (2nd ed.). Philadelphia: Lippincott.

Davis, G., & White, T. (2000). Planning an osteoporosis education program for older adults in a residential setting. *Journal of Gerontological Nursing, 26*(1), 16–23.

Dimant, J., Kaplan, N., Finkelstein, R., & Gearhart, S. A. (1990). *Proceedings of NYOAS Best Practices Conference on Promotion of Mobility Independence in Long-Term Care Facilities, New York State Department of Health and Hunter/Mount Sinai Geriatric Education Center.* Crown Nursing Home Associates.

Ettinger, W. (2003a). Local joint, tendon, and bursa disorders. In M. Beers & R. Berkow (Eds.), *The Merck manual of geriatrics* (3rd ed., pp. 489–493). Whitehouse Station, NJ: Merck Research Laboratories.

Ettinger, W. (2003b). Rheumatic diseases. In M. Beers & R. Berkow (Eds.), *The Merck manual of geriatrics* (pp. 499–503). Whitehouse Station, NJ: Merck Research Laboratories.

Finkel, M., Cohen, M., & Mahoney, H. (2001). Treatment options for the menopausal woman. *Nurse Practitioner, 26*(2), 5–15.

Flynn, M. (2000). *Arthritis.* Baltimore: Johns Hopkins Medical Institutions.

Gerhart, T. (2003). Fractures. In M. Beers & R. Berkow (Eds.), *The Merck manual of geriatrics* (Chap. 22). Whitehouse Station, NJ: Merck Research Laboratories.

Gornisiewicz, M., & Moreland, L. (2001). Rheumatoid arthritis. In L. Robbins, C. Burckhardt, & R. Dehoratius (Eds.), *Clinical care in the rheumatic diseases* (pp. 89–96). Atlanta, GA: Association of Rheumatology Health Professionals.

Greendale, G., Wells, B., Marcus, R., & Barrett-Connor, E. (2000). How many women lose bone mineral density while taking hormone replacement therapy? *Archives of Intestinal Medicine, 160*(20), 3065–71.

Gregg, E., Pereira, M., & Caspersen, C. (2000). Physical activity, falls, and fractures among older adults: A review of epidemiologic evidence. *Journal of the American Geriatrics Society, 48*(8), 883–893.

Gunningberg, L., & Lindholm, C. (2000). The development of pressure ulcers in patients with hip fractures: Inadequate nursing documentation is still a problem. *Journal of Advanced Nursing, 31*(5), 1155–1164.

Hall, S. E., Williams, J., Goldswain, P. R., & Criddle, R. A. (2000). Hip fracture outcomes: Quality of life and functional status in older adults living in the community. *Australian and New Zealand Journal of Medicine, 30*(3), 327–332.

Hartford Institute for Geriatric Nursing. (1999). *Best practices in care for older adults.* New York: New York University, John A. Hartford Foundation Institute for Geriatric Nursing.

Hausdorff, J., Rios, D., & Edelber, H. (2001). Gait variability and fall risk in community-living older adults: A 1-year prospective study. *Archives of Physical Medicine and Rehabilitation, 82*(8), 1050–1056.

Hayes, K. (2001). Physical modalities. In L. Robbins, C. Burckhardt, & R. Dehoratius (Eds.), *Clinical care in the rheumatic diseases* (pp. 185–189). Atlanta, GA: Association of Rheumatology Health Professionals.

Hollinger, L., & Patterson, R. (1992). Key aspects of elder care: Managing falls and cognitive impairment. In S. Funk, E. Tornquist, M. Champagne, & R. Weise (Eds.), *A fall prevention program for the acute care setting.* New York: Springer.

Huether, S., & McCance, K. (2000). *Understanding pathophysiology.* St. Louis, MO: Mosby.

Hwang, M. Y., Glass, R., & Moher, J. (1999a). Falling and the elderly. *Journal of the American Medical Association, 281*(20), 1962.

Hwang, M. Y., Glass, R., & Moher, J. (1999b). Living with arthritis. *Journal of the American Medical Association, 282*(20), 1982.

Hwang, M. Y., Glass, R., & Moher, J. (1999c). Prevent hip fracture. *Journal of the American Medical Association, 282*(14), 1396.

Ignatavicius, D., & Workman, M. L. (2002). *Medical-surgical nursing: Critical thinking for collaborative care* (4th ed.). Philadelphia: W.B. Saunders.

John A. Hartford Foundation Institute for Geriatric Nursing. (2003). *Best nursing practices in care for older adults: Incorporating essential geriatric content into baccalaureate and staff development education: A curriculum guide, 4e,* New York: New York University, The Steinhardt School of Education, Division of Nursing, The John A. Hartford Foundation Institute for Geriatric Nursing.

Johnson, C. (1999). Exercise programs for fitness and health for geriatrics. *Journal of the American Academy of Nurse Practitioners, 11*(4), 147–150.

Johnson, M., Kramer, A., Lin, M., Kowalsky, J., & Steiner, J. (2000). Outcomes of older persons receiving rehabilitation for medical and surgical conditions compared with hip fracture and

stroke. *Journal of the American Geriatrics Society, 48*(11), 1389–1397.

Kamel, H., Razuman, S., & Shareeff, M. (2000). The activities of daily vision scale: A useful tool to assess fall risk in older adults with vision impairment. *Journal of the American Geriatrics Society, 48*(11), 1474–1477.

Karlson, E., Mandl, L., Aweh, G., Sangha, O., Liang, M., & Grodstein, F. (2003). Total hip replacement due to osteoarthritis: The importance of age, obesity, and other modifiable risk factors. *American Journal of Medicine, 114*(2), 93–98.

Kase, E., & Ostrov, B. (2001). Intricacies in the diagnosis and treatment of gout. *Patient Care, 33*–47. Retrieved November, 2002, from www.patientcare.com.

Keller, C., Fullerton, J., & Mobley, C. (1999). Supplemental and complementary alternatives to hormone replacement therapy. *Nurse Practitioner, 24*(3), 187–198.

Kerr, L. D. (2003). Inflammatory arthritis in the elderly. *Mount Sinai Journal of Medicine, 70*(1), 23–26.

Kessenich, C. (2000). Update on osteoporosis in elderly men. *Geriatric Nursing, 21*(5), 242–244.

Kleerekoper, M. (1999). Protecting bone mass with fundamentals and drug therapy. *Geriatrics, 54*(7), 38–43.

Knutsson, S. (1999). An evaluation of patients' quality of life before, 6 weeks and 6 months after total hip replacement. *Journal of Advanced Nursing, 30*(6), 1349–1359.

Lawson, M. (2001). Evaluating and managing osteoporosis in men. *Nurse Practitioner, 26*(5), 26–49.

Leboff, M., Bermas, B., Dunaif, A., Gharib, S., & Fairchild, D. (2000). *Osteoporosis: Guide to prevention, diagnosis and treatment.* Retrieved February 18, 2002, from www.guidelines.gov/VIEWS/summary.

Lewis, T., Tesh, A., & Lyles, K. (1999). Caring for the patient with Paget's disease of the bone. *Nurse Practitioner, 24*(7), 52–65.

Lie, L. (2000). Staying current with osteoporosis. Medscape Conference Summaries from the American Academy of Family Practitioners (AAFP) 52nd Annual Scientific Assembly, September 20–24. Dallas, TX.

Love-McClung, B. (1999). Using osteoporosis management to reduce fractures in elderly women. *Nurse Practitioner, 24*(3), 26–42.

Lozada, C., & Altman, R. (2001). Osteoarthritis. In L. Robbins, C. Burckhardt, & R. Dehoratius (Eds.), *Clinical care in the rheumatic diseases* (pp. 113–119). Atlanta, GA: Association of Rheumatology Health Professionals.

Mahoney, J., Palta, M., Johnson, J., Park, S., & Sager, M. (2000). *Temporal association between hospitalization and rate of falls after discharge.* Retrieved November 28, 2002, from http://archinte.ama-assn.org/issues/v160n18/abs/ioi90801.html.

Manolagas, S. (2003). Aging and the musculoskeletal system. In M. Beers & R. Berkow (Eds.), *The Merck manual of geriatrics.* Whitehouse Station, NJ: Merck Research Laboratories.

Masten, Y., & Gary, A. (1999). Is anyone listening? Does anyone care? Menopausal and postmenopausal health risks, outcomes, and care. *Nurse Practitioner Forum, 10*(4), 195–200.

McCance, K., & Mourad, L. (2000). Alterations in musculoskeletal function. In S. Huether & K. McCance (Eds.), *Understanding pathophysiology* (pp. 1031–1074). St. Louis, MO: Mosby.

McConnell, E. (2001). Myths and facts about gout. *Nursing, 2001, 31*(5), 73.

Meiner, S. (2001). Gouty arthritis: Not just a big toe problem. *Geriatric Nursing, 22,* 132–134.

Messier, S., Loeser, R., & Mitchell, M. (2000). Exercise and weight loss in older adults with knee osteoarthritis: A preliminary study. *Journal of the American Geriatrics Society, 48*(9), 1062–1072.

Metter, E., Lynch, N., Conwit, R., Lindle, R., Tobin, J., & Hurley, B. (1999). Muscle quality and age: Cross-sectional and longitudinal comparisons. *Journals of Gerontology Series A: Biological Sciences and Medical Sciences Online, 54*(5), B207–218.

Miller, D. (2001). Pharmacologic interventions in the 21st century. In L. Robbins, C. Burckhardt, & R. Dehoratius (Eds.), *Clinical care in the rheumatic diseases* (pp. 169–177). Atlanta, GA: Association of Rheumatology Health Professionals.

Minor, M., & Westby, M. (2001). Rest and exercise. In L. Robbins, C. Burckhardt, M. Hannan, & R. Dehoratius (Eds.), *Clinical care in rheumatic disease* (2nd ed., pp. 179–184): Association of Rheumatology Health Professionals.

Murphy, S. L. (2000). Deaths: Final data for 1998. *National Vital Statistics Reports, 48*(11). Hyattsville, MD: National Center for Health Statistics.

National Center for Injury Prevention and Control (NCIPC). Centers for Disease Control and Prevention. (2003). *Falls and hip fractures among older adults.* Atlanta. Retrieved November, 2003, from www.cdc.gove/ncipc/factsheets/falls/htm.

National Institute of Arthritis and Musculoskeletal and Skin Diseases. (2001). *National Institutes of Health, health topics: Questions and answers about hip replacement.* Retrieved November, 2002, from www.niams.nih.gov/hi/topics/hip/hiprepqa.htm.

National Institute of Arthritis and Musculoskeletal and Skin Diseases. (2002a). *National Institutes of Health, health topics: Handout on health: Rheumatoid arthritis.* Retrieved November, 2002, from www.niams.nih.gov/hi/topics/arthritis/rahandout.htm.

National Institute of Arthritis and Musculoskeletal and Skin Diseases. (2002b). *National Institutes of Health, health topics: Questions and answers about arthritis and rheumatic diseases.* Retrieved November, 2002, from www.niams.nih.gov/hi/topics/arthritis/artrheu.htm.

National Institute of Arthritis and Musculoskeletal and Skin Diseases. (2003). *National Institutes of Health. Topics: Questions and answers about gout.* Retrieved November, 2002, from www.niams.nih.gov/hi/topics/gout/gout.htm.

National Osteoporosis Foundation. (2002). *Physician guide to osteoporosis prevention and treatment.* Washington, DC: Author.

NIH Consensus Development Panel on Osteoporosis Prevention, Diagnosis, and Therapy. (2000). Retrieved November 29, 2002, from www.consensus.nih.gov/cons/lll/lll_htm.

Pace, B. (2001). Hip fractures. *JAMA, 285*(21), 2814.

Paget Foundation. (2002a). *General information about Paget's disease.* Retrieved July 29, 2003, from www.paget.org?Register/index.asp?page=QA/disease_bone.htm.

Paget Foundation. (2002b). *Two types of drugs, bisphosphonates and calcitonin, are approved by the U.S. Food and Drug Administration (FDA) for the treatment of Paget's disease.* Retrieved July 29, 2003, from www.paget.org/Register/index.asp.

Paget Foundation. (2003). *Bisphosphonates fact sheet.* Retrieved July 29, 2003, from www.paget.org/Information/FactSheet/bisfact.html.

Patrick, L., Leber, M., Scrim, C., Gendron, I., & Eisener-Parche, P. (1999). A standardized assessment and intervention protocol for managing risk for falls on a geriatric rehabilitation unit. *Journal of Gerontological Nursing, 25*(4), 40–46.

Popovic, J. (1999). National Hospital Discharge Survey: Annual summary with detailed diagnosis and procedure data. National Center for Health Statistics. *Vital Health Statistics, 13*(151), 23, 154.

Raisz, L. (2003). Metabolic bone disease. In M. Beers & R. Berkow (Eds.), *The Merck manual of geriatrics* (3rd ed., pp. 472–486). Whitehouse Station, NJ: Merck Research Laboratories.

Reginato, A. M., & Reginato A. J. (2001). Periarticular rheumatic diseases. In L. Robbins, C. Burckhardt, C. Hannan, & M. Dehoratius (Eds.), *Clinical care in rheumatic diseases.* Atlanta: Association of Rheumatology Health Professionals.

Resnick, B. (2001). Promoting health in older adults: A four-year analysis. *Journal of the American Academy of Nurse Practitioners, 13*(1), 23–33.

Robbins, L., Burckhardt, C., Hannan, M., & Dehoratius, R. (Eds.). (2001). *Clinical care in the rheumatic diseases.* Atlanta, GA: Association of Rheumatology Health Professionals.

Robinson, S. (1999). Transitions in the lives of elderly women who have sustained hip fractures. *Journal of Advanced Nursing, 30*(6), 1341–1348.

Rubenstein, L. (2001). *Falls and balance problems.* Retrieved February 13, 2001, from www.americangeriatrics.org/edicatopm/forum/falling.shtml.

Sturrock, R. (2000). Gout: Easy to misdiagnose. *British Medical Journal, 320,* 132–133.

Tinetti, M. (2003). Chronic dizziness and postural instability. In M. Beers & R. Berkow (Eds.), *The Merck manual of geriatrics* (Chap. 19). Whitehouse Station, NJ: Merck Research Laboratories.

Twiss, J., Waltman, N., Ott, C., Gross, G., Lindsey, A., & Moore, T. (2001). Bone mineral density in postmenopausal breast cancer survivors. *Journal of the American Academy of Nurse Practitioners, 13*(6), 276–284.

Ullom-Minnich, P. (1999). *Prevention of osteoporosis and fractures.* Retrieved May 3, 2001, from www.aafp.org/afp/990700/194.html.

U.S. Department of Health and Human Services. (2000). *Healthy people 2010. Summary of objectives.* Retrieved from www.health.gov/healthy-people//Document/HTML/Volume1/02arthritis.htm.

U.S. Food and Drug Administration (FDA), Center for Drug Evaluation and Research. (2003). *Questions and answers for estrogen and estrogen plus progestin therapies for postmenopausal women.* Retrieved November, 2002, from www.fda.cder/drug/infopage/estrogens_progestins/Q&.

Wener, M. (2001). Diagnostic laboratory tests and imaging. In L. Robbins, C. Burckhardt, & R. Dehoratius (Eds.), *Clinical care in the rheumatic diseases* (pp. 37–45). Atlanta, GA: Association of Rheumatology Health Professionals.

Willson, H. (2000). Factors affecting the administration of analgesia to patients following repair of a fractured hip. *Journal of Advanced Nursing, 31*(5), 1145–1154.

Wilson, B., Shannon, M., & Stang, C. (2003). *Nurse's drug guide 2003.* Upper Saddle River, NJ: Prentice Hall Health.

Workman, M. L. (2000). Immune mechanisms in rheumatic disease. *Nursing Clinics of North America, 35*(1), 175–188.

Writing Group for the Women's Health Initiative. (2002). Risks and benefits of estrogen plus progestin in healthy postmenopausal women. *JAMA, 288,* 321–333.

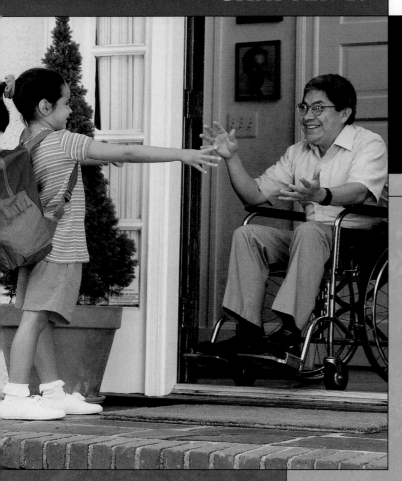

CHAPTER 19

The Endocrine System

CHAPTER OBJECTIVES

Upon completion of this chapter, the reader will be able to:

- Describe age-related changes that affect endocrine function.

- Describe the impact of age-related changes on endocrine function.

- Identify risk factors to health for the older person with an endocrine problem.

- Describe unique presentation of diabetes and thyroid problems in the older person.

- Define appropriate nursing interventions directed toward assisting older adults with endocrine problems to develop self-care abilities.

- Identify and implement appropriate nursing interventions to care for the older person with endocrine problems.

KEY TERMS

beta cells 617
blood glucose 601
euthyroid 629
glycosylated hemoglobin 608
Graves' disease 629
Hashimoto's disease 629
hyperthyroidism 626
hypothyroidism 626
ketones 607
nephropathy 612
neuropathy 608
retinopathy 611

MediaLink

Additional resources for this chapter can be found on the Student CD-ROM accompanying this textbook and on the Companion Website at **www.prenhall.com/tabloski**. Click on Chapter 19 to select the activities for this chapter.

CD-ROM

- Animations/Video
  Diabetes Mellitus
  Endocrine System A & P
- NCLEX Review
- Case Studies
- Tools

COMPANION WEBSITE

- Audio Glossary
- Additional NCLEX Review
- Case Study
- MediaLink Applications

The endocrine glands control the body's metabolic processes. The endocrine and metabolic control systems offer many of the greatest opportunities for preventing the disabilities associated with aging (Solomon, 2003). Endocrine glands respond to specific signals by synthesizing and releasing hormones into the circulation that affect cells with appropriate receptors and trigger specific cellular responses and activities. Most hormones operate via a feedback system that maintains an optimal internal environment or homeostasis within the body (McCance & Huether, 2001). Two major endocrine problems of importance to gerontological nursing are diabetes mellitus and thyroid disease. Thyroid disease is common, often undiagnosed, and easily treated in people of all ages. Early detection prevents unnecessary disability and loss of function. Diabetes mellitus is common, and normalization of **blood glucose** levels may minimize the devastating vascular and neurologic complications that often occur (Solomon, 2003). Knowledge of endocrine function and metabolism and an understanding of normal changes associated with aging is crucial for gerontological nurses in order to interpret signs and symptoms of illness and advise older persons on health promotion activities (Figure 19-1 ■).

Diabetes Mellitus

Diabetes mellitus (DM) is highly prevalent and increasing in persons over 65, particularly in racial and ethnic minorities (California Healthcare Foundation/American Geriatrics Society, 2003). DM is classified as type 1 (the result of a lack of insulin production) and type 2 (the result of insulin resistance). Between 1980 and 2000, the prevalence of diagnosed DM increased in all age groups. People from age 65 to 74 had the highest prevalence, followed by people 75 years of age or older (Centers for Disease Control, 2004). As Figure 19-2 ■ illustrates, in 2000 the prevalence of diagnosed DM among people ages 65 to 74 (15.43 per 100) was about 13 times that of people less than 45 years of age (1.19 per 100). As many as 25% of older adults are diagnosed with DM in some ethnic groups.

In general, age-specific prevalence of diagnosed DM is higher for African Americans and Hispanics than for Caucasians. Among those less than 75 years of age, Black women have the highest prevalence. Across almost all sex and ethnic categorizations, prevalence is highest among those 65 to 74 years of age (except Hispanic men, where prevalence increases slightly after age 75) (Centers for Disease Control, 2004). Figure 19-3 ■ illustrates the age-specific prevalence of diagnosed DM by race/ethnicity in the United States in 2002.

The reasons for the increased incidence of DM in minorities are poorly understood. In the United States, about 25% of all adults with DM and most children and adolescents are minorities. Further, minorities are more likely to develop microvascular complications and to have more lower limb amputations than Caucasians (National Institute of Diabetes and Digestive and Kidney Diseases [NIDDK], 2004). It is believed that both genetic and environmental factors can contribute to the development of DM. Research is ongoing to attempt to identify factors that may account for these disparities.

Older adults often bear the greatest burden of diabetes. The statistics in Box 19-1 indicate the need for improving the quality of healthcare provided to older people with DM.

COMPLICATIONS OF DIABETES MELLITUS

DM affects people of all ages; however, the disease can be particularly serious in the older person because of the many complications that can develop. Poor glycemic control may synergistically interact with normal changes of aging and other coexisting

FIGURE ☐ **19-1**

Normal changes of aging in the endocrine system.

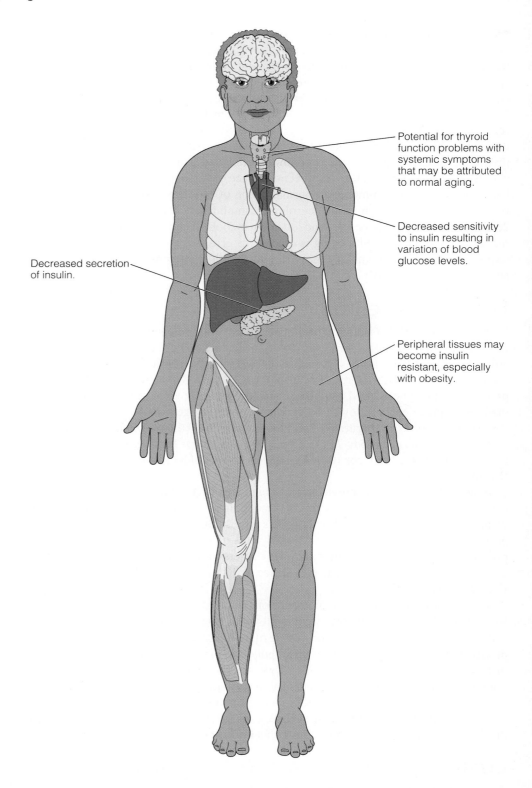

Potential for thyroid function problems with systemic symptoms that may be attributed to normal aging.

Decreased sensitivity to insulin resulting in variation of blood glucose levels.

Decreased secretion of insulin.

Peripheral tissues may become insulin resistant, especially with obesity.

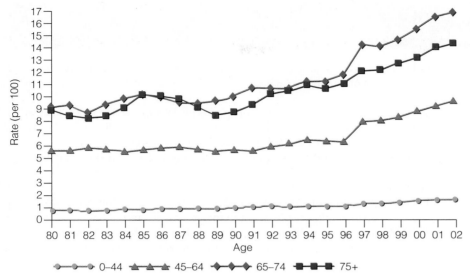

FIGURE ▢ 19-2

Prevalence of diagnosed diabetes in the United States by age, 1997–2002.

Source: Centers for Disease Control, 2004.

diseases to accelerate diabetes complications (Blair, 1999). About 41% of the population with diabetes is over the age of 65. Older people have higher rates of diabetes than younger people (National Academy on an Aging Society, 2000). Optimizing glucose control and decreasing risk factors for microvascular, macrovascular, and neurologic complications can improve the quality and quantity of life for patients of all ages. Complications that can develop due to poor glycemic control include the following:

- Eye disease leading to loss of vision or even blindness
- Kidney failure
- Heart disease
- Nerve damage that may cause a loss of feeling or pain in the hands, feet, legs, or other parts of the body (peripheral neuropathies)
- Stroke
- Poor wound healing due to impaired immune response and poor tissue perfusion in peripheral vascular disease

The diagnosis of DM can shorten the average life span up to 15 years. Additionally, DM leads to higher death rates from other illness such as pneumonia, influenza, and heart disease. Care of persons with DM in the United States is estimated to cost more

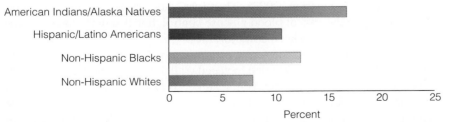

FIGURE ▢ 19-3

Age-adjusted total prevalence of diabetes in people 20 years or older by race/ethnicity, United States, 2002.

Source: 1999–2001 National Health Interview Survey and 1999–2000 National Health and Nutrition Examination Survey estimates projected to year 2002. 2002 outpatient database of the Indian Health Service, Centers for Disease Control, 2004.

<table>
<tr><td>

BOX 19-1   **Older Adults and the Burden of Diabetes**

- Currently 1 out of 5 older adults (18.7%) have DM. The prevalence rates are 29.4% for older Mexican Americans, 27.3% for African Americans, and 27% for American Indians.
- The high price of direct care of older persons with DM exceeded $32 billion in 1997. The majority of these costs were paid by Medicare and Medicaid and by co-payments and deductibles assumed by older persons themselves.
- Kidney disease and nerve damage caused by DM can result in end-stage renal disease requiring dialysis and lower extremity amputation. Diabetes-related lower extremity amputations are common among older patients. Sixty-four percent of amputations among older persons with DM occur in those over the age of 65.
- Diabetes is the sixth leading cause of death for persons 65 and older and a major contributor to heart disease, the leading cause of death for this age group.
- The death rate is higher among older persons with diabetes than among those without diabetes.

</td></tr>
</table>

Source: Centers for Disease Control, 1999.

than $105 billion annually, including direct and indirect costs such as disability, lost work productivity, and premature death (NIDDK, 2004). Although diabetes affects just 6% of the U.S. population (over 16 million people), more than 1 of every 19 U.S. healthcare dollars is spent on diabetes (National Academy on an Aging Society, 2000). By 2025, over 20 million Americans are expected to have diabetes.

PATHOPHYSIOLOGY OF DM

DM can be caused by defective insulin secretion or use, resulting in abnormally high levels of blood glucose and damage or destruction to many organs in the body, including the eyes, kidneys, blood vessels, and nervous system. The nurse plays a key role in monitoring blood glucose levels, organizing and participating in screening activities, and providing ongoing assessment for early signs of complications in older patients with DM. Older patients with DM have higher rates of premature death, functional disability, and coexisting illnesses such as hypertension, coronary heart disease, and stroke than other older adults. More than 50% of nontraumatic amputations in the United States occur in patients with DM. With proper foot care, many of these amputations could be prevented. Older persons with DM are also at greater risk from depression, cognitive impairment, urinary incontinence, falls, and persistent pain (California Healthcare Foundation, 2003). Therefore, older people require attention and emphasis not only in the area of blood glucose control, but also in the area of identification and treatment of DM-related comorbidities.

It has been recommended that the terms *insulin-dependent diabetes mellitus* and *not–insulin-dependent diabetes mellitus* be replaced with the terms *type 1 diabetes mellitus* and *type 2 diabetes mellitus,* using Arabic numerals rather than Roman numerals (American Diabetes Association, 2001). This recommendation was made to improve communications between healthcare providers and patients, to reduce confusion and chance of error resulting from the use of Roman numerals, and to eliminate the artificial designation that occurs from the linkage with the use or nonuse of insulin, as both types of DM may be treated using insulin therapy.

Type 1 DM develops due to B-cell destruction and results in a lack or underproduction of insulin in the body. Type 1 DM can be the result of (1) autoimmune disease in which cell-mediated destruction of the B cells in the pancreas occurs, or (2) idiopathic DM that occurs for no apparent reason. Regardless of cause, patients with type 1 DM are insulin dependent and at risk for ketoacidosis.

Type 2 DM, the most prevalent form of diabetes in all age groups, results from a combination of insulin resistance and an insulin secretory defect. The insulin secretion is insufficient to compensate for the insulin resistance, which occurs in response to decreased insulin effectiveness in stimulating glucose uptake by skeletal muscle and failure to inhibit hepatic glucose production. The body attempts to compensate for rising blood glucose levels by producing more insulin. In some cases, this is adequate and the person does not go on to develop DM. In others, genetic influences may play a role, and heightened insulin production results in hyperinsulinemia. This leads to further insulin resistance, characterized by visceral/abdominal obesity, hypertension, hyperlipidemia, and coronary artery disease (Barzilai, 2003). Autoimmune destruction of B cells does not occur, ketoacidosis seldom occurs spontaneously, and insulin treatment is often not needed for survival.

RISK FACTORS FOR DEVELOPMENT OF DIABETES MELLITUS

Patients with type 2 DM are often overweight and have higher percentages of body fat. In some patients, weight may be normal, but the waist-to-hip ratio is increased (greater than 1) as a result of upper body obesity. These patients may go undiagnosed for years because the hyperglycemia develops gradually (Caughron & Smith, 2002). Blood glucose levels will decrease and may return to normal when the patient loses weight. A recent study demonstrated that lifestyle modification may delay or prevent the development of type 2 DM in high-risk individuals. In a study of 3,234 persons of both sexes, a 58% reduction in blood glucose concentrations resulted after participants started eating a lower fat diet (less than 25% of caloric intake) and engaging in moderate exercise three times per week (National Diabetes Education Program, 2003).

Risk factors for the development of type 2 DM include:

- Age over 45 (the risk of DM increases with age).
- Overweight (body mass index greater than 25) and having a waist-to-hip ratio approaching 1.
- African American, Hispanic or Latino American, Asian American or Pacific Islander, or American Indian ethnicity.
- Parents or siblings with DM.
- Blood pressure above 140/90.
- Low levels of high-density lipoprotein (less than 40 for men and less than 50 for women) (good cholesterol) and high levels of triglycerides (above 250 mg/dl).
- Diabetes occurrence while pregnant or giving birth to a large baby (over 9 lbs).
- Sedentary lifestyle and exercise less than three times per week.

(National Diabetes Education Program, 2003)

Because older people at risk for development of type 2 DM are at greater risk of cardiovascular disease and other health problems, appropriate screening is indicated. One third of people with DM remain undiagnosed. Finding and treating DM early can improve health outcomes. Fasting plasma glucose should be measured periodically as part of routine health screening in older people at high risk for DM. Early identification of DM may lessen or prevent long-term complications. Terms such as "a touch of diabetes" or "blood sugars running a little too high" should be avoided so that diagnosis is clear and appropriate interventions can be instituted as soon as possible (National Diabetes Education Program, 2003).

> ### Practice Pearl
>
> Your patient is at risk for diabetes if he or she reports being tired or hungry, losing weight, urinating frequently, or having blurry vision, slow-healing cuts, and numb or tingling feet. A referral to the primary healthcare provider for a blood glucose test is indicated.

DIAGNOSTIC CRITERIA

When an older person is identified as high risk for diabetes, appropriate testing includes a fasting plasma glucose (FPG) level or a 2-hour oral glucose tolerance test (OGTT). The FPG is performed by obtaining a blood sample and measuring the person's blood glucose after an overnight fast (8 to 12 hours). The 2-hour OGTT is performed after an overnight fast by measuring the person's blood glucose immediately before and 2 hours after drinking a 75-g glucose solution. The diagnostic criteria are listed in Table 19-1.

Although the 2-hour OGTT is more sensitive for diagnosing DM, it is not always practical because the older person has to drink a sugary solution after an all-night fast and then wait 2 hours for retesting. For that reason, the OGTT is not recommended for routine clinical use (American Diabetes Association, 2001). However, the FPG test is not as sensitive and, if used alone, will miss accurate diagnoses in up to 17% of patients with DM. Patients and their families should be informed regarding the benefits and limitations of both testing procedures (National Diabetes Education Program, 2003). Persons with prediabetes or impaired glucose tolerance are at higher risk of developing DM. Older patients who have random blood glucose levels (obtained when nonfasting) above 160 mg/dl should be referred for further testing and diagnostic evaluation of DM (American Diabetes Association, 2001). Use of glucocorticoids, some diuretics, peritoneal dialysis, infection, or an acute event such as myocardial infarction can also elevate blood glucose levels. Elevated blood glucose levels obtained from older persons in these circumstances should not be considered diagnostic of DM.

TABLE 19-1

Diagnostic Criteria for Diabetes

Test	Value	Diagnosis
FPG*	<110 mg/dl	Normal
FPG	110–125 mg/dl	Prediabetes
FPG	>126 mg/dl	Diabetes
OGTT**	2-hr value <140 mg/dl	Normal
OGTT	2-hr value 140–199 mg/dl	Prediabetes
OGTT	2-hr value >200 mg/dl	Diabetes

* FPG Fasting plasma glucose test
** OGTT Oral glucose tolerance test

Drug Alert !

Use of glucocorticoids or diuretics can greatly and suddenly increase blood glucose levels both in older patients with DM and in those without DM.

Screening should be followed by a history, physical examination, and comprehensive geriatric assessment including nutritional status, functional capabilities, and psychosocial issues. Some symptoms of a diabetic condition in the older person include anorexia, incontinence, falls, pain intolerance, and cognitive or behavioral changes (Berenbeim, Parrott, Purnell, & Pennachio, 2001). Older patients with DM may complain of symptoms of hyperglycemia (usually above 200 mg/dl), including polydipsia (excessive thirst), weight loss, polyuria (excessive urination), polyphagia (excessive hunger), blurred vision, fatigue, nausea, and fungal and bacterial infections (Barzilai, 2003). Older women may complain of perineal itching due to vaginal candidiasis. Additionally, older women with DM may experience frequent urinary tract infections.

Once DM is diagnosed, the physician will determine whether the patient has the type 1 or type 2 form. The majority of older people have type 2 DM with gradual onset of symptoms and obesity. The patient with type 1 DM is typically younger than 40, is lean, exhibits a rapid onset of symptoms, and may have ketonuria. However, type 1 DM can occur at any age and in obese persons. The onset symptoms of hyperglycemia in the older adult with type 1 DM may occur more slowly and without the presence of **ketones**, making an accurate diagnosis difficult. When the older adult reports rapid onset of weight loss, polyuria, polydipsia, and polyphagia with elevated blood glucose levels, the nurse should consider an underlying problem such as pancreatic cancer (Blair, 1999).

Table 19-2 presents the typical history and onset of symptoms common to type 1 and type 2 DM.

The initial physical examination should include blood pressure measurement (including orthostatic changes), weight, dilated retinal examination by an ophthalmologist or eye specialist, cardiovascular examination for evidence of cardiac or peripheral

TABLE 19-2

Typical History of Symptom Onset in Type 1 and Type 2 Diabetes Mellitus

Type 1	Type 2
Sudden onset, severe symptoms	Gradual onset, less severe symptoms
Polyuria, polyphagia, polydipsia	Atypical presentation: weight loss, depression, gastrointestinal problems, incontinence
Weight loss with normal or increased appetite	Gradual weight loss, decreased appetite
Orthostatic hypotension (secondary to dehydration)	Normal blood pressure with orthostatic changes, hyperlipidemia
Blurred vision	Attributes vision changes to aging
Fatigue/weakness	Attributes fatigue/weakness to aging
Nausea/vomiting	Decreased appetite may make presentation more vague
Vaginal itching	Recurrent vaginitis, urinary tract infection, fungal skin infections
Ketones in urine	Protein in urine
Dry, flaky skin	Slow-healing skin ulcerations
Sensation usually intact	Parasthesias

vascular disease, and neurologic examination to rule out any peripheral or autonomic **neuropathy** (American Diabetes Association, 2001). Fundoscopic examination may reveal the presence of microaneurysms, hemorrhages, exudates, or increased intraocular pressure indicative of glaucoma. Peripheral pulses, capillary filling, and warmth of extremities should be assessed to indicate the presence of macrovascular pathology. Mental status, deep tendon reflexes, and ability to detect peripheral sensation are key components of the neurologic examination. Smoking status and a visual foot examination (without shoes and socks) is recommended for every older person with DM initially and at every subsequent clinical visit to the healthcare provider. Patients who smoke cigarettes should be counseled to discontinue smoking. Those ready to undertake smoking cessation should be referred to ongoing support groups and counseling centers. Patients with diabetes who are overweight should be counseled regarding weight loss.

The following laboratory tests are recommended:

- Thyroid function tests (thyroid-stimulating hormone)
- Urinalysis to test for albuminuria, serum creatinine for renal function
- Electrocardiogram if patient has not had one within 10 years
- Fasting lipid profile to assess cardiovascular risk
- **Glycosylated hemoglobin** (HbA_{1c})

(Diabetes Guidelines Work Group, 1999)

The HbA_{1c} is not specific for diagnosing diabetes; however, elevated HbA_{1c} levels confirm the degree of estimated blood glucose control over the last 3 months. The HbA_{1c} measures how much glucose attaches to the hemoglobin in the red cells. As the average life of a red cell is about 4 months, the test summarizes how high the glucose levels have been during the life of the cell. Figure 19-4 ■ illustrates the relationship between the HbA_{1c} level and average blood sugar readings. The ideal HbA_{1c} goal is less than 7.0%. Levels of 8.0% or greater indicate the need to adjust the treatment plan (Diabetes Guidelines Work Group, 1999).

An in-depth foot examination should include the presence of protective sensation, vascular status, skin integrity, and foot structure. Approximately 15% of all patients with DM will develop a foot or leg ulcer during the course of their disease (Halpin-Landry & Goldsmith, 1999). Patients with DM have sensory, motor, and autonomic neuropathies; lower extremity peripheral vascular disease; impaired host defenses

FIGURE ■ 19-4

The relationship between the HbA_{1c} level and average blood sugar readings.

AIC Level	Blood Glucose Test Average
12	300
11	270
10	240
9	210
8	180
7	150
6	120
5	80

Source: NIDDK, 2004.

against infection; and delayed wound healing. When a diabetic ulcer occurs, ischemia, neuropathy, and infection delay healing and raise the risk of complications.

A monofilament or a tuning fork can be used to assess for the presence of protective sensation that can alert the patient to the development of a blister or foot ulcer. It is recommended that a visual examination of the diabetic foot be conducted at each healthcare encounter and a more in-depth inspection be done annually. Saving the diabetic foot and preventing amputation requires the following:

- Identification of feet at risk
- Prevention of foot ulcers
- Treatment of foot ulcers
- Prevention of recurrence of foot ulcers

(NIDDK, 2004)

The older patient can be classified as high or low risk depending on the outcome of the foot examination. High-risk patients should have their foot status followed more closely, be taught preventive self-care of the feet, and be referred to therapeutic shoes and footwear. A small mirror placed on or near the floor (like those in a shoe store) can assist older persons to monitor and inspect their own feet. After sitting in a chair, they should remove their shoes and socks and raise their feet in front of the mirror to inspect the heels, toes, and dorsal aspects. Older patients with DM should not attempt to cut their own toenails because of the risk of cutting their skin. Rather they should see the podiatrist on a regular basis for toenail care and cutting. Figure 19-5 ▢ indicates the procedure for foot inspection and monofilament use for sensory foot examination.

Patients who can sense that their foot is being touched with the filament have protective sensation. Additional nursing assessments include using a 128-cps tuning fork to assess vibratory sensation in the feet and checking peripheral pulses including the doralis pedis, posterior tibial, popliteal, and femoral. Loss of vibration and diminished pulses may indicate early findings in neuropathy and circulatory impairment. When protective sensation is lost and the skin is broken, whether by an ulcer or a blister, bacteria and fungi can enter the skin. The patient with neuropathy may not feel the infection until it is well established. Peripheral vascular disease makes healing less likely (NIDDK, 2004).

Practice Pearl

Foot care in the patient with DM includes hygiene and protection. It is important to lubricate dry areas with lotion, carefully dry moist areas (between toes), and care for the nails. Patients with DM should not cut their own toenails and are urged to see the podiatrist regularly and use an emery board to keep nails short and smooth between visits.

In addition to the history and physical examination, assessment of the patient with DM includes the following components:

- Nutritional assessment
- Medication review
- Functional assessment
- Psychosocial assessment
- Gait and balance evaluation

FIGURE ■ 19-5

Foot inspection and monofilament use for sensory foot examination.

The sensory testing device used to complete a foot examination is a 10-gram (5.07 Semmes-Weinstein) nylon filament mounted on a holder that has been standardized to deliver a 10-gram force when properly applied. Research has shown that a person who can feel the 10-gram filament in the selected sites is at reduced risk for developing ulcers.

- The sensory examination should be done in a quiet and relaxed setting. The patient must not watch while the examiner applies the filament.
- Test the monofilament on the patient's hand so he or she knows what to anticipate.
- The five sites to be tested are indicated on the screening form.
- Apply the monofilament perpendicular to the skin's surface (see diagram A below).
- Apply sufficient force to cause the filament to bend or buckle (see diagram B below)
- The total duration of the approach, skin contact, and departure of the filament should be approximately 1½ seconds.
- Apply the filament along the perimeter and *not on* an ulcer site, callus, scar, or necrotic tissue. Do not allow the filament to slide across the skin or make repetitive contact at the test site.
- Press the filament to the skin such that it buckles at one of two times as you say "time one" or "time two." Have patients identify at which time they were touched. Randomize the sequence of applying the filament throughout the examination.

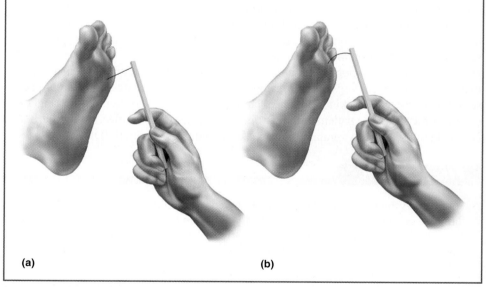

(a)   **(b)**

Source: National Diabetes Education Program, 2003.

Complications of DM can develop at an accelerated rate in older patients because of poor glycemic control. The principal goals of therapy are to enhance quality of life, decrease chance of complications, improve self-care through education, and maintain or improve general health status (California Healthcare Foundation, 2003). The approach the nurse selects should be individualized and take into account life expectancy, coexisting illness, functional capability, level of independence, and economic and social considerations.

Goals of Management

The goals of management of DM in the older person include control of hyperglycemia and its symptoms; prevention, evaluation, and treatment of macrovascular and microvascular complications; DM self-management through education; and maintenance or improvement of general health status (California Healthcare Foundation, 2003). The goals must reflect the fact that older adults with DM have varying degrees of frailty, differences in underlying chronic conditions, varying degrees of DM-related comorbidity, and highly variable life expectancies. In general, the more functional the older person and the longer the life expectancy, the more aggressively the DM will be treated by the healthcare provider to decrease the probability of DM-related complications. If an older patient is close to death, then multiple insulin injections and frequent (4 to 6 times/day) blood glucose monitoring may not be justified (Mooradian, McLaughlin, Boyer, & Winter, 1999). A less aggressive approach may be indicated because long-term complications of hyperglycemia are not relevant.

For highly functional older patients with good vision, manual dexterity, and cognitive function, a more aggressive management plan can be implemented with support from the primary healthcare provider, the nurse, and the family. Aggressive glycemic control decreases microvascular complications of DM, but also increases the risk of hypoglycemic episodes. Older people who live alone, those with cognitive or physical deficits, or those with serious underlying chronic illnesses are more likely to suffer serious consequences from hypoglycemic episodes, including falls, disorientation, metabolic problems, and dehydration.

The goals of therapy for the highly functional older person include:

- A fasting blood glucose level between 100 and 120 mg/dl.
- A postprandial glucose level of less than 180 mg/dl.
- An HbA_{1c} under 8%.

The goals of therapy for the older patient with advanced microvascular complications (neuropathy or **retinopathy**), cognitive deficits, serious associated cardiovascular problems, frailty, or underlying serious illness are more conservative and include the following:

- A fasting glucose level of less than 140 mg/dl
- A postprandial glucose level of less than 200 to 220 mg/dl
- An HbA_{1c} under 10%

(Berenbeim et al., 2001)

Figure 19-6 ■ illustrates a glucometer used to test the blood sugar. Equipment and techniques vary. An older person with visual impairment should use a glucometer with a large number display for accuracy.

Older patients should be taught to perform blood glucose testing and to keep track of their readings using a daily log. This log will provide feedback to the older patient and guide day-to-day choices regarding exercise, food, and medication. The finger or forearm is pricked with a lancet, and a drop of blood is placed on a test strip and read by the machine. The normal readings and treatment goals (70 to 140 mg/dl) should be clearly written in the log book for easy referral. Newer glucometers have large digital readouts, making them easier for older patients to read. A sample daily diabetes record in Figure 19-7 ■ illustrates the kind of information to be recorded and shared with the healthcare provider.

A glucometer with a large visual display.

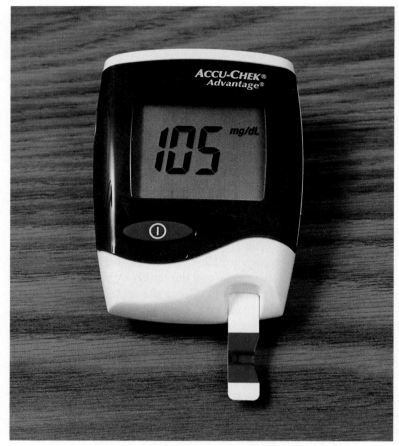

Source: International Hospital Federation, 2004, www.hospitalmanagement.net.

Controlling DM in the older person requires intervention in three areas: weight management, appropriate use of medications, and prevention of complications. There is an increased obesity and lipid abnormality risk independent of glycemic control in type 2 DM. The low-density lipoprotein (LDL) goal for older adults is less than 100 mg/dl. A second goal is to raise high-density lipoprotein (HDL) to greater than 45 mg/dl in men and greater than 55 in women. Control of hypertension reduces the progression rate of diabetic **nephropathy,** cardiovascular disease, and cerebrovascular disease. Desired blood pressure is below 130/80. Postural blood pressure should be monitored in older adults to prevent falls and dizziness during and immediately after changes in position (American Diabetes Association, 2001).

WEIGHT MANAGEMENT

Maintenance of near-normal blood glucose levels, achievement of optimal serum lipid levels, provision of adequate caloric intake to attain or maintain normal weight, prevention and treatment of complications, and improvement of overall health through optimal nutrition comprise the nutrition goals for the older patient with DM (American Diabetes Association, 2001). For obese older patients with DM, weight loss is encouraged. Insulin sensitivity increases when obese patients begin to lose weight. When insulin sensitivity is improved, medication doses may be lowered and blood glucose levels are more responsive to medications. A registered dietitian can give advice on

FIGURE ▢ 19-7

Sample daily diabetes record.

Daily Diabetes Record										
Week Starting _____										
	Other Blood Glucose	Breakfast Blood Glucose	Medicine	Lunch Blood Glucose	Medicine	Dinner Blood Glucose	Medicine	Bedtime Blood Glucose	Medicine	Notes: (Special events, sick days, exercise)
Monday										
Tuesday										
Wednesday										
Thursday										
Friday										
Saturday										
Sunday										

Source: NIDDK, 2004.

meal planning that is consistent with the cultural, social, and energy requirements of the older person. The recommendations should also address associated risk factors such as elevated lipids, protein and calcium requirements, and sodium restrictions. Ideally, the patient with DM should attempt to keep blood glucose levels stable throughout the day by eating smaller portions of carbohydrates and fats at mealtime and scheduling snacks during peak times of insulin or oral hypoglycemic medication action. The Food Guide Pyramid is a good starting point for educating the older person regarding healthy eating (see Chapter 5 for more information on nutrition and diabetes ⊂⊃).

Patients with diabetes should be encouraged to eat at regular times and never skip meals. Snacks should be taken at the same time each day. Older patients with DM should eat a variety of foods to keep the meal plan interesting and to meet nutritional needs. Once the older patient becomes skilled at choosing healthy foods that are consistent with nutritional needs and blood glucose control, nutritional status and overall health often improve. A sample daily menu for the older patient with DM is included in Figure 19-8■.

Additional nutritional guidelines for patients with DM include:

- **Eat less fat.** Avoid fried foods. Choose baked, broiled, grilled, or steamed foods to reduce fat. Choose reduced-fat dairy products. Limit fat to less than 30% of total calories, saturated fat to less than 10% of calories, and monounsaturated fat to between 10% and 15% of calories.

FIGURE ■ 19-8

A sample daily menu for the older patient with DM.

Meal	Food Example
Breakfast	
3 carbohydrate servings	½ grapefruit
0–1 meat servings	½ cup cooked oatmeal
0–1 fat servings	1 cup low-fat milk
Lunch	
3–4 carbohydrate servings	1 cup chicken noodle soup
2–3 meat servings	1 oz sliced chicken or turkey
0–1 fat servings	1 slice whole wheat bread
	1 serving of fresh fruit
Afternoon Snack	
1 carbohydrate serving	1 low-fat granola bar or 1 cup cereal with low-
0–1 fat servings	fat milk
Evening Meal	
3–4 carbohydrate servings	1 slice whole wheat bread with 1 pat of
3–4 meat servings	margarine
1–2 fat servings	1 cup vegetable of choice
	3–4 oz lean meat or fish
	½ cup low-fat cottage cheese or yogurt
	1 serving of fresh fruit
Evening Snack	
2 carbohydrate servings	1 cup low-fat milk
1 fat serving	1 serving low-calorie cookie (ginger snap)

Source: Blair, 1999.

- **Eat less sugar.** Read the labels on jars, cans, and food packages before buying them. If one of the first four ingredients is dextrose, sucrose, corn sweeteners, honey, molasses, or sugar, try to find a less sweetened substitute. Try to avoid highly sweetened cereal, cakes, pastries, and candy.
- **Eat less salt.** Taste food before salting it. Use additional spices when cooking food. Cut down on processed foods and salty snacks. Try to consume no more than 3 g of sodium daily. For persons with hypertension, the goal should be 2 g or less.
- **Eat foods with higher fiber.** High-fiber foods improve glycemic control and decrease hyperinsulinemia. As foods high in fiber take longer to be digested and absorbed, postprandial hyperglycemia is decreased and medications can work more effectively. Try to consume 20 to 35 g dietary fiber from soluble and insoluble fiber sources daily.
- **Avoid or reduce alcohol.** Alcohol can cause problems for people with DM. In addition to adding empty calories, it can interact with diabetic medications. An occasional drink can be incorporated into meal plans with the guidance of a dietitian. It is recommended that patients with DM consume no more than two drinks per day for men and no more than one drink per day for women (one alcoholic beverage is a 12 oz beer, 5 oz wine, or 1.5 oz distilled spirits). Alcohol must be consumed with food to prevent hypoglycemia, and calories from alcohol must be calculated as part of the total caloric intake and are best substituted for fat calories (Centers for Disease Control, 1999).

Physical exercise slows the progression of DM, improves weight control, and maintains overall function. Regular physical activity is encouraged for all older people with DM. Strenuous exercise should be avoided because of the risk of injury, retinal detachment, or vitreous hemorrhage (Berenbeim et al., 2001). Additionally, patients taking insulin who engage in strenuous physical exercise may suffer from hypoglycemia, primarily because absorption from the injection site increases (Barzilai, 2003). Older patients taking insulin should check their blood glucose levels before exercising and eat additional carbohydrates if their glucose levels are below 100 mg/dl prior to exercise. Monitoring blood glucose before and after exercise helps to identify when changes in insulin or food intake are necessary to learn how the glycemic response changes as the result of exercise. The goal is to adjust the insulin and food regimen to allow safe participation in exercise that is consistent with the older person's desires. To avoid hypoglycemia, the patient should have carbohydrate foods available during and after exercise. The older person should avoid exercise if fasting glucose levels are greater than 250 mg/dl (American Diabetes Association, 2001).

Older patients with DM should receive a detailed medical evaluation before beginning an exercise program, including medical history, physical examination, diagnostic studies, and screening for heart disease (American Diabetes Association, 2001). The healthcare provider may obtain a graded exercise test or radionuclide stress test to assess cardiac function. Recommended exercises include walking, swimming, bicycling, rowing, chair exercises, arm exercise, and other non–weight-bearing exercises. Because of the risk of ulceration and bone fracture, older patients with peripheral neuropathy should avoid strenuous exercise such as prolonged walking, treadmill use, jogging, or step exercise (American Diabetes Association, 2001).

Walking or swimming three times a week for 30 minutes is a good way to keep or get active. An older person who has not been physically active should begin gradually. If there is doubt about strength and endurance, advice from the physical therapist and primary healthcare provider is helpful. The older person should choose a form of exercise that is acceptable and safe. If walking is chosen, a safe place to walk and good footwear are essential. When older people walk outside during the winter months in northern climates, they risk falling on ice or snow. Additional hazards include uneven sidewalks, cold weather, and criminal activity. Some older adults engage in mall walking. Usually malls are warm, are well lighted, and have security personnel so they are ideal places for older people to engage in physical activity. As they grow in strength, older persons are encouraged to add a minute or two of activity to their daily exercise. Older people who are already active should be encouraged to maintain and even increase their activity levels. If they experience pain, shortness of breath, or dizziness, they should stop and wait until the feeling subsides. Recurrent symptoms of exercise intolerance such as shortness of breath, chest pain, and excessive fatigue should be evaluated by the healthcare provider because underlying undiagnosed heart disease may be responsible for these symptoms.

Gerontological nurses may encourage older patients to begin walking by educating them and their families regarding the benefits of regular activity. Education enables persons with DM to participate more actively in their treatment and prevention of complications. Diabetes education should be presented simply and in a straightforward manner and should continue over time. As time progresses, the instruction defines and addresses the individual needs of the older person and his or her family (National Diabetes Education Program, 2003). For example, the nurse may educate the older person regarding the benefits of walking.

Walking is one of the easiest ways to be active. It can be done almost anywhere and anytime. The older person should purchase a good pair of walking shoes and enjoy the following benefits:

- Getting more energy
- Reducing stress
- Improving sleep
- Toning muscles
- Controlling appetite
- Increasing the number of calories burned daily
- Preventing complications of diabetes

(National Diabetes Education Program, 2003)

The walking program should be integrated into the older person's schedule in a way that will work best for him or her. The nurse should recommend the following actions:

- Choose a safe place to walk. Find a partner or exercise group to walk with you. You and your partner should be at about the same level of fitness so you can walk together and engage in pleasant conversation.
- Wear shoes with thick flexible soles that cushion your step and absorb shock. (Figure 19-9 ■ illustrates factors to be considered when an older patient with DM is being fitted for shoes.)
- Wear clothes that keep you dry and comfortable. Dress in layers so that you can remove your jacket or sweatshirt when you get warmed up.
- Think of your walk in three parts. Walk slowly for 5 minutes, and subsequently increase your speed for 5 minutes. Slow your pace at the end of your walk for 15 minutes to cool down.
- Try to walk at least 3 to 5 times per week. Add 2 to 3 minutes per week to the walk.

FIGURE ■ 19-9

Guidelines for footwear assessment.

Improper or poorly fitting shoes are major contributors to diabetes foot ulcerations. Counsel patients about appropriate footwear. All patients with diabetes need to pay special attention to the fit and style of their shoes and should avoid pointed-toe shoes or high heels. Properly fitted athletic or walking shoes are recommended for daily wear. If off-the-shelf shoes are used, make sure that there is room to accommodate any deformities.

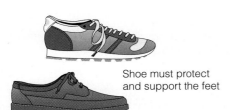
Shoe must protect and support the feet

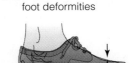
Shoe must accomodate foot deformities

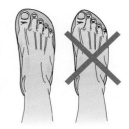
Shoe shape must match foot shape

High-risk patients may require therapeutic shoes, depth-inlay shoes, custom-molded inserts (orthoses), or custom-molded shoes, depending on the degree of foot deformity and history of ulceration.

Source: National Diabetes Education Program, 2003.

■ Start slowly to avoid stiff muscles and joints. Work your way up gradually and increase distance and pace slowly. Engage in warm-up exercises. Figure 19-10■ illustrates warm-up exercises, and Figure 19-11■ gives guidelines for how to build up to 30 minutes of brisk walking 5 days a week.

(NIDDK, 2004)

The nurse should help the older patient to set realistic goals and not to be discouraged if progress proceeds more slowly than anticipated. Beginning a regular activity program involves a major lifestyle modification. Most older patients will need ongoing support and encouragement before they finally incorporate this healthy habit into their lifestyle.

MEDICATIONS USED TO CONTROL DIABETES MELLITUS

Oral hypoglycemic drugs are used for type 2 DM only. Single or combination drugs can achieve good glycemic control and have been used successfully for years. However, newer drugs have emerged during the last 10 years. Each medication addresses a different glycemic problem, and they can be used as monotherapy or in combination with other drugs.

Oral antidiabetic drugs include the antihyperglycemic drugs (biguanides, alpha-glucosidase inhibitors, and thiazolidinediones) and oral hypoglycemic drugs (sulfonylureas and meglitinide). The oldest class of oral hypoglycemic drugs is the sulfonylureas, and these drugs have been improved over the last 20 years to increase effectiveness. These second-generation sulfonylureas stimulate the **beta cells** in the pancreas to secrete insulin. They are effective drugs, but sometimes can stimulate the release of too much insulin, resulting in hypoglycemia. Hypoglycemia occurs most often with long-acting sulfonylureas (glyburide). Sulfonylurea-induced hypoglycemia can be severe and last or

FIGURE ■ 19-10

Warm-up exercises to prepare the older person with diabetes for walking.

Before you start to walk, do the stretches shown here. Remember not to bounce when you stretch. Perform slow movements and stretch only as far as you feel comfortable.

Side Reaches

Reach one arm over your head and to the side. Keep your hips steady and your shoulders straight to the side. Hold for 10 seconds and repeat on the other side.

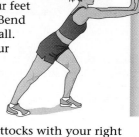

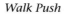

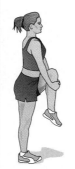

Knee Pull

Lean your back against a wall. Keep your head, hips, and feet in a straight line. Pull one knee to your chest, hold for 10 seconds, then repeat with the other leg.

Walk Push

Lean your hands on a wall with your feet about 3–4 feet away from the wall. Bend one knee and point it toward the wall. Keep your back leg straight with your foot flat and your toes pointed straight ahead. Hold for 10 seconds and repeat with the other leg.

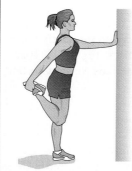

Leg Curl

Pull your right foot to your buttocks with your right hand. Keep your knee pointing straight to the ground. Hold for 10 seconds and repeat with your left foot and hand.

Source: NIDDK, 2004.

recur for days after treatment is stopped. All older patients treated with sulfonylureas who develop hypoglycemia should be closely monitored in the hospital for 2 to 3 days (Barzilai, 2003). An additional adverse effect is that weight gain occurs in many older patients taking these drugs. The extended-release formulations offer the advantage of simplifying dosing to once a day. Because they contain sulfa, they should not be used by patients who are sulfa-allergic.

Metformin is a biguanide introduced in 1994 that improves insulin sensitivity by enhancing glucose uptake and use by the muscles (Coyle, 2003). Additional benefits include mild weight loss and favorable changes in lipid profiles for patients with high lipid levels. Gastrointestinal side effects are common during initial dosing but are usually mild and resolve spontaneously. Metformin should not be used by patients over 80 or those with renal insufficiency (serum creatinine above 1.4 in women and above 1.5 in men) (Coyle, 2003). In contrast with oral antihyperglycemics, these drugs rarely cause hypoglycemia and may be safer for older persons (Barzilai, 2003).

Alpha-glucosidase inhibitors decrease postprandial hyperglycemia by slowing digestion and delaying intestinal absorption of carbohydrates. These drugs are helpful in older patients who exhibit baseline blood glucose levels in the normal range but become hyperglycemic immediately after eating a meal. The major side effects of these drugs are gastrointestinal and include flatulence and bloating, so many patients wish to discontinue taking these medications (Coyle, 2003). Sometimes starting at a low dose and slowly titrating up to the therapeutic dose will minimize adverse effects.

Thiazolidinediones were introduced in 1997 with the introduction of troglitazone (Rezulin). This drug was withdrawn in 2000 after it was associated with several deaths and liver transplants resulting from hepatotoxicity (Coyle, 2003). Since then, two new thiazolidinediones have been approved. These drugs enhance insulin sensitivity through activation of intracellular receptors and also suppress hepatic glucose production. Absolute contraindications include active liver disease (alanine aminotransferase (ALT) more than 2.5 times the upper limit of normal) and congestive heart failure (New York Heart Association class III or IV) (Coyle, 2003). Regular monitoring of liver function tests is recommended at baseline and every 2 months for the first year and periodically thereafter. An additional side effect is weight gain (Coyle, 2003).

The final class of oral hypoglycemics is meglitinides. Drugs in this class are insulin secretagogues and act by stimulating insulin release in response to a meal. Although

A sample walking program

Walking right is very important.

FIGURE ■ 19-11

A sample walking program.

	Warm Up Time	Fast Walk Time	Cool Down Time	Total time
Week 1	Walk slowly 5 min.	Walk briskly 5 min.	Walk slowly 5 min.	15 min.
Week 2	Walk slowly 5 min.	Walk briskly 8 min.	Walk slowly 5 min.	18 min.
Week 3	Walk slowly 5 min.	Walk briskly 11 min.	Walk slowly 5 min.	21 min.
Week 4	Walk slowly 5 min.	Walk briskly 14 min.	Walk slowly 5 min.	24 min.
Week 5	Walk slowly 5 min.	Walk briskly 17 min.	Walk slowly 5 min.	27 min.
Week 6	Walk slowly 5 min.	Walk briskly 20 min.	Walk slowly 5 min.	30 min.
Week 7	Walk slowly 5 min.	Walk briskly 23 min.	Walk slowly 5 min.	33 min.
Week 8	Walk slowly 5 min.	Walk briskly 26 min.	Walk slowly 5 min.	36 min.
Week 9 & Beyond	Walk slowly 5 min.	Walk briskly 30 min.	Walk slowly 5 min.	40 min.

Walk with your chin up and your shoulder held slightly back.
Walk so that the heel of your foot touches the ground first. Roll your weight forward.
Walk with your toes pointed forward.
Swing your arms as you walk.

If you walk less than three times per week, increase the fast walk time more slowly.

Source: NIDDK, 2004.

they are considered rapid-onset drugs, their duration of action is short and they must be taken with each meal for maximum effect. They should not be taken without food, in the event that a patient skips a meal or ingests a meal that is very low in carbohydrate content (Coyle, 2003).

Some patients take combination drugs such as glyburide-metformin (Glucovance), glipizide-metformin (Metaglip), and rosiglitazone-metformin (Avandamet). These drugs simplify the dosing requirements and may be less expensive in some cases. They combine drugs with different mechanisms of action to achieve better basal glucose levels and prevent postprandial peaks. However, the use of combination drugs incurs more risk in the older patient. Should an adverse effect occur, it may not be clear which drug in the combination is responsible. Extra caution and monitoring are needed to prevent hypoglycemia and ensure success with combination medications. Table 19-3 illustrates the commonly used medications, and starting and maximum doses.

Insulin

Insulin is used alone in type 1 DM and may be used alone or in combination with oral hypoglycemic medications in type 2 DM (Coyle, 2003). Although most patients with type 2 DM will not need insulin, it may be used in patients whose diabetes cannot be adequately controlled with oral agents alone. Insulin is injected subcutaneously with special insulin syringes. The 0.5-ml syringes are preferred by older patients who inject doses of 50 U or less, because these syringes facilitate the accurate measurement of smaller insulin doses. A multiple-dose insulin injection device (e.g., Novolin Pen) uses

TABLE 19-3

Commonly Used Medications and Recommended Starting and Maximum Doses

Medication	Starting Dose	Maximum Dose
Second-Generation Sulfonylureas		
Glyburide (Micronase, DiaBeta)	2.5 mg daily	20 mg daily
Glipizide (Glucotrol)	2.5 mg daily	40 mg daily
Glipizide Controlled Release (Glucotrol XL)	2.5 mg daily	20 mg daily
Metformin (Biguanide)		
Metformin (Glucophage)	500 mg daily with food	2,500 mg daily
Metformin Extended Release (Glucophage XR)	500 mg daily with food (evening meal)	2,000 mg daily
Alpha-Glucosidase Inhibitors		
Acarbose (Precose)	25 mg with first bite of each meal	300 mg
Miglitol (Glyset)	25 mg with first bite of each meal	300 mg
Thiazolidinedione		
Rosiglitazone (Avandia)	4 mg daily	8 mg
Pioglitazone (Actos)	15 mg daily	45 mg
Meglitinide		
Repaglinide (Prandin)	0.5 mg before each meal	16 mg
Nateglinide (Starlix)	120 mg before each meal	360 mg

Source: Coyle, 2003.

Insulin	Duration of Action	TABLE 19-4
Short-Acting		Available Insulins and Duration of Action
Regular	3–6 hours	
Lispro (Humalog)	1–2 hours	
Aspart (NovoLog)	1–2 hours	
Intermediate-Acting		
NPH	18–24 hours	
Lente	18–24 hours	
Long-Acting		
Ultralente	24–36 hours	
Glargine (Lantus)	24 hours	
Premixed Combinations		
50/50 NPH-Regular Mixture	Up to 24 hours	
70/30 NPH-Regular Mixture	Up to 24 hours	
75/25 Humalog Mix—NPH—Lispro	Up to 24 hours	
70/30 NovoLog Mix—NPH—NovoLog	Up to 24 hours	

Source: Barzilai, 2003; Coyle, 2003; epocrates.com, 2004.

a cartridge containing several days' dosage. The accuracy and ease of use of the insulin pen is ideal for some older patients. Insulin should be refrigerated but never frozen. Most insulin is stable at room temperature, but it should not be stored near a heat source or transported in an overheated car or trunk (Barzilai, 2003). For patients with visual difficulties, magnifying glasses can be helpful or the medication can be drawn up by the visiting nurse or a family member. Prefilled syringes should be used within a week.

As with oral hypoglycemics, the insulin regimen should mimic normal physiology with control of both basal and postprandial glucose levels. Long-acting insulin controls blood glucose levels and uses glucose as a fuel long after the meal has been digested (basal insulin). Short-acting insulin satisfies the need for insulin after meals or ingestion of food and is usually injected around mealtime. Newer insulins are made from recombinant DNA and do not require extraction from the pancreas of animals. NPH, Lente, Ultralente, and Regular Insulin are still available but are being used less often (Coyle, 2003). Lispro (Humalog) and aspart (NovoLog) are the newest rapid-acting insulins with onset of action within 15 minutes. They are usually injected immediately prior to eating a meal several times daily. Longer acting insulins such as glargine (Lantus) are designed to release insulin evenly throughout the day and control basal glucose levels. Patients who take Lantus experience less overnight hypoglycemia compared to those using NPH (Coyle, 2003).

Mixtures of insulin preparations with different onsets and durations of action are often given in a single injection to simplify the dosing and better control blood glucose levels. These insulin combinations are more suitable for patients with type 2 DM because patients with type 1 DM are totally reliant on insulin and would lose the ability to make individual dose adjustments based on food consumption and metabolic demands imposed by exercise (Coyle, 2003).

Table 19-4 lists the available insulins and duration of action. Caution and careful monitoring are indicated during the initial dosing period. The major determinant of the

TABLE 19-5

Food and Liquids for Low Blood Glucose Levels[*]

Food Item	Amount
Sugar packets	2 to 3
Fruit juice	1/2 cup (4 oz)
Soda pop (not diet)	1/2 cup (4 oz)
Hard candy	3 to 5 pieces
Sugar or honey	3 teaspoons
Glucose tablets	2 to 3

[*]About 10–15 grams of carbohydrate.

Source: Centers for Disease Control, 1999.

onset and duration of action is the rate of insulin absorption from the injection site, and this can vary widely among patients (Barzilai, 2003).

Hypoglycemia as a Complication of Insulin Treatment

Hypoglycemia can be caused by too high a dose of insulin, missing a meal or eating a smaller meal, unplanned exercise, or the onset of illness that alters metabolic need. Older patients should be taught to recognize the symptoms of hypoglycemia, including feeling nervous, shaky, sweaty, or excessively fatigued. The signs may be mild at first, but may progress rapidly to confusion, passing out, or having seizures as blood levels continue to drop. Older patients should test their blood glucose levels if they experience these symptoms. If it is less than 60 to 70 mg/dl, they should treat themselves right away. If they are unable to test their glucose levels, they should treat it anyway. The usual treatment recommendation is to eat 10 to 15 g of carbohydrates right away. Table 19-5 indicates examples of food or liquids with this amount of carbohydrate.

After ingesting 10 to 15 g of carbohydrate, the older person should wait 15 minutes and test the blood glucose level again. More carbohydrates may need to be ingested. This process should be repeated until the blood glucose is above 70 mg/dl or the signs of hypoglycemia have resolved. Patients must be cautioned that eating the foods on this list will keep the blood glucose level up for only about 30 minutes. If the next meal or snack is a long way off, they should eat something more substantial like crackers with peanut butter or a slice of cheese or meat. All patients with DM should carry an identification card that identifies them as having diabetes and wear a medical bracelet or necklace. Family members, caregivers, and close friends should be taught to administer glucagon with an easy-to-use injection device as part of an emergency kit. Glucagon is available by prescription and is injected like insulin. If no one is available to help and the symptoms do not subside, the older person should be instructed to call for emergency assistance and hospital evaluation. They should not attempt to drive themselves to the hospital as confusion or loss of consciousness from low glucose levels may occur.

Morning Hyperglycemia

The dawn phenomenon refers to the normal tendency of blood glucose levels to rise in the early morning before breakfast. This normal phenomenon is exaggerated in older patients with type 1 and type 2 diabetes. The liver may produce increased glucose as a result of a midnight surge of growth hormone. In some patients, nocturnal hypoglycemia may be followed by a marked increase in fasting blood glucose with an increase in plasma ketones (Somogyi phenomenon) (Barzilai, 2003).

Injection Site Reactions

At the injection site, local fat atrophy or allergic reactions can occur. Pain and burning at the injection site may last for a few hours, followed by redness, itching, and induration. These reactions usually disappear on their own as the body becomes desensitized to the insulin. Injection sites should be routinely rotated to prevent fat atrophy.

EFFECT OF ACUTE ILLNESS

Should an older patient with DM experience an acute illness such as pneumonia or urinary tract infection, hyperglycemia can be the result. However, if the patient has lost his or her appetite or is vomiting, continuing to take the same dose of oral hypoglycemics or insulin can result in hypoglycemia. If the patient is hospitalized or in a long-term care facility, the nurses will routinely check blood glucose levels and "cover" the patient with a sliding scale of insulin until the acute illness resolves and the blood glucose levels stabilize. The physician may request that hypoglycemic drugs be withheld during an acute condition associated with decreased food intake or persistent nausea and vomiting. The effects of surgical procedure (anesthesia, surgical trauma, emotional stress) can markedly increase blood glucose levels. Every attempt should be made by the nurse and other members of the healthcare team to regulate medications and oral intake to prevent dangerous variations in blood glucose levels.

Patients and their families should be instructed to call their healthcare provider if any of the following conditions occur:

- Unable to keep food or liquids down or eat normally for over 6 hours
- Severe diarrhea
- Unintentional weight loss of 5 lb
- Oral temperature over 101°F
- Blood glucose levels lower than 60 mg/dl or over 300 mg/dl
- Presence of large amounts of ketones in the urine
- Difficulty breathing
- Feeling sleepy or unable to think clearly

(Centers for Disease Control, 1999)

NONKETOTIC HYPERGLYCEMIC-HYPEROSMOLAR COMA

Nonketotic hyperglycemic-hyperosmolar coma (NKHHC) is a complication of type 2 DM that has a high mortality rate (Barzilai, 2003). It usually develops after a period of symptomatic hyperglycemia during which fluid intake is inadequate to prevent extreme dehydration from osmotic diuresis. Symptoms of hyperglycemia include dry mouth, extreme thirst, excessive urination, fatigue, blurred vision, weight loss, nausea, abdominal pain, and vomiting. NKHHC can occur in some older patients with undiagnosed or untreated type 2 DM when they receive drugs that impair glucose tolerance such as glucocorticoids or drugs that increase fluid loss such as diuretics. Older persons with severe dementia may also be at risk because the decreased thirst and hunger drive may prevent them from eating and drinking adequate amounts of fluid and nutritious foods.

NKHHC may begin as mild confusion and progress to coma or seizures. Laboratory studies reveal hyperglycemia (above 500 mg/dl), hyperosmolarity, and metabolic acidosis. Serum sodium and potassium levels are usually normal, but blood urea nitrogen (BUN) and serum creatinine levels are increased. As the average fluid deficit is greater than 10 L, acute circulatory collapse is common. Widespread thrombosis is a frequent finding on autopsy and may lead to disseminated intravascular coagulation (DIC) (Barzilai, 2003). Treatment must begin immediately and intravenous fluids are needed to expand the intravascular volume, stabilize blood pressure, and improve circulation and urine flow. Insulin treatment is not always necessary, because adequate hydration may decrease blood glucose levels.

DIFFICULTIES IN CARING FOR OLDER PATIENTS WITH DM

Six geriatric syndromes were selected by the California Healthcare Foundation/ American Geriatrics Society panel based on literature review and expert opinions (2003). These syndromes represent areas where gerontological nurses can intervene and collaborate with other healthcare professionals to improve the quality of care provided to older patients with DM. They include:

1. **Polypharmacy.** Older patients with DM may require several medications to manage their overall health problems, including elevated blood glucose levels, hypertension, hyperlipidemia, and other associated conditions. Nurses should perform a careful and accurate drug assessment at each visit and document whether the patient is taking the medications as ordered. Patients and their families should be provided with information describing the expected benefits, risks, and potential side effects of each medication.

2. **Depression.** Older adults with DM are at an increased risk for depression that may be undetected and untreated. A depression screen should be performed using a standardized screening instrument (for example, the Geriatric Depression Scale) and periodically thereafter. Symptoms of depression should be clearly noted on the chart, and drug therapy or counseling begun as needed. Progress toward symptom relief should be noted in the chart.

3. **Cognitive impairment.** Older adults with DM are at increased risk for cognitive impairment. Subtle or unrecognized cognitive impairment may interfere with the patient's ability to manage this complicated disease. Therefore, screening for cognitive impairment on the initial visit using a standardized assessment instrument (Mini-Mental State Examination) is needed and should be repeated periodically thereafter. Any increased difficulty with self-care or failure of self-management should be aggressively investigated. Caregivers should be consulted (with the patient's permission) and involved with the ongoing education and management plan to successfully manage DM in the patient with cognitive impairment.

4. **Urinary incontinence.** Older women with DM are at increased risk of urinary incontinence. Urinary incontinence should be assessed initially and periodically thereafter. Older age and disease-associated conditions that can contribute to urinary incontinence include polyuria, neutrogenic bladder, atrophic vaginitis, urinary tract infection, and vaginal candidiasis.

5. **Injurious falls.** Falls in older people are associated with higher rates of morbidity, mortality, and functional decline. Older persons with DM are at increased risk for injurious falls because of higher rates of frailty and functional disability, visual impairment, peripheral neuropathy, hypoglycemia, and polypharmacy. Fall risk screening should be done initially and periodically

thereafter. Risk factors should be noted and addressed by the healthcare team to prevent injurious falls.

6. **Pain.** Older persons with DM are at risk for neuropathic pain, which often goes untreated. Older patients should be screened for persistent pain initially and periodically thereafter. Patients with persistent pain should be monitored, treated, and provided with appropriate therapy with results of treatment noted in the patient's chart.

GENERAL HEALTH PROMOTION FOR THE OLDER PERSON WITH DIABETES

Coordinated care is essential in the management of the older patient with DM. Treatment emphasizes dietary modification, exercise, weight reduction, and appropriate use of medication as described in this chapter. At each visit, the patient's progress should be evaluated by the nurse and problems identified and reviewed. The plan should be revised and reassessed on an ongoing basis.

Older persons with DM and their families should be taught self-management skills including self-monitoring for signs of hypoglycemia, blood glucose monitoring skills and medication adjustment, nutrition management, and development and maintenance of a physical activity plan. Older persons with DM should receive the influenza vaccine every fall. The pneumococcal vaccine is recommended at age 65. Revaccination is suggested if the patient is over the age of 65 and the initial vaccine was given over 5 years ago and the patient was under 65 at that time.

The nurse should counsel patients with DM regarding smoking cessation, psychosocial function and depression screening, sexuality and erectile dysfunction, urinary incontinence, falls, presence of pain or neuropathy, and foot and skin assessment. Referral to a certified diabetes educator may be indicated for additional education and self-management skills consistent with the National Standards for Diabetes Patient Education Programs. Podiatry and dental consultation should be scheduled as needed. An annual comprehensive dilated eye and visual examination is recommended by an opthalmologist so that microvascular complications can be detected and treated early to prevent vision loss.

At each visit, the older patient is weighed and has blood pressure recorded. The feet and skin are carefully examined. Any irritation, ulceration, deformity, or loss of sensation is carefully noted and referred for treatment. It is recommended that laboratory tests be obtained as indicated in Table 19-6.

TABLE 19-6

Recommended Laboratory Testing and Frequency for Older Persons With Diabetes

Test	Frequency	Action
HbA$_{1c}$	Every 3 months	Ideal goal <7.0%. Action suggested at >8.0%.
Fasting/random blood glucose	As needed	Compare lab results with home glucometer readings.
Fasting lipid profile	Annually	Cardiovascular risk reduction if indicated.
Urinalysis	Annually	Refer if albuminuria is present.
Electrocardiogram	Every 5–10 years	
Thyroid function	As needed	Thyroid palpation and TSH

Source: Diabetes Guidelines Work Group, 1999.

HOPE FOR THE FUTURE

Continuous subcutaneous insulin infusion pumps are being used more widely. These small devices (about the size of a beeper) can be programmed to deliver an individualized basal dose of insulin and can be bolused by the patient before a meal to control the postprandial glucose levels. A small tube connects to a subcutaneous catheter usually placed in the abdomen. Patients wearing the pumps must be motivated to perform frequent self-monitoring of blood glucose levels and be able to calculate the need for the insulin bolus depending on the size and content of their meal. Usually four to six finger sticks to test blood glucose are needed daily to ensure appropriate dosing and prevent hypo- or hyperglycemia (Coyle, 2003).

In the future, inhaled insulin will replace the need for frequent subcutaneous injections. An implantable insulin pump is being developed that will be programmed to measure blood glucose levels and release an appropriate insulin dose in response. Transplantation of islet cell from one human pancreas to another is also being tested. Despite the possibilities for improvement of future treatment, nurses should work with older patients to prevent DM from developing through rigorous lifestyle modification including diet, exercise, weight loss, and reduction of cardiac risk factors. After diagnosis, these same lifestyle modifications will improve the effect of medications, delay or prevent secondary complications, preserve strength and function, and improve the quality of life for the older person.

Thyroid Disorders

The prevalence of thyroid disease rises with age. **Hypothyroidism** is much higher in women than in men of all ages, and is higher in older persons living in institutions than in older community-residing persons (Solomon, 2003). The prevalence of **hyperthyroidism** in older people is similar to the rates in the general population. Approximately 5% to 10% of persons over 65 have hypothyroidism, and 0.2% to 2% have hyperthyroidism. When the thyroid is functioning well, the nurse will observe an older patient who is functioning well metabolically. When thyroid dysfunction is present, and insufficient or excessive amounts of thyroid hormone are produced, the nurse will see dramatic effects in the cardiovascular system, hematologic system, and central nervous system. Because thyroid dysfunction often occurs gradually, the signs and symptoms may be imperceptible to the patient and family and may be attributed to normal changes of aging. Hypothyroidism is characterized by a generalized reduction in metabolic function that most often manifests as a slowing of physical and mental activity. The complaints may vary from asymptomatic, mild, moderate, or severe, and depend on a variety of factors such as the patient's age, general health status, cognitive abilities, and rate at which the disease develops (Burman, 2000). As older patients do not complain of classic symptoms of thyroid disease, their complaints may be attributed to other causes. The necessary testing is often not done, leaving the condition undiagnosed for long periods of time. This can result in expensive and unnecessary testing, inappropriate use of healthcare resources, and prolonged suffering for the patient (American Association of Clinical Endocrinologists, 2002). Undiagnosed thyroid disease can have a profound effect on the body, making early and accurate diagnosis and treatment a necessity.

NORMAL ANATOMY AND PHYSIOLOGY

The thyroid is an endocrine gland that produces thyroxine (T_4) and triiodothyronine (T_3), two hormones that play a key role in regulating the body's energy levels and metabolic function. Normally, thyrotropin-releasing hormone (TRH) is produced by the hypothalamus, stimulating the anterior pituitary gland to produce thyroid-stimulating hormone

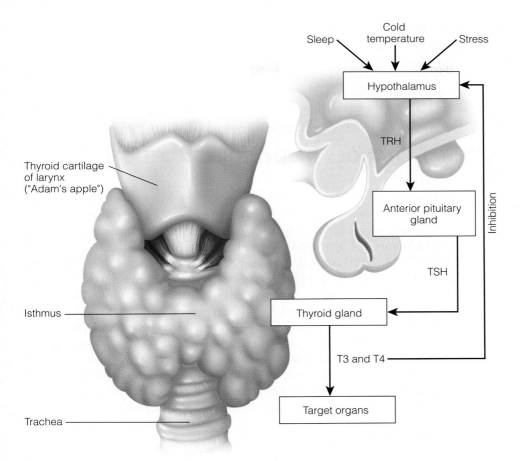

FIGURE ■ **19-12**
Physiological function of the thyroid gland.

(TSH). This in turn stimulates the thyroid to produce T4 and T3. Additionally, TSH increases carbohydrate, protein, and lipid metabolism and stimulates cell proliferation, thus affecting many systems of the body (Burman, 2000). High levels of T4 and T3 provide negative feedback to the pituitary gland and hypothalamus, decreasing the production of TSH and TRH. If free T4 and T3 levels are low, feedback to the pituitary gland and hypothalamus stimulates increased production of TRH and TSH, which stimulates the thyroid to produce more hormone. More than 99% of T4 and T3 is bound to thyroxine-binding globulin (TBG) and albumin, leaving only a small amount free to influence metabolic effect. Figure 19-12■ illustrates the physiology of the normally functioning thyroid gland.

Practice Pearl

Deficient amounts of thyroid hormones stimulate TSH secretion, whereas excess levels inhibit TSH secretion. Therefore, an older person with hypothyroidism will have an elevated TSH, and an older person with hyperthyroidism will have an abnormally low TSH level.

Both T3 and T4 rely on an adequate supply of iodine from the diet that is taken up by the gland from the circulating blood. T4 comprises the main hormone produced by the thyroid (about 80%); T3 is formed from T4 and is the active form of hormone, but much less is directly produced (20%). Once T4 and T3 are released into the circulation, they are bound by plasma proteins including TBG and albumin. T3 and T4 are inactive when bound to circulating proteins, and only the free fraction is able to bind to specific thyroid hormone receptors in peripheral tissue and stimulate biological activity. The bound hormones form a circulating reservoir of T3 and T4 that is available to the body to use as needed for regulating metabolic activity.

NORMAL CHANGES OF THYROID FUNCTION WITH AGING

Thyroid function is significantly altered with aging, and the thyroid gradually loses function and undergoes atrophy. The gland becomes more nodular, especially in areas with low iodine levels in the food and water. Fortunately, only about 2% of thyroid nodules are cancerous, and the presence of hypothyroidism and thyroid nodules rises dramatically with age (Solomon, 2003). Additionally, thyroid antibody levels rise with age, making it difficult to discern at what levels these antibodies indicate thyroiditis. Although the production of T4 decreases about 30% between young adulthood and old age, the serum T4 levels remain unchanged because of a decreased use of the hormone by tissue (Solomon, 2003). The body's decrease in use of T4 correlates with the age-related decline in lean body mass, indicating a compensatory mechanism with decreased production resulting from decreased need for thyroid hormone rather than thyroid failure. Serum T3 levels decrease slowly with age, while the average serum TSH levels rise with age. Although the prevalence of hyperthyroidism is similar for younger and older persons, the presentation of hyperthyroidism is often different in elderly adults, making it difficult to detect.

THYROID FUNCTION TESTING

Thyroid function tests help to diagnose and detect the presence of thyroid disease. With laboratory testing, thyroid disease is detectable at early stages, before significant loss of function occurs in the older person. The American Thyroid Association recommends initially checking free T4 and TSH levels to test thyroid function. Serum TSH level remains the best test of thyroid function because TSH is central to the negative-feedback system, small changes in serum thyroid function cause major changes in TSH secretion, and the most advanced measurement methods can detect both elevation and lowering of TSH levels and are capable of reliably measuring values below 0.1 mU/L (Ladenson et al., 2000). Total serum T4 levels, measured by radioimmunoassay, have high sensitivity with elevated readings exhibited in approximately 90% of older patients with hyperthyroid disease and decreased T4 levels in 85% of patients with hypothyroid disease. Interpretation of T3 levels can be more misleading because diminished peripheral conversion of T4 to T3 contributes to low serum T3 levels. Therefore, T3 levels are low in only 50% of hypothyroid patients. The presence of nutritional deficiencies and acute illnesses such as cirrhosis, uremia, or malnutrition can slow peripheral conversion (Supit & Peiris, 2002). With thyroid disorders occurring so commonly, these tests are often obtained in the clinical setting. Test results must be interpreted in relationship to the older person's overall health status, presence of diagnosed illnesses, and medications taken. Table 19-7 lists common laboratory tests of thyroid function and interpretation of abnormal findings.

Additional thyroid function tests may be ordered by the primary healthcare provider or endocrinologist to make an accurate diagnosis in patients with atypical or complicated presentation of thyroid disease. Although expensive, these tests can yield valuable information. They should be reserved for older patients with multiple systemic illnesses, mul-

TABLE 19-7

Common Laboratory Tests of Thyroid Function

	Normal Value	Value in Hypothyroidism	Value in Hyperthyroidism
TSH	0.32–5.0 mU/ml	↑ Usually >10–20	↓ Usually low (<0.30) or undetectable
Free T4	4.5–12 µg/dl	↓ decreased	↑ increased
Free T3	75–200 ng/dl	Normal	↑ increased

tiple medications, and atypical presentations. These tests include T3-resin uptake (T3RU), an assessment of binding in both thyroxine and triiodothyronine; thyroglobulin levels (Tg), a measure of circulating thyroglobulin, a useful marker for thyroid cancer; thyroid autoantibody levels which are elevated in 95% of patients with autoimmune thyroiditis (Hashimoto's thyroiditis); iodine 131 uptake, useful in differentiating a hyperfunctioning thyroid (**Graves' disease**) from a nonfunctioning gland (subacute thyroiditis); and radioactive iodine scan or sonogram, which provides a functional picture of the thyroid and is useful in the evaluation of thyroid nodules.

HYPOTHYROIDISM

Hypothyroidism is relatively common and can be caused by dysfunction of the thyroid gland (primary), pituitary (secondary), or hypothalamus (tertiary). The most common cause of primary hypothyroidism is Hashimoto's thyroiditis, an autoimmune disease with subtle onset and minimal symptoms while the thyroid gland undergoes progressive inflammatory destruction. Hypothyroidism may also be caused by factors that negatively affect the synthesis of thyroid hormones such as iodine deficiency or excess and inherited defects in thyroid hormone biosynthesis (Burman, 2000). The cause of **Hashimoto's disease** is unknown, but it is accompanied by elevated levels of antithyroglobulin or antimicrosomal antibodies (Kuritzky, 2001). Patients with Hashimoto's disease will progress to hypothyroidism because the chronic inflammation will result in scarred, nonproductive glandular tissue that cannot produce thyroid hormone.

Subclinical hypothyroidism is a condition in which the serum TSH level is between the upper limits of normal (between 5 mU/L and 15 mU/L) and the free T4 is within the normal range, but below the mean of the **euthyroid** older population (Solomon, 2003). Approximately 17% of patients over the age of 60 with subclinical hypothyroidism progress to overt hypothyroidism over a 1-year period (Burman, 2000). Many of these older patients have no clinical signs or symptoms of hypothyroidism and usually careful monitoring of laboratory values and ongoing assessment for debilitating signs and symptoms of hypothyroidism is indicated. The serum TSH measurement may need to be repeated in patients with concurrent illnesses because it may be subnormal during the illness and elevated during the recovery phase in response to the body's metabolic demands (Solomon, 2003).

In more than 95% of older patients, hypothyroidism is caused by primary dysfunction of the thyroid gland (Burman, 2000). Factors associated with the increased risk of developing hypothyroidism include older age, female gender, a history or diagnosis of thyroid disease including goiter, thyroid nodules, thyroiditis, hyperthyroidism, treatment of head or neck cancer with external radiation or iodine 131, family history of thyroid disease, diagnosis of nonthyroid autoimmune disease, and certain medications (Burman, 2000; Kuritzky, 2001). Medications associated with hypothyroidism include lithium, amiodarone, sulfonylureas, salicylates, furosemide, phenytoin, rifampin, and radioactive contrast dyes (Burman, 2000).

Older patients with goiter or enlarged thyroid glands detected through physical examination are euthyroid with the goiter representing a proliferation of thyroid tissue in response to inadequate serum levels of T3. Patients with goiter will often undergo thyroid function tests, antithyroid antibody tests, and thyroid scans to rule out Graves' disease, nodular goiter, hypothyroidism, or some other thyroid dysfunction (Kuritzky, 2001).

Effects of Hypothyroidism

Thyroid hormone deficiency results in a reduction in the metabolic rate. The onset of symptoms is usually gradual, and the patient can present with a wide range of symptoms. It is easy to attribute symptoms like constipation, fatigue, depression, and decreased hearing to aging when hypothyroidism may be responsible (Kuritzky, 2001). Typical symptoms include the following:

- Fatigue
- Increased need for sleep
- Muscle aches
- Dry skin
- Bradycardia
- Increased cholesterol levels (elevations in LDL)
- Ataxia and balance difficulties
- Hearing loss
- Depression
- Cold intolerance
- Hair loss
- Voice changes
- Hypothermia
- Periorbital swelling
- Decreased appetite and weight loss

(Burman, 2000; Kuritzky, 2001)

Hypothyroidism can cause a variety of symptoms associated with all of the major body systems. Neurologic symptoms include headache, vertigo or tinnitus, relaxation of the deep tendon reflexes, psychiatric disorders, cognitive deficits, and visual disturbances. Sensory disorders include numbness, tingling, and paresthesias. All older patients with symptoms of depression should have their thyroid function evaluated before treatment is begun. Cardiovascular effects of hypothyroidism can mimic heart failure with cardiac enlargement and decreased contractility of cardiac muscle. Pulse rate and stroke volume are diminished. These changes may be difficult to detect, especially if the older patient is being treated with a beta-blocker for hypertension. Musculoskeletal changes attributed to hypothyroidism include generalized muscle fatigue, cramps, myalgias, joint effusions, and pseudogout. Osteoporosis may be aggravated by hypothyroidism as the growth of new bone can be inhibited. Gastrointestinal effects of hypothyroidism include constipation and gaseous distention as a result of prolonged gastric emptying and intestinal transit. Achlorhydria and pernicious anemia occur more frequently in older patients with hypothyroidism. The manifestations of hypothyroidism are diverse and numerous. Thyroid hormone is important for normal metabolic functioning (Burman, 2000).

The evaluation of thyroid function in chronically ill older patients may be confusing. Many illnesses, medications, and treatments can affect thyroid function tests, and these abnormal values do not reflect abnormal thyroid function. This syndrome has been named *euthyroid sick syndrome* and can result from illness, hospitalization, and starvation as the body attempts to decrease metabolic rates and compensates by decreasing TSH levels with corresponding low free T4 levels. The chronically ill or hospitalized patient with abnormal thyroid function tests should be evaluated by a clinical endocrinologist (American Association of Clinical Endocrinologists, 2002).

Older patients with hypothyroidism have fewer symptoms than younger patients (Solomon, 2003). Most often, the older patient will present with chronic, nonspecific complaints. The patient may fall, exhibit poor coping patterns, lose mental function, exhibit new-onset incontinence, and become less mobile. Physical findings are often difficult to interpret. Complications of hypothyroidism include hypertension and hyperlipidemia. Untreated hypothyroidism may lead to myxedema coma, a life-threatening emergency. In myxedema, mental confusion progresses to stupor and coma and is accompanied by hyponatremia, hypoglycemia, or hypercapnia. Treatment of myxedema coma involves hospitalization in the intensive care unit with the patient receiving large intravenous doses of thyroid hormones supplemented by intravenous adrenal corticosteroids. Additional interventions are needed to treat hyponatremia, hypoglycemia, and respiratory failure, if present (Solomon, 2003).

Diagnosis of Hypothyroidism

Hypothyroidism is diagnosed by precise measurement of serum TSH and T4 levels. In primary hypothyroidism, the TSH is elevated and free serum T4 levels are below normal. The free serum T3 level has little value because it is normal in about one third of older patients with hypothyroidism and because low T3 levels are associated with acute illness and inadequate caloric intake (Solomon, 2003). An older patient with chronic thyroiditis may have an atrophic, normal, or enlarged thyroid gland, but thyroid autoantibodies are positive in 95% of these patients, making high titers a valuable diagnostic tool. Thyroid nodules or sudden enlargement of the thyroid requires thyroid scans or ultrasounds (American Association of Clinical Endocrinologists, 2002).

The thyroid is examined first with a visual inspection of the neck to identify any enlargements or irregularities. The nurse observes the neck using tangential lighting and stands a foot or two away to identify any shadows. Asking the patient to swallow will accentuate any irregularities during movement. The nurse begins to palpate the thyroid by placing fingers on the trachea at either side of the larynx and moving them gently up and down. The patient is asked to swallow to assess symmetry during movement. The nurse palpates underneath the muscles on either side of the trachea to ensure that the entire gland has been examined, and places a finger gently over the larynx to palpate the isthmus, the part of the thyroid that crosses over the larynx and forms the center of the butterfly-shaped gland. It should feel soft and spongy without nodules or irregularities. Giving the patient a sip or two of water may make it easier for the older patient to swallow.

A comprehensive health assessment and history may suggest the development of hypothyroidism. However, because the symptoms are vague and many older patients experience few symptoms, laboratory assessment of thyroid function is required to confirm the diagnosis.

Treatment and Nursing Management of Hypothyroidism

The goals of therapy are to relieve symptoms and to provide sufficient thyroid hormone to decrease raised serum TSH levels to the normal range. The treatment of hypothyroidism should be tailored to meet the needs of the patient. Long-standing untreated hypothyroidism is a risk factor for coronary artery disease. The older patient with heart disease may need cardiac stress testing and complete cardiovascular risk assessment before treatment is begun. Thyroid hormone replacement should be started cautiously because in some older patients, an increase in levels of thyroid hormones can increase myocardial oxygen demand and result in myocardial infarction, angina, and cardiac arrhythmia (Sidani, 2001; Solomon, 2003). If cardiac symptoms develop or worsen, therapy should be stopped pending evaluation of the symptoms.

The treatment of choice is T4 replacement with levothyroxine sodium. The average dose for patients over 65 years of age is 0.075 to 0.1 mg/day by mouth. If the patient has coronary artery disease, the initial dose should only be 0.0125 to 0.025 mg/day. The dose should be increased gradually (0.025 mg) over 4-week intervals and the serum TSH level monitored to assess the effectiveness of treatment. If the TSH levels are below normal, the dose of levothyroxine should be decreased. If the TSH levels are above normal, the dose should be increased slowly until the TSH is normal. Close monitoring of blood levels, overall function, cardiac status, and cognitive function is indicated during the initial period. After the TSH has stabilized in the normal range, thyroid function should be assessed every 6 to 12 months by an appropriate health assessment and laboratory testing (Burman, 2000). Overly suppressed TSH levels indicate that the patient is at increased risk for osteoporosis; however, T4 replacement with carefully monitored TSH levels has not been associated with decreased bone density (Kuritzky, 2001).

Several brands and generic preparations of levothyroxine sodium are now available. Although no one preparation appears distinctly superior to another, many patients experience a change in thyroid status when switching brands; therefore, it is best to maintain patients on the same preparation they have been taking during the initial titration period. As the half-life of levothyroxine is one week, dose adjustments will not be immediately apparent. If it is necessary to change from one brand to another, a dose adjustment may be needed. Reevaluation of thyroid status is indicated because some preparations are more bioavailable than others (Burman, 2000). Since levothyroxine has a narrow therapeutic range, small differences in absorption can produce subclinical or clinical hypothyroidism (American Association of Clinical Endocrinologists, 2002). The two most popular brand names are Synthroid and Levoxyl, with Levoxyl priced at about 30% less in retail cost to the patient (Epocrates.com, 2004; Kuritzky, 2001).

Oral levothyroxine should be taken on an empty stomach at the same time every day. Drugs that can decrease the absorption of levothyroxine and cause harmful drug interactions should be taken several hours after the levothyroxine has been taken. Drugs that interfere with levothyroxine absorption include aluminum hydroxide, calcium preparations, cholestyramine, colestipol, iron preparations, and sucralfate (American Association of Clinical Endocrinologists, 2002; Burman, 2000). Other drugs such as anticonvulsants and antitubercular agents (rifampin) may accelerate levothyroxine metabolism, necessitating a higher replacement dose (American Association of Clinical Endocrinologists, 2002). The nurse should carefully monitor the patient's medications on an ongoing basis to prevent harmful drug interactions.

The American Thyroid Association recommends screening every 5 years by measuring serum TSH for all men and women over age 35. For those with risk factors for thyroid disease, the serum TSH level should be checked more often and as indicated by the presence of new or unexplained symptoms of decreased metabolism. Screening of thyroid function should be performed in populations that have a high incidence of thyroid dysfunction because of disease state, drug therapy, or other predisposing factor, and when early intervention is crucial to prevent irreversible pathology once the diagnosis of hypothyroidism is made (American Association of Clinical Endocrinologists, 2002). The TSH assay is the screening method of choice for identifying hypothyroidism.

HYPERTHYROIDISM

Hyperthyroidism, or thyrotoxicosis, is the result of excess thyroid hormone with metabolic overstimulation of body function. The prevalence of hyperthyroidism in the older person is similar to that of the general population (about 2%) (Solomon, 2003). Hyperthyroidism in the older patient is often due to Graves' disease or toxic goiter, an autoimmune disorder associated with the production of immunoglobulins that attach to and stimulate the TSH receptor, leading to sustained thyroid overactivity (Cobin, Weisen, & Trotto, 1999). Older people are prone to the development of toxic nodular goiters, abnormal growths within the thyroid gland that can secrete excessive amounts of TSH. Additionally, hyperthyroidism may be medication induced as a result of taking amiodarone, a cardiac drug containing iodine that deposits in tissue and delivers iodine to the general circulation over long periods. Hyperthyroidism may also result from overtreatment with levothyroxine. Less common causes include pituitary tumors, pituitary resistance to thyroid hormones, and malignancies such as thyroid cancer (Cobin et al., 1999). Regardless of the cause, hyperthyroidism is the result of high levels of thyroid hormones, especially T_3 and to a lesser extent T_4 as the peripheral tissue will convert excess T4 to T3 (Solomon, 2003).

Signs and Symptoms of Hyperthyroidism

Hyperthyroidism in the older patient is even more difficult to assess than hypothyroidism because older patients exhibit fewer and different signs and symptoms than do younger adults. Only about 25% of hyperthyroid patients over the age of 65 exhibit classic symptoms (Solomon, 2003). The severity of signs and symptoms relates to duration of the illness, magnitude of the hormone excess, and age of the patient (American Association of Clinical Endocrinologists, 2002). Common clinical features of hyperthyroidism in the older person may include the following:

- Cardiac arrhythmias and tachycardia
- Tremor
- Weight loss and appetite changes
- Sleep disturbances
- Changes in vision, photophobia, diplopia, eye irritation
- Fatigue and muscle weakness

In the older patient, the most common presentation of hyperthyroidism is tachycardia, weight loss, fatigue, and weakness or apathy. Decreased appetite is common. Because of decreases in baseline heart rate with age, tachycardia should be interpreted as a resting heart rate greater than 90 beats per minute. Most often, the thyroid is not enlarged or easily palpated. Some of the classic symptoms of hyperthyroidism commonly exhibited in younger persons are rather uncommon in the older person, including feelings of nervousness and anxiety, hyperactive deep tendon reflexes, heat intolerance with excessive sweating, diarrhea or frequent bowel movements, and enlarged thyroid (Solomon, 2003).

Cardiac symptoms are experienced by 27% of older persons with hyperthyroidism. New-onset atrial fibrillation, heart failure, and angina are common presentations. Because cardiac disease is common in the older person, underlying hyperthyroidism may not be suspected. Gastrointestinal symptoms may be confused with malignancy or other bowel disease. Other commonly overlooked symptoms of hyperthyroidism in the older person include depression (called apathetic thyroidism), myopathy, and osteoporosis (Solomon, 2003).

Thyroid storm is a rare, life-threatening situation that can occur when a physical illness is superimposed on an older person with hyperthyroidism. Extreme tachycardia, fever, nausea, vomiting, heart failure, and changes in mental status or level of consciousness in a patient with hyperthyroidism should be immediately reported to the physician. Emergency treatment will be required. Treatment includes large doses of propylthiouracil and intravenous propranolol to slow the heartbeat to 90 to 110 beats per minute. Intravenous glucocorticoid and oral ipodate sodium are also given to decrease inflammation and lower serum T3 levels (Solomon, 2003).

Diagnosis of Hyperthyroidism

A comprehensive health history and physical assessment should be performed with emphasis on weight and blood pressure, pulse rate and rhythm, thyroid palpation, neuromuscular examination, eye examination, vision assessment, and cardiovascular assessment. The TSH is the best screening test for hyperthyroidism, and subnormal or undetectable values are considered to be diagnostic (Solomon, 2003). Serum T4, T3, and thyroglobulin levels are on average lower in older patients with hyperthyroidism than in younger patients, but are not considered diagnostic of the disease. Ultrasound and radioisotope scans are needed when nodules are detected by palpation. Fine-needle aspiration may be done to rule out malignancies. Thyroid cancer is rare over the age of 60 and should be suspected when masses are painless and rapidly growing, the gland is hard and fixed, lymph nodes are palpable, and hoarseness or vocal cord paralysis is present as indication of laryngeal nerve involvement.

Treatment and Nursing Management of Hyperthyroidism

The prognosis for hyperthyroidism is excellent with treatment, usually leading to euthyroid or hypothyroidism with supplementation of levothyroxine (Solomon, 2003). The treatment of choice for most older persons is ingestion of radioactive sodium iodide (^{131}I). It is easy to administer and avoids the option of surgery with all the complications related to anesthesia and hospitalization. No consensus exists on the appropriate dose of ^{131}I for hyperthyroidism. One option is to administer a low dose and monitor for return to euthyroid state; another option is to administer a single large dose intended to produce hypothyroidism and treat with levothyroxine to achieve normal thyroid function. The large dose option may provide the patient with more years of well-being because the relief of hyperthyroidism is faster and more reliable (Solomon, 2003).

Drugs other than ^{131}I may be used to treat hyperthyroidism under the following circumstances: (1) ^{131}I is refused by the patient; (2) to control symptoms before the administration of ^{131}I; or (3) to deplete the thyroid gland of stored hormone in order to prevent hyperthyroidism or "dumping" of hormone into the blood after treatment with ^{131}I (Solomon, 2003). These drugs are designed to block thyroid hormone production. The remission rates are variable, but relapses are frequent (American Association of Clinical Endocrinologists, 2002). Propylthiouracil (PTU) is given initially at 150 to 300 mg/day in divided doses every 8 hours. Based on signs and symptoms and serum hormone levels that are monitored every 2 months the dose of PTU may be decreased to 100–150 mgm/daily. Methimazole can be given as a single daily dose, usually starting at 15 to 40 mg/day. The dose is monitored and changed every 1 to 2 months as needed based on symptoms. Side effects of propylthiouracil and methimazole are dose related and include skin rash, nausea, hepatitis, and arthritis. The most serious side effect is granulocytopenia. Patients should be warned to stop taking the medications and to seek medical attention when a sore throat or generalized infection occurs (Cobin et al., 1999).

Propranolol and other beta-blockers can help to manage symptoms of hyperthyroidism, including atrial fibrillation. Although it protects the heart from the effects of excessive thyroid hormone, it can cause adverse effects such as hypotension, heart failure, and bronchospasm. It will conceal the symptoms of thyrotoxicosis, but does not affect thyroxine levels or readings on thyroid function tests.

When hyperthyroidism is due to subacute thyroiditis, Hashimoto's disease, or radiation damage, the only effective treatment is to administer beta-blockers and closely observe the patient's function and cardiac status for complications. Antithyroid drugs are ineffective because they do not decrease the uncontrolled output of hormone from the damaged thyroid follicles (Solomon, 2003).

Another therapeutic option for hyperthyroidism is surgery to remove a significant portion of the thyroid gland. This procedure is usually a last option for older patients and reserved for those with suspicious nodules, those allergic or intolerant of antithyroid drugs, and those with symptoms so severe that they cannot wait for ^{131}I to become effective (Cobin et al., 1999).

NURSING DIAGNOSES ASSOCIATED WITH ENDOCRINE PROBLEMS

Nursing diagnoses associated with older patients with endocrine problems are diverse and depend upon the older person's severity of illness and success of treatment. For older persons with type 2 DM and obesity, *imbalanced nutrition: more than body requirements* is appropriate. All older patients with DM should be diagnosed as at *risk for infection* and *risk for sensory/perceptual alterations: tactile*. As DM requires many lifestyle modifications and therapeutic interventions, effect of therapeutic regimen (family, community, and individual) should be assessed and ineffective patterns noted. Noncompliance to any aspect of diet, exercise, medication, or other self-care strategy should be assessed.

Patient-Family Teaching Guidelines

DIABETES MELLITUS

Education of the older patient and his or her family should focus on disease management principles, lifestyle modification, and promotion of health and safety. The goal is to assist patients to acquire and maintain the knowledge, skills, and behaviors to successfully manage their disease.

Without comprehension of the relationship between home blood glucose readings, meal planning, and physical activity, older patients with diabetes will be hindered in their ability to achieve optimal blood glucose control and are at higher risk for long-term complications.

1. I have diabetes. What can I do to stay healthy?

General goals of health maintenance for older persons with diabetes include:

- Achieving and maintaining near normal blood glucose levels by balancing food intake and medication with physical activity.
- Achieving optimal serum lipid levels.
- Providing adequate calories for attaining and maintaining reasonable weight.
- Preventing and treating the acute and long-term complications of diabetes (damage to the eyes, kidneys, nerves, and heart).
- Improving overall health through optimum nutrition.

RATIONALE:

Older people with DM are at increased risk for morbidity and mortality related to microvascular and macrovascular complications. Education regarding prevention of complications is crucial.

(continued)

2. I have just been diagnosed with diabetes. What are the most important things for me to know?

Important things to know include:

a. The relationship of food and meals to blood glucose levels, medication, and activity including action, side effects, timing, and interactions of all medications.

- Recognition, causes, treatment, and prevention of hypo- and hyperglycemia.
- Benefits of control.
- Importance of lifestyle modification.
- Use of glucagon if appropriate.
- Use of blood glucose meter and establishment of blood glucose target with guidelines for reporting high or low levels.
- Disposal of lancets and other contaminated materials.

b. Basic food and meal plan guidelines—referral to the dietitian if necessary.

c. Consistent times each day for meals and snacks.

d. Recognition, prevention, and treatment of hypoglycemia.

e. Sick day management.

f. Self-monitoring of blood glucose.

g. Complication prevention and recognition.

- Self foot care and podiatry consultation.
- Need for yearly eye examination.
- Impact of lipids and need for yearly lipid evaluation.
- Need for blood pressure control and establishment of regular monitoring schedule.
- Identification of symptoms; treatment and methods for preventing kidney disease, peripheral vascular disease, cardiovascular disease, periodontal disease, and peripheral neuropathy.
- Need for pneumococcal vaccine and annual flu immunization.

RATIONALE:

Older patients and their families can become overwhelmed when they realize that managing this disease will affect every aspect of their lives and daily activities. Making a list and providing one or two key points of information on each of the items to the left will assist patients and their families in the management of diabetes and prevention of diabetic complications.

3. What are some things I will need to know over time?

As you and your family become more familiar with the management of DM and blood glucose levels, additional content beyond basic meal planning is needed. As you make changes in your weight, exercise regimen, medications, and functional status, we will schedule follow-up sessions and focus on increasing your knowledge, skills, and flexibility to improve the quality of your life. Additional content may include:

- Sources of essential nutrients and their effect on blood glucose and lipid levels.
- Label reading and grocery shopping guidelines.
- Dining out and restaurant guidelines.
- Modifying fat intake.
- Use of sugar-containing foods, and dietetic foods and sweeteners.
- Alcohol guidelines.
- When to modify blood glucose testing schedules for glucose patterning and increased control.
- Adjusting mealtimes.
- Adjusting food for exercise.

RATIONALE:

As older patients become more sophisticated in the management of diabetes, they will be ready to adapt the basic principles to accommodate a more flexible lifestyle. This information will be helpful for the patient who has mastered the basics.

- Special occasions and holidays.
- Travel and schedule changes.
- Vitamin and mineral supplementation.

Older patients with thyroid problems may be noted to have *sleep deprivation, fatigue, risk for activity intolerance, ineffective thermoregulation,* and *risk for imbalanced body temperature.* Because of the many signs and symptoms manifested by the older person with endocrine problems, the gerontological nurse should focus on principles of disease management, health promotion, safety, and patient and family coping.

Patient-Family Teaching Guidelines

THYROID CONDITIONS

Education of the older patient and his or her family should focus on disease management principles, lifestyle modification, and promotion of health and safety. The goal is to assist patients to acquire and maintain the knowledge, skills, and behaviors to successfully manage their disease.

1. I have just been diagnosed with a thyroid problem. What should I know about my thyroid?

People live long and healthy lives with thyroid problems. The essential knowledge for you to understand about your thyroid disorder includes:

- Understanding the relationship between the thyroid hormones and the body's metabolic rate.
- Correctly identifying the body's reaction to excess or deficient thyroid hormone levels (signs and symptoms of hypo- or hypermetabolic state).
- Preventing or delaying complications resulting from hypo- or hyperthyroidism.
- Participating in the plan of care and improving your disease management skills.

RATIONALE:

Older people with thyroid problems are at risk for the development of fatigue or anxiety, sleep disorders, changes in their weight, and other vague symptoms that may be falsely attributed to normal changes of aging. Education regarding prevention of complications is crucial.

2. What are some things I need to know right away?

Some basic information that you need to begin to manage your thyroid problem includes:

- The importance of taking thyroid medication daily and avoiding other drugs that are known to interact with thyroid medications.
- Awareness of the signs and symptoms of thyroid disease such as appetite changes, fatigue, cardiovascular symptoms, change in bowel movement, weight changes, and mood changes.
- Need for careful ongoing monitoring of TSH by the healthcare provider and importance of keeping appointments.
- Need to tell all healthcare providers about the diagnosis and treatment of hypo- or hyperthyroidism.
- Importance of not changing brand of levothyroxine without careful monitoring of thyroid function.

RATIONALE:

As with diabetes, the older patient may be overwhelmed at the amount of information needed to manage this newly diagnosed disease. Making a list of important items and listing one or two key points under each item may ease the patient's and family's anxiety. Make sure the patient knows that you are available to answer any questions that arise in the future.

Care Plan

A Patient With Chest Pain R/T Hypothyroid

Case Study

Mrs. Jones is an 82-year-old woman who presents in the emergency department with complaints of fatigue, palpitations, and intermittent chest pain. She is highly functional and lives alone with support of her daughter who lives close by and visits regularly. She denies nausea or vomiting. Physical examination reveals her lungs are clear, her blood pressure is 150/96, and pulse is 96 and irregular. Mrs. Jones's skin is clammy and she has trouble lying still for the electrocardiogram because she feels the need to move about. Her pulse oximetry is 99% on room air. Laboratory values reveal a TSH of 0.1 and a T4 of 19. The electrocardiogram reveals atrial fibrillation. Mrs. Jones has a regular care provider but has not seen her physician for about 6 months. She states she has never had any problems with her heart before.

Applying the Nursing Process

ASSESSMENT

Mrs. Jones is in need of emergency evaluation and stabilization of her cardiac status. New-onset atrial fibrillation, elevated pulse rate and blood pressure, and abnormal laboratory values need immediate attention. Intermittent chest pain and atrial fibrillation could indicate a myocardial infarction in progress.

DIAGNOSIS

Appropriate nursing diagnoses for Mrs. Jones may include the following:

- *Ineffective tissue perfusion and decreased cardiac output* based upon her rapid heart rate and new-onset atrial fibrillation
- *Fatigue and activity intolerance* based upon her cardiac status
- *Fear and anxiety* related to her altered metabolic and cardiac status
- *Pain, acute*

EXPECTED OUTCOMES

The expected outcomes for Mrs. Jones may include the following:

- Mrs. Jones's vital signs and cardiac rhythm will gradually return to normal.
- She will report no further chest pain.

A Patient With Chest Pain R/T Hypothyroid

- She will report decreased levels of anxiety.
- She will begin to establish a therapeutic relationship with the nurse.

PLANNING AND IMPLEMENTATION

The main issue is to decrease Mrs. Jones's heart rate and stabilize her cardiac status. An intravenous line should be established and a cardiologist consulted. Laboratory values reveal the patient is in a metabolic hyperthyroid state because her TSH is low. Her increased metabolic drive has triggered increases in systolic blood pressure, increased heart rate, and myocardial irritability. She is at risk for embolic stroke because of her atrial fibrillation. Her cardiac situation should improve spontaneously once the atrial refractory period is lengthened. The cardiologist may use a beta-blocker to slow the heart rate.

Mrs. Jones will need reassurance and a calm approach. She may wish her daughter to be called in for additional support. Instructions should be delivered in a reassuring manner with appropriate use of calming touch.

EVALUATION

The nurse hopes to work with the emergency department team to stabilize Mrs. Jones's medical condition and rule out myocardial infarction. Once stabilized, Mrs. Jones can be admitted to the hospital. The nurse will consider the plan a success based on the following criteria:

- Mrs. Jones will demonstrate knowledge of her condition and medications.
- Mrs. Jones and her family will identify safe living arrangements and a plan for rehabilitation if needed after hospital discharge.
- She will institute advance directives by establishing a living will or naming a healthcare proxy.
- A family meeting will be held to discuss Mrs. Jones's overall health.

Ethical Dilemma

Change the previous scenario slightly to reflect that Mrs. Jones has been taking levothyroxine for many years because she was diagnosed with hypothyroidism years ago. Lately, she reports she has been having trouble remembering things and often takes her medicine three or four times a day because "if one pill is good, then three or four are probably better." When informed of this, Mrs. Jones's daughter replies in anger, "OK. That's it. You're going to a nursing home. I'd rather have you safe than dead." Mrs. Jones is devastated and begins to cry uncontrollably.

Mrs. Jones's autonomy is in conflict with her daughter's beneficence or need to do good for her mother. The nurse should try to defuse the emotionally charged situation by urging both Mrs. Jones and her daughter not to say anything in anger or make any immediate decisions. With team involvement and appropriate safeguards, there may be a way to offer Mrs. Jones more support with her medication management and home safety while satisfying her daughter's concerns regarding her mother's safety. A social worker referral and early discharge planning with identification of additional resources is needed.

(continued)

A Patient With Chest Pain R/T Hypothyroid *(continued)*

Critical Thinking and the Nursing Process

1. What strategies can a gerontological nurse use to educate older people about the need for lifestyle modification when they are unaware that they are at risk for development of type 2 DM?

2. Examine your own nutrition and exercise habits. Do you have risk factors for development of type 2 DM? Are you setting a good example for your patients?

3. How can you increase your colleagues' level of suspicion regarding symptoms relating to hypo- and hyperthyroidism when the signs and symptoms are vague and atypical in the older person?

4. Imagine that you have been diagnosed with type 1 DM and have to be reliant on insulin injections for the rest of your life. What thoughts go through your head? What fears do you have? What kinds of support would make you feel better?

5. Discuss with a colleague the importance of genetics and lifestyle in the development of type 2 DM. Try to reach some agreement on which of these factors is most crucial to the development of type 2 DM in the older person.

■ Evaluate your responses in Appendix B. ⬭

EXPLORE MediaLink

NCLEX review, case studies, and other interactive resources for this chapter can be found on the Companion Website at **http://www.prenhall.com/tabloski**. Click on Chapter 19 to select the activities for this chapter. For animations, video tutorials, more NCLEX review questions, and case studies, access the accompanying CD-ROM in this textbook.

Chapter Highlights

■ The endocrine glands control the body's metabolic processes. The endocrine and metabolic control systems offer many of the greatest opportunities for preventing the disabilities associated with aging.

■ Two major endocrine problems of importance to gerontological nursing are diabetes mellitus and thyroid disease.

■ Thyroid disease is common, often undiagnosed, and easily treated in people of all ages. Early detection prevents unnecessary disability and loss of function.

■ Diabetes mellitus is common, and normalization of blood glucose levels may minimize the devastating vascular and neurologic complications that often occur.

■ Knowledge of endocrine function and metabolism is crucial for gerontological nurses to interpret signs and symptoms of illness and advise older persons on health promotion activities.

- Type 1 DM develops due to B-cell destruction and results in a lack or underproduction of insulin in the body. Patients with type 1 DM are insulin dependent and at risk for ketoacidosis.

- Type 2 DM, the most prevalent form of diabetes in all age groups, results from a combination of insulin resistance and an insulin secretory defect.

- The prevalence of thyroid disease rises with age. Hypothyroidism is much higher in women than in men of all ages, and is higher in older persons living in institutions than in community-residing elderly adults.

- Symptoms of hyperthyroidism and hypothyroidism are vague and can be debilitating, affecting many body systems. Detection and treatment of thyroid problems can improve quality and length of life.

References

American Association of Clinical Endocrinologists. (2002). AACE clinical practice guidelines for the evaluation and treatment of hyperthyroidism and hypothyroidism. *Thyroid Guidelines Task Force, 1–23.*

American Diabetes Association. (2001). Clinical practice recommendations. *Diabetes Care, 24* (S1–S1320).

Barzilai, N. (2003). Disorders of carbohydrate metabolism. In M. Beers & R. Berkow (Eds.), *Merck manual of geriatrics.* Internet Edition Merck & Co. Retrieved February 14, 2003, from http://www.merck.com/pubs/mm.

Berenbeim, D., Parrott, M., Purnell, J., & Pennachio, D. (2001). How to manage diabetes in the older patient. *Patient Care/*January 30. Retrieved August 9, 2002, from www.patientcareonline.com.

Blair, E. (1999). Diabetes in the older adult. *Advance for Nurse Practitioners, 7*(7), 33–36.

Burman, K. (2000). *Clinical management of hypothyroidism.* Retrieved September 14, 2001, from www.medscape.com.

California Healthcare Foundation/American Geriatrics Society Panel on Improving Care for Elders with Diabetes. (2003). *Journal of the American Geriatrics Society, 51*(5), S5265–5280.

Caughron, K., & Smith, E. (2002). Definition and description of diabetes mellitus. Selected guidelines. *Southern Medical Journal, 95*(1), 35–49.

Centers for Disease Control. (1999). *Special focus: Healthy aging.* Retrieved August 19, 2000, from www.cdc.gov/nccdphp.

Centers for Disease Control. (2004). *Diabetes public health resource: Statistics.* Retrieved November 11, 2004, from http://www.cdc.gov/diabetes/statistics/prev/national.

Cobin, R., Weisen, M., & Trotto, N. (1999). Hypothyroidism, hyperthyroidism, hyperparathyroidism. *Patient Care, 9,* 185–206.

Coyle, C. (2003). Current management of diabetes mellitus in adults. *Advance for Nurse Practitioners, 11*(5), 33–38.

Diabetes Guidelines Work Group. (1999). *Massachusetts guidelines for adult diabetes care.* Boston: Massachusetts Department of Public Health, Massachusetts Health Promotion Clearinghouse.

Epocrates.com. (2004). Drug and formulary reference. Retrieved October 14, 2004, from www.epocrates.com.

Halpin-Landry, J., & Goldsmith, S. (1999). Feet first. Diabetes care. *American Journal of Nursing, 99*(2), 26–34.

Kuritzky, L. (2001). Hypothyroidism. *American Journal for Nurse Practitioners,* May, 26–41.

Ladenson, P., Singer, P., Ain, & K., Bagchi, N., Bigos, S., Levy, E., Smith, S., & Daniels, G. (2000). American Thyroid Association guidelines for detection of thyroid dysfunction. *Archives of Internal Medicine, 160,* 1573–1575.

McCance, K., & Huether, S. (2001). *Pathophysiology: The biologic basis for disease in adults and children.* St. Louis, MO: Mosby.

Mooradian, A., McLaughin, S., Boyer, C., & Winter, J. (1999). Diabetes care for older adults. *Diabetes Spectrum, 12*(2), 70–77.

National Academy on an Aging Society. (2000). *Diabetes, A drain on US resources,* 6. Retrieved May 13, 2001, from www.agingsociety.org.

National Diabetes Education Program. (2003). *Four steps to control your diabetes for life.* Retrieved August 16, 2004, from www. ndep.nih.gov/diabetes/control/4steps.htm.

National Institute of Diabetes and Digestive and Kidney Diseases (NIDDK). National Diabetes Information Clearinghouse. (2004). *Diabetes overview.* Retrieved August 16, 2004, from www.diabetes.NIDDK.NIH.gov.

Sidani, M. (2001). Thyroid disorders in the elderly. *Female Patient, 26,* 27–32.

Solomon, D. (2003). Metabolic and thyroid disorders. In M. Beers & R. Berkow (Eds.), *Merck manual of geriatrics.* Rahway, NJ: Merck.

Supit, E., & Peiris, A. (2002). Interpretation of laboratory thyroid function tests for the primary care physician. *Southern Medical Journal, 95*(5), 481–485.

CHAPTER 20

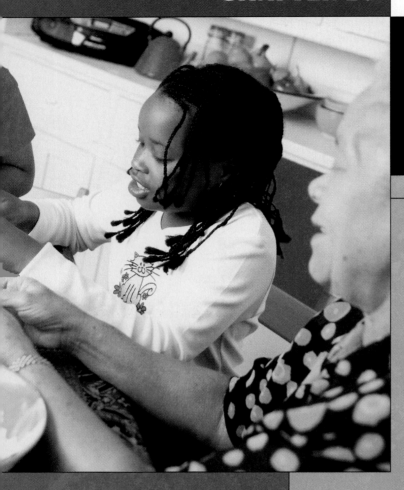

The Gastrointestinal System

CHAPTER OBJECTIVES

Upon completion of this chapter, the reader will be able to:

- Describe age-related changes that affect gastrointestinal function.

- Describe the impact of age-related changes of gastrointestinal function.

- Identify risk factors to health for the older person with gastrointestinal problems.

- Describe unique presentation of gastrointestinal problems in the older person.

- Define appropriate nursing interventions directed toward assisting the older adult with gastrointestinal problems to develop self-care abilities.

- Identify and implement appropriate nursing interventions to care for the older person with gastrointestinal problems.

MediaLink

Additional resources for this chapter can be found on the Student CD-ROM accompanying this textbook and on the Companion Website at **www.prenhall.com/tabloski**. Click on Chapter 20 to select the activities for this chapter.

CD-ROM
- Animations
    Cirrhosis
    *Gastroesophageal Reflux
       Disease*
    Gastrointestinal A&P
- NCLEX Review

- Case Studies
- Tools

COMPANION WEBSITE
- Audio Glossary
- Additional NCLEX Review
- Case Study
- MediaLink Applications

KEY TERMS

achalasia 649
Clostridium difficile 665
Crohn's disease 665
diverticula 662
diverticulitis 664
diverticulosis 662
dyspepsia 660
dysphagia 646
endoscopy 655
fissures 669
gastric volvulus 662
gastritis 656
gastroesophageal reflux
   disease 649
hemorrhoids 669

The gastrointestinal (GI) tract is responsible for four major functions relating to food ingestion: digestion, absorption, secretion, and motility. The GI tract begins at the mouth and ends at the rectum and includes the accessory organs of digestion, the liver, gallbladder, and pancreas. Throughout life, the GI tract is constantly remodeling with the endothelial lining shedding and regenerating every 24 to 48 hours. Ingested food, partially degraded by chewing in the mouth, enters the stomach where it is churned and mixed with acid, mucus, enzymes, and other secretions, beginning the process of digestion. After the food passes from the stomach to the small intestine, the liver and pancreas secrete enzymes to further break it down into protein, fat, and carbohydrates for easy absorption and metabolic use. These substances pass through the walls of the small intestine into the blood vessels and lymphatic system where they are transported to the liver for processing and storage. The peristaltic movements of the intestine are regulated by hormones and by the autonomic nervous system. The autonomic innervation is controlled by centers in the brain and local stimuli mediated by networks of nerve fibers within the walls of the GI tract (McCance & Huether, 2001).

Unabsorbed food continues into the large intestine, and fluid is absorbed and transported to the kidneys for elimination as urine. Under normal circumstances, the colon absorbs approximately 1 to 2 L of water per day. Solid waste and fiber are transported to the rectum and held for elimination. When the rectum is distended with stool, a signal is sent to relax the anal sphincter and triggers the urge to defecate. Normal bowel continence is dependent upon the individual's ability to recognize rectal distention and to delay defecation. Figure 20-1 ■ illustrates the normal configuration of the GI tract.

Normal Changes of Aging

Figure 20-2 ■ illustrates the normal changes of aging related to the gastrointestinal tract. Biological changes in GI function that occur in older persons result from the physical, mental, and psychological changes of aging and other factors associated with aging, such as immobility, impaired fluid balance, neuromuscular disorders, endocrine and metabolic problems, and the effects of medications. Age-related changes in the gastrointestinal system begin before age 50 and continue gradually throughout life (McCance & Huether, 2001). These changes include:

- Changes in the mouth, including loss of teeth, periodontal disease, decline in sense of taste and smell, and decreases in salivary secretion.
- Decreased esophageal motility.
- Diminished gastric motility with increased stomach-emptying time.
- Diminished capacity of the gastric mucosa to resist damage from factors such as nonsteroidal anti-inflammatory drugs (NSAIDs) and *Helicobacter pylori*.
- Achlorhydria or insufficient hydrochloric acid in the stomach.
- Decreased production of intrinsic factor leading to pernicious anemia.
- Decreased intestinal absorption, motility, and blood flow.
- Decreased pancreas size with duct hyperplasia and lobular fibrosis.

FIGURE ▇ 20-1

Normal configuration of the GI tract.

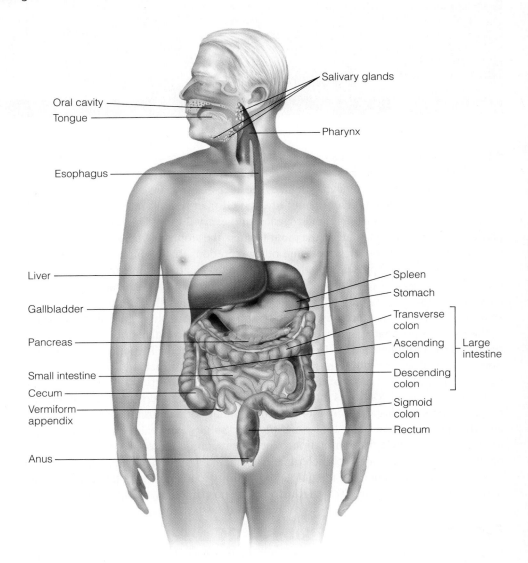

- Salivary glands
- Oral cavity
- Tongue
- Pharynx
- Esophagus
- Liver
- Spleen
- Stomach
- Gallbladder
- Transverse colon
- Pancreas
- Ascending colon
- Large intestine
- Small intestine
- Descending colon
- Cecum
- Vermiform appendix
- Sigmoid colon
- Rectum
- Anus

- Increased incidence of cholelithiasis (gallstones) and decreased production of bile acid synthesis.
- Decreased liver size and blood flow.
- Decreased thirst and hunger drive due to cognitive changes or psychological conditions such as depression.
- Increased medication use and possible adverse drug reactions.

(Horowitz, 2004; McCance & Huether, 2001)

Medications with great potential to affect the GI tract include the anticholinergics (antidepressants, neuroleptics, antihistamines, antiparkinsonian agents), antihypertensives (calcium channel blockers, ACE inhibitors, diuretics), iron and calcium supplements, aluminum-containing antacids, opiates, and laxatives (Camilleri, Lee, Viramontes, Bharucha, & Tangalos, 2000). See Chapter 6 for further information relating to medication use and the GI tract. ▭

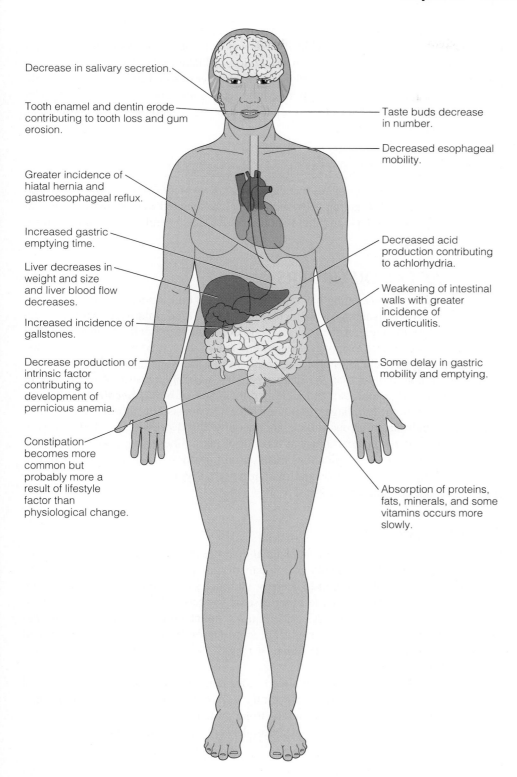

FIGURE 20-2

Normal changes of aging related to the gastrointestinal tract.

Decrease in salivary secretion.

Tooth enamel and dentin erode contributing to tooth loss and gum erosion.

Greater incidence of hiatal hernia and gastroesophageal reflux.

Increased gastric emptying time.

Liver decreases in weight and size and liver blood flow decreases.

Increased incidence of gallstones.

Decrease production of intrinsic factor contributing to development of pernicious anemia.

Constipation becomes more common but probably more a result of lifestyle factor than physiological change.

Taste buds decrease in number.

Decreased esophageal mobility.

Decreased acid production contributing to achlorhydria.

Weakening of intestinal walls with greater incidence of diverticulitis.

Some delay in gastric mobility and emptying.

Absorption of proteins, fats, minerals, and some vitamins occurs more slowly.

Older patients with diseases of the GI tract and visceral organs are much more likely than younger adults to present atypically. For instance, older patients with peptic ulcer disease exhibit impaired visceral pain perception and take longer to recognize and report pain. This often leads to delayed diagnosis, longer hospital stay, and higher probability of mortality due to perforation (Moore & Clinch, 2004). Additionally, older people will also exhibit changes in GI function as the result of other illnesses (diabetes, neurologic illness, vascular disorders).

Common Disorders in Aging

Because of the large functional reserve capacity of most of the GI tract, aging alone has very little impact on GI function. However, aging is associated with an increased prevalence of many GI disorders, and these should be evaluated carefully and not be attributed to normal aging.

ESOPHAGEAL DISORDERS

In healthy older persons, aging has only minor effects on esophageal motor and sensory function. Upper esophageal sphincter pressure and the amplitude of peristalsis decrease slightly with age, but these changes do not significantly affect function. Older patients with significant esophageal disorders usually have underlying systemic diseases, including vascular or neurologic problems. Gastroesophageal reflux appears to be more common in older than in younger persons, possibly because of weakening of the lower esophageal sphincter and increased incidence of **hiatal hernia**. Many drugs can cause injury to the esophagus, including NSAIDs, potassium chloride, tetracycline, quinidine, alendronate, ferrous sulfate, and theophylline (Horowitz, 2004). Older people are at risk for esophageal injury as a result of taking these drugs. They should be advised to swallow these medications in an upright position, drink at least 8 oz of water when taking any medication, and remain in an upright position for 30 minutes to prevent reflux into the esophagus.

DYSPHAGIA

Dysphagia is the most common esophageal disorder in older people (Borum, 2004). Dysphagia is defined as difficulty in any part of the process involved with swallowing solid foods or liquids. Whether acute or chronic, the condition affects oral intake and is usually indicative of some other disease process. The act of swallowing involves approximately 50 muscles and requires intact oropharyngeal anatomy and unimpaired nerve conduction, permitting coordination between the respiratory and digestive systems. From start to finish, a single swallow takes about 20 seconds (Dahlin, 2004).

An estimated 50% of institutionalized older persons have identifiable signs and symptoms of dysphagia. This is especially common in patients with neurologic problems. One third of conscious acute stroke patients admitted to the hospital had signs and symptoms of dysphagia (Davies, 1999). The normal swallow consists of three stages:

1. **Oral stage.** Food is prepared for transfer from the mouth to the oropharynx. Patients need to be able to chew, have the desire to eat, and be able to see or smell the food. The food is mixed with saliva and forms a bolus for swallowing. When

the bolus is pushed to the back of the mouth, the soft palate is raised, and coordinated muscular movements occur in the pharynx and larynx to move the bolus downward.

2. **Pharyngeal stage.** The bolus is propelled into the esophagus, and the larynx moves upward under the base of the tongue to prevent food from entering. The epiglottis lowers to protect the airway. This phase takes about a second in the normal swallow.

3. **Esophageal stage.** The bolus is propelled toward the stomach by peristalsis. This phase can take 8 to 20 seconds depending on the consistency of the food, the strength of the peristaltic movements, and the patient's position and anatomy.

Figure 20-3 ■ illustrates the anatomy of the oral cavity and the esophagus.

Any of the phases of normal swallowing may be disrupted in patients with dysphagia. For instance, a patient may have poor tongue control and thus experience delay in initiating the swallow reflex. The bolus of food may be poorly prepared for swallowing, and the food may collect in the pharynx and spill over into the trachea. Poor dentition may contribute to chewing problems. Psychotropic drugs may cause excessive lethargy or oversedation. Lack of saliva may make food excessively dry and difficult to swallow. Most often, older patients will experience more than one probable cause for dysphagia (Dahlin, 2004; Davies, 1999).

Patients at Risk for Dysphagia
Signs and symptoms observable in older patients at risk for dysphagia include the following:

- Reports from the older person or his or her family that swallowing food or medications is difficult
- Difficulty in controlling food or saliva in the mouth (drooling, dribbling)
- Facial droop, open mouth
- Dementia, frailty, confusion, extreme lethargy, decreased level of consciousness
- Inability to sit in an upright position and maintain trunk position for a reasonable length of time

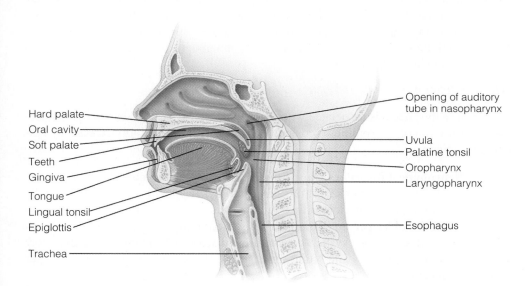

FIGURE ■ **20-3**

Anatomy of the oral cavity and the esophagus.

Hard palate
Oral cavity
Soft palate
Teeth
Gingiva
Tongue
Lingual tonsil
Epiglottis
Trachea

Opening of auditory tube in nasopharynx
Uvula
Palatine tonsil
Oropharynx
Laryngopharynx
Esophagus

- Choking or coughing while eating or drinking
- Increased nasal or oral congestion or secretion after a meal
- Weak voice, cough, and tongue movements
- Slurred speech
- Change in voice during meal (wet, gurgling, or hoarse voice)
- Recurrent upper respiratory infections or pneumonia
- Retention or pocketing of food in mouth
- Oral thrush
- Refusal to open mouth or accept a large bite of food
- Unexplained weight loss

(Dahlin, 2004; Kayser-Jones & Pengilly, 1999)

Early detection of dysphagia is vital because its complications can be life threatening. Aspiration of food or fluid into the respiratory tract can cause choking, airway obstruction, hypoxia, and aspiration pneumonia. Risk factors associated with nursing home residents and dysphagia include the following:

- **Residents not positioned properly.** Eating while in an upright position (90-degree angle) helps prevent choking and aspiration. Residents who are confined to bed should not be fed in the semireclined position.
- **Residents fed inappropriate food and liquid.** Thin food and liquids such as tea, juice, water, and clear broth are difficult for older people with dysphagia to swallow. Thin liquids quickly drain into the esophagus before the swallow reflex is triggered. Thickened liquids slow the swallow process, give the older person time to prepare for the swallow, and help prevent aspiration and dehydration.
- **Residents fed quickly with large bites of food.** Residents with dysphagia must be fed slowly and given small bites of food to minimize the risk of choking and aspiration. Some residents are labeled as "combative" or "resistive" to the person feeding them and are noted to turn their heads and constantly push away the spoon. These residents may be protecting themselves from choking because they need extra time to swallow the food remaining in their mouths.
- **Residents labeled as "difficult" or "uncooperative."** Busy and overburdened staff may feel the slow and difficult pace of eating is purposeful behavior and the resident is attempting to cause them to be frustrated. The older person may be at risk for use of additional medications (psychotropic, antianxiety, or sedatives). Weight loss may be the inevitable result.

(Kayser-Jones & Pengilly, 1999)

Because dysphagia is associated with underlying illness or disorders, the older person with multiple comorbidities is considered to be at risk for aspiration. Causes of dysphagia include:

1. **Neurological disorders.** Any disease that affects neuromuscular function, including movement or sensation, may cause dysphagia. Stroke, especially in the midbrain or the anterior cortical areas, is the most common cause of dysphagia in the older person. Parkinson's disease, multiple sclerosis, brain tumors, and central nervous system degenerative diseases (Alzheimer's disease) may cause dysphagia by inhibiting movements of the tongue, pharynx, or upper esophagus.

2. **Muscular disorders.** Disorders such as muscular dystrophy, myasthenia gravis, and extreme frailty at the end of life may cause dysphagia by inhibiting muscular function.

3. **Anatomical abnormalities.** Abnormalities such as tumors, esophageal scarring, outpouchings of the esophageal wall, and premature closure of the upper esophageal sphincter may restrict the passage of the food bolus and trap the bolus in the esophagus. In a condition known as **achalasia**, a neurogenic esophageal disorder of unknown cause, esophageal peristalsis is impaired and the lower esophageal sphincter fails to relax, trapping food in the esophagus. **Zenker's diverticulum** is an outpouching of the posterior pharyngeal wall immediately above the upper esophageal sphincter. Esophageal **strictures** or localized narrowing of the esophagus can develop in persons with long-standing **gastroesophageal reflux disease** due to acid reflux into the unprotected esophagus causing erosion and scarring. Strictures can also result from swallowing caustic agents (bleach, lye) and certain drugs such as doxycycline, tetracycline, clindamycin, NSAIDs, and alendronate (McCance & Huether, 2001).

Drug Alert

Older patients should be advised to swallow their medication with a full 8 oz of water and remain upright for 30 minutes to decrease the risk of reflux and formation of esophageal erosion, stricture, and scarring.

Nursing Assessment of Dysphagia

Often, the gerontological nurse is aware that the patient has a swallowing disorder based on the signs and symptoms previously presented. In other cases, the nurse must carefully observe the older patient at rest and during the process of eating and drinking. Speech and occupational therapists can assist the nurse and provide valuable professional opinions during the assessment process. The following questions should be included in a dysphagia assessment:

- Have you ever choked while eating or drinking? If so, how recently? Does choking occur frequently?
- Does your mouth feel dry? Do you have enough saliva to chew your food easily?
- Do you have problems with drooling or controlling saliva?
- Does food ever fall out or get stuck in your mouth?
- Do you ever spit up food after a meal?
- Do you feel the need to clear your throat frequently?
- Do you have problems sitting upright during mealtime?

If the answer to any of these questions is positive, the gerontological nurse should notify the primary care provider and request a formal swallowing evaluation by the speech pathologist. A bedside evaluation may be carried out with the older person drinking a variety of liquids (thin to thickened) and observed for swallowing functionality. In some cases, videofluoroscopic radiographic evaluation of the swallowing process is conducted. The patient drinks a chalklike radiopaque solution, and the movement of the oropharyngeal structures is evaluated. A report is issued that notes any anatomical abnormalities, abnormal movements, or esophageal scarring or strictures.

This information helps the interdisciplinary team determine how best to meet the older person's nutrition needs and prevent aspiration.

> ### Practice Pearl
>
> The chalk mixture is constipating, and the nurse should carefully monitor bowel function after the procedure to prevent fecal impaction.

Residents at risk for aspiration should have a notation made on the nursing care plan to inform all involved with the patient's care regarding this risk and appropriate interventions to facilitate safe eating and drinking. Nurses and others caring for the patient should follow these guidelines:

- Try to minimize distractions during eating. Provide a pleasant and calm environment during mealtime.
- Try to use consistent feeding techniques with notations as to the older person's likes, dislikes, eating and drinking habits, and consumption patterns.
- Make sure the older patient is properly positioned and supported during mealtime.
- Try to maintain the upright position for at least 1 hour after eating.
- Ensure the patient has swallowed one bite before giving another. Do not try to rush. The patient may become resistive.
- Monitor the patient's respirations. A change in breathing pattern or rate can signal the onset of aspiration.
- Provide oral hygiene before and after the meal. A clean, fresh, odor-free mouth will stimulate the patient's appetite. Ensure dentures are in place and in good repair.
- Plan meals at times when the patient is rested. Present meals to persons with dementia according to routine.
- Offer food and liquid consistencies according to the speech pathologist's and dietitian's recommendations. Do not overly thicken liquids. The older person will resist "chewing" juice or liquids (rightly so).
- Keep conversation to a minimum and focus attention on the task at hand. For instance, "Now here's a bite of vegetables. Chew them slowly and let me know when you are ready to swallow." Assess mental status to ensure the patient can understand instructions and follow commands.
- Instruct all persons who assist the patient with feeding in the appropriate techniques. Nurses' assistants should feed no more than two or three patients at mealtime and they should sit comfortably at the same level as the patient.
- Never engage in forceful feeding techniques. Everyone has times when they are not hungry and do not feel like eating. Forcing an older patient to eat may set the stage for a power struggle at the next meal.

(Geronurse online, 2004; Kayser-Jones & Pengilly, 1999)

Ongoing monitoring of weight, functional status, and patient satisfaction during mealtime should be carefully recorded in the patient's record. Periodic swallowing evaluation is recommended every 6 months, after a significant change in the patient's condition, or with the onset or return of signs and symptoms of dysphagia. If the patient is unable to tolerate oral feeding, the alternatives may include administration of total parenteral nutrition or placement of a gastric tube for administration of liquid nourishment. Total parenteral nutrition is discussed in detail in Chapter 5. ⊂▭▭ Nasogastric tubes (tubes placed through the nose and down the throat into the stomach) should be avoided because they increase the risk of aspiration, interfere with swallow recovery, and may be uncomfortable for the patient. The head of the bed should be elevated at least 30 degrees during continuous feeding of liquid nourishment through a gastric tube and for 1 hour after intermittent feeding to prevent regurgitation and aspiration (Dahlin, 2004).

Nursing Diagnoses Related to Dysphagia

Nursing diagnoses related to dysphagia include the following:

- *Impaired swallowing*
- *Feeding self-care deficit*
- *Risk for fluid volume imbalance (deficient fluid volume)*
- *Ineffective airway clearance*
- *Risk for aspiration*
- *Altered dentition (if appropriate)*

Related factors identified by the North American Nursing Diagnosis Association (2003) include the following:

- *Neuromuscular impairment*
- *Decreased strength or excursion of muscles involved in mastication*
- *Perceptual impairment*
- *Mechanical obstruction (edema, tracheostomy tube, tumor)*
- *Fatigue*
- *Limited awareness*
- *Reddened, irritated oropharyngeal cavity*

Nursing Outcomes Related to Caring for Older Patients With Dysphagia

Nursing sensitive outcomes that would indicate an appropriate nursing intervention include no new aspiration events; adequate food and fluid intake to maintain weight and body functions; maintenance of good skin turgor; normal or improving hemoglobin, hematocrit, and serum albumin levels; patient and family satisfaction with oral intake and meals; maintenance of good oral hygiene; and patient's report or observation that the patient possesses appropriate levels of energy. See the Best Practices feature on pages 652 and 653 for aspiration prevention guidelines.

GASTROESOPHAGEAL REFLUX DISEASE

Gastroesophageal reflux disease (GERD) involves reflux of gastric contents into the esophagus. Many people occasionally experience heartburn, but for some, it is a frequent and continual problem. In the United States, symptoms of GERD occur daily in about 7% of adults and monthly in 44% of adults. GERD occurs more frequently in men than in women. The incidence in older people is thought to be about the same as the incidence in the general population (Borum, 2004). Older adults are more at risk for GERD complications because of prolonged esophageal acid exposure over a period of years. Additionally, the higher frequency of hiatal hernia, decreased saliva volume, and use of drugs that reduce lower esophageal sphincter tone may contribute to the development and progression of GERD in older adults (Ray, Secrest, Ch'ien, & Corey, 2002).

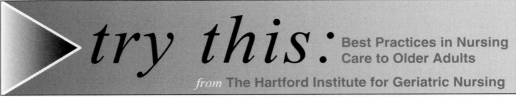

try this : Best Practices in Nursing Care to Older Adults

from The Hartford Institute for Geriatric Nursing

Issue Number 20, Fall 2004

Series Editor: Marie Boltz, APRN, MSN, GNP

Preventing Aspiration in Older Adults with Dysphagia

By: *Norma A. Metheny, RN, PhD, FAAN*

WHY: Aspiration (the misdirection of oropharyngeal secretions or gastric contents into the larynx and lower respiratory tract) is common in older adults with dysphagia and can lead to aspiration pneumonia, a leading cause of death in this population (Langmore et al, 1998).

TARGET POPULATION: Dysphagia is common in persons with neurologic diseases such as stroke, Parkinson's disease, and dementia. The older adult with one of these conditions is at even greater risk for aspiration because the dysphagia is superimposed on the slowed swallowing rate associated with normal aging (Marik & Kaplan, 2003). Conditions that suppress the cough reflex (such as sedation) further increase the risk for aspiration.

BEST PRACTICES: ASSESSMENT AND PREVENTION

ASSESSMENT

Aspiration:

Although aspiration during swallowing is best detected by procedures such as video-fluoroscopy or fiberoptic endoscopy, clinical observations are also important. Symptoms to look for include:

- Sudden appearance of respiratory symptoms (such as severe coughing and cyanosis) associated with eating, drinking, or regurgitation of gastric contents.
- A voice change (such as hoarseness or a gurgling noise) after swallowing.
- Small-volume aspirations that produce no overt symptoms are common and are often not discovered until the condition progresses to aspiration pneumonia.

Aspiration Pneumonia:

- Older persons with pneumonia often complain of significantly fewer symptoms than their younger counterparts; for this reason, aspiration pneumonia is under-diagnosed in this group (Marrie, 2000).
- Delirium may be the only manifestation of pneumonia in elderly persons (Marrie, 2000).
- An elevated respiratory rate is often an early clue to pneumonia in older adults; other symptoms to observe for include fever, chills, pleuritic chest pain and crackles (Marrie, 2002).
- Observation for aspiration pneumonia should be ongoing in high-risk persons.

PREVENTION OF ASPIRATION DURING HAND FEEDING:

There is little research-based information regarding specific strategies to prevent aspiration during the feeding of dysphagic individuals (Loeb et al, 2003). However, the following actions may be of some benefit.

- Provide a 30-minute rest period prior to feeding time; a rested person will likely have less difficulty swallowing.
- Sit the person upright in a chair; if confined to bed, elevate the backrest to a 90-degree angle.
- Slightly flexing the person's head to achieve a 'chin-down' position is often helpful in reducing aspiration (Shanahan et al, 1993). Swallowing studies may be needed to determine which individuals are most likely to benefit from this position.
- Adjust rate of feeding and size of bites to the person's tolerance; avoid rushed or forced feeding.
- Alternate solid and liquid boluses.
- Vary placement of food in the person's mouth according to the type of deficit. For example, food may be placed on the right side of the mouth if left facial weakness is present.
- Determine the food viscosity that is best tolerated by the individual. For example, some persons swallow thickened liquids more easily than thin liquids.
- Minimize the use of sedatives and hypnotics since these agents may impair the cough reflex and swallowing.
- Evaluate the effectiveness of cueing, redirection, task segmentation and environmental modifications (minimizing distractions) as alternatives to hand feeding. (See Try This: Assessing Mealtime Behavior in Persons with Dementia.)

PREVENTION OF ASPIRATION DURING TUBE FEEDING:

Persons who aspirate oral feedings are also likely to aspirate tube feedings, either by nasogastric or gastrostomy tubes (Feinberg et al, 1996; Finucane et al, 1999; Siddique et al, 2000). Therefore, there is a growing trend to avoid the use of tube feedings merely as a means to prevent aspiration. Nonetheless, there are instances in which tube feedings are needed, especially during periods of acute illness. When tube feedings are necessary, the following activities may help to minimize aspiration:

- Keep the bed's backrest elevated to at least 30° during continuous feedings; for intermittently tube-fed persons, maintain a head elevated position for one to two hours afterward. There is evidence that a sustained supine position (with the head of the bed flat) increases the probability for aspiration pneumonia (Drakulovic et al, 1999).
- When the tube-fed person is able to communicate, ask if any of the following signs of gastrointestinal intolerance are present: nausea, feeling of fullness, abdominal pain or cramping. These signs are indicative of slowed gastric emptying that may, in turn, increase the probability for regurgitation and aspiration of gastric contents.
- Measure gastric residual volumes every 4 to 6 hours during continuous feedings and immediately before each intermittent feeding. This assessment is especially important when the tube-fed person is unable to communicate signs of gastrointestinal intolerance. Although there is no convincing research-based information regarding how much gastric residual volume is 'too much,' a persistently elevated amount (such as greater than 200 ml) should raise concern (McClave et al, 2002).
- A prokinetic agent (such as metoclopramide or erythromycin) may be prescribed to alleviate persistently slowed gastric emptying (McClave et al, 2002).
- Placement of the feeding tube in the distal duodenum or proximal jejunum may be prescribed if persistently slowed gastric emptying is a problem (McClave et al, 2002). The efficacy of this action is controversial (Lazarus et al, 1990).
- Results from a recent study suggest that pump-assisted feedings are associated with fewer aspiration events than are gravity–controlled feedings in bedridden patients with gastrostomy tubes (Shang et al, 2004).

PREVENTION OF ASPIRATION PNEUMONIA BY ORAL CARE:

Missing teeth and poorly fitted dentures predispose to aspiration by interfering with chewing and swallowing. Infected teeth and poor oral hygiene predispose to pneumonia following the aspiration of contaminated oral secretions (Terpening et al, 2001). Results from a recent study suggest that tube feeding in elderly persons is associated with significant pathogenic colonization of the mouth, more so than that observed in those who received oral feedings (Leibovitz et al, 2003).

There is evidence that providing weekly dental care and cleaning the elder person's teeth with a toothbrush after each meal lowers the risk of aspiration pneumonia (Yoneyama et al, 2002).

References:

1. Amella, E.A. & Lawrence, J.F. (2004) Assessing Mealtime Behavior in Persons with Dementia *Try This: Best Practices in Nursing Care to Older Adults*, New York: The Hartford Institute for Geriatric Nursing, New York University, Division of Nursing.
2. Ariumi, S., Morita, T., Mizuno, Y., Ohsawa, T., Akagawa, Y., Hashimoto, K., & Sasaki, H. (2002). Oral care reduces pneumonia in older patients in nursing homes. *Journal of the American Geriatrics Society, 50*(3), 430-433.
3. Drakulovic, M. B., Torres, A., Bauer, T. T., Nicolas, J. M., Nogue, S., & Ferrer, M. (1999). Supine body position as a risk factor for nosocomial pneumonia in mechanically ventilated patients: a randomised trial. *Lancet, 354*(9193), 1851-1858.
4. Feinberg, M. J., Knebl, J., & Tully, J. (1996). Prandial aspiration and pneumonia in an elderly population followed over 3 years. *Dysphagia, 11*, 104-109.
5. Finucane, T. E., Christmas, C., & Travis, K. (1999). Tube feeding in patients with advanced dementia: a review of the evidence. *Journal of American Medical Association, 282*(14), 1365-1370.
6. Langmore, S. E., Terpenning, M. S., Schork, A., Chen, Y., Murray, J. T., Lopatin, D., & Loesche, W. J. (1998). Predictors of aspiration pneumonia: How important is dysphagia? *Dysphagia, 13*(2), 69-81.
7. Lazarus BA, Murphy JB, Culpepper L: Aspiration associated with long-term gastric versus jejunal feeding: a critical analysis of the literature. *Archives of Physical Medicine & Rehabilitation.* 71(1):46-53, 1990 January
8. Leibovitz, A., Plotnikov, G., Habot, B., Rosenberg, M., & Segal, R. (2003). Pathogenic colonization of oral flora in frail elderly patients fed by nasogastric tube or percutaneous enterogastric tube. *Journal of Gerontology Series A-Biological Sciences & Medical Sciences, 58*(1), 52-58.
9. Loeb, M. B., Becker, M., Eady, A., & Walker-Dilks, C. (2003). Interventions to prevent aspiration pneumonia in older adults: a systematic review. *Journal of the American Geriatrics Society, 51*(7), 1018-1022.
10. Marik, P. E., & Kaplan, (2003) D. Aspiration pneumonia and dysphagia in the elderly. *Chest. 124*(1), 328-336.
11. Marrie, T. J. (2000). Community-acquired pneumonia in the elderly. *Clinical Infectious Disease, 31*(40), 1066-1078.
12. Marrie, T. J. (2002). Pneumonia in the long-term care facility. *Infection Control and Hospital Epidemiology, 23*(3), 159-164.
13. McClave, S. A., DeMeo, M. T., DeLegge, M. H., DiSario, J. A., Heyland, D. K., Maloney, J. P., Metheny, N. A., Moore, F. A., Scolapio, J. S., Spain, D. A., & Zaloga, G. P. (2002). Consensus statement. North American Summit on Aspiration in the Critically Ill Patient: consensus statement. *Journal of Parenteral & Enteral Nutrition, 26*(6 Suppl), S80-5.
14. Shanahan, T. S., Logemann, J. A., Rademaker, A. W., et al. (1993). Chin-down posture effect on aspiration in dysphagic patients. *Archive of Physical Rehabilitation, 74*, 736-739.
15. Shang, E., Geiger, N., Sturm, J. et al. (2004). Pump-assisted enteral nutrition can prevent aspiration in bedridden percutaneous endoscopic gastrostomy patients. *Journal of Parenteral and Enteral Nutrition, 28*(3), 180-183.
16. Siddique, R., Neslusan, C. A., Crown, W. H., et al. (2000). A national inpatient cost estimate of percutaneous endoscopic gastrostomy associated aspiration pneumonia. *American Journal of Managed Care, 6*(4), 490-496.
17. Terpenning, M. S., Taylor, G. W., Lopatin, D. E., Kerr, C. K., Dominguez, L., & Loesche, W. J. (2001). Aspiration pneumonia: dental and oral risk factors in an older veteran population. *Journal of the American Geriatrics Society, 49*(5), 557-63.
18. Yoneyama, T., Yoshida, M., Ohrui, T., Mukaiyama, H., Okamoto, H., Hoshiba, K., Ihara, S., Yanagisawa, S., Ariumi, S., Morita, T., Mizuno, Y., Ohsawa, T., Akagawa, Y., Hashimoto, K., & Sasaki, H. (2002). Oral care reduces pneumonia in older patients in nursing homes. *Journal of the American Geriatrics Society*, 50(3), 430-433

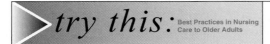

try this: Best Practices in Nursing Care to Older Adults

A series provided by
The Hartford Institute for Geriatric Nursing
(hartford.ign@nyu.edu)
www.hartfordign.org

Hiatal hernias, or diaphragmatic hernias that allow a small portion of the stomach to slide into the chest, are common in older people and are usually asymptomatic.

Those with thyroid disease, diabetes, scleroderma, or connective tissue disorders may develop esophageal motility problems and heighten their risk for GERD. In the majority of patients with GERD, the cause of the problem is not overproduction of acid, but length and frequency of esophageal acid exposure (Ray et al., 2002). In healthy persons, the contractile motions in the esophagus move substances quickly out of the esophagus into the stomach, and these clearance mechanisms limit the amount of time that the esophageal tissues are exposed to reflux. The longer the reflux is in contact with the unprotected esophageal lining, the greater the opportunity for esophageal injury, erosion, and scarring.

The symptoms of GERD include heartburn (sensation of burning in the substernal or sternal area), indigestion, belching, hiccups, and regurgitation of gastric contents into the mouth (sour mouth). The heartburn will typically worsen with lying flat or bending over. Chest pain can be so severe and persistent that it is sometimes confused with cardiac pain or angina. The older person may seek emergency evaluation because he or she fears the onset of a heart attack. Erosive esophagitis occurs when the caustic gastric contents remain in contact with the esophageal mucosa and begin to cause damage to the esophageal lining. Chronic laryngeal irritation can cause voice hoarseness, wheezing, bronchitis, asthma, and aspiration pneumonia. Symptoms may be worsened by eating large meals, using certain medications, eating foods and drinking beverages high in fat or caffeine, using tobacco and alcohol, reclining after eating, and obesity (Borum, 2004). Drugs that may worsen reflux symptoms include those listed in Box 20-1.

In addition to physical consequences, GERD is associated with psychosocial consequences. Some patients may be fearful of eating out or attending social events because stress and certain foods may trigger symptoms. Because the symptoms of GERD may be heightened when the patient is lying flat, sleep is often disrupted (Ray et al., 2002). Complications from untreated GERD include esophagitis, bleeding, scarring, and stricture formation. Barrett's esophagus occurs in about 10% to 15% of older patients with GERD and results when chronic acid exposure causes the cells lining the esophagus to become inflamed, with cellular changes considered to be pre-

---

BOX 20-1 **Drugs That May Worsen Reflux Symptoms**

Alendronate	Nonsteroidal anti-inflammatory agents
Anticholinergics	Phentolamine
Caffeine and alcohol	Potassium supplements
Calcium channel blockers	Progesterone
Codeine and opioid narcotics	Prostaglandins
Dopamine	Quinidine
Estrogen	Sedatives and hypnotics
Glucagon	Tetracycline
Nicotine	Theophylline
Nitrates	

Source: Epocrates.com, 2004; Ray et al., 2002; Reuben et al., 2002.

cancerous for development of adenocarcinoma. Hemorrhage can occur from deep erosions and ulcerations resulting in anemia, black tarry stools, or vomiting of bright red blood.

Nursing Assessment of Gastroesophageal Reflux Disease

The patient's report of symptoms, past medical history, medications, and dietary and sleep habits are the most useful sources of information to diagnose GERD. The nurse should question the patient about characteristics of the symptoms, onset, duration, frequency, aggravating and alleviating factors, and prior methods of treatment and symptom control. Generally, pain resulting from GERD can be distinguished from cardiac pain because esophageal pain worsens after a large meal, worsens after lying down, often is accompanied by belching and regurgitation, and is relieved by antacids. Referral to the primary care provider for a thorough cardiac evaluation is necessary to rule out cardiac disease and will confirm the chest discomfort as GERD. Patients with atypical pain, weight loss, or anemia should be referred to a gastroenterologist for diagnostic testing. The most frequently used diagnostic test is the barium swallow. Upper **endoscopy** is the best method to assess mucosal injury. Acid perfusion tests are usually not necessary and require the placement of an esophageal probe above the esophageal sphincter to collect esophageal contents. Esophageal contents with a pH less than 4 verify reflux of stomach acids (Borum, 2004). Most often, the patient's diagnosis is based upon signs and symptoms and improvement of symptoms with treatment.

Treatment Goals for Gastroesophageal Reflux Disease

The goal of treatment is to control symptoms and heal esophageal mucosal injury. Many healthcare providers recommend lifestyle changes first to avoid the use of medications, or they may recommend lifestyle changes along with the prescription of medications to maximize the treatment effects. Lifestyle modifications include those listed in Box 20-2.

Medications Used to Manage Gastroesophageal Reflux Disease

Over-the-counter antacids buffer the gastric pH and are widely available. The cost is reasonable, but side effects may include diarrhea, constipation, altered mineral metabolism, and acid-base disturbances. Magnesium-containing antacids can cause diarrhea and should be used with caution in older patients with renal dysfunction, including chronic or acute renal failure, because of the potential for hypermagnesemia and related toxicity. Aluminum-containing antacids can cause constipation, osteomalacia, hypophosphatemia, and related toxicity (Borum, 2004).

Histamine$_2$ receptor agonists decrease acid production by inhibiting histamine stimulation of the parietal cells. They are now available over-the-counter at lower strength than the prescription medication. These medications are potent inhibitors of gastric acid secretion and are generally well tolerated in older people with a low incidence of side effects. Risk factors for side effects include advanced age, hepatic or renal impairment, and diagnoses of additional medical conditions. Cimetidine, a drug available without prescription, has the greatest chance for adverse effects, including erectile dysfunction, gynecomastia, confusion, agitation, anxiety, and depression, and should be used with caution. Further, cimetidine inhibits the cytochrome P-450 oxidase system, increasing the probability of interactions with other medications. See Chapter 6 for further information related to the P-450 oxidase system and the potential for drug interactions. ⊂▭ More general side effects

BOX 20-2	**Lifestyle Modifications to Control Symptoms of Gastroesophageal Reflux Disease**

- Elevate the head of the bed 6 to 10 inches on wooden blocks.
- Reduce portion sizes so the stomach is not overfilled.
- Avoid foods that increase reflux such as chocolate, cola, certain spices, onions, garlic, and citrus fruits.
- Drink 6 to 8 oz of water with all medications.
- If you are taking medications daily (prescription or over-the-counter) ask your healthcare provider if they can be contributing to your symptoms of GERD.
- Stop drugs that promote reflux (if possible).
- Avoid tight-fitting clothes and girdles.
- Decrease fat, alcohol, and caffeine intake.
- Avoid supine position immediately after eating. Stay upright for 1 to 3 hours after a meal.
- Avoid lying on right side when reclining as this position encourages reflux.
- Avoid vigorous exercise within 1 hour after meals.
- Lose weight if indicated.
- Stop smoking.

of histamine blockers include headache, diarrhea, and constipation. Clinically significant interaction between H_2 blockers and other medications may occur because of an alteration in absorption, metabolism, or excretion of these drugs due to inhibition of gastric acid production.

Practice Pearl

Older persons taking H_2 blockers may not absorb enteric-coated medications because they lack the gastric acid necessary to dissolve the protective coating. The nurse should obtain a complete medication history (including over-the-counter medications) before the dosage of any medication is altered.

Proton pump inhibitors suppress acid secretion by inhibiting the hydrogen/potassium adenosinetriphosphatase pump at the parietal cell. The effect is dose related. In the older person, the acid-reducing effect of the medication and the duration of action and bioavailability are increased. However, these drugs are usually well tolerated in the older person, with healing and rate of adverse reactions similar to those in younger people. Common side effects of proton pump inhibitors include atrophic **gastritis**, headache, diarrhea and constipation, dizziness, rash, cough, backache, and abdominal pain (Borum, 2004; epocrates.com, 2004; Reuben et al., 2002).

Other medications besides acid-suppression agents can help control the symptoms of GERD, including promotility agents that enhance esophageal clearance and gastric emptying. However, these drugs are considered second-line treatments because of the prevalence of adverse effects, including abdominal cramping, diarrhea, gynecomastia, galactorrhea, fatigue, drowsiness, and movement disorders (tremor, rigidity, and tardive dyskinesia).

The mucosal protectant agent sucralfate aids in mucosal healing by reducing direct tissue exposure to acid. Sucralfate works locally by forming an adherent complex that coats the ulcer site and protects it from further injury from acid, pepsin, and bile salts. It is minimally absorbed, but bowel function should be carefully monitored as it may cause constipation. Sucralfate should be used with caution in older patients with renal impairment because of the potential for aluminum absorption and associated toxicity. Further, sucralfate can reduce the absorption of other drugs, including quinolone antibiotics, phenytoin, and warfarin (Borum, 2004). Older patients taking these drugs should have drug levels carefully monitored if sucralfate is added to the medication regimen.

Misoprostol, a combination drug that has an antisecretory and mucosal protective effect, is a synthetic prostaglandin E analogue. It is indicated only for prophylactic treatment in older patients taking NSAIDs (Borum, 2004). It has been shown to prevent NSAID-induced damage to the gastric mucosa but does not protect against duodenal ulcers. The major side effects are diarrhea (13% to 40% of patients) and abdominal pain (7% to 20%). The severity of these side effects is sometimes improved with dose reduction. The older patient should be instructed to report the onset of diarrhea or abdominal pain immediately to prevent dehydration and associated secondary problems. Table 20-1 lists medications used to manage GERD.

TABLE 20-1

Medication Management of Gastroesophageal Reflux Disease

Drug	Initial Dose	Maximum Dose	Formulation
Antacids			
(Tums, Rolaids, Mylanta)	1–2 tbs or tablets prn before meals and bedtime		Chewable, liquid
Histamine Blockers			
Cimetidine	400–800 mg bid	2× initial dose	Tablets, liquid
Famotidine	20 mg bid × 6 wks	2× initial dose	Tablets
Nizatidine	150 mg bid	2× initial dose	Tablets
Ranitidine	150 mg bid	2× initial dose	Tablets, liquid
Proton Pump Inhibitors			
Esomeprazole	20 mg qd × 4 wks	_____	Delayed release tablets
Lansoprazole	15 mg qd × 8 wks	60 mg	Delayed release tablets
Omeprazole	20 mg qd × 4–8 wks	_____	Tablets
Mucosal Protective Agents			
Sucralfate	1 g qid 1 hr before meals and bedtime	4 g/day	Oral suspension
Antisecretory/Mucosal Protective Agent			
Misoprostol	100–200 µg po qid	800 µg/day	Tablets
Prokinetic Agents			
Bethanechol	25 mg qid	50 mg qid	Tablets, injection
Metoclopramide	5 mg qid	15 mg qid	Tablets, injection syrup

Source: Data from Epocrates.com, 2004; Ray et al., 2002; Reuben et al., 2002.

To minimize adverse effects, medications are usually begun at a low dose and then "stepped up" until symptoms resolve. If symptoms persist after 6 to 8 weeks of treatment, the older patient should return to the primary care provider for further evaluation. The underlying problem may be more serious than initially determined, and further testing may be needed. If the patient's symptoms are controlled, therapy at the initial dose is usually continued for about 8 weeks to allow complete healing. However, some patients will relapse and require long-term maintenance therapy to prevent future recurrences and return of symptoms. Maintenance therapy should consist of the least costly, most convenient, and most effective (desired effect achieved without troubling side effects) drug for the patient (Ray et al., 2002).

Older patients with GERD and with Barrett's esophagus require aggressive treatment with proton pump inhibitors and regular endoscopic examination. Surgery may be required if esophageal erosion does not reverse with treatment. The surgery of choice is Nissen fundoplication and involves closing any hiatal hernia and restoring an antireflux barrier by creating a pressure gradient in the distal esophagus. The surgery is usually 85% successful. The most common side effect is dysphagia and inability to belch or vomit. Increasingly, Nissen fundoplication is being performed laparoscopically as an alternative to major surgery (Borum, 2004).

Nursing Diagnoses Related to Older Patients With Gastroesophageal Reflux Disease

Nursing diagnoses related to GERD include the following:

- *Impaired swallowing*
- *Impaired skin integrity*
- *Impaired social interaction* (if appropriate)
- *Sleep pattern disturbance* (if appropriate)
- *Acute or chronic pain*

Nurse Sensitive Outcomes Related to Care of Older Patients With Gastroesophageal Reflux Disease

Nurse sensitive outcomes that would indicate an appropriate nursing intervention include positive relief of signs and symptoms, no significant side effects of medications, sustained progress on lifestyle modification plan, and adequate nutrition as measured by weight and nutritional markers.

GASTRIC DISORDERS

Gastric disorders occurring in the older person will exhibit different signs and symptoms, complications, and treatment options (Borum, 2004). Symptoms may be more vague and less specific than those of younger adults, are more likely to be attributed to changes of aging, and may be diagnosed and treated in the more severe stage of the disease progression. Common gastric disorders include gastritis, hiatal hernias, ulcers, and stomach tumors.

Gastritis

Gastritis, or inflammation of the gastric mucosa, is classified by the severity of the mucosal inflammation, the site of involvement, and the inflammatory cell type. Erosive (hemorrhagic) gastritis may be caused by ingestion of substances that irritate the gastric mucosa such as NSAIDs, alcohol, radiation therapy, gastric trauma, or ischemia as a result of arterial insufficiency or circulatory problems. Diagnosis is based upon endoscopic appearance of the stomach lining, and biopsy is usually not necessary to confirm the diagnosis. Antral gland gastritis (type B) is the most common form of gastritis and is associated with *H. pylori* and duodenal ulcers. Fundic gland gastritis (type A) is associated with diffuse severe mucosal atrophy and the presence of pernicious anemia. Treatment of gastritis is directed at the underlying cause, including reducing factors contributing to the inflammatory process, acid neutralization and suppression (with antacids, H_2 blockers, proton pump inhibitors), protection of the gastric mucosa (sucralfate), and antibiotic therapy to eradicate *H. pylori* (Borum, 2004). Older patients with severe gastritis may be diagnosed with anemia and require transfusion, careful ongoing monitoring of hemoglobin and hematocrit levels, and periodic evaluation of stool for occult blood testing.

Peptic and Duodenal Ulcer Disease

In the United States, about 10% of adults have peptic ulcer disease. The specific incidence in older people is unknown, but hospitalization, morbidity, and mortality rates from peptic ulcer disease are higher for older persons than the general population (Borum, 2004). **Peptic ulcer disease** is defined as an excoriated area of the gastric mucosa (peptic ulcer) or first few centimeters of the duodenum (duodenal ulcer) that penetrates through to the muscularis mucosae. Duodenal ulcers are more common than gastric ulcers. Bleeding from duodenal ulcers occurs more frequently in older patients (Borum, 2004). Chronic or slow upper gastrointestinal bleeding may present with anemia, melena (black, tarry stools), or a positive fecal occult blood test. Upper gastrointestinal endoscopy is required for evaluation of the cause of upper gastrointestinal bleeding (Ali & Lacy, 2004).

H. pylori is an important factor in the development of ulcers, and the prevalence of *H. pylori* infections increases with age. In the United States, about 70% to 90% of patients with gastric ulcers and 90% to 100% of patients with duodenal ulcers are infected with *H. pylori*. Although nearly all patients with *H. pylori* will develop gastritis, only 15% develop peptic ulcer. Eradication of *H. pylori* is associated with more rapid ulcer healing and decrease in recurrence rates (Borum, 2004).

NSAID use increases the incidence of peptic ulcer disease, especially early in treatment (during the first 3 months). Higher doses of NSAIDs, history of peptic ulcer disease, and concurrent use of anticoagulants (warfarin, aspirin) predispose older patients to larger ulcers. These patients often do not experience abdominal pain. The first signs of peptic ulcer disease may be serious gastrointestinal bleeding episodes requiring emergency evaluation, treatment, and transfusion. Defensive factors to protect the stomach lining, such as the production of a mucous-bicarbonate barrier, are overwhelmed by the production of acid-induced aggressive factors, resulting in the penetration of the mucous barrier and allowing tissue injury. The strength of the mucous barrier is dependent upon the production of prostaglandin, and older persons have decreased prostaglandin concentrations in the stomach and duodenum (Borum, 2004). These factors contribute to the development of peptic and duodenal ulcers in older people and are a key reason why the use of NSAIDs in older people often results in GI side effects and problems.

Zollinger-Ellison syndrome is characterized by gastric hypersecretion and peptic ulceration caused by a gastrin-producing tumor (gastrinoma) of the pancreas or duodenal wall. The continuous high gastrin output stimulates the parietal cells to produce acid. The onset of Zollinger-Ellison syndrome is usually between the ages of 30 and 50, but one third of the patients developing this syndrome are over the age of 60 (Borum, 2004). Peptic ulcer occurs in 95% of patients with Zollinger-Ellison syndrome with persistent symptoms that progress and do not respond to drug treatment. For these patients, referral to a gastroenterologist for additional testing and assessment of gastrin levels is indicated. Treatment may include tumor removal and surgical resection for older patients without surgical risk or treatment with omeprazole. Gastric acid production and levels are carefully monitored.

Signs and Symptoms of Peptic and Duodenal Ulcer Disease. In older people, the classic signs and symptoms of peptic ulcer disease are rare. The classic sign of abdominal pain occurs in only 35% to 50% of older patients. When pain is present, it is often vague and diffuse throughout the abdomen. Often the presenting sign is blood loss and iron deficiency anemia. **Dyspepsia** (indigestion with bloating, early satiety, abdominal distention, or nausea) is a common symptom but often is not vigorously investigated and is attributed to normal changes of aging. Complications, including bleeding, perforation, and gastric outlet obstruction, occur in about 50% of patients over the age of 70 with a high mortality rate (Borum, 2004).

Nursing Diagnosis of Peptic and Duodenal Ulcer Disease. The patient's report of symptoms, past medical history, use of medications, and dietary habits are the most useful sources of information to diagnose peptic ulcer disease. The nurse should question the patient about characteristics of the symptoms, onset, duration, frequency, aggravating and alleviating factors, and prior methods of treatment and symptom control. A history of anemia or occurrence of new-onset anemia should be aggressively investigated by the healthcare provider. Generally, pain resulting from peptic ulcer disease is described as dyspepsia localized in the epigastric area, occurring hours after a meal (on an empty stomach), and relieved by food or antacids. Abdominal pain that awakens the patient at night can be a symptom of peptic ulcer disease. Referral to a gastroenterologist for an upper endoscopy or x-ray is the best method to diagnose ulcer disease. Upper endoscopy is the most sensitive and specific test for assessing abnormalities in the upper GI tract. Biopsies can be taken, if needed, during the procedure. Gastric ulcers are often difficult to distinguish from stomach cancer, and biopsy is required to eliminate the possibility of malignancy. For the very frail or those with cognitive impairment, symptomatic treatment with antiulcer medications may be tried to assess if troublesome symptoms can be reduced and quality of life improved without invasive testing or treatment. Avoidance of all medications associated with gastric ulcers is indicated.

The morbidity and mortality rates from peptic ulcer disease have increased significantly in older patients. These trends are thought to be related to the increased use of NSAIDs among older patients. It was hoped that the introduction of cyclooxygenase (COX-2) inhibitors (celecoxib) would decrease this trend; however, recent evidence indicates the use of these medications may be associated with increased risk of stroke and heart attack and casts doubt on the continued utility of these medications. Concurrent use of antiulcer drugs with traditional NSAIDs is not likely to prevent the formation of peptic ulcers (Borum, 2004).

Treatment Goals for Peptic and Duodenal Ulcer Disease. Older patients should discontinue the use of all NSAIDs, alcohol, tobacco, and caffeine. Alcohol stimulates acid secretion, and tobacco and caffeine delay healing. Eating small frequent meals and avoiding offending foods is helpful to relieve symptoms. The goal of treatment is to promote healing of the gastric mucosa through the use of lifestyle modification and medications that neutralize acid, inhibit gastric acid secretion, improve gastric mucosal defense mechanisms, and eradicate the presence of *H. pylori*.

TABLE 20-2

Laxatives by Category

Type	Action	Examples
Bulk laxatives	Increase stool bulk and urge to defecate with adequate fluid intake	Metamucil, Citrucel, FiberCon
Stool softeners	Surfactant wetting agent	Colace, Surfak
Lubricants	Lubricate stool surface	Mineral oil
Saline	Hypertonic increase in stool water content	Milk of magnesia, Fleet Phospho-Soda
Stimulants	Increase colonic peristalsis	Dulcolax, Ex-Lax, senna, Senokot
Osmotic agents	Hypertonic increase in stool water content	Sorbitol, lactulose
Enemas and suppositories	Local rectal stimulants	Fleet enemas, glycerine suppositories

Data from Epocrates.com, 2004; Reuben et al., 2002; Thomas et al., 2003.

Medications used are listed in Table 20-2, and are similar to those used in the treatment of GERD. In older patients with documented *H. pylori* infection, the use of antisecretory drugs combined with antibiotic results in more rapid duodenal ulcer healing. Although no standard therapy exists, triple or quadruple therapy regimens are advocated based on efficacy, tolerability, compliance, and cost (Borum, 2004). Usually two or three antibiotics are combined with a proton pump inhibitor. Monotherapy (use of only one antibiotic) is not recommended because of its limited effectiveness and potential for stimulating antimicrobial resistance. The most effective combination for eradicating *H. pylori* includes oral lansoprazole 30 mg bid, clarithromycin 500 mg bid, and amoxicillin 1,000 mg bid for 2 weeks. Ranitidine bismuth citrate 400 mg po bid for 4 weeks and clarithromycin 500 mg Po tid for 2 weeks may also be effective. Surgery is reserved for older ulcer patients without comorbidities who do not respond to treatment or who have potential for serious complications (perforation, hemorrhage) (Borum, 2004). Recurrence of ulcers following eradication of *H. pylori* is not usually due to recurrent *H. pylori* infection. Among the factors that can contribute to ulcer formation are NSAID use, smoking, and continued acid hypersecretion (Wollner, 2004).

Nursing Diagnoses Related to Older Patients With Peptic and Duodenal Ulcer Disease. Nursing diagnoses related to peptic ulcer disease include the following:

- *Risk for imbalanced nutrition*
- *Risk for infection*
- *Impaired tissue integrity*
- *Sleep pattern disturbance* (if appropriate)
- *Fatigue* (if appropriate)
- *Risk for activity intolerance* (if appropriate)
- *Acute or chronic pain*

Nurse Sensitive Outcomes Related to Care of Older Patients With Peptic Ulcer Disease. Nurse sensitive outcomes that would indicate an appropriate nursing intervention include positive relief of signs and symptoms, no significant side effects of medications, sustained progress on lifestyle modification plan, adequate nutrition as measured by weight and nutritional markers, and resolution of ulcer disease as evidenced by tissue healing and stable hemoglobin and hematocrit levels.

Gastric Volvulus

Gastric volvulus, or a turning, twisting, or telescoping of the stomach into or onto itself, occurs more commonly in older adults than in younger adults because of relaxation of the ligaments supporting the stomach. A complete twist can lead to strangulation of the blood supply and tissue death and is considered a surgical emergency. Symptoms include acute pain localized to the abdomen or chest, shock and hypotension, abdominal distention, an inability to vomit, and dyspnea. Emergency evaluation is needed, and an x-ray of the abdomen reveals an "upside-down stomach" (Borum, 2004). Treatment is always surgical, and mortality rate is as high as 60%.

LOWER GASTROINTESTINAL TRACT DISORDERS

The lower GI tract is composed of the colon and the rectum. The function of the lower GI tract is affected by metabolic or endocrine disorders, lifestyle and environmental factors, neurologic disorders or injury, and many medications. Many older people experience problems or dysfunction of the lower GI tract.

Anatomy and Physiology

The main functions of the colon and rectum are the storage and passing of feces. Fecal storage is enhanced by the ability of the colon to stretch and adapt to the amount of fecal matter contained within. Rhythmic colonic contractions and peristaltic waves, known as mass movements, regulate the progression of stool and allow water to be absorbed, thus decreasing stool volume. Normally, the colon absorbs approximately 1 to 2 L of water each day. There are both intrinsic and extrinsic innervations to the colon. The intrinsic nervous system regulates motility in response to immediate factors such as distention and intraluminal irritants. The extrinsic nervous system originates from the autonomic nervous system and regulates colonic motility (McCrea, 2003). Bowel continence and controlled defecation are dependent upon the ability of the older person to sense fullness and accurately identify contents in the rectum and to coordinate function of the internal and external anal sphincters (Wald, 2004). The anal canal is 3 to 5 cm long and is formed by circular muscles known as the internal and external anal sphincters. The internal sphincter is smooth muscle and under autonomic control, while the external sphincter is under voluntary control. Figure 20-4 ■ illustrates the anatomy of the lower GI tract.

Normal Changes of Aging

Colonic motility and transit in healthy older persons are similar to those in younger persons; however, aging is associated with diminished anal sphincter tone and strength (Wald, 2004). The structural weakening of colonic muscle may contribute to the development of **diverticula**, or saclike mucosal projections through the muscle wall. Older persons with the presence of diverticula are diagnosed with **diverticulosis**. Several factors can alter colonic function and lead to alterations in the lower bowel function, including diagnosis with a metabolic or endocrine disorder, lifestyle and environmental factors such as insufficient fiber or fluid in the diet, neurologic disorders or injury, mobility problems, cognitive impairment or mood disorders, and many medications. These factors may make the older person more susceptible to fecal incontinence, constipation, or diarrhea.

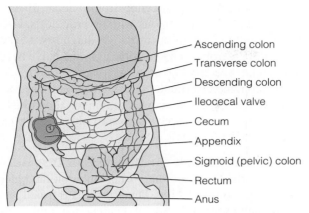

Source: National Digestive Disease Information Clearinghouse, 2003.

FIGURE ■ 20-4

The lower digestive tract.

In the healthy older adult, the large intestine does not experience major changes with regard to colonic motility. Although 50% of nursing home residents suffer from fecal incontinence, this is commonly caused by chronic constipation, fecal impaction, laxative use, and mobility or neurologic disorders. There is, however, a slight decrease in the older person's ability to recognize rectal wall distention and this may play a role in the pathogenesis of constipation (Horowitz, 2004). Dementia, depression, chronic pain, and lack of mobility may further compound the problem and contribute to the development of fecal incontinence over time.

Common Lower Gastrointestinal Disorders

The major lower gastrointestinal disorders in older persons are constipation, diarrhea, abdominal pain, rectal bleeding, and fecal incontinence. Lower GI disorders that occur more commonly in the older person than in younger persons include diverticular disease, colonic ischemia, antibiotic-associated diarrhea and colitis, and fecal incontinence. Additionally, inflammatory bowel diseases occur in all age groups, and new onset is common in the older person (Wald, 2004).

Diverticular Disease

Diverticula are acquired saclike mucosal projections that protrude through the muscular layer of the GI tract. They can potentially trap feces, become inflamed and infected, and rupture. Usually diverticula are found in the sigmoid and descending colon where blood vessels penetrate to the submucosa (Wald, 2004). In the United States, diverticular disease occurs in about 50% of persons over the age of 65. Lifestyle-related factors include inadequate intake of dietary fiber. A low-fiber diet increases the density of the stool with increases in intraluminal pressure, forcing the saclike projections of the colon wall through the muscular layers of the colon.

Bleeding may occur from rupture of the penetrating arteriole contained within the mucosal diverticula and is usually painless. Although 10% to 20% of older patients continue to bleed chronically, bleeding usually stops spontaneously unless the older person is taking medications that increase clotting times such as anticoagulants. Usually, diverticula are asymptomatic and occur commonly in the older person. Older persons with diverticulosis or diverticula without inflammation should be urged to increase dietary fiber to prevent complications such as diverticulitis (Wald, 2004).

Diverticulitis is an infection from colonic diverticula. Diverticulitis develops in 15% to 25% of older persons with diverticulosis, and the probability of infection increases with the length of time from diagnosis. Diverticulitis is caused when normal bowel flora (aerobic and anaerobic gram-negative bacilli) overgrow and flourish in the diverticular pouch when stool becomes entrapped, causing inflammation. With inflammation, the diverticular opening becomes obstructed and a pouch forms, trapping the infection. Fever, leukocytosis, pain, or abdominal tenderness may be indicators of diverticulitis, but the very old or frail older person may exhibit none of these classic symptoms (Wald, 2004).

Nursing Assessment for Diverticular Disease. The gerontological nurse should perform a careful abdominal examination on the older patient with complaints of abdominal pain or discomfort. Diverticulosis is usually asymptomatic; however, the older person may experience mild abdominal pain in the lower left quadrant, cramping, and bloating. Occasional constipation or diarrhea may also be symptomatic of diverticulosis. Diverticulitis usually presents more dramatically with symptoms of abdominal pain (severe at times), cramping (usually on the left side), fever, nausea or vomiting, and disturbed bowel habits such as constipation, diarrhea, and watery stools with flatus.

Examination of the abdomen for abnormal peristaltic waves and auscultation of bowel sounds should always precede palpation because palpation may stimulate or alter peristaltic movement. Hyperactive bowel sounds, rebound tenderness, or the presence of an abdominal mass may indicate a bowel obstruction or perforation and require immediate referral and medical attention. The older patient or caregiver should be questioned as to the time and nature of the last normal bowel movement. Diarrhea and fecal oozing may accompany bowel obstruction and complicate recognition of the problem. Some older patients and caregivers may confuse rectal oozing with diarrhea and administer antidiarrheal medications, further compounding the problem. Rectal bleeding is usually not present.

Most often, a gastroenterologist will obtain an abdominal computerized tomography (CT) scan or ultrasound to assess colonic wall thickness and extraluminal structures for suspected diverticulitis. Invasive studies such as barium enema and colonoscopy should be delayed until the inflammation and infection resolve with treatment because of the increased risk of bowel perforation. Surgery may be recommended for some older patients who fail to respond to medical therapy within 72 hours, for those with repeated attacks of diverticulitis, and for the immunocompromised older patient (including those on chemotherapy, chronic steroid users, and those with diabetes mellitus). Emergency surgery is required for generalized peritonitis, persistent bowel obstruction, and uncontrollable GI bleeding (Wald, 2004).

Practice Pearl

When palpating the abdomen of an older person with abdominal discomfort or pain, always begin with very light palpation and warm hands in an area as remote from the area of pain as possible. Deep palpation or cold hands can trigger intense pain, causing the patient to become uncooperative and resist further examination attempts.

Goals of Treatment. The goal of treatment is to eliminate the bacterial infection that is the source of pain and inflammation. Mild infections may be treated with oral antibiotics on an outpatient basis, whereas severe infections may require hospitalization with intravenous antibiotics. Sometimes a liquid diet progressing to a low-fiber diet may be suggested to allow the colon to rest and heal (Wald, 2004).

To prevent recurrence of diverticulitis and manage diverticular disease, the nurse may suggest the following interventions:

- Eat more fiber and drink plenty of fluids (try to drink 8 full glasses of water per day). This will decrease intraluminal pressure and soften the consistency of the stool.
- Do not ignore the urge to have a bowel movement. Holding stool in the colon and rectum longer will encourage further water absorption, causing stool to become drier, more compact, and more difficult to pass. Older persons who regularly resist the urge to have a bowel movement will, over time, become unaware of the need and may suffer from chronic constipation.
- Exercise regularly (walking, swimming, etc.) to aid digestion and increase colonic peristalsis.
- Avoid foods that precipitate painful attacks. Some foods with seeds, such as popcorn, sesame seeds, and poppy seeds, can become trapped in the diverticula and trigger an infection and inflammatory response.

Inflammatory Bowel Disease

Inflammatory bowel disease includes **ulcerative colitis** and **Crohn's disease**. The age of onset for these diseases occurs at two points in life: first in the 20s and then again between the ages of 50 and 80. The reasons for the differences in the age of occurrence and causes of these diseases are unknown (Wald, 2004).

Ulcerative Colitis. Ulcerative colitis is a chronic inflammatory process that affects the superficial layers of the wall of the colon in a continuous distribution. Pathological changes to the epithelial lining of the colon include inflammatory changes such as widespread ulceration, epithelial necrosis, depletion of goblet cells, and leukocyte infiltration. The incidence and prevalence of ulcerative colitis is roughly the same in older and younger persons and commonly occurs after the age of 65 (Wald, 2004).

The major signs and symptoms of ulcerative colitis include bloody diarrhea, left lower quadrant abdominal pain, and weight loss. Systemic manifestations may also occur and include uveitis and arthralgia. Diagnosis is made by referral to a gastroenterologist for sigmoidoscopy, colonoscopy, and rectal mucosa biopsy. Stool samples may be obtained and cultured or examined for toxins indicating the presence of pathogens such as *Salmonella, Shigella,* and **Clostridium difficile** in older patients with recent history of antibiotic use. Although part of the normal bowel flora, *C. difficile* diarrhea can occur when antibiotics allow overgrowth of the *C. difficile* bacterium. *C. difficile* produces a toxin that is irritating to the lining of the bowel and results in inflammation and a frothy diarrhea.

Toxic megacolon may occur in the older patient as a result of chronic ulcerative colitis. Symptoms of toxic megacolon include abdominal distention, fever, colonic dilatation, and rapid deterioration. The risk of developing colorectal cancer increases substantially in older patients with ulcerative colitis. Annual colonoscopy with biopsy to detect mucosal dysplasia (premalignant lesions in ulcerative colitis) is recommended in older patients diagnosed with toxic megacolon (Wald, 2004).

Goals of Treatment for Inflammatory Bowel Disease. Treatment is based on the extent and severity of the disease. For older patients with severe ulcerative colitis or toxic megacolon, hospitalization for administration of intravenous corticosteroids may be necessary. For older patients with moderate disease, oral corticosteroids are used to decrease inflammation. Prednisone 40 to 60 mg per day may be given initially and then tapered to 20 mg every morning as symptoms resolve. To avoid adverse effects from long-term corticosteroid use, the dose of prednisone should be tapered by 5 mg per week as long as symptoms do not recur. Long-term corticosteroid use may cause or induce hyperglycemia in patients with diabetes, induce steroid psychosis or acute delirium, accelerate osteoporosis, and worsen heart failure and hypertension. Corticosteroid retention enemas may be used for patients with left-sided disease; however, approximately 60% of rectal corticosteroid may be absorbed and systemic effects may occur (Wald, 2004).

Sulfasalazine, olsalazine, or mesalamine (5-ASA drugs) are often given with oral corticosteroids; however, adverse effects occur in up to 30% of patients. Adverse effects are dose related and include nausea, anorexia, diarrhea, headache, and rash. Treatment should be maintained indefinitely for older patients who can tolerate these drugs. The usual maintenance dose of sulfasalazine is 1 g po bid (Wald, 2004).

Surgery may be necessary for functional older patients with acute disease, when drug therapy fails, and when multiple precancerous lesions are detected. The most common surgical procedure is subtotal colectomy and ileostomy.

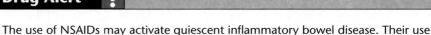

Drug Alert !

The use of NSAIDs may activate quiescent inflammatory bowel disease. Their use should be avoided in these patients unless absolutely necessary.

Crohn's Disease. Crohn's disease is a chronic inflammatory process that usually affects the terminal ileum or colon and is characterized by inflammation, linear ulcerations, and granulomas. The inflammatory process affects all layers of the bowel and can often result in scarring and fibrosis. Unlike ulcerative colitis, Crohn's disease exhibits "skip areas" or areas where normal bowel exists between areas of inflammation (Wald, 2004).

Signs and symptoms of Crohn's disease in the older person are similar to those in younger people but may be less dramatic and include diarrhea, fever, abdominal pain, and weight loss. The diagnosis is confirmed by barium enema or colonoscopy when visualization of the colon reveals discontinuous or skip areas of ulceration and inflammation followed by areas of healthy bowel. Abdominal CT scans are being used more to diagnose Crohn's disease as they are noninvasive and identify abnormalities of the colon wall more easily. A complete blood count may confirm leukocytosis or elevated white cell count and elevated sedimentation rate as a result of the inflammatory process. If the disease is long-standing or severe, the older patient may exhibit signs of systemic illness such as hypoalbuminemia or anemia due to chronic blood loss and malabsorption syndromes. Treatment is based on the extent, severity, distribution, and complications. Drug therapy includes all the drugs used for ulcerative colitis. In some older patients, antibiotics are used to supplement treatment (Wald, 2004). Unlike ulcerative colitis, Crohn's disease is not cured by surgery. For older patients who are candidates for surgery, complications of Crohn's disease such as abscesses and fistulas may be treated by colectomy or ileostomy to prevent peritonitis.

Benign and Malignant Tumors

Benign colorectal tumors and polyps are present in 75% of persons over the age of 50 (Tompkins, 2004). Most benign tumors are polyps. Predisposing factors include age, diet, family history, and prior diagnosis of polyps. Most polyps are asymptomatic, but occasionally rectal bleeding can occur. Diagnosis is usually confirmed by sigmoidoscopy, colonoscopy, or barium enema. During colonoscopy, polyps can be removed for biopsy.

Malignant tumors or colorectal cancer is second only to lung cancer as the most common malignancy in the United States and the most common cancer occurring after the age of 65 (Tompkins, 2004). Age is a critical risk factor and incidence doubles every 5 years after the age of 45. Adenocarcinoma accounts for 95% of all colorectal cancers. Predisposing factors include family history, inflammatory bowel disease, and history of colorectal tumors. In early stages, colorectal cancer is asymptomatic and diagnosis is most often made by barium enema or endoscopy. Later stage tumors may be accompanied by change in bowel habits, abdominal pain, abdominal mass, onset of anemia, rectal bleeding, and weight loss. Carcinoembryonic antigen levels may be elevated in patients with cancer of the colon as well as those with benign conditions. Therefore, it cannot be considered a diagnostic tool but it may be used to follow the effectiveness of treatment and management of those diagnosed with colon cancer (Tompkins, 2004). As with most cancers, early diagnosis and treatment of colorectal cancer improves outcomes and survival rates.

Surgical resection of the primary tumor is needed to prevent perforation, bleeding, and obstruction of the bowel. Segmental resection, subtotal colectomy, or colostomy may be performed, depending on the stage and extent of the disease and the older patient's underlying health status. About 25% of patients with colorectal cancer develop hepatic metastases, and adjuvant chemotherapy is frequently used as a treatment in these patients. Radiation therapy can ease the pain of recurrent rectal cancer, and laser therapy has been used to reduce inoperable rectal tumors and prevent obstruction (Tompkins, 2004). For end-stage patients with bowel obstruction, nasogastric tubes can be used to relieve distention and prevent the vomiting of fecal material.

Annual fecal occult blood testing increases detection of colorectal tumors in the early and curable stage and improves long-term survival. Sigmoidoscopy and colonoscopy have been established as cost-effective screening tools. Initial screening should begin at age 50 and be repeated every 10 years until the age of 85. If polyps are identified, the procedures should be repeated every 3 to 5 years (Ali & Lacy, 2004).

Antibiotic-Associated Colitis and Diarrhea

Diarrhea that occurs during or shortly after the administration of antibiotics is caused by a cytotoxin produced by *C. difficile,* an organism that is part of the normal bowel flora but overgrows as a result of elimination of other bowel organisms during antibiotic treatment. This cytotoxin produces inflammation in the bowel and epithelial necrosis resulting in diarrhea and pseudomembranous colitis. *C. difficile*–induced diarrhea and colitis are more common in older people receiving treatment in hospitals or residing in nursing homes and may indicate underlying frailty and the presence of acute and chronic illnesses. The organism can also be spread on the hands of staff providing care to the older person. Nosocomial transmission and environmental contamination with the organism are common. Risk factors for the acquisition of *C. difficile* include recent surgery, spending time in the intensive care unit, nasogastric or gastric intubation, and extended hospital stays. Although most antibiotics are associated with the development of *C. difficile* infection, cephalosporins, extended-spectrum pencillins (ampicillin), and clindamycin are implicated most often (Wald, 2004).

Practice Pearl

Careful hand washing done on a regular basis is the best way to stop the spread of nosocomial infections like *C. difficile*. It is easier and safer to prevent an infection than to cure one.

The signs and symptoms of *C. difficile* infection range from mild diarrhea to severe colitis often associated with pseudomembranes that adhere to necrotic colonic tissue. Typically, the patient passes watery nonbloody diarrhea, complains of lower abdominal pain and cramping, and exhibits a low-grade fever. In severe cases and in those who are not treated, dehydration, hypotension, and colonic perforation may occur. The stools have a characteristic odor that many nurses over time recognize as associated with this infection.

Diagnosis is confirmed by stool analysis and examination by enzyme-linked immunoassay or stool culture. Often several stool samples are necessary to diagnose the condition. Flexible sigmoidoscopy can confirm the presence of gray pseudomembranous tissue but should be performed only as a last resort on the most seriously ill patients because of the invasive nature of the procedure and the risk of perforation (Wald, 2004). Usually barium enemas and abdominal CT scans are not useful.

Treatment includes metronidazole 250 mg by mouth qid for 7 to 10 days. Refractory cases are treated with vancomycin 125 mg by mouth qid for 7 to 14 days. Metronidazole is about as effective as vancomycin in mild to moderate cases and much less expensive, making it the drug of choice under these circumstances. Fever usually resolves within 24 hours, and diarrhea decreases over 4 to 5 days. Antidiarrhea drugs should not be used because they expose the colonic tissue to the toxin for longer periods of time and place the patient at risk for the development of necrotic tissue and pseudomembranes. Aggressive nursing interventions to prevent dehydration should be implemented, including frequently assessing pulse and blood pressure, assessing postural blood pressure if the patient is ambulatory, establishing a schedule to offer the patient oral fluids (water, juice, and the beverage of choice) every 15 to 30 minutes, monitoring urinary output and skin turgor, and notifying the primary care provider of imminent dehydration so that intravenous fluids may be initiated if necessary. If the older person is receiving diuretics, these drugs should be held until the diarrhea subsides as they may exacerbate dehydration.

Relapse rates average 20% to 25% after successful treatment with metronidazole or vancomycin. Older patients who relapse are likely to continue with higher relapse rates over time. Relapses can be treated successfully with another course of metronidazole or vancomycin. Patients who are prone to relapse should avoid the offending antibiotic if possible. *Lactobacillus acidophilus* 500 mg qid or eating yogurt with active acidophilus culture may be helpful to recolonize the bowel with normal flora and prevent overgrowth by *C. difficile* (Wald, 2004).

Constipation

Constipation is a common problem in older people and affects up to 20% of those residing in the community and 50% to 75% of nursing home residents. The number of persons reporting constipation increases with age. Constipation means different things to different people, and many older adults feel that a daily bowel movement is necessary for good health. Approximately 60% of older people in the community report taking laxatives, and 24% to 37% report chronic constipation (Prather, 2004). However, constipation is not defined by presence of daily stool passage, but rather as two or fewer stools per week, straining at stool, or difficult passage of hard feces, often with fecal impaction and feeling of incomplete evacuation (Howard, West, & Ossip-Klein, 2000; Prather, 2004). Factors contributing to constipation include dehydration, side effects of medication, insufficient fiber intake, cognitive impairment, and immobility. Presence of physical illness can also predispose an older person to constipation, including metabolic and endocrine disorders (diabetes, hypothyroidism, chronic renal failure), muscular dystrophy, neurologic disorders (spinal cord injury, multiple sclerosis, Parkinson's disease, cerebrovascular accident, Alzheimer's disease), and recent abdominal surgery (McCrea, 2003). Obstructive disorders are also associated with constipation and include **rectal prolapse**, presence of a tumor, and megacolon resulting from chronic constipation and storage of large amounts of feces in the colon over time. Surgical adhesions and hernias sometimes inhibit transport of stool, causing constipation and obstruction. Constipation can lead to abdominal discomfort, loss of appetite, and nausea and vomiting.

> ## Drug Alert !
>
> Drugs known to cause constipation include all of those with anticholinergic side effects (antidepressants, neuroleptics, antihistamines, antiparkinsonian agents), some antihypertensive agents (calcium channel blockers, ACE inhibitors, diuretics), iron supplements, calcium supplements, aluminum-containing antacids, benzodiazepines, antiarrhythmics, and opiates. The nurse should carefully monitor bowel function in patients taking these medications.

The major complication of constipation is fecal impaction, which can result in intestinal obstruction, colonic ulceration, overflow incontinence with leakage of stool around the obstructing feces, and paradoxical diarrhea (Prather, 2004). Urinary incontinence, urinary tract infection, and urinary retention are also associated with fecal impaction. Excessive straining to pass stool is associated with syncope, transient ischemic attacks, **hemorrhoids**, anal **fissures**, and rectal prolapse. Over time, older patients with chronic constipation and straining at stool will dread having a bowel movement and may ignore the need to defecate, further compounding the problem.

Nursing Assessment of Constipation.   When assessing an older person with constipation, the gerontological nurse should carefully evaluate the complaint. It is important to understand the older person's beliefs about bowel habits and frequency of bowel movements. The older person should be questioned as to the basis of the complaint of constipation, such as frequency of bowel movement (fewer than three per week), consistency of stool (hard or difficult to pass), presence of excessive straining, or feeling of fullness in the rectum after completing a bowel movement. The presence of bright red blood on the stool or toilet tissue may indicate bleeding from internal or external hemorrhoids or perhaps a more serious underlying condition such as a rectal fissure or tumor. This information should be reported to the primary healthcare provider for further investigation and diagnosis.

A careful review of the older person's medications, medical conditions, level of exercise, fluid and fiber, and psychological status (somatization, anxiety, and depression) is indicated. The nursing assessment should also include an abdominal examination with auscultation of bowel sounds and palpation to detect the presence of large amounts of stool in the colon. The rectum may be examined digitally for the presence of hard impacted stool in the rectal vault. The primary healthcare provider may, when appropriate, seek further diagnostic testing such as barium enema, colonoscopy, or x-ray of the abdomen.

A multidisciplinary approach is needed for management of constipation in older patients, with the primary care provider assessing predisposing and underlying diseases and side effects of medication, and the nurse addressing nutrition and hydration issues, monitoring bowel function, and administering laxatives as needed. Nursing management of constipation involves education of older patients so that they understand the importance of fluid and fiber intake, exercise, and avoidance of medications that can cause constipation. Older people should be aware that changes in bowel function occur naturally with change in routine such as travel, hospitalization, illness, stress, taking pain medication, or other transitory conditions.

Constipation is often relieved by adequate hydration, increased mobility, fiber supplementation (20 to 35 g/day), and use of laxatives. One nursing study reported that laxatives can sometimes be discontinued for an older person with bran intake that reached 25 g daily (Howard et al., 2000). A bran mixture that significantly reduces laxative use for older patients includes 3 cups unsweetened applesauce, 2 cups coarse wheat bran, and 1 1/2 cups unsweetened prune juice. Administering 4 tablespoons per day (2 before breakfast and 2 before supper) will stimulate natural bowel movements and decrease dependence on laxatives (Smith & Newman, 1989). Fiber should be consumed as wheat or oat bran, fruits, vegetables, or nuts. When fiber intake is increased, excessive gas may be initially present but this annoying problem usually resolves as the body becomes accustomed to the change. It is recommended to increase fiber intake slowly with 5 g daily, adding small increments until the desired results are achieved with good tolerance and minimal gas and bloating. Contraindications to use of the fiber mixture include bowel obstruction, severe dysphagia, dietary restriction to low-fiber diet, and limited fluid intake. Lack of sufficient fluid intake with increased fiber diets or use of fiber supplements is associated with impaction, bowel obstruction, and large amounts of dry stool accumulating in the colon. The older person should be instructed in techniques of bowel training and urged not to delay the urge to have a bowel movement and to take advantage of the natural defecation reflex that usually occurs about 30 minutes after a meal.

Laxatives. When lifestyle modification has failed, the primary care provider may prescribe a laxative. These agents can be divided into several categories based on pharmacological action. Table 20-2 illustrates these agents by category.

Bulk laxatives contain soluble and insoluble fibers that absorb water (in states of adequate hydration) into the intestinal tract and increase stool mass. The increased mass will stimulate colonic peristalsis. Bulk laxatives are contraindicated in the presence of intestinal obstruction or when peristaltic activity is compromised (paralytic ileus). Stool softeners should be limited to patients who complain of straining at stool, painful defecation with the presence of hemorrhoids, or anal fissures. Stool softeners are sometimes used to facilitate bowel movements and prevent constipation in high-risk patients (postoperative abdominal surgery). Osmotic laxatives draw water into the colon by osmotic pressure. If the osmotic laxative is metabolized by bacteria in the colon, production of gases may lead to flatulence, abdominal bloating, or cramping. Magnesium-containing products should not be used in older persons with chronic renal failure, and sodium agents should be avoided in the presence of congestive heart failure and hypernatremia (Thomas, Goode, & LaMaster, 2003). Laxatives containing senna increase peristalsis and secretion of water into the bowel. These agents tend to be more harsh than other agents and can sometimes cause unpleasant cramping. Suppositories and enemas are usually reserved for those patients who have not responded to the other laxatives, and are invasive and sometimes uncomfortable for the older patient; therefore, they should be used as a last resort. Enemas are the treatment of choice if colonic fecal impaction is suspected. Plain tap water or sodium phosphate enemas are recommended. Soapsud enemas produce mucosal damage and cramping and should be avoided. Because rectal volumes increase with age, the enema should be administered slowly to prevent cramping and should generally contain about 150−300 milliliters or 5−10 fluid ounces of solution. After the initial blockage has been passed or removed manually, a second enema may be needed to remove additional stool that has moved into the proximal colon (Prather, 2004). As this procedure is uncomfortable and unpleasant, fecal impaction should be avoided by paying close attention to the older person's bowel function.

For drug-induced constipation, the best action is to seek advice from the primary care provider as to whether the offending medication may be discontinued. Some drugs (verapamil) cause more constipation than others, and the primary care provider may wish to substitute a less constipating antihypertensive agent if the older patient experiences problems with constipation. However, when the medication cannot be discontinued (for example, opioids for pain), a careful bowel management plan is needed to prevent constipation and fecal impaction. Opioids inhibit gastric emptying time and decrease peristaltic movements. About 50% of older people taking opioids report symptoms of constipation. Correction of constipation associated with opioid use requires a senna or osmotic laxative to overcome the strong opioid effect. Stool softeners and bulking agents alone are inadequate because of the opioid-related constipation resulting from slowed gut motility. A prophylactic bowel regimen should be initiated whenever an older person is started on an opioid pain medication to prevent fecal impaction (Thomas et al., 2003). Fecal impactions high in the rectum or in the sigmoid can lead to nausea and vomiting, anorexia, pain, obstruction, perforation, and fecal peritonitis.

Diarrhea

Diarrhea is defined as abnormally loose stool accompanied by a change in frequency or volume (Prather, 2004). As with constipation, diarrhea is a subjective symptom and careful nursing assessment is required. The nurse should assess for the presence of urgency, cramping, bloating, incontinence, pain on defecation, and blood in the stool. A history of gastric tube feeding or recent antibiotic use may suggest the presence of *C. difficile*.

The incidence of diarrhea in the older person is unknown, but older people may be more susceptible to diarrhea because of hypochlorhydria or achlorhydria when taking gastric acid-suppressing drugs, increased use of antibiotics, and decreased mucosal immune function (Prather, 2004). The likelihood of morbidity and mortality increases with persistent diarrhea. In nursing homes, outbreaks of *Escherichia coli* infections have been documented with three times the morbidity and mortality occurring in younger persons. The higher mortality rate (16% to 35%) occurs mostly because the older person is more susceptible to the harmful effects of fluid loss, dehydration, and hypovolemia (Prather, 2004).

Diarrhea of less than 2 weeks' duration is considered acute; diarrhea occurring longer than 4 weeks is defined as chronic. Most diarrhea in the older person is acute and self-limited. Causes include infection (viral, bacterial, or parasitic), medications and drug changes, and food intolerances. Acute bloody diarrhea needs immediate medical evaluation. Causes include ischemia, diverticulitis, or inflammatory bowel disease. Viruses responsible for infectious diarrhea include the Norwalk virus and rotavirus. Both viruses are spread by the fecal-oral route and have caused epidemic diarrhea in nursing homes. Toxic diarrhea can result from food poisoning (*Salmonella, Staphylococcus aureus, E. coli*) or ingestion of contaminated food. Careful hand washing and food preparation in sanitary conditions are required to prevent infectious diarrhea in the older person.

Chronic diarrhea may occur as a result of tumors, surgery, and medications. Almost all drugs can cause diarrhea. Commonly associated drugs include NSAIDs, magnesium-containing antacids, antiarrhythmics, beta-blockers, quinidine, colchicine, and digoxin (Prather, 2004). If the pattern of diarrhea suggests lactose intolerance (diarrhea after ingestion of dairy products), a trial lactose-free diet or treatment with lactase can be tried and bowel function carefully monitored. Older patients who are immunosuppressed, such as those receiving chemotherapy or those diagnosed with HIV/AIDS (10% of patients with

HIV/AIDS are older people), may experience chronic diarrhea secondary to bowel infections caused by giardiasis, microsporidiosis, and *Mycobacterium avium-intracellulare* (Prather, 2004).

Nursing Evaluation. Evaluation should focus on quantifying the nature of the stool, frequency of passage, and presence of associated symptoms. Overflow diarrhea can occur as a result of fecal impaction, and the date of the last normal bowel movement should be carefully identified. Older patients at risk for dehydration will require aggressive fluid replacement, including frequent offerings of oral fluids, consultation with the primary healthcare provider to temporarily hold diuretics, and perhaps administration of intravenous fluids. Hospitalization may be required for complete evaluation and treatment.

Nursing Assessment of Diarrhea. Nursing assessment should include a careful examination of the abdomen, including visual examination for bloating or excessive peristaltic movements, auscultation of bowel sounds, palpation to identify masses or rebound tenderness, and digital rectal examination to determine presence of impacted stool. Older patients with recent antibiotic use, those who have experienced recent foreign travel, and those who may have been exposed to food poisoning should have stool collected for culture and analysis. A plain abdominal x-ray (kidneys, ureter, bladder) may indicate the presence of an intestinal obstruction or fecal impaction.

If toxin-producing and infectious diarrhea are not suspected, antidiarrheal agents can be administered. However, administration of these drugs in the presence of toxins and infectious agents can lead to colon damage and systemic adverse effects by allowing the toxic substance to remain in the bowel for longer periods of time and thus to be absorbed into the general circulation. Soluble fiber (Metamucil) adds bulk to the stool and is sometimes helpful to slow bowel movements in persons requiring bulk. Kaopectate, Pepto-Bismol, and Imodium A-D can be administered after each loose stool in divided doses. Lomotil should be avoided because of significant atropine-like side effects (Prather, 2004).

Fecal Incontinence

Fecal incontinence is embarrassing and can cause an older person to severely limit social activity. Approximately 5% of the community-residing elderly and 50% of the institutionalized elderly suffer from fecal incontinence (Prather, 2004). Continence requires adequate sensation and ability to discriminate between feces and flatus, coordination of internal and external anal sphincters, and adequate pelvic floor muscles to retain stool in the rectum. Sometimes mobility problems, severe depression, or cognitive impairment may inhibit the older patient's motivation and ability to remain continent. Immobilized and functionally impaired older persons may be unable to suppress the urge to defecate and suffer fecal incontinence while waiting for assistance to use the bedpan or toilet. A regular toileting program, administration of a high-fiber diet, elimination of medications associated with diarrhea, and treatment of infections are appropriate interventions for older persons with fecal incontinence.

Hemorrhoids and Rectal Bleeding

Hemorrhoids and colorectal cancer are the most common causes of rectal bleeding (Tompkins, 2004). Hemorrhoids are varicose veins of the anorectal junction and are separated as internal or external if they protrude through the anus (Schulz, 2004). Although hemorrhoids have been commonly thought to develop as a result of straining and constipation, hemorrhoids may actually develop because of sliding of the lining of the anal canal (Ali & Lacy, 2004). A thrombosed external hemorrhoid is a localized clot that forms in the vein of an external hemorrhoid or arises from a ruptured blood vessel (Schulz, 2004). Thrombosed hemorrhoids appear bluish in color and may be painful.

Hemorrhoids tend to be asymptomatic in the early stages but may bleed over time. Bleeding is usually scant and involves bright red blood on toilet tissue. External hemorrhoids may be easily seen, but internal hemorrhoids require visualization by sigmoidoscopy or colonoscopy because they cannot be reliably felt with a digital examination. Any rectal bleeding should be referred to a gastroenterologist for an accurate diagnosis and followed up with endoscopic examination to rule out malignancy.

Treatment of hemorrhoids depends on size. Grade 1 hemorrhoids are those that do not prolapse. Grade 2 hemorrhoids reduce spontaneously after prolapse. Grade 1 and 2 hemorrhoids may be treated with rubber banding, high-fiber diet, and bulking agents such as psyllium. Heavy lifting and straining at stool should be avoided as they can worsen prolapse. Sitz baths and suppositories with benzocaine can relieve symptoms. Sclerotherapy, cryosurgery, and laser therapy may also be effective options for some older patients. Hemorrhoidectomy should be reserved for those patients with persistent symptoms who have not been helped by nonsurgical techniques (Ali & Lacy, 2004).

Rectal prolapse or passage of the rectum through the anus is common in older persons, affecting women more than men (Schulz, 2004). The main symptom is protrusion of the rectum with the passage of stool or upon standing. Continued rectal prolapse can lead to fecal incontinence, and surgical repair may be necessary. Conservative therapy includes instruction on avoiding heavy lifting and prolonged standing and prevention of constipation and straining at stool.

Liver and Biliary Disorders

With aging, the liver is more susceptible to the effects of drugs and other toxins. An older person with liver disease may present with vague and ambiguous symptoms, including fatigue, weight loss, anorexia, and malaise. The older patient with viral **hepatitis** may complain of nausea, fatigue, and loose stools. Acute hepatitis A is much less common in the older person than in younger persons, and more than 70% of older persons possess immune antibodies indicating they have had a previous infection. Acute hepatitis B and C are also less common in the older person than the younger person. If an older person is infected with the hepatitis virus, the likelihood the disease will become chronic is heightened and poorer clearance of the virus results from treatment. For example, in younger patients with hepatitis B, 5% to 15% of acute cases become chronic, compared with 43% in older persons (Luxon, 2004). Older patients who have abnormal liver function tests, who have a history of intravenous drug use, who have recently traveled in third world countries, or who engage in unsafe sexual practices should consult a gastroenterologist for further evaluation and treatment.

Hepatic cysts are common in the older person and are usually benign. If a cyst enlarges and causes discomfort, excision or draining may be necessary. Hemangioma, a common benign liver tumor, is found in about 5% of older persons. Benign tumors and cysts are usually asymptomatic and are often found when a CT scan or ultrasound is done for another reason. Liver function tests are usually normal. Typically no treatment is required; however, for patients with complaints of abdominal discomfort, the cysts may be aspirated under local anesthesia as needed for comfort.

Metastatic carcinoma is the most common form of liver cancer, and many cancers metastasize to the liver. In the United States, the incidence of liver cancer is highest in persons 50 to 70 years of age (Castells, 2004). Primary liver cancer or hepatocellular cancer rates are higher in parts of the world where the incidence of viral hepatitis is higher. In most cases, the tumor develops in cirrhosis resulting from hepatitis B or C infection. The 5-year probability of a patient with cirrhosis developing hepatocellular carcinoma is about 20%. Other predisposing factors include excessive alcohol and tobacco use.

Only 20% of older patients with hepatocellular cancer will have symptoms at the time of diagnosis. These symptoms usually include jaundice, variceal bleeding, ascites, right upper quadrant abdominal pain, weight loss, or an enlarged liver. Liver function tests are usually abnormal with increased serum bilirubin levels, elevated serum alkaline phosphatase, and decreased serum albumin concentrations. Definitive diagnosis follows after abdominal ultrasound, CT scan, and liver biopsy (Castells, 2004).

Treatment is determined by the tumor stage and the older person's functional status. Small tumors (less than 4 cm) may be treated with percutaneous hepatic injection with ethanol under ultrasound control. This treatment often results in complete tumor necrosis. Other options include tumor embolization, chemotherapy, and immunotherapy (Castells, 2004). Many of these treatments are experimental, and effect on the patient's survival has not been clearly established. Surgical resection is usually restricted to highly functional older patients with solitary tumors that have not metastasized. Liver transplantation may be curative for nonmetastasized tumors, but most centers will not perform liver transplantation in patients over 65, especially if they have coexisting medical conditions (Castells, 2004). Regardless of treatment, the gerontological nurse should provide holistic care including careful attention to pain and symptom control, nutritional issues, skin care, emotional support for the patient and family, and issues relating to death and dying.

In the United States, gallbladder cancer is the fourth most common GI cancer. The mean age of diagnosis is about 76 years (Castells, 2004). Bile duct cancer, usually adenocarcinoma, is more common in men. The average age of diagnosis is around 60 years. Adenocarcinoma also accounts for 80% of all gallbladder cancers (more common in women), and gallstones are present in 85% of cases. Symptoms include intermittent vague pain in the upper right quadrant. Later in the progression of the disease, jaundice and weight loss are common. Abdominal ultrasound and CT provide definitive diagnosis.

The prognosis for cure is poor with only 5% of older patients experiencing 5-year survival. Radical cholecystectomy is the treatment of choice for nonmetastasized tumors of the gallbladder. Radiation therapy and chemotherapy are ineffective (Castells, 2004). Whipple operation (radical resection of the bile duct and pancreatoduodenectomy) provides some promising benefit for bile duct cancer with 5-year survival rates about 20% to 30%, but patients over the age of 70 have a high surgical risk (Castells, 2004). As previously mentioned, the gerontological nurse should address issues of symptom palliation and death and dying.

Gallstones

The incidence of gallstones rises with age. About one third of persons over 70 have gallstones (Tompkins, 2004). Typical symptoms include right upper quadrant pain, gas, distention, and nausea and vomiting. Acute cholecystitis, a complication of gallstones, is characterized by increased local tenderness, fever, and increased white blood count. If a gallstone migrates into the common bile duct, blockage and pancreatitis can result with increases in serum amylase levels (Tompkins, 2004). Surgery should be performed within 2 or 3 days from the onset of symptoms of acute cholecystitis, especially after several acute attacks.

Ultrasound visualizes gallstones in 95% of cases, and abdominal CT scans will diagnose biliary problems. Treatment includes laparoscopic cholecystectomy, stone dissolution by chenodeoxycholic acid, and extracorporeal shock wave lithotripsy (Ali & Lacy, 2004). Many older persons decide to avoid aggressive treatment for gallstones and instead manage their symptoms by avoiding high-fat and other foods that cause them pain or distress.

Pancreatitis

Acute pancreatitis occurs more frequently and is more severe in older persons than in younger persons. Factors that increase risk include gallstone, medications, alcohol abuse, and cancer. Drugs increasing the risk of pancreatitis include estrogen, furosemide, ACE inhibitors, and mesalamine. Diagnosed hyperlipidemia and hypercalcemia also increase the risk. Typical presenting symptoms are epigastric pain, nausea, and vomiting. Serum amylase, lipase, bilirubin, and alkaline phosphatase levels may be elevated. Abdominal ultrasonography or CT scanning should be done to confirm the diagnosis (Ali & Lacy, 2004).

Treatment for acute pancreatitis includes nasogastric suction, pain management, hyperalimentation, and fluid replacement. In 90% of older persons, acute pancreatitis is self-limiting and conservative measures are sufficient.

Chronic pancreatitis results in weight loss, diarrhea, diabetes, and presence of persistent pain. Diagnosis is based on symptoms and specialized testing. All older patients with chronic pancreatitis must refrain from alcohol (Tompkins, 2004). Surgical treatment may be necessary when conservative measures fail.

Pancreatic cancer accounts for 5% of all cancer deaths in the United States (Ali & Lacy, 2004). Painless jaundice, pruritus, and weight loss are common presenting symptoms. The prognosis of pancreatic cancer is poor (Ali & Lacy, 2004).

Endoscopic Gastrointestinal Procedures

Upper or lower gastrointestinal endoscopic procedures can be done to view body cavities with fiberoptic tubing. Conventional x-rays cannot identify color changes, bleeding, or vascular malformations. Endoscopy allows biopsy of abnormalities, allows stent placement, and helps surgeons determine if surgery is needed (Waye, 2004).

Esophagogastroduodenoscopy visualizes the upper gastrointestinal tract. Inspection of the esophagus to the duodenum is indicated for evaluation of the esophageal and gastric areas and provides information on upper gastrointestinal bleeding. Therapeutic indications include dilating esophageal strictures, vaporizing gastric and esophageal neoplasms, endoscopic injection therapy or thermal coagulation of upper gastrointestinal bleeding, sclerotherapy for esophageal varices, and removal of polyps. Older patients are at risk of complications due to lowered oxygen intake during the passage of the tube. Using a small-caliber endoscopic tube and administering additional oxygen during the procedure may help these patients (Waye, 2004).

Before endoscopy, food and drink may be restricted to allow the stomach to empty, and a strong laxative is taken to clean the bowel for colonoscopy preparation. Because transient bacteremia may occur during endoscopy, older patients at high risk for infection (those with valvular heart disease or artificial heart valves) should receive antibiotics (usually ampicillin or gentamicin) before the procedure (Waye, 2004).

Most endoscopies are performed while the patient is consciously sedated. Usually benzodiazepines are given for relaxation. Midazolam is given for conscious sedation. Aggressive cleansing protocols are difficult for some older patients to tolerate. Harsh cathartics can result in dehydration in an older person, and adequate fluid intake must be maintained during preparation for the procedure.

A sigmoidoscopy permits inspection of the rectum and distal sigmoid colon, and most of the descending colon. The flexible sigmoidoscope (about 60 cm in length) may be used to evaluate the left side of the colon where two thirds of neoplasms appear (Waye, 2004). Polyps are usually not removed during examination with the flexible sigmoidoscope. Sedation is not required, and one or two phosphate enemas cleanse the bowel adequately. The patient usually lies on the left side during the procedure.

Colonoscopy allows visual examination of the entire colon. Colonoscopy is indicated for routine testing or when anemia is present, positive fecal occult blood testing is noted, or polyps are suspected. Screening in asymptomatic older people should begin at age 50 and continue every 10 years. No data indicate at what age screening should be stopped, but some geriatricians recommend screening of highly functional older persons until the age of 85 (Waye, 2004). Colonoscopy allows the removal of colonic polyps and evaluation of bleeding sites with electrocautery treatment. Strictures may be dilated and stents may be placed in strictures resulting from malignant growths to prevent bowel obstruction. Contraindications to colonoscopy include fulminant colitis, acute diverticulitis, perforated bowel, and recent myocardial infarctions (Waye, 2004).

The colon must be cleansed to allow complete visualization. Typical preparation is 1 or 2 days of a liquid diet and administration of a cathartic the night before the procedure. Even the smallest amount of feces in the colon can hide important details and compromise the examination. Two doses of sodium phosphate should be administered. Older patients with cardiovascular or renal instability should be carefully monitored. The nurse should consult with the gastroenterologist who is to perform the procedure and the primary care provider regarding the administration of regularly scheduled medications.

Complications from colonoscopy when performed by a skilled clinician are minimal. Colonoscopy is a relatively safe procedure and reliable results are valuable for accurate diagnosis. Risk of colonic perforation and excessive bleeding is low. Complications from sedative use include arrhythmias, aspiration, and rarely cardiac arrest (Waye, 2004). Patients should be instructed to bring a friend or relative to the procedure because they will be unable to drive for at least 24 hours after the administration of the sedation. The older person will usually receive a smaller dose of the sedating drug but still may be lethargic and sleepy for 24 hours.

Nursing Diagnoses for Older Patients With Gastrointestinal Tract Problems

Nursing diagnoses (North American Nursing Diagnosis Association, 2003) for problems associated with the gastrointestinal tract include the following:

- *Imbalanced nutrition: less than body requirements* for those with anorexia
- *Risk for infection* for those undergoing endoscopic examination and needing antibiotic prophylaxis
- *Constipation and perceived constipation*
- *Diarrhea*
- *Bowel incontinence*
- *Risk for constipation*
- *Ineffective tissue perfusion: gastrointestinal tract*
- *Risk for aspiration*
- *Impaired oral mucous membrane*
- *Social isolation* (if appropriate)
- *Noncompliance* (if appropriate)

- *Ineffective health maintenance*
- *Toileting self-care deficit*
- *Acute or chronic pain disturbance*
- *Nausea*

The nurse should educate older persons and their families regarding the causes, prevention, and treatment of gastrointestinal diseases.

Patient-Family Teaching Guidelines

GASTROINTESTINAL DISEASE

The following are guidelines that the nurse may find useful when instructing older persons and their families about gastrointestinal problems.

1. How can I prevent gastrointestinal disease?

Many people experience heartburn, constipation, diarrhea, and other problems with the gastrointestinal tract as they get older. Some problems are common and will go away on their own such as occasional constipation or diarrhea. Other problems are more serious and require further investigation such as blood in the stool and change in normal elimination patterns. Some suggestions for general health of the gastrointestinal tract include the following:

- Know your family history. Do you have a blood relative with polyps in the colon, colon cancer, Crohn's disease, or diverticulitis? If so, you may be more at risk than others without a family history.
- Eat a balanced diet that is high in fiber and low in fat.
- Maintain a normal weight.
- Stop smoking or using tobacco products.
- Decrease the size of portions at mealtime and avoid lying down for 2 to 3 hours after eating.
- Ask your healthcare provider to provide you with occult blood stool testing cards every year, and begin having colonoscopies at age 50 and periodically thereafter.
- Take medications with 8 oz of water and sit upright for 20 minutes after taking them.
- Limit the use of nonsteroidal anti-inflammatory agents such as ibuprofen because they can interfere with the protective covering in the stomach and cause ulcers.

RATIONALE:

Many of the problems that develop in the gastrointestinal tract are preventable with healthy lifestyle choices and early disease prevention. Older patients should be encouraged to preserve GI function by making healthy lifestyle choices.

2. If I already have gastrointestinal disease is there anything I can do to stop it?

Yes. Take medications prescribed by your healthcare provider and begin lifestyle changes immediately. Also carry out all suggestions previously discussed. If your doctor prescribes medication for you, take it exactly as directed. Report any worsening of your condition or new symptoms to your doctor or nurse. Avoid straining at stool and heavy lifting if you have hemorrhoids. Drink plenty of fluids and try to get daily exercise. With treatment and lifestyle changes, most gastrointestinal problems can be successfully treated.

RATIONALE:

Most older persons who already have diseases or problems of the GI tract will have improvement in symptoms by following treatment suggestions and making healthy lifestyle choices. It is important to stress to older patients and families that it is never too late to work toward good health.

(continued)

Patient-Family Teaching Guidelines, *cont.*

3. Is there anything else I should do to make the most of living with gastrointestinal disease?

Yes. Exercise to keep your muscles fit and strong, eat a healthy diet, control your weight, and see your healthcare provider on a regular basis. Screening tests, no matter how unpleasant, save lives. Your healthcare provider can give you specific instructions that will help you to lead a long and healthy life.

RATIONALE:

Following general health promotion principles and engaging in periodic screening are good ideas for everyone.

Care Plan

A Patient With GERD

Case Study

Mrs. Stein is an overweight 67-year-old woman who is complaining of heartburn that she has had on and off for over a year. She has seen the commercial on television warning people that they could have serious problems with erosive esophagitis if they do not take an expensive prescription drug to ease the symptoms.

Specifically, she says the pain is worse when lying flat after a big meal. The symptoms include nausea at times, and the burning is worse when she has her evening glass of wine. Other medications include ibuprofen 200 mg three times a day for arthritis and one of the bisphosphonates (Fosamax) for osteoporosis.

Applying the Nursing Process

ASSESSMENT

The gerontological nurse should carefully question Mrs. Stein regarding the nature of her symptoms. How consistently are they occurring? Has she noticed a pattern with certain foods? Have the symptoms become worse since taking the ibuprofen and bisphosphonate? What is her pattern of alcohol use? Does she drink alcoholic beverages in addition to her evening glass of wine? What has she done to make it better? Has she had any weight loss or gain? Does she see her healthcare provider regularly? Does she have any other diagnosed illnesses? A complete nursing assessment is indicated.

A Patient With GERD

DIAGNOSIS

The current nursing diagnoses for Mrs. Stein include the following:

- *Intermittent chronic pain syndrome*
- *Occasional nausea*

EXPECTED OUTCOMES

The expected outcomes for the plan of care specify that Mrs. Stein will:

- Become aware of the harmful effects of alcohol, ibuprofen, and Fosamax on esophageal function.
- Use weight loss techniques to begin gradual weight reduction.
- Develop a therapeutic relationship with the nurse to begin a variety of lifestyle modifications that will improve her GI symptoms and health status in general.
- Agree to see a gastroenterologist for further diagnosis of her GI symptoms.

PLANNING AND IMPLEMENTATION

The following nursing interventions may be appropriate for Mrs. Stein:

- She should be weighed to establish a baseline weight. If previous weights are documented, the baseline weight can be compared with previous readings. Over 2 or 3 lb of unintentional weight loss could be significant even in an overweight older person. A careful review of her eating habits and preferences will assist the nurse in this area.
- Mrs. Stein may be advised to discontinue use of ibuprofen as chronic heartburn can result in damage to the lining of the esophagus, including inflammation, ulcers, bleeding, and scarring. Further risks include formation of peptic erosion or ulcer with slow blood loss. The pain will be dulled by the pain-relieving qualities of the medication.
- Mrs. Stein should be carefully questioned as to how she takes her Fosamax. It is to be taken on an empty stomach with a full 8 oz of water. Additionally, she must sit upright or stand for 30 minutes to prevent esophageal reflux and erosion.

As the pain has persisted for Mrs. Stein for about a year and she has risk factors for gastroesophageal reflux disease and peptic ulcer formation, with the patient's permission, the nurse should contact the primary care provider and report the change in condition and the information gathered in the nursing assessment. Mrs. Stein and her family should schedule an appointment with the healthcare provider for further evaluation. If the nurse has access to screening cards for fecal occult blood testing, Mrs. Stein should gather the specimens at home and bring them with her for analysis at the next appointment. This will provide valuable information at the time of the visit.

In the meantime, the patient should be instructed to:

- Avoid foods that seem to make her situation worse (such as wine).
- Decrease the size of portions at mealtime.

(continued)

A Patient With GERD *(continued)*

- Avoid lying down for 2 to 3 hours after eating.
- Elevate the head when resting or sleeping.
- Take an antacid for symptom relief.

EVALUATION

The nurse hopes to work with Mrs. Stein over time to provide support and improve overall health and function. The nurse will consider the plan a success based on the following criteria:

- Mrs. Stein will agree to meet with a social worker to assess caregiver strain, the situation in the home, and the need for supportive services.
- A family meeting will be held to discuss Mrs. Stein's overall health.
- She will begin to decrease her alcohol consumption at bedtime and report improvement in GI symptoms.
- She will begin a gradual weight reduction program to decrease her GI symptoms and enjoy a general improvement in overall health status.

Ethical Dilemma

On the way out the door, Mrs. Stein tells the nurse that her 80-year-old husband is ill with dementia and she is exhausted caring for him. He is incontinent and often soils himself. She has to constantly clean him and is unsure how long she can keep providing his care without assistance. When the nurse offers to have Elder Services come to the home and do an assessment for assignment of home services, Mrs. Stein refuses. She states, "I can't have strangers in my home right now. It's a mess and I'm too exhausted to clean." How should the nurse respond?

The issue here is the conflict between Mrs. Stein's autonomy (the right to determine her husband's care and control entry into her home) and beneficence (what is in Mrs. Stein's and her husband's best interest). Clearly, further information and involvement of the healthcare team are needed. On the surface, it seems to make sense to allow Mrs. Stein more time to organize her life and seek treatment for herself. However, her husband's dementia may be progressive and irreversible and therefore the likelihood of improvement may not be realistic. Should something happen to Mrs. Stein, who would care for her husband? Is there a family member who can help? Why has Mrs. Stein not gotten help thus far? Would she be willing to meet with the social worker and explore these issues further?

The nursing code of ethics supports the patient's right to self-determination and believes that nurses will and must play a primary role in implementing this right. The nurse should identify and mobilize mechanisms in place within Mr. and Mrs. Stein's support network and community. Mrs. Stein is trying to act responsibly but, by not accepting help, she may be denying her husband and herself of much needed physical and psychosocial support services.

A Patient With GERD

Critical Thinking and the Nursing Process

1. What reaction have you observed when a physician or nurse recommends that an older person undergo a colonoscopy as a health maintenance measure?
2. When working with older patients experiencing GI problems, what barriers to lifestyle modification suggestions can you anticipate?
3. What is the perception of society in general regarding older persons and bowel function? Discuss this with your classmates to see if you can understand why some older people are "bowel obsessed" and overly concerned about bowel function.

- Evaluate your responses in Appendix B.

EXPLORE MediaLink

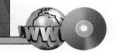

NCLEX review, case studies, and other interactive resources for this chapter can be found on the Companion Website at **www.prenhall.com/tabloski**. Click on Chapter 20 to select the activities for this chapter. For animations, video tutorials, more NCLEX review questions, and case studies, access the accompanying CD-ROM in this textbook.

Chapter Highlights

- The gastrointestinal tract performs four major functions: digestion, absorption, secretion, and motility.

- Gastrointestinal problems are common in older persons and range from mild, self-limiting problems to serious problems requiring immediate attention and intervention.

- Comorbid illness and polypharmacy also can contribute to gastrointestinal problems and exacerbate normal changes of aging. Frail older persons and those residing in nursing homes may be most at risk for adverse events and experience worse outcomes as a result of adverse events.

- Changes in bowel habits, swallowing disorders, unintentional weight loss, melena, rectal bleeding, and abdominal pain are all examples of significant abnormalities in the GI system that require careful investigation and should not be attributed to normal aging.

- The risk of colorectal cancer and peptic ulcer disease secondary to NSAID use rises rapidly with age.

- Dysphagia is the most common esophageal disorder of the older person and is estimated to occur in up to 50% of institutionalized older persons. Swallowing difficulties can be successfully assessed and risk of aspiration pneumonia minimized by the gerontological nurse.

- Gastroesophageal reflux disease can cause chest pain, exacerbate asthma and insomnia, and negatively affect quality of life. An integrated approach involving lifestyle modification, pharmacological therapy, and referral to specialists if needed can greatly improve the older patient's comfort level, ability to eat, and overall quality of life.

- Constipation and diarrhea are common motility disorders that result in malnutrition, social isolation, and fluid and electrolyte imbalances. Medications are often implicated as causative factors of motility disorders.

- Diverticulosis increases with age. Complications include bleeding, diverticulitis, and perforation. Inflammatory bowel disease may present for the first time after the age of 65.

- The rate and incidence of GI malignancies rises with age, and the presenting symptoms may be more vague in the older person than in the younger adult. Most GI malignancies are more successfully treated with early detection.

- Beginning at age 50, yearly occult blood testing and colonoscopy every 10 years are recommended. While the colonoscopy itself is relatively safe, the preparation and bowel cleansing routine can be difficult. Older people with respiratory and cardiac problems may need additional supervision and monitoring of fluid and electrolyte status.

References

Ali, A., & Lacy, B. (2004). Abdominal complaints and gastrointestinal disorders. C. Landefeld, R. Palmer, M. Johnson, C. Johnston, & W. Lyons, (Eds), In *Current geriatric diagnosis and treatment.* New York: Lange Medical Books/McGraw-Hill.

Ariumi, S., Morita, T., Mizuno, Y., Ohsawa, T., Akagawa, Y., Hashimoto, K., & Sasaki, H. (2002). Oral care reduces pneumonia in older patients in nursing homes. *Journal of the American Geriatrics Society, 50*(3), 430–433.

Arnella, E. A., & Lawrence, J. F. (2004). Assessing mealtime behavior in persons with dementia. *Try this: Best practices in nursing care to older adults.* New York: Hartford Institute for Geriatric Nursing, New York University, Division of Nursing.

Aronson, B. (2000). Applying clinical practice guidelines to a patient with complicated gastroesophageal reflux disease. *Gastroenterology Nursing, 23*(4), 143–147.

Bartz, S. (2003). Gastrointestinal disorders in the elderly. *Annals of Long-Term Care, 11*(7), 33–39.

Borum, M. (2004). Esophageal disorders. In M. Beers & R. Berkow (Eds.), *Merck manual of geriatrics.* Retrieved January 18, 2004, from www.merck.com.

Camilleri, M., Lee, J., Viramontes, B., Bharucha, A., & Tangalos, E. (2000). Insights into the pathophysiology and mechanisms of constipation, irritable bowel syndrome and diverticulosis in older people. *Journal of the American Geriatrics Society, 48,* 1142–1150.

Castells, A. (2004). Gastrointestinal tumors. In M. Beers & R. Berkow (Eds.), *Merck manual of geriatrics.* Retrieved January 22, 2004, from www.merck.com.

Dahlin, C. (2004). Oral complications at the end of life. *American Journal of Nursing, 104*(7), 40–47.

Davies, S. (1999). Dysphagia in acute strokes. *Nursing Standard, 13*(30), 49–54.

DiPalma, J. (2002). Approach to the diagnosis and management of constipation. *Sessions in Primary Care, 5,* 7–8.

Drakulovic, M. B., Torres, A., Bauer, T. T., Nicolas, J. M., Nogue, S., & Ferrer, M. (1999). Supine body position as a risk factor for nosocomial pneumonia in mechanically ventilated patients: A randomised trial. *Lancet, 354*(9193), 1851–1858.

Epocrates.com. (2004). Epocrates essentials, drug information program. Retrieved November 13, 2004, from www.epocrates.com.

Feinberg, M. J., Knebl, J., & Tully, J. (1996). Prandial aspiration and pneumonia in an elderly population followed over 3 years. *Dysphagia, 11,* 104–109.

Finucane, T. E., Christmas, C., & Travis, K. (1999). Tube feeding in patients with advanced dementia: A review of the evidence. *Journal of the American Medical Association, 282*(14), 1365–1370.

Garnett, W. (2000). *Irritable bowel syndrome.* Power-Pak C.E., Power-Pak Communications, Retrieved July 29, 2001, from www.powerpak.com.

Geronurse Online. (2004). *Mealtime difficulties.* Retrieved September 9, 2004, from www.geronurseonline.org.

Gibson, C., Opalka, P., Moore, C., Brady, R., & Mion, L. (1995). Effectiveness of bran supplement on the bowel management of elderly rehabilitation patients. *Journal of Gerontological Nursing, 21*(10), 21–30.

Herbert, S. (1996). A team approach to the treatment of dysphagia. *Nursing Times, 82*(50), 26–34.

Hope, A., & Down, E. (1986). Dietary fiber and fluid in the control of constipation in a nursing home population. *Medical Journal of Australia, 144,* 306–307.

Horowitz, M. (2004). Aging and the gastrointestinal tract. In M. Beers & R. Berkow (Eds.), *Merck manual of geriatrics.* Retrieved August 4, 2004, from www.merck.com.

Howard, L., West, D., & Ossip-Klein, D. (2000). Chronic constipation management for institutionalized older adults. *Geriatric Nursing, 21*(2), 78–82.

Kayser-Jones, J., & Pengilly, K. (1999). Dysphagia among nursing home residents. *Geriatric Nursing, 20*(2), 77–84.

Kosta, J., & Mitchell, C. (1998). Current procedures for diagnosing dysphagia in elderly clients. *Geriatric Nursing, 19*(4), 195–199.

Langmore, S. E., Terpenning, M. S., Schork, A., Chen, Y., Murray, J. T., Lopatin, D., & Loesche, W. J. (1998). Predictors of aspiration pneumonia: How important is dysphagia? *Dysphagia, 13*(2), 69–81.

Lazarus, B. A., Murphy, J. B., & Culpepper, L. (1990). Aspiration associated with long-term gastric versus jejunal feeding: A critical analysis of the literature. *Archives of Physical Medicine and Rehabilitation, 71*(1), 46–53.

Leibovitz, A., Plotnikov, G., Habot, B., Rosenberg, M., & Segal, R. (2003). Pathogenic colonization of oral flora in frail elderly patients fed by nasogastric tube or percutaneous enterogastric tube. *Journal of Gerontology Series A—Biological Sciences and Medical Sciences, 58*(1), 52–58.

Loeb, M. B., Becker, M., Eady, A., & Walker-Dilks, C. (2003). Interventions to prevent aspiration pneumonia in older adults: A systematic review. *Journal of the American Geriatrics Society, 51*(7), 1018–1022.

Luxon, B. (2004). Liver and biliary disorders. In M. Beers & R. Berkow (Eds.), *Merck manual of geriatrics.* Retrieved September 16, 2004, from www.merck.com.

Marik, P. E., & Kaplan, D. (2003). Aspiration pneumonia and dysphagia in the elderly. *Chest, 124*(1), 328–336.

Marrie, T. J. (2000). Community-acquired pneumonia in the elderly. *Clinical Infectious Disease, 31*(40), 1066–1078.

Marrie, T. J. (2002). Pneumonia in the long-term care facility. *Infection Control and Hospital Epidemiology, 23*(3), 159–164.

McCance, K., & Huether, S. (2001). *Pathophysiology: The biologic basis for disease in adults and children.* St. Louis, MO: Mosby.

McClave, S. A., DeMeo, M. T., DeLegge, M. H., DiSario, J. A., Heyland, D. K., Maloney, J. P., et al. (2002). North American Summit on Aspiration in the Critically Ill Patient: Consensus statement. *Journal of Parenteral and Enteral Nutrition, 26*(Suppl. 6), S80–85.

McCrea, L. (2003). *Anatomy and physiology of constipation. New approaches to the management of constipation.* Symposium highlights, Medical Association Communications, Wrightstown, PA.

Metheney, N. (2004). Preventing aspiration in persons with dysphagia. *Try this: Best practices in nursing care to older adults. Vol. 20, Fall.* New York: Hartford Institute of Geriatric Nursing, New York University.

Moore, A., & Clinch, D. (2004). Underlying mechanisms of impaired visceral pain perception in older people. *Journal of the American Geriatrics Society, 52,* 132–136.

National Digestive Disease Information Clearinghouse. (2003). Your digestive system and how it works. Retrieved February 6, 2004, from www.digestive.NIDDK.NIH.gov.

North American Nursing Diagnosis Association. (2003). *Nursing diagnoses: Definitions and classifications.* Philadelphia: Author.

Prather, C. (2004). Constipation, diarrhea and fecal incontinence. In M. Beers & R. Berkow (Eds.), *Merck manual of geriatrics.* Retrieved August 16, 2004, from www.merck.com.

Ray, S., Secrest, J., Ch'ien, A., & Corey, R. (2002). Managing gastroesophageal reflux disease. *Nurse Practitioner, 27*(5), 36–50.

Reuben, D., Herr, K., Pacala, J., Potter, J., Pollock, B., & Semla, T. (2002). *Gastrointestinal diseases: Geriatrics at your fingertips.* Malden, MA: Blackwell.

Schiller, L. (2002). The pathophysiology of constipation. *Sessions in Primary Care, 5,* 5–6.

Schulz, J. (2004). Anorectal disorders. In M. Beers & R. Berkow (Eds.), *Merck manual of geriatrics.* Retrieved January 15, 2004, from www.merck.com.

Shanahan, T. K., Logemann, J. A., Rademaker, A. W., Pauloski, B. R., & Kahrilas, P. J. (1993). Chin-down posture effect on aspiration in dysphagic patients. *Archives of Physical Medicine and Rehabilitation, 74,* 736–739.

Shang, E., Geiger, N., & Sturm, J. (2004). Pump-assisted enteral nutrition can prevent aspiration in bedridden percutaneous endoscopic gastrostomy patients. *Journal of Parenteral and Enteral Nutrition, 28*(3), 180–183.

Siddique, R., Neslusan, C. A., Crown, W. H., Crystal-Peters, J., Sloan, S., Farup, C., et al. (2000). A national inpatient cost estimate of percutaneous endoscopic gastrostomy associated aspiration pneumonia. *American Journal of Managed Care, 6*(4), 490–496.

Smith, D., & Newman, D. (1989). The bran solution. *Contemporary Long Term Care, 12,* 66.

Terpening, M. S., Taylor, G. W., Lopatin, D. E., Kerr, C. K., Dominguez, L., & Loesche, W. J. (2001). Aspiration pneumonia: Dental and oral risk factors in an older veteran population. *Journal of the American Geriatrics Society, 49*(5), 557–563.

Thomas, D., Goode, P. S., & LaMaster, K. (2003). Clinical consensus: The constipation crisis in long-term care. *Supplement to the Annals of Long-Term Care, (S),* October, 2–12.

Tompkins, R. (2004). Acute abdomen and surgical gastroenterology. In M. Beers & R. Berkow (Eds.), *Merck manual of geriatrics.* Retrieved January 22, 2004, from www.merck.com.

Van Gerpen, R. (2003). Colorectal cancer. *Massachusetts Report on Nursing, Sept.,* Vol. 9, 18–23.

Wald, A. (2004). Lower gastrointestinal tract disorders. In M. Beers & R. Berkow (Eds.), *Merck manual of geriatrics.* Retrieved January 22, 2004, from www.merck.com.

Waye, J. (2004). Endoscopic gastrointestinal procedures. In M. Beers & R. Berkow (Eds.), *Merck manual of geriatrics.* Retrieved January 20, 2004, from www.merck.com.

Wollner, T. (2004). Eradicate *H. pylori* with effective treatment regimens. *Nurse Practitioner, 29*(6), 40–44.

Yoneyama, T., Yoshida, M., Ohrui, T., Mukaiyama, H., Okamoto, H., Hoshiba, K., et al. (2002). Oral care reduces pneumonia in older patients in nursing homes. *Journal of the American Geriatrics Society, 50*(3), 430–433.

CHAPTER 21

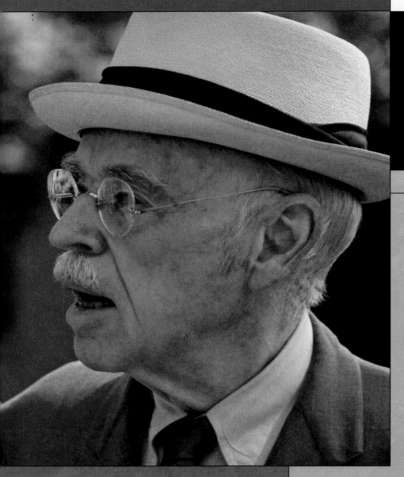

The Hematologic System

CHAPTER OBJECTIVES

Upon completion of this chapter, the reader will be able to:

- Describe age-related changes that affect hematologic function.

- Describe the impact of age-related changes on hematologic function.

- Identify risk factors to health for the older person with hematologic problems.

- Describe the unique presentation of hematologic problems in the older person.

- Define appropriate nursing interventions directed toward assisting older adults with hematologic problems to develop self-care abilities.

- Identify and implement appropriate nursing interventions to care for the older person with hematologic problems.

KEY TERMS

MediaLink

Additional resources for this chapter can be found on the Student CD-ROM accompanying this textbook and on the Companion Website at **www.prenhall.com/tabloski**. Click on Chapter 21 to select the activities for this chapter.

CD-ROM
- NCLEX Review
- Case Studies
- Tools

COMPANION WEBSITE
- Audio Glossary
- Additional NCLEX Review
- Case Study
- MediaLink Applications

The hematologic system is responsible for many functions in the body and serves as a medium of exchange between the outside environment and the body's cells. The main function of the circulating blood is to carry oxygen and nutrients to and remove carbon dioxide and waste products from the internal organs and peripheral tissue. Additionally, blood transports other substances such as hormones, proteins, solutes, water, and medications to sites where they are needed. Blood contributes to homeostasis by regulating the acid-base balance, thus maintaining a constant internal body environment. Blood consists of red blood cells, white blood cells, **platelets**, and **plasma**. Plasma accounts for about 55% of the blood, and blood volume accounts for 7% of total body weight (Berne & Levy, 2000). Blood volume in adults is about 6 quarts (5.5 L). Older patients with diseases associated with blood and blood-forming organs may experience health problems that range from minor disruptions in functional ability to major life-threatening problems (LeMone & Burke, 2004).

Erythrocytes, or red blood cells (RBCs), have a life span of about 120 days. They are flexible concave disks that arise from stem cells in the **bone marrow**. Erythrocytes are composed of **hemoglobin**, a protein that binds with oxygen to form oxyhemoglobin. Old RBCs are destroyed in the spleen, liver, bone marrow, and lymph nodes by **phagocytes** that save and reuse key materials from the destroyed RBCs, including proteins and iron. The number of circulating RBCs remains fairly stable under normal conditions, but illness, blood loss, toxic substances, and nutritional deficiencies can decrease the number of circulating cells and result in **anemia**. Anemia occurs whenever the hemoglobin content of the blood is insufficient to satisfy body demands (LeMone & Burke, 2004). Erythropoiesis, or the production of RBCs, is regulated by erythropoietin, a hormone secreted by the kidneys that stimulates the cells in the bone marrow. Erythropoietin is released by the kidneys in response to hypoxia and stimulates the bone marrow to produce RBCs. This process usually takes about 5 days to reach a maximum and will result in the release of a higher percentage of reticulocytes or immature RBCs in the circulation (LeMone & Burke, 2004).

Practice Pearl

Anemia is a sign and symptom of disease—not a disease itself. When an older person is diagnosed with anemia, the underlying condition should be diagnosed before the anemia is corrected.

Normally, about 4,000 to 10,000 **leukocytes**, or white blood cells (WBCs), are present in a microliter of blood. The function of WBCs is to protect the body and form a defense against invading microorganisms. The WBCs include granulocytes (65%), lymphocytes (30%), and monocytes (5%). The granulocytes are composed mostly of neutrophils (60% to 70%), eosinophils (4%), and basophils (1%). Granulocytes and monocytes (immature macrophages) are produced in the bone marrow, and lymphocytes are produced in the lymph nodes, spleen, and thymus. The function of the granulocytes and monocytes is to engage in phagocytosis and help the body to fight off infections by surrounding and dissolving invading microorganisms. The B lymphocytes are responsible for humoral and cell-mediated immunity. When stimulated by an antigen (a foreign protein or allergen), some lymphocytes are transformed into plasma cells to release antibodies. Antibodies are carried by the bloodstream to the site of infection and will bind with foreign proteins to destroy or neutralize their biological functions (Berne & Levy, 2000).

Platelets are small cell fragments that reside in bone marrow. When mature, they enter the circulation as platelets. Platelets are essential for blood coagulation and control bleeding. The spleen holds about one third of the platelets in reserve for use in the body. A platelet lives approximately 10 days, after which it dies and is removed by macrophages (McCance & Huether, 2001).

In humans, there are four major types of blood groups: O, A, B, and AB. These groups differ by the nature of the antigens (A and B) present on the RBCs. Persons with blood type A have A antigens present, those with type B have B antigens, those who are type AB have both antigens, and those who are type O have neither antigen. ABO antibodies develop in the serum of persons whose RBCs lack the corresponding antigen. These antibodies are called anti-A and anti-B. Persons with blood type A have anti-B antibodies, and persons with blood type B have anti-A antibodies. Because plasma of persons with blood types A, B, and AB has no antibodies to group O red blood cells, people with group O blood are called universal donors. Conversely, persons with AB blood are called universal recipients, because their plasma has no antibodies to antigens in the other three groups (Berne & Levy, 2000). A third antigen on the red blood cell is D. People who are Rh positive have the D antigen, and those who are Rh negative do not have this antigen. The presence of these antigens and antibodies may cause ABO and Rh incompatibilities unless the appropriate blood type is administered during transfusion. An acute hemolytic transfusion reaction can occur when an ABO incompatibility results when an antigen-antibody of the recipient reacts to blood of the donor who has a different antigen.

Normal Changes of Aging

Most of the changes of aging in the hematologic system are the result of reduced capacity of the bone marrow to produce RBCs quickly when disease or blood loss has occurred. However, without major blood loss or the diagnosis of a serious illness, the bone marrow changes are not clinically significant. Figure 21-1☐ illustrates the normal changes of aging in the hematologic system.

At about age 70, the amount of bone marrow in the long bones begins to decline steadily. Additional changes of aging in the hematologic system include the following:

- The number of stem cells in the marrow is decreased.
- The administration of erythropoietin to stimulate use of iron to form RBCs is less effective in older persons than in younger persons.
- Lymphocyte function, especially cellular immunity, appears to decrease with age.
- Platelet adhesiveness increases with age.
- Average hemoglobin and **hematocrit** values decrease slightly with age but remain within normal limits.

Many functions of the hematologic system remain constant in healthy older persons, including RBC life span, total blood volume, RBC volume, total lymphocyte and granulocyte counts, and platelet structure and function (Berne & Levy, 2000; Friedman, 2004; McCance & Huether, 2001).

Common Disorders in Aging

With aging, several common disorders can occur in the hematologic system. Most common of these disorders is anemia, a condition often falsely attributed to normal aging.

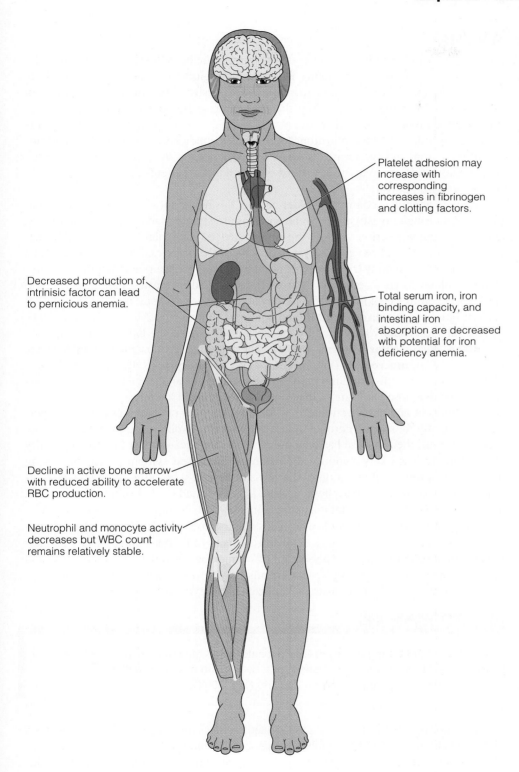

Platelet adhesion may increase with corresponding increases in fibrinogen and clotting factors.

Decreased production of intrinisic factor can lead to pernicious anemia.

Total serum iron, iron binding capacity, and intestinal iron absorption are decreased with potential for iron deficiency anemia.

Decline in active bone marrow with reduced ability to accelerate RBC production.

Neutrophil and monocyte activity decreases but WBC count remains relatively stable.

ANEMIA

Anemia, or insufficient hemoglobin content to meet the body's needs, is defined as decreases in the number of circulating RBCs or hemoglobin resulting from blood loss, impaired production of RBCs, or increased RBC destruction. Anemia is common in older persons. Although old age alone does not increase the chances of developing anemia, many chronic illnesses that occur with aging can be responsible. Chronic disorders such as kidney disease, nutritional deficiencies, medication use, chronic infections or inflammation, and endocrine disorders are associated with various types of anemia (Friedman, 2004). As many as one third of hospitalized patients have anemia (Blackwell & Hendrix, 2001).

Although anemia is common in older people, it is never normal and it requires complete and thorough investigation. Some anemias are simply markers of chronic illness, and others indicate serious underlying illness such as malignant neoplasms. All anemias result in a loss of oxygen-carrying capacity of the blood and produce generalized tissue hypoxia. The body tries to compensate by raising the heart and respiratory rates, shunting blood to vital organs away from the skin, and increasing blood viscosity to supply oxygen to hypoxic tissues. The physiological results may include skin pallor, chronic fatigue, dyspnea on exertion, and bone and joint pain (LeMone & Burke, 2004).

Anemias are usually classified by measuring the size of the RBCs and computing the **mean corpuscular volume (MCV)**. The resulting groups include **microcytic** (smaller RBCs), **macrocytic** (larger RBCs), and **normocytic** (RBCs of normal size). However, some anemias fall into more than one category, and sometimes an older person may be diagnosed with more than one type or a mixed anemia.

Symptoms of anemia are similar for older and younger people; however, older persons, especially those with chronic illness and mobility problems, may not experience symptoms until their disease has become more severe because they are not physically active and are less likely to notice the troubling signs and symptoms accompanying anemia. Symptoms include fatigue, shortness of breath, worsening of angina, and developing or worsening of peripheral edema. Dizziness and mental status changes such as confusion, depression, agitation, and apathy may also occur as symptoms of anemia, especially in the frail older adult who is less likely to be physically active and to exhibit the more common musculoskeletal and cardiac symptoms. Pallor, usually less noticeable in the older person and persons of color, may be noticed in the oral mucosa and conjunctiva (Friedman, 2004). Severe anemia may result in tachycardia, palpitations, systolic murmurs, and angina with ischemic changes evident on electrocardiogram.

Practice Pearl

Judicious blood testing in hospitalized patients would minimize anemia resulting from blood loss for laboratory testing, especially in intensive care patients and others subjected to frequent blood drawing (Toy, 2004).

Evaluation of the older person with suspected anemia should begin with laboratory tests including measurement of hemoglobin, hematocrit, red blood cell count and indices, reticulocyte count, white blood cell count and differential, and platelet count. A man is considered anemic with a hemoglobin concentration below 13 g/dl, and the cutoff for a woman is below 12 g/dl. Hemoglobin concentrations will be artificially higher in a dehydrated older person and in those who smoke cigarettes or live at high altitudes. Hemoglobin concentrations are 0.5 to 1.0 g/dl lower in African Americans of both sexes (Toy, 2004).

TABLE 21-1

Laboratory Tests to Determine Anemia

Test	Purpose	Normal Value
Transferrin	Regulates iron absorption and transport. *Increased* in iron deficiency anemia due to hemorrhage and acute hepatitis. *Decreased* in anemia of chronic disease and protein deficiency.	240–480 mg/dl
Serum iron	Transferrin bound iron. Used in combination with transferrin test and TIBC. Serum iron levels vary throughout the day and are higher in the morning.	Men: 75–175 µg/dl Women: 65–165 µg/dl
Total iron-binding capacity (TIBC)	Reflects the transferrin content of the serum. When the body is deficient in iron (iron deficiency anemia), the TIBC is increased.	250–450 mg/dl
Serum ferritin	An iron compound found in the intestinal mucosa, spleen, and liver. Contains >20% iron and is essential for **hematopoiesis**. Indicates adequacy of iron stores. *Increased* in iron overload, acute hepatitis, and chronic inflammatory disorders. *Decreased* in iron deficiency anemia.	Men: 18–270 ng/ml Women: 18–160 ng/ml
Mean corpuscular volume (MCV)	Index for classifying anemias on size of the red cell. Indicates whether the RBC is normocytic, microcytic, or macrocytic. *Decreased* MCV in iron deficiency anemia. *Increased* with B_{12} and folic acid deficiency. *Normal* in anemia of chronic disease.	Men: 84–96 fl Women: 76–96 fl
Mean corpuscular hemoglobin concentration (MCHC)	A measure of the average hemoglobin concentration in the RBCs. A decreased MCHC signifies that a unit volume of packed RBCs contains less hemoglobin than normal.	27–32 pg
Reticulocyte count	Reticulocytes are immature cells in the RBC cycle and last 1–2 days in the circulation before the RBC matures. *Increased* in hemolytic anemia, leukemia, sickle cell anemia, and after acute hemorrhage. *Decreased* in iron deficiency and aplastic anemia, untreated pernicious anemia, anemia of chronic disease, and bone marrow disease.	Men: 0.5%–1.5% of total RBCs Women: 0.5%–2.5% of total RBCs

Important laboratory tests to determine anemia and their normal values are listed in Table 21-1.

Microcytic Anemias

Anemias are classified as microcytic if the MCV is less than 80 fl. In older people, microcytic anemias can result from iron deficiency and thalassemia minor (a result of inadequate globin synthesis). Anemia of chronic disease can be microcytic but is more commonly normocytic, especially early in the disease process (Friedman, 2004). Iron deficiency anemia is characterized by small, pale RBCs and eventual depletion of iron stores. The body cannot synthesize hemoglobin without iron, and gradually the number of RBCs decreases. Serum ferritin levels usually accurately reflect bone marrow iron stores; however, these may remain normal early in the process before iron stores are depleted. The reticulocyte count is usually decreased. Serum ferritin levels of less than 10 µg/L are highly diagnostic of iron deficiency (Friedman, 2004).

> **Practice Pearl**
>
> Serum ferritin concentrations can be falsely elevated in patients with liver damage or certain cancers (Blackwell & Hendrix, 2001).

Iron deficiency can occur as the result of acute blood loss (from surgery or trauma) or chronic blood loss (from gastrointestinal bleeding, hemorrhoids, or cancer). It may also result from inadequate dietary intake of iron or malabsorption of iron. In menstruating women, blood loss is the most common cause of iron deficiency; however, in men or postmenopausal women, the first site to consider for possible blood loss is the gastrointestinal tract. Excessive blood donation and frequent phlebotomies (patients who are on warfarin or hospitalized) are causes that are often overlooked (Blackwell & Hendrix, 2001).

Once the cause of the iron deficiency has been identified, oral iron therapy is the preferred treatment. Stool should be tested for occult blood, and additional gastrointestinal testing (colonoscopy or barium studies) may be necessary. Iron therapy should never be recommended for an older person with iron deficiency anemia without identifying the reason for occult blood loss. Correcting the symptom without knowing the underlying cause of the problem can mask the symptoms of serious disease like cancer.

The usual treatment is ferrous sulfate 325 mg daily. Enteric-coated and sustained-release formulations should be avoided, because they are poorly absorbed. A single daily dose of ferrous sulfate reduces the risk of constipation and gastric irritation. Increasing the dose only minimally increases iron absorption; however, the nurse should carefully monitor the older person taking iron supplements and report new-onset constipation and symptoms of gastrointestinal distress. Therapeutic response is monitored by measuring the serum hemoglobin, hematocrit, and ferritin levels in about 2 months, and it may take up to a year to fully replenish iron stores in the marrow (Friedman, 2004).

Thalassemia is an inherited disorder of hemoglobin synthesis in which parts of the hemoglobin molecular chain are missing or defective. As a result the RBC is fragile, hypochromic, and microcytic. Thalassemia occurs mostly in persons of Mediterranean (Greek or Italian) descent, but may be found in persons of Asian or African descent (LeMone & Burke, 2004). The disease is usually diagnosed in infancy or childhood, and most undiagnosed adults will have the disease in a milder form that may go unnoticed until late in life. The diagnosis is made by a hematologist using serum electrophoresis. Iron replacement is not indicated and may result in iron overload (Friedman, 2004).

Normocytic Anemia

The most common types of normocytic anemia in the older person are anemia of chronic disease, hemolytic anemia, and aplastic anemia. Anemia in which the MCV is 30 to 100 fl is considered normocytic as the RBCs are of normal size. Normocytic anemia is usually caused by concurrent chronic illness (heart, respiratory, or renal disease, or malignancy), and anemia of chronic disease is the most common type of normocytic anemia.

Anemia of chronic disease is usually associated with malnutrition or conditions such as chronic infection or inflammation, cancer, renal insufficiency, chronic liver disease, endocrine disorders, and malnutrition. These diseases influence RBC production in the following manner:

- **Chronic infection and inflammation.** After 4 to 8 weeks of illness, anemia may result from slightly decreased erythropoietin production, decreased RBC survival, and impaired transport of iron to the bone marrow. The reticulocyte count is low, serum iron is normal or slightly reduced, and serum ferritin is normal or elevated. When the underlying disease is treated and the infection or inflammation resolves, the anemia disappears.
- **Renal insufficiency.** This anemia results from decreased erythropoiesis and decreased RBC survival. Serum iron stores are normal. In hemodialysis patients, injections of erythropoietin may reverse the anemia. In nondialysis patients, erythropoietin is not as effective because erythropoietic inhibitors can accumulate. Erythropoietin is given intravenously to hemodialysis patients and subcutaneously to nondialysis patients with renal failure in an attempt to produce more prolonged bone marrow stimulation (Friedman, 2004).
- **Chronic liver disease.** Normocytic anemia results from decreased RBC production and survival. Large quantities of alcohol are toxic to the bone marrow and the liver as well as other organs of the body. The result is decreased serum iron levels and total iron-binding capacity. Treatment is aimed at stopping the progression of or correcting the underlying liver disease.
- **Malnutrition.** When essential nutrients such as folic acid and vitamin C are missing, RBC production decreases, resulting in a normocytic anemia. Nutritional deficiencies can also result from malabsorption disorders or heightened need for nutrients when nutritional intake is adequate.
- **Malignancies.** Cancer in the later stages is nearly always accompanied by anemia of chronic disease. Chemotherapy can suppress bone marrow function and contribute to decreased appetite, nausea and vomiting, and nutritional deficiencies leading to inadequate caloric, protein, and vitamin intake. Erythropoietin injected subcutaneously is sometimes used to treat anemia and fatigue in older patients with nonmyeloid cancers.

Diseases associated with anemia of chronic disease include:

- Acute infections—bacterial, fungal, or viral.
- Chronic infections—osteomyelitis, infective endocarditis, chronic urinary tract infection, tuberculosis, or chronic fungal disease.
- Inflammatory disorders—rheumatoid disease, systemic lupus erythematosus, burns, severe trauma, and acute and chronic hepatitis.
- Malignancy—carcinoma, myeloma, lymphoma, leukemia.
- Chronic renal failure.

(Rasul & Kandel, 2001)

Hemolytic anemia is also a normocytic anemia that can occur at any age, but it becomes more common with aging. When the **hemolysis** or premature destruction of RBCs increases, the body compensates by increasing production of immature RBCs in the bone marrow, resulting in increased numbers of circulating reticulocytes in the blood. The causes of increased RBC destruction may be associated with increased autoimmune antibodies, inherited enzyme deficits (G6PD deficiency), infections such as syphilis, leukemia, Hodgkin's disease and non-Hodgkin's lymphoma, trauma, mechanical factors (prosthetic heart valves), burns, exposure to toxic chemicals and venoms, and drugs (Friedman, 2004; LeMone & Burke, 2004).

Drugs capable of causing hemolytic anemia include ibuprofen, l-dopa, penicillin, drugs classified as cephalosporins, tetracycline, acetaminophen, aspirin, erythromycin, hydralazine, hydrochlorothiazide, insulin, isoniazid, methadone, phenacetin, procainamide, quinidine, rifampin, streptomycin, sulfonamides, and triamterene (Epocrates.com, 2004; Friedman, 2004). Increased destruction results in increased levels of unconjugated bilirubin. The indirect Coombs' test is used to detect antibody of complement on the RBC. Hemolysis usually stops quickly when the drug is withdrawn (Friedman, 2004).

All hemolytic anemias require folic acid treatment because this vitamin is used up with increased bone marrow production of RBCs. Folic acid is absorbed from the intestine and is found in green leafy vegetables, fruits, cereals, and meats. Deficiencies are often found in chronically undernourished persons. When the cause of the hemolytic anemia cannot be found, prednisone is sometimes used to treat this idiopathic autoimmune hemolysis. More commonly, the identifying drug can be identified. Drug-induced hemolysis is usually treated by simply discontinuing the responsible drug.

Aplastic anemia is not very common and is usually a disease of adolescents and young adults, but it can occur in old age. The cause of aplastic anemia is unknown in the majority of cases, but this anemia may sometimes develop as a result of damage to the cells in the bone marrow by radiation or chemical substances (benzene, arsenic, chloramphenicol, and chemotherapeutic agents). The overall mortality rate is greater than 50%. In this disorder the reticulocyte count is low, and the bone marrow function is suppressed and hypoplastic and does not produce adequate numbers of RBCs. Treatment involves discontinuation of all medications and administration of ongoing blood transfusions. Bone marrow transplantation is usually not effective in patients over the age of 65 (Friedman, 2004).

Macrocytic Anemias

Anemias are classified as macrocytic if the MCV is greater than 100 fl. The most common cause of macrocytic anemia in the older person is B_{12} or folate deficiency. Vitamin B_{12} deficiencies can occur when the amount of the vitamin in the diet is inadequate or, more commonly, when sufficient amounts are not absorbed from the gastrointestinal tract. Failure to absorb vitamin B_{12} from the gastrointestinal tract is called pernicious anemia and results from a lack of intrinsic factor. About 12% of older people have low serum vitamin B_{12} levels (<300 pg/ml). Neurologic damage, such as neuropathies, paresthesias, and cognitive impairment, may occur before the anemia is discovered. Additional causes of macrocytic anemia include hypothyroidism, chronic liver disease, and drugs such as chemotherapeutic agents and anticonvulsants (Friedman, 2004).

Pernicious anemia results when an older person lacks the needed intrinsic factor to absorb vitamin B_{12}. As only about 1% of older persons lack intrinsic factor, a more common cause of low serum vitamin B_{12} results from the inability to split vitamin B_{12} from proteins in food. This inability may be the result of a deficiency of hydrochloric acid or pancreatic enzymes. Other causes of B_{12} deficiency include gastrectomy, small bowel disease, *Helicobacter pylori* infection, prolonged use of antacids, intestinal bacterial overgrowth, cachexia, and adherence to a strict vegetarian diet (Friedman, 2004).

The signs and symptoms of B_{12} deficiency may take years to develop and are often subtle. Mental status may be affected, and cognitive impairment, depression, mania, and other psychiatric syndromes may develop. Neurologic findings will include peripheral neuropathies, numbness and tingling in the extremities, and ataxia and difficulty walking and maintaining balance. Unfortunately, correcting the B_{12} deficiency does not usually reverse or improve mental status but may halt the progression of the symptoms. Laboratory tests used to detect low levels of B_{12} may not be abnormal until the older person becomes overtly anemic. In addition to a large MCV, leukopenia and thrombocytopenia may occur.

The diagnosis of vitamin B_{12} deficiency has traditionally been based on low serum vitamin B_{12} levels, usually less than 200 pg/ml, along with clinical evidence of disease. However, studies indicate that older patients tend to present with neurologic effects and cognitive disorders in the absence of anemia. Furthermore, measurements of metabolites such as methylmalonic acid and homocysteine have been shown to be more sensitive in the diagnosis of vitamin B_{12} deficiency than measurement of serum B_{12} levels alone (Oh & Brown, 2003).

Drug Alert

The widespread use of gastric acid–blocking agents may contribute to the eventual development of vitamin B_{12} deficiency because these medications neutralize the acidic environment that is needed to break down and release vitamin B_{12} bound to the ingested food. When caring for an older patient on long-term acid suppression therapy, methylmalonic acid and homocysteine levels should be monitored periodically.

The Schilling test was once relied upon to determine if the digestive tract is capable of absorbing an adequate amount of vitamin B_{12} to maintain health, and the test provided information as to whether the patient would require parenteral B_{12} supplementation. However, the Schilling test is complex, radiolabeled vitamin B_{12} is difficult to obtain, and interpretation of test results can be problematic in patients with renal insufficiency (Oh & Brown, 2003). In the Schilling test, the patient swallows a capsule containing a small amount of radioactive vitamin B_{12}. Two hours later, the patient receives an intramuscular injection of normal nonradioactive vitamin B_{12}. This injection forces any radioactive vitamin B_{12} the patient has absorbed through the gastrointestinal tract into the urine. Following the injection, all urine is collected for a 24-hour period. A complete urine collection is essential for the accuracy of the Schilling test. The amount of vitamin B_{12} the body was able to absorb is calculated from the amount of B_{12} excreted in the 24-hour urine. The information obtained in the Schilling test is now unnecessary because evidence points to a B_{12} absorption pathway independent of intrinsic factor, and studies have shown that oral replacement is equal in efficacy to intramuscular therapy. Regardless of the test result, successful treatment can still be achieved with oral replacement therapy (Oh & Brown, 2003).

For those with pernicious anemia, treatment usually consists of lifelong B_{12} replacement. Because most clinicians are generally unaware that oral vitamin B_{12} therapy is effective, the traditional treatment for B_{12} deficiency has been intramuscular injections. The usual intramuscular dose is 1,000 µg/day for the first week, then 1,000 µg/week for 4 weeks, and then 1,000 µg/month for life. Although the daily requirement of vitamin B_{12} is approximately 2 µg, the initial oral replacement dosage consists of a single daily dose of 1,000 to 2,000 µg. This high dose is required because of the variable absorption of oral vitamin B_{12} in smaller doses. The oral replacement should be taken on an empty stomach. It has been shown to be safe, cost-effective, and well tolerated by patients (Oh & Brown, 2003). Approximately 1 month of treatment is needed to correct the anemia. Treatment with folic acid alone may improve the anemia, but it will not prevent further decline or improve existing neurologic changes associated with the B_{12} deficiency (Friedman, 2004). Folic acid supplementation may mask an occult vitamin B_{12} deficiency and further exacerbate or initiate neurologic disease (Oh & Brown, 2003).

Folic acid deficiency produces laboratory results similar to those found with B_{12} deficiency. Serum folate levels will measure below 4 ng/ml, and B_{12} levels are normal in early folate deficiencies. Folate deficiency is not common in the healthy older person but may be found in older people with malabsorption syndromes, poor nutrition, alcoholism, and underlying malignancies. Foods high in folate include liver, orange juice, cereals, whole grains, beans, nuts, and dark green leafy vegetables like spinach. Chronic use of certain drugs such as triamterene, trimethoprim, anticonvulsants, and nitrofurantoin can also cause folic acid deficiency by blocking folic acid metabolism. It usually takes about 6 months to deplete the folic acid from body storage (Kado et al., 2004).

Laboratory testing usually reveals a macrocytic RBC and low serum folate levels (<2 ng/ml) or low RBC folate levels (<100 ng/ml). However, RBC folate levels are a more stable marker and more clinically reliable. Treatment consists of folic acid 1 mg/day by mouth (Friedman, 2004).

Drug Alert !

In older patients with macrocytic anemia due to a B_{12} deficiency, treatment with folic acid alone may correct the anemia but will not prevent or reverse neurologic damage as a result of the B_{12} deficiency.

Sickle Cell Anemia

Sickle cell anemia is an inherited disease in which the RBCs are crescent shaped. As a result, they tend to form small clots and clump together. These clots give rise to recurrent painful episodes called sickle cell crises. Symptoms of sickle cell disease begin at about 4 months of age. Complications of the disease include lung disease, kidney and liver failure, gallstones, joint destruction, blindness, neurologic symptoms, and stroke. Approximately 1 out of every 500 African Americans has sickle cell disease, and about 1 in 12 has the trait or carries the gene that can cause the disease if he or she has a child with another carrier. In the past, death from organ failure occurred between the ages of 20 and 40 years in most persons with sickle cell disease. Now with better management, patients are living into their 50s and 60s. Persons with sickle cell disease should avoid infection, consume a balanced diet, avoid dehydration, and avoid stress as these factors can precipitate a sickle cell crisis (Medline Plus, 2004).

TRANSFUSIONS

Many older people gradually adjust to being anemic by conserving energy and adopting sedentary lifestyles. Some care providers attribute lack of energy to aging and fail to diagnose anemia. Therefore, severe anemias may be present for long periods of time and avoid detection. Severe anemia can lead to myocardial infarction, falls, confusion, and other serious complications. When quick reversal of anemia is indicated, a transfusion may be needed. There is no agreement among clinicians on when a transfusion is needed, but when the older patient's hematocrit is below 30% and he or she is experiencing symptoms such as shortness of breath or chest pain, a blood transfusion may be needed (Toy, 2004).

Older patients are subject to fluid overload and are at risk for acute heart failure. Therefore, the physician may request transfusion with packed red blood cells (most of the plasma removed) to reduce the volume to be transfused. By administering packed red blood cells, anemia can be improved and volume replacement is not required. Signs of fluid overload include elevated systolic blood pressure, jugular vein distention, crackles, dyspnea, tachycardia, peripheral edema, cyanosis, and headache. Early detection and physician notification allows more time for the implementation of appropriate treatments including discontinuation of further intravenous fluids and administration of diuretics.

Most transfusions for older people are given slowly over a 4-hour period. If several units of packed cells are to be infused, often a diuretic (20 mg furosemide) is given orally between units to prevent fluid overload and congestive heart failure. Older people may have more fragile veins, and venous access may be more difficult. Therefore, older people are at increased risk for infiltration. The IV site should be carefully secured and frequently observed for signs of infiltration including bruising, swelling, and accumulation of fluid into the soft tissue surrounding the site. The gerontological nurse should carefully monitor the older patient's vital signs and urinary output during the transfusion process.

As with all transfusions, the patient's blood type must match the donor's. To prevent transfusion errors and potentially fatal hemolytic reactions, the blood will be tested by type and crossmatch each time the patient requires a transfusion. The hemolytic reaction that can occur when a patient receives an incompatible blood transfusion is life threatening, and every precaution must be taken both in the laboratory and at the bedside to ensure that the patient and the blood type are correctly identified and matched. Hemolytic reactions can progress to oliguria, renal failure, and disseminated intravascular clotting with uncontrolled hemorrhage.

CHRONIC MYELOPROLIFERATIVE DISORDERS

Chronic myeloproliferative disorders are characterized by abnormal proliferation of one or more hematopoietic processes and become more common with age. These classic disorders include primary thrombocythemia, polycythemia vera, and myelofibrosis.

Thrombocythemia is characterized by an increased number of circulating platelets in the blood. Older patients with thrombocythemia are more likely to exhibit uncontrolled bleeding with hemorrhage or develop clot formation. The average age of diagnosis is 60 years, and it is more common in women. Symptoms are absent or vague and may include headache, visual disturbances, and burning pain and erythema of the hands and feet. Accurate diagnosis requires bone marrow aspiration. Usually, the treatment includes administration of hydroxyurea to suppress platelet formation, and the goal is to keep the platelet count below 400,000/μl. Older persons with thrombocythemia are at significantly increased risk of thrombosis, and careful monitoring of platelet levels and symptoms is indicated (Tefferi, 2004).

Polycythemia vera is a chronic stem cell disorder characterized by an increase in hemoglobin concentration and uncontrolled production of mature RBCs. Approximately 90% of persons with this disease are diagnosed after age 60. The condition is relatively rare but is most common in Caucasian men of European Jewish ancestry (LeMone & Burke, 2004). Symptoms of the disease are absent initially but later progress to findings common in hypervolemia, including headache, dizziness, hypertension, visual disturbances, weight loss, and night sweats. Itching after bathing is a common complaint. Complications include thrombosis (20% of cases) and transformation to acute leukemia after 10 to 20 years of disease diagnosis. Phlebotomy significantly decreases the risk of thrombosis. About 500 ml of blood may be removed daily until the hematocrit is below 45% in men and 42% in women. Hydroxyurea can decrease the risk of thrombosis and can supplement phlebotomy in older persons. Gentle bathing, use of soft towels, and starch baths may decrease postbathing pruritus (Tefferi, 2004).

Myelofibrosis is a chronic disease characterized by bone marrow fibrosis (scarring of the bone marrow), splenomegaly, and teardrop-shaped RBCs. It is usually diagnosed at about age 60. The cause is unknown, and the liver and spleen become enlarged as the disease progresses. Symptoms include weight loss, pallor, abdominal distention, fatigue, low-grade fever, and night sweats. The diagnosis is made by examination of a peripheral blood smear and bone marrow biopsy. Survival time after diagnosis is about 3 to 5 years. There is no specific treatment, but blood transfusions can eliminate symptoms of anemia, and administration of erythropoietin may stimulate RBC production. In younger persons, allogeneic bone marrow transplantation may be effective, but this intervention is usually not indicated in the older person. For seriously ill patients, palliative care with attention to pain and symptom control is indicated. Splenectomy can improve symptoms and may be indicated in some patients (Tefferi, 2004).

HEMATOLOGIC MALIGNANCIES

Hematologic malignancies arise when immature lymphoid and myeloid cells are over-produced with associated bone marrow failure. Large numbers of immature WBCs accumulate in the bone marrow, liver, spleen, lymph nodes, and central nervous system, and eventually cause failure. Acute leukemia is primarily a disease of children and elderly adults (Friedman, 2004). The incidence of acute leukemia is equal in men and women over the age of 50 (LeMone & Burke, 2004). In most cases, the cause of acute leukemia is unknown. Predisposing factors include exposure to chemical agents such as benzene, genetic factors, viruses, immune disorders, certain antineoplastic drugs, and radiation exposure (LeMone & Burke, 2004). An increased incidence of leukemia has been noted in the atomic bomb survivors of Hiroshima and Nagasaki, radiologists, and patients receiving radiation therapy. Careful monitoring of radiation exposure is mandatory for all healthcare workers caring for patients receiving radiation treatments or diagnosis by x-ray.

Acute leukemia presents dramatically in children with high fevers, but in the older person the onset is more insidious with weakness, pallor, and acute confusion. Often the liver, spleen, and lymph nodes are enlarged. The WBC court may or may not be elevated. Diagnosis is confirmed by bone marrow aspiration. The prognosis is poor without treatment. Advanced age, bleeding, and concurrent diagnosed chronic illness are indicators of poor prognosis. Treatment consists of a combination of drugs designed to inhibit WBC production, including vincristine, prednisone, anthracycline, and asparaginase. Most older patients experience relapse within one year. Bone marrow transplantation is rarely used for patients over 65 (Friedman, 2004).

Infections are the major cause of morbidity and mortality. The lack of mature WBCs to fight infection compromises the ability to fight disease. Acute leukemia in older patients is most often fatal within 1 to 2 years. The risks and benefits of aggressive chemotherapy must be discussed with the older person and the family so they can make an informed decision about treatment choices. Palliative care with emphasis on pain and symptom control and hospice care (when and if appropriate) will enhance the quality of life of the older person.

Chronic leukemia usually progresses more slowly than acute leukemia. Chronic lymphoid leukemia (CLL) is primarily a disease of older persons and accounts for 25% to 40% of all leukemias. CLL is characterized by a proliferation and accumulation of small, abnormal mature lymphocytes in the bone marrow, peripheral blood, and body tissues. These cells are usually unable to produce adequate antibodies to maintain normal immune function (LeMone & Burke, 2004). Men are affected twice as often as women and the majority are over the age of 60. The cause of CLL is unknown, but there is a predisposition in some families, and the Epstein-Barr virus has also been suggested as a possible cause. Common symptoms include fatigue, malaise, rapid worsening of coronary artery disease, and decreased exercise tolerance. Enlarged lymph nodes occur in the cervical, axillary, and supraclavicular areas. The spleen may also be enlarged as the disease progresses.

As with acute leukemia, infections and fever are frequent complications of CLL. The diagnosis of CLL requires repeated measurement of sustained lymphocytosis and examination of the bone marrow. The 5-year survival rate is about 50%, and 25% to 30% of patients with CLL live 10 years of more. Older patients with CLL have a heightened risk of developing a second malignancy. Although CLL is very responsive to chemotherapy and radiation, early treatment has not been shown to increase survival; therefore, treatment should not be started until the patient manifests symptoms of weight loss, night sweats, fever, or enlarged lymph nodes. Oral alkylating agents combined with prednisone provide effective treatment (Mortimer & McElhaney, 2004). As the disease progresses, older patients will increasingly require nutritional support, pain control, skin care, and emotional support from the gerontological nurse.

Multiple myeloma is a malignancy that results from the overproduction and accumulation of immature plasma cells in the bone marrow, lymph nodes, spleen, and kidneys. Multiple myeloma is more common after the age of 50 and occurs more frequently in African Americans. It occurs equally in men and women (Friedman, 2004).

Bone pain in the lower back or ribs is the most common early symptom of multiple myeloma. Additional symptoms include bone fractures, pallor, weakness, fatigue, dyspnea, and palpitations. Bruising and excessive bleeding from trauma are common. Renal disease occurs in about 50% of patients, including urinary tract infections, calcium or uric acid calculi, and dehydration. Most patients have a normocytic anemia and osteolytic bone lesions or osteoporosis, monoclonal proteins *(Bence Jones protein)* in blood serum, and increased plasma cells in the bone marrow. Treatment involves administration of steroids, chemotherapy, and radiation therapy for localized tumors and to relieve back pain from osteolytic lesions.

Autologous transplantation with peripheral blood stem cells is being used for people up to age 70 and older, depending on functional status. All older patients should be urged to stay as active as possible to counteract bone demineralization and the deconditioning common with prolonged bed rest. All infections, fevers, and night sweats should be reported to the healthcare provider and treated aggressively and promptly. Fluid intake should be 2 to 3 L/day to increase urinary output and increase the excretion of calcium, uric acid, and other metabolites. There is no cure for multiple myeloma. The disease is progressive, with death occurring 2 to 5 years from diagnosis (LeMone & Burke, 2004). Palliative care with the emphasis on pain management and symptom control, referral to hospice (if and when appropriate), and emotional support will be needed by the patient and family.

LYMPHOMAS

A malignant lymphoma is a neoplastic tumor affecting the lymphoid tissue. The disease is diagnosed by the presence of excess lymphocytes and progressive enlargement of the lymph nodes. The major types of lymphoma are Hodgkin's disease and non-Hodgkin's lymphoma. These diseases have differences in origin, patterns of spread, and clinical presentation.

Hodgkin's Disease

Hodgkin's disease occurs most often in people between the ages of 15 and 35 or over age 50. It is more common in men than women and usually presents as one or more painlessly enlarged lymph nodes. Other symptoms include persistent fever, night sweats, fatigue, weight loss, malaise, pruritus, and anemia (LeMone & Burke, 2004).

The diagnosis is made by lymph node biopsy. Additional testing includes computerized tomography (CT) scans, magnetic resonance imaging (MRI), splenectomy, and liver biopsy (Friedman, 2004). Treatment of the disease depends on the stage, but older people usually receive chemotherapeutic drugs for 6 to 8 months.

Non-Hodgkin's Lymphoma

Malignant disorders that originate from lymphoid tissue but are not diagnosed as Hodgkin's disease are classified as non-Hodgkin's lymphoma. Non-Hodgkin's lymphoma can begin with one node and spread throughout the lymphatic system and then metastasize to bones, the central nervous system, and the gastrointestinal tract. Because of the more systemic nature of non-Hodgkin's lymphoma, the prognosis is generally poorer than the prognosis of an older patient with Hodgkin's lymphoma. The risk of acquiring the disease increases with age. The cause is unknown, but those with impaired immune systems abnormalities or taking phenytoin are more at risk.

In non-Hodgkin's lymphoma, the normal lymphoid tissue is replaced by malignant cells leading to infection and immunodeficiency. Tumors can also form in the spleen, liver, and gastrointestinal tract. Symptoms include cervical or inguinal lymph node enlargement. Diagnosis is made by lymph node biopsy, bone marrow aspiration, blood testing, and chest x-ray. Chemotherapy is used to treat intermediate and high-grade lymphomas but does not prolong survival time in early disease. Aggressive chemotherapy in older persons with comorbidities can be extremely difficult, resulting in disability and inability to engage in self-care. Older patients with early disease are closely monitored for progressive problems, and radiation can be used to treat enlarged lymph nodes. The gerontological nurse should provide ongoing pain control, symptom management, nutritional guidance, and counseling during the treatment and recuperative phases of the illness.

Both lymphomas are curable with radiation and intensive chemotherapy; however, aggressive treatment in the older person with comorbidities is often difficult and may not be tolerated. Older people living alone may need assistance with activities of daily living, nutrition, and pain and symptom control during the required 6 months of aggressive treatment (Friedman, 2004).

Nursing Assessment of Older Patients With Hematologic Abnormalities

A complete review of the older person's past medical history and current health status is needed to assess the situation of a person with anemia or other blood disorders. The complaints of an older person with anemia or a blood disorder may be vague and often confused with normal changes of aging or symptoms of chronic disease. Any complaints of fatigue, shortness of breath, loss of appetite, weight loss, mental status changes, bruising, and activity intolerance should be carefully investigated. The nurse can play a key role in advising the older person to seek treatment and report symptoms to the healthcare provider. Anemia and other blood disorders can be caused by nutritional problems, blood loss, chronic illness, medications, or a variety of other factors that may respond to treatment.

The nurse can begin by gathering the following information:

- Diagnosis of any concurrent chronic or progressive illness such as cancer or heart or kidney disease
- Medication listing, including over-the-counter and herbal remedies

- History of surgery or trauma
- Baseline level of function and activity level and documentation of change of status
- Lifestyle factors that can be related to the older person's status, including smoking, alcohol use, depression, obesity, poor nutrition, and sedentary lifestyle
- Family history and diagnosed blood disorders in first-degree relatives
- Occupational exposures during the patient's work career to chemicals or pollutants

Because anemia is a sign of disease and not an actual disease itself, further investigation and careful assessment of the person with vague symptoms of fatigue, activity intolerance, and weakness should always be carried out. The skin should be examined for pallor, bruising, and poor turgor. The axillary, cervical, and inguinal areas should be checked for lymphadenopathy. The liver and spleen should be palpated for enlargement. The presence of rashes, urticaria, and itching should be noted. Balance and endurance should be observed and documented. Although there is no single recommended test of endurance, the nurse can observe the older person walking in a protected environment for several minutes and then assess for the presence of increased heart and respiratory rate, irregular respiratory or cardiac rate, weakness, and decreasing pulse oximetry after exercise. As depression can contribute to and be a result of chronic illness, the older person should be carefully screened for depression (see Chapter 7 for further information ⚬▭⚬).

Referral to a health provider for a complete health assessment is indicated for older patients who might be experiencing anemia. A complete physical examination, electrocardiogram, test of thyroid function, and complete blood count with differential are indicated. Older patients with a decreased WBC count should be protected from infection and placed in reverse isolation if necessary until their WBC count returns to normal.

Nursing diagnoses as defined by NANDA (2004) that may be associated with an older person experiencing anemia or other hematologic problems include the following:

- *Activity intolerance*
- *Risk for falls*
- *Risk for poisoning: drug toxicity*
- *Risk for infection*
- *Changes in the immune system*
- *Altered nutrition: less than body requirements*
- *Depression*
- *Impaired skin integrity*
- *Ineffective breathing pattern*
- *Anxiety*
- *Hopelessness*

Some nursing interventions that may be appropriate for the older person with hematologic problems include:

- Providing support and teaching for the patient and family.
- Protecting the skin from dryness, cracking, and injury.
- Providing teaching and administration of medications to relieve nausea and vomiting.
- Encouraging recreational and diversional activities consistent with the patient's general functional ability.
- Advising and referral regarding nutritional intake.
- Assessing and treating pain with appropriate pharmacological and nonpharmacological techniques.

- Treating associated symptoms, including constipation, diarrhea, and dry mouth.
- Involving the multidisciplinary team to address physical, social, psychological, and spiritual needs.

Nurse sensitive outcomes include lessening of symptom severity, increased effectiveness of cardiac pump, improvement of vital signs, improvement of ambulation and endurance, improvement of nutritional status, discontinuation of toxic medication, improvement in quality of life and overall functional ability, and improvement of depressive symptoms. If serious underlying disease is found during the investigation of the older person with anemia or other hematologic problems, the nurse can provide support during aggressive therapy and palliative care, with hospice referral if appropriate.

HYPERCOAGULABILITY AND ANTICOAGULATION

Deep vein thrombosis (DVT) and pulmonary embolism can lead to myocardial infarction and stroke, and the incidence increases with age. Hospitalized older patients are more at risk due to impaired mobility, surgical interventions, and orthopedic procedures. The older person is more at risk because of three components:

1. Abnormalities in the vessel walls caused by trauma, atherosclerosis, or intravenous medication administration
2. Abnormalities within the circulating blood and hypercoagulability seen with coagulation disorders, some cancers, and hormone (estrogen) use
3. Stasis of blood flow secondary to immobility, age, or heart failure

(Becker, 2004; McCance & Huether, 2001)

The major danger associated with DVT is that a portion of the thrombus will embolize to the lungs, causing pulmonary embolism (McCance & Huether, 2001). It is estimated that each year, DVT affects 2 million Americans, and pulmonary embolism affects 600,000 with approximately 10% dying from complications (Nadeau & Varrone, 2003). Aggressive therapy is needed to treat DVT because it is a potentially life-threatening situation. Anticoagulation and bed rest are critical to prevent movement of the clot to the lungs, heart, or brain where it can block vital circulation.

The clinical manifestations of DVT include edema, skin discoloration, and pain. The hallmark of DVT is the rapid onset of unilateral leg swelling with pitting edema. The diagnosis is made with Doppler ultrasonography, plethysmography, or venogram.

> **Practice Pearl**
>
> In older persons with heart failure and dependency edema, both legs will be swollen. Edema from a DVT is unilateral.

Preventive approaches are individualized to minimize the risk factors that can predispose to DVT. Specific conditions warranting prevention include:

- **Orthopedic procedures.** Examples include total hip replacement, traumatic hip fracture, and total knee replacement. For total hip replacement, the incidence of DVT without prophylaxis is 25%; for traumatic hip fracture, about 50%; and for total knee replacement, as high as 60%.

- **Atrial fibrillation.** Older persons with atrial fibrillation can form thrombi within the atria that can enter the general circulation and cause stroke. Transesophageal echocardiography identifies patients at risk for thromboembolism.
- **Acute myocardial infarction.** The risk of DVT in post–myocardial infarction patients approaches 20%. Older patients with heart failure, recurrent angina, or ventricular arrythmias are most at risk.
- **Ischemic stroke.** In patients with stroke and paralyzed lower extremities, the incidence of DVT is 40%.

(Becker, 2004).

Nursing interventions designed to prevent DVT formation include:

- Identifying patients at risk, including those with a history of DVT, clotting disorders, heart failure, orthopedic surgery, and other risk factors.
- Getting patients up and walking as soon as possible after surgery or injury.
- Changing the position of bed-bound patients every 2 hours to prevent circulatory compromise.
- Urging patients at risk for DVT to wear fitted support stockings, avoid stasis, maintain adequate hydration, elevate legs during periods of rest, and perform meticulous skin care to keep skin clean and intact.
- Urging the use of intermittent pneumatic compression boots postoperatively until patients are ambulatory.
- Administering anticoagulants as prescribed.

There are many anticoagulants and each has distinct uses. In general, drugs given intravenously, such as heparin or the fibrinolytic agents, are used short term for hospitalized patients. Oral drugs, such as warfarin and antiplatelet drugs, are used long term for outpatients. Low-molecular-weight heparins, administered subcutaneously, are used in both settings (Becker, 2004). Drugs are given for prevention and treatment of thrombotic conditions.

Laboratory tests to monitor efficacy and to determine the dosage of medications are usually done every 3 to 4 days of therapy. They include the prothrombin time (PT) and the partial thromboplastin time (PTT). The PT, a measure of the time required for a firm fibrin clot to form after reagents are added to the blood sample, is the standard mea-sure of efficacy. It is commonly reported in an international normalized ratio (INR) because the World Health Organization urged the adoption of a standardized reagent so that all laboratories would report standardized results. Warfarin will prolong the INR. The higher the INR, the longer it takes the blood to clot. Guidelines suggest various target INR measurements and duration of therapy. The PTT is used to evaluate the time required for a firm fibrin clot to form after phospholipid reagents are added to the specimen. Heparin will prolong the PTT.

Anticoagulant Medications

Heparin is the most widely used anticoagulant. It accelerates the inhibitory interaction between hemostatic proteins and clotting factors. Unfractionated heparin is used in older patients to prevent and to treat venous or arterial thromboembolism.

Low-dose heparin therapy (500 U subcutaneously every 8 to 12 hours) is prophylactic therapy for DVT in patients who have the following:

- Orthopedic surgery
- Acute myocardial infarction
- Ischemic stroke with lower extremity paralysis
- Congestive heart failure

High-dose heparin therapy (intravenous administration) to maintain a PTT (1.5 to 2.5 times control) is indicated in the following patients:

- Those with DVT, pulmonary embolism, or unstable angina
- Those receiving thrombolytic therapy
- Those receiving perioperative care who are on warfarin therapy

(Becker, 2004; Reuben et al., 2003)

The most common adverse effect of heparin is hemorrhage. Other adverse effects include thrombocytopenia, alopecia, and skin necrosis. The risk of bleeding increases with increased dosage. Other risk factors include older age, low body weight, recent trauma or surgery, and performance of invasive procedures with concurrent use of aspirin. Mild bleeding can be handled by reducing the dose, and severe bleeding requires discontinuation of the heparin (Becker, 2004).

Low-molecular-weight heparins are used for DVT prophylaxis and in the treatment of DVT with acute coronary syndromes such as unstable angina and myocardial infarction. Low-molecular-weight heparins can be given intravenously or subcutaneously. Because of the predictable bioavailability, dose-independent clearance rates, and a more stable anticoagulant response, these drugs have been increasingly used in the clinical setting (Nadeau & Varrone, 2003). They do not prolong the PTT, and the predictable antithrombotic response eliminates the need for laboratory monitoring and dose adjustment. However, as a precaution, the older patient receiving low-molecular-weight heparins should be carefully monitored for signs of excessive bleeding.

Warfarin is frequently used for anticoagulation in the prevention or treatment of DVT. It is rapidly absorbed from the gastrointestinal tract, reaches maximal serum concentration in about 90 minutes, and takes up to 7 days to reach stable serum levels on fixed doses (Reuben et al., 2003). Warfarin interacts with many substances, and older patients taking the medication should be instructed to report any changes in their medication regimen to their healthcare providers so that INRs can be monitored and warfarin dosage adjusted in response. Table 21-2 lists substances that affect warfarin response.

Hepatic clearance of warfarin declines with age. The older person is more likely to experience bleeding complications, so the drug is usually started at lower doses. Frequent monitoring is required to safely titrate dosage during the induction period.

TABLE 21-2

Substances That Affect Warfarin Response

These agents **increase** the INR in conjunction with warfarin.	Alcohol (binge)	Phenytoin
	Allopurinol	Propoxyphene
	Amiodarone	Selective serotonin reuptake inhibitors
	Antibiotics	
	Acetaminophen	Tamoxifen
	Aspirin	Vitamin E
	Corticosteroids	
	Omeprazole	
These agents **decrease** the INR in conjunction with warfarin.	Alcohol (moderate)	Estrogen
	Barbiturates	Rifampin
	Carbamazepine	Sucralfate
	Cholestyramine	Vitamin K

Source: Epocrates.com, 2004; Reubens et al., 2003.

TABLE 21-3

Indications for Anticoagulation With Target International Normalized Ratios

Condition	Target INR	Duration of Therapy
Orthopedic surgery	2.0–3.0	7–10 days postoperatively or until patient is ambulatory
Deep vein thrombosis	2.0–3.0	At least 3 months
Pulmonary embolism	2.0–3.0	At least 6 months
Atrial fibrillation	2.0–3.0	Indefinitely for chronic atrial fibrillation and at least 3 weeks before and 4 weeks after cardioversion
Mechanical heart valve	2.5–3.5	Indefinitely
Acute myocardial infarction	2.0–3.0	1–3 months

Source: Epocrates.com, 2004; Reubens et al., 2003.

Table 21-3 lists anticoagulation indications for conditions with target INRs.

Contraindications to warfarin therapy include patients with bleeding disorders, frequent fallers at risk for intracranial bleeding, and those who are not compliant with dosage adjustments and laboratory testing. Some surgeons will request that warfarin be held for four doses prior to surgery to decrease the risk of intraoperative bleeding.

Excessively high INRs (3.5 and over) should be reported immediately to the healthcare provider or anticoagulation clinic so that dosage adjustment and possible action to reduce the INR reading can be accomplished. For INRs between 3.5 and 5, the usual recommendation is to omit the next dose and lower the maintenance dose. For INRs between 5 and 9, the recommendation may be to omit the next several doses and restart at a lower dose. Some healthcare providers recommend administration of vitamin K 1.0 to 2.5 mg by mouth. For INRs over 9 with or without bleeding, the warfarin would probably be discontinued and vitamin K given orally or intravenously until the INR returns to normal levels.

Protamine sulfate is indicated in the treatment of heparin overdosage. Protamine sulfate should be administered by very slow intravenous injection over a 10-minute period in doses not to exceed 50 mg. All serious or significant bleeding requires emergency treatment and evaluation for an older patient taking any anticoagulant. Signs of bleeding may occur as blood in the urine or stool, vomiting of blood, nosebleeds, blood in the sputum, bleeding gums, bruising out of proportion to or in the absence of injury, fatigue, severe headache, and loss of vision or weakness on one side of the body. All patients taking warfarin should be instructed to take the medication as ordered, regularly monitor INR levels, check for interactions before starting any new medications, recognize dietary sources of vitamin K and ingest stable amounts, and recognize the signs of bleeding and the need to seek treatment (Nadeau & Varrone, 2003).

Platelet Antagonists

Platelets participate in the thrombotic process by adhering to abnormal surfaces, aggregating to form a plug, and triggering the coagulation cascade. Aspirin irreversibly inhibits platelet aggregation by blocking enzymes in the clotting process and impairing prostaglandin metabolism. Aspirin is used for primary and secondary prevention of myocardial infarction and stroke and is used with other antiplatelet agents (clopidogrel or ticlopidine) after the placement of intracoronary stents (Becker, 2004).

Ticlopidine is a potent inhibitor of platelet aggregation by impairing platelet adhesion and inhibiting platelet release action. Ticlopidine has been used in the treatment of transient ischemic attacks, strokes where aspirin was already being taken, unstable angina, and cardiac stent placement. Side effects include two serious conditions: neutropenia and thrombocytopenic purpura. Clopidogrel reduces the risk of myocardial infarction and recurrent myocardial infarction among older patients with atherosclerotic vascular disease. It has a more favorable side-effect profile than ticlopidine, and the longer half-life requires only once-a-day dosing (Becker, 2004).

Nursing Assessment of the Older Patient With Hypercoagulability

Older persons at risk for hypercoagulability and DVT formation include those with atherosclerosis, circulating blood abnormalities, and slowing of blood flow. Immobility and orthopedic surgery greatly increase the risk of DVT formation, and the older person should be assisted to ambulate as soon as possible after surgery. Postoperative nursing care involves use of compression stockings, intermittent pneumatic compression boots, early and consistent ambulation of older patients, maintenance of adequate hydration, and careful administration of anticoagulants. Postoperative and chronic pain should be carefully assessed and treated to prevent the hazards of immobility.

Practice Pearl

The older patient who says "It only hurts when I move, so I don't need any pain medication" is at risk for immobility and DVT formation.

Older patients receiving anticoagulation medications require careful and ongoing nursing assessment of frank or occult bleeding and laboratory examination of clotting times. Older persons taking warfarin should report any bleeding or medication changes immediately to the healthcare provider.

The following nursing diagnoses as defined by NANDA (2004) may be associated with an older person experiencing potential hypercoagulability:

- *Activity intolerance*
- *Risk for falls and injury*
- *Risk for poisoning: drug toxicity*
- *Risk for infection*
- *Potential alterations in risk control (inability to recognize signs and symptoms of bleeding)*
- *Risk for nonadherence to laboratory monitoring procedures*

Nurse sensitive outcomes may include the following:

- Lessening of symptom severity
- Increased effectiveness of cardiac pump
- Improvement of vital signs
- Improvement of ambulation and endurance
- Improvement of mobility
- Discontinuation of toxic medication
- Adherence to monitoring and laboratory requirements

Many older patients with anemia lack sufficient energy to carry out their daily activities and suffer from functional impairment, including cognitive and mood impairment. The gerontological nurse may find that many older patients and their families lack knowledge regarding the significance, assessment, and treatment of anemia in later life. The patient-family teaching guidelines in the following feature will assist the nurse in the education of older patients and their families regarding anemia.

Patient-Family Teaching Guidelines

THE OLDER PATIENT WITH ANEMIA

The following are guidelines that the nurse may find useful when instructing older persons and their families about anemia, the most common hematologic problem experienced by older people.

1. How do I know if I have anemia?

There is no one main symptom of anemia. Often the symptoms are vague and may be noticed as fatigue, lack of energy, shortness of breath on physical exertion, pale skin color, memory problems, and worsening of other problems like heart or lung conditions.

RATIONALE:

Often the symptoms of anemia develop gradually and are attributed to normal changes of aging. The nurse can help the older patient and his or her family to examine current function and make a comparison to previous functional ability to identify changes over time.

2. What are the most common causes of anemia?

Anemia is caused by either an underproduction of red blood cells or excessive loss or destruction of red blood cells. Iron deficiency is common in older people who have had blood loss due to injury or surgery. Unexplained blood loss should be investigated to make sure there is not hidden bleeding in the stomach or intestinal tract. Some medications can cause red blood cells to be broken down and destroyed, causing anemia. Sometimes red blood cells are not formed quickly enough to replace the ones that live a natural life span. The bone marrow slows production because of chronic illness in the heart, lungs, or kidneys. Sometimes a nutritional deficiency is responsible. Whatever the cause, it is important to pinpoint the kind of anemia and treat the cause.

RATIONALE:

Most people attribute anemia to iron deficiency or nutritional problems; however, the causes of anemia in the older person are diverse and varied. It is often necessary to think beyond the obvious and simple causes of anemia.

3. What kinds of tests is my healthcare provider likely to order to diagnose anemia?

The most basic test is a complete blood count with differential. This test gives a measure of the number of circulating red blood cells and the types and numbers of other cells, including white blood cells and platelets. Sometimes iron studies are performed and vitamin B_{12} and folate levels examined, depending on the kind of anemia suspected. If the physician suspects bleeding in the stomach or intestine, an endoscopy or examination of the stomach or colon with a small tube and camera may be performed. Because anemia is not a disease itself but a symptom of some other condition, a careful search for the cause is indicated.

RATIONALE:

Older patients and their families should be instructed that finding the cause of the anemia is as important as treating the anemia and a variety of tests may be ordered to pinpoint the cause of the problem. To treat an anemia in the older person without knowing the cause is inappropriate and may mask the symptoms of serious underlying diseases or health problems.

(continued)

Patient-Family Teaching Guidelines, *cont.*

4. How often should I ask my healthcare provider to check my blood for the presence of anemia?

Healthy older people should be checked for anemia every year. A complete blood count may be ordered and stool checked for occult bleeding. Those with chronic conditions, recent injury or trauma, or symptoms should be checked more frequently.

RATIONALE:

Regular health maintenance and disease detection in the healthy older person is indicated yearly to diagnose and treat diseases early and improve chances of success. Healthy older patients and those with chronic conditions should be urged to have blood testing, fecal occult stool testing, and colonoscopy/sigmoidoscopy on a regular basis.

5. What can I do to prevent anemia?

Eat a balanced diet, keep active, avoid taking unnecessary medications, and report any fatigue or loss of energy to your healthcare provider. Taking a once-a-day multivitamin can help. There is no need to take iron pills unless you are instructed to do so by your healthcare provider. Be sure to report any gastrointestinal distress, black stools, or red blood in the stool to your health-care provider immediately.

RATIONALE:

General good health, regular exercise, and avoidance of medications will help promote overall health (including hematologic health) at all ages and stages of life. A multivitamin will help to ensure adequate vitamin intake when an occasional meal is skipped. Usually iron replacement is not necessary in an older person who has not had recent surgery or trauma. Taking iron unnecessarily can cause gastrointestinal problems and constipation.

Care Plan

A Patient With a Bleeding Disorder

Case Study

Mr. Thayer is a 78-year-old man who has been diagnosed with chronic atrial fibrillation. He is receiving warfarin therapy for anticoagulation to prevent pulmonary embolism from his decreased cardiac output. His INR goal is 2.5 to 3.5. He is usually quite responsible with his warfarin regimen and monitoring requirements. He recently has not been feeling well and calls the clinic office to report he has a nosebleed that he cannot stop.

A Patient With a Bleeding Disorder

Applying the Nursing Process

ASSESSMENT

The nurse should conduct a brief focused history of the bleeding event over the phone. A patient's assessment of bleeding is often subjective and influenced by anxiety, so it would be helpful to accurately assess how long the bleeding has occurred and the approximate quantity of blood. The nurse may ask, "Is it gushing? Is it trickling? Is it soaking a handkerchief? Is it soaking a towel?" Large amounts of blood and uncontrolled bleeding need immediate attention and may constitute a medical emergency. Smaller amounts of blood may be controlled with ice packs to the nose, pressure on the external nose, and sitting upright to avoid swallowing blood.

Upon further questioning, Mr. Thayer reports he has been taking an antibiotic that was prescribed when he went to the local hospital emergency department because he had a bad cold. The nurse knows that many antibiotics can interact with warfarin and cause the INR to be elevated. An elevated INR means that the patient is at risk for uncontrolled bleeding. Additionally, Mr. Thayer may have taken other medications such as aspirin or cold and flu preparations that can interact with warfarin.

DIAGNOSIS

The current nursing diagnoses for Mr. Thayer include the following:

- *Anxiety* related to uncontrolled nasal bleeding
- *Risk for aspiration* related to nosebleed
- *Potential complication: hemorrhage* related to uncontrolled nosebleed secondary to insufficient clotting factors
- *Altered activity levels* due to hypovolemia and possible anemia as the result of excessive bleeding
- *Activity intolerance*
- *Risk for falls*
- *Risk for poisoning: drug toxicity* due to drug reactions between warfarin and many other medications
- *Risk for infection*
- *Ineffective breathing pattern*

EXPECTED OUTCOMES

The expected outcomes for the plan of care specify that Mr. Thayer will:

- Become aware of the harmful effects of drug interactions on clotting time.
- Call his healthcare provider who is responsible for his anticoagulation regimen and report changes in the medication regimen when he begins taking an antibiotic or any other new medication (his healthcare provider could have altered his warfarin dose and requested extra INR monitoring during the period he was taking the antibiotic).
- Seek immediate medical help and attention for his nosebleed if it is assessed to be of a serious nature.
- Agree to establish a therapeutic relationship with the nurse and develop a mutually acceptable plan to work toward these outcomes.

(continued)

A Patient With a Bleeding Disorder *(continued)*

PLANNING AND IMPLEMENTATION

Some nursing interventions that may be appropriate for Mr. Thayer include:

- Providing support and teaching for the patient and family.
- Urging him to contact his healthcare provider for an INR reading as soon as possible.
- Teaching Mr. Thayer about any dose adjustment in warfarin that may be required as a result of his INR reading.
- Involving the multidisciplinary team to address physical, social, psychological, and spiritual needs.

EVALUATION

The nurse hopes to work with Mr. Thayer over time and formulate a mutually agreeable plan to achieve the identified outcomes. The nurse will consider the plan a success based on the following criteria:

- Mr. Thayer will become more compliant and responsive to his warfarin regimen and dose adjustments based on regularly scheduled INR readings.
- A family meeting will be held to discuss Mr. Thayer's overall health and psychosocial function.
- Mr. Thayer will verbalize an understanding of the many possible drug interactions between warfarin and other medications and report all changes in his medication regimen to his healthcare provider.

Ethical Dilemma

Mr. Thayer admits he does not always adhere to his medication regimen. Lately he and his wife have been arguing, and he reports: "I just don't care if I live anymore." It is not a cognitive or financial problem, but perhaps represents depression due to marital stress. The nurse suggests further evaluation with a geriatric social worker, but he refuses.

The nurse realizes that Mr. Thayer sounds as if he is truly depressed. Assuming he has no suicidal ideation or plan to harm himself or his wife, the principle of autonomy must be honored. However, the nurse realizes that depressed older patients often lack the will and energy to engage in behaviors that will improve depressive symptoms.

The nurse should stress to Mr. Thayer that failure to take his medication can result in serious adverse health events such as stroke. His depression may be transient, but a devastating stroke will adversely impair his function and self-care for the rest of his life. Perhaps Mr. and Mrs. Thayer would agree to a joint session with the social worker, or Mr. Thayer might engage in a short-term trial of an antidepressant. The nurse could attempt to set some short-term goals with Mr. Thayer and encourage him to identify some actions to reach those goals. Support, encouragement, and ongoing monitoring of this patient's depression and medication regimen will be required.

A Patient With a Bleeding Disorder

Critical Thinking and the Nursing Process

1. What physical, emotional, and environmental factors make Mr. Thayer more at risk for stroke?
2. The INR obtained on Mr. Thayer was 5.4. What safety measures should the nurse implement while this patient has an elevated INR?
3. What nutritional modifications should be made, if any?
4. What additional support is needed from members of the interdisciplinary healthcare team?

- Evaluate your responses in Appendix B.

EXPLORE MediaLink

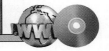

NCLEX review, case studies, and other interactive resources for this chapter can be found on the Companion Website at **http://www.prenhall.com/tabloski**. Click on Chapter 21 to select the activities for this chapter. For animations, video tutorials, more NCLEX review questions, and case studies, access the accompanying CD-ROM in this textbook.

Chapter Highlights

- The hematologic system is responsible for many functions, including the transport of oxygen and nutrients to and the removal of carbon dioxide and waste products from the peripheral tissue.

- Disturbances to the hematologic system are common in the older person, and often the symptoms are vague and attributed to normal aging.

- Anemia or a decrease in the number of red blood cells can be the result of nutritional problems, drug toxicity, chronic illness, and metabolic disorders. Because anemia is a sign, not a diagnosis, further evaluation of the older person with anemia is always indicated.

- White blood cell production can be affected by disorders of the bone marrow, lymph nodes, spleen, and thymus. When lymphocyte formation is impaired, the older person will have problems with humoral and cell-mediated immunity and will be unable to mount an effective immune response.

- Platelet adhesiveness increases with age. Older persons are at risk for the development of deep vein thrombosis and pulmonary embolism, especially after suffering a traumatic injury, in the presence of atherosclerosis, or with changes within the blood clotting factors. With proper administration, monitoring, and support, anticoagulation therapy can be a lifesaving intervention for older people.

■ Many functions of the hematologic system remain constant in healthy older persons, including RBC life span, total blood volume, RBC volume, total lymphocyte and granulocyte counts, and platelet structure and function. Average hemoglobin and hematocrit values decrease slightly with age, but remain within normal limits.

References

Becker, R. (2004). Hypercoagulability and anticoagulation. In M. Beers & R. Berkow (Eds.), *Merck manual of geriatrics*. Retrieved September 14, 2004, from www.merck.com.

Berne, R., & Levy, M. (2000). Blood and hemostasis. In *Principles of physiology* (3rd ed.). Boston: Mosby.

Blackwell, S., & Hendrix, P. (2001). Common anemias. *Clinical Reviews, 11* (3), 53–64.

Epocrates.com. (2004). *Adverse drug events—hemolytic anemia*. Retrieved September 14, 2004, from www.epocrates.com.

Friedman, M. (2004). Aging and the blood; Anemias; Hematologic malignancies; Lymphomas. In M. Beers & R. Berkow (Eds.), *Merck manual of geriatrics*. Retrieved September 14, 2004, from www.merck.com.

Kado, D., Karlamangla, A., Huang, M., Troen, A., Rowe, J., Selhub, J., & Seeman, T. (2004). *Homocysteine versus the vitamins folate, B_6 and B_{12} as predictors of cognitive function and decline in older high functioning adults: Macarthur studies of successful aging.* Retrieved December 6, 2004, from ars.usda.gov.

Kaesberg, P. (2004). Cancer. In M. Beers & R. Berkow (Eds.), *Merck manual of geriatrics*. Retrieved December 6, 2004, from www.merck.com.

LeMone, P., & Burke, K. (2004). *Medical-surgical nursing: Critical thinking in client care* (3rd ed.). Upper Saddle River, NJ: Prentice Hall Health.

McCance, K., & Huether, S. (2001). *Pathophysiology: The biologic basis for disease in adults and children* (4th ed.). St. Louis, MO: Mosby.

Medline Plus. (2004). *Medical encyclopedia: Sickle cell anemia*. U.S. National Library of Medicine and the National Institutes of Health. Retrieved September 14, 2004, from www.nlm.nih.gov.

Mortimer, J., & McElhaney, J. (2004). Cancers in the geriatric population. In C. Landefeld, R. Palmer, M. Johnson, In C. Johnston, & W. Lyons, (Eds.). *Current geriatric diagnosis and treatment*. New York: Lange Medical Books/McGraw-Hill.

Nadeau, C., & Varrone, J. (2003). Treat DVT with low molecular weight heparin. *Nurse Practitioner, 28*(10), 22–29.

North American Nursing Diagnosis Association (NANDA). (2004). *Nursing diagnoses: Definitions and classifications*. Philadelphia: Author.

Oh, R., & Brown, D. (2003). Vitamin B_{12} deficiency. *American Family Physician, March 1, 67*(5). Retrieved December 6, 2004, from www.aafp.org.

Rasul, I., & Kandel, G. (2001). An approach to iron deficiency anemia. *Canadian Journal of Gastroenterology, 15*(11), 739–747.

Reuben, D., Herr, K., Pacala, J., Pollick, B., Potter, J., & Semla, T. (2003). *Geriatrics at your fingertips*. Malden, MA: American Geriatrics Society, Blackwell.

Tefferi, A. (2004). Chronic myeloid disorders. In M. Beers & R. Berkow (Eds.), *Merck manual of geriatrics*. Retrieved December 6, 2004, from www.merck.com.

Toy, P. (2004). Anemia. In C. Landefeld, R. Palmer, M. Johnson, C. Johnston, & W. Lyons, (Eds.). *Current geriatric diagnosis and treatment*. New York: Lange Medical Books/McGraw-Hill.

CHAPTER 22

The Neurologic System

Ann C. Hurley, RN, DNSC, FAAN, FGSA
Ladislav Volicer, MD, PhD, FGSA, FAAN
Ellen K. Mahoney, RN, DNSC, FGSA

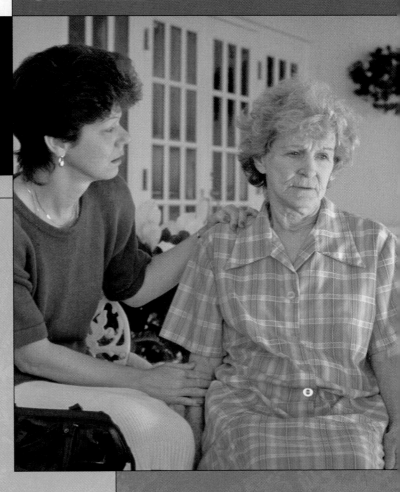

CHAPTER OBJECTIVES

Upon completion of this chapter, the reader will be able to:

- Describe Alzheimer's disease and related progressive dementias.
- Discuss the stages of Alzheimer's disease and implications for nursing care.
- Describe a contextual model to direct behavioral and pharmacological interventions for behavioral symptoms of Alzheimer's disease.
- Discuss Parkinson's disease in terms of diagnosis, treatment strategies, and nursing interventions.
- Define cerebrovascular accident (CVA)/stroke.
- Discuss CVA/stroke in terms of high-risk patients, treatment, and nursing implications.
- Discuss nursing interventions for seizures.
- Discuss the difference between epilepsy and seizures.
- Define seizure classifications.

MediaLink

Additional resources for this chapter can be found on the Student CD-ROM accompanying this textbook and on the Companion Website at **www.prenhall.com/tabloski**. Click on Chapter 22 to select the activities for this chapter.

CD-ROM
- Animations/Videos
    Alzheimer's Disease
    Epilepsy
    Neurologic System A&P
    Parkinson's Disease
- NCLEX Review

- Case Studies
- Tools
COMPANION WEBSITE
- Audio Glossary
- Additional NCLEX Review
- Case Study
- MediaLink Applications

KEY TERMS

The human nervous system controls consciousness, cognition, ethics, and behavior through processes in the central and peripheral nervous system. Each mature brain has 100 billion neurons, several miles of axons and dendrites, and more than 10^{15} synapses. The neurologic disorders arise from pathological processes and are manifested as individual symptoms, as a defined syndrome that includes several symptoms, or as a specific disease entity. From the perspective of directing nursing care, the neurologic conditions fall into the categories of memory, movement, **seizure disorders,** and stroke.

Understanding the clusters of symptoms surrounding the neurologic disorders in general and in specific neurologic diseases and their impact on elderly patients is important to plan and provide nursing care. Because of the uniqueness of specific symptoms, this chapter is organized around the primary neurologic conditions. Several general commonalities are directly related to planning and providing nursing care. The neurologic disorders presented in this chapter are:

- **Acquired.** An individual may be born with a genetic predisposition, but the disorder develops during the life span. Many are typically neurodegenerative diseases of elderly adults.
- **Progressive.** Currently there are no preventive or curative interventions or mechanisms to halt the basic pathological processes that cause the symptomatology, although some experimental therapeutics may be effective in years to come.
- **Chronic.** In the absence of cure, patients and their families must manage these conditions for many years, making these diseases family disorders.

Neurologic disorders also lead to disease-specific consequences and predispose to other complications. Nursing care is paramount to manage aversive symptoms, prevent avoidable complications, help the patient maintain independence within the context of disease progression, and help the patient and family manage an incurable disease. Many patients with neurologic disorders are also elderly. Persons who developed neurologic disorders in their youth are living longer today, and well into old age. Furthermore, many neurologic conditions develop in older persons.

Normal Changes of Aging

Advances in conquering many infectious diseases, improved public health, discovery of new medications, and application of technology to healthcare have resulted in decreased numbers of otherwise premature deaths and have delayed dying from various chronic diseases. As a result, persons are living longer and are exposed to age-related chronic conditions. Although elderly adults in general are in better health than decades ago, many are still dependent and frail (Wunderlich & Koehler, 2001). Normal age-related changes occur in all body systems. Normal and abnormal changes directly affect patients' nursing care needs. Changes in the senses, such as alterations in vision, hearing, taste, touch, and kinesthesia, influence care of the elderly patient. When the person has a neurologic disorder, the impact is magnified (see Figure 22-1 ■).

Vision changes result in overall decreased visual acuity and decrements in depth perception, color discrimination, and adaptation to changes in light levels. Hearing problems and decrements in high-tone and high-frequency sounds, voice discrimination, consonants, or increase in sound threshold may progress to loss of hearing. Loss of taste buds leading to inability to taste food can result in decreased appetite and weight loss. Diminished tactile sensation can lead to loss of hobbies or accidental injury or burns. Loss of kinesthesia sense can lead to falls.

Dementia

Dementia is a symptom of several acquired, progressive, life-limiting disorders that erase memory and the person's usual way of being in the world. The person with dementia has both a chronic illness and a terminal illness, first losing the ability to independently perform activities of daily living and finally becoming completely dependent in all aspects of self-care. Since the disease can affect different areas of the brain and different levels of the cortex, there is no uniform course and no predictability.

Growing old is the biggest risk factor for developing **Alzheimer's disease (AD)**. By the year 2011, 13% of Americans will be over the age of 65, and one in 100 will be over age 85 (Borson, Bartels, Colenda, Gottlieb, & Meyers, 2001). AD is a major age-related chronic condition since it affects the most rapidly growing segment of the population, persons over the age of 85 (Hurley & Wells, 1999). About 47% of persons age 85 and older may get AD (Evans et al., 1989), and about 4 million Americans had AD in 1998 (Klein & Kowall, 1998). The annual number of incident cases in the United States is expected to reach 959,000 in 2050 (Hebert, Beckett, Scherr, & Evans, 2001). AD lasts from 2 to 20 years, with an average duration of 8 years (Mahoney, Volicer, & Hurley, 2000a). Thus, in the next 50 years, millions of persons will suffer from AD, develop related complications, require care for long-standing or age-related chronic problems, and require nursing care.

AD requires a variety of nursing interventions and an interdisciplinary approach. The following characterizations about AD should be considered when planning and providing care.

- There is currently no medicine or technology that prevents or cures AD. Symptomatic nursing care is the primary intervention for this relentlessly progressive neurologic disorder.
- AD is both a life-limiting and a chronic illness. Caregivers require expertise in long-term care and end-of-life care. Due to the nature of AD, family caregivers also require supportive care.
- AD predisposes persons to develop challenging behavioral and psychiatric symptoms. Care targeted at alleviating symptoms and teaching patients and caregivers about the effects of AD is necessary to promote comfort and reduce feelings of distress.
- Persons with AD are cared for in a variety of settings, including their own homes, hospitals and nursing homes, congregate living facilities, and hospice settings to provide palliative care.
- AD is a family disease. All generations are affected (e.g., grandchildren who cannot understand why a grandparent has forgotten their name, and adult children or relatives who must provide caregiving services).

FIGURE 22-1

Normal changes of aging in the neurologic system.

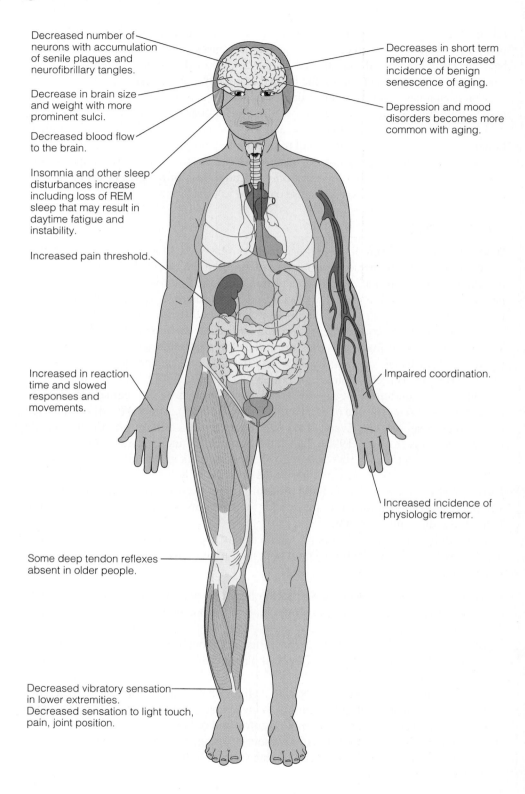

Decreased number of neurons with accumulation of senile plaques and neurofibrillary tangles.

Decrease in brain size and weight with more prominent sulci.

Decreased blood flow to the brain.

Insomnia and other sleep disturbances increase including loss of REM sleep that may result in daytime fatigue and instability.

Increased pain threshold.

Increased in reaction time and slowed responses and movements.

Some deep tendon reflexes absent in older people.

Decreased vibratory sensation in lower extremities. Decreased sensation to light touch, pain, joint position.

Decreases in short term memory and increased incidence of benign senescence of aging.

Depression and mood disorders becomes more common with aging.

Impaired coordination.

Increased incidence of physiologic tremor.

- AD is a public health problem. The effects of growing numbers of persons with AD raise many caregiving concerns, including costs of care.
- Persons with AD and their families depend on nursing for promoting independence and autonomy, preventing avoidable complications, providing comfort, and promoting quality of life.

PROGRESSIVE DEMENTIAS

Dementia is an acquired syndrome that causes progressive loss of intellectual abilities, such as memory, as well as **aphasia**, **apraxia**, and loss of **executive function**. Dementing disorders are characterized by gradual onset plus continuing cognitive decline that is not due to other brain disease. Screening tests can identify persons who should be referred for a complete diagnostic workup (Boustani et al., 2003). Early diagnosis of dementia is the goal of a diagnostic workup, which is done to exclude potentially reversible causes and initiate therapy as early as possible. Short-term memory impairment is usually the first symptom of dementia. Clinical diagnosis of dementia requires (1) loss of an intellectual ability with impairment severe enough to interfere with social or occupational functioning and (2) ruling out delirium. **Delirium** must be ruled out because cognitive impairment caused by delirium may be reversible. The development of delirium may indicate decreased reserve capacity of the brain and may signal an increased risk for dementia (Expert Consensus Panel, 2004).

Mild cognitive impairment is another risk factor for dementia. Persons with mild cognitive impairment have complaints and objective evidence of memory problems, but do not have deficits in activities of daily living or in other cognitive functions and do not meet the diagnostic criteria for dementia. Although mild cognitive impairment refers to a transitional state between normal aging and dementia (Arnaiz et al., 2004), it is associated with an increased risk of death, greater decline in cognitive abilities, and incident AD (Bennett et al., 2002), with an annual conversion rate of 8.3% to AD (Larrieu et al., 2002). Elderly persons with mild cognitive impairment who are depressed are at greater risk of converting to AD (Modrego & Ferrandez, 2004).

Dementia may be caused by more than one mechanism, even in the same individual. An autopsy examination is necessary to confirm the diagnosis. The most common combinations are AD with **vascular dementia** and AD with Lewy bodies. Clinically, progressive dementia symptoms are similar, especially in the later stages of the disease. Persons may differ in the onset and severity of a particular symptom. For example, **hallucinations** may occur early in **dementia with Lewy bodies** and only later in AD. In addition, there is no uniform progression of symptoms (i.e., the symptoms do not appear at a consistent time or in the same order).

ALZHEIMER'S DISEASE

Neuropathological criteria for AD include presence of two abnormal structures: neuritic plaques and neurofibrillary tangles. The plaques and tangles each contain a specific protein that may play a role in pathogenesis of AD. Beta-amyloid protein is present in the plaques, and the tau protein is found in the tangles. AD disrupts the three processes that keep neurons healthy: (1) communication, (2) metabolism, and (3) repair. As a result, nerve cells are destroyed or die, causing memory failure, personality changes, problems carrying out activities of daily living, and other deficits. Although the definitive diagnosis is provided only after histopathological confirmation at autopsy, the clinical diagnosis can be made from history, physical examination, and neuropsychological testing (Ala, Mattson, & Frey, 2003).

The majority of cases of AD result from complex interactions between genetic and environmental factors. To date, mutations in genes on chromosomes 1, 14, and 21 have been shown to cause AD, but these genes are responsible for fewer than 5% of the AD cases (McConnell, 1999). Unlike the rare causative mutations, alleles or variants of these other genes act as risk or susceptibility factors. The most robust risk factor for developing AD is the ε4 allele of the apolipoprotein (APOE) on chromosome 19 (Pericak-Vance et al., 1997; Roses, 1997). There are three common APOE alleles (ε2, ε3, and ε4). Individuals with one copy of the ε4 allele are about 2 to 4 times more likely to develop AD compared to persons who have the ε3/ε3 genotype, while ε4 homozygotes are 5 to 30 times more likely to do so (Farrer, Cupples, et al., 1995; Farrer et al., 1997). Although these observations have raised the possibility of using APOE genotyping in a predictive manner to help evaluate risk, its use in asymptomatic individuals is not recommended (Brodaty et al., 1995; Farrer, Brin, & Elsas, 1995; Post et al., 1997; Relkin, Kwon, Tsai, & Gandy, 1996; Relkin, 1996) due to the possibility of psychological harm or discrimination in an environment where no preventive treatments are yet available.

There is high interest in seeking genetic testing (Green, Clarke, Thompson, Woodard, & Letz, 1997), and Caucasians have expressed the greatest interest in and endorsed more reasons for seeking genetic testing for AD (Hipps, Roberts, Farrer, & Green, 2003). Survey research with relatives of persons with AD using hypothetical scenarios found that perceived advantages of AD genetic testing largely outweighed perceived disadvantages. The most important reasons cited were to inform later life decisions and plan for future care (Roberts, 2000). Results from the first randomized controlled clinical trial to offer APOE testing to asymptomatic adult children of patients with AD found similar motivating factors for seeking genetic susceptibility testing (Roberts et al., 2003; Roberts et al., 2004).

Epidemiological studies have implicated several nongenetic risk factors for AD. The strongest of these include age, gender, race, head injury, and environmental exposures (McConnell, Sanders, & Owens, 1999). Combining estimates of genetic risk and environmental risk provides a higher degree of precision in estimating an individual's lifetime risk for developing AD (McConnell et al., 1999).

VASCULAR DEMENTIA

Diagnostic criteria for vascular dementia are an abrupt onset of dementia, focal neurologic findings (abnormal reflexes or nerve functions), low-density areas (indicating vascular changes in the white matter), or presence of multiple strokes in computerized tomography (CT) or magnetic resonance imaging (MRI) scans. Other criteria include fluctuation of impairment, unchanged personality, emotional lability, and a temporal relation between a stroke and development of dementia.

LEWY BODY DISEASE

Dementia with Lewy bodies, also called diffuse Lewy body disease, may be confused with delirium and differs from AD (Marui, Iseki, Kato, Akatsu, & Kosaka, 2004). Clinical features of dementia with Lewy bodies persist over a long period and progress to severe dementia. Autopsy confirmation reveals round structures, called Lewy bodies, and Lewy neuritis in specific systems throughout the brain stem, diencephalon, basal ganglia, and neocortex (Duda, 2004). These Lewy bodies are also present in **Parkinson's disease**, but in that condition they are limited to subcortical areas of the brain.

FRONTOTEMPORAL DEMENTIA

Frontotemporal dementia, which includes **Pick's disease**, is diagnosed on the basis of personality changes and the presence of frontal brain area atrophy in neuroimaging studies (CT scan or MRI). Personality changes observed in frontotemporal dementia are similar to changes induced by damage of frontal lobes by other causes (injury, stroke) and include behavioral disinhibition, loss of social or personal awareness, or disengagement with apathy. Atrophy of the brain frontal and temporal lobes, and proliferation of nonneuronal glial cells in these areas, characterize pathological findings in frontotemporal dementia. Pick's disease is characterized by two specific neuropathological findings on autopsy: (1) Pick's bodies inside nerve cells, and (2) ballooned nerve cells.

Alzheimer's Disease

No treatments currently available reverse or stop the advancement of the pathological processes of progressive dementia, but some drugs may temporarily reverse or slow the progression of clinical symptoms. Because early studies had found that AD was less common among women taking hormone replacement therapy (HRT) (Paganini-Hill & Henderson, 1996; Yaffe, Sawaya, Lieberburg, & Grady, 1998), the HRT hypothesis posited that the abrupt decline in estrogen production in postmenopausal women may be associated with AD and thus could be mitigated by HRT. The administration of estrogen to postmenopausal women with AD was not found to decrease the rate of dementia progression, nor to improve global, cognitive, or functional outcomes in women with mild to moderate AD (Mulnard et al., 2000). Because of recent studies (Writing Group for the Women's Health Initiative Investigators, 2002), HRT is no longer recommended for prevention of cardiovascular disease (Grady et al., 2002). However, there is higher prevalence of AD in women, suggesting a link between gonadal hormone levels and AD. Some studies reported that HRT decreased the risk for or delayed the onset of AD in postmenopausal women (Zandi et al., 2002). However, more recent studies dispute this finding and instead report increased risk to older women taking estrogen plus progestin or estrogen therapy alone for postmenopausal symptoms. These findings support the conclusion that the risks of estrogen outweigh the benefits. Currently, the use of HRT to prevent or delay the onset of dementia is not recommended (Shumaker et al., 2003).

Other medications, vitamins, and herbal remedies have been examined for use to prevent or slow the progression of AD. Because persons using nonsteroidal anti-inflammatory drugs (NSAIDs) for treating arthritis were found to have lower rates of AD, epidemiological studies were conducted and found that long-term use of NSAIDs may protect against AD (In't Veld, et al., 2001). A large randomized clinical trial is being conducted to test the hypothesis that NSAID use in elderly persons with a family history of AD may protect against AD. In epidemiological studies, the drug group statins, when given to reduce cholesterol levels, has been found to reduce the risk of AD (Buxbaum, Geoghagen, & Friedhoff, 2001). Administration of vitamin E to patients with AD delayed the loss of functional abilities, temporarily preserved independence in activities of daily living, and delayed institutionalization (Sano et al., 1997). Delay in the progression of dementia was also observed after administration of ginkgo biloba extract, which may also prevent toxic effects of free radicals (Oken, Storzbach, & Kaye, 1998). Further research is required to determine optimal dosage and drug combinations.

There is a group of drugs, cholinesterase inhibitors (ChEI therapy), that slow the progression of AD symptoms. The ChEI hypothesis is that preventing the destruction of acetylcholine (a neurotransmitter) by inhibiting the acetylcholinesterase enzyme

MediaLink

Alzheimer's Disease Video

that destroys acetylcholine should result in decreasing symptoms of cognitive improvement. ChEI has been found to have a cognitive and functional benefit in the early stage of AD, lesser clinical benefit as the disease progresses, but a beneficial effect by delaying admission to nursing homes (Lopez et al., 2002). In general, ChEI therapy by cholinesterase enhancers such as donepezil (Aricept), rivastigmine (Exelon), and galantamine (Reminyl) may keep the patient in the early stage of AD for an additional 6 to 12 months. Donepezil has been found to be beneficial with good drug tolerability for use in patients with moderate to severe AD (Feldman et al., 2001).

Donepezil has been found to stabilize or retard the decline of cognitive and functional impairment and to improve problematic behaviors of dementia (Smith, 2003). Rivastigmine has been found effective in treating cognitive and behavioral symptoms in AD and in Lewy body dementia (Farlow, 2003). In general, for this class of medication, doses should be titrated to the highest therapeutic dose tolerated, but as slowly as necessary to decrease the development of gastrointestinal or other side effects. Nausea may be reduced by administering the ChEI on a full stomach, and intermittent antiemetics may be required.

The newest class of medication used for AD is based on the hypothesis that overstimulation of the N-methyl-d-aspartate (NMDA) receptor by glutamate causes neuronal degeneration induced by beta-amyloid. The drug, memantine, is an antiglutamatergic treatment that protects against beta-amyloid–induced neurotoxicity. It has been used in Europe since 1978 as an all-purpose neurological tonic, and officially used as a dementia drug in Germany since 1989. It received approval from the U.S. Food and Drug Administration in 2003. Memantine-treated animals have had reductions in neuronal degeneration (Miguel-Hidalgo, Alvarez, Cacabelos, & Quack, 2002). In a clinical trial, memantine was found to reduce clinical deterioration in patients with moderate to severe AD (Reisberg et al., 2003).

STAGES OF ALZHEIMER'S DISEASE AND IMPLICATIONS FOR NURSING CARE

There are differences in the pathological processes detected by histopathological examination at autopsy and clinical symptoms observed across the progressive dementias. However, for planning nursing care, differences in clinical symptoms are subtle. Since AD is the most prevalent of the progressive dementias, it is used in the remainder of this chapter to illustrate nursing care needs.

As a chronic illness, AD may require 20 years of home care, assisted living, or long-term institutional care with an array of community and acute care services to maintain independence, prevent excess disability, ensure safety, and manage medical complications. Even with the finest efforts of caregivers, the disease progresses and creates dependency in activities of daily living and ultimately results in death if the care recipient has not died from another cause (Hurley, Volicer, & Mahoney, 1996). Figure 22-2 ■ depicts the progressive decline observed in AD.

The hallmark of AD is the cognitive symptom of memory loss. As AD worsens, other deficits appear and symptoms develop. Several classification systems have been proposed to describe stages commonly observed in the dementing diseases. In general, symptoms are clustered into four stages: mild, moderate, severe, and terminal (Volicer & Hurley, 1998). These symptoms and their consequences make planning and providing care complex during all the progressive stages and in all settings.

At the Time of Diagnosis

Both the patient and primary family caregivers must understand the clinical diagnosis of AD and receive advice regarding early-stage issues (Drickamer & Lachs, 1992).

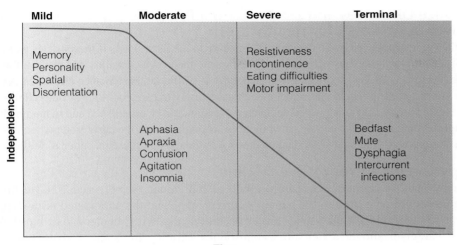

Source: Volicer, Brandeis, & Hurley, 1998.

FIGURE ■ 22-2

Progressive decline observed in AD.

While the patient still has decision-making capacity, the clinician should initiate discussions about desired treatment modalities, selecting a healthcare proxy (power of attorney for healthcare), and informing the proxy about desired care to be provided when unable to make those decisions later in the disease (Rempusheski & Hurley, 2000). The patient may benefit from cognitive-enhancing medications (discussed earlier), which should be initiated as soon after the diagnosis as possible and may keep the patient in the early stage of AD for an additional 6 to 12 months. Referrals should be made to the local Alzheimer's Association for support groups, services, and assistance locating other community services such as the Program of All Inclusive Care for the Elderly (PACE). The patient may benefit from being in a support group with other persons who have early-stage AD. There are also specific family support groups, such as for working spouses and adult children.

In this stage there is a need to balance safety with autonomy. Caregivers need to address and resolve issues of not driving, not leaving the person home alone, and providing the least restrictive protective physical environment.

Without infantilizing persons with AD, strategies used to prevent injury to toddlers may be modified to provide a *safer* physical environment (Hurley et al., 2004). There is no completely *safe* physical environment (Warner, 1998). Persons with AD are taller and stronger than toddlers and may have retained implicit memory for how to exit their home. To make the home safer and decrease the chances of falls, fires, burns, and getting lost, the caregiver (with another person such as the visiting nurse or occupational therapist) should tour the home to identify safety issues and develop a plan to rectify them. At entrances and exits, the caregiver should put a slide bolt lock at the top or bottom of exit doors where it is the least noticeable, lock sliding glass doors using a wooden dowel in the runner at the bottom, and use a motion sensor (which is especially useful at night to wake the caregiver if the care recipient gets confused and walks toward an exit door). In the kitchen, it is important to remove knobs from the stove, remove medicine from the counter, reset water temperature to below 120°F, remove scissors and knives from counters and drawers, disable the garbage disposal and instant hot water, remove cleaning and other toxic items, remove outdated foods from the refrigerator, and unplug small electrical appliances when they are not being used. In all rooms, clutter should be removed. Clutter is a safety issue because the person with dementia will not understand what it is and may trip over it.

MediaLink ❧ Program of All Inclusive Care for the Elderly (PACE)

Advance Directives and Establishing a Proxy (Power of Attorney for Healthcare)

Families will struggle to make decisions about care in the later stages if these issues were not discussed when persons with AD still could make their own decisions and plan for the future. Persons with AD should be given an opportunity to establish advance directives. As early as practicable, they should select a healthcare proxy to carry out their wishes (Rempusheski & Hurley, 2000). Educated decision making should be established and maintained throughout the progressive course, with the roles changing from the early stage when patients can represent themselves, to later stages when their proxy presents patients' wishes.

Preparing for a Progressive Decline

Progression of AD does not occur uniformly in all individuals (see Figure 22-2). Health teaching should be geared to the patient's current stage and the anticipated issues. In the early stage, care planning may center on interventions for memory loss, but the family caregiver should anticipate that insomnia (leading to unattended nocturnal **wandering**) might soon become an issue. As the disease progresses, the role of the caregiver becomes more active to compensate for the patient's cognitive losses and the development of behavioral symptoms. Families will need support from their professional caregivers as they make and live through some of the most difficult decisions of their lives—selecting life-prolonging treatments that may also increase discomfort, or choosing care that will provide comfort but may be seen as hastening death.

After receiving the diagnosis, AD caregivers may go through five stages of grief, as described by Kubler-Ross (1969, 1986). The caregiver may deny that there is anything wrong, and follow this stage with overinvolvement, in which the caregiver will want to be present in all aspects of the patient's life. The caregiver may appear to look more like a patient. The patient is well groomed and looks well cared for, but the caregiver is exhausted from providing that care. The third stage involves anger at the patient (usually concurrent with behavior disorders). The fourth stage is guilt, and the fifth stage is acceptance. See Chapter 11 for further discussion. ⊂▭⊃

Effect of the Disease on the Person

The appearance of behavioral symptoms is a common consequence (Mahoney, Hurley, Smith, & Volicer, 1992; Mahoney, Volicer, & Hurley, 2000b) and creates an imperative for nursing interventions to prevent, alleviate, or minimize these symptoms. Management of behavioral symptoms is as central to care of the person with dementia as pain management is to cancer. However, the various etiologies of the symptoms, their variability, and their appearance and disappearance at different times during the progressive stages of disease make their management complex. Figure 22-3 ■ illustrates the relationship between behavioral symptoms and the social, caregiving, physical, and medical treatment environments.

The AD process directly causes cognitive impairment. Progressive dementia in combination with the person's underlying personality may lead to **delusions** and hallucinations as well as mood disorders and functional impairment. This may impose numerous challenges for caregivers, such as patients' dependence for activities of daily living, inability to initiate meaningful activities, anxiety, and **spatial disorientation**. These core and secondary symptoms often cause peripheral symptoms. Processes at each level influence the next level in a comprehensive way. Thus, delusions may result in spatial disorientation, anxiety, and dependence in activities of daily living. The mood disorder **depression** may lead to anxiety and inability to initiate meaningful activities. Similarly, spatial disorientation may lead to **elopement**, combativeness, interference with other residents, and **agitation**. Inability to initiate meaningful activities may lead to apathy, repetitive vocalization, agitation, and insomnia.

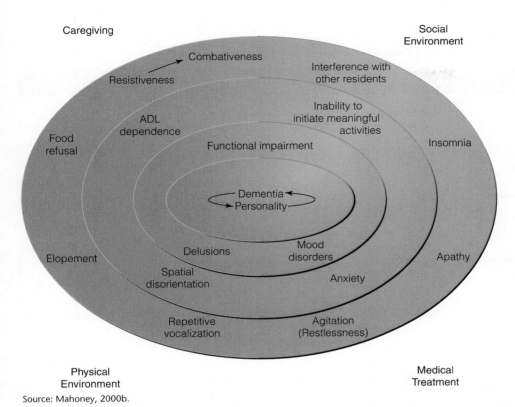

Caregiving

Social Environment

Combativeness

Resistiveness

Interference with other residents

Inability to initiate meaningful activities

ADL dependence

Food refusal

Functional impairment

Insomnia

Dementia
Personality

Elopement

Delusions

Mood disorders

Apathy

Spatial disorientation

Anxiety

Repetitive vocalization

Agitation (Restlessness)

Physical Environment

Medical Treatment

Source: Mahoney, 2000b.

FIGURE ■ 22-3

Contextual framework for understanding challenging behaviors.

The four quadrants surrounding the model in Figure 22-3 direct symptom management. The caregiving environment and caregiving strategies, especially a nonpharmacological approach to manage symptoms (Volicer, Mahoney, & Brown, 1998), establish the tone for nursing care. The social environment provides caregiving in a milieu that recognizes and accommodates the special needs of persons with dementia and can range from a one-on-one interaction to a special care unit (Volicer & Simard, 1996). The physical environment emphasizes the importance of environmental design, both as a treatment for dementia and a "crutch" to help compensate for cognitive and functional deficits (Zeisel, Hyde, & Shi, 1999). Medical treatment ensures that physical problems, related or unrelated to dementia, are addressed (Volicer, 1996; Volicer, Hurley, & Camberg, 1999).

The overall approach is first on prevention. If known triggers result in problematic behaviors, the caregiver should remove those stimuli. Secondly, nurses should provide and suggest behavioral strategies (Table 22-1). When nonpharmacological strategies have been instituted and the patient still suffers from symptoms, pharmacological interventions should be added to the care plan (Table 22-2). Medications are given for the benefit of the patient and for no other reason.

AD causes patients to act in ways that make them uncomfortable, are distressing to their caregivers, and would embarrass them if they had their normal faculties. Nurses and other caregivers need to assess symptoms and intervene to prevent troublesome behaviors or to minimize those that are inevitable, while providing opportunities for success and pleasure. Discussion of the 12 core, primary, and peripheral symptoms follows.

Functional Impairment

Functional impairment is a primary consequence of dementia and has both cognitive and physical components. The physical component may result from the underlying dementia,

TABLE 22-1

Management Guidelines for Alzheimer's Disease

Issue/Condition	Goal	Treatment
• **Recent injury,** e.g., unwitnessed fall • **Discomfort or pain,** e.g., undertreated arthritis • **Physical complications,** e.g., urinary tract infection • **Uncomfortable environment,** e.g., too hot or too cold	1. Eliminate physical and medical causes	• Individualized care • Analgesic medication given liberally and possibly prophylactically before routine physical care • Comfortable environment
• **Frustrating interaction** • **Chaotic environment** • **Overly complex task request** • **Nothing to occupy time** • **Patterns,** e.g., time of day (fatigue), after a certain drug administration (untoward effect), before meals (hungry) • **Events,** e.g., change in physical or caregiving environment	2. Remove immediate precipitants and eliminate, reduce, or compensate for "triggers"	• Never say "no" • Calm environment • Avoid stress • Provide meaningful activities • Give rest breaks • Trial of drug "holiday" or discontinue drug • Caregiver and environmental continuity
• **Dementia** • **Mood disorders (depression)** • **Delusions or hallucinations** • **Functional impairment** • **Anxiety** • **Dependence in activities of daily living** • **Inability to initiate meaningful activities** • **Spatial disorientation**	3. Treat core and/or primary or secondary symptoms that may be the cause of the behavior	• Cholinesterase inhibitors • Correct amount of assistance (to preserve independence/prevent excess disability without overtaxing ability) • Nonpharmacological approaches and medications as needed

other comorbid conditions, or disuse. Improving or supporting functional ability will have a positive effect on multiple behavioral consequences of dementia. The pathological processes of dementing illnesses cause receptive and expressive aphasia and similar problems with reading and writing. It is important to continue to talk with persons who have AD and to use other interventions of cueing, reminiscence, favorite familiar music, environmental modification, and stimulus control to facilitate communication.

Practice Pearl

Provide verbal prompts one at a time to decrease the chances of the patient becoming confused. Even when verbal language is lost, nonverbal communication by way of tone of voice, smiling, and body language may be comforting. It is important to avoid any pressure to perform and to allow persons with dementia to continue with patterns that give a sense of security. Fatigue, nonroutine activities, alcohol, and a high-stimulus environment should be avoided because they increase functional impairment.

TABLE 22-2

Useful Medications for Patients With Alzheimer's Disease

Drug Class	Name	Dose Range (mg)/ Frequency*	Comments
Selected Antidepressant Medications			
Selective serotonin reuptake inhibitors	Fluoxetine (Prozac)	10 – 40/qam	Desired dose for a person with AD may vary from traditional range, e.g., Block (2001) recommends 25–100 mg/day for sertraline dose.
	Fluvoxamine (Luvox, Faverin)	50 – 300/qhs	
		20 – 50/qam/hs	
	Paroxetine (Paxil)	50 – 200/qam/hs	
	Sertraline (Zoloft)	20 – 40/qam	
	Citalopram (Celexa)		
Other	Mirtazapine (Remeron)	15 – 45/qhs	Trazodone and mirtazapine may be useful in patients who suffer from insomnia.
	Nefazodone (Serzone)	50 – 300/bid	
	Trazodone (Desyrel)	50 – 600/tid, hs (up to 300 mg)	
	Venlafaxine (Effexor)	25 – 75/bid–tid	
Selected Drugs Used in Treatment of Delusions and Hallucinations			
Typical neuroleptics	Haloperidol (Haldol)	0.5 – 1/qd–tid	Half-lives range from 4 (thioridazine) to 30 (olanzapine) hours. Do not give a drug with a long half-life for an intermittent symptom of short duration.
	Thioridazine (Mellaril)	10 – 40/qd–tid	
	Loxapine (Loxitane)	5 – 10/bid–tid	
Atypical neuroleptics	Risperidone (Risperdal)	0.25 – 1/qd–bid	
	Olanzapine (Zyprexa)	2.5 – 10/qd	
	Quetiapine (Seroquel)	25 – 100/bid–tid	
Selected Medications to Treat Anxiety			
Benzodiazepines	Lorazepam (Ativan)	0.5 – 1/bid–tid	Side effects are sedation, impaired motor coordination, akathisia, risk of falls, memory loss, respiratory or central nervous system depression, and paradoxical reaction. Must be tapered slowly.
	Alprazolam (Xanax)	0.25 – 0.5/tid	
	Oxazepam (Serax)	10 – 20/tid–qid	
	Clonazepam (Klonopin)	0.25 – 0.5/bid	
Azaspirone	Buspirone (BuSpar)	5 – 20/tid	Side effects are headache, nausea, drowsiness, and lightheadedness.

* qd = once a day, bid = twice a day, tid = three times a day, qid = four times a day, qam = every morning, qhs = every evening.

Apraxia interferes with the ability to follow a command such as "wash your face." However, patients with AD may be able to wash their face if handed a washcloth, or to continue an activity such as eating if someone helps them get started. **Agnosia** causes functional impairment and predisposes to safety hazards, such as putting inedible things into the mouth or pouring water into a toaster. Persons with AD may not recognize the bathroom or remember how to use the toilet. If the functional consequences of agnosia and apraxia decrease self-care independence, the nurse should use multiple channels to overcome the deficit. To maintain independence in toothbrushing, the nurse could say, "Here is your toothbrush. Brush your teeth. Smell the toothpaste. Taste the toothpaste." The nurse then might show his or her own teeth and point to the patient's mouth. If the patient does not take the toothbrush and begin brushing, he or she may need help getting started. The nurse should put the brush in the patient's hand, guide the toothbrush to the mouth, and initiate the procedure.

Physical impairment may result from specific brain pathology. If the person has vascular dementia, the infarcts may have caused weakness of an extremity, exaggerated deep tendon reflexes, or caused gait abnormalities. Persons with diffuse Lewy body disease may exhibit Parkinsonian symptoms that affect posture, balance, and gait. AD may result in abnormal reflexes, seizures, myoclonic jerks and rigidity, loss of the ability to walk, and loss of ability to stand. The hazards of immobility, when combined with neuromotor deterioration, create a double jeopardy for the person with dementia.

Interventions for physical impairment should be targeted to maintain the highest level of functional capacity for as long as possible and to restore capacity that may be remediable. Often patients are restrained for no reason other than a belief that the person may fall (Hamers, Gulpers, & Strik, 2004). Some general guidelines to retard physical impairment include the following:

1. Prevent excess disability. To prevent immobility, provide assisted ambulation versus allowing the person to remain on bed rest.
2. Treat other conditions that lead to physical decline. If pain interferes with walking, be sure prn pain relief is ordered and provided.
3. Identify and respond rapidly to acute changes in function. Be alert to symptoms suggesting an infection in order to make an early diagnosis.
4. Adapt care to accommodate neuromotor changes secondary to the progression of dementia. Compensate for changes in muscle tone and reflexes that affect posture, balance, range of motion, and ability to cooperate with care. Establish a preventive program to assess mobility, prevent falls, promote proper positioning, and implement environmental adaptations, such as redesigning furniture or introducing appropriate assistive devices (Trudeau, 1999b).

> ### Practice Pearl
>
> An individualized assessment should be conducted to develop specific interventions to prevent excess disability, create a therapeutic environment, actualize functional potential, and promote dignity.

Mood Disorders

Depression may be a core consequence of AD and cause secondary and peripheral symptoms such as agitation and inability to initiate meaningful activities. Depression is difficult to diagnose since many of its clinical signs also result from other complications of dementia (e.g., insomnia and agitation), and many patients cannot respond to most standardized assessment instruments or express sadness. Caregivers should be alert for changes in appetite, disinterest and **anhedonia**, sleep abnormality, and fatigue.

> ### Practice Pearl
>
> The treatment of depression in AD requires long-term administration of antidepressants.

Delusions and Hallucinations

Paranoid delusions are common psychotic symptoms in AD and were first described by German neurologist Alois Alzheimer in 1906. A study of 228 patients with AD reported that 52% showed evidence of delusions or hallucinations, most with only delusions (80%), some with both (18%), and a few with only hallucinations (2%) (Hirono et al., 1998). Delusions and hallucinations may also be caused by delirium induced by drugs, electrolyte imbalance, hyperglycemia, urinary tract infection, seizure disorder, hypothyroidism, and Parkinson's disease. Delusions in AD may be due to (1) an intercurrent confusional state (delirium), (2) an interaction of dementia and personality, (3) a separate mental disorder that coexists with the dementia, or (4) a disinhibition of cortical functions resulting in "released" symptomatology.

The nursing role is to attempt to control the consequences of delusions and hallucinations. Nonpharmacological approaches targeted to presumed causes should be initiated and evaluated (Volicer, Mahoney, & Brown, 1998). If delusions and hallucinations are causing other behavioral problems, pharmacological treatment may be necessary (see Table 22-2). Very potent and effective neuroleptic medications for treatment of delusions and hallucinations are available, but they should be avoided unless absolutely necessary.

Practice Pearl

Delusions and hallucinations should not be treated when they are pleasant and comforting, such as the "happy confabulator" who is mentally living in an earlier happy time of life with a long-dead spouse. Environmental interventions such as turning off the television set or covering a mirror may prevent distressing delusions and hallucinations when the patient fears another person in the room.

Dependence in Activities of Daily Living

Persons with AD will need varying degrees of assistance depending on their retained capacities and deficits. The goal is to preserve and promote functional independence. The nurse should determine the best time for activities of daily living and develop a preventive care plan to avoid potential problems. For maintaining continence as long as possible, a prompted voiding plan should be established. There are many ways to encourage independence. To assist with dressing, it is helpful to use garments that are easy to put on (jogging clothes, sneakers with Velcro closures), lay out the clothes, provide a verbal prompt, and repeat if necessary. When assistance is needed, the nurse should provide what is necessary to prevent stressing the patient, but not so much as to cause excess disability.

Practice Pearl

Not all dependence in activities of daily living is attributable to dementia. Preventing avoidable decrements in capacity can be accomplished by knowledgeable caregivers. Since there may be other reasons for decreased ability to carry out daily activities, a complete assessment should be done. For example, new incontinence may be related to a urinary tract infection, which when treated may reverse the incontinence.

Inability to Initiate Meaningful Activities

Inability to initiate meaningful activities, although easy to overlook, affects persons with dementia and their caregivers. This inability has roots in functional impairment and depression, and its effects are far-reaching. Lack of meaningful activity may result in apathy or agitation for the person with dementia, and frustration and burden for the caregiver. Involvement with meaningful activity is important for maintenance of functional abilities and social involvement—providing a feeling of success and accomplishment, improving mood, and reducing disruptive behaviors. Even in the very late stage of dementia, persons can enjoy activities such as **Snoezelen**, relaxation induced by providing pleasing sensory stimuli in a multisensory environment (Brown, 1999; Chitsey, Haight, & Jones, 2002) or music (Hanser, 1999).

> **Practice Pearl**
>
> Since the person with dementia cannot initiate meaningful activities, caregivers must select appropriate activities that match the person's capacity and provide pleasure.

Anxiety

Anxiety may be a primary disorder or a symptom of depression. It may result from delusions, hallucinations, or functional impairment. Environmentally focused and behavioral interventions should be used before prescribing anxiolytics (Table 22-2). The nurse should plan specific interventions to minimize stress level, enhance feelings of trust and safety, and promote stability by providing a daily routine with few variations. Diversional activities such as music therapy (Hanser, 1999), reminiscence (Spector, Orrell, Davies, & Woods, 2003), structured sensory stimulation (Trudeau, 1999a), Snoezelen (Brown, 1999), or simulated presence therapy (Camberg et al., 1999) should be provided.

> **Practice Pearl**
>
> Anxiety is an unpleasant symptom. Caregivers must identify and treat anxiety before it channels the person's energy into defensive behaviors.

Spatial Disorientation

Even when persons with AD have no eyesight problem, space and location may be distorted, objects may be interpreted incorrectly, or directions may be misunderstood. Spatial disorientation may cause misunderstanding of the environment and lead to the development of fear, anxiety, suspicions, illusions, delusions, and safety problems such as getting lost. In the early stage of dementia, the person may become confused when in an unfamiliar place. In the later stages, the person can become confused when in previously familiar places.

Two basic concepts, pop-up cues and environmental landmarks, can guide interventions. A pop-up (contrasting color should be used, such as a red wall in the bathroom) can help when a person does not use a white toilet in a white bathroom or will not sit on a blue chair in front of a blue wall. Landmarks capitalize on long-standing memory and use objects that are associated with the years the individual best remembers. Personal effects associated with specific rooms should be used as orientation devices.

> **Practice Pearl**
>
> Specific color-cued interventions should be targeted for individuals in their environment. The same furniture should be kept in the same place, and no changes should be made in room decorations except to simplify rooms and remove clutter.

Elopement

Caregivers are justifiably fearful that their care recipient will wander away and become lost, get injured, or die. Elopement is a potential problem in all settings. Community-dwelling AD patients are more likely to wander if they have severe cognitive impairment, exhibit more than one challenging behavior, and spend long periods alone (Logsdon et al., 1998). Other risk factors include a darkened or unfamiliar environment, boredom, stress, tension, lack of control, lack of exercise, and nocturnal delirium.

In designing prevention strategies, the primary care provider should ask caregivers two questions: (1) Is the patient ever left alone? (2) Is the patient registered with the Alzheimer's Association Safe Return Program? Safe Return is a national program that helps to find and return registered AD patients and helps guide the family through elopement (Silverstein & Flaherty, 1996). You can call 888-572-8566 to register a patient in the national database for a reasonable fee. The caregiver fills out a form, supplies a photograph, and selects an identification product (e.g., bracelet, wallet card, or information sewed into clothing). Since 1993, over 78,000 persons have been registered and the program has helped locate and return more than 6,400 individuals.

> **Practice Pearl**
>
> It is important to remove the precipitants of elopement such as unmet physical needs, boredom, easy exit, or reminders stimulating leaving. Safe walking activities provide exercise, offer social interaction, fill time, and use energy. Exits should be locked. The caregiver must not leave cues to leaving, such as car keys or coats, by the door.

Resistiveness to Care

Resistiveness to care is common during the middle to late stages of dementia and stresses both patients and caregivers (Mahoney et al., 1999). If unmanaged, it is also a major reason for institutionalization and the use of psychotropic medications and restraints (Potts, Richie, & Kaas, 1996). Resistiveness to care occurs during interactions among care recipient, caregiver, and their environment. At times, simply responding with a relaxed and smiling manner may achieve calm and functional behavior. A time-out with a pleasant distraction should divert the patient's attention from the disturbing stimulus.

> **Practice Pearl**
>
> There are no medications to directly prevent or treat resistiveness to care. Core consequences and secondary symptoms of AD that may lead to resistiveness can be managed by behavioral or pharmacological interventions (Tables 22-1 and 22-2). Because resistiveness occurs intermittently for short periods, a medication with a long duration and poor side-effect profile should not be used.

Since the neurologic conditions are chronic, patients and families manage the disorder for their entire lives. Nursing interventions can often be incorporated into activities of daily living.

Food Refusal

Specific issues related to food refusal occur during each of the progressive stages of AD as a consequence of primary or secondary symptoms. In all stages, changes in environment and disruption of usual routines can be upsetting, so mealtime rituals and consistency are helpful. One aspect of short-term memory loss for persons with AD is that they forget yesterday's menu and their most recent meal or snack. Caregivers may become bored with preparing the same food every day, but each meal and snack is a new experience for the person with AD. Mealtimes should be a focal point of the day, and other activities can be built around structured eating times. The primary caregiver should know the individual's current likes and dislikes, his or her level of physical activity and degree of independence, and how to make eating pleasant and nutritious to provide adequate calories, nutrition, and hydration. A nourishment plan should specify which foods will be provided and how they will be prepared, identify the best eating areas, and establish routines for the eating process.

The person with AD may have age-related changes in the sense of taste which can lead to decreased appetite and decreased food intake. Often persons with AD develop a fondness for sweet food. See Table 22-3 for recommendations for preventing food refusal.

The amount and type of food and beverages should be limited to prevent too much visual stimulation or too many choices, which can be overwhelming. It is best to use foods that are easily handled, chewed, and swallowed. Since persons with AD tend to lose weight later in the disease, caloric density should be maximized, unless they are above ideal weight. Use of finger foods (sandwiches) is one way to address misperception or inability to use a knife, fork, or spoon. In the terminal stage, when patients are bedfast, mute, dysphagic, and subject to infections, eating difficulties can become very problematic (Volicer et al., 1989). Choking may appear in the severe to terminal stage and may be prevented or at least minimized by avoiding thin liquids, feeding the person in a sitting position or keeping the head of the bed at a 90-degree angle, and using foods

TABLE 22-3

Preventing and Breaking the Cycle of Behaviors Used to Refuse Food in the Later Stages of Alzheimer's Disease

Patient Behaviors	Suggested Approaches for Staff
Passive	**Provide Sensory Stimulation**
Unaware of environment	*Auditory:* "Hello. Here's your breakfast. It smells good."
	Olfactory: Aroma of food product, e.g., freshly baked bread.
	Visual: Smile and make eye contact.
	Tactile: Move hand over patient's hand to take spoon.
	Taste: Put small amount of sweet food on lips for patient to lick.
No involvement with feeder	Hold hand and make eye contact.
"Kisses the spoon"	Place food on patient's lips for him or her to lick off.
Defensive	**Gently Encourage**
Averts head	Say patient's name; engage; say, "Here's some pudding."
Closes mouth	Smile and say, "Open."
Clamps down on eating tool	Stroke cheek and say, "Eat."
Will not swallow	Stroke throat and say, "Swallow."
Active Opposition	**Do Not Force; Distract; Wait**
Pushes utensil or feeder away	Distract from utensil; try again.
Spits out food	Stop; wait.
Screams "no!"	Stop; wait; distract; come back later.

Source: Mahoney, 2000a.

in which the bolus has sufficient moisture content to help passage through the pharynx and facilitate swallowing (Frisoni, Franzoni, Bellelli, Morris, & Warden, 1998).

> ## Practice Pearl
>
> If a person likes a food, the caregiver should serve it. The same meals and snacks can be served until the person cannot eat them or does not want to eat them. Some medications can be eliminated if they alter the taste of food, take away appetite, or interfere with the ability to use eating utensils.

Insomnia

Insomnia in elderly adults is discussed in Chapter 8, but AD may present more difficulties with insomnia since it causes death of nerve cells in many areas of the brain, including the suprachiasmatic nucleus. Cell loss in the suprachiasmatic nucleus leads to abnormalities of circadian rhythms in persons with AD. Retrospective evaluation of persons with autopsy-confirmed AD found that disturbances of circadian rhythms were present in 56% of patients, and the average time of onset of these disturbances was several months before the diagnosis of AD (Jost & Grossberg, 1996). Circadian rhythm disruption leads to changes of sleep, body temperature, melatonin secretion, and possibly other physiological functions.

When persons with AD experience insomnia, several strategies may be used. Lifestyle changes should be explored to establish proper sleep hygiene. Activities inconsistent with maintaining high-quality sleep and daytime alertness should be avoided, such as irregular use of daytime naps, extended amount of time in bed, irregular sleep-wake schedules, or inactivity. It is important to avoid using products that interfere with sleep (caffeine, nicotine, and alcohol), scheduling exercise close to bedtime, engaging in exciting or emotionally upsetting activities close to bedtime, and having a poor sleep environment, such as an uncomfortable bed or a bedroom that is too bright, stuffy, hot, cold, or noisy (Bootzin, Epstein, & Wood, 1991).

> ## Practice Pearl
>
> Insomnia places a burden on persons with AD and their caregivers — depriving family caregivers of their sleep and precipitating institutionalization of the person with AD dementia. In an institution, residents suffering from insomnia may disturb the sleep of other residents.

> ## Drug Alert !
>
> All persons with AD are choline deficient, and anticholinergic drugs have the potential to worsen the symptoms of AD. It is essential to be wary of over-the-counter sleeping medications that may contain an anticholinergic component or other drugs that may have anticholinergic properties.

Apathy and Agitation

Apathy and agitation are likely to occur as AD worsens and persons experience more functional and cognitive decline. Persons with AD are unable to make sense of their environment, to filter the stimulation that comes their way, and to handle the stress of what is happening to them. **Engagement**, the opposite of apathy, involves attention to and participation in the external environment such as involvement in a conversation or other meaningful activities. Persons with AD need help to become active and interested in what is going on around them. It is common for persons with AD to have bouts of apathy followed by agitation. By uncovering the causes, it is easier to treat agitation before it escalates into assaultive or even violent behavior.

Treatment for agitation and apathy is central to promoting psychological well-being specific for persons with dementia (Volicer et al., 1999). Worsening of AD over time restricts the capacity to express emotions. As persons with AD lose their ability to express their emotions verbally, they resort to other, primarily nonverbal, means of communication. Caregivers control the environment and can communicate emotionally with persons who have AD (Raia, 1999).

> **Practice Pearl**
>
> The right amount of stimulation will promote pleasure and prevent apathy without inciting agitation. The nurse should identify appropriate activities and help the older person become engaged with them and assess causes and management of overstimulation (too many visitors or television set).

Pharmacological Interventions

Pharmacotherapy is indicated only when nonpharmacological interventions do not prevent or alleviate challenging behaviors. Prevention or treatment of challenging behaviors is critical to patients' overall well-being since behavioral dysregulation can be associated with functional impairment (Schultz, Ellingrod, Turvey, Moser, & Arndt, 2003). In all cases, medications are prescribed to promote the patient's comfort and for no other reason. Two traditional principles of geriatric nursing—start low and go slow, and monitor treatment continuously—must be followed. Exactly which medication to select is dependent on the patient's clinical condition and the balance between the desired action and side-effect profile. For example, capitalizing on the hypnotic side effect of trazodone for a depressed patient who also has insomnia uses one medication to treat two problems (see Table 22-2).

> **Practice Pearl**
>
> Although it is always important to consider the patient first when developing nursing interventions for persons with a neurologic disorder, these conditions are family disorders because they affect the entire family. Families will be stressed and in crisis as a result of their loved one's dementia and symptoms.

Late-Stage Issues

There often comes a time when the family cannot manage home care any longer and must seek institutionalized long-term care. This difficult decision carries dual concerns: (1) finding an appropriate facility, and (2) managing the guilt of transferring care to another. Many assisted-living facilities have **dementia special-care units**. When the person's needs overwhelm home or assisted-living care, a skilled nursing facility will be required. An ideal skilled nursing facility provides for basic safety needs, meets overall health needs, and promotes quality of life in daily living. The nurse can help the family by suggesting questions to ask the nursing director (Table 22-4).

TABLE 22-4

How Nurses Can Help Families Choose a Nursing Home

Issues	Questions to Ask the Medical Director, Nursing Director, and Administrator
Safe physical environment	Is the unit locked? Are there protected inside and outdoor wandering paths? How is elopement prevented? How are falls prevented? Are physical or chemical restraints ever used? What types of assistive devices are used?
Dementia health	How often does a physician or nurse practitioner routinely visit each resident? What memory-enhancing medications are typically used? What cognitively enhancing activities are used?
Overall health	What drugs and treatment are available for other medical conditions without being transferred from the unit? from the nursing home? How are chronic pre-existing and other new problems assessed and managed? What is the procedure if acute care is needed? Where is terminal care provided? Is hospice available on the unit?
Knowledgeable and available staff	What kinds of staff training programs are there? How often are they provided? What percent of staff attend? What percent of nursing assistants are certified? What percent of nursing assistants are certified in dementia care? What special consultants are available? How many hours of direct nursing care does each resident receive each 24 hours? How many full-time equivalent registered nurses are there per resident?
Quality-of-life issues	What programs are there to maintain physical functioning (toileting, feeding assistance, ambulation)? What is the pain management program? How much time in each 24-hour period do residents spend outside their bedrooms? What are the ongoing activities and daily events?
Support services	What types of family support groups are there and how frequently do they meet? What family education programs are provided?
Interdisciplinary team approach	How are individual resident's care plans developed, evaluated, revised, and shared with the family? How frequently does the team evaluate each resident's care plan? Is there a system to include family input?

Source: Hurley & Volicer, 2002.

Practice Pearl

Too much information can be overwhelming. The nurse should teach what the patient and family will need to know tomorrow, not next year.

Family caregivers must be supported in dealing with their guilt at "failing" the person with AD. The nurse can help by stating, "You have done such a fine job of caregiving. Look at the nursing home staff. It takes a team of nurses working three shifts a day, seven days a week to do what you have been doing." The nurse should reiterate that AD will continue to worsen and the patient will continue to decline. The family may confront four issues: (1) Should cardiopulmonary resuscitation (CPR) be attempted? (2) Will the person be transferred to an acute care facility? (3) Should a feeding tube be used? (4) How should life-threatening infections be managed?

Do Not Resuscitate. For persons with late-stage Alzheimer's disease, CPR should not be offered. If the person does not have an advance plan stipulating either CPR or do not resuscitate (DNR), the DNR decision should be discussed with the surrogate decision maker. DNR does not present an ethical dilemma as clinicians recognize both the futility (Awoke, Mouton, & Parrott, 1992) and adverse effects (Applebaum, King, & Finucane, 1990) of CPR on long-term care patients in general, and its use is low (Duthie et al., 1993). Resuscitation for an unwitnessed cardiac arrest in this population has a very low probability of restoring life (Duthie et al., 1993). Patients who survive and are discharged back to their long-term care unit are invariably in a much more advanced stage of dementia than they were before the arrest. A DNR order would spare the few patients who survive the resuscitation event from living in an uncomfortable state for the remainder of their lives. If the definition of success is to restore patients to their previous functional capacity, no matter how limited, there is no place for resuscitation attempts when patients with AD have a cardiac or respiratory arrest. Although healthcare workers may understand that CPR is futile in late-stage AD, the family may not. Education should be provided to families who make the ultimate decision about DNR for persons who do not have the capacity to do so for themselves.

Transfer to an Acute Care Site. There are many reasons why older adults in general and persons with AD in particular are transferred from a long-term care facility to a hospital, and often these reasons are not patient care centered. One team of researchers found that transfers to the hospital were influenced by an insufficient number of adequately trained staff to administer and monitor intravenous therapy, lack of diagnostic services, and pressure from staff and family (Kayser-Jones, Wiener, & Barbaccia, 1989). Another team found that nurses influenced the decision to transfer dying residents because of insufficient knowledge of resident or family preferences, lack of technological and personnel resources in the nursing home, and concerns about liability (Bottrell, O'-Sullivan, Robbins, Mitty, & Mezey, 2001). Staffing in nursing homes is less than ideal (Harrington et al., 2000), and staffing problems may further contribute to hospitalization of patients with AD. Many long-term care sites do not accept patients with advanced AD. In this case, the patient may qualify for hospice, which is paid for by Medicare.

Once in the hospital, elderly adults with dementia are at risk for complications such as delirium, being tube-fed, relocation stress, and dying. Delirium superimposed on AD was found in 8 of 20 elderly adults with documented dementia (Fick & Foreman, 2000). It is estimated that anywhere from 14% to 80% of all elderly patients hospitalized for the treatment of an acute physical illness experience an episode of delirium (Foreman, Wakefield, Culp, & Milisen, 2001). The problems of delirium during an acute phase of illness are well documented, but the long-term outcomes, or the results of an entire episode of delirium, are lacking (Foreman et al., 2001). It is not known how the hospital-induced delirium episode affects an already frail individual's cognitive and physical functioning long term. Refer to the Best Practices feature for information on rating delirium.

When discussing the issue of transferring, healthcare providers have to help the family understand the differences between reversing an acute care problem in an otherwise healthy individual and extending the dying process in a person with AD. For instance, coronary bypass surgery might extend the life of a patient who has severe coronary disease. However, living on a long-term care unit without perceiving the stresses of the world and receiving care in a low-stimulus environment may be clinically advantageous. Cataract surgery may be advocated to allow patients the ability to connect visually with their environment. However, patients with AD will be at risk of removing an intraocular lens because, unless restrained, they would be likely to rub their eyes. A transfer to an acute care unit means that patients will be cared for by staff who may be experts in critical care but not in dementia care. Transferring AD patients to acute units also predisposes them to translocation stress (Dehlin, 1990).

According to Holzer and Warshaw (2002, p. 192), "Traditional patterns of caring for elderly patients in an acute care hospital in which the nursing staff bathes, toilets, feeds, and grooms these patients without ensuring that they can perform these tasks by themselves may contribute to a lack of independence. In addition, enforced bed rest, use of sedating drugs, indwelling bladder catheters, physical restraints, and medications that lead to acute confusional states contribute to the loss of independence of these patients." When Fick and Foreman (2000) examined the consequences of undetected delirium in 20 hospitalized AD patients, they found that 12 patients were incontinent, 3 on admission and 9 with new incontinence that developed after admission. Patients with pneumonia were more likely to experience decline in their activities of daily living if hospitalized than comparable patients with similar severity of illness treated in the skilled nursing facility (Gillick, 2002). Almost one third of older adults hospitalized for acute medical or surgical illness decline in their ability to perform daily activities (Holzer & Warshaw, 2002). Thus, hospital-acquired decrements last beyond hospitalization.

On acute care units there is an increased potential for the use of restraints, which can predispose patients to increased delirium and the complications of immobility. A vicious circle of events leading to increased iatrogenesis can be set in motion. The issue of using restraints to deliver technology the patient cannot understand is complex. One could argue that the patient will forget being restrained and the long-term benefit outweighs the short-term requirement of being in restraints. However, because patients with AD appear to live in the present, the stress associated with being restrained is not outweighed by the ability to deliver technology. Patients with late-stage AD have a reduced life span, which needs to be considered when asking if the burden is outweighed by the benefit.

Feeding Tube. The "need" for feeding tubes may be avoided by promoting eating and preventing food refusal. Caregivers should sit and make eye contact, chat, and make eating an important and pleasurable component of long-term institutional care (Burger, Kayser-Jones, & Bell, 2001; Kayser-Jones & Schell, 1997). More than one third of severely cognitively impaired nursing home residents in the United States have feeding tubes (Mitchell, Teno, Roy, Kabumoto, & Mor, 2003). Even though patients with AD may refuse food, turn away when food is offered, push the spoon or hand away, or spit out food, they can be successfully fed by hand (Volicer et al., 1989).

Even patients with advanced AD can revert to natural feeding after tube feeding (Volicer, Rheaume, Riley, Karner, & Glennon, 1990). An individualized care plan, based on the patient's target body weight and functional eating abilities, should be developed by an interdisciplinary team, including a nurse, dietitian, and physician (Frisoni et al., 1998). Natural feeding can begin with the tube in place until the patient's eating is reestablished. Then the tube may be removed. Skillful hand feeding should continue, and a program of functional feeding using the patient's remaining skills should be initiated. To promote independence, the caregiver may place a hand over the patient's hand, take a large spoon, place a small amount of sweetened food such as applesauce on the tip of the spoon, move it to the patient's mouth, and follow steps outlined in Table 22-3.

Permanent tube feeding is not recommended for persons with advanced AD, even those who choke on food and liquids. Tube feeding does not prevent aspiration, improve functioning or quality of life, increase comfort, or promote weight gain (Finucane, Christmas, & Travis, 1999). One widely held misconception about tube feeding is that

To rate delirium and distinguish delirium from other types of cognitive impairment, The Hartford Institute for Geriatric Nursing Try This Assessment Series (2001) recommends use of the Confusion Assessment Method (CAM) (Inouye, S., van Dyck, Alessi, et al., 1990). The CAM includes two parts. Part 1 is an assessment instrument that screens for overall cognitive impairment. Part 2 includes only those four features that distinguish delirium. The tool can be administered in less than 5 minutes. It closely correlates with DSM-IV criteria for delirium.

The Confusion Assessment Method Instrument

1. *Acute onset* Is there evidence of an acute change in mental status from the patient's baseline?
2A. *Inattention* Did the patient have difficulty focusing attention, for example, being easily distractible, or having difficulty keeping track of what was being said?
2B. *If present or abnormal* Did this behavior fluctuate during the interview, that is, tend to come and go or increase and decrease in severity?
3. *Disorganized thinking* Was the patient's thinking disorganized or incoherent, such as rambling or irrelevant conversation, unclear or illogical flow of ideas, or unpredictable switching from subject to subject?
4. *Altered level of consciousness* Overall, how would you rate this patient's level of consciousness? (alert [normal]; vigilant [hyperalert, overly sensitive to environmental stimuli, startled very easily]; lethargic [drowsy, easily aroused]; stupor [difficult to arouse]; coma [unarousable]; uncertain)
5. *Disorientation* Was the patient disoriented at any time during the interview, such as thinking that he or she was somewhere other than the hospital, using the wrong bed, or misjudging the time of day?
6. *Memory impairment* Did the patient demonstrate any memory problems during the interview, such as inability to remember events in the hospital or difficulty remembering instructions?
7. *Perceptual disturbances* Did the patient have any evidence of perceptual disturbances, for example, hallucinations, illusions, or misinterpretations (such as thinking something was moving when it was not)?
8A. *Psychomotor agitation* At any time during the interview did the patient have an unusually increased level of motor activity such as restlessness, picking at bedclothes, tapping fingers, or making frequent sudden changes of position?
8B. *Psychomotor retardation* At any time during the interview did the patient have an unusually decreased level of motor activity such as sluggishness, staring into space, staying in one position for a long time, or moving very slowly?
9. *Altered sleep-wake cycle* Did the patient have evidence of disturbance of the sleep-wake cycle, such as excessive daytime sleepiness with insomnia at night?

The Confusion Assessment Method Diagnostic Algorithm

Feature 1: *Acute Onset and Fluctuating Course*

This feature is usually obtained from a family member or nurse and is shown by positive responses to the following questions: Is there evidence of an acute change in mental status from the patient's baseline? Did the (abnormal) behavior fluctuate during the day, that is, tend to come and go, or increase and decrease in severity?

Feature 2: *Inattention*

This feature is shown by a positive response to the following question: Did the patient have difficulty focusing attention, for example, being easily distractible, or having difficulty keeping track of what was being said?

Feature 3: *Disorganized Thinking*

This feature is shown by a positive response to the following question: Was the patient's thinking disorganized or incoherent, such as rambling or irrelevant conversation, unclear or illogical flow of ideas, or unpredictable switching from subject to subject?

Source: Adapted from Waszynski, C. M. (2002). Confusion Assessment Method (CAM) in *Try This: Best Practices in Care for Older Adults.* New York: New York University, The Steinhardt School of Education, Division of Nursing, The John A. Hartford Foundation Institute for Geriatric Nursing.

it is ordinary care like spoon feeding. However, tube feeding does not resemble eating or drinking in any way (Ahronheim, 1996; Huang & Ahronheim, 2000). Although some family members and healthcare workers may fear that the patient will "starve to death," patients who are cognitively intact and dying have reported that they often do not feel thirsty and hungry (McCann, Hall, & Groth-Juncker, 1994). Body functions are shutting down during the dying process, and food and liquids are no longer necessary (Smith, 1998). In fact, dehydration is beneficial during the dying process because it decreases the sensation of pain and prevents edema and excessive respiratory secretions. Dehydration also decreases the incidence of vomiting and diarrhea. The only consequence of dehydration that may lead to discomfort is dryness of the mouth, lips, or eyes, which can be prevented or alleviated by moisturizing spray, swabs or salve, or ice chips.

Treatment of Infections. Infections are an inevitable consequence of advanced AD because of several risk factors that cannot be avoided, such as changes in immune function, incontinence, decreased mobility, and aspiration (Volicer, Brandeis, & Hurley, 1998). Infections may be treated by the administration of oral antibiotics that are as effective as parenteral antibiotics and do not require restraints to prevent removal of an intravenous catheter. However, the effectiveness of antibiotic treatment is diminished in the terminal stage of AD when infections become recurrent. Pneumonia is the most common cause of death in individuals with dementia, reflecting the limited effectiveness of antibiotic therapy in this patient population. Antibiotics are not necessary to maintain comfort of the patient during an infectious episode because comfort can be maintained by administration of analgesics and antipyretics.

In summary, successfully caring for the person with dementia requires the humane, empathetic, and skillful application of evidence-based interventions. "Good endings" are possible. Caregivers can provide the education, guidance, and support needed to appropriately care for AD patients, who may live for 20 years or more from the onset of symptoms (Hurley & Volicer, 2002).

Parkinson's Disease

Parkinsonism is a group of symptoms and signs in which there are variable combinations of tremor, rigidity, bradykinesia, and a disturbance in gait and posture. Parkinson's disease (PD) is a chronic, progressive neurologic disorder in which idiopathic Parkinsonism appears without other widespread neurologic symptoms, such as cognitive impairment. PD symptoms are caused by the loss of nerve cells in the pigmented substantia nigra pars compacta and the locus coeruleus in the midbrain. In PD, Lewy bodies are present in the basal ganglia, brain stem, spinal cord, and sympathetic ganglia. PD is considered an extrapyramidal syndrome because of the anatomical structures involved and the resulting symptoms of tremor, **chorea**, and **dystonia**.

> ### Practice Pearl
>
> PD may progress to PD with dementia, and the nurse will be caring for a patient with two characteristic groups of neurologic symptoms, including movement and memory disorders.

Similar to Alzheimer's disease, PD is a disorder for which the risk increases dramatically with age. PD occurs at similar rates in all ethnic groups, is equally distributed in males and females, and has a prevalence of 1 to 2 per 1,000 persons in the general population, which increases to 2% of adults over age 65. The exact cause of PD is unknown, but it is hypothesized that exposure to environmental toxins or a genetic predisposition lead to PD. The disease can be induced in primates by chemical exposure leading to death of nigrostriatal neurons, depletion of dopamine in the basal ganglia, and Parkinsonism. First-degree relatives of patients are twice as likely to develop PD as are controls. Currently, there is no exact diagnostic test for PD. It is considered a disease of exclusion, that is, the diagnosis is made when all other causes of chronic Parkinsonism are ruled out.

The pathology of PD is related to the loss of the dopaminergic cells situated deep in the midbrain in the substantia nigra (the black substance so named because of the melanin seen in those neurons). The human brain is able to compensate for loss of up to 85% of these cells, but the remaining cells are not able to provide the neurotransmission necessary to prevent the symptoms of PD (Moore, Cicchetti, & Isacson, 2001). Neurotransmission that takes place at the nerve terminals produces dopamine, which is necessary to initiate movement. Thus, therapy directed to correct **dopamine** deficiency currently drives the pharmacological bases of treatment. Pharmacological intervention by administration of levodopa, the metabolic precursor of dopamine provides symptomatic relief of symptoms, particularly bradykinesia.

Although the replacement hypothesis sounds like a straightforward solution, two factors complicate the issue. First, the active medication must pass into the brain through the blood-brain barrier. Because the enzyme dopa decarboxylase in the intestinal mucosa converts ingested levodopa to dopamine, most is lost before it even enters the general circulation. Thus, levodopa is combined with a peripheral dopa-carboxylase inhibitor. The combination of medication is available commercially as Sinemet in formulations of 1:10 and 1:4 ratios. A common starting dose is 25/100 mg carbidopa/levodopa three times daily and increased gradually to 25/250 mg up to four times daily. To maximize absorption and facilitate crossing the blood-brain barrier, Sinemet should be taken on an empty stomach. The nurse should incorporate timing of the administration of Sinemet into the patient's care plan. Both the patient and caregiver should be taught that this medication should be taken 1 hour before or 2 hours after a meal. Nursing interventions should be planned to minimize potential side effects of nausea and vomiting. The patient may experience postural hypotension. The nurse needs to teach strategies to prevent falling, such as sitting on the side of the bed before standing or holding onto a table when arising from a chair.

The second issue related to levodopa therapy is that the patient may at times appear to have developed a drug-induced tolerance. However, the patient's symptoms can vary widely despite constant levels of the drug in the peripheral circulation and in the brain. During the "off" time, the drug becomes ineffective and the patient may freeze up momentarily and lose mobility. During the "on" time, side effects such as involuntary and hyperactive movements and dystonia occur. The exact pathogenesis of this on-off phenomenon is unknown, but the patient and family need to be prepared for this possibility, which can revert to normal action of the drug and symptom management.

The anticholinergics are another class of medications used for symptomatic treatment of PD. These drugs are prescribed to relieve tremors. The nurse needs to be vigilant in managing the side effects of dry mouth, constipation, blurred vision, and urinary retention. Because PD is a movement disorder, a vision problem can further increase the risk of falling. In elderly men, urinary retention could complicate symptoms of an enlarged prostate. Another drug, amantadine, alone or in combination with an anticholinergic drug, may help by potentiating the release of endogenous dopamine. However, this benefit may be transitory. Another class of medications are dopamine agonists, which directly stimulate the dopamine receptors, such as Permax (Parkinson Study Group, 2000). Dopamine agonists are often initiated in early PD before starting levodopa and are also used in combination with levodopa through the progressive course of PD. Thus, because of the on-off effects of levodopa, some patients are tried on other medications at the onset of symptoms.

Surgery for PD has been tried with destructive neurosurgical procedures of unilateral posteroventral pallidotomy or thalamotomy. Although some positive but incomplete responses have been reported in patients on the side contralateral to the procedure, bilateral procedures have a higher morbidity and are generally discouraged. Brain stimulation surgery, such as thalamic stimulation, has a lower morbidity than ablative surgery. Exploratory surgery in the form of transplantation of fetal midbrain dopaminergic cells has been explored, but because of the ethical issues involved, there has been limited experimentation. Currently, there is lack of evidence from clinical trials to recommend surgery for PD (Stowe et al., 2003).

Nursing care should be directed to helping the patient manage Parkinsonism—that is, to design individualized interventions to promote mobility, prevent falls, and preserve independence for as long as possible. In the early stage, the patient may have mild symptoms on one side only, which are inconvenient but not disabling, and changes in posture, walking, and facial expression (masklike, as originally described by English physician James Parkinson). In the middle stages, patients often will have difficulty rising from bed or chair, tend to assume a flexed posture when standing, and have difficulty initiating walking. They lean forward increasingly to "get started." They may walk with small shuffling steps with no arm swing, have an unsteady gait especially on turning, and have difficulty in stopping. Some patients walk at an increased speed to prevent themselves from falling to counteract their abnormal center of gravity because of moving forward to initiate walking. In the very late stage, the patient cannot stand or walk, becomes cachectic, and requires constant nursing care.

Nurses should assess fall risk (Gray & Hildebrand, 2000) using an agreed upon assessment measure such as the functional reach test (Behrman, Light, Flynn, & Thigpen, 2002). Based on the patient's retained capacity, the nurse should develop a plan to include the patient and family. An interdisciplinary approach to care is important. The nurse should be part of a team that includes the occupational therapist to help retain skills and promote independence in activities of daily living (Deane, Ellis-Hill, Playford, Ben-Shlomo, & Clarke, 2001; Gauthier, Dalziel, & Gauthier, 1987). Exercise is another way to preserve independence (Baatile, Langbein, Weaver, Maloney, & Jost, 2000).

MediaLink

Tremor Video

Stroke

A stroke is a sudden loss of consciousness followed by paralysis. Stroke is a leading cause of death in the United States, and annually 12 in each 10,000 Americans have a stroke. The pathology typically is caused by hemorrhage into the brain, an embolus or thrombus that occludes an artery, or rupture of an extracerebral artery causing subarachnoid hemorrhage. Immediate treatment is targeted to lifesaving techniques, prevention of extension of the stroke, and early treatment using a plasminogen activator. Stroke is an emergency, and the benefits of reducing further morbidity have to be balanced with risks of increasing the possibility of intracerebral hemorrhage. An adequate airway needs to be established and maintained with ventilation and oxygenation provided as needed. The nurse assesses for neurologic status using the Glasgow Coma Scale (Ingersoll & Leyden, 1994), vital signs, papillary responses, respiratory patterns, and sensory and motor responses to verbal, tactile, and painful stimulation (Crosby & Parsons, 1989). An experienced team needs to make the decision about movement of the patient and transport.

After an acute stroke, the patient is typically transferred to an emergency department. Usually the National Institutes of Health (NIH) Stroke Scale (Figure 22-4 ■) is used to gauge the degree of cerebral infarction by determining level of consciousness. Also used are performance and examination tests of gaze, visual fields, facial palsy, motor strength, **ataxia**, sensation, language, dysarthria, and extinction or inattention (Brott et al., 1989). The NIH Stroke Scale is considered to be a valid and reliable clinical examination scale to determine stroke severity (Muir, Weir, Murray, Povey, & Lees, 1996). If thrombolytic therapy is not contraindicated, then often recombinant tissue plasminogen activator (rt-PA) will be administered within 3 hours to treat the acute ischemic stroke (Tanne et al., 2002). However, not all patients treated with rt-PA therapy have positive outcomes. The occurrence of symptomatic intracerebral hemorrhage after rt-PA therapy is a catastrophic event, and most of those who survive are discharged to a long-term care facility versus home (Schlegel et al., 2004).

For those stroke survivors who are able to return home, the physical, cognitive, and emotional sequelae place great burdens on the patient and family. Many of their postdischarge needs are ameliorable to nursing interventions. An examination of community-dwelling stroke survivors found that the most commonly reported interventions were directed toward ensuring continuity of care between the hospital and home, family care, and modifying risk factors (McBride, White, Sourial, & Mayo, 2004). Structured nursing interventions during the rehabilitative period have resulted in better functional status, less depression, and higher self-perceived health, self-esteem, and dietary adherence (Nir, Zolotogorsky, & Sugarman, 2004).

Although the prognosis is grave, many patients survive and rehabilitation becomes the cornerstone of nursing care. The major issues for older persons who survive a stroke have to do with activity limitations across multiple domains (basic and instrumental activities of daily living), psychological distress, and communication difficulties. In contrast to AD, which worsens, stroke survivors' conditions often improve with rehabilitation. However, persons who experience a stroke associated with small vessel disease are at risk for both motor and cognitive impairment problems (Mok et al., 2004), thus underscoring the importance of preventing strokes by promoting good cardiovascular health.

Although the onset of stroke is precipitous, the risk factors have often developed over the years. Stroke prevention is best accomplished by prudent heart living. Prevention activities include maintaining normal blood pressure, not smoking, exercising, and maintaining normal weight. The nurse has an important role in prevention and health education. These interventions should begin in the formative years in elementary school.

FIGURE ■ 22-4

National Institutes of Health (NIH) Stroke Rating Scale.

Patient Identification ___ ___ - ___ ___ ___ - ___ ___ ___   Pt. Date of Birth ___ ___ /___ ___ /___ ___

Hospital _____ (___ ___ - ___ ___)   Date of Exam ___ ___ /___ ___ /___ ___

Interval: [ ] Baseline [ ] 2 hours post treatment [ ] 24 hours post onset of symptoms ±20 minutes
      [ ] 7–10 days [ ] 3 months [ ] Other _____ (___ ___)

Time: ___ ___ : ___ ___ [ ] am [ ] pm   Person Administering Scale _____

Administer stroke scale items in the order listed. Record performance in each category after each subscale exam. Do not go back and change scores. Follow directions provided for each exam technique. Scores should reflect what the patient does, not what the clinician thinks the patient can do. The clinician should record answers while administering the exam and work quickly. Except where indicated, the patient should not be coached (i.e., repeated requests to patient to make a special effort).

Instructions	Scale Definition	Score
1a. Level of Consciousness: The investigator must choose a response if a full evaluation is prevented by such obstacles as an endotracheal tube, language barrier, or orotracheal trauma/bandages. A 3 is scored only if the patient makes no movement (other than reflexive posturing) in response to noxious stimulation.	0 = **Alert;** keenly responsive. 1 = **Not alert;** but arousable by minor stimulation to obey, answer, or respond. 2 = **Not alert;** requires repeated stimulation to attend, or is obtunded and requires strong or painful stimulation to make movements (not stereotyped). 3 = Responds only with reflex motor or autonomic effects or totally unresponsive, flaccid, and flexic.	_____
1b. LOC Questions: The patient is asked the month and his/her age. The answer must be correct—there is no partial credit for being close. Aphasic and stuporous patients who do not comprehend the questions will score. 2. Patients unable to speak because of endotracheal intubation, orotracheal trauma, severe dysarthria from any cause, language barrier, or any other problem not secondary to aphasia are given a 1. It is important that only the initial answer be graded and that the examiner not "help" the patient with verbal or nonverbal cues.	0 = **Answers** both questions correctly. 1 = **Answers** one question correctly. 2 = **Answers** neither question correctly.	_____
1c. LOC Commands: The patient is asked to open and close the eyes and then to grip and release the non-paretic hand. Substitute another one step command if the hands cannot be used. Credit is given if an unequivocal attempt is made but not completed due to weakness. If the patient does not respond to command, the task should be demonstrated to him or her (pantomime), and the result scored (i.e., follows none, one, or two commands). Patients with trauma, amputation, or other physical impediments should be given suitable one-step commands. Only the first attempt is scored.	0 = **Performs** both tasks correctly. 1 = **Performs** one task correctly. 2 = **Performs** neither task correctly.	_____

Source: National Institutes of Health, 2003, www.stroke-site.org/stroke_scales/stroke_scales.html.

(continued)

FIGURE ■ **22-4** (continued)

| Patient Identification __ __ - __ __ __ - __ __ __ | Pt. Date of Birth __ __/__ __/__ __ |

Hospital _____ (__ __ - __ __)   Date of Exam __ __/__ __/__ __

Interval: [ ] Baseline [ ] 2 hours post treatment [ ] 24 hours post onset of symptoms ±20 minutes
    [ ] 7–10 days [ ] 3 months [ ] Other _____ (__ __)

Instructions	Scale Definition	Score
2. Best Gaze. Only horizontal eye movements will be tested. Voluntary or reflexive (oculocephalic) eye movements will be scored, but caloric testing is not done. If the patient has a conjugate deviation of the eyes that can be overcome by voluntary or reflexive activity, the score will be 1. If a patient has an isolated peripheral nerve paresis (CN III, IV or VI), score a 1. Gaze is testable in all aphasic patients. Patients with ocular trauma, bandages, pre-existing blindness, or other disorder of visual acuity or fields should be tested with reflexive movements, and a choice made by the investigator. Establishing eye contact and then moving about the patient from side to side will occasionally clarify the presence of a partial gaze palsy.	0 = **Normal.** 1 = **Partial gaze palsy**; gaze is abnormal in one or both eyes, but forced deviation or total gaze paresis is not present. 2 = **Forced deviation**, or total gaze paresis not overcome by the oculocephalic maneuver.	_____
3. Visual: Visual fields (upper and lower quadrants) are tested by confrontation, using finger counting or visual threat, as appropriate. Patients may be encouraged, but if they look at the side of the moving fingers appropriately, this can be scored as normal. If there is unilateral blindness or enucleation, visual fields in the remaining eyes are scored. Score 1 only if a clear-cut asymmetry, including quadrantanopia, is found. If patient is blind from any cause, score 3. Double simultaneous stimulation is performed at this point. If there is extinction, patient receives a 1, and the results are used to respond to item 11.	0 = **No visual loss.** 1 = **Partial hemianopia.** 2 = **Complete hemianopia.** 3 = **Bilateral hemianopia** (blind including cortical blindness).	_____
4. Facial Palsy: Ask—or use pantomime to encourage—the patient to show teeth or raise eyebrows and close eyes. Score symmetry of grimace in response to noxious stimuli in the poorly responsive or non-comprehending patient. If facial trauma/bandages, orotracheal tube, tape, or other physical barriers obscure the face, these should be removed to the extent possible.	0 = **Normal** symmetrical movements. 1 = **Minor paralysis** (flattened nasolabial fold, asymmetry on smiling). 2 = **Partial paralysis** (total or near-total paralysis of lower face). 3 = **Complete paralysis** of one or both sides (absence of facial movement in the upper and lower face).	_____
5. Motor Arm: The limb is placed in the appropriate position: extend the arms (palms down) 90 degrees (if sitting) or 45 degrees (if supine). Drift is scored if the arm falls before 10 seconds. The aphasic patient is encouraged using urgency in the voice and pantomime, but not noxious stimulation. Each limb is tested in turn, beginning with the non-paretic arm. Only in the case of amputation or joint fusion at the shoulder, the examiner should record the score as untestable (UN), and clearly write the explanation for this choice.	0 = **No drift**; limb holds 90 (or 45) degrees for full 10 seconds. 1 = **Drift**; limb holds 90 (or 45) degrees, but drifts down before full 10 seconds; does not hit bed or other support. 2 = **Some effort against gravity**; limb cannot get to or maintain (if cued) 90 (or 45) degrees, drifts down to bed, but has some effort against gravity. 3 = **No effort against gravity**; limb falls. 4 = **No movement.** UN = **Amputation** or joint fusion, explain: _____ **5a. Left Arm** **5b. Right Arm**	_____ _____

FIGURE ■ 22-4 *(continued)*

Patient Identification ___ ___ - ___ ___ ___ - ___ ___ ___   Pt. Date of Birth ___ ___ /___ ___ /___ ___

Hospital _____ (___ ___ - ___ ___)   Date of Exam ___ ___ /___ ___ /___ ___

Interval: [ ] Baseline [ ] 2 hours post treatment [ ] 24 hours post onset of symptoms ±20 minutes

   [ ] 7–10 days [ ] 3 months [ ] Other _____ (___ ___)

Instructions	Scale Definition	Score
6. **Motor Leg:** The limb is placed in the appropriate position: hold the leg at 30 degrees (always tested supine). Drift is scored if the leg falls before 5 seconds. The aphasic patient is encouraged using urgency in the voice and pantomime, but not noxious stimulation. Each limb is tested in turn, beginning with the non-paretic leg. Only in the case of amputation or joint fusion at the hip, the examiner should record the score as untestable (UN), and clearly write the explanation for this choice.	0 = **No drift**; leg holds 30-degree position for full 5 seconds. 1 = **Drift**; leg falls by the end of the 5-second period but does not hit bed. 2 = **Some effort against gravity**; leg falls to bed by 5 seconds, has some effort against gravity. 3 = **No effort against gravity**; leg falls to bed immediately. 4 = **No movement.** UN = **Amputation** or joint fusion, explain: _____ 6a. **Left Leg** 6b. **Right Leg**	_____
7. **Limb Ataxia:** This item is aimed at finding evidence of a unilateral cerebellar lesion. Test with eyes open. In case of visual defect, ensure testing is done in intact visual field. The finger-nose-finger and heel-shin tests are performed on both sides, and ataxia is scored only if present out of proportion to weakness. Ataxia is absent in the patient who cannot understand or is paralyzed. Only in the case of amputation or joint fusion, the examiner should record the score as untestable (UN), and clearly write the explanation for this choice. In case of blindness, test by having the patient touch nose from extended arm position.	0 = **Absent.** 1 = **Present in one limb.** 2 = **Present in two limbs.** UN = **Amputation** or joint fusion, explain:	_____
8. **Sensory:** Sensation or grimace to pinprick when tested, or withdrawn from noxious stimulus in the obtunded or aphasic patient. Only sensory loss attributed to stroke is scored as abnormal and the examiner should test as many body areas (arms [not hands], legs, trunk, face) as needed to accurately check for hemisensory loss. A score of 2, "severe or total sensory loss," should only be given when a severe or total loss of sensation can be clearly demonstrated. Stuporous and aphasic patients will, therefore, probably score 1 or 0. The patient with brainstem stroke who has bilateral loss of sensation is scored 2. If the patient does not respond and is quadriplegic, score 2. Patients in a coma (item 1a=3) are automatically given a 2 on this item.	0 = **Normal**; no sensory loss. 1 = **Mild-to-moderate sensory loss;** patient feels pinprick is less sharp or is dull on the affected side; or there is a loss of superficial pain with pinprick, but patient is aware of being touched. 2 = **Severe to total sensory loss;** patient is not aware of being touched in the face, arm, and leg.	_____

(continued)

FIGURE ☐ **22-4** *(continued)*

Patient Identification ___ ___ - ___ ___ ___ - ___ ___ ___   Pt. Date of Birth ___ ___/___ ___/___ ___

Hospital _____ (___ ___ - ___ ___)   Date of Exam ___ ___/___ ___/___ ___

Interval: [ ] Baseline [ ] 2 hours post treatment [ ] 24 hours post onset of symptoms ±20 minutes
          [ ] 7–10 days [ ] 3 months [ ] Other _____ (___ ___)

Instructions	Scale Definition	Score
9. **Best Language:** A great deal of information about comprehension will be obtained during the preceding sections of the examination. For this scale item, the patient is asked to describe what is happening in the attached picture, to name the items on the attached naming sheet, and to read from the attached list of sentences (see the following page). Comprehension is judged from responses here, as well as to all of the commands in the preceding general neurological exam. If visual loss interferes with the tests, ask the patient to identify objects placed in the hand, repeat, and produce speech. The intubated patient should be asked to write. The patient in a coma (item 1a=3) will automatically score 3 on this item. The examiner must choose a score for the patient with stupor or limited cooperation, but a score of 3 should be used only if the patient is mute and follows no one-step commands.	0 = **No aphasia;** normal. 1 = **Mild-to-moderate aphasia;** some obvious loss of fluency or facility of comprehension, without significant limitation on ideas expressed or form of expression. Reduction of speech and/or comprehension, however, makes conversation about provided materials difficult or impossible. For example, in conversation about provided materials, examiner can identify picture or naming card content from patient's response. 2 = **Severe aphasia;** all communication is through fragmentary expression; great need for inference, questioning, and guessing by the listener. Range of information that can be exchanged is limited; listener carries burden of communication. Examiner cannot identify materials provided from patient response. 3 = **Mute, global aphasia;** no usable speech or auditory comprehension.	_____
10. **Dysarthria:** If patient is thought to be normal, an adequate sample of speech must be obtained by asking patient to read or repeat words from the attached list. If the patient has severe aphasia, the clarity of articulation of spontaneous speech can be rated. Only if the patient is intubated or has other physical barriers to producing speech, the examiner should record the score as untestable (UN), and clearly write an explanation for this choice. Do not tell the patient why he or she is being tested.	0 = **Normal.** 1 = **Mild-to-moderate dysarthria;** patient slurs at least some words and, at worst, can be understood with some difficulty. 2 = **Severe dysarthria;** patient's speech is so slurred as to be unintelligible, in the absence of or out of proportion to any dysphasia, or is mute/anarthric. UN = **Intubated** or other physical barrier, explain: _____	_____
11. **Extinction and inattention (formerly Neglect):** Sufficient information to identify neglect may be obtained during the prior testing. If the patient has severe visual loss preventing visual double simultaneous stimulation, and the cutaneous stimuli are normal, the score is normal. If the patient has aphasia but does appear to attend to both sides, the score is normal. The presence of visual spatial neglect or anosognosia may also be taken as evidence of abnormality. Since the abnormality is scored only if present, the item is never untestable.	0 = **No abnormality.** 1 = **Visual, tactile, auditory, spatial, or personal inattention** or extinction to bilateral simultaneous stimulation in one of the sensory modalities. 2 = **Profound hemi-inattention or extinction to more than one modality;** does not recognize own hand or orients to only one side of space.	_____

FIGURE ■ **22-4** *(continued)*

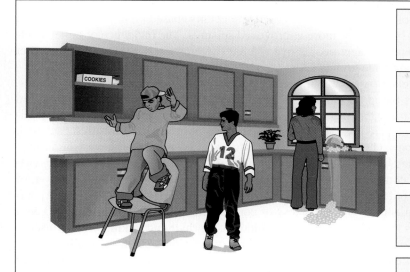

You know how.

Down to earth.

I got home from work.

Near the table in the dining room.

They heard him speak on the radio last night.

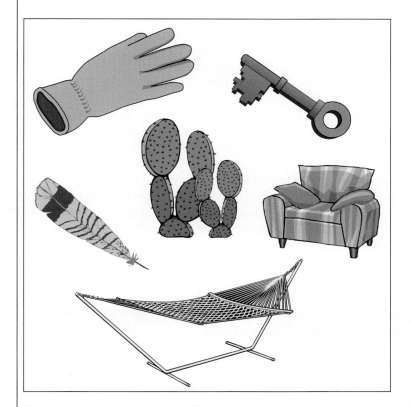

MAMA

TIP-TOP

FIFTY-FIFTY

THANKS

HUCKLEBERRY

BASEBALL PLAYER

Pictures, words, and sentences used to score item 9 of the Stroke Rating Scale.

Seizures

Seizure is an abnormal, abrupt release of electrical activity in the brain. A seizure can cause a variety of symptoms (e.g., spasticity, flaccidity) based on the area of the brain affected. **Epilepsy** is two or more unprovoked seizures. The incidence of epilepsy increases with advanced age; people over 75 are twice as likely to develop new-onset epilepsy as all adult age groups under 65.

Seizures are classified as either generalized, partial (focal), or unclassified seizures. Classification is based on the area of the brain that the electrical activity originated from, regardless if it then spreads to other areas. In generalized seizures, both hemispheres of the brain are involved. There are six types of generalized seizures, each with separate symptoms: (1) Tonic-clonic seizures (also called grand mal) have a duration of 2 to 5 minutes and begin with a period of rigidity and stiffening (extension) of the muscles and loss of consciousness. The second phase entails rhythmic jerking (flexion) of the extremities, but this may not always occur. (2) Absence seizures (petit mal) are common in children and involve brief loss of consciousness, as if daydreaming. (3) Myoclonic seizures last only a few seconds and involve rhythmic jerking of the muscles. (4) A tonic seizure, like the first phase of the tonic-clonic seizure, entails rigidity. (5) Clonic seizure involves repetitive motor activity (e.g., lip smacking). (6) An atonic seizure is sudden loss of muscle tone.

Partial (focal) seizures occur in only one hemisphere of the brain and are either complex or simple. Complex partial seizures are 1 to 3 minutes in duration and involve loss of consciousness and automatisms. During a simple partial seizure the patient remains conscious and often feels an aura (e.g., ringing in ears) before the seizure takes place. The patient can have autonomic changes or unilateral movement of a limb. Determining the type of seizure is important to choose the appropriate medication. Table 22-5 lists the preferred antiseizure drug based on type of seizure.

There are several nursing interventions when caring for a patient with a history of seizures. It is the nurse's responsibility to obtain an accurate patient history, including age of seizure onset and frequency of attacks. In addition, the nurse should inquire about the dates and duration of the seizures as well as medication name, dosage, and frequency. It is important for the nurse to be aware of the medication dose, as many patients are not initially given a high enough dose.

If a patient has a seizure, the most important responsibility of the nurse is to prevent injury of the patient. Suction equipment should be kept by the patient's bedside so that an oral airway may be obtained and aspiration prevented. In addition, patients should be placed on their side during a seizure to prevent aspiration. If necessary, the head-tilt-chin method can be used to obtain an airway. Although it is rare for patients to die during a seizure, the chief causes of death are asphyxiation and suffocation due to turning of the face during the postictal unconscious phase. If there is time to place an air-

TABLE 22-5

Type of Seizure and Preferred Drug

Type of Seizure	Preferred Drug
Partial (focal), simple	Phenytoin (Dilantin), carbamazepine (Tegretol)
Partial (focal), complex	Phenytoin (Dilantin), carbamazepine (Tegretol)
Tonic-clonic	Phenytoin (Dilantin), carbamazepine (Tegretol)
Absence	Ethosuximide (Zarontin)
Myoclonic	Valproic acid (Depakene), clonazepam (Klonopin)

way before the seizure begins, this can be done. However, once the seizure has begun nothing should be put in the mouth, as this can create an airway obstruction and cause injury to the oral mucosa. Oxygen and intravenous access should always be made available. Oxygen is used if the patient experiences signs of hypoxia (change of skin color), and intravenous access is needed in case emergency medication must be administered. Side-rail pads are used to prevent injury to the patient.

A seizure that lasts more than 10 minutes or groups of seizures that occur in rapid succession and last a combined time of 30 minutes are **status epilepticus**, a neurologic emergency. In the event of status epilepticus the physician should be notified, an airway should be established, and oxygen should be given. If an intravenous access is not already available, one should be started and the patient should receive 0.9% sodium chloride. The physician may prescribe medications to cease the motor movement (intravenous diazepam, lorazepam, or valproate) followed by a medication to prevent recurrence (Dilantin or Cerebyx). Vital signs should be closely monitored during the entire event. If the patient needs to be transported, only padded carts should be used because there is a great risk of a fall with the use of a wheelchair.

Patient-family education is an important intervention of the nurse. Patients and families should be provided with audiovisual aids they may review at their own pace (e.g., handouts and videotapes). Identifying and avoiding precipitating factors associated with seizures should be taught, such as alcohol withdrawal, stress, and lack of sleep. It is important to emphasize taking medication correctly and the dangers of not adhering to the prescribed self-care regimen. The family should be taught what to do in the event of a seizure (lay the patient on his or her side, surround with soft objects, and do not place anything in the mouth) and how long to wait before taking the patient to the emergency department as a possible status epilepticus. The patient should be taught to keep a seizure calendar (including date, time, duration, and specific descriptions) to assist with the treatment program.

Many older patients and their families are fearful of memory loss and the possibility of developing AD. The patient-family teaching guidelines in the following feature will assist the nurse in the education of patients and families regarding memory loss in later life.

Patient-Family Teaching Guidelines

FORGETFULNESS OR MEMORY PROBLEMS

1. Sometimes I forget things. Should I be worried that I'm developing Alzheimer's disease?

A lot of people forget things and experience memory lapses. Sometimes this is serious and sometimes it is not. Serious changes in memory accompanied by changes in personality, behavior, or the ability to care for oneself often accompany the diagnosis of dementia. Symptoms of dementia include asking the same question repeatedly; getting lost or disoriented in a familiar environment; being unable to follow directions; becoming disoriented to time and place; neglecting personal safety, hygiene, and nutrition; and being unable to manage personal affairs and finances. Alzheimer's disease is one of the many types of dementia.

RATIONALE:

Nurses can greatly assist older patients and families to distinguish between benign senescence of aging (memory loss that does not affect a person or the ability to remain safe and independent) and the more serious memory loss of dementia. Supplying concrete examples of serious symptoms may help.

(continued)

Patient-Family Teaching Guidelines, *cont.*

2. What causes dementia or serious memory problems?

Dementia has many causes, some of which are reversible by treatment and some of which are permanent and progressive. Some reversible conditions that may cause dementia include high fever, dehydration, vitamin deficiencies, poor nutrition, side effects of medications, thyroid conditions, head injuries, and undiagnosed serious illness like urinary tract infection or pneumonia. Sometimes older people who are depressed, bored, or worried can have memory problems. Seeing a doctor as soon as possible after the detection of memory problems can assist in the diagnosis and treatment of these reversible conditions.

RATIONALE:

Many older persons and their families will try to cover up or hide memory problems because they are fearful. The nurse should reassure them that seeking medical attention can be beneficial as some memory problems are correctable.

3. How is the diagnosis of Alzheimer's disease confirmed?

Your doctor will carry out a complete medical, neurologic, psychiatric, and social evaluation of your health status. Information will be gathered about your medical history, use of medications, diet, past medical problems, and general health and function. A family member should accompany you if you have problems relating specific information regarding your symptoms or past medical history. Tests of blood and urine will also be done. A CT scan may be done to examine the brain. It usually takes one or two visits to gather all of the information needed for an accurate diagnosis.

RATIONALE:

It is important to prepare the older person and the family for the intensive examinations and questioning that are needed to diagnose Alzheimer's disease. Because there are so many causes of memory problems in the older person, the diagnosis is careful and other potential causes must be ruled out or eliminated.

4. How is Alzheimer's disease treated?

In the early and middle stages of Alzheimer's disease, drugs like donepezil (Aricept) and galantamine (Reminyl) are used to delay the worsening of the disease and the progression of symptoms. Medications are also used for behavioral problems like agitation, anxiety, depression, and sleep disorders. Careful use of drugs is important, and nurses will keep track of symptoms to make sure that they are improving as a result of medication administration. General healthcare like diet, exercise, social activities, and memory aids such as calendars, lists of important phone numbers, and other notes about day-to-day activities can help improve the quality of life of older persons with dementia.

RATIONALE:

At the present, there is no cure for Alzheimer's disease but treatment is possible and can improve an older person's quality of life even in the face of this serious and debilitating illness.

5. What can I do to prevent dementia?

The research shows that people who remain active and engaged in life stimulate their bodies and brains to continue to function effectively. Develop hobbies and interests, enjoy your life, exercise to remain or become fit, eat a balanced diet, avoid smoking and heavy drinking, do not take unnecessary drugs, avoid stress and anxiety, and stay connected with at least one other person on a daily basis. Some physical and mental changes occur with age in healthy people; however, dementia is a disease and not a normal part of aging. Report any memory problems to your physician or nurse and seek an accurate diagnosis as soon as possible to identify reversible causes.

RATIONALE:

General health promotion activities will help to prevent disabling illness and comorbidities that can hasten or exacerbate the symptoms of memory loss or dementia. Minimizing threats to good health is always an appropriate intervention.

Care Plan

A Patient With a Neurological Disorder

Case Study

Mr. Dalton is a 75-year-old man who has been admitted to the hospital. He fell in his home and suffered a fractured left hip and had an open reduction with internal fixation this morning. When Mr. Dalton first arrived, he was quiet and pleasant but now he is agitated, attempting to get out of bed, yelling, and throwing his sheets on the floor. The nurse attempts to reason with him and reassure him, but he is not responding.

Applying the Nursing Process

ASSESSMENT

The nurse suspects Mr. Dalton is delirious or suffering a transient organic mental syndrome that has an acute onset and poses a common and serious problem in older patients with hip fracture. Systematic determination of an older person's mental status is of major importance for early recognition and treatment of delirium. The nurse knows that delirium can be caused by any of the following factors:

- Medications
- Anesthesia
- Electrolyte imbalance
- Pain
- Sleep disturbance
- Underlying dementia (diagnosed or undiagnosed)

A complete assessment of each of these factors using standardized assessment instruments is indicated while the patient is protected from injury.

DIAGNOSIS

Nursing diagnoses that may be appropriate for Mr. Dalton include the following:

- *Acute confusion*
- *Previously altered thought processes* (if previously diagnosed with cognitive impairment)
- *Risk for imbalanced fluid volume* (overhydration or dehydration)
- *Risk for injury* (due to falls)
- *Impaired verbal communication*
- *Impaired physical mobility*
- *Delayed surgical recovery*
- *Acute pain*

(continued)

A Patient With a Neurological Disorder *(continued)*

- *Anxiety*
- *Fear*

EXPECTED OUTCOMES

The expected outcomes for the plan of care specify that Mr. Dalton will:

- Begin to exhibit resolution of his symptoms of delirium.
- Be free from injury.
- Experience correction of the underlying mechanisms causing his delirium.
- Receive consultation, assessment, and treatment from appropriate members of the interdisciplinary team, including physicians, nurses, physical therapists, dietitians, social workers, and others as appropriate to resolve and improve his delirium.

PLANNING AND IMPLEMENTATION

The following nursing interventions may be appropriate for Mr. Dalton:

- Establish a therapeutic relationship by being present and using gentle touch and a soft voice for communication.
- Review all current medications.
- Evaluate basic laboratory studies (complete blood count, serum electrolytes, and urinalysis).
- Provide supportive and restorative care.
- Treat behavioral symptoms.
- Correct sensory deficits (place glasses and hearing aids if used by the patient).
- In consultation with the physician, consider further testing as appropriate that may include chest radiology, blood culture, drug levels, serum B_{12}, thyroid function tests, pulse oximetry, electrocardiogram, brain imaging, lumbar puncture, or electroencephalogram.
- Administer medications as ordered by the physician (haloperidol 0.5 to 2.0 mg or lorazepam 0.5 to 2.0 mg by mouth every 4 to 6 hours).
- Reassure and educate family.

EVALUATION

The nurse will consider the plan a success based on the following criteria:

- Mr. Dalton will return to normal cognitive and physical function.
- He will be free from injury.
- He will cooperate with a rehabilitation program and be discharged to home or a rehabilitation facility (as appropriate).

Ethical Dilemma

Mr. Dalton's daughter requests that he be restrained to prevent falls. She has seen patients with waist restraints and feels the use of this device will keep her father safe from injury. The nurse wishes to be responsive to the daughter's request, but professional standards indicate that restraints can worsen delirium and injure the patient. The ethical dilemma involves threats to the patient's and surrogate's autonomy versus benefi-

A Patient With a Neurological Disorder

cence or the desire to do no harm. The nurse should educate and inform the daughter regarding the risks of entrapment and strangulation that accompany the use of restraints. Agitation and anxiety can be exacerbated as the patient fights to free himself from the restraints, and larger doses of medication may be needed to reduce symptoms. Physical restraints should be used cautiously (if at all) and only as a last resort. Additionally, a delirious physically restrained patient will need constant observation to prevent injury, entrapment, and strangulation.

Critical Thinking and the Nursing Process

1. How would you explain the diagnosis of Alzheimer's disease to a family?
2. What resources are available in your community or professional setting to assist older patients and their families caring for a loved one with dementia?
3. Identify three major changes you would like to see implemented in your clinical agency that would facilitate the care of older persons with dementia.
4. Caring for older persons with cognitive impairments (dementia and delirium) can be stressful for nurses and other healthcare providers. What types of support services and resources in the clinical setting would assist you to provide the highest quality care to older patients with cognitive impairments?

■ Evaluate your responses in Appendix B. ⊂⊐

EXPLORE MediaLink

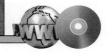

NCLEX review, case studies, and other interactive resources for this chapter can be found on the Companion Website at **http://www.prenhall.com/tabloski**. Click on Chapter 22 to select the activities for this chapter. For animations, video tutorials, more NCLEX review questions, and case studies, access the accompanying CD-ROM in this textbook.

Chapter Highlights

■ The nursing care of patients with neurologic disorders often involves care of a person with both a memory and a movement disorder, thus the nursing diagnosis *alteration in cognition and movement.*

■ Secondary symptoms appear at various stages of illness and may resolve only because the person's condition has worsened and the individual no longer has the physical capacity to express the symptom (e.g., elopement because the person can no longer walk) or sign (e.g., elevated temperature because the elderly person is too frail to mount a typical fever response).

■ Some secondary symptoms cause more suffering than does the primary disorder.

■ Neurologic disorders are very amenable to nursing interventions. While focusing on care rather than cure, nurses can attend to quality-of-life issues, prevent suffering, and promote positive coping.

References

Ahronheim, J. C. (1996). Nutrition and hydration in the terminal patient. *Clinics in Geriatric Medicine, 12,* 379–391.

Ala, T. A., Mattson, M. D., & Frey, W. H. (2003). The clinical diagnosis of Alzheimer's disease without the use of head imaging studies. A cliniconeuropathological study. *Journal of Alzheimer's Disease, 5(6),* 463–465.

Applebaum, G. E., King, J. E., & Finucane, T. E. (1990). The outcome of cardiopulmonary resuscitation initiated in nursing homes. *Journal of the American Geriatrics Society, 38,* 197–200.

Arnaiz, E., Almkvist, O., Ivnik, R. J., Tangalos, E. G., Wahlund, L. O., Winblad, B., et al. (2004). Mild cognitive impairment: A cross-national comparison. *Journal of Neurology, Neurosurgery & Psychiatry, 75,* 1275–1280.

Awoke, S., Mouton, C., & Parrott, M. (1992). Outcomes of skilled cardiopulmonary resuscitation in a long-term care facility: Futile therapy? *Journal of the American Geriatrics Society, 40,* 593–595.

Baatile, J., Langbein, W. E., Weaver, F., Maloney, C., & Jost, M. B. (2000). Effect of exercise on perceived quality of life of individuals with Parkinson's disease. *Journal of Rehabilitation Research & Development, 37,* 529–534.

Behrman, A. L., Light, K. E., Flynn, S. M., & Thigpen, M. T. (2002). Is the functional reach test useful for identifying falls risk among individuals with Parkinson's disease? *Archives of Physical Medicine & Rehabilitation, 83,* 538–542.

Bennett, D. A., Wilson, R. S., Schneider, J. A., Evans, D. A., Beckett, L. A., Aggarwal, N. T., et al. (2002). Natural history of mild cognitive impairment in older persons. *Neurology, 59,* 198–205.

Block, S. D. (2001). Perspectives on care at the close of life. Psychological considerations, growth, and transcendence at the end of life: The art of the possible. *Journal of the American Medical Association, 285,* 2898–2906.

Bootzin, R. R., Epstein, D., & Wood, J. M. (1991). Stimulus control instructions. In P. J. Hauri (Ed.), *Case studies in insomnia* (pp. 19–28). New York: Plenum.

Borson, S., Bartels, S. J., Colenda, C. C., Gottlieb, G. L., & Meyers, B. (2001). Geriatric mental health services research: Strategic plan for an aging population: Report of the Health Services Work Group of the American Association for Geriatric Psychiatry. *American Journal of Geriatric Psychiatry, 9,* 191–204.

Bottrell, M. M., O'Sullivan, J. F., Robbins, M. A., Mitty, E. L., & Mezey, M. D. (2001). Transferring dying nursing home residents to the hospital: DON perspectives on the nurse's role in transfer decisions. *Geriatric Nursing, 22,* 313–317.

Boustani, M., Peterson, B., Hanson, L., Harris, R., Lohr, K. N., & U.S. Preventive Services Task Force. (2003). Screening for dementia in primary care: A summary of the evidence for the U.S. Preventive Services Task Force. *Annals of Internal Medicine, 138,* 927–937.

Brodaty, H., Conneally, M., Gauthier, S., Jennings, C., Lennox, A., & Lovestone, S. (1995). Consensus statement on predictive testing for Alzheimer disease. *Alzheimer Disease & Associated Disorders, 9,* 182–187.

Brott, T., Adams, H. P., Olinger, C. P., Marler, J. R., Barsan, W. G., Biller, J., et al. (1989). Measurements of acute cerebral infarction: A clinical examination scale. *Stroke, 20,* 864–870.

Brown, E. J. (1999). Snoezelen. In L. Volicer & L. Bloom-Charette (Eds.), *Enhancing the quality of life in advanced dementia* (pp. 168–185). Philadelphia: Taylor & Francis.

Burger, S. G., Kayser-Jones, J., & Bell, J. P. (2001). Food for thought. Preventing/treating malnutrition and dehydration. *Contemporary Long-Term Care, 24,* 24–28.

Buxbaum, J. D., Geoghagen, N. S., & Friedhoff, L. T. (2001). Cholesterol depletion with physiological concentrations of a statin decreases the formation of the Alzheimer amyloid Abeta peptide. *Journal of Alzheimer's Disease, 3,* 221–229.

Camberg, L., Woods, P., Ooi, W. L., Hurley, A., Volicer, L., Ashley, J., et al. (1999). Evaluation of simulated presence: A personalized approach to enhance well-being in persons with Alzheimer's disease. *Journal of the American Geriatrics Society, 47,* 446–452.

Chitsey, A. M., Haight, B. K., & Jones, M. M. (2002). Snoezelen: A multisensory environmental intervention. *Journal of Gerontological Nursing, 28,* 41–49.

Crosby, L., & Parsons, L. C. (1989). Clinical neurologic assessment tool: Development and testing of an instrument to index neurologic status. *Heart and Lung, 18,* 121–129.

Deane, K. H., Ellis-Hill, C., Playford, E. D., Ben-Shlomo, Y., & Clarke, C. E. (2001). Occupational therapy for patients with Parkinson's disease. *Cochrane Database of Systematic Reviews:* CD002813.

Dehlin, O. (1990). Relocation of patients with senile dementia: Effects on symptoms and mortality. *Journal of Clinical and Experimental Gerontology, 12,* 1–12.

Drickamer, M. A., & Lachs, M. S. (1992). Should patients with Alzheimer's disease be told their diagnosis. *New England Journal of Medicine, 326,* 947–951.

Duda, J. E. (2004). Pathology and neurotransmitter abnormalities of dementia with Lewy bodies. *Dementia & Geriatric Cognitive Disorders, 17,* 3–14.

Duthie, E., Mark, D., Tresch, D., Kartes, S., Neahring, J., & Aufderheide, T. (1993). Utilization of cardiopulmonary resuscitation in nursing homes in one community: Rates and nursing home characteristics. *Journal of the American Geriatrics Society, 41,* 384–388.

Evans, D. A., Funkenstein, H. H., Albert, M. S., Scherr, P. A., Cook, N. R., Chown, M. J., et al. (1989). Prevalence of Alzheimer's disease in a community population of older persons: Higher than previously reported. *Journal of the American Medical Association, 262,* 2551–2556.

Expert Consensus Panel. (2004). Treatment of agitation in older persons with dementia. Expert Knowledge Systems. Alexopoulos, G., Silver, J., Kahn, D., Frances, A., & Carpenter, D. (Eds). Retrieved December 13, 2004, from www.psychguides.com.

Farlow, M. R. (2003). Update on rivastigmine. *Neurologist, 9(5),* 230–234.

Farrer, L. A., Brin, M., & Elsas, L. (1995). Statement on use of apolipoprotein E testing for Alzheimer disease. *Journal of the American Medical Association, 247,* 1627–1629.

Farrer, L. A., Cupples, L., Haines, J. L., Hyman, B., Kukull, W. A., Mayeux, R., et al. (1997). Effects of age, sex and ethnicity on the association between apolipoprotein E genotype and Alzheimer disease: A meta-analysis. *Journal of the American Medical Association, 278,* 1349–1356.

Farrer, L. A., Cupples, L. A., van Duijn, C. M., Kurz, A., Zimmer, R., Muller, U., et al. (1995). Apolipoprotein E genotype in patients with Alzheimer's disease: Implications for the risk of dementia among relatives. *Annals of Neurology, 38,* 797–808.

Feldman, H., Gauthier, S., Hecker, J., Vellas, B., Subbiah, P., Whalen, E., et al. (2001). A 24-week, randomized, double-blind study of donepezil in moderate to severe Alzheimer's disease. *Neurology, 57,* 613–620.

Fick, D., & Foreman, M. (2000). Consequences of not recognizing delirium superimposed on dementia in hospitalized elderly individuals. *Journal of Gerontological Nursing, 26,* 30–40.

Finucane, T. E., Christmas, C., & Travis, K. (1999). Tube feeding in patients with advanced dementia: A review of the evidence. *Journal of the American Medical Association, 282,* 1365–1370.

Foreman, M. D., Wakefield, B., Culp, K., & Milisen, K. (2001). Delirium in elderly patients: An overview of the state of the science. *Journal of Gerontological Nursing, 27*(4), 13–20.

Frisoni, G. B., Franzoni, S., Bellelli, G., Morris, J., & Warden, V. (1998). Overcoming eating difficulties in the severely demented. In L.Volicer & A. Hurley (Eds.), *Hospice care for patients with advanced progressive dementia* (pp. 48–67). New York: Springer.

Gauthier, L., Dalziel, S., & Gauthier, S. (1987). The benefits of group occupational therapy for patients with Parkinson's disease. *American Journal of Occupational Therapy, 41,* 360–365.

Gillick, M. R. (2002). Do we need to create geriatric hospitals? *Journal of the American Geriatrics Society, 50,* 174–177.

Grady, D., Herrington, D., Bittner, V., Blumenthal, R., Davidson, M., Hlatky, M., et al. (2002). Cardiovascular disease outcomes during 6.8 years of hormone therapy: Heart and estrogen/progestin replacement study follow-up (HERS II). *Journal of the American Medical Association, 288,* 49–57.

Gray, P., & Hildebrand, K. (2000). Fall risk factors in Parkinson's disease. *Journal of Neuroscience Nursing, 32,* 222–228.

Green, R. C., Clarke, V. C., Thompson, N. J., Woodard, J. L., & Letz, R. (1997). Early detection of Alzheimer disease: Methods, markers, and misgivings. *Alzheimer Disease & Associated Disorders, 11,* (Suppl.5), 1–5.

Hamers, J. P. H., Gulpers, M. J. M., & Strik, W. (2004). Use of physical restraints with cognitively impaired nursing home residents. *Journal of Advanced Nursing, 45,* 246–251.

Hanser, S. B. (1999). Music therapy with individuals with advanced dementia. In L.Volicer & L. Bloom-Charette (Eds.), *Enhancing the quality of life in advanced dementia* (pp. 141–167). Philadelphia: Taylor & Francis.

Harrington, C., Kovner, C., Mezey, M., Kayser-Jones, J., Burger, S., Mohler, M., et al. (2000). Experts recommend minimum nurse staffing standards for nursing facilities in the United States. *The Gerontologist, 40,* 5–16.

Hebert, L. E., Beckett, L. A., Scherr, P. A., & Evans, D. A. (2001). Annual incidence of Alzheimer disease in the United States projected to the years 2000 through 2050. *Alzheimer Disease & Associated Disorders, 15,* 169–173.

Hipps, Y. G., Roberts, J. S., Farrer, L. A., & Green, R. C. (2003). Differences between African Americans and Whites in their attitudes toward genetic testing for Alzheimer's disease. *Genetic Testing, 7,* 39–44.

Hirono, N., Mori, E., Ishii, K., Ikejiri, Y., Imamura, T., Shimomura, T., et al. (1998). Hypofunction in the posterior cingulate gyrus correlates with disorientation for time and place in Alzheimer's disease. *Journal of Neurosurgery and Psychiatry, 64,* 552–554.

Holzer, C., & Warshaw, G. A. (2002). Perioperative care and hospital care. In R. J. Ham, P. D. Sloane, & G. A. Warshaw (Eds.), *Primary care geriatrics, A care-based approach* (4th ed., pp. 183–197). St. Louis, MO: Mosby.

Huang, Z. B., & Ahronheim, J. C. (2000). Nutrition and hydration in terminally ill patients: An update. *Clinics in Geriatric Medicine, 16,* 313–315.

Hurley, A., Volicer, L., & Mahoney, E. (1996). Progression of Alzheimer's disease and symptom management. *Federal Practitioner,* (Suppl. 1)(13), 16–22.

Hurley, A. C., Gauthier, M. A., Horvath, K. J., Harvey, R., Smith, S. J., Trudeau, S. A., et al. (2004). Promoting safer home environments for persons with Alzheimer's disease. *Journal of Gerontological Nursing, 30*(6), 43–51.

Hurley, A. C., & Volicer, L. (2002). Alzheimer's disease. It's okay, Mama, if you want to go, it's okay. *Journal of the American Medical Association, 288,* 2324–2332.

Hurley, A. C., & Wells, N. (1999). Past, present, and future directions for Alzheimer research. *Alzheimer Disease and Associated Disorders, 13* (Suppl. 1), S6–S10.

Ingersoll, G. L., & Leyden, D. B. (1994). The Glasgow Coma Scale for patients with head injuries. *Critical Care Nurse, 7*(5), 26–32.

Inouye, S., van Dyck, C., Alessi, C., Balkin, S., Siegal, A., & Horwitz, R. (1990). Clarifying confusion: The confusion assessment method. A new method for the detection of delirium. *Annals of Internal Medicine, 113*(12), 941–948.

In't Veld, B. A., Ruitenberg, A., Hofman, A., Launer, L. J., van Duijn, C. M., Stijnen, T., et al. (2001). Nonsteroidal antiinflammatory drugs and the risk of Alzheimer's disease. *New England Journal of Medicine, 345,* 1515–1521.

Jost, B. C., & Grossberg, G. T. (1996). The evolution of psychiatric symptoms in Alzheimer's disease: A natural history study. *Journal of the American Geriatrics Society, 44,* 1978–1981.

Kayser-Jones, J., & Schell, E. (1997). The mealtime experience of a cognitively impaired elder: Ineffective and effective strategies. *Journal of Gerontological Nursing, 23*(7), 33–39.

Kayser-Jones, J. S., Wiener, C. L., & Barbaccia, J. C. (1989). Factors contributing to the hospitalization of nursing home residents. *Gerontologist, 29,* 502–510.

Klein, A., & Kowall, N. (1998). Alzheimer's disease and other progressive dementias. In L.Volicer & A. C. Hurley (Eds.), *Hospice care for patients with advanced progressive dementia* (pp. 3–28). New York: Springer.

Kubler-Ross, E. (1969). *On death and dying.* London: MacMillan.

Kubler-Ross, E. (1986). *Death: The final stage of growth.* New York: Simon & Schuster.

Larrieu, S., Letenneur, L., Orgogozo, J. M., Fabrigoule, C., Amieva, H., Le Carret, N., et al. (2002). Incidence and outcome of mild cognitive impairment in a population-based prospective cohort. *Neurology, 59,* 1594–1599.

Logsdon, R. G., Teri, L., McCurry, S. M., Gibbons, L. E., Kukull, W. A., & Larson, E. B. (1998). Wandering: A significant problem among community-residing individuals with Alzheimer's disease. *The Journal of Gerontology, 53,* P294–P299.

Lopez, O. L., Becker, J. T., Wisniewski, S., Saxton, J., Kaufer, D. I., & DeKosky, S. T. (2002). Cholinesterase inhibitor treatment alters the natural history of Alzheimer's disease. *Journal of Neurology, Neurosurgery & Psychiatry, 72,* 310–314.

Mahoney, E. K., Hurley, A. C., Volicer, L., Bell, M., Gianotis, P., Harsthorn, M., et al. (1999). Development and testing of the resistiveness to care scale. *Research in Nursing and Health, 22,* 27–38.

Mahoney, E. K., Volicer, L., & Hurley, A. C. (2000a). Introduction. In E. K. Mahoney, L. Volicer, & A. C. Hurley (Eds.), *Management of challenging behaviors in dementia* (pp. 1–9). Baltimore: Health Professions Press.

Mahoney, E. K., Volicer, L., & Hurley, A. C. (2000b). *Management of challenging behaviors in dementia.* Baltimore: Health Professions Press.

Mahoney, M. A., Hurley, A., Smith, S., & Volicer, L. (1992). Advance management preferences: The nurse's role in surrogate decision making about life sustaining interventions. In G. B.White (Ed.), *Ethical dilemmas in nursing practice* (pp. 45–58). Kansas City, MO: American Nurses Association.

Marui, W., Iseki, E., Kato, M., Akatsu, H., & Kosaka, K. (2004). Pathological entity of dementia with Lewy bodies and its differentiation from Alzheimer's disease. *Acta Neuropathologica, 108,* 121–128.

McBride, K. L., White, C. L., Sourial, R., & Mayo, N. (2004). Postdischarge nursing interventions for stroke survivors and their families. *Journal of Advanced Nursing, 47,* 192–200.

McCann, R., Hall, W., & Groth-Juncker, A. (1994). Comfort care for terminally ill patients. The appropriate use of nutrition and hydration. *Journal of the American Medical Association, 272,* 1263–1266.

McConnell, L. M. (1999). Understanding genetic testing for Alzheimer disease: Medical and epidemiological background. *Genetic Testing, 3,* 21–27.

McConnell, L. M., Sanders, G. D., & Owens, D. K. (1999). Evaluation of genetic tests: APOE genotyping for the diagnosis of Alzheimer disease. *Genetic Testing, 3,* 47–53.

Miguel-Hidalgo, J. J., Alvarez, X. A., Cacabelos, R., & Quack, G. (2002).

Neuroprotection by memantine against neurodegeneration induced by beta-amyloid(1-40). *Brain Research, 958,* 210–221.

Mitchell, S. L., Teno, J. M., Roy, J., Kabumoto, G., & Mor, V. (2003). Clinical and organizational factors associated with feeding tube use among nursing home residents with advanced cognitive impairment. *Journal of the American Medical Association, 290,* 73–80.

Modrego, P. J., & Ferrandez, J. (2004). Depression in patients with mild cognitive impairment increases the risk of developing dementia of Alzheimer type: A prospective cohort study. *Archives of Neurology, 61*(8), 1290–1293.

Mok, V. C., Wong, A., Lam, W. W., Fan, Y. H., Tang, W. K., Kwok, T., et al. (2004). Cognitive impairment and functional outcome after stroke associated with small vessel disease. *Journal of Neurology, Neurosurgery & Psychiatry, 75,* 560–566.

Moore, A. E., Cicchetti, F., Hennen, J., & Isacson, O. (2001). Parkinsonian motor deficits are reflected by proportional A9/A10 dopamine neuron degeneration in the rat. *Experimental Neurology, 172,* 363–376.

Muir, K. W., Weir, C. J., Murray, G. D., Povey, C., & Lees, K. R. (1996). Comparison of neurological scales and scoring systems for acute stroke prognosis. *Stroke, 27,* 1817–1820.

Mulnard, R. A., Cotman, C. W., Kawas, C., van Dyck, C. H., Sano, M., Doody, R., et al. (2000). Estrogen replacement therapy for treatment of mild to moderate Alzheimer disease: A randomized controlled trial. Alzheimer's Disease Cooperative Study. *Journal of the American Medical Association, 283,* 1007–1015.

Nir, Z., Zolotogorsky, Z., & Sugarman, H. (2004). Structured nursing intervention versus routine rehabilitation after stroke. *American Journal of Physical Medicine & Rehabilitation, 83,* 522–529.

Oken, B. S., Storzbach, D. M., & Kaye, J. A. (1998). The efficacy of ginkgo biloba on cognitive function in Alzheimer's disease. *Archives of Neurology, 55,* 1409–1415.

Paganini-Hill, A., & Henderson, V. W. (1996). Estrogen replacement therapy and risk of Alzheimer disease. *Archives of Internal Medicine, 156,* 2213–2217.

Parkinson Study Group. (2000). A randomized controlled trial comparing pramipexole with levodopa in early Parkinson's disease: Design and methods of the CALM-PD Study. *Clinical Neuropharmacology, 23,* 34–44.

Pericak-Vance, M. A., Bass, M. P., Yamaoka, L. H., Gaskell, P. C., Scott, W. K., Terwedow, H. A., et al. (1997). Complete genomic screen in late-onset familial Alzheimer disease. *Journal of the American Medical Association, 278,* 1237–1241.

Post, S. G., Whitehouse, P. J., Binstock, R. H., Bird, T. D., Eckert, S. K., Farrer, L. A., et al. (1997). The clinical introduction of genetic testing for Alzheimer disease. An ethical

perspective. *Journal of the American Medical Association, 277,* 832–836.

Potts, H. W., Richie, M. F., & Kaas, M. J. (1996). Resistance to care. *Journal of Gerontological Nursing, 22,* 11–16.

Raia, P. (1999). Habilitation therapy: A new starscape. In L. Volicer & L. Bloom-Charette (Eds.), *Enhancing the quality of life in advanced dementia* (pp. 38–55). Philadelphia: Taylor & Francis.

Reisberg, B., Doody, R., Stoffler, A., Schmitt, F., Ferris, S., Mobius, H. J., et al. (2003). Memantine in moderate-to-severe Alzheimer's disease. *New England Journal of Medicine, 348,* 1333–1341.

Relkin, N. R. (1996). Apolipoprotein E genotyping in Alzheimer's disease. National Institute on Aging/Alzheimer's Association Working Group. *Lancet, 347,* 1091–1095.

Relkin, N. R., Kwon, Y. J., Tsai, J., & Gandy, S. (1996). The National Institute on Aging/Alzheimer's Association recommendations on the application of apolipoprotein E genotyping to Alzheimer's disease. *Annals of the New York Academy of Sciences, 802,* 149–176.

Rempusheski, V. F., & Hurley, A. C. (2000). Advance directives and dementia. *Journal of Gerontological Nursing, 26*(10), 27–33.

Roberts, J. S. (2000). Anticipating response to predictive genetic testing for Alzheimer's disease: A survey of first-degree relatives. *The Gerontologist, 40,* 43–52.

Roberts, J. S., Barber, M., Brown, T. M., Cupples, L. A., Farrer, L. A., LaRusse, S. A., et al. (2004). Who seeks genetic susceptibility testing for Alzheimer's disease? Findings from a multisite, randomized clinical trial. *Genetics in Medicine, 6,* 197–203.

Roberts, J. S., LaRusse, S. A., Katzen, H., Whitehouse, P. J., Barber, M., Post, S. G., et al. (2003). Reasons for seeking genetic susceptibility testing among first-degree relatives of people with Alzheimer disease. *Alzheimer Disease & Associated Disorders, 17,* 86–93.

Roses, A. D. (1997). Genetic testing for Alzheimer disease: Practical and ethical issues. *Archives of Neurology, 54,* 1226–1229.

Sano, M., Ernesto, C., Thomas, R. G., Klauber, M. R., Schafer, K., Grundman, M., et al. (1997). A controlled trial of selegiline, alpha-tocopherol, or both as treatment for Alzheimer's disease. *New England Journal of Medicine, 336,* 1216–1222.

Schlegel, D. J., Tanne, D., Demchuk, A. M., Levine, S. R., Kasner, S. E., & Multicenter rt-PA Stroke Survey Group. (2003). Prediction of hospital disposition after thrombolysis for acute ischemic stroke using the National Institutes of Health Stroke Scale. *Archives of Neurology, 61,* 1061–1064.

Schultz, S. K., Ellingrod, V. L., Turvey, C., Moser, D. J., & Arndt, S. (2003). The influence of cognitive impairment and behavioral

dysregulation on daily functioning in the nursing home setting. *American Journal of Psychiatry, 160,* 582–584.

Shumaker, S., Legault, C., Rapp, S., Thal, L., Wallace, R., Ockene, J., Hendrix, S., et al. (2003). Estrogen plus progestin and the incidence of dementia and mild cognitive impairment in postmenopausal women. *Journal of the American Medical Association, 289,* 2651–2662.

Silverstein, N. L., & Flaherty, G. (1996). Deadly mix: Dementia and wandering. *Gerontologist, 36,* 156–157.

Smith, D. R. (2003). Update on Alzheimer drugs. *Neurologist, 9,* 225–229.

Smith, S. J. (1998). Providing palliative care for the terminal Alzheimer patient. In L. Volicer & A. Hurley (Eds.), *Hospice care for patients with advanced progressive dementia* (pp. 247–256). New York: Springer.

Spector, A., Orrell, M., Davies, S., & Woods, R. T. (2003). Reminiscence therapy for dementia. *Cochrane Library:* CD001120.

Stowe, R. L., Wheatley, K., Clarke, C. E., Ives, N. J., Hills, R. K., Williams, A. C., et al. (2003). Surgery for Parkinson's disease: Lack of reliable clinical trial evidence. *Journal of Neurology, Neurosurgery & Psychiatry, 74,* 519–521.

Tanne, D., Kasner, S. E., Demchuk, A. M., Koren-Morag, N., Hanson, S., Grond, M., et al. (2002). Markers of increased risk of intracerebral hemorrhage after intravenous recombinant tissue plasminogen activator therapy for acute ischemic stroke in clinical practice: The Multicenter rt-PA Stroke Survey. *Circulation, 105,* 1679–1685.

Trudeau, S. A. (1999a). Bright eyes: A structured stimulation intervention. In L. Volicer & L. Bloom-Charette (Eds.), *Enhancing the quality of life in advanced dementia* (pp. 93–106). Philadelphia: Taylor & Francis.

Trudeau, S. A. (1999b). Prevention of physical limitations in advanced Alzheimer's disease. In L. Volicer & L. Bloom-Charette (Eds.), *Enhancing quality of life for persons with advanced Alzheimer's disease* (pp. 80–90). Philadelphia: Taylor & Francis.

Volicer, L. (1996). Clinical issues in advanced dementia. In S. B. Hoffman & M. Kaplan (Eds.), *General care programs for people with dementia* (pp. 59–75). Baltimore: Health Professions Press.

Volicer, L., Brandeis, G. H., & Hurley, A. C. (1998). Infections in advanced dementia. In L. Volicer & A. Hurley (Eds.), *Hospice care for patients with advanced progressive dementia* (pp. 29–47). New York: Springer.

Volicer, L., & Hurley, A. C. (1998). *Hospice care for patients with advanced progressive dementia.* New York: Springer.

Volicer, L., Hurley, A., & Camberg, L. (1999). A model of psychological well being in advanced dementia. *Journal of Mental Health and Aging, 5*(4), 83–94.

Volicer, L., Mahoney, E., & Brown, E. J. (1998). Nonpharmacological approaches to the management of the behavioral consequences of advanced dementia. In M. Kaplan & S. B. Hoffman (Eds.), *Behaviors in dementia: Best practices for successful management* (pp. 155–176). Baltimore: Health Professions Press.

Volicer, L., Rheaume, Y., Riley, M. E., Karner, J., & Glennon, M. (1990). Discontinuation of tube feeding in patients with dementia of the Alzheimer type. *American Journal of Alzheimer's Care and Related Disorders and Research, 5,* 22–25.

Volicer, L., Seltzer, B., Rheaume, Y., Karner, J., Glennon, M., Riley, M. E., et al. (1989). Eating difficulties in patients with probable dementia of the Alzheimer type. *Journal of Geriatric Psychiatry and Neurology, 2*(4), 169–176.

Volicer, L., & Simard, J. (1996). Establishing a dementia special-care unit. *Nursing Home Economics, 3*(1), 12–19.

Warner, M. L. (1998). *The complete guide to Alzheimer's-proofing your home.* West Lafayette, IN: Purdue University Press.

Writing Group for the Women's Health Initiative Investigators. (2002). Risks and benefits of estrogen plus progestin in healthy postmenopausal women: Principal results from the Women's Health Initiative randomized controlled trial. *Journal of the American Medical Association, 288,* 321–333.

Wunderlich, G. S., & Koehler, P. O. (2001). *Improving the quality of long-term care.* Washington, DC: National Academy Press.

Yaffe, K., Sawaya, G., Lieberburg, I., & Grady, D. (1998). Estrogen therapy in postmenopausal women: Effects on cognitive function and dementia. *Journal of the American Medical Association, 279,* 688–695.

Zandi, P. P., Carlson, M. C., Plassman, B. L., Welsh-Bohmer, K. A., Mayer, L. S., Steffens, D. C., et al. (2002). Hormone replacement therapy and incidence of Alzheimer disease in older women: The Cache County Study. *Journal of the American Medical Association, 288,* 2123–2129.

Zeisel, J., Hyde, J., & Shi, L. (1999). Environmental design as a treatment for Alzheimer's disease. In L. Volicer & L. Bloom-Charette (Eds.), *Enhancing quality of life in advanced dementia* (pp. 206–222). Philadelphia: Taylor & Francis.

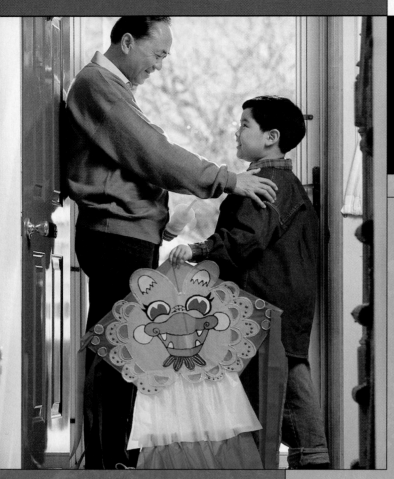

CHAPTER 23

The Immune System

Gail A. Harkness, DRPH, RN, FAAN

CHAPTER OBJECTIVES

Upon completion of this chapter, the reader will be able to:

- Explain the importance of the immune system in the maintenance of health.
- Define the three characteristics that are unique to the immune system.
- Identify factors that affect proper immune system function.
- Identify the similarities, differences, and interactions between the humoral immune response and the cellular immune response.
- Explain the pathology that underlies illnesses associated with the four types of excessive immune responses (hypersensitivity).
- Discuss the unique characteristics associated with HIV infection in the older person.
- Relate the care of the patient with a rheumatoid disorder to the pathology involved.
- Describe the susceptibility of the older person to infections.
- Identify nursing interventions that can be effective in improving immune status in the older person.

KEY TERMS

MediaLink

Additional resources for this chapter can be found on the Student CD-ROM accompanying this textbook and on the Companion Website at **www.prenhall.com/tabloski**. Click on Chapter 23 to select the activities for this chapter.

CD-ROM
- Animation/Video
    AIDS
    EpiPen
- NCLEX Review
- Case Studies

- Tools

COMPANION WEBSITE
- Audio Glossary
- Additional NCLEX Review
- Case Study
- MediaLink Applications

Three major biological defense mechanisms protect the human body from injurious chemicals, foreign bodies, microorganisms, and parasites. The first line of defense is the **anatomical and biochemical barrier** provided by the skin and mucous membranes. The second line of defense is **mechanical clearance** that prevents substances from entering the body or assists in expelling them, such as sloughing of the skin, actions of the respiratory cilia and mucous secretions, vomiting, defecation, and urination. If these external barriers are breached, the inflammatory response is evoked immediately at the site of entry. Fluids, cells, and body secretions attempt to isolate, neutralize, destroy, and remove the invaders by surrounding the affected area. The first two lines of defense target all invaders, and therefore are nonspecific defense mechanisms (Huether & McCance, 2001).

The third line of defense is the **immune response**, a highly complicated, integrated system that is controlled by a complex communication mechanism. The immune system is briefly reviewed here. Anatomy and physiology or pathophysiology textbooks should be accessed for more detailed information.

The Immune System

Although the immune response occurs more slowly, it has the capability to confer long-term and, sometimes, permanent protection against living organisms such as bacteria, viruses, and parasites. It also protects the body from its own cancer cells. It is composed of a diverse group of structures, including cells that are carried throughout the body by the blood and lymphatic fluids. Structures include the thymus gland, red bone marrow, spleen, lymph nodes, lymph vessels, lymphatic tissues, and skin. The immune system identifies anything that is not a normal part of the body, and attacks and destroys the invader. However, the normal tissues of the body are left undisturbed. In this process, invaders can be blocked from entering the body, chemically neutralized, or destroyed.

Multiple factors affect the individual's immune system. First are the internal characteristics of the individual such as age, gender, and inherited genetic sequence. These factors cannot be modified. However, factors such as nutritional status and existence of underlying disease are potentially modifiable. External factors also can have a substantial effect upon a person's immune system. These include environmental pollutants, radiation, ultraviolet light, and drugs. The intensity and effectiveness of the immune response depends upon the combined effects of these factors. Occasionally, the immune system needs to be suppressed, such as after organ transplantation. Also, a person's immune system may overreact to a substance, and allergies or hypersensitivities result.

Among the multiple theories of aging, there are three major immune theories: the autoimmune theory, the immune deficiency theory, and the immune dysregulation theory (Digiovanna, 2000). The autoimmune theory postulates that as a person ages, the ability of the immune system to differentiate between invaders and normal tissues diminishes. Therefore, immune cells begin to attack normal body tissues, causing conditions that are often associated with aging, such as arthritis in joints. The immune deficiency theory states that with increasing age, the immune system is no longer able to defend the body from foreign invaders, and detrimental changes result. The immune dysregulation theory states that multiple changes in the immune system disrupt the regulation between the multiple components of the immune process. The result is progressive destruction of the body cells. Proponents of the immune theories of aging cite the decline in immune response, the association of this decline with specific diseases such as cancer, and the increased production of substances that attack body tissues as arguments in favor of their theory (Digiovanna, 2000).

CHARACTERISTICS UNIQUE TO THE IMMUNE SYSTEM

Three characteristics are unique to the immune system: **self-recognition**, **specificity**, and **memory** (Digiovanna, 2000). In self-recognition (tolerance), the immune system differentiates between substances that are normal constituents of a person's body and those that are not. **Antigens** are a wide range of substances that are identified as "nonself" and stimulate an immune response. Antigens are large protein or polysaccharide molecules found on the surfaces of living cells such as viruses, bacteria, fungi, or parasites. They are also on environmental substances such as pollen and foods, and on drugs, vaccines, transfusions, and transplanted tissues. Some types of cancer cells have surface molecules that are identified as foreign, and these will also stimulate an immune response.

Self-antigens on body cells will not stimulate an immune reaction. These are found on the surface of almost every cell of the body. These self-antigens are called **histocompatibility antigens**, or human leukocyte antigens (HLA antigens). Each person has HLA proteins on his or her body cells that are different from all other people. Exceptions occur with genetically identical twins. With some abnormalities, however, the immune system will attack self-antigens and an autoimmune condition will occur.

Specificity means that the immune response reacts only to one antigen. Each time a new antigen is identified, a different immune response is stimulated. For example, an immune response against chickenpox will not confer immunity to any other disease. The immune response results in production of antigen-specific glycoprotein molecules called antibodies that attach to the antigen and render it harmless.

Memory means that the immune system has the capacity to develop long-lasting protection against specific invaders. A residual set of cells that are specific to the antigen remain in the body, to be stimulated when the antigen presents itself at a later time. Each successive time the antigen is encountered will stimulate a quicker and more intense reaction by the immune system.

TYPES OF IMMUNITY

Natural immunity, or innate resistance, is not produced by the immune response. One type of natural immunity that is present at birth is specific to the human species. For example, humans are resistant to many diseases of animals, such as canine distemper. Other natural immunity is specific to the characteristics of the human individual. Natural passive immunity results from the passage of the mother's antibodies across the placental barrier into the circulation of the fetus. This provides transitory immunity for the first 3 to 6 months when infant mortality is the greatest.

Acquired active immunity results from stimulation of the body's immune system to destroy or neutralize foreign substances, usually microorganisms. It occurs after an agent is introduced into the body, either from the environment or through immunization, producing either an illness or an inapparent illness. Immunity is most durable if the person actually acquires the infectious disease, although severe or fatal complications can result from some infections. It is also possible for a recovered person to become a carrier of microorganisms and transmit them to others unknowingly. Immunizations, vaccines, or toxoids produce artificially acquired active immunity. Boosters may be given periodically to maintain immunity.

Acquired passive immunity is obtained by introducing a serum that contains specific antibodies into a person who is susceptible to the disease. Because the person receives antibodies that have been formed elsewhere, there is no direct stimulation of the person's own immune system. The immunity that is acquired is temporary (passive) and rarely lasts longer than a few weeks. Administration of gamma globulin to prevent hepatitis A in exposed people is an example.

COMPONENTS OF THE IMMUNE RESPONSE

White blood cells are primarily associated with both inflammation and the immune response. The three primary types of white blood cells are granulocytes, monocytes, and **lymphocytes**. Granulocytes ingest and digest debris and foreign material throughout the body and release powerful chemicals such as histamine and heparin that assist in the inflammatory process. Monocytes become large phagocytic cells, or **macrophages**, when stimulated by chemicals released by the body, and play an important part in inflammation.

Lymphocytes are the primary cells concerned with the development of immunity. Of all white blood cells, only lymphocytes have the ability for self-recognition, specificity, and memory. They arise from undifferentiated stem cells in the bone marrow, liver, and spleen. To become mature cells that can elicit an immune response, lymphocytes must pass through lymphoid tissue in various parts of the body. In doing so, they are committed to one of two types of lymphocytes. Cells destined to become B lymphocytes (B cells) migrate through the bone marrow to mature. When mature B lymphocytes come in contact with antigens, they are stimulated to become mature plasma cells and secrete antibodies to counteract the antigen. This reaction is called the **humoral immune response**. Cells destined to become T lymphocytes (T cells) migrate through the thymus gland when the person is very young. When mature T lymphocytes come in contact with antigens, the lymphocyte attacks the antigen directly. This reaction is called the **cell-mediated immune response**.

Humoral Immune Response

The humoral immune response is initiated when an antigen binds with **antibody** receptors on the surface of the mature B cell. This triggers a sequence of events, including assistance from helper T cells, resulting in production of plasma cells that secrete antibodies (immunoglobulin molecules). These antibodies are specific to the antigen that initially bound to the B-cell surface receptors. Also, memory cells are produced that live for months or years and can react swiftly when the antigen once again presents itself.

There are five classes of **immunoglobulins**: IgG, IgA, IgM, IgE, and IgD (Table 23-1). The classes of immunoglobulins differ in antigenic properties, structure, and function. The antibodies function in a number of ways to enhance the removal of antigens from the body. These functions are precipitation, agglutination, neutralization, opsonization, and complement activation.

Antibodies and antigens bind together (agglutination) to form large insoluble complexes (immune complexes) that fall out of body fluids (precipitation) (Figure 23-1 ■).

TABLE 23-1

Characteristics of Immunoglobulins

Class	Characteristics
IgG	Approximately 75% to 80% of total; four subclasses Present in serum, interstitial fluid, and amniotic fluid Crosses placenta; protects newborns Responsible for most of the antibody functions; activates complement Enhances phagocytosis
IgA	Approximately 15% of total; two subclasses Present in serum, tears, saliva, and body secretions from the pulmonary system, vagina, gastrointestinal tract, and other areas Prevents attachment and invasion of pathogens through mucosal membranes Passes to neonate through breast milk
IgM	Approximately 10% of total; largest immunoglobulin Present in serum; activates complement First antibody produced during the initial response to antigen Forms antibodies for ABO blood antigens
IgD	Less than 1% present in serum and umbilical cord Located on surfaces of developing B lymphocytes Action is relatively unknown
IgE	Less than 1% of circulating antibodies Present in serum and tissues Principal antibody in allergic reactions; combats parasitic infestations

Phagocytic cells, such as macrophages, can find these complexes easier and then engulf and destroy them. Antibodies also can inactivate an antigen (neutralization) by binding with it before it can interact with body cells. Some antibodies can coat the foreign antigen (opsonization) and make it more susceptible to phagocytosis. Many bacteria produce toxins that can harm people. Antibodies produced against these toxins function as

FIGURE ■ 23-1

Antigen-antibody reaction.

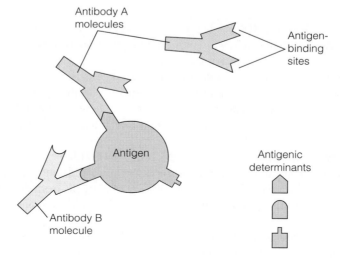

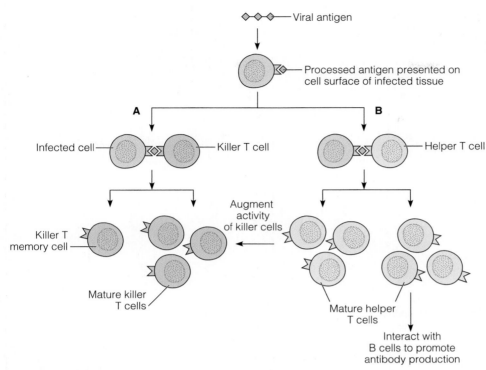

Viral antigen

Processed antigen presented on cell surface of infected tissue

A

B

Infected cell — Killer T cell

Helper T cell

Augment activity of killer cells

Killer T memory cell

Mature killer T cells

Mature helper T cells

Interact with B cells to promote antibody production

Source: National Institute of Allergy and Infectious Diseases, 2003.

FIGURE ■ 23-2

Various mechanisms of the primary immune response.

antitoxins that neutralize the bacterial toxins. Antibodies also protect people against some viral infections by preventing the attachment and entrance of viral cells into body cells. Neutralized viral particles may agglutinate or be ingested and destroyed by phagocytes. However, many viruses do not circulate in the bloodstream where antibodies are plentiful. Instead, they enter cells and spread by cell-to-cell contact (Huether & McCance, 2001).

The antigen-antibody complexes also trigger the complement system, which consists of approximately 20 plasma proteins that normally circulate inactivated in the bloodstream. When activated, they enhance inflammation, draw other cells to the antigen site, and increase destruction of abnormal cells.

The body has many weapons when mounting a primary immune response. Figure 23-2 ■ illustrates various immune responses when a virus is threatening to invade the body's defenses.

PRIMARY AND SECONDARY IMMUNE RESPONSES

The characteristic of memory is involved in both primary and secondary immune responses (Figure 23-3 ■). The first exposure to the foreign antigen results from active infection or immunization, and a **primary immune response** is begun. A latent period occurs initially, during which no antibodies can be detected. After approximately 5 days, IgM antibodies can be detected in the blood. It is followed by lesser amounts of IgG antibodies. During this time the person's immune system is activated or "primed," and memory cells are produced. If the immune process is effective and the infection is removed, the circulating antibodies will gradually be broken down and destroyed.

FIGURE ◼ 23-3

Primary and secondary immune response.

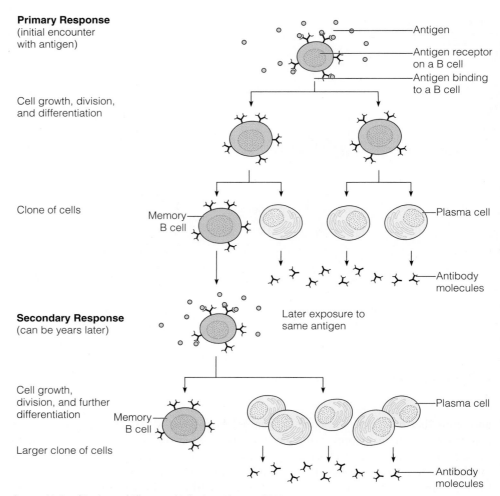

Primary Response
(initial encounter with antigen)

—Antigen

—Antigen receptor on a B cell

—Antigen binding to a B cell

Cell growth, division, and differentiation

Clone of cells

Memory B cell

Plasma cell

—Antibody molecules

Secondary Response
(can be years later)

Later exposure to same antigen

Cell growth, division, and further differentiation

Memory B cell

Larger clone of cells

Plasma cell

—Antibody molecules

Source: National Institute of Allergy and Infectious Diseases, 2003.

With a second exposure, however, the **secondary immune response** is evoked. Due to presence of memory cells, there is a more rapid production of large amounts of antibodies than occurred in the primary immune response. IgG is the predominant type of antibody associated with the secondary immune response, although IgM is also produced. The production of these antibodies is immediate, and high levels may last for several years. The characteristics of the primary and secondary response allow clinicians to determine the individual's stage of an infectious disease by evaluating a series of antibody titers for a specific antigen.

CELL-MEDIATED IMMUNE RESPONSE

During the process of maturation in the thymus gland, T cells begin producing several types of new proteins that become attached to the surface of the T cell. Most of these become specialized receptors called T cell antigen receptors (TCRs). Mature T cells have tens of thousands of TCRs on their surface that respond to only one foreign antigen (specificity). Other proteins, called CD proteins, result from a "cluster of differentiation" process. While TCRs recognize the specific antigen being presented, CD proteins along with HLA proteins (self-antigens) assist in the binding of the antigens to the T cells. Prior to presentation, the macrophages have engulfed and processed the antigen. The entire T cell then binds to the foreign antigen in multiple areas on the surface of the cell.

The two major types of mature T cells are helper T (Th) cells and cytotoxic (Tc) cells. Helper (Th) cells have CD4 proteins on their surface. When presented with an antigen, helper T cells produce signaling substances such as interleukin, interferon, and tumor necrosis factor. These stimulate other T cells and B cells in such a way that inflammation and other body activities are promoted. Cytotoxic (Tc) cells have CD8 proteins on their surface to promote binding; they attack and destroy cells that contain foreign antigens.

The humoral and cell-mediated immune responses are complex and interdependent. While some antigens can stimulate B cells to become plasma cells and produce antibodies independently, other antigens cannot stimulate either B cells or T cells independently to evoke the immune response. First, the antigen must interact with antigen-presenting cells such as the macrophage or macrophage-like cells in body tissues. A highly regulated communication system with a series of positive and negative feedback systems regulates and coordinates the immune response so that normal body tissues are not injured. These regulatory functions can be affected by aging and disease.

Changes in Immunity With Aging

Generally, aging is associated with physiological changes that cause stiffness or rigidity and decreased levels of functioning in many systems. As a result, it is difficult to differentiate age changes that are occurring simultaneously in organs throughout the body from specific changes in the immune system. Aging results in lifetime accumulative effects of environmental exposures, such as sunlight, radiation, pesticides, and other chemicals, as well as a lifetime of exposure to illness and stress.

These factors contribute in varying ways to decreased immune functioning. Older individuals, therefore, have more variation in the effectiveness of their immune system than younger people. Data comparing immune function between the young and old are often conflicting. Some older people show relatively little change, and others are severely compromised. There is a trend, however. As the age of a population increases, the proportion of people with declining humoral and cellular immune function increases (National Institute of Allergy and Infectious Diseases and National Cancer Institute, 2003). Within the individual, there is a decrease in the speed, strength, and duration of both the immune response and the regulation of immune activities (Digiovanna, 2000).

A decreased ability to respond to antigenic stimulation by B lymphocytes is a common characteristic of the aging immune system. Although the secondary immune response of the humoral (B cell) immune system may be normal due to the presence of memory cells, the response to new antigens is decreased. More antigenic material may be needed to prompt antibody production, and the production is slower. A lower peak antibody concentration may occur, and antibody levels decline faster as the person ages. As a result, risk of an insufficient humoral immune system response increases with the age at which antigens are first encountered.

Over time, the secondary immune response may also show changes. The number of B cells in the circulation decreases in some individuals. As a result, tissues are slower to repair and are more vulnerable to disease, especially infections. A decline in the production of IgE leads to a decrease in allergic or **hypersensitivity** reactions. An increase in antibody production that reacts against the person's own body cells also may occur, contributing to the development of autoimmune diseases such as rheumatoid arthritis. All changes in B cells develop slowly until the age of 60, when they begin to occur more rapidly. Therefore, vaccinations should be given by the age of 60 to have the greatest effectiveness.

There is consensus among investigators that normal aging, when no pathological conditions exist, is associated with diminished proliferative responses by T lymphocytes when exposed to some antigens. This is regarded as a key age-related factor in the gradual reduction in effectiveness of the immune system (Digiovanna, 2000; U.S. National Library of Medicine, 2002). A decrease in T-cell proliferation leads to reductions in all the subsequent parts of the immune response. Cell secretions such as interleukin-2 decline. Helper T cells (CD4) and cytotoxic T cells (CD8) are often reduced in their ratio to other T cells. There is a slower response to delayed hypersensitivity reactions, and regulation of the immune system is impaired. As a result, the incidence of infectious diseases, cancer, and autoimmune diseases increases. A summary of age-related changes in the immune system is found in Box 23-1. Figure 23-4 ■ illustrates the structures of the immune system and normal changes associated with aging.

FACTORS AFFECTING AGING OF THE IMMUNE SYSTEM

Many factors directly or indirectly associated with aging can affect the immune system. These factors include stress, diagnosis with comorbidities, exercise, and nutrients in the diet.

Stress

Older people are at a higher risk for acute and chronic diseases in which the aging immune system may have a role. It is generally believed that the stress response, resulting in sympathetic nervous system stimulation and hormonal changes, can suppress the immune system in older adults. In some illnesses, such as respiratory infections, a short-term change in immune function may be all that is required to increase susceptibility. However, since chronic diseases often take years to develop, it may also take many years of stress-induced

---

BOX 23-1 Aging Influences on the Immune System

- Overall decrease in:
  - Speed and strength of the immune response.
  - Neuroendocrine regulation of immune activities.
- Decrease in humoral immunity:
  - B-cell response to new antigenic stimulation decreases.
  - Number of B cells in the circulation decreases.
  - Decline in the production of IgE.
  - Increase in antibody production against self; contributes to development of autoimmune diseases.
  - Decrease is slow until the age of 60, then occurs more rapidly.
- Decrease in cellular immunity:
  - The key factor in the gradual reduction in effectiveness of the immune system is diminished proliferative responses by T lymphocytes.
  - Reductions in all the subsequent parts of the immune response occur.
  - Cell secretions such as interleukin-2 decline.
  - Helper T cells (CD4) and cytotoxic T cells (CD8) are often reduced in their ratio to other T cells.
  - There is slower response to delayed hypersensitivity reactions.
  - Regulation of the immune system is impaired.

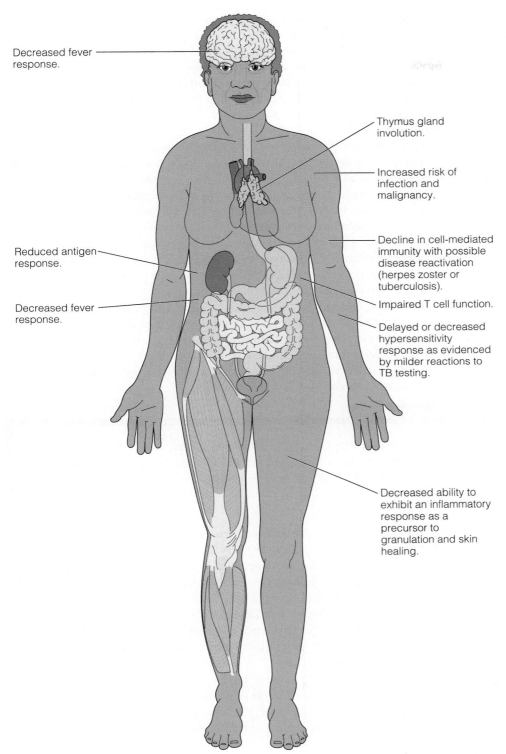

Normal changes of aging in the immune system.

Decreased fever response.

Thymus gland involution.

Increased risk of infection and malignancy.

Decline in cell-mediated immunity with possible disease reactivation (herpes zoster or tuberculosis).

Reduced antigen response.

Impaired T cell function.

Decreased fever response.

Delayed or decreased hypersensitivity response as evidenced by milder reactions to TB testing.

Decreased ability to exhibit an inflammatory response as a precursor to granulation and skin healing.

alterations of the immune system to affect the progress and severity of chronic diseases such as cardiovascular disease or cancer.

The cumulative effect of stress over time most likely contributes to the physical aging of the immune system and associated effects upon health (Burleson et al., 2002; McEwen, 1998). Individuals who characteristically react more strongly to stress may have greater stress-related effects over the course of their lives. Older people often have increased psychosocial stressors such as caring for an infirm spouse or partner. Investigators have reported high levels of stress, dysphoria, and social isolation among caregivers of dementia patients. The stress that accompanies this kind of caregiving has been equated to multiple and severe long-term stressors, and detrimental effects have been documented (Kiecolt-Glaser, Glaser, Gravenstein, Malarkey, & Sheridan, 1996). However, every individual has a different exposure to the type, frequency, intensity, and duration of stressful events in everyday life. This is a major factor in the heterogeneity demonstrated in the variation of effectiveness of immune systems in older people.

An increase in the amount of stress perceived by individuals is generally associated with poorer cellular immunity. However, this relationship is modified by the amount and type of coping used by the individual (Kiecolt-Glaser et al., 1996). Coping styles are likely to differ among individuals, even when faced with a similar stressful situation. Stowell, Kiecolt-Glaser, and Glaser (2001) studied the effects of coping on a measure of proliferation of the immune system following antigenic challenge. *Active coping* was defined as taking direct actions to eliminate or circumvent the stressor. Conversely, *avoidance coping* was defined as denial, disengagement, and giving up. The investigators concluded that active coping can have positive effects on immune function, particularly at high stress levels.

> ### Practice Pearl
>
> If older adults have assistance with stress-inducing events, such as death of a spouse, for a period of approximately 6 months after the event, resolution and stabilization of the immune system is likely to occur.

Comorbidity

The central nervous system, the immune system, and the endocrine system are interrelated. Aberrations in one system can adversely affect another system. Lymphocytes have receptors on their surface for many neuroendocrine hormones that consequently have regulatory effects on the lymphocytes. Mood, stress, depression, and mental illness influence the immune system. For example, patients with schizophrenia have increased presence of autoantibodies and decreased immune responses to antigens. Patients with systemic lupus erythematosus, an autoimmune disease, are associated with a psychosis that has symptoms similar to those seen in patients with schizophrenia (U.S. National Library of Medicine, 2002). Several feedback systems between the central nervous and immune systems exist. For example, antigen induces the production of interleukin-1, which increases levels of glucocorticoids. The glucocorticoids in turn inhibit the production of interleukin-1. Hypnosis has been found to modify the immune response, such as to suppress allergic responses (Tricerri et al., 1999).

Exercise

Exercise may prevent or slow the age-related decline in the immune response, particularly the decline in cell-mediated immunity. However, there is scant literature on the effects of exercise training on the immune response in the older person. Although some studies have found increased T-cell function in highly conditioned older persons compared with controls, results have been mixed. Long-term exposure to physical activity may be required to obtain a positive immune response in the older person. Other lifestyle factors, such as nutrition, are associated with physical activity and may have an effect on the immune response.

Both physical activity and nutrition may be compromised in the frail older person. Chin et al. (2000) investigated the effects of a 17-week physical exercise regimen combined with enriched foods on the cellular immune response in frail older persons. The exercises in the randomized controlled trial focused on skills training, and the foods were enriched with micronutrients that have a high prevalence of deficiency in older people. The study did not find any effect from micronutrients on cellular immune response, although blood levels of the nutrients increased. However, the data did suggest that a moderately intensive, comprehensive, and individualized exercise program may prevent or slow the age-related decline in the cellular immune response.

Tai chi is a moderate Chinese exercise that has beneficial effects upon the immune system as well as other body systems. Various studies in China have found that practicing tai chi has an impact upon circulating levels of IgG and IgM. Results of Li, Hong, and Chan's study (2001) indicated that tai chi is beneficial to cardiorespiratory function, mental control, flexibility, balance control, and muscle strength as well as the immune system. Tai chi improved muscle strength and reduced the risk of falls in the older person.

Nutrients

Deficiencies of vitamins and trace elements are observed in almost one third of all older persons. Nine micronutrients have been identified as contributing to the cellular immune response. They are vitamins A, C, E, B_6, folate, iron, copper, selenium, and zinc (Chandra, 1997; McClain, McClain, Barve, & Boosalis, 2002). A number of studies have suggested that supplements containing micronutrients that approximate the recommended dietary allowances improve delayed-type hypersensitivity and assist in preventing infections (Buzina et al., 1998).

Mild zinc deficiency is prevalent in the older population. Several studies have evaluated zinc supplementation and its effect upon the immune system. Supplementation improved selected components of the cellular immune system and decreased respiratory infections (Girodon et al., 1999; High, 2001). Zinc should be administered with caution, however. High doses of zinc can cause toxicity, copper deficiency, and immunosuppression.

A year's supply of micronutrients is relatively inexpensive. Since there is no evidence that the recommended daily allowances given for prolonged periods have any toxic or adverse consequences, many clinicians feel that supplements in modest amounts can be recommended for all older individuals. Hopefully, the maximum physiological and health benefit would be obtained with the least risk of toxicity. The exact types and optimum amounts have not yet been determined.

Excessive Immune Responses

Excessive responses of the immune system result from an increase in the normal activities of the immune system. Hypersensitivity and **autoimmunity** are types of excessive responses. Overreaction of the immune system is believed to result from interplay between environmental factors and the genetic makeup of the individual. For instance, type 1 diabetes is thought to be an autoimmune disease where misguided T cells attack the beta cells in the pancreas and eventually destroy their ability to produce insulin. Figure 23-5 ▇ illustrates the pathological process.

The pathological process of misguided T cells attacking beta cells in the pancreas.

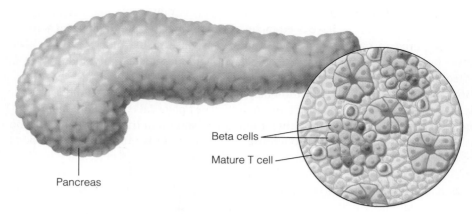

Beta cells

Mature T cell

Pancreas

Source: National Institute of Allergy and Infectious Diseases, 2003.

HYPERSENSITIVITY

Hypersensitivity is either an excessive response to antigen stimulation or a normal response that is inappropriate. It usually does not occur on the first exposure to the antigen when the primary immune response occurs (sensitization). Reexposure to the antigen and initiation of the secondary immune response can stimulate hypersensitive reactions in predisposed individuals. The four types of hypersensitivity are characterized by a specific humoral or cell-mediated response. Types I, II, and III are primarily reactions of the humoral immune system (B cells). Type IV hypersensitivity is a response of the cellular immune system (T cells). There is a complex interrelationship between some hypersensitivity reactions and several autoimmune diseases. Characteristics of the four types of hypersensitivity and the diseases associated with each type are found in Table 23-2.

Type I Hypersensitivity

Type I hypersensitivities are immediate and may be life threatening. Reactions normally occur within 15 to 30 minutes after exposure to an antigen (allergen). Manifestations vary in severity, but often include hives, localized swelling, tightening of the throat, shortness of breath, wheezing, tachycardia, and hypotension. Anaphylactic allergic reactions leading to shock can occur.

Asthma is a common hypersensitivity type I problem that is often underdiagnosed and suboptimally treated in the older person (Huss et al., 2001). The prevalence of asthma increases steadily with age; however, it is not identified well in older adults. The symptoms

TABLE 23-2

Characteristics and Diseases Associated With the Four Types of Hypersensitivity

Type	Action	Diseases
Type I	Immediate reaction: IgE mediated local or systemic allergic response	Anaphylaxis; atrophic disorders
Type II	Cytotoxic reactions: IgG and/or IgM mediated destruction of cells	Drug and transfusion reactions
Type III	Immune complex reactions: IgM or IgG mediated formation of antigen-antibody complexes	Serum sickness, Arthus reactions
Type IV	Cell-mediated reactions: mediated by sensitized T cells	Allergic contact dermatitis; delayed hypersensitivity reactions

are often attributed to other diseases of the respiratory system such as congestive heart failure, chronic obstructive pulmonary disease, and other pulmonary disorders, especially chronic bronchitis. Patients with asthma are more likely to have had symptoms earlier in life. Older people also may have less awareness of symptoms. Asthma medications may aggravate coexisting medical conditions, and some drugs commonly used for the older person (aspirin and beta-blockers) may adversely influence asthma (Buttaro, Trybulski, Bailey, & Sandberg-Cook, 2003). Interventions should be aimed at identifying allergens that precipitate attacks and reducing them in the home (Huss et al., 2001).

Type II Hypersensitivity

Type II hypersensitivities also occur within 15 to 30 minutes of exposure. Examples of this type of reaction include transfusion reactions, drug reactions, myasthenia gravis, thyroiditis, and autoimmune hemolytic anemia (Copstead & Banasik, 2000). Autoimmune thyroiditis can result in both hyperthyroidism and hypothyroidism. Other than hypothyroidism, none of these conditions are particularly prevalent disorders in the older person. Hypothyroidism does occur in women over 60 years of age, and often the symptoms are subtler than in younger people. As a result, thyroid-stimulating hormone (TSH) screening is recommended in this age group. If older adults require thyroid hormone replacement medications, a low dose should be given initially. After the dose has stabilized, periodic TSH measurements are required. Also, patients should be aware that supplementation is lifelong.

Type III Hypersensitivity

Type III hypersensitivity is characterized by a failure to remove antigen-antibody complexes from the circulation and tissues. The subsequent inflammatory reaction can lead to cell and tissue injury. The underlying cause may be a persistent low-grade infection by a viral or bacterial agent; chronic exposure to an environmental antigen from molds, plants, or animals; or an autoimmune process. For example, glomerulonephritis typically occurs about 10 to 14 days after an infection by a *Streptococcus* bacterial organism. The immune complex is deposited in the glomerular capillary wall of the kidney with resulting proteinuria, hematuria, hypertension, oliguria, and red cell casts in the urine. This may lead to acute or chronic renal failure.

Systemic lupus erythematosus is another example of a type III hypersensitivity reaction caused by autoantibody production. The prevalence of the disease is considered to be underreported (Lupus Foundation of America, 2001). Antibodies are formed against nuclear DNA and RNA throughout the body. The resulting inflammatory response causes a cycle of cell damage and further formation of antigen-antibody immune complexes that are deposited in connective tissues. The signs and symptoms vary significantly since any organ of the body can be involved. Lesions of the skin, mucosal ulcerations, nephritis, restrictive pulmonary disease, retinal changes, neuritis, and gastrointestinal ulceration are but a few. Progressive use of anti-inflammatory agents, systemic corticosteroids, and immunosuppressives can decrease symptoms and increase the person's quality of life.

Rheumatoid arthritis is believed to be another example of type III hypersensitivity that affects the older person. About 1% of all adults have rheumatoid arthritis, and it is more frequent in women. Peak incidence is between the fourth and sixth decade of life. A number of theories exist to explain the etiology, all related to components of the immune system and the development of autoimmunity.

There does seem to be a genetic predisposition to rheumatoid arthritis. It is two to three times more common in women with a familial history. Pathological changes occur initially in the synovial tissue of joints. Antibodies form against the person's own IgG, and the resulting complex is identified as foreign. The inflammatory process, stimulated by infiltrating T cells, gradually destroys articular cartilage. Bone erosion occurs, causing swelling, pain, and loss of motion. The freely movable joints of the hands, wrists, ankles, and feet are the most commonly affected, in a symmetrical pattern. Characteristic ulnar deviations lead to swan neck deformities of the hands. The elbows, knees, and shoulders may also be involved. Eventually, proper functioning of the joints becomes impossible and crippling deformities occur.

Rheumatoid arthritis is a chronic, fluctuating, systemic disease, and widespread damage can occur. Fibrous materials everywhere in the body can be attacked. Along with specific joint pain, patients are chronically tired and may complain of generalized

---

BOX 23-2 Nursing Diagnoses and Interventions for Rheumatic Disorders

Nursing Diagnosis: Pain related to inflammatory process and advancing disease process.

Outcome: Pain decreased below current level or relieved. Incorporation of pain relief measures into daily life.

Interventions:

- Measure the level of pain on a pain scale; observe for subjective changes.
- Provide a variety of nonpharmacological comfort measures:
    - Heat or cold
    - Massage
    - Position change
    - Supportive equipment
    - Relaxation techniques
    - Diversion activities
- Encourage verbalization.
- Administer anti-inflammatory analgesics and antirheumatic medications on an individualized plan.
- Encourage exercise routine while protecting joints.
- Teach pathophysiology of pain.

Nursing Diagnosis: Activity intolerance or fatigue related to disease process.

Outcome: Increased tolerance for daily activities.

Interventions:

- Assist in development of an activity/rest/sleep schedule.
- Explain the relationship of the disease to fatigue.
- Encourage use of energy-saving techniques.
- Encourage adequate nutrition.
- Encourage adherence to medication and treatment plans and evaluate effects.

Nursing Diagnosis: Impaired physical mobility caused by disease process or surgical intervention.

Outcome: Achieves and maintains optimal mobility.

Interventions:

- Encourage independence in mobility.
    - Assess need for physical or occupational therapy.
    - Develop a routine exercise program, including range of motion, strengthening, and endurance exercises along with rest periods.
    - Use appropriate ambulatory devices.
    - Explain importance of supportive shoes.

aching. Prolonged inactivity increases stiffness and swelling. As the disease progresses, activities such as climbing stairs and opening jars become difficult. A low-grade fever, weight loss, and depression are common. Cardiac, pulmonary, and ophthalmic manifestations may occur in later stages of the disease. Drug therapy often consists of a combination of non-steroidal anti-inflammatory drugs (NSAIDs), antirheumatic drugs, and glucocorticoids. A summary of the care of patients with rheumatic disorders is found in Box 23-2. A thorough discussion of rheumatoid arthritis can be found in Chapter 18 of this text. ▭

- Assess environmental barriers.
- Refer to community health agency for assistance.

Nursing Diagnosis: Self-care deficit related to loss of motion and fatigue.

Outcome: Becomes independent in self-care using necessary resources.

Interventions:
- Assist patient and family in identifying factors that interfere with self-care activities, and ways to ameliorate problems.
- Develop goals and a plan for meeting self-care needs.
  - Protect joints.
  - Conserve energy.
  - Simplify activities.
- Assess need for assistive devices and instruct on their safe use.

Nursing Diagnosis: Body image disturbance related to changes in mobility and dependency.

Outcome: Takes an active part in improving self-concept.

Interventions:
- Assess concerns about body image.
- Encourage expression of feelings about deformities with support and concern.
- Teach strategies for improving body image (how to dress, apply makeup, improve hygiene).
- Assist significant others to understand the impact of the limitations and solicit their help in identifying methods to promote a positive body image.

Nursing Diagnosis: Impaired skin integrity related to altered peripheral perfusion.

Outcome: Skin remains intact.

Interventions:
- Assess skin color, pulses, capillary refill, sensation, and temperature.
- Discourage use of nicotine products.
- Avoid exposure to cold and protect extremities in cold environment.
  - Wear natural fiber clothing.
  - Use lanolin-based ointments.
- Monitor complaints of numbness and tingling.
- Encourage routine skin care.
- Promote adequate nutrition.

Type IV Hypersensitivity

Type IV hypersensitivity is also called delayed hypersensitivity. Tissue is damaged as a result of a delayed T-cell reaction to an antigen. The reaction normally occurs within 1 to 14 days after exposure, although it is often slower in older persons. Contact hypersensitivity such as dermatitis from a latex allergy, tuberculin reactions, and transplant rejections are examples. In people with multiple sclerosis, a variety of studies have documented abnormalities in both B cells and T cells.

Deficient Immune Responses

Deficient immune responses occur when there is a functional decrease in one or more components of the immune system. These are either primary or secondary immunodeficiency disorders.

PRIMARY IMMUNODEFICIENCY DISORDERS

Primary immunodeficiency disorders are either congenital or acquired, and are not attributed to other causes.

HIV/AIDS

Infection with the human immunodeficiency virus (HIV) and the resulting acquired immunodeficiency syndrome (AIDS) is the best example of a primary immunodeficiency disorder. The hallmark of this infection is a decrease in cellular (T cell) immunity. Helper T (CD4) cells are primarily affected by the virus. These T cells mediate between the antigen presenting cells (macrophages) and other B and T cells. HIV is an example of an emerging infectious disease that jumped from animal to human, probably in the 1950s. It is a chronic disease spread primarily through sexual contact with an infected person. The widespread organ involvement associated with the infection has caused much human suffering and death. Extensive information regarding the pathophysiology, interventions, and outcomes associated with HIV infection can be found in pathophysiology and medical-surgical textbooks and in medical journals. Only the effects of HIV infection in the older person are described here.

The mean age of patients who are first detected with HIV and who are diagnosed with AIDS is progressively increasing over time (Manfredi, 2002). This is due to a number of factors. Survival rates have improved due to advances in diagnostic resources, antiviral treatment, and prophylaxis. The senior population is increasing and so are their expectations regarding their sex lives. Male sexual function has been enhanced by medications such as sildenafil citrate (Viagra). Research continues into medications to enhance female sexual drive and response. The sexually permissive baby boomers are about to enter the ranks of the older population. Some older persons continue their risky sexual behaviors and pay little attention to preventive measures, believing that HIV infection is not an issue in their age group.

Older people have been compared to teenagers in their knowledge of HIV. They have not known people who have suffered from HIV/AIDS, and so they have little knowledge, personal awareness, or interest in preventing the disease. However, many senior centers now have AIDS awareness programs that provide information about HIV prevention and safe sex. Klein et al. (2001) studied the HIV/AIDS prevention education needs of older adults. A need for concisely presented, accurate information appropriate for their age group was clearly demonstrated. The print media, such as the health section of newspapers, and the Internet were suggested as particularly valuable resources.

In the early stages of the HIV epidemic, the major route of transmission in older adults was through receipt of contaminated blood and blood products. Since effective blood screening has been implemented, this type of transmission has decreased substantially. However, the risk of infection through exposure to HIV by the more traditional methods has increased. Increasing numbers of older persons are contacting HIV infection through heterosexual and homosexual activities, and through intravenous drug use.

HIV infection in the older person is most likely underdiagnosed and underreported. Healthcare workers often do not take sexual histories of older patients, nor do they recommend HIV testing. Symptoms of HIV infection, such as memory loss and weight loss, are often treated as symptoms of other common age-related health problems, such as Alzheimer's disease (Szirony, 1999).

In general, the older person has not fared as well as the younger person with HIV infection. Older people have lower CD4 cell counts, are more ill at the initial diagnosis, have more comorbidity, are characterized by a more aggressive course of the disease, and have a higher risk of death from the disease (Chen, Ryan, & Ferguson, 1998; Wellons et al., 2002). It is believed that these characteristics are due to delayed diagnosis, chronic coexisting health problems, and the age-related impairments in T-cell immunity.

Antiretroviral therapy, which typically contains at least three antiretroviral medications, holds promise for treatment of older people with HIV infection. When compared to younger people, older patients in one study had somewhat better virological responses and similar immunological responses to antiretroviral therapy. Older patients had fewer interruptions in the therapy and were able to tolerate and adhere to the therapy regimen relatively well. Failure of an older patient to respond to antiretroviral therapy should not be attributed to age alone (Wellons et al., 2002). The prognosis for seniors diagnosed with HIV today is good. Although they live fewer years after diagnosis, they can still live long productive lives (Marcus, 2002). Care of the older patient with an HIV infection is presented in Box 23-3.

Nursing Diagnoses and Interventions: The Older Patient With an HIV Infection	**BOX 23-3**

Nursing Diagnosis: Knowledge deficit related to preventing transmission of HIV.
Outcome: Knows how to prevent the spread of HIV infection.
Interventions:
- Instruct patient, family, and friends on preventing transmission of HIV.
  - Avoid sexual contact with multiple partners.
  - Use condoms if the partner's HIV status is uncertain.
  - Avoid oral contact with genitals.
  - Avoid sexual practices that can cause injury to tissue.
  - Avoid sex with people at high risk.
  - Do not use intravenous recreational drugs.

Nursing Diagnosis: Risk for infection due to immunodeficiency.
Outcome: Infections do not occur.
Interventions:
- Monitor for symptoms of new infection.
  - A body temperature of 37.8°C or 100°F.
  - White blood cell count and differential.
  - Classic symptoms may not be present in the elderly person.

(continued)

- Instruct patient, family, or caregiver in ways to prevent infection.
- Administer antimicrobial therapy as prescribed.
- Encourage adequate nutrition.
- Use strict aseptic techniques for any invasive procedure.

Nursing Diagnosis: Altered thought processes and sensory-perceptual alterations related to CNS infection or other complications.

Outcome: Communication in a lucid manner.

Interventions:

- Assess mental status and sensory changes.
- Monitor for drug interactions, infections, nutrition and electrolyte imbalances, depression, and other associated conditions.
- Create an environment that will minimize disorienting stimuli.
- Orient to changes in the environment.
- Help obtain a power of attorney if necessary to handle legal and financial matters.
- Assess self-care deficits.

Nursing Diagnosis: Self-care deficit related to factors such as mental changes, neurologic impairment, and depression.

Outcome: Becomes independent in self-care using necessary resources.

Interventions:

- Assist patient and family in identifying factors that interfere with self-care activities, and ways to ameliorate problems.
- Encourage adherence to antiviral medications.
  - Take steps to avoid medication errors due to memory loss.
- Develop goals and a plan for meeting self-care needs.
- Assess need for assistive devices and instruct on their safe use.

Nursing Diagnosis: Potential for poisoning from drug toxicity.

Outcome: Tolerates medication regimen.

Interventions:

- Encourage adherence to antiviral drug therapy.
- Explain dosage, route of administration, action, and side effects of all medications.
- Instruct when to discontinue drugs and call for assistance.
- Keep list of medications and time of administration.

Nursing Diagnosis: Social isolation related to fear of AIDS, rejection by family and withdrawal from social activities, and fear of infecting others.

Outcome: Contacts with people are maintained.

Interventions:

- Observe for behaviors that suggest isolation, such as hostility, depression, withdrawal, feelings of rejection, or loneliness.
- Encourage maintenance of important personal relationships.
- Encourage visitors and telephone calls.
- Encourage diversional activities such as reading, watching TV, or crafts.
- Educate patient, family, and friends about how HIV is transmitted.
- Refer to support groups and community resources.

SECONDARY IMMUNODEFICIENCY DISORDERS

Secondary immunodeficiency disorders are a consequence of other disorders or treatment regimens. Many factors can lead to the development of secondary immunodeficiency disorders, including physical, nutritional, environmental, psychosocial, and pharmacological factors (Table 23-3). For example, an excessive neuroendocrine secretion of corticosteroids in response to stress can lead to increased susceptibility to infectious disease and cancer. Low levels of corticosteroids may enhance autoimmune diseases. People who have high levels of physical and psychosocial stress, limited social support, depression, and bereavement show decreased immune functioning (Copstead & Banasik, 2000). Older people are often exposed to these types of stressors.

The stress of surgery, including the effects of anesthesia, can decrease the number of both B and T cells, and the deficiency can last for up to one month. This is particularly true for removal of the spleen, a structure of the immune system. Diabetes mellitus, cirrhosis, severe trauma and burns, malignancies, and severe infections are associated with secondary immune deficiencies. Medications, such as the cancer pharmacotherapeutic drugs, also cause a state of general immunosuppression. Others, such as antibiotics, anticonvulsants, antihistamines, and steroids, affect various mechanisms of the immune system. X-rays can destroy the rapidly proliferating cells of the immune system. Malnutrition can lead to protein and other deficiencies that impair immune function. Many

TABLE 23-3

Effects of Selected Medications and Therapy on the Immune System

Drug	Action on Immune System
Antibiotics in high doses	Bone marrow suppression: aplastic anemia
Chloramphenicol	Leukopenia
Gentamicin sulfate	Agranulocytosis
Streptomycin	Leukopenia, pancytopenia
Penicillin	Agranulocytosis
Antithyroid drugs	Agranulocytosis, leukopenia
Nonsteroidal anti-inflammatory drugs (NSAIDs) in high doses	Prostaglandin synthesis/release inhibited Agranulocytosis, leukopenia
Adrenal corticosteroids Prednisone	Immunosuppression
Cancer chemotherapeutic drugs (cytotoxic drugs)	Immunosuppression
Alkylating agents	Leukopenia, agranulocytosis
Cyclosporine	Decreased T-cell function, leukopenia
Antimetabolites	Immunosuppression
Fluorouracil	Leukopenia, eosinophilia
Mercaptopurine	Leukopenia, pancytopenia
Methotrexate	Leukopenia, aplastic bone marrow
Ionizing radiation	Suppression of stem cell division; pancytopenia

Source: Adapted from Smeltzer, S. C., & Bare, B. B. (2004). *Brunner & Suddarth's textbook of medical-surgical nursing* (10th ed., p. 1340). Philadelphia: Lippincott.

of these factors affect older persons, many of whom already have a decreased ability to reproduce new cells of the immune system (Copstead & Banasik, 2000).

Susceptibility to Infections

Infections are one of the most frequently encountered problems in the older population. Although specific relationships between an aging or compromised immune system and infection are not clear, the decline in responsiveness of the immune system to harmful foreign invaders leads to an increase in the incidence and severity of infections. Sometimes they are difficult to diagnose. The febrile response that signals infections may be blunted in the older person. Medications commonly taken may also decrease the normal fever response. The baseline body temperature in older people is approximately 1°F lower than the normal temperature in younger people. Therefore, a rise in body temperature may not be immediately evident. Any temperature of 37.8°C or 100°F when other symptoms are present may indicate an infection. Other classic signs and symptoms of infection, such as redness, swelling, and pain, may also be altered.

> **Practice Pearl**
>
> A body temperature of 37.8°C or 100°F, combined with other symptoms, may often herald an infection in the older person.

PNEUMONIA

Pneumonia is a leading cause of death in people over 65 years of age. It is the most common hospital-associated infection, and it has the highest mortality rate of all **nosocomial infections**. The combination of pneumonia and influenza causes the greatest number of deaths. *Streptococcus pneumoniae* (pneumococcus) remains the single most common cause of pneumonia in the older person, and it increases with age. It accounts for approximately 40% to 60% of the cases. Pneumococcal pneumonia may occur as a primary illness or as a complication of a chronic disease. *S. pneumoniae* is a common resident of the human upper respiratory tract, and has been isolated in up to 70% of healthy adults.

Clearance of foreign invaders by the action of mucous production and cilia is less effective in the older person. As part of the aging process, there is a loss of both alveolar ducts and the surrounding elastic tissue. Demineralization of bones in the chest and a decreased effectiveness of the respiratory musculature further predispose the older person to lower respiratory infections. Under these conditions, pneumonia can occur following aspiration of microorganisms into the lungs. A serious complication of pneumonia is the development of bacteremia in 20% to 25% of those infected (Chan & Fernandez, 2001).

The signs and symptoms of pneumonia in older people are likely to be atypical. Often the classic signs of fever, productive cough, chest pain, and leukocytosis are muted, and the diagnosis may be missed. Instead, other symptoms such as general deterioration, lethargy, falls, changes in mental status and orientation, anorexia, gastrointestinal symptoms, and tachycardia may signal the onset. Older people who live alone are particularly at risk of advanced illness since no one may be present to notice early changes in their general function. Underlying conditions may also mask the symptoms of pneumonia. For example, purulent sputum or slight changes in respiratory symptoms may be the only sign of pneumonia in patients with chronic obstructive pulmonary disease. Chest x-rays may determine whether chronic congestive heart failure or other processes are involved.

To prevent serious complications, all people 65 years of age and older should receive pneumococcal vaccine. Antibody response is often lower in the older person and may decline after 5 to 10 years. Revaccination is occasionally recommended (Reuben et al., 2004). Yearly influenza immunizations are also highly recommended for the older person. The only contraindication is an allergy to eggs. Over 90% of the deaths during previous U.S. influenza epidemics were attributed to pneumonia as a complication of influenza. The vaccine reduces influenza-related morbidity and mortality by 70% to 90% among vaccinated individuals (Fune, Shua-Haim, Ross, & Frank, 1998).

> ### Practice Pearl
>
> All people 65 and over should receive an initial dose of pneumococcal vaccine at age 65, and a yearly influenza immunization. Pneumococcal vaccine immunization can be repeated every 6 to 7 years (Reuben et al., 2004).

Refer to the following Best Practices feature for recommendations regarding immunization practices for older adults.

URINARY TRACT INFECTION

Urinary tract infection is one of the most common problems in older adults, especially in women. It is important to differentiate between asymptomatic bacteriuria and symptomatic infection. The prevalence of urinary bacteriuria increases with age. It is found in approximately 1% of young women and increases to approximately 20% among women over the age of 70 years. It is found in approximately 10% of men over 70 (Fune et al., 1998). Asymptomatic bacteriuria generally is not treated. Adverse reactions, reinfection, and the development of resistant organisms can occur.

Symptomatic infections usually include urinary frequency, urgency, and suprapubic or flank pain. Fever may or may not occur. As with other infections in the older person, the presenting symptoms may vary. Mental status may change, falls may occur, and a decline in activities of daily living may be noticed. Generalized observations such as these may signal a smoldering urinary tract infection. All older people who are symptomatic should be treated promptly. A short course of oral antibiotic therapy is often effective. However, hospitalization may be required for those who have hypotension, dehydration, or signs of sepsis. Intravenous antibiotics may be required.

Bladder dysfunction, a hypertrophied prostate gland, the relaxation of pelvic musculature, and other coexisting illnesses increase the incidence of infection. Indwelling catheters will eventually become infected, even with a closed drainage system. Long-term catheterization should be avoided whenever possible.

BACTEREMIA

Microorganisms can be introduced into the bloodstream as a complication of pneumonia, urinary tract infections, infection of skin and soft tissues, and other infectious

The Hartford Institute for Geriatric Nursing *Try This* assessment series (2004) recommends the following Best Practices regarding immunizations for the older adult. It is imperative to screen for immunization histories during patient office visits, as well as hospital admissions, and offer vaccination as indicated. It is vital to screen healthcare staff on a pre-employment basis, and keep them informed and immunized at regular intervals.

For the Older Adult Patient

1. Always attempt to obtain the patient's immunization history. Ask the family for assistance if the patient cannot provide reliable information. Old medical records or computer records may indicate prior vaccinations. Pay attention to any history of neurologic or hypersensitivity reactions.
2. Educate the patient on vaccine-preventable diseases and the importance of vaccination. Patients and patients' families oftentimes have misconceptions or lack of information regarding immunization. Offer vaccination as indicated.
3. Provide clear documentation of vaccination provided to minimize risk of unnecessary duplication.
4. Follow the following guidelines recommended by the U.S. Department of Health and Human Services:
   - Provide influenza vaccine annually, starting October and ending February.
   - Provide pneumococcal vaccine once after the age of 65 with a revaccination after 5 years if diseases such as chronic renal failure, chronic immunosuppression, malignancies, and functional or anatomic asplenia are present.
   - Provide tetanus-diphtheria toxoid (Td) as a booster shot every 10 years to those who have completed the immunization series during childhood or teen years. If the patient has never been vaccinated, administer 0.5 mg intramuscularly twice with a 1 to 2 month interval and an additional dose 6 to 12 months later. Again, previous neurologic or hypersensitivity reactions are an absolute contraindication.

Hospital Immunization Protocols

Work with hospital administration to develop a system that:

1. Screens for immunization, upon admission, of the older adult.
2. Educates new admissions about immunization.
3. Incorporates immunization history and standing physician orders into the electronic medical record.
4. Tracks healthcare staff immunizations and ensures adequate compliance.
5. Provides immunization education and screening to the community at large.
6. Provides personal immunization records for the older adult patient.

Source: Adapted from Kennedy, R. D., & Cullamar, K. (2004). Immunizations for the Older Adult. *Try This: Best Practices in Care for Older Adults 21*. New York: New York University, The Steinhardt School of Education, Division of Nursing, The John A. Hartford Foundation Institute for Geriatric Nursing.

processes. The urinary tract is the most common source of bacteremia, followed by the respiratory tract. Perirectal abscesses are frequently missed and can be a source of infection. Once in the bloodstream, microorganisms are disseminated to other organs throughout the body. Increased age and associated illness contribute to a poorer prognosis, and mortality rates are between 15% and 40%. Gram-negative rods, such as *Escherichia coli, Proteus* species, and *Klebsiella* species, are the most common microorganisms. *Staphylococcus aureus* is the most common gram-positive organism and is associated with 50% mortality.

As with most infections in the older person, the clinical clues vary. Often the older person becomes confused and agitated, with altered mental status. Decreased consciousness may occur. Fever, while usually present, may be low grade. Blood cultures confirm the diagnosis, and immediate antibiotic treatment is essential. Septic shock is a serious complication.

TUBERCULOSIS

Tuberculosis still remains a worldwide problem. It is a chronic pulmonary and extra-pulmonary infectious disease that is acquired through exposure to *Mycobacterium tuberculosis.* It spreads from person to person by airborne transmission. The number of cases of tuberculosis is highest in people over 65 years of age, with the exception of those who are infected with HIV. The majority of active cases occur through reactivation of a dormant infection in an older person who has not been effectively treated in the past. Older persons are also at increased risk of initial infection, particularly those who are chronically ill or debilitated and residing in nursing homes.

Typical symptoms of hemoptysis, fever, and night sweats are less common in the older person. Pleural effusion may be the only direct manifestation of tuberculosis, although signs of confusion and altered mental status are common. Disseminated disease to lymph nodes, bones, kidneys, gastrointestinal tract, and skin may cause delay in diagnosis. Due to the blunted immune system and delayed reactivity in many older people, a two-step Mantoux method of administering the tuberculin test is preferred. This reduces the likelihood of interpreting a booster reaction as a recent infection. Refer to Chapter 16 for guidelines on interpretation of the Mantoux test. ⊂▭⊃

Infection should be differentiated from active disease. Those with a latent infection may be treated with daily isoniazid (INH) for 6 to 12 months to prevent development of the disease. Active disease should be treated aggressively with a combination of drugs over a long period. Directly observed therapy is often recommended to increase compliance with the rather complicated medication regimen.

SKIN INFECTIONS

As the skin becomes thinner and less elastic with age, the older person becomes more susceptible to injury and breakdown of tissue. Peripheral neuropathy with decreased sensation and circulation may lead to abrasions, burns, and stasis ulcers. Reduced physical activity, malnutrition, dehydration, and other systemic illnesses are also predisposing factors. Immobilized people who are convalescing at home are at high risk for the development of pressure ulcers. Any interruption of skin integrity leads to infection, especially with organisms that are a part of the normal skin flora.

Erysipelas, a superficial cellulitis of the skin caused by group A streptococcus, usually affects the lower extremities or the face (Figure 23-6 ▪). Any illness that compromises skin integrity, such as diabetes mellitus or alcohol abuse, may increase the risk of this infection. The involved area is bright red and raised with well-defined borders. Skin infections such as this can predispose the individual to bacteremia and septic shock. Although antibiotic treatment is effective, the most important method of therapy is prevention. Necrotizing fasciitis, although uncommon, can cause extensive invasion of the subcutaneous tissues. Immediate surgical intervention and appropriate antibiotic treatment are required.

The reactivation of the herpes zoster (varicella) virus that has lingered in nerve tissue for years following chickenpox infection can lead to shingles. Approximately 9 per 1,000 people over 60 years of age acquire the illness each year (Fune et al., 1998). Vesicular lesions occur along spinal nerves, most frequently affecting T3 to L2 nerves and the fifth cranial nerve. Extreme discomfort may occur. Early treatment with acyclovir or other antiviral medications should begin within 72 hours after appearance of the rash. This treatment reduces acute pain and shortens the period of infectivity. Otherwise, treatment is largely supportive with administration of analgesics and topical

FIGURE ☐ 23-6

Erysipelas, a superficial cellulitis of the skin caused by group A streptococcus.

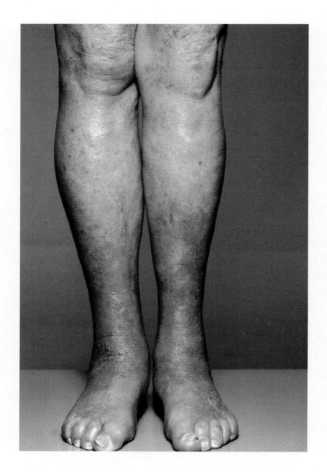

cleansing. Occasionally, chronic pain develops that will require longer term analgesics and possibly antidepressants.

NURSING ASSESSMENT

Multiple factors underlie immune problems in the older person. Therefore, a health history and physical examination are essential. The key assessment areas include the following factors:

- Age
- Nutrition
- Recent infections
- Immunization status
- Allergies
- Disorders and diseases
    - Autoimmune disease
    - Neoplastic disease
    - Chronic illness
    - Surgery
- Pain
- Medications
- Blood transfusions
- Lifestyle, stress, and other factors

NURSING INTERVENTIONS TO IMPROVE IMMUNE STATUS

Nursing interventions that can improve immune status in the older person include the following:

- Consider older people who are under substantial stress at high risk for conditions associated with a decreased immune status.
- Encourage laboratory testing for hormone levels associated with stress to identify older people at high risk.
- Assist people in identifying active, positive coping strategies, especially following stressful events.
- Educate the person, family, and friends about the effects of stress.
- Administer pneumococcal vaccine at or prior to the age of 65 with revaccination as recommended by the primary care provider.
- Stress the importance of obtaining yearly influenza immunizations.
- Encourage daily vitamin and mineral supplements.
- Encourage all older persons to develop an exercise plan appropriate for their physical status.
- Encourage community senior centers to offer education about HIV infection.
- Screen for HIV infection in older people.
- Encourage older adults to seek advice from healthcare professionals when symptoms occur.

The nurse will often engage in teaching older patients and families about prevention of infectious disease like influenza. Refer to the following patient-family teaching guidelines.

Patient-Family Teaching Guidelines

PREVENTION OF INFLUENZA

The following are guidelines that the nurse may find useful when instructing older persons and their families about preventing the flu (adapted from NIH, 2000).

1. Can the flu be prevented?

A flu shot greatly reduces your chances of getting the flu. No vaccine is completely effective, but studies show that older people who get the flu shot are 70% less likely to be hospitalized and 85% less likely to die as a result of getting the flu.

    The flu is highly contagious and spreads easily from person to person. It is caused by viruses that infect the nose, throat, and lungs. When you are out in crowded places like church or the mall, try to avoid contact with people who are coughing and sneezing. Wash your hands often and do not put things found in public places in or near your mouth. The flu can be life threatening in an older person or a person with other chronic illness like diabetes or diseases of the kidneys, liver, heart, or lungs.

RATIONALE:

Administration of yearly influenza vaccine and avoiding contact with persons infected with the flu are effective preventive measures.

(continued)

Patient-Family Teaching Guidelines, *cont.*

2. Who should get a flu shot?

The Centers for Disease Control (a part of the federal government) recommends the following people receive flu shots each year because these persons are categorized as high risk for serious illness and complications from the flu:

- People over the age of 65
- Residents of nursing homes and other long-term care facilities where older persons live in close contact
- Adults with chronic heart or lung disease
- Adults with diabetes or with kidney, liver, heart, or lung disease
- Healthcare workers in contact with people in high-risk groups
- Caregivers or people who live with someone in a high-risk group

RATIONALE:

Persons in these high-risk groups are at risk for life-threatening complications from the flu, including hospitalization, development of pneumonia and sepsis, and death. Healthcare workers are less likely to develop a serious case of the flu but may inadvertently spread the flu virus from person to person by transmitting the virus carried in their noses and throats.

3. Will my insurance cover the cost of the shot?

The cost of the flu shot is covered by Medicare. Many private health insurance plans also pay for the flu shot. You can get a flu shot at your doctor's office or you may receive it from your local health department or at flu shot clinics sponsored by some drug or department stores.

RATIONALE:

It makes sense for insurance companies and Medicare to cover the cost of flu shots as they greatly reduce costs by preventing hospitalization, treatment of serious complications, and death.

4. When is the best time to get the flu shot?

In the United States, the flu season usually starts in December and ends in April. The best time to get the flu shot is between mid-September and mid-November. It takes about 1 to 2 weeks to develop immunity after you receive the flu shot.

RATIONALE:

Although the impact and start of the flu season vary from year to year, it is always best to plan ahead and make sure high-risk older patients are immunized by mid-November.

5. What about side effects of the flu shot?

The vaccine is made from killed flu viruses, so you cannot possibly get the flu. The vaccine is grown in eggs, so people who are severely allergic to eggs should not get the flu shot. Some people (fewer than one third who get the flu shot) report soreness, redness, or swelling in the arm where the flu shot was given. These side effects can last up to 2 days and usually are controlled with acetaminophen.

RATIONALE:

The danger of getting the flu is far greater than the danger of getting a flu shot. Reassurance and education can empower some older persons to request and receive the flu shot.

6. What are the symptoms of the flu?

Flu causes fever, chills, dry cough, sore throat, runny nose, headache, muscle ache, and fatigue. Usually symptoms are worse than symptoms of a cold or upper respiratory infection. If you get the flu, make sure to rest, drink plenty of fluids, and take acetaminophen to control aches and fever. Call your doctor or primary healthcare provider if:

- Your fever (usually over 100°F) lasts for more than a few days.
- You are diagnosed with heart, lung, liver, or kidney problems.
- You are taking drugs to fight off cancer or other drugs that weaken your body's immune response.
- You feel sick and do not seem to be getting better.

RATIONALE:

If serious side effects or complications of the flu develop, early treatment improves the chance of success.

Patient-Family Teaching Guidelines

- You have a cough with phlegm.
- You or someone caring for you is worried about your condition.

7. How is the flu treated?

Because the flu is caused by a virus, antibiotics (only effective against bacterial infections) are not an effective treatment. The four drugs approved to treat the flu include:

- Amantadine (Symmetrel)
- Rimantadine (Flumadine)
- Zanamivir (Relenza)
- Oseltamivir (Tamiflu)

These drugs must be taken within 48 hours of the onset of symptoms, so it is important to call your doctor or primary healthcare provider if you think you have the flu. These drugs shorten the duration of the illness and prevent complications like pneumonia. They are only available by prescription and are not right for everyone. Other drugs may be given to make you feel better, including cough medication and antibiotics should you develop a bacterial pneumonia as a complication of the flu.

RATIONALE:

Early treatment with an antiviral medication can ease the symptoms and prevent complications in high-risk persons. High-risk patients should contact their doctor quickly if symptoms of the flu are detected during flu season.

Care Plan

A Patient With Joint Pain from an Autoimmune Disease

Case Study

On the first home visit to Mrs. Ryan for a health assessment, the visiting nurse notes that the patient walks with difficulty and complains of pain in her knee joints. Mrs. Ryan is an 83-year-old woman who has enjoyed good health all her years. She has had rheumatoid arthritis for years and no other medical problems. She gets some pain relief from daily naproxen (Aleve) but does not ambulate much during the day, spending her time on the couch. She states, "I just don't like to move around much now. My darn knees hurt too much so I mostly sit here on my couch and rest." Family members shop for her and visit weekly, but the apartment seems dirty and disorganized and there is spoiled food in the refrigerator.

On examination, the nurse finds warm, swollen knees with little active range of motion (ROM). Passive ROM produces pain after 30 degrees flexion. Mrs. Ryan denies

(continued)

A Patient With Joint Pain from an Autoimmune Disease *(continued)*

weight loss, but her clothing fits her loosely, indicating she may have recently lost a significant amount of weight. She also has a bruise on her left hip that she cannot explain. The rest of the examination is negative.

Applying the Nursing Process

ASSESSMENT

The nurse should assess whether Mrs. Ryan has seen her healthcare provider for evaluation of her rheumatoid arthritis recently. The presence of warm swollen knees, weight loss, and bruising (from a possible fall) might indicate an exacerbation of this chronic illness. A complete functional assessment, dietary history, medication assessment, and safety inventory in the home are needed.

DIAGNOSIS

Current nursing diagnoses for Mrs. Ryan may include the following:

- *Chronic pain in knee joints* (related to progression of rheumatoid arthritis)
- *Limited ROM*
- *Altered activity level*
- *Risk for imbalanced nutrition: less than body requirements*
- *Constipation* (potentially as a result of immobility and dehydration)
- *Urinary incontinence* (potentially as a result of pain on movement)
- *Deficient fluid volume* (related to possible dehydration)
- *Risk for disuse syndrome* (related to immobility and pain on movement)
- *Social isolation*
- *Risk for loneliness*
- *Caregiver role strain*
- *Impaired walking*
- *Activity intolerance*
- *Adult failure to thrive*
- *Risk for falls*

PLANNING AND IMPLEMENTATION

Appropriate nursing interventions for Mrs. Ryan may include the following:

- Referral to members of the interdisciplinary team, including social worker, physical therapist, occupational therapist, nutritionist, and primary care provider
- Consultation with primary care provider about pain evaluation and possible referral to a rheumatologist
- Development of a home safety plan including improving fall risk and food safety measures
- Gaining additional services for Mrs. Ryan to ease caregiver strain, including meals-on-wheels and homemaker services
- Requesting a family meeting to clarify care issues, identify involved family members, and clarify end-of-life goals, values, and advance directives

A Patient With Joint Pain from an Autoimmune Disease

EXPECTED OUTCOMES

The expected outcomes for Mrs. Ryan may include the following:

- Mrs. Ryan's pain will be decreased with active and passive exercises, use of topical rubs, heating pads, and optimum doses of appropriate medications, including NSAIDs, methotrexate, sulfasalazine, corticosteroids, or other medications as recommended by the rheumatologist to prevent further joint destruction.
- Mrs. Ryan will maintain mobility, strengthen muscles, prevent deformity, and minimize the risk of falls and injury.
- Mrs. Ryan's home environment will be free of barriers to mobility, and she will begin appropriate use of mobility assistive devices, such as a cane or walker.
- Caregiver strain will be eased and family involvement improved.
- The healthcare team will arrange for ongoing support and evaluation of progress.

EVALUATION

The nurse hopes to work with Mrs. Ryan over time to provide support and improve overall health and function. The nurse will consider the plan a success based on the following criteria:

- Mrs. Ryan will agree to meet with a social worker to assess caregiver strain, the situation in the home, and the need for supportive services.
- A family meeting will be held to discuss Mrs. Ryan's overall health.
- Mrs. Ryan will arrange an appointment with her primary healthcare provider for further assessment and evaluation of her rheumatoid arthritis.
- She will improve her nutrition and establish and maintain a normal healthy weight.
- She will not exhibit further unexplained bruising and will remove safety hazards from her home.
- Advance directives will be established with healthcare goals and appropriate levels of treatment specified.

Ethical Dilemma

The visiting nurse requested permission from Mrs. Ryan to contact her son and daughter-in-law who live in a nearby town and visit her on weekends. She granted permission, but warned: "My son and his wife are fed up with me. I'm afraid to be a burden on them and I never ask them for anything. I'm afraid they'll put me in a nursing home and I could never stand that." When the nurse reached Mrs. Ryan's son at work, he agreed to a family meeting but said, "I can't schedule a long meeting. I'm busy at work and Mom is requiring more and more help. I want her to be safe, but I can't do any more for her. Let's just pursue nursing home placement. Is this meeting really necessary?" The nurse responded that it was necessary and the meeting would last one hour or less. The ethical dilemma for Mrs. Ryan and her family involved patient autonomy and self-determination (her wish to remain home and endure the risk) versus her family's wish for nursing home placement and safety (beneficence). At first, the family was reluctant to become involved, but during the family meeting at which the social worker was present, they learned the plan of care

(continued)

A Patient With Joint Pain from an Autoimmune Disease *(continued)*

for improvement of home safety and nutritional status. Once the visiting nurse had completed the visits, the family was able to continue support of Mrs. Ryan, encouraging her to prevent deformity, increase muscle strength, and improve her range of motion. Taking a regular dose of pain medication (acetaminophen) and using a topical pain-relieving rub twice daily controlled her pain, allowing her to become more active in the home.

Critical Thinking and the Nursing Process

1. Why is the treatment of rheumatoid arthritis more complicated in the older person?
2. When teaching an older person about HIV prevention and safe sex practices, what information would you include?
3. What factors place older people at risk for developing nosocomial infections in hospitals and long-term care facilities?
4. Identify behaviors you have observed during your clinical experiences that place older persons at risk for the development of nosocomial infections.

■ Evaluate your responses in Appendix B. ⊂▣⊃

EXPLORE MediaLink

NCLEX review, case studies, and other interactive resources for this chapter can be found on the Companion Website at **http://www.prenhall.com/tabloski**. Click on Chapter 23 to select the activities for this chapter. For animations, video tutorials, more NCLEX review questions, and case studies, access the accompanying CD-ROM in this textbook.

Chapter Highlights

- The three major biological defense mechanisms are:
  - Anatomical and biochemical barrier of skin and mucous membranes
  - Mechanical clearance
  - Immune response
- Self-recognition, specificity, and memory are the three characteristics that are unique to the immune system.
- Immunity can be natural or acquired. Acquired immunity can be either active or passive.
- Lymphocytes are the white blood cells primarily concerned with immunity.
- The humoral immune response is initiated when an antigen binds with antibody receptors on the surface of mature B cells. This results in production of plasma cells that secrete one of five types of antibodies.

- The first exposure to foreign antigen results in production of antibodies in about 5 days. With a second exposure, there is a more rapid production of large amounts of antibodies.

- The cell-mediated immune response is characterized by the entire T cell binding to the foreign antigen in multiple areas on the surface of the cell.

- Immune changes with aging result in a decrease in functioning of both B cells and T cells. The primary deficit is in the proliferation of T cells in the body.

- Stress, comorbidity, exercise, and nutrition all affect immune system function.

- Hypersensitivity and autoimmunity are overreactions or abnormal reactions of the immune system. Rheumatoid disorders are autoimmune reactions.

- Deficient immune responses occur when there is a functional decrease in one or more components of the immune system. Susceptibility to infections is common. HIV is a primary immunodeficiency disease.

- Secondary immune deficiencies include physical, nutritional, environmental, psychosocial, and pharmacological factors.

- Pneumonia, urinary tract infections, bacteremia, tuberculosis, and skin infections are common in the older person.

- A variety of nursing interventions can improve immune status. Relieving stress, encouraging positive coping strategies, exercise, diet supplements, immunizations, and HIV teaching and screening are a few.

References

Burleson, M. H., Poehlmann, K. M., Hawkley, L. C., Ernst, J.M., Berntson, G. G., Malarkey, W. B., et al. (2002). Stress-related immune changes in middle-aged and older women: 1-year consistency of individual differences. *Health Psychology, 21*(4), 321–331.

Buttaro, T. M., Trybulski, J., Bailey, P. P., & Sandberg-Cook, H. (2003). *Primary care: A collaborative practice* (2nd ed.). St. Louis, MO: Mosby.

Buzina, S. K., Buzina, R., Stavijenic, A., Grgic, Z., Jusic, M., Sapunar, J., et al. (1998). Ageing, nutritional status and immune response. *International Journal of Vitamin and Nutritional Research, 68* (36), 133–141.

Chan, E. D., & Fernandez, E. (2001). The challenge of pneumonia in the elderly: Part I. *Journal of Respiratory Diseases, 22*(3), 139–148.

Chandra, R. K. (1997). Graying of the immune system: Can nutrient supplements improve immunity in the elderly? *Journal of the American Medical Association, 277*(17), 1398–1399.

Chen, H. X., Ryan, P. A., & Ferguson, R. P. (1998). Characteristics of acquired immunodeficiency syndrome in older adults. *Journal of the American Geriatrics Society, 46*(2), 153–156.

Chin, A., Paw, M. J. M., DeJong, N., Pallast, E. G. M., Kloek, G. C., Schouten, E. G., & Kok, F. J. (2000). Immunity in frail elderly: A randomized controlled trial of exercise and enriched foods. *Medicine & Science in Sports & Exercise, 32*(12), 2005–2011.

Copstead, L. C., & Banasik, J. L. (2000). *Pathophysiology, biological and behavioral perspectives* (2nd ed., pp. 184–218). Philadelphia: Saunders.

Digiovanna, A. G. (2000). *Human aging, Biological perspectives* (2nd ed., pp. 46–47, 312–326). New York: McGraw-Hill.

Fune, L., Shua-Haim, J. R., Ross, J. S., & Frank, E. (1998). Infectious diseases in the elderly. *Clinical Geriatrics, 6*(3), 31–50.

Girodon, F., Galan, P., Monget, A. L., Boutron-Ruault, M., Brunet-Lecomte, P., Preziosi, P., et al. (1999). Impact of trace elements and vitamin supplementation on immunity and infections in institutionalized elderly patients: A randomized controlled trial. Geriatric network. *Archives of Internal Medicine, 159*(7), 748–754.

Girodon, F., Lonbard, M., & Galan, P. (1997). Effect of micronutrient supplementation on infection in institutionalized elderly subjects: A controlled trial. *Annals of Nutrition and Metabolism, 41*(2), 98–107.

Hartford Institute for Geriatric Nursing, Division of Nursing, New York University. (2004). *Immunizations for the older adult, 21,* Fall. Retrieved August 14, 2004, from www.hartfordign.org.

Huether, S.E., & McCance, K. L. (2001). *Understanding pathophysiology* (2nd ed., pp. 125–150). St. Louis, MO: Mosby.

High, K. P. (2001). Nutritional strategies to boost immunity and prevent infection in elderly individuals. *Clinical Infectious Diseases, 33*(11), 1892–1900.

Huss, K., Naumann, R. L., Mason, P. L. J., Nanda, J. R., Huss, R. W., Smith, C. M., & Hamilton, R. G. (2001). Asthma severity, atopic status, allergen exposure, and quality of life in elderly persons. *Annals of Allergy & Asthma Immunology, 86*(5), 524–530.

Kiecolt-Glaser, J. K., Glaser, R., Gravenstein, S., Malarkey, W. B., & Sheridan, J. (1996). Chronic stress alters the immune response to influenza virus vaccine in older adults. *Proceedings of the National Academy of Sciences, 93,* 3043–3047.

Klein, S. J., Nokes, K. M., Devore, B. S., Holmes, J. M., Wheeler, D. P., & St. Hilaire, M. B. (2001). Age appropriate HIV prevention messages for older adults: Findings from focus groups in New York State. *Journal of Public Health Management Practice, 7*(3), 11–18.

Li, J. X., Hong, Y., & Chan, K. M. (2001). Tai chi: Physiological characteristics and beneficial effects on health. *British Journal of Sports Medicine, 35*(3), 148–156.

Lupus Foundation of America. (2001). *Late onset lupus fact sheet.* Retrieved December 20, 2004, from www.lupus.org/education/lateonset.html.

Manfredi, R. (2002). HIV disease and advanced age: An increasing therapeutic challenge. *Drugs Aging, 19*(9), 647–669.

Marcus, M. B. (2002). Aging of AIDS. *U.S. News and World Report, 133*(6), 40.

McClain, C. J., McClain, M. S., Barve, S., & Boosalis, M .G. (2002). Trace metals and the elderly. *Clinical Geriatric Medicine, 18*(4), 801–818.

McEwen, B. S. (1998). Protective and damaging effects of stress mediators. *New England Journal of Medicine, 338*(30), 171–179.

National Institute of Allergy and Infectious Diseases and National Cancer Institute. (2003). *Understanding the immune system: How it works* (NIH Publication No. 03-5423). Washington, DC: U.S. Department of Health and Human Services.

National Institute of Health (2000) Age Page: What to do about flu. http//www.NIApublications. org. downloaded 8/14/2002.

Reuben, D., Herr, K., Pacala, J., Pollock, B., Potter, J., & Semla, T. (2004). *Geriatrics at your fingertips.* Malden, MA: American Geriatrics Society, Blackwell.

Smeltzer, S. C., & Bare, B. B. (2004). *Brunner & Suddarth's textbook of medical-surgical nursing* (10th ed., p. 1340). Philadelphia: Lippincott.

Stowell, J. R., Kiecolt-Glaser, J. K., & Glaser, R. (2001). Perceived stress and cellular immunity: When coping counts. *Journal of Behavioral Medicine, 24*(4), 323–339.

Szirony, T. A. (1999). Infection with HIV in the elderly population. *Journal of Gerontological Nursing, 25*(10), 25–31.

Tricerri, A., Guidi, L., Frasca, D., Costanzo, M., Errani, A., Riccioni, M., et al. (1999). Characteristics of gastric-vein lymphocytes with regard to the immune response to *Helicobacter pylori. Scandinavian Journal of Gastroenterology, 34*(8), 757–764.

U.S. National Library of Medicine and National Institutes of Health. (2002). *Aging changes and immunity.* Retrieved December 20, 2004, from www.nlm.nih.gov/medlineplus/ency/article/004008.htm.

Wellons, M. F., Sanders, L., Edwards, L. J., Bartlett, J. A., Heald, A. E., & Schmader, K. E. (2002). HIV infection: Treatment outcomes in older and younger adults. *Journal of the American Geriatrics Society, 50*(4), 603–607.

CHAPTER 24

Multisystem Problems: Caring for Frail Elders With Comorbidities

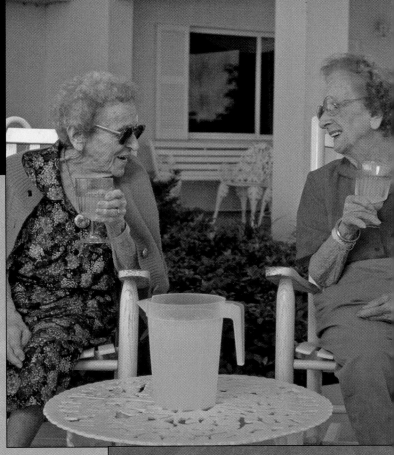

CHAPTER OBJECTIVES

Upon completion of this chapter, the reader will be able to:

- Describe age-related changes that affect overall health and function and that contribute to frailty.

- Describe the impact of age-related changes, including organ function and presence of comorbidities.

- Identify risk factors of health for the older person at risk for acute care hospitalization.

- Describe causes and unique presentation of frailty in the older person.

- Define appropriate nursing interventions directed toward assisting older adults with frailty to regain baseline function.

- Identify and implement appropriate nursing interventions to care for the older person with multisystem problems.

KEY TERMS

adverse drug events 803
confusion 795
frail 788
futile therapy 807
geriatric cascade 788
iatrogenesis 792

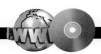

MediaLink

Additional resources for this chapter can be found on the Student CD-ROM accompanying this textbook and on the Companion Website at **www.prenhall.com/tabloski**. Click on Chapter 24 to select the activities for this chapter.

CD-ROM
- NCLEX Review
- Case Studies
- Tools

Companion Website
- Audio Glossary
- Additional NCLEX Review
- Case Study
- MediaLink Applications

Comprehensive nursing care of the older adult is incomplete unless the perspective of the entire person is considered. This book focuses on the nursing interventions appropriate for each body system in isolation from other systems. However, gerontological nurses often care for older people who have multisystem problems or comorbidities. The purpose of this chapter is to describe special needs of frail older persons with multiple comorbidities, the risk factors associated with functional decline, problems encountered during hospitalization, and methods to avoid these problems and improve care. The medical comorbidities complicate the nursing assessment and treatment of medical conditions and place the frail older person at risk for poor outcomes because of the atypical presentation of disease, delays in the initiation of treatment, need for multiple pharmacological interventions, and diminished organ reserve capacity that inhibits the physiological and psychological responses to stressors. Often, the term **frail** is used to describe an older person with diagnosed chronic illness, loss of organ function, diagnosis of recurrent acute illness, and social risk factors such as poverty, social isolation, and functional or cognitive decline. A frail older person exhibits dependence in one or more activities of daily living and is diagnosed with three or more comorbid conditions and one or more geriatric syndromes (including dementia, delirium, depression, incontinence, falls, osteoporosis, gait disturbance, or pressure ulcers) (Lichtman, 2003). Frailty has also been defined as the presence of three or more of the following criteria:

- Unplanned weight loss (10 lb in the last year)
- Weakness
- Poor endurance and energy
- Slowness
- Low activity

(Young, 2003)

Frailty is an important concept for gerontological nurses and other healthcare providers caring for older people because:

- The frail older adult is the largest consumer of healthcare, community services, and long-term care.
- The number of older persons over the age of 85 is increasing rapidly in the United States, and the prevalence of frailty increases dramatically with age.
- Nurses and other healthcare professionals are interested in identifying frail older persons to initiate specialized geriatric services to meet their needs, including geriatric assessment, multidisciplinary care, and specialized geriatric services (Fried et al., 2001).

Risks of Frailty

A frail older person is at high risk for dependency, institutionalization, falls, injuries, hospitalization, slow recovery from illness, and mortality. The frail older adult is most in need of and most likely to benefit from specialized geriatric services (Fried, 1994; Fried et al., 2001). The very old (85+), those with physical frailty and cognitive impairment, and those dependent on formal and informal supports to maintain health, function, and autonomy are most at risk for decline. Often the frail older person will suffer a rapid decline and decompensation as a result of acute illness or worsening of a chronic condition. This phenomenon of decline has been termed the **geriatric cascade** and results from the interaction of the frail older person, acute illness, and the stress of institutional care (Fretwell, 1998). Frailty independently predicts poor health outcomes, with frail older people having a sixfold higher mortality rate (18%) over a 7-year period (Fried et al., 2001). Intensive, individualized nursing interventions must be instituted immediately when a frail older person is institutionalized with an acute illness or exacerbation of a chronic illness to prevent the geriatric cascade and return the older person to levels of baseline function.

The Paths to Frailty

It has been hypothesized (Albert, Im, & Raveis, 2002) that older persons can become frail by one or more of three pathways:

- Changes of aging and loss of organ reserve and function in the very old
- Diagnosis with several chronic illnesses, each of which alone and in combination with others can cause harmful effects on overall physiological function
- Existence in harmful social and psychological environments

Figure 24-1 ■ illustrates the interrelationship between the causes of frailty.

In this model of frailty, each of the factors not only directly influences the onset and severity of frailty, but also influences all other factors in the model. For instance, the diagnosis of diabetes mellitus is known to accelerate systemic aging. Older patients with diabetes are more at risk for heart disease, stroke, and micro- and macrovascular decline, thus illustrating the interrelationship between chronic illness and physiological changes of aging. Age also directly affects the prognosis when an acute or chronic illness is diagnosed. For instance, older people are more at risk for death and adverse outcomes when they are diagnosed with influenza or pneumonia. These very old patients (85+) are more likely to die and suffer morbid events, especially during acute care hospitalization. Table 24-1 describes the age-related changes and loss of organ reserve that can contribute to the onset of frailty in the older adult.

Many of these changes are not disease specific. It may be that a critical mass of physiological changes leads to frailty rather than any one change (Fried, 1994; Fried et al., 2001). Individuals age at different rates and have varying degrees of compensatory abilities to overcome these age-related declines. Further, aging is affected by genetics, lifestyle, diet, physical activity, and comorbid conditions. In general, physiological aging causes a linear decline in the homeostatic reserve of organ systems (Bailes, 2000).

FIGURE ■ **24-1**

Causes of frailty.

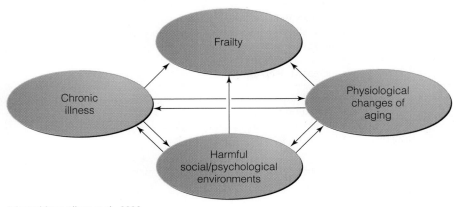

Adapted from Albert et al., 2002.

TABLE 24-1

Physiological Changes of Aging and Contribution to Frailty

Age-Related Change	Contribution to Frailty
Integumentary System • Thinning of the dermis • Decrease in eccrine and apocrine glands • Loss of subcutaneous fat • Decrease in collagen	Potential for: • Skin tears, bruising, laceration, injury, and infection • Hypo/hyperthermia • Decubitus ulcers • Decreased wound healing
Musculoskeletal System • Decreased bone density • Reduction in muscle mass/strength • Decreased range of motion in joints	Potential for: • Falls • Injury from falls • Gait disorders • Hazards from immobility • Deconditioning
Neurologic System • Increases in reaction time • Slowing of coordinated movements • Deterioration of balance mechanisms • Decreased sense of vibration, proprioception • Decreased sensation (touch, taste, hearing, vision) • Diminished deep sleep	Potential for: • Falls • Generalized confusion during illness • Increased time for learning/adapting to new situations and circumstances • Inability to protect self from injury • Increased susceptibility to medications • Weight changes due to changes in taste and appetite
Cardiovascular System • Decreased arterial compliance • Deterioration of baroreceptor response • Impaired diastolic filling • Degeneration of conduction tissue • Absence of ischemic pain accompanying myocardial infarction	Potential for: • Increased risk of conduction disturbances, tachyarrhythmias • Increased risk of hypotension with dehydration • Decreased heart rate in response to stress • Increased risk of postural hypotension • Increased risk of systolic hypertension and ventricular hypertrophy
Immune System • Decreases in immune response	Potential for: • Atypical presentation of disease • Delayed or incomplete healing • Infections resulting from more serious pathogens • Increased susceptibility to infectious disease • Increases in rate of cancer and autoimmune diseases
Respiratory System • Decreased oxygenation of tissues • Decreased lung capacity • Decreased pulmonary function	Potential for: • Respiratory failure under anesthesia • Respiratory depression in response to drugs • Increased risk for aspiration and infection • Decreased cough reflex • Increased sleep apnea
Renal System • Decreased renal function • Decrease in number of nephrons • Decreased glomerular filtration rate and creatinine production	Potential for: • Toxic drug reactions • Increased renal thresholds for glucose, electrolytes • Overhydration or dehydration

TABLE 24-1 *(continued)*

Physiological Changes of Aging and Contribution to Frailty

Age-Related Change	Contribution to Frailty
Gastrointestinal System • Decreased blood supply to intestines • Decrease in liver function • Delayed gastric motility and emptying • Decreased gastric acid production	Potential for: • Toxic drug reactions • Digestive disorders/malabsorption syndrome • Dysphagia • Gastrointestinal bleeding • Gastroesophageal reflux disease, gastric and peptic ulceration • Diarrhea/constipation • Fecal incontinence
Endocrine • Decreased/increased secretion and action of insulin • Changes in secretion and action of thyroid hormone	Potential for: • Hypo/hyperglycemia • Hypo/hyperthyroidism
Hematopoietic • Decline in active bone marrow • Decreased number of red blood cells • Reduced ability to accelerate red blood cell production	Potential for: • Anemia • Decline in phagocytosis and ability to fight pathogens

Source: Adapted from Bailes, 2000; Fried et al., 2001.

While organ function may remain within normal limits and homeostatic mechanisms remain intact in many older persons, under periods of stress (including acute illness or exacerbation of chronic illness) the older body is less able to compensate because of declines in physiological function and reserve.

It is hypothesized that several additional factors may affect the care of the frail older person, including decline in organ function that often prohibits aggressive treatment of illness, patient and family preference, pre-existing diagnosis of other diseases that already have a negative impact on quality of life, and ageism in the healthcare system with older people seen as less desirable candidates for aggressive interventions (Rosenthal, Kaboli, Barnett, & Sirio, 2002). The inevitable outcome is that older patients may not be offered or receive the same curative treatments as middle-aged or young patients, thus contributing to the higher mortality and morbidity rates based on age alone. Because of the variability in aging and uniqueness of each person's compensatory ability, chronological age should never serve as a sole marker for making treatment decisions. Given the varying rates of aging between individuals and the heterogeneity of the aging process, a particular older patient may have many, some, or no age-related problems or comorbidities (National Institute on Aging & National Cancer Institute, 2004). Fundamental mechanisms of the body decline progressively at different rates with age, giving way to a gradual incapacity for maintenance and repair. Older adults without adequate social support or financial resources, or who have depression, cognitive impairment, or progressive apathy will progress on a path of functional decline that may be irreversible and lead to death in some cases even though they appear to be physiologically fit (Robertson & Montagnini, 2004). Optimum care is achieved by an overall understanding of the older patient's current health problems, past health history, baseline levels of physical and cognitive function, financial and family support systems, and expectations and goals of care.

SOCIAL AND PSYCHOLOGICAL ENVIRONMENTS AS CONTRIBUTORS TO FRAILTY

Poverty, social isolation, depression, and cognitive impairment can undermine access to adequate healthcare, assistive technologies, motivation for self-care, and environmental modifications designed to encourage and maintain functional independence. Harmful social and psychological environments can directly influence frailty and compound the effects of chronic illness and physiological changes of aging, thus completing the model of interdependency of factors (Albert et al., 2002).

Common Diagnoses Associated With Frailty in the Older Adult

Chronic conditions and diseases such as diabetes, cardiovascular diseases, osteoporosis, and arthritis are major causes of frailty and disability in late life. Risks for disease and frailty increase with age and can be exacerbated by poor lifestyle choices and poverty (National Institute on Aging, 2005). Table 24-2 depicts common diagnoses and the mechanism by which each contributes to frailty in an older person.

CUMULATIVE EFFECT OF COMORBIDITIES

Often a frail older person will be diagnosed with several underlying chronic conditions and develop an acute condition that disrupts the stability of the chronic conditions. For instance, a person with a mild cognitive impairment might develop a urinary tract infection and might become more confused as a result of the infection. This confusion may limit the older person's ability to recognize or communicate the urinary symptoms. As a result, the urinary tract infection may go undiagnosed or untreated, leading to sepsis or pyelonephritis. Other common atypical presentations of illness in frail older persons include falls, loss of appetite, delirium, dehydration, atypical pain, dizziness, incontinence, sleep disturbances, and failures of self-care (Amella, 2004). (See Chapter 2 for information on atypical presentation of disease in the older person. ⊂⊃) Often, treatment is delayed because nurses and other healthcare providers do not recognize the importance of subtle changes in the frail older person's function. This delay in treatment can make the acute illness more difficult to treat.

> **Practice Pearl**
>
> Older persons with cognitive impairment cannot adequately report symptoms of acute or chronic illness. Careful assessment of changes from baseline function, vital signs, and information from reliable caregivers is crucial.

The frail older person is more at risk for poor treatment outcomes and even death because of the interaction between normal changes of aging and common illnesses associated with age (Rosenthal et al., 2002). Comorbidity and functional status are important factors in determining medical therapy and nursing interventions. Careful monitoring of the patient's status and effectiveness of the overall plan of care is indicated because frail older persons with poor function are at increased risk of toxicity from multiple medications, **iatrogenesis** or adverse outcomes of therapeutic inter-

TABLE 24-2

Common Diagnoses and Contribution to Frailty

Diagnosis	Contribution to Frailty
Asthma	Toxicity of treatment, especially chronic steroid use contributing to risk of osteoporosis, elevated blood glucose levels, decreased immune response, increased risk of pulmonary infection, and decreased activity levels. Inability to engage in aerobic exercise and meet oxygen demands.
Cancer	Toxicity of treatment, anorexia, pain, systemic and metastatic nature of the disease.
Chronic obstructive pulmonary disease/emphysema	Decreased levels of blood oxygenation, chronic acute lung infections and need for antibiotic treatment, chronic fatigue and decreased activity levels.
Chronic renal failure	Potential for drug toxicity, fluid overload, dependency edema, pleural effusion, electrolyte and metabolic abnormalities.
Chronic liver disease	Potential for drug toxicity, metabolic and digestive abnormalities.
Cognitive and mood disorders	Inability to engage in self-care activities, lack of motivation for rehabilitation, toxic side effects of medications, including tardive dyskinesia and movement disorders associated with use of psychotropic medications.
Diabetes	Malabsorption, metabolic disorders, end organ damage, decreased immune response, use of multiple medications, increased risk of cardiovascular disease, potential for hyper/hypoglycemia, and exercise intolerance.
Bone fractures	Pain, toxic effects of pain medication, decreased mobility with associated risks, functional impairment, risks of surgery for open reduction, risks of hospitalization with eventual placement in long-term care facility.
Inflammatory bowel disease	Malabsorption; nutritional deficiencies; risk for dehydration; potential toxic effects of medications, including antidiarrheals, steroids, and antibiotics; risk for bowel obstruction, surgery, and hospitalization.
Cardiovascular disease	Potential for treatment with many medications, including antihypertensives, cholesterol-lowering agents, diuretics, and others with risk for dehydration, metabolic and electrolyte imbalance, and other systemic adverse effects; potential for fatigue and activity intolerance.
Musculoskeletal disease	Pain and potential toxic effects of pain medications, including gastrointestinal bleeding, lethargy, liver failure, and renal impairment; functional impairment, decreased mobility, and associated risks; risks of chronic inflammation and medications associated with treatment; risk of injury, surgery, and treatment.

Source: Data from Robertson & Montagnini, 2004; National Institute on Aging, 2005; Saltvedt et al., 2002.

ventions, and poor treatment outcomes when receiving nursing and medical treatment for acute illness. To meet the special needs of older patients during hospitalization, every effort should be made to correctly diagnose all vague symptoms and problems; treat all relevant diseases; assess the effect of current changes in the older person's health status, including the effect of the acute illness on other diagnosed chronic illnesses; and prevent complications of hospitalization (nosocomial infections, falls, delirium, polypharmacy, nutritional deficiencies) (Saltvedt, Mo, Fayers, Kaasa, & Sletvold, 2002).

PATHWAYS TO FRAILTY

Fried and colleagues (2001) studied frail older adults and showed linkages between disease states and the mechanisms that lead to those states, or causal pathways. One thread followed nutritional deficiencies that can reduce vision, leading to falls and serious

FIGURE ■ 24-2

Fried's Scientific
Explanation of the Cycle
of Frailty.

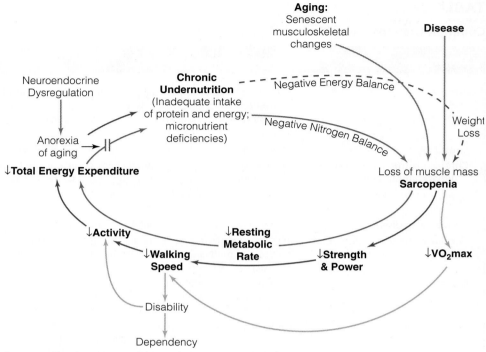

Source: Fried et al., 2001.

injury. Another looked at how disease combinations like arthritis and visual impairment, heart disease and arthritis, or stroke and high blood pressure may magnify each other's symptoms and hasten the onset of dependency. These factors combined with weight loss, loss of muscle mass, and decreased strength and energy can all lead to inactivity, decreased total energy expenditure, anorexia, and neuroendocrine dysregulation that contributes to undernutrition and negative energy balance. This vicious cycle will eventually produce frailty in the older adult (Figure 24-2 ■).

According to Young (2003, p. 2), "Functional status varies considerably among older adults, with a substantial portion remaining independent in daily function throughout their lives and continuing to volunteer or work, the majority needing some assistance with instrumental activities after the age of 85, and a portion of frail elderly who are disabled." Many older people who have chronic conditions and disabilities are not frail and lead active, productive lives. However, some meet the description of frailty and are more disabled, requiring assistance with activities of daily living. Approximately 41 million older Americans with chronic conditions require assistance daily. In general, older people with lower incomes are more likely to have conditions that are more difficult or costly to treat. African Americans are more likely than Caucasians to have limitations in activities of daily living when chronically ill. Older African American men and women with arthritis are more likely to have activity limitations than other older people (National Academy on an Aging Society, 1999). Nearly 60% of older African Americans report high blood pressure, and a growing number of older African Americans and Hispanics are reporting diabetes. "An image emerges of a subgroup of older adults whose health is marginal and whose lives are in delicate balance" (Young, 2003, p. 3). Frail older adults are at risk for any number of adverse events that can be caused by a variety of stressors, some seemingly benign. For instance, an upper respiratory infection that may cause only minor inconvenience to a middle-aged or young adult may cause delirium, falls, **confusion**, dehydration, incontinence, and institutionalization in the frail older adult. Capacity to fight disease and achieve full recovery may be more difficult in frail older adults.

While the number of Americans with chronic conditions is expected to increase significantly over the next several years and the prevalence of chronic conditions is also increasing, there is a simultaneous decline in the functional limitations associated with these chronic conditions. It is possible that chronic conditions are being more widely diagnosed and treated, thereby reducing their ability to cause functional limitations. Noninvasive or minimally invasive testing and screening procedures are leading to earlier diagnosis of osteoporosis, heart disease, vascular problems, cancer, and other disabling illnesses. Prescription drugs and technologies in development have the potential to contribute further to these trends (Bishop, 2003).

Some older adults with chronic conditions remain active and independent whereas others decline into frailty and dependence (Bennett & Flaherty-Robb, 2003). Several factors can affect the chronic illness trajectory:

- Some conditions are more disabling than others. For instance, a cognitive impairment may have a greater impact upon an older person's function than does osteoarthritis.
- Many chronic conditions, such as osteoporosis and hypertension, are controllable with medications. Disabling effects and progression of symptoms may be controlled or halted.
- Many older adults have health insurance, prescription drug coverage, access to healthcare, social support, and adequate financial resources to manage their chronic conditions while maintaining functional ability.

(Bennett & Flaherty-Robb, 2003; Bishop, 2003)

TRAJECTORIES OF FUNCTIONAL DECLINE

Lunney, Lynn, Foley, Lipson, and Guralnik (2003) studied over 14,000 older adults from four regions of the United States to observe and document various patterns of functional decline. Frail older adults and individuals at the end of life exhibit four distinct trajectories of functional decline:

1. **Sudden death.** Physical function is optimal and a massive unpredictable event such as accident or trauma, heart attack, or stroke occurs suddenly, resulting in immediate death. Approximately 16% of study participants experienced sudden death.
2. **Diagnosis with a terminal illness.** Physical function is optimal and a terminal illness such as cancer is diagnosed with gradual, progressive, linear decline over a short and predictable period of time. Twenty-one percent of study participants experienced death from a terminal illness.
3. **Organ failure.** Physical function gradually declines with entry and re-entry into the healthcare system with periods of return home between hospital stays, resulting in a downhill trajectory with periods of plateau. Twenty percent experienced death from organ failure.
4. **Frailty.** Lingering, expected deaths occur with a long, gradual downhill progression of already diminished physical function. Twenty percent experienced death with a frailty trajectory.

(Glaser & Strauss, 1968; Lunney et al., 2003)

Patients who die suddenly will not need health services, but it is likely that their survivors and loved ones will need supportive bereavement services. The majority of older Americans will experience one of the other end-of-life trajectories and will require varying clinical approaches with differing types of health services. The patients who are diagnosed with terminal illness and who endure short-term expected death with a predictable loss of function are the only group of patients who are likely to meet the requirements for hospice care and thus access supportive services. Those who experience entry and re-entry trajectories and frailty are likely to require, but may not have access to, supportive services because of steadily diminishing reserve capacity to cope with inevitable but unpredictable acute health challenges (Lunney et al., 2003).

FRAILTY AND EMOTIONAL HEALTH

Chronic conditions and frailty also negatively affect emotional health. New-onset depression is frequent in older patients with significant chronic illnesses. The negative impact of these illnesses on function is increased by the presence of depression (Robertson & Montagnini, 2004). Women with chronic conditions are more likely to rate their health as poor, and older African American women provide the least positive assessment of their emotional well-being (National Academy on an Aging Society, 1999). With the cost of healthcare rising each year, the United States already faces the challenge of providing appropriate and accessible healthcare to all persons. It is important to consider not only how to achieve this goal, but also how to recognize that different groups of older and chronically ill persons have different healthcare needs. The focus of healthcare for the frail older person will move beyond the medical model to include how to mobilize necessities for daily care, including medications, provision of nutritious meals, transportation to healthcare appointments, and home maintenance and safety (Young, 2003).

Americans can improve their chances for a healthy old age by simply taking advantage of recommended preventive health services and by making healthy lifestyle changes. About 70% of the physical decline that occurs with aging is related to modifiable factors such as smoking, poor nutrition, physical inactivity, and failure to use preventive and screening services (National Center for Chronic Disease Prevention and Health Promotion, 1999). The challenge for healthcare professionals is to encourage people at all stages of life to reduce their chances of disability and chronic illness by undertaking healthy lifestyle changes. This strategy will increase the number of healthy years an older person is expected to live. Improvements in lifestyle choices may lead to future declines in disability rates (Bishop, 2003).

FRAILTY, COMORBIDITIES, AND FUNCTIONAL STATUS

Chronic diseases like diabetes, cardiovascular disease, osteoporosis, and arthritis are major causes of frailty and disability in late life (National Institute on Aging, 2005). The established goal of the National Institute on Aging is to "add life to years" and to educate professionals and support research that establishes specific, practical ways to reduce disability and promote functional independence in later life. Risks for chronic illness and disability increase with age, and the onset of symptoms can be accelerated by lifestyle choices and other behavioral and social factors.

Many older people who have chronic conditions and disabilities lead active, productive lives, but some are more disabled and require assistance with activities of daily living. About 41 million Americans with chronic conditions require daily assistance. Heart failure, cancer, and Alzheimer's disease represent a significant burden of care.

Nurses often provide care to older persons in a variety of settings with these diagnoses. It is difficult for older patients and their families to receive specialty care without giving up accountability for comprehensive care (Kagan, 2004). The growing number of older people with longer survival times with multiple chronic diseases illustrates the need to have expert nurses educated regarding issues of holistic geriatric care. This shifting epidemiology will dramatically alter the nature of care as these patients will increasingly require specialized physical and behavioral treatment across community and institutional settings. Finely tuned therapies, sophisticated levels of interdisciplinary care, and careful coordination characterize the healthcare that will be provided to persons with heart failure, cancer, and Alzheimer's disease as well as other chronic illnesses (Kagan, 2004).

Cancer

Increasing age is directly associated with increasing rates of cancer, corresponding to an 11-fold increased incidence in persons over the age of 65. Despite these statistics, very few older persons enter into chemotherapy clinical trials. Limited information is available regarding the efficacy of various treatments such as surgery, chemotherapy, and radiation in this age group. The course of cancer treatment has shifted from relatively high mortality risks to patterns of chronic remission and recurrence in many of the most common malignancies, particularly solid tumors, with the advent of therapies that use multiple treatment modalities and collaborative care (Kagan, 2004). Chronological age does not always predict the physical response of the individual to cancer treatment, but rather the presence of comorbidities. Very old and frail patients often cannot tolerate aggressive chemotherapy, and less aggressive treatment regimens should be instituted. For those highly functional older persons with potential life expectancy exceeding predicted survival time, aggressive treatment should be offered (Lichtman, 2003).

Signs and symptoms of frailty in a person with cancer include cachexia or wasting syndrome, functional and cognitive decline, serum albumin less than 2.5 g/100 dl, recurrent diagnoses with secondary infections (pneumonia, skin infections, urinary tract infection), and unremitting pain.

Cardiovascular Disease

Cardiovascular disease is the most common cause of hospitalization and death in the older population. The underlying cause is most often coronary atherosclerosis, which occurs not only as a result of aging processes but also from the cumulative effect of poor personal health habits such as smoking, obesity, sedentary lifestyle, and poorly controlled hypertension (McCance & Huether, 2001). Separating the effects of aging from the effects of pathology is difficult and requires more ongoing study.

In the past, heart disease was thought to be a male problem. Healthcare providers are just beginning to understand that heart disease greatly affects older women, who comprise the majority of older people. One in nine women between the ages of 45 and 64 has some form of cardiovascular disease, ranging from coronary artery disease to stroke or renal vascular disease. By the time a woman reaches 65, she has a one in three chance of developing cardiovascular disease. A number of studies show that African American women are at even greater risk than these averages.

- One third of all deaths of American women each year are attributable to heart disease. Heart disease kills more women each year than cancer, accidents, and diabetes combined.

- All forms of cardiovascular disease kill nearly 500,000 American women a year. Stroke alone kills 88,000.
- Myocardial infarction, commonly known as a heart attack, kills 244,000 women a year.
- Forty percent of women with heart disease will eventually die of it.

(HealthSquare, 2004)

Men are much more likely to be stricken with heart disease in their prime middle years, whereas women tend to get it 10 to 20 years later. For most women, it is only after menopause that heart disease becomes a problem. A woman of 60 is about as likely to get heart disease as a man of 50. By the time they are in their 70s, men and women get heart disease at equal rates. Statistics reflect an encouraging trend. Better understanding of preventive measures and increasing sophistication in diagnosis and treatment have resulted in decreasing rates of heart disease in both men and women. In the 1980s, death rates from heart disease went down 27% for White women and 22% for African American women (HealthSquare, 2004).

A new emphasis on prevention and treatment of heart disease includes lower blood pressure goals and guidelines including lower levels for those with diabetes (see Chapter 19 ⊂▭⊃), new guidelines for lowering lipid levels, a greater understanding of the role of obesity on development of heart disease, use of less invasive surgical procedures to relieve arterial blockages and prevent restenosis, new drugs for the prevention and treatment of heart failure, and increasingly aggressive measures to prevent and treat the complications and disabilities associated with stroke. Indicators of frailty in a person with cardiovascular problems might include frequent hospitalization despite optimal treatment, functional decline, elevations in blood urea nitrogen and creatinine levels, fluctuating vital signs and daily weights, persistent angina or shortness of breath even at rest, cognitive or financial problems that inhibit access to appropriate medications and treatments, and indications of drug toxicity from medications needed to sustain life and cardiovascular function.

Alzheimer's Disease

An estimated 4.5 million Americans have Alzheimer's disease, according to sampling in an ethnically diverse population and the 2000 U.S. Census (Hebert et al., 2003). By 2050, this number could grow to an estimated 13.2 million Americans. A person with Alzheimer's disease will live an average of 8 years and as many as 20 years or more from the onset of symptoms (U.S. Congress Office of Technology Assessment, 2003). Half of all nursing home residents have Alzheimer's disease, and the average cost for nursing home care ranges from $42,000 to $70,000 per resident per year (MetLife, 2004; National Nursing Home Survey, 2003). The average lifetime cost of caring for an individual with Alzheimer's disease is $174,000 (Ernst & Hay, 2003).

When cognitive capacity is impaired due to the diagnosis of Alzheimer's disease or another irreversible neurodegenerative dementia, care and treatment decisions become even more difficult. Virtually all patients with dementia have unremitting disease courses inevitably leading to death (Marson, Dymek, & Geyer, 2001). The treatment preferences of persons with dementia are often made by family members on behalf of the patient or upon predetermined wishes such as living wills. In reality, however, treatment choices may not be so simple. There are many factors to consider such as burden of treatment, chance of success of the intervention, relief of symptoms, reduction of a family's burden of care, level of understanding and commitment on the part of families, and level of acuity of the setting in which the care is provided.

Advanced age is the biggest risk factor for the development of Alzheimer's disease. One in 10 persons over the age of 65 and nearly half of those over 85 have the disease

(Alzheimer's Association, 2004). Because life expectancy in the United States is increasing and persons over 85 represent the fastest growing segment of the population, need for care of people with Alzheimer's disease may become even more problematic over the next several decades. While more than 7 of 10 people with Alzheimer's disease live at home, the need for long-term care is nearly inevitable in the later stages of dementia to supply respite for family caregivers and to provide a comfortable and safe environment and symptomatic treatment (Alzheimer's Association, 2004; Hurley, Volicer, & Volicer, 1996).

Nearly 87% of nursing home residents with dementia exhibit one or more behavioral problems, including agitation, aggression, wandering, and sleep disorders. Delusions and hallucinations are common in all stages of dementia as the person loses contact with reality and can no longer function in his or her environment. A misplaced pair of eyeglasses may trigger a confrontation as the dementia victim accuses the caregiver of hiding the glasses or just trying to make things more difficult. The average family caregiver is usually a woman (wife, daughter, or daughter-in-law) about 60 years of age. Alzheimer's caregivers report significant physical and mental health problems, including sleep disturbances, anxiety, depression, backache, arthritis, indigestion, hypertension, and high cholesterol. Institutionalization often becomes necessary when caregivers are exhausted and can no longer provide care to their family member. For every elder in a nursing home, two others with similar needs are living in the community (Bishop, 2003).

Half of all nursing home residents have Alzheimer's disease, and approximately one fourth of elderly nursing home residents will be hospitalized during a 1-year period. Most hospitalizations will occur in the first 3 months of residence in the nursing facility. Seventy percent of nursing home residents are hospitalized in the year preceding their death; 20% require two hospitalizations and 10% have three or more hospitalizations (Malone & Danto-Nocton, 2004).

Nursing home residents admitted to hospitals are at risk for poor outcomes based on advanced age; lack of baseline laboratory data; higher baseline levels of functional and cognitive impairment; potential for information and communication errors regarding treatments, medications, and goals of treatment during the transfer process; and diagnoses with many comorbidities. During the hospital stay the nursing facility resident is at risk for delirium, restraints, functional decline, pressure ulcers, and medication changes that may or may not be adequately communicated to the nursing home upon discharge.

Musculoskeletal Problems

Changes in bone and muscle are associated with functional disability in later life. Osteoporosis, osteoarthritis, and age-related loss of muscle mass force many older people to become functionally dependent, suffering weakness, falls, fractures, and other problems related to immobility. Older patients diagnosed with musculoskeletal problems are at risk for frailty because weakness and immobility will compound recovery from surgery, acute illness, or chronic illness. Loss of bone and muscle mass may make position change more difficult, complicate early ambulation attempts after surgery, necessitate the use of bedpans and catheters, and delay trips to the bathroom, thus facilitating urinary and fecal incontinence. The older person is also at risk for falls and significant injury resulting from these falls. Signs of frailty in an older person with musculoskeletal problems may include decreased stamina and physical deconditioning, shortness of breath on exertion, history of falls, dizziness, weakness, poor vision or hearing, cognitive or mood impairment inhibiting judgment and preparation for movement, and diagnoses with comorbidities such as cardiovascular or neurologic disease.

Diabetes

Older persons with diabetes are at risk for frailty because of the complicated nature of managing and treating diabetes and its association with other diseases and problems such as cardiovascular disease and declines in neural, renal, immune, and sensory function (see Chapter 19 ⬭). When acute illness is diagnosed in an older person with diabetes, often eating patterns are disrupted, new medications are added, and activity levels are changed. All of these factors can greatly affect the patient's blood glucose levels and medication regimen. Because of declines in the immune system's ability to protect against infection, older adults with diabetes are more at risk for urinary tract infection, otitis media, development of peripheral ulcers, cholecystitis, and respiratory infection. When antibiotics are used in older persons with diabetes, they are usually prescribed at higher doses for longer periods of time to ensure complete eradication of the offending organism. These higher doses place the person at risk for medication side effects and drug interactions, including development of antibiotic-associated diarrhea, fungal infections, decreases in renal excretion of all prescribed medications, and development of hypo- or hyperglycemia. Older persons with diabetes may be considered frail if they exhibit any of the following characteristics: frequent need for treatment of severe hypo- or hyperglycemia indicating poor regulation and control, frequent diagnosed secondary infections, fluctuating vital signs and weight, presence of cognitive or functional impairment, financial and social problems inhibiting access to appropriate medications or treatment, and diagnosis with comorbidities complicating the assessment and treatment of the diabetes.

LONG-TERM CARE

Factors in the long-term care environment may exacerbate behavioral problems. Maintaining the emotional and relational well-being of those with dementia depends on caregivers who see dignity even in those severely affected by their condition. Overly restrictive institutional care facilities designed to protect vulnerable persons with dementia are capable of myriad abuses of power (Post, 1995; Post et al., 2001). With the best intentions, an efficient nursing staff may actually reinforce the resident's dependence (National Institutes of Health, 2000). Many long-term care facilities are understaffed. Nurses and nursing assistants may save time by "doing for" residents rather than encouraging residents to do more for themselves. Nurses should address problem behaviors using social and environmental modifications and creative activities, thereby preserving independence and self-esteem. Drugs for behavioral control should be used cautiously and only for specific purposes such as depression, psychosis, anxiety, and sleep disturbances (Martin & Whitehouse, 1990). Polypharmacy and overmedication are serious problems inherent in the care of patients with dementia.

Behavioral approaches include training caregivers in therapeutic responses to resistiveness to care, use of calming music, therapeutic touch, and other nonpharmacological responses appropriate for each particular patient (Tabloski, Remington, & McKinnon-Howe, 1995). Long-term care facilities should provide residents with safe areas to walk, access to protected outside areas, access to common rooms where activities can be enjoyed 24 hours a day, and more privacy in individual rooms. Sleep disturbances are common when two elderly residents share the same room and one resident requires frequent staff supervision and monitoring. Long-term care facilities should shift their focus of care delivery to become more resident-centered and construct systems of care that enhance quality of life for individuals with dementia.

Post (1995) described effective quality of life for persons with dementia to include:

1. Adjustment to and coping with the experience of increasing forgetfulness prior to the point of forgetting that one forgets.
2. Attainment of optimal emotional-behavioral conditions in the more advanced stages.
3. Avoidance of treatment-induced agitation, fear, and pain.

According to Post (1995, p. 99), "Because memories and sense of self are lost to the ravages of the disease, the existential moment assumes paramount importance. When care providers can establish a system of care that enhances positive adjustment and a relatively calm emotional life, life becomes more worth living for the dementia victim." The nurse can greatly improve the quality of a person's life by providing a safe and consistent environment, predictable pleasures and things to look forward to, avoidance of pain and invasive interventions when possible, and abundant and generous reassurance and support in times of stress.

Long-term care facilities support daily living activities for frail older people with limited functional abilities, and this objective is conceptually different from the objectives of other healthcare facilities. However, occupancy rates in nursing homes have been falling, as have the number of private-pay residents (Bishop, 2003). According to Bishop, two factors may be responsible for this trend: (1) Nursing homes are reorienting themselves more toward postacute care and intensive rehabilitation and somewhat away from services provided to the traditional long-term care resident. (2) Other care settings are emerging in the marketplace for elders with disabilities who can pay for their own care. Many of these financially able elders will choose to purchase home care services or move to upscale assisted-living facilities rather than live in nursing homes. Therefore, the average nursing home resident is becoming more frail with increasing financial and physical dependency.

MAKING TREATMENT DECISIONS

The healthcare of persons with dementia or other frailty is complicated. The dying process is often prolonged and accompanied by ethical questions about when and under what circumstances to withhold or withdraw treatment (Hurley et al., 1996). In general, the provision of care for the seriously ill long-term care resident should honor the resident's preferences, reflect the needs and wishes of families, be consistent with accepted public policy, and not inflict undue burden or harm to the resident without a reasonable chance of success. Although treatment decisions must be cost indifferent, fairness demands that treatments should be provided for those patients most likely to benefit and begin to be discouraged from patients with slim or no chance of benefit (Clancy & Brody, 1995; Government Accounting Office, 2002). Ineffective treatments, delivered by clinicians who are rewarded on a fee-for-service basis and requested by distraught families and patients, strain limited resources within the healthcare system and produce suffering on the part of patients who may already have poor quality of life.

Palliative care can be provided to seriously ill patients at any time during the disease process (see Chapter 11 ⬚). Unlike hospice, which is a system of care that is intended for individuals close to death, palliative care can be delivered for extended periods and throughout all phases of the treatment process. Palliative care emphasizes development of a therapeutic relationship by the provision of stable healthcare providers, alleviation of pain and management of troublesome symptoms, respite for families, reduction in use of acute care hospitals for death and unnecessary hospitalization, and increases in patient and family satisfaction with healthcare delivery (City of Hope & American Association of Colleges of Nursing, 2003).

The demand for newer and more expensive services and treatments continues to grow, while the equitable delivery of high-quality healthcare at reasonable cost remains an unresolved challenge in the American healthcare system (Paris, Reardon, & Browne, 2003). Healthcare providers are often reticent to discuss advance directives and treatment options within the context of dementia or other forms of frailty with healthy patients. For instance, a person may be perfectly willing to undergo a serious operation when he or she has coping abilities and mental faculties to deal with pain, spend time in a hospital away from family and friends, and participate in rehabilitation with eventual return to home. Any person who has had a serious operation knows that the experience is stressful and difficult, and most patients cannot wait to be discharged to home. The same serious operation carries a more significant burden for a patient with dementia or physical frailty. Nurses providing care to older persons with dementia or physical frailty should be experts in pain assessment and treatment techniques, address safety issues, administer medications carefully while being alert for adverse effects, and involve the interdisciplinary healthcare team as much as possible from the moment of admission to develop and facilitate treatment goals and a discharge plan.

Cognitively impaired and physically frail patients become even more confused with social isolation, exposure to narcotic pain medications and drugs used for anesthesia, and changes in their usual care routine. They are less able to participate in rehabilitation after surgery. Dementia patients and others with aphasia are much less likely to verbalize pain and request pain medications.

Often, physical and chemical restraints are needed to control agitation in patients with dementia or delirium. A dementia patient will often have a hand restrained to protect intravenous lines, drains, and oxygen tubing from being removed. One can only imagine how frightening this must be to an already confused and seriously ill older patient. The "do everything" philosophy, nurtured in medical and nursing schools and encouraged by a litigious culture, promotes aggressive cure-oriented treatment (Post et al., 2001). Many times, significant others and families do not realize that they have the options of choosing less aggressive care that may be more appropriate for the frail older person who is at risk for adverse treatment outcomes. Nurses can play a key role in educating families, providing support, and involving the interdisciplinary team.

ACUTE ILLNESS AND HOSPITALIZATION

Common causes of hospitalization include pneumonia, influenza, heart failure, ischemic heart disease, urinary tract infection, hip fracture, digestive disorders, and dehydration (Malone & Danto-Nocton, 2004). Additional facts about hospitalization include:

- Older persons account for 36% of all hospitalizations and 50% of hospital revenues.
- About 66% of Americans die in hospitals, and over 80% of the deaths occur in persons 65 years of age or older.
- About one fourth of patients who died in hospitals were perceived by their families to have moderate or severe pain at the end of life.
- In the year before death, nearly all older Americans are hospitalized, accounting for 20% of all Medicare expenditures.

(Landefeld, 2004; SUPPORT, 1995)

Hospital care is associated with increased use of medications, invasive procedures, diagnostic testing requiring food and fluid restriction, nosocomial infections, and occurrence of adverse events and poor outcomes to hospitalized elderly patients. Over 770,000 people are injured or die each year in hospitals from **adverse drug events** costing up to $5.6 million per hospital (Agency for Healthcare Research and Quality, 2001). Psychological decompensation or delirium occurs in nearly 20% of older people during acute care hospitalization. Risk factors for delirium include immobility, medications, iatrogenesis, illness, narcotic medications, sensory deprivation, and social isolation. Delirium independently contributes to functional decline, higher rates of postoperative complications, and longer lengths of hospital stay as compared to nondelirious postoperative patients (Milisen et al., 2004).

Adverse drug events can be minimized by implementing preventive strategies. Use of computerized entry systems, monitoring of prescriptions by a clinical pharmacist, and identification of the correct patient and drug using bar-code technology are methods that have been shown to decrease the frequency of medication errors. Adverse drug events can result from the following errors:

- Missed dose (7%)
- Wrong technique (6%)
- Illegible order (5%)
- Duplicate therapy (5%)
- Drug-drug interaction (5%)
- Equipment failure (1%)
- Inadequate monitoring (1%)
- Preparation error (1%)

(Agency for Healthcare Research and Quality, 2001)

Drug Alert !

Medications that can cause delirium through intoxication or withdrawal include anesthetics, analgesics, antiasthmatics, anticonvulsants, antihypertensives, antimicrobials, antiparkinsonian medications, corticosteroids, gastrointestinal H_2 blockers, muscle relaxants, hypnotics, and psychotropic medications.

Some evidence suggests that sensory deprivation experienced by patients placed in windowless hospital rooms is associated with higher rates of delirium (McCusker et al., 2001). Additional factors include not wearing hearing aids or eyeglasses, separation from personal objects, and lack of clocks and calendars. Falls can occur when older people are moving about in unsafe environments and trying to ambulate with intravenous poles on slippery or wet floors without appropriate footwear. Very old patients may arrive at the hospital in later and more severe stages of illness, may have other diagnosed chronic illness, may have sensory or cognitive impairment, and may be less able to adapt to their new environment. Thus, they are more at risk from adverse events and poor outcomes during hospitalization. Entering the hospital from a nursing home is associated with many of the attributes (including cognitive impairment) predicting poor outcomes during hospitalization (Fretwell, 1998). Nursing home residents are more at risk for adverse events, and nurses are required to provide special monitoring of their progress. Delirium and functional decline should be recognized as signs of the failure or side effects of the treatment regimen and of inadequate efforts to maintain function (Landefeld, 2004).

Common problems experienced by nursing home residents before, during, and after hospitalization are listed in Table 24-3. To facilitate better care of hospitalized nursing

TABLE 24-3

Common Problems Relating to Hospitalization Experienced by Nursing Home Residents

Time Period	Examples
Upon transfer to the hospital	Incomplete data regarding baseline cognitive and physical function
	New care providers
	Lack of clarity regarding predetermined wishes and code status
	Vague reports of signs and symptoms prompting the hospital transfer
During hospitalization	Delirium, physical and chemical restraints, urinary catheters, decubitus ulcers, malnutrition, functional decline, medication changes, falls
Upon return to the nursing home	Poor communication from the hospital regarding new diagnoses, medications, treatments
	Loss of function from illness/hospital experience
	Congestive heart failure from overhydration and aggressive fluid replacement
	Indwelling catheter still in place
	Nosocomial infection diagnosed upon return

Source: Adapted from Malone & Danto-Nocton, 2004.

home residents, the nurse should attempt to communicate with the nursing home staff and gain as much information as possible. Hospital and nursing home nurses can work together to develop a standardized transfer database to include all necessary information and keep open lines of communication to better meet the needs of nursing home residents requiring acute care.

Two general issues should be considered in caring for older persons in the hospital: (1) determining the goals of care and (2) designing and implementing strategies to achieve those goals (Landefeld, 2004). Failure to address these issues leads to frustration on the part of patients, families, and caregivers. Setting realistic goals is an important opportunity for caregivers to engage in open and honest conversations with patients and families. For instance, if a very old and frail patient suffers a major heart attack, the family may benefit from honest information about chances for survival, opportunities for and chances of success in rehabilitation, and possibility of returning to the prior living situation. The family may have different goals, and by engaging in conversation and development of a therapeutic and trusting relationship, the plan of care will have more chance of success. The goal may be to provide aggressive intervention including invasive testing and surgery, modified interventions such as drug administration and minimally invasive procedures, or comfort care in which pain and symptom control are the predominant issues. Table 24-4 illustrates goals and levels of care. Code status and goals of care should be discussed, clarified, and clearly noted on the chart as early as possible during the hospital admission process. Disagreements between family, patient, and caregivers are red flags that signal trouble during the caring process. The multidisciplinary team can be mobilized to help resolve conflicts.

Aggressive care is usually appropriately delivered to older persons with high functional ability, satisfactory quality of life, high rehabilitation potential, and the ability to endure and cooperate with the demands of therapy. Modified aggressive treatment is usually appropriate for older persons with higher degrees of frailty or multiple comorbidities who still have sufficient reserve capacity to respond to the treatment. Palliative care is appropriate for all older persons and can be delivered alone or in conjunction with aggressive or modified care. Hospice care is delivered to those with a life expectancy of 6 months or less. Age alone should not dictate the appropriate level

TABLE 24-4

Goals and Levels of Care

Level of Intervention	Goal	Examples of Intervention
Aggressive	Extension of life	Aggressive chemotherapy, invasive testing, radical surgery
Modified	Extension of life with consideration of the burden of treatment	Management of illness with medications, minimally invasive surgery, and noninvasive testing
Palliative care	Patient comfort with life extension as secondary goal	Pain management, symptom control, gentle rehabilitation, holistic care
Hospice	Comfortable death	Pain management, holistic care, symptom control

of care. The older person's predetermined wishes in conjunction with his or her underlying degree of frailty and the professional opinions of members of the healthcare team are the key factors.

Proposed screening tests for relevant comorbid conditions upon hospital admission include:

- Mental status testing to quantify the older person's baseline mental status and to identify cognitive deficits that may interfere with the ability to provide informed consent or to participate in the treatment and rehabilitation plan.
- Depression testing to quantify the older person's baseline level of depression, to identify patients needing referral for counseling or treatment with antidepressants, and to identify patients who may lack motivation, incentive, and drive to participate in the plan of care.
- Activities of daily living to identify previous level of function and baseline status. This is helpful information to be considered in discharge planning.
- Social support to identify family, friends, and religious and spiritual advisors who can assist and support the older person during illness and recovery.
- Presence of comorbidities, including heart disease, lung disease, chronic renal insufficiency, hypertension, diabetes, malignancy, collagen disorders, arthritis, visual impairment, and autoimmune disorders. If the patient is capable, he or she should be asked for permission to obtain and review old medical records from other hospitalizations or healthcare clinics.
- Nutrition measures, including weight, height, bone mass index, serum albumin, and cholesterol, to provide valuable information and predict responses to drug therapy and aggressive treatment.
- Polypharmacy information regarding the medications taken by the older person to prevent duplication of prescriptions during hospitalization, to avoid interactions, and to predict compliance with the discharge plan.
- End-of-life preferences. Has the older person established a living will or named a healthcare proxy? Is the older person still able to state the kind of treatment he or she would like during this hospitalization and illness?

(Adapted from Lichtman, 2003)

The Hartford Institute for Geriatric Nursing (1999) offers resources for several types of nursing tools used to clinically assess an older person's health status and monitor the effectiveness of treatments and nursing interventions. The *Try This* series is available online at the Gerontological Nurse Website, and many of the tools and assessment parameters have been offered thoughout this book. Tools for assessment of mood, memory, delirium, falls, medications, urinary incontinence, and other geriatric problems are included at this Website along with information on interpretation of results. Many of these tools will assist the nurse to meet the special needs of frail older patients by providing a systematic way to conduct a nursing assessment, diagnose problems, guide the treatment of disease, assess the effect of treatment on health status and function, and prevent complications of hospitalization.

Hospitalization also provides the opportunity for nurses to assess health promotion and disease prevention measures in older persons. For instance, older persons who smoke should be advised to discontinue smoking and be provided with information about smoking cessation programs available in the community. Influenza, pneumococcal, and tetanus vaccines can be administered if needed. Nutritional problems can be addressed. The management of comorbid conditions can be assessed and medication and treatment regimens modified if needed. For instance, an older person admitted to the hospital for a heart condition may have consistently elevated blood glucose levels and may need adjustments in antidiabetic medications and diet. Unsafe behaviors such as excessive alcohol intake, unsafe driving in the presence of cognitive or visual impairment, and history of falling can be screened for and addressed by the nurse and the interdisciplinary healthcare team. Older people without advance directives should be urged to identify healthcare proxies or complete a living will during hospitalization. The social worker can be consulted to collect information and coordinate the needed resources.

Many hospitals have established acute care of the elderly (ACE) units to provide specialized care to older persons and decrease the risks of adverse events during hospitalization. An ACE unit is based on four key concepts:

1. A safe environment with uncluttered halls to promote mobility, carpeted floors to decrease glare, raised toilet seats to improve continence, and a common lounge area to promote socialization and decrease isolation
2. Patient-centered interdisciplinary care guided by nurse-driven protocols to address key nursing issues such as mobility, skin care, nutrition, and continence
3. Discharge planning with the goal of returning the older patient to his or her former living status
4. Careful medical and nursing interventions to prevent adverse outcomes and avoid iatrogenic problems

ACE units have been shown to prevent functional decline, decrease length of stay, and decrease nursing home placement. Additionally, ACE units have demonstrated improvement in the process of care, including increased implementation of nursing care plans to promote independent function, increased physical therapy consults, and greater satisfaction among patients, caregivers, physicians, and nurses (Counsell, S., et al., 2000; Landefeld, 2004).

Assessing Treatment Burden

The most significant quality-of-life concern arises from the burdens that life-extending treatment can impose on people with frailty or dementia. The caregiver must examine the potential of an intervention from the very ill or disoriented person's point of view. Will the treatment be interpreted as assault or torture? Will it prolong a life with significant behavioral or physical problems? Are there indications that the dementia patient is refusing treatment by continued attempts to remove dialysis and feeding tubes (Post,

1995)? Therapeutic interventions that impose considerable burdens on the person with dementia should not be tolerated in a humane and just healthcare system and are considered to be **futile therapy**.

Hospital care is often rushed and fragmented among many specialists, each with a limited view and perspective of the overall patient and family situation. Burdensome interventions may result in distressing conditions, including pressure ulcers, constipation, pain, and shortness of breath (Mitchell, Kiely, & Hamel, 2003). However, legitimate concerns exist when advocating that dying residents receive their care in the long-term care facilities that have become their homes. Given the uneven history of care in long-term care facilities, lower nurse-to-patient ratios, and the fact that long-term care facilities exist with the objective of providing assistance to residents to compensate for functional and cognitive disabilities, the transfer to an acute care hospital may be appropriate (Post et al., 2001). Persons with end-stage dementia and physical frailty are in need of a rational approach to care at the end of life.

The cascade of illness or functional decline is the hypothesized pathway of development of complications during illness (Fretwell, 1998). For instance, hospitalization may trigger functional decline from falls, incontinence, not eating, and increased confusion. The medical interventions resulting from these conditions include use of physical and chemical restraints, placement of nasogastric tubes, and use of indwelling urinary catheters. Iatrogenesis and medical complications of these interventions include increased risk of thrombophlebitis, development of decubitus ulcers, aspiration pneumonia, urinary tract infection, and increased confusion or delirium. If the cascade of illness is able to progress unabated, an older person who is admitted to the hospital with mild confusion and stable chronic illness could progress to serious illness, functional decline, nursing home placement, or even death as a result of the hospitalization.

Ethical standards that guide healthcare decision making at the end of life support the self-determination of the patient (assuming the patient has made these known before becoming cognitively impaired) or best interests of the patient (in the case of the patient who did not execute advance directives before becoming impaired) (Veatch, 1989; 2000). An ethical dilemma that may arise is whether a patient should be treated for a secondary problem, such as infection, if death is pending. For instance, a patient with severe dementia may develop pneumonia during the late stages of disease. The administration of antibiotics may resolve the pneumonia, but may not be justified for a patient who is suffering from dementia. In rare cases, antibiotics may improve patient comfort (as in treatment of bladder infections). A study of dementia patients showed there were no differences in observed discomfort before, during, or after an infectious episode regardless of whether they were treated aggressively with antibiotics or managed palliatively with antipyretics and analgesics (Hurley, Volicer, Camberg, Ashley, & Woods, 1999).

PALLIATIVE CARE

The use of valuable social and financial resources on inappropriate or futile medical care depletes healthcare resources, drives up costs, and results in less money that could be spent on providing appropriate healthcare treatment and quality-of-life enhancement for older persons who may improve as a result of such treatment. Palliative care improves the quality of life of patients and their families when facing the problems associated with life-threatening illness. This is achieved through prevention and relief from suffering; early identification, impeccable assessment, and treatment of pain; and recognition and treatment of other physical, psychosocial, and spiritual problems (World Health Organization, 2002). Figure 24-3 ■ illustrates the key concepts associated with palliative care.

FIGURE ■ 24-3

Elements of palliative care.

Palliative Care Incorporates

Disease prevention
Symptom control
Life extension efforts

Reflecting the unique needs of
the individual

Although most physicians and nurses oppose active euthanasia or "mercy killing," there is no ethical or legal mandate involved with honoring the patient's or family's refusal of treatment or recommending against disproportionately burdensome treatment or treatment that will not benefit the patient (American Nurses Association, 1985). The *Code for Nurses* delineates the nursing profession's opposition to nurse participation in active euthanasia but does not negate the obligation of the nurse to provide proper and ethically justified end-of-life care which includes the promotion of comfort and the alleviation of suffering, adequate pain control, and, at times, forgoing life-sustaining treatments.

Common reasons for withholding or withdrawing aggressive treatment include patient choice, excessively burdensome care, potential for further reduction in quality of life, prolongation of the dying process, and acknowledgment that the disease progression will inevitably result in death, and treatment is likely to be ineffective (Lesage & Latimer, 1998). Healthcare professionals may find it difficult to stop life-sustaining treatment because they have been educated to "do everything possible" to support life. Although life-sustaining treatments may be appropriate for some patients with frailty and dementia, such treatments may only prolong suffering of other patients. Palliative treatments such as surgery, radiation, or chemotherapy may be appropriate in that they relieve pain and suffering, but the benefit of these treatments should outweigh the burdens to ensure they are morally and ethically justified. Treatments designed to prolong life so that families have time to gather and say goodbye are most likely justifiable, but treatments designed to prolong life for family convenience (e.g., the family is going on vacation and does not want to deal with a funeral now) are most likely morally unjustifiable, especially when significant pain and suffering are involved with life extension.

Healthcare providers can practice preventive ethics to promote an environment where early identification of issues and anticipation of possible dilemmas may avert potential areas of conflict (Forrow, Arnold, & Parker, 1993). The thoughtful healthcare provider will be able to anticipate where patient and family values may be in conflict with societal and professional values. As always, conflict resolution and communication skills are the key to clarifying goals and avoiding misrepresentation (Reigle & Boyle, 2000).

Healthcare treatments for coexisting diseases should be modified early in the course of care for the person with dementia. Because dementia shortens the life span, some interventions designed to reduce long-term risk factors can be avoided. For instance, limiting the food choices of a patient with dementia who has high cholesterol and urging a cardiac prudent diet may lead to weight loss, frustrate the patient, and prove to be a source of conflict with caregivers. Sometimes aggressive treatment of disease can place the patient with dementia at risk for side effects and injury. For example, it is counterproductive to strive for low blood glucose levels in a patient with dementia because of the increased danger of hypoglycemic reactions (Volicer, Volicer, & Hurley, 1993).

Some interventions routinely carried out in long-term care facilities are less likely to be successful or appropriate for patients who are physically frail or have dementia. Older persons who die in nursing homes with advanced frailty and dementia are not recognized as having a terminal condition and do not receive care that promotes palliation and comfort at the end of life. Potentially manageable symptoms (pain, shortness of breath, fever, and constipation) are not uncommon among residents dying with advanced frailty and dementia. Markers of poor quality care such as development of pressure ulcers, use of physical restraints, and treatment with antipsychotic medications are also common among dementia patients at the end of life (Mitchell, Kiely, & Hamel, 2003). High-risk interventions that are commonly carried out and are associated with limited chance of therapeutic success include cardiopulmonary resuscitation, tube feeding, intravenous therapy, fluid restriction, and invasive laboratory testing (Mitchel, Kiely, & Hamel, 2003; Volicer et al., 1993). Invasive medical treatments often upset the patient's emotional-behavioral adjustment, either because such treatments cannot be understood by the recipient or because the extension of life will add to mental and physical suffering (Post, 1995). Further, the failure to aggressively assess and treat pain in the patient with dementia is morally inappropriate. Patients with dementia often cannot express pain. A carefully trained nurse is needed to provide high-quality palliative care.

Professional integrity is foremost in the caring relationship, and patients and families have the right to this level of care. Palliative care can begin on the day the resident is admitted to the long-term care facility and can be applied throughout the course of illness to ensure comfort. Palliative care can enhance quality of life as patients and families adapt to the changes brought about by the disease progression. If the patient is eligible for hospice, the patient and family should be offered that option. The caregiver is responsible for ensuring that the patient and family fully understand the options available so they can make informed decisions.

When ethical dilemmas cannot be resolved through the usual care planning and communication process, the ethics committee should be consulted. All healthcare institutions should have access to an ethics committee to provide a forum for reflection and discussion of values, to build a moral community, and to attempt to meet the needs of the patient and family through group process and consensus. Ethics committees often validate or provide options regarding ethical dilemmas and support the care team in relation to already planned options (City of Hope & American Association of Colleges of Nursing, 2003).

Conclusion

Older persons who are diagnosed with comorbidities, functional deficits, disadvantaged resources, and lack of organ system reserve are at risk for poor outcomes and adverse events when receiving healthcare. Gerontological nurses have the potential to improve the quality of life across settings by conducting effective and holistic nursing assessments, facilitating access to programs and services, educating and empowering older patients and their families, participating in and leading multidisciplinary health teams, serving as advocates and influencing the development of public policy and reform of legislation to improve long-term healthcare, and conducting and applying research related to aging (Young, 2003). By avoiding stereotypes, thinking holistically, using the most current and appropriate medical treatments, and trying to minimize the burden of treatment, the nurse can greatly contribute to the health and well-being of many older persons.

Nurses in all settings should practice according to the following guidelines:

- Be aware of drug interactions. Polypharmacy and drug toxicity are key problems for older persons.
- Remember that the presentation of illness is less dramatic and more vague than in other age groups. Key signs and symptoms of heart disease, infection, gastrointestinal

problems, depression, and cancer may not be accompanied by the classic signs and symptoms seen in younger adults. Aggressively investigate falls, weight loss, confusion, fatigue, decline in functional ability, and incontinence.

■ Conduct holistic nursing assessments when caring for frail older adults and those with comorbidities. Use valid and reliable assessment tools on admission and periodically thereafter to monitor the effect of treatments and interventions.

■ Seek to access and provide the most intensive services to those considered the most frail and those diagnosed with multiple comorbidities. The comprehensive services provided by a multidisciplinary team can benefit the older adult with acute and chronic needs and deliver a full range of services across settings.

■ Practice ethically according to professional standards. Try to establish advance directives and identify end-of-life preferences. Educate and empower older patients and families so that they can make more informed treatment decisions, avoid futile care, and refuse interventions that are excessively burdensome, painful, and invasive.

■ Promote healthy aging in all clinical settings. Establishing a healthy lifestyle at any age will prevent or delay the onset of disability, make the pharmacological treatment of chronic illness more effective, and improve or maintain functional ability.

■ Recognize and treat pain in older persons, including those with dementia or other disabilities that preclude them from adequately expressing their pain.

■ Become expert at providing end-of-life care to the seriously ill and dying patient. The nurse can help provide a comfortable death that is free from pain and troubling symptoms in a supportive, caring environment.

■ Seek continuing education programs and pursue advanced degrees. Keep current by reading journals. Collaborate with experts in nursing and other health professions, and advocate to improve care and services for older persons with health needs.

(Amella, 2004; Mezey & Fulmer, 1998; Young, 2003; Nurses Improving the Care of the Hospitalized Elderly (NICHE) project. See the Hartford Institute for Geriatric Nursing Website) www.hartfordign.org.

Patient-Family Teaching Guidelines

PLANNING FOR HOSPITALIZATION

The nurse will often teach older persons and their families about planning for a hospital stay for surgery or treatment of an illness. The following guidelines may help an older person at risk for adverse outcomes to have a safer and more effective hospitalization experience.

1. What should I consider when planning to enter the hospital next week for treatment of my illness?

Bring complete medical records with you to the hospital. Ask your doctor for a copy of your most recent laboratory values, your last physical examination, and an accounting of your past medical history including all hospitalizations, surgical interventions, invasive testing, and so on. Also bring a list of your current medications and dosing schedule, all of your contact information, contact information for your healthcare proxy, insurance information, and living will (if you have one).

RATIONALE:

The more information shared with the hospital providers, the less likely the chance of errors, including adverse drug events. Carrying as much information to the hospital as possible will facilitate a smooth admission and decrease the risk of iatrogenesis.

Patient-Family Teaching Guidelines

2. What should I tell the nurses at the hospital when I am admitted?

Tell them why you are there and what goals you would like to accomplish. Also tell them if you have allergies to food or medication, problems walking, bowel or bladder problems, sleep problems, chronic pain, or other important issues relating to your care. If you wear a hearing aid or glasses, please let the nurses know. Answer all of their questions as openly and honestly as you can. Your family or significant other can help, if you wish.

RATIONALE:

Sharing information about daily function and goals of treatment will assist the nurses in planning safe, effective, and appropriate nursing care. This information is crucial to development of an individualized nursing care plan.

3. What personal items should I bring with me?

Bring good walking slippers, a bathrobe, medical records, a book if you are a reader, a CD player for music, a small amount of money for incidental purchases, and pictures of your family. Avoid bringing valuable jewelry and large or bulky items. Ask your friends to send flowers when you go home instead of to the hospital because they can be difficult to carry out and can clutter up a small hospital room.

RATIONALE:

Good planning and bringing a few personal items can make the hospital experience more enjoyable. Large items and valuables present storage and safety problems. They should be left at home if possible.

4. Besides my family, who should I notify regarding my hospitalization?

You may want to let some close friends know and notify them of your visiting preferences. Some hospitalized patients like to have visitors and others prefer phone calls or cards. If you are religious, you should notify your priest, minister, or rabbi.

RATIONALE:

Sometimes lots of visitors and phone calls can be exhausting to an older patient during the hospital experience. Helping older persons think about the number and types of visitors they would like ahead of time can head off potential problems and hurt feelings.

5. How can I prepare myself to come back to my home after my hospitalization?

Your nurse and social worker will work with you and your family from the moment you are admitted so that you will be able to return to your previous level of function and living arrangement. Some older people find that after treatment for an illness or an operation they are too weak to go directly home, and a short stay at a rehabilitation facility may be indicated. You should discuss these options with your nurse, physician, and social worker when you reach the hospital.

RATIONALE:

The older person and family may need warning that a direct return to home may not be possible after hospitalization for surgery or serious illness. A short-term stay in a rehabilitation unit may be needed. Some patients and families may investigate these options and other discharge options beforehand, thus easing the transition and hospital discharge.

6. I am worried that they will hitch me up to a machine and if something goes wrong, I will be a burden to my family.

Discuss the goals of your hospitalization and your fears with your healthcare providers and your family. Your predetermined wishes are critical to your care and will be clearly noted on your chart. If you do not have a current healthcare proxy, you will be asked to name one when you reach the hospital in the unlikely event that you will be unable to make decisions for yourself.

RATIONALE:

Having a valid and current advance directive in place is a benefit for all involved. A discussion before the hospital admission allows time to come to agreement and verbalize preferences. Even if an advance directive is in place already, repeating the discussion and reinforcing preferences is advantageous to all involved.

Care Plan

Nursing Care of a Frail Older Person

Case Study

Mr. Krane is an 84-year-old man who has just been admitted to the acute care hospital from the emergency department. He is a nursing home resident with the following medical problems: moderate Alzheimer's disease, history of falls with injury, atrial fibrillation, and fever of unknown origin. The emergency department notes that he has a low-grade temperature, and a chest x-ray reveals a possible area of consolidation in the right lower lobe. Mr. Krane is restless, irritable, and agitated. He was held in the emergency department for 8 hours because there were several victims of a motor vehicle accident brought in for treatment of trauma shortly after he arrived. The environment was chaotic because of the trauma victims. Mr. Krane has an intravenous line in his left arm and an indwelling urinary catheter. He has not eaten a full meal since he came to the hospital. His daughter is his only living relative and she lives out of state. The social worker is attempting to contact her and has left several messages on her telephone answering machine. Code status is unknown.

Applying the Nursing Process

ASSESSMENT

The gerontological nurse should immediately assess Mr. Krane's comfort level. He is agitated and has endured a long stay in the emergency department. If his diet order has not been specified by the admitting physician, the nurse should contact the physician immediately and obtain an order for a regular or no-added-salt diet. Mr. Krane should be asked what kind of food he likes, if he has allergies or food intolerances, and what assistance he needs while eating. The nurse may wish to call the nursing home staff and request information regarding Mr. Krane's nutritional status and dietary preferences. It is hoped that food will improve his irritability and level of comfort. An additional assessment priority is patient safety. As Mr. Krane has a history of falls, a fall prevention program should be immediately instituted. The next priority is to assess what medications he usually takes and when the last doses were administered. As he has been diagnosed with atrial fibrillation, he is most likely on warfarin, and every effort should be made to keep his dosing schedule intact to prevent the increased risk of stroke. Additional medications to treat his dementia and pneumonia may have been ordered and should be obtained from the pharmacy as quickly as possible.

Nursing Care of a Frail Older Person

DIAGNOSES

The current nursing diagnoses for Mr. Krane include the following:

- *Imbalanced body temperature*
- *Chronic confusional state*
- *Risk for falls*
- *Imbalanced nutrition, less than body requirements*
- *Ineffective tissue perfusion: cardiopulmonary*
- *Social isolation*
- *Risk for impaired skin integrity*
- *Impaired mobility*

EXPECTED OUTCOMES

The expected outcomes for the plan of care specify that Mr. Krane will:

- Not suffer injury or adverse outcomes during his hospital stay.
- Receive appropriate medications to manage his acute and chronic illness.
- Return to the nursing home at approximately the same level of baseline function.
- Receive appropriate care consistent with his and his family's specified values and expected outcomes.

PLANNING AND IMPLEMENTATION

The following nursing interventions may be appropriate for Mr. Krane:

- A fall prevention plan will be instituted with measures to include lowering the bed to the lowest position, placing the call light within easy reach, instructing Mr. Krane to call for assistance when needed, asking him not to attempt to leave the bed without assistance, and placing him in a room close to the nurses' station in order to routinely observe him.
- If Mr. Krane is on warfarin, he is at increased risk for injury from falls due to increased clotting times as a result of anticoagulation therapy. Careful monitoring of his international normalized ratio is warranted, especially with the addition of new medications.
- Non-pharmacological measures to improve his agitation will include approaching him calmly, calling him by name, decreasing noise and light (he is probably overstimulated from his emergency department stay), and playing calm music.
- As Mr. Krane is at high risk for the development of delirium, careful monitoring of his cognition and level of consciousness is warranted. Appropriate parameters include mental status changes, inattention, evidence of disorganized thinking, and altered level of consciousness. The nurse should carefully note Mr. Krane's baseline level of function so changes can be detected early. Psychoactive medications should be avoided if at all possible, and behavioral and environmental interventions should be utilized to manage agitation and improve sleep.
- Mr. Krane should wear his glasses and hearing aids during the day to improve his communication ability. Food and fluid intake should be monitored.

(continued)

Nursing Care of a Frail Older Person *(continued)*

EVALUATION

The nurse will consider the plan a success based on the following criteria:

- Mr. Krane and his family will specify an advance directive noting the appropriate level of healthcare interventions and outcomes desired.
- The patient will maintain his weight and nutritional status.
- He will receive appropriate medications to resolve his pneumonia without toxic side effects or drug interactions.
- Mr. Krane will be discharged from the hospital to the nursing home at his previous level of function.

Ethical Dilemma

During Mr. Krane's hospitalization for pneumonia, he is found to have a suspicious lesion on his lung. A CT scan reveals it is most likely the result of lung cancer. The daughter states, "I'd like to have it removed so that Dad can live out his natural life." Mr. Krane is unsure if he wants the operation, but if his daughter thinks it is necessary, he will go along with it. Mr. Krane's pulmonologist notes that there is very little chance that a lung resection will improve his prognosis or improve the quality or length of his life.

The nurse should consult with the social worker and physician regarding the need to consult the ethics committee. Disputes about appropriate care for frail older persons with dementia can be emotional and require the input of the multidisciplinary team. Assuming that the daughter has her father's best interests at heart, she may need education and support to reconsider her decision. Additionally, Mr. Krane should be assessed for his ability to make decisions regarding his own medical care. Even with the diagnosis of dementia, Mr. Krane may have an understanding of his situation and be able to state his preferences and fears. When conflict arises regarding treatment decisions, it is often unclear who should make the final decision. The patient, the family member, the physician, and other members of the healthcare team all may have opinions regarding the best course of action. The ideal situation is to begin a dialogue until consensus can be reached and all parties are satisfied with the decision. Ethics committees usually have members who are experts in the mechanics of conflict resolution. It is hoped that early involvement of this committee will lead to satisfactory resolution of the conflict regarding Mr. Krane's treatment plan.

Critical Thinking and the Nursing Process

1. Imagine that you will be admitted to a hospital for a surgical procedure. If hospital procedure allowed you to bring only five personal items, what items would you select?
2. Choose a classmate and engage in a civilized debate of the following issue: Older people with dementia should or should not receive the same medical and nursing interventions as those without dementia. Argue one point of view for 5 minutes and then switch sides to argue the opposite point of view.

Nursing Care of a Frail Older Person

3. What are the advantages and disadvantages of having special units for caring for acutely ill hospitalized older patients?

4. What suggestions can you make to improve the nursing care provided to older patients during transfer between the hospital and nursing home?

■ Evaluate your responses in Appendix B. ▭

EXPLORE MediaLink

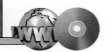

NCLEX review, case studies, and other interactive resources for this chapter can be found on the Companion Website at **www.prenhall.com/tabloski**. Click on Chapter 24 to select the activities for this chapter. For animations, video tutorials, more NCLEX review questions, and case studies, access the accompanying CD-ROM in this textbook.

Chapter Highlights

■ Multisystem problems and comorbidities complicate the delivery of care to older persons. The frail and the very old are especially at risk for adverse events and poor outcomes as the result of acute illness, exacerbation of chronic illness, and hospitalization.

■ Nursing home residents are the most at risk for adverse outcomes based on their extreme frailty and high degree of cognitive impairment.

■ Hospital care can be improved for older persons. Multidisciplinary teams, patient-centered care, ACE units, and careful assessment and monitoring all increase the chances of success during hospitalization.

■ Pain management, advance care planning, treatment cessation, and resource allocation are all issues of organizational ethics.

■ Accreditation bodies such as the Joint Commission on Accreditation of Healthcare Organizations are increasingly monitoring for evidence of organization commitment and involvement in addressing the ethical dimensions of care.

■ To address the provision of fair and equitable long-term care, healthcare professionals and policymakers should begin public education and awareness campaigns; enhance professional education and staff development regarding delivery of palliative care; establish policies and procedures within long-term care facilities to support timely, comprehensive, and compassionate care; and advocate for funding of clinical research to evaluate the benefits and burdens of medical interventions related to caring for the frail elderly with dementia in the long-term care facility.

References

Agency for Healthcare Research and Quality. (2001). *Reducing and preventing adverse drug events to decrease hospital costs* (AHRQ Publication No. 01-0020). Retrieved September 19, 2004, from www.ahrq.gov/qual/aderia/aderia.htm.

Albert, S., Im, A., & Raveis, V. (2002). Public health and the second 50 years of life. *American Journal of Public Health, 92*(8) 1–3.

Alzheimer's Association. (2004). *Fact sheet, Alzheimer's disease.* Retrieved July 19, 2004, from www.alz.org.

Amella, E. (2004). Presentation of illness in older adults. *American Journal of Nursing, 104*(10), 40–51.

American Association of Retired Persons. (1999). *Baby boomers envision retirement.* Retrieved October 4, 2003, from research.aarp.org.

American Nurses Association. (1985). *Code for nurses with interpretive statements.* Kansas City, MO: American Nurses Publishing.

Bailes, B. (2000). Perioperative care of the elderly surgical patient. *American Association of Operating Room Nurses Journal, August.* Retrieved August 16, 2004, from www.aorn.org/journal.

Bennett, J., & Flaherty-Robb, M. (2003). Issues affecting the health of older citizens: Meeting the challenge. *Online Journal of Issues in Nursing, 8*(2), 1–12. Retrieved December 12, 2004, from www.nursingworld.org/ojin/topic21/tpc21_1.htm.

Bishop, C. (2003). Long-term-care needs of elders and persons with disability. In D. Blumenthal, M. Moon, M. Warshawsky, & C. Boccuti (Eds.), *Long-term care and Medicare policy.* Washington, DC: National Academy of Social Insurance.

Chrvala, C., & Bulger, R. (1999). *Leading health indicators for Healthy People 2010.* Washington, DC: Institute of Medicine, National Academy Press.

City of Hope & American Association of Colleges of Nursing. (2003). *ELNEC graduate curriculum.* End of Life Nursing Care at the End of Life. Education Consortium, Nat'l Cancer Institute, Bethesda, MD.

Clancy, C. M., & Brody, H. (1995). Managed care. Jekyll or Hyde? *Journal of the American Medical Association, 27,* 338–339.

Counsell, S., Holder, C. Liebenauer, L., Palmer, R., Fortunsky, R, Kresevic, D., Quinn, L. et al., (2000). Effects of a multicomponent intervention on functional outcomes and process of care in hospitalized older patients: A randomized controlled trial of acute care for elders (ACE) in a community hospital. *Journal of the American Geriatrics Society, 48*(12), 1572–1581.

Ernst, R., & Hay, J. (2003). The U.S. economic and social costs of Alzheimer's disease. *American Journal of Public Health, 84*(8), 1261–1264.

Forrow, L., Arnold, R. M., & Parker, L. S. (1993). Preventive ethics: Expanding the horizons of clinical ethics. *Journal of Clinical Ethics, 9,* 287–294.

Fretwell, M. (1998). Acute hospital care for frail older patients. In W. Hazzard, E. Bierman, J. Blass, W. Ettinger, & J. Halter (Eds.), *Principles of geriatric medicine and gerontology.* New York: McGraw-Hill.

Fried, L. (1993). The epidemiology of frailty: The scope of the problem. In H. M. Perry, J. E. Morley, & R. M. Coe (Eds.), *Aging, musculoskeletal disorders and care of the frail elderly* (pp. 3–16). New York: Springer.

Fried, L. (1994). Frailty. In W. Hazzard, E. Bierman, J. Blass, W. Ettinger, & J. Halter (Eds.), *Principles of geriatric medicine and gerontology.* New York: McGraw-Hill.

Fried, L., Tangen, C., Walston, J., Newman, A., Hirsch, C., Gottdiener, J., et al. (2001). Frailty of older adults: Evidence for a phenotype. *Journals of Gerontology: Biological Sciences and Medical Sciences, 56A*(3), M146–156.

Glaser, B., & Strauss, A. (1968). *A time for dying.* Chicago: Aldine.

Government Accounting Office. (2002). *Long-term care. Aging baby boom generation will increase demand and burden on federal and state budgets* (GAO-02-544T). Washington, DC: U.S. Government Printing Office.

Hartford Institute of Geriatric Nursing, (1999). Try This Series, Retrieved Sept 19, 2004, from www. Hartfordign.org/resources/education/trythis.html.

HealthSquare. (2004). Women's Health heart disease. Retrieved September 19, 2004, from www.healthsquare.com/fgwh/wh1ChI2.htm.

Hebert, L., Scherr, P., Bienias, J., Bennett, D., & Evans, D. (2003). Alzheimer disease in the U.S. population. *Archives of Neurology, 60,* 1119–1122.

Hurley, A., Volicer, B., & Volicer, L. (1996). Effect of fever-management strategy on the progression of dementia of the Alzheimer type. *Alzheimer Disease and Associated Disorders, 10*(1), 5–10.

Hurley, A., Volicer, L., Camberg, L., Ashley, J., & Woods, P. (1999). Measurement of observed agitation in patients with dementia of the Alzheimer type. *Journal of Mental Health and Aging, 5*(2), 117–133.

Izaks, G., & Westendorp, R. (2003). Ill or just old? Towards a conceptual framework of the relation between aging and disease. *BMC Geriatrics, 3*(7), 1–6. Retrieved February 18,

2004, from www.biomedcentral.com/1471-2318/3/7.

Kagan, S. (2004). *The advanced practice nurse in an aging society. The 2004 sourcebook for advanced practice nurses.* Lippincott Williams & Wilkins. Philadelphia, PA. Retrieved 9/21/2004. www.tnpj.com.

Kapp, M. (1992). *Geriatrics and the law* (2nd ed.). New York: Springer-Verlag.

Landefeld, C. (2004). Hospital care. In C. Landefeld, R. Palmer, M. Johnson, C. Johnston, & W. Lyons (Eds.), *Current geriatric diagnosis and treatment.* New York: Lange Medical Books.

Lesage, P., & Latimer, E. (1998). An approach to ethical issues. In N. MacDonald (Ed.), *Palliative medicine: A case-based approach.* New York: Oxford University Press.

Lichtman, S. (2003). Guidelines for the treatment of elderly cancer patients. *Cancer Control, 10*(6), 445–453.

Luchins, D. J., & Hanrahan, P. (1993). What is appropriate health care for end-stage dementia? *Journal of the American Geriatrics Society, 41*(8), 25–30.

Lunney, J., Lynn, J., Foley, D., Lipson, S., & Guralnik, J. (2003). Patterns of functional decline at the end of life. *Journal of the American Medical Association, 289*(18), 2387–2392.

Malone, M., & Danto-Nocton, E. (2004). Improving the hospital care of nursing facility residents. *Annals of Long-Term Care, 12*(5), 42–49.

Marson, D., Dymek, M., & Geyer, J. (2001). Informed consent and competency. *Neurologist, 7,* 317–326.

Martin, R., & Whitehouse, P. (1990). Evaluation of dementia. *Neurology, 40,* 439–443.

McCance, K. L., & Huether, S. E. (2001). *The biologic basis of disease in adults and children.* St. Louis, MO: Mosby.

McCusker, J., Cole, M., Abrahamowicz, M., Han, L., Podoba, J., & Ramman-Haddad, L. (2001). Environmental risk factors for delirium in hospitalized older people. *Journal of the American Geriatrics Society, 49,* 1327–1334.

MetLife. (2004). General News: Press Release. Nursing home costs average $70,080 per year in U.S. 2004 MetLife Mature Market Institute Survey. Retrieved September 19, 2004, from www.metlife.com.

Mezey, M., & Fulmer, T. (1998). Quality care for the frail elderly. *Nursing Outlook, 46*(6), 291–292.

Milisen, K., Foreman, M., Wouters, B., Driesen, R., Godderis, J., Abraham, I., & Broos, P. (2004). Documentation of delirium in elderly patients with hip fracture. *Journal of Gerontological Nursing, 28*(11), 23–29.

Mitchell, S., Kiely, D., & Hamel, M. (2003). Dying with advanced dementia in the nursing home. *Archives of Internal Medicine, 164,* 321–326.

National Academy on an Aging Society. (1999). *Public policy and aging report.* Retrieved August 14, 2001, from www.agingsociety.org.

National Center for Chronic Disease Prevention and Health Promotion. (1999). *Leading causes of death.* Washington, DC: Centers for Disease Control.

National Institute on Aging. (2005). *Portfolio for progress: Reducing disease and disability.* Retrieved January 9, 2005, from www.nia publications.org/pubs/portfolio/html/reducing.htm.

National Institute on Aging & National Cancer Institute. (2004). *Working group 3: Effects of comorbidity on cancer.* Retrieved August 16, 2004, from www.nia.nih.gov/health.

National Institutes of Health. (2000). *Progress report on Alzheimer's disease.* Alzheimer's Disease Education and Referral Center, Rockville, Maryland.

National Nursing Home Survey. (2003). *Long term care cost.* Washington, DC: U.S. Government Printing Office.

Office of Technology Assessment. (2003). *Alzheimer's disease impact.* Washington, DC: U.S. Congress Printing Office.

Paris, J., Reardon, F., & Browne, J. (2003). An economic, ethical, and legal analysis of problems in critical care medicine. In R. Irwin, F. Cerra, & J. Rippe, (eds) Hagerstown, MD: *Intensive care medicine* (5th ed.). Lippincott.

Post, L., Mitty, E., Bottrell, M., Dubler, N., Hill, T., Mezey, M., & Ramsey, G. (2001). Guidelines for end-of-life care in nursing facilities: Principles and recommendations. *NAELA Quarterly,* vol. no. 14(2) Spring, 24–30.

Post, S. (1995). *The moral challenge of Alzheimer disease.* Baltimore: Johns Hopkins University Press.

Reigle, J., & Boyle, R. (2000). Ethical decision-making skills. In A. B. Hamric, J. A. Spross, & C. M. Hanson (Eds.), *Advanced nursing practice: An integrative approach* (2nd ed.). Philadelphia: W. B. Saunders.

Robert Wood Johnson Foundation. (1996). *Chronic illness and the health care system.* Retrieved August 17, 2002, from www.rwjf.org.

Robertson, R., & Montagnini, M. (2004). Geriatric failure to thrive. *American Family Physician, 70*(2), 343–350.

Rosenthal, G., Kaboli, P., Barnett, M., & Sirio, C. (2002). Age and risk of in-hospital death: Insights from a multihospital study of intensive care patients. *Journal of the American Geriatrics Society, 50,* 1205–1212.

Saltvedt, I., Mo, E., Fayers, P., Kaasa, S., & Sletvold, O. (2002). Reduced mortality in treating acutely sick, frail older patients in a geriatric evaluation and management unit. A prospective randomized trial. *Journal of the American Geriatrics Society, 50,* 792–798.

SUPPORT. (1995). A controlled trial to improve care for seriously ill hospitalized patients. The study to understand prognoses and preferences for outcomes and risks of treatment. *Journal of the American Medical Association, 274*(20), 1591–1598.

Tabloski, P., Remington, R., & McKinnon-Howe, L. (1995). The relationship between music and agitation in cognitively impaired nursing home residents. *American Journal of Alzheimers Disease Research and Practice, Jan/Feb*(10), 1–6.

U.S. Congress, Office of Technology Assessment. (2003). *Alzheimer's Disease,* OTA-BA 94-3676, Washington, DC., Supt. of Docs, US Govt Printing Office:

Veatch, R. M. (1989). *The patient as partner: A theory of human-experimentation ethics.* Bloomington and Indianapolis: Indiana University Press.

Veatch, R. M. (2000). *Transplantation ethics.* Washington, DC: Georgetown University Press.

Volicer, L., Volicer, B., & Hurley, A. (1993). Is hospice care appropriate for Alzheimer patients? *Caring, 11,* 50–55.

World Health Organization. (2002). *National cancer control programmes: Policies and managerial guidelines* (2nd ed.). Geneva, Switzerland: Author.

Young, H. (2003). Challenges and solutions for care of frail older adults. *Online Journal of Issues in Nursing, 8*(2), Manuscript 4. Retrieved December 12, 2004, from www.nursingworld. org/ojin/topic21/tpc21_4.htm.

PHOTO CREDITS

CHAPTER 1
Page 16: Ron Chapple/Getty Images,
Inc.–Taxi
Page 54: Michal Heron/Pearson Education/
PH College

CHAPTER 3
Page 27: Michal Heron/Pearson Education/
PH College

CHAPTER 4
Page 84: Owen Franken/Stock Boston

CHAPTER 5
Page 110: Michal Heron/Pearson Education/
PH College
Page 126: Michal Heron/Pearson Education/
PH College

CHAPTER 6
Page 155: Michal Heron/Pearson Education/
PH College

CHAPTER 7
Page 188: © Dorling Kindersley

CHAPTER 8
Page 227: Carolin Hansa
Page 228: © Dorling Kindersley
Page 230: Pearson Education/PH College
Page 233: John Childers
Page 224: Shirley Zeiberg/Pearson
Education/PH College

CHAPTER 9
Page 249: Skjold/Pearson Education/
PH College

CHAPTER 10
Page 271: Pearson Education/PH College

CHAPTER 11
Page 293: Michal Heron/Pearson Education/
PH College
Page 296: Michal Heron/Pearson Education/
PH College

CHAPTER 12
Page 328: Pearson Education/PH College
Page 334: Custom Medical Stock Photo,
Inc.

CHAPTER 13
Page 365: Trish Gant © Dorling Kindersley

CHAPTER 14
Page 383: Bill Burlingham/Pearson
Education/PH College

CHAPTER 15
Page 421: Michal Heron/Pearson Education/
PH College

CHAPTER 16
Page 501: CORBIS–NY
Page 459: Teri Stratford/Pearson Education/
PH College

CHAPTER 17
Page 517: Bill Irwin/Pearson Education/PH
College

CHAPTER 18
Page 558: John M. Daugherty/Photo
Researchers, Inc.
Page 562: L. Samsuri/Custom Medical
Stock Photo, Inc.
Page 565: James Stevenson/Photo
Researchers, Inc.
Page 551: Michal Heron/Pearson Education/
PH College

CHAPTER 19
Page 600: Pearson Learning Photo Studio

CHAPTER 20
Page 642: Trish Gant © Dorling Kindersley

CHAPTER 21
Page 684: Michal Heron/Pearson Education/
PH College

CHAPTER 22
Page 711: Michal Heron/Pearson Education/
PH College

CHAPTER 23
Page 778: Custom Medical Stock Photo,
Inc.
Page 754: Silver Burdett Ginn

CHAPTER 24
Page 787: Michal Heron/Pearson Education/
PH College

2005–2006 NANDA-APPROVED NURSING DIAGNOSES

Activity Intolerance

Activity Intolerance, Risk for

Adaptive Capacity: Intracranial, Decreased

Adjustment, Impaired

Airway Clearance, Ineffective

Anxiety

Anxiety, Death

Aspiration, Risk for

Attachment, Parent/Infant/Child, Risk for Impaired

Body Image, Disturbed

Body Temperature: Imbalanced, Risk for

Bowel Incontinence

Breastfeeding, Effective

Breastfeeding, Ineffective

Breastfeeding, Interrupted

Breathing Pattern, Ineffective

Cardiac Output, Decreased

Caregiver Role Strain

Caregiver Role Strain, Risk for

Communication, Readiness for Enhanced

Communication: Verbal, Impaired

Confusion, Acute

Confusion, Chronic

Constipation

Constipation, Perceived

Constipation, Risk for

Coping: Community, Ineffective

Coping: Community, Readiness for Enhanced

Coping, Defensive

Coping: Family, Compromised

Coping: Family, Disabled

Coping: Family, Readiness for Enhanced

Coping (Individual), Readiness for Enhanced

Coping, Ineffective

Decisional Conflict (Specify)

Denial, Ineffective

Dentition, Impaired

Development: Delayed, Risk for

Diarrhea

Disuse Syndrome, Risk for

Diversional Activity, Deficient

Dysreflexia, Autonomic

Dysreflexia, Autonomic, Risk for

Energy Field Disturbance

Environmental Interpretation Syndrome, Impaired

Failure to Thrive, Adult

Falls, Risk for

Family Processes, Dysfunctional: Alcoholism

Family Processes, Interrupted

Family Processes, Readiness for Enhanced

Fatigue

Fear

Fluid Balance, Readiness for Enhanced

Fluid Volume, Deficient

Fluid Volume, Deficient, Risk for

Fluid Volume, Excess

Fluid Volume, Imbalanced, Risk for

Gas Exchange, Impaired

Grieving, Anticipatory

Grieving, Dysfunctional

Grieving, Risk for Dysfunctional

Growth, Disproportionate, Risk for

Growth and Development, Delayed

Health Maintenance, Ineffective

Health Seeking Behaviors (Specify)

Home Maintenance, Impaired

Hopelessness

Hyperthermia

Hypothermia

Identity: Personal, Disturbed

Infant Behavior, Disorganized

Infant Behavior: Disorganized, Risk for

Infant Behavior: Organized, Readiness for Enhanced

Infant Feeding Pattern, Ineffective

Infection, Risk for

Injury, Risk for

Knowledge, Deficient (Specify)

Knowledge (Specify), Readiness for Enhanced

Latex Allergy Response

Latex Allergy Response, Risk for

Lifestyle, Sedentary

Loneliness, Risk for

Memory, Impaired

Mobility: Bed, Impaired

Mobility: Physical, Impaired

Mobility: Wheelchair, Impaired

Nausea

Neurovascular Dysfunction: Peripheral, Risk for

Noncompliance (Specify)

Nutrition, Imbalanced: Less than Body Requirements

Nutrition, Imbalanced: More than Body Requirements

Nutrition, Imbalanced: More than Body Requirements, Risk for

Nutrition, Readiness for Enhanced

Oral Mucous Membrane, Impaired

Pain, Acute

Pain, Chronic

Parenting, Impaired

Parenting, Readiness for Enhanced

Parenting, Risk for Impaired

Perioperative Positioning Injury, Risk for

Poisoning, Risk for

Post-Trauma Syndrome

Post-Trauma Syndrome, Risk for

Powerlessness

Powerlessness, Risk for

Protection, Ineffective

Rape-Trauma Syndrome

Rape-Trauma Syndrome: Compound Reaction

Rape-Trauma Syndrome: Silent Reaction

Religiosity, Impaired

Religiosity, Readiness for Enhanced

Religiosity, Risk for Impaired

Relocation Stress Syndrome

Relocation Stress Syndrome, Risk for

Role Conflict, Parental

Role Performance, Ineffective

Self-Care Deficit: Bathing/Hygiene

Self-Care Deficit: Dressing/Grooming

Self-Care Deficit: Feeding

Self-Care Deficit: Toileting

Self-Concept, Readiness for Enhanced

Self-Esteem, Chronic Low

Self-Esteem, Situational Low

Self-Esteem, Risk for Situational Low

Self-Mutilation

Self-Mutilation, Risk for

Sensory Perception, Disturbed (Specify: Visual, Auditory, Kinesthetic, Gustatory, Tactile, Olfactory)

Sexual Dysfunction

Sexuality Patterns, Ineffective

Skin Integrity, Impaired

Skin Integrity, Risk for Impaired

Sleep Deprivation

Sleep Pattern Disturbed

Sleep, Readiness for Enhanced

Social Interaction, Impaired

Social Isolation

Sorrow, Chronic

Spiritual Distress

Spiritual Distress, Risk for

Spiritual Well-Being, Readiness for Enhanced

Spontaneous Ventilation, Impaired

Sudden Infant Death Syndrome, Risk for

Suffocation, Risk for

Suicide, Risk for

Surgical Recovery, Delayed

Swallowing, Impaired

Therapeutic Regimen Management: Community, Ineffective

Therapeutic Regimen Management, Effective

Therapeutic Regimen Management: Family, Ineffective

Therapeutic Regimen Management, Ineffective

Therapeutic Regimen Management, Readiness for Enhanced

Thermoregulation, Ineffective

Thought Processes, Disturbed

Tissue Integrity, Impaired

Tissue Perfusion, Ineffective (Peripheral)

Tissue Perfusion, Ineffective (Specify: Renal, Cerebral, Cardiopulmonary, Gastrointestinal, Peripheral)

Transfer Ability, Impaired

Trauma, Risk for

Unilateral Neglect

Urinary Elimination, Impaired

Urinary Elimination, Readiness for Enhanced

Urinary Incontinence, Functional

Urinary Incontinence, Reflex

Urinary Incontinence, Stress

Urinary Incontinence, Total

Urinary Incontinence, Urge

Urinary Incontinence, Risk for Urge

Urinary Retention

Ventilation, Impaired Spontaneous

Ventilatory Weaning Response, Dysfunctional

Violence: Other-Directed, Risk for

Violence: Self-Directed, Risk for

Walking, Impaired

Wandering

ANSWERS TO CRITICAL THINKING EXERCISES

Chapter 1

1. Thinking about your own aging is a great way to face your fears, realize your hopes, and prepare for the future. This exercise will not only help you to prepare for your own aging, but also allow you to be more effective when working with older patients.

2. Your actions in youth will form the foundations of health in old age. Your lifestyle now will be crucial to your function as you get older. If you are engaging in choices that will compromise your health in old age, make changes today. The earlier you make positive changes, the better.

3. Some common themes you might discover include strength of character, zest for life, positive outlook, avoidance of bad health habits, ability to form at least one loving and caring relationship with another, and genetic hardiness.

4. Often geriatric care is not perceived as glamorous or a good recruitment technique. Pictures showing student nurses caring for babies are more popular than pictures showing nurses with older people. Hopefully, this will change in the future and many more students will want to work with older people and make contributions to improving their health and quality of life.

Chapter 2

1. You may be pleasantly surprised at what you may hear from your older patients and older people in your family and community. By spending time getting to know an older person "up close and personal" most often, younger people begin to realize and appreciate diversity and richness in aging. Try to understand the older person's circumstances today in light of past decisions and actions.

2. Because many health care professionals (including nurses) are educated in isolation from other health care professionals, the understanding and appreciation of the various professional roles is often not truly understood by others. Our professional role as gerontological nurses is evolving and we are assuming more responsibility daily in response to the complex health care needs of our patients. Take every opportunity you can to educate others if they have misconceptions about the role of gerontological nurses.

3. Some of your colleagues from other professions and even some nurses themselves feel trapped in the medical model. The role of nursing may be viewed too narrowly. Educate others about the use of nursing diagnosis and the ways its use complements and enriches the medical diagnosis and validates the nurses' actions specified on the nursing care plan. The nursing diagnosis is holistic and usually defines the older person's reaction to their illness, identifies immediate or possible nursing problems, and lists health promotion activities. The medical diagnosis usually is focused on an actual or potential disease process.

4/5. Many nurses choose to work with older patients because they want to help people and improve the quality of their lives. The nurse's holistic focus can enrich the interdisciplinary team perspective. The nurse can provide input whether the topic is health and wellness, spirituality, nutrition, coping and stress, or any other number of related subjects. A multidisciplinary team requires the input of nursing to function efficiently and effectively.

Chapter 3

1. This older patient should be reassured by the healthcare team that no one will go against his wishes if he becomes impaired near the time of death. The social worker and other members of the interdisciplinary team should meet with the family and patient and carefully document Mr. Turner's preferences in the medical record.

2. Mrs. Lee is considered an elder at risk. A referral to the Area Council on Aging is needed. A social worker will perform an assessment. If Mrs. Lee is considered unsafe to live alone or a threat to others, a guardian will be appointed to help her make decisions to get help in her home or move to a more supportive living environment.

3. Explain the importance of protecting the patient's confidential records from unauthorized viewing by others. Ask your colleague to voluntarily discuss this issue with the supervisor. If the behavior continues to occur, you may be required by workplace policy to report these confidentiality lapses to someone in authority.

Chapter 4

1. You may be amazed at both the culturally competent and the culturally incompetent interventions you find listed now that your awareness has been raised.

2. Many clinicians are unaware of their own stereotypes on aging. The nurse you interview may deny that age plays a factor in thinking about culture and care planning, but it may become apparent that the nurse is influenced by unconscious attitudes and beliefs.

3. Truth telling is a great topic to investigate as it will incorporate many different underlying cultural values and beliefs, including legitimate role of the patient and provider, hope, reliance and trust in authority, faith in the future, and so on.

4. Many students are surprised to find that they are from a specific cultural background. Most of us have been influenced by the beliefs and attitudes of our parents and grandparents who may have immigrated from other parts of the world. Interview some older people in your family to discover your own roots.

5. Most older people will welcome the opportunity to talk with you about their beliefs and values. You will be the wiser.

6. Family and community support systems vary according to basic beliefs about life, death, health, suffering, role of elders, and so on. This examination will clarify some key concepts regarding various cultures. If you have traveled to other countries, this is a plus. International travel will open your eyes to differences and commonalities between that culture and the American culture.

Chapter 5

1. Risk factors for undernutrition can include depression, multiple chronic illnesses, immobility, advanced age, and other factors included in Box 5-5. Appropriate nursing interventions are presented in Box 5-8. Some risk factors are modifiable and others are not. The nurse is urged to try to come up with novel and creative solutions to maintain good nourishment in the older person.

2. Nutrition and hydration concerns for a homebound older person with arthritis include:

- Ability to shop for or obtain groceries and prepare meals (grasping utensils, cutting, standing, carrying dishes or containers).
- Effect of any pain or discomfort on appetite.
- Effect of medications on nutrition, taste perception, digestion.
- Potential for voluntary fluid restriction to limit need to travel to bathroom.
- Poor access to fluids due to potential immobility.

Careful monitoring by the nurse and creative approaches are needed for this older person at risk for undernutrition.

3. Nursing interventions appropriate for a cognitively impaired nursing home resident with no documentation on ability to self- or hand-feed include:

- Provide mealtime assistance to assess ability to self-feed.
- Assess for need to provide finger foods or one food item and proper utensil singly.
- Cue appropriately.
- Allow adequate unhurried time to feed.
- Minimize environmental distractions during mealtime.
- Assist with proper positioning for feeding.
- Assess for any difficulties with swallowing.
- Obtain food preferences from family or significant others.
- Encourage family to visit at mealtime and assist with feeding.

Be sure to ask all three shifts to observe the resident's eating pattern as the pattern may vary according to meal, time of day, level of fatigue, staffing, and other factors.

4. Nursing interventions appropriate for an older person in long-term care at risk for dehydration include:

- Obtain fluid preferences.
- Prompt to drink fluids at regular intervals throughout the day.
- Educate resident of need to drink to a schedule and not wait for thirst.
- Offer larger volumes of fluid with snacks and medication passes.
- Flag meal trays or room door to alert staff to leave fluids at bedside table within reach. Offer non-spillable drinking containers if needed.
- Monitor for signs and symptoms of dehydration.

Document the fluids preferred by the resident in the nursing care plan. Offer the desired fluid frequently, but remember to vary the choice. Variety is the spice of life!

5. Appropriate nursing assessment for an older person with new dentures and weight loss might include:

- Assess fit and comfort of dentures and check for oral pain and alterations in mucosal integrity. Refer back to dentist if indicated.
- Assess for alteration in taste perception due to dentures.
- Conduct diet history and assess for texture modifications and other diet changes or omissions, which may account for nutrition deficit of calories and other nutrients. Specifically assess protein intake since many high-protein foods, such as meats, can be difficult to chew and therefore may be avoided.

- Assess the older person's ability to care for the dentures and keep them clean. Poor oral hygiene can detract from appearance, cause bad breath, and make the older person dread placing the teeth in his or her mouth.
- Monitor the older person's weight. Even a slight weight loss (5 to 10 lb) can cause the dentures to slip, cause pain and irritation, and inhibit ability to chew. Be proactive and urge the patient to revisit the dentist if weight changes.

Once your patient adjusts to the new dentures, you may note improvements in appearance, nutritional intake, self-confidence, and rate of smiling. Frequent modifications may be needed in the adjustment period, but it is worth it.

Chapter 6

1. Many healthcare professionals have no idea of the cost of the medications they are prescribing. Even with a drug benefit or discount card, the copayment may be extremely expensive, especially when the patient is taking many medications.

2. Often the older patient's medication regimen is changed but the medical record is not updated. This can lead to confusion and errors.

3. Some older patients take their medications by size or color (e.g., "the big white one is for my joints and the little yellow one is for my heart"). This can be an unsafe and risky practice for an older person taking many medications. Colors and shapes may change when generic brands of the same medication are used.

4. Some students are surprised to discover that anyone can become confused when taking a complicated medication regimen. Even young and middle-aged persons can make errors.

Chapter 7

1. Remember to consider the physical, psychological, spiritual, and social causes in your list. Compare your list with your classmates' lists and see if there is any commonality in your perspectives.

2. Older persons with poor vision or hearing may misinterpret normal conversations and events in daily life. These mistakes can be frightening to the older person who is "seeing" things that are not there and "hearing" things that have not been said.

3. Because many older persons live alone, they can successfully conceal the amount of alcohol they consume. A person who is still working may be missed from work due to excessive alcohol intake, but the flexible schedule in re-

tirement allows the older person to sometimes escape detection from others.

4. The older person may be unwilling to admit mental health problems. A stigma against mental health problems and fear of seeing a psychiatrist or psychologist may cause the older person to conceal feelings of depression or anxiety.

5. Public education, continued education of health professionals, and evidence-based protocols can all enhance the mental health of older persons.

Chapter 8

1. Excessive alcohol consumption can disrupt normal sleep patterns and result in further problems such as daytime sleepiness, hangovers, dehydration, and falls. Excessive alcohol consumption is a high-risk behavior in an older person.

2. Mrs. Johnson may be lonely, depressed, experiencing chronic pain, or physically ill. As she has recently had a complete physical examination and health assessment that was within normal limits, it is most likely that she is experiencing a psychological problem that may be discovered with a complete nursing assessment. A Mini-Mental State Examination and a depression screen would be a good place to start.

3. Proper diet, exercise, appropriate recreational activities, and alcohol avoidance may be behaviors Mrs. Johnson would carry out if she believes they will allow her to live independently and stay out of a nursing home. Sleep hygiene measures and establishment of a satisfactory nighttime ritual may be appropriate interventions for this patient.

4. While the nurse is establishing a therapeutic relationship with Mrs. Johnson, it is important to convey that she is a valuable person with a potentially serious problem and that she can regain control of her situation and achieve satisfactory sleep. A values clarification will help this patient to begin thinking about long-term goals and how she wishes to spend the rest of her life. Asking Mrs. Johnson what is important to her and what actions she is willing to take to maintain these values is a good place to start. If she values independence and wishes to remain living in her own apartment, she may be more likely to engage in behaviors that are health promoting.

5. The nurse should inform Mrs. Johnson that taking a sleep medication is indicated for short-term use only (usually less than 2 weeks) and that a long-term solution to her problem is indicated. If she is depressed or in pain, treatment of these conditions may improve her sleep patterns. Taking any medication with alcohol increases the risk of an adverse drug event and should be avoided.

Chapter 9

1. A chronic degenerative joint problem generates pain because bone surfaces come in contact with one another and produce an inflammatory response. This inflammatory response includes increased fluid in the joint, swelling, and pain signals transmitted to the brain.

2. Mr. Adams may be lonely and depressed while experiencing chronic pain. As he recently had a complete physical examination and health assessment that was within normal limits, it is likely that he is experiencing depression as a result of social isolation and fears for his future independence that may be discovered with a complete nursing assessment. A depression screen would be a good place to start.

3. Proper diet, exercise, and appropriate recreational and social activities may be behaviors Mr. Adams would carry out if he believes they will allow him to live independently. His inability to obtain needed groceries is of concern. His ability to climb stairs should be improved, or alternative living situations should be explored.

4. While the nurse is establishing a therapeutic relationship with Mr. Adams, it is important to convey to him that it is very risky to take acetaminophen on a regular basis and consume any amount of alcohol. The probability of hepatic failure is greatly increased in older persons who ingest alcohol. If he values independence and wishes to remain living in his own apartment, he may be more likely to engage in behaviors that are health promoting.

Chapter 10

1. Many caregivers experience anger directed towards the abuser. Caring for a frail older person who has been mistreated can trigger a variety of emotions. Although painful, try to identify your emotions, record them, and discuss them with an advisor or mentor. Identifying and discussing your emotional response can prevent stress and burnout.

2. Every community is different. Each has strengths and weaknesses that may indirectly contribute to elder mistreatment. Does your community have services for stressed caregivers? Are there services to monitor older adults at risk for self-neglect? Make a list of strengths and weaknesses in your community and begin to advocate for services to older people by addressing weaknesses.

3. Sometimes older patients are treated harshly in the clinical setting by stressed caregivers. This cannot be excused or tolerated. Nurses and nurse's assistants may scold older patients, neglect their psychological and physical needs, or touch them harshly. This may result in emotional distress, anxiety, and skin tears and bruising.

Be alert for such incidents and report them to your instructor or the charge nurse immediately.

4. Stressed family caregivers are at high risk for mistreating the older adults they care for. Engaging in healthy lifestyle habits and good coping mechanisms can help. Suggestions might include arranging for respite to engage in daily exercise, prayer, or meditation; listening to music; having someone to trust and confide in to receive needed support; and involving others as much as possible so as not to "go it alone." A caregiver who can maintain good emotional and physical health is an asset.

Chapter 11

1. Many nurses and nursing assistants are experts in pain assessment and will pick up on verbal and nonverbal cues when working with their patients. Others are less expert and may not be able to identify relevant factors such as grimacing, avoidance of moving about, refusal of care, and so on. Start to identify the clinical experts.

2. Some students have not faced their own feelings about death and dying. Sometimes they have not faced the loss of a loved one in their own families and are relatively unfamiliar with the death and dying process. Films, stories, role-playing, and other techniques help prepare the student to face death in the clinical setting and provide appropriate end-of-life care.

3. Journaling is a technique that helps us to sort out and record feelings and emotions as we progress through growth and developmental processes. Keeping a small journal by your bed allows you to record a few observations regarding the day's experiences and the emotional responses to those experiences. Later, when rereading the journal, you may be surprised at your responses and how you have grown in insight and strength over time.

4. Identifying key people to help you is important because you may need to seek them out for support now or in the future. Often, the first time you see a patient die who is in your care stimulates feelings of sadness, remorse, and inadequacy. Having someone you can talk to openly and honestly about your feelings is important. Try not to repress your feelings or turn away from your emotions. You will become stronger by addressing your fears and emotions.

Chapter 12

1. Intrinsic factors such as age, nutritional status, genetic predisposition, and degree of sun damage will all be important to identify. Extrinsic factors such as medication use, degree of dryness, and temperature of the environment will also have an impact. Considering both sets of factors will improve your management of dermatological problems.

2. Good nutrition forms the basis for many areas of health, including dermatological health. Poor fluid intake can cause skin dryness and flakiness. Poor protein intake can cause dull, thin skin and many other skin problems both now and in the future.

3. Many healthcare facilities have protocols and procedures for skin care based on habit, tradition, provider and staff preference, or trial and error. If you find discrepancies between current guidelines and clinical practices, bring in a copy of current guidelines from the Agency for Healthcare Research and Quality Website to key decision makers. Become a change agent.

4. Often despite the best efforts of staff, older patients are overly positioned on their backs and thus can develop skin breakdown on the coccyx and other bony prominences. Pillows, rolled blankets, wedge cushions, and other positioning aids can assist patients to comfortably use alternative positions.

Chapter 13

1. Many people are uncomfortable with others giving them oral care. This exercise will increase your sensitivity toward the feelings of your older dependent patient.

2. It is natural to feel sad when caring for someone with oral cancer and perhaps feel anger toward things the older person may have done to develop the disease. However, many older people began smoking before the risks were clearly known, and your patient may have tried many times to "kick" this addictive habit. The best bet is to assist your patients to quit smoking and urge others never to start while caring for patients with oral cancer.

3. Many nursing home patients rely on Medicaid for reimbursement and are financially indigent. Reimbursement rates are lower for dental care, and many patients cannot manage the copayments. It is distressing to realize you are caring for a patient with unmet needs and be unable to locate a dental provider. Advocate for your patient and try to locate providers who can assist older nursing home residents with dental needs.

4. The aid should be spoken to immediately and informed that the approach was not appropriate. The nurse can role-model appropriate behavior such as using a pleasant tone, smiling, explaining the reason for the intervention, and returning at a later time if the resident refuses to cooperate at this time.

Chapter 14

1. Appropriate interventions to the nurse may be completely unacceptable to the older person. For instance, a pet who is always underfoot is a fall hazard. From the per-spective of the nurse, the pet should be eliminated from the home. However, the older person may rely on the friendship and companionship of the pet and feel socially isolated and lonely if the pet were to be forced from the home. Therefore, each suggestion should be discussed and a mutually agreed upon plan instituted.

2. Each nurse should report safety hazards as they occur in the clinical setting. Many hazards exist in hospitals and nursing homes, including dangling wires, wet floors, uneven surfaces, medical equipment crowding the walkways, and uneven lighting in hazardous areas. The nurse should be prepared to call upon housekeeping services to quickly clean up spills and leaks that could cause frail older persons to fall and endure injury.

3. The problem may be reframed to be more positive. For instance, the nurse might say, "Instead of seeing a cane as a sign of weakness, think of it this way. The cane indicates a person with a vision problem who is getting around independently. Instead of a sign of weakness, it is a sign of self-sufficiency."

4. Assess the lighting in your dining area, the degree of contrast, and the help available to older persons with vision problems. You may find areas for improvement.

5. You may find that wearing gloves somewhat separates you from fully experiencing your environment. This is a reasonable emotional response to the situation.

6. Often, nurses only touch patients in a clinical and professional manner. Older patients may feel "touch deprived" or miss the caring and loving touch from others.

Chapter 15

1. The underlying process of atherosclerosis has not been changed by invasive procedures. Changing diet and exercise can help atherosclerosis to be reversed. Rehabilitation also provides support for smoking cessation and stress reduction.

2. When a nurse knows a patient, even subtle changes are more apparent. The patient may be developing decreased cardiac output, which may be evident in levels of energy or mood. If a patient develops sudden confusion or change in function, this will be more obvious to a person who knows that patient. The patient is also more likely to trust the person giving health information.

3. Rehabilitation programs provide socialization, group support, monitoring during activity progression, and stress reduction techniques. There is much more to a good rehabilitation program than exercise.

4. Older persons who live alone and have heart failure need to learn self-management of their condition. This

includes medication management, daily weights, healthy food choices, and knowing when to call the healthcare provider to report changes in condition. Learning all these things will require ongoing support. Meals-on-wheels may be required to provide balanced nutrition. Adult day health programs might be appropriate to provide socialization and assessment.

5. Rehabilitation programs that would be ideal for people of all ages include socialization, cooking classes, exercise that is like a dance class, and stress reduction through meditation.

Chapter 16

1. There are community programs (sponsored by the American Lung Association, for example) that can assist older persons to quit smoking. There are also pharmacological (nicotine patches, bupropion) and nonpharmacological techniques (relaxation, counseling) to help older people to quit. Try to identify resources in your clinical and community setting to assist your patients.

2. The best advice is not to start at all. Smoking is addictive and it is often very difficult to quit. Smoking will yellow your teeth, cause premature wrinkles, and make your breath smell stale. Further, cigarettes are very expensive and a waste of money that could be spent on clothing or entertainment. Stress the immediate negative impact of smoking because sometimes teenagers cannot contemplate long-term negative health outcomes.

3. Portable oxygen use improves the quality of life and daily function of older people with chronic lung disease. Unfortunately, there is added expense and difficulty in the maintenance and use of the equipment. Newer oxygen tanks are smaller and easier to use, so encourage their use if appropriate.

Chapter 17

1. Human sexuality is a complex subject, and discussing it with older adults requires great sensitivity on the part of the nurse. It is important to recognize one's own practice limits and to know when a referral to another healthcare provider is needed. It is equally important to know when a referral is not needed and when a concern can be addressed with knowledge base. By becoming comfortable with your own feelings toward sexuality, you will be better able to counsel and support your older patients.

2. Nurses have a wealth of knowledge and a powerful array of skills that should not be underestimated. Sometimes, accurate information and an empathetic listener are all the intervention that is needed. The person who makes ageist or negative remarks about sexuality in old

age is probably misinformed. There are many societal stereotypes about sexuality, especially in old age. Provide accurate information about the need for and enjoyment of sexual activity in older people.

3. Ask your colleagues in your clinical setting if they have advisors, counselors, resources, or educational materials for older persons with sexual problems. There may be more materials available for men with erectile dysfunction problems because of educational campaigns initiated by pharmaceutical manufacturers. You may have to search more widely for information for older women.

4. Many of the things that enhance sexual activity for the older adult are similar to those used by other age groups such as soft lighting, background music, and romantic food and beverages. Urge older adults to conserve energy before sexual activity so that they do not become fatigued, to take pain medications to ease arthritic aches, to use appropriate positioning techniques to enhance pleasure, and to keep lubricants and other sexual aids handy so they can be used when needed. Sexual activity between consenting adults is fun and should be enjoyed, so urge them to approach each encounter without anxiety performance and to keep an open mind.

Chapter 18

1. Nursing considerations include patient safety (they are more at risk for fracture as the result of a fall), prevention of further bone loss (daily calcium intake and use of an antiresorptive if appropriate), and ongoing medical assessment (bone density scans every other year). Aggressive nursing intervention is needed to prevent unnecessary injury and disability as the result of further bone loss.

2. Remove clutter, secure scatter rugs, make sure there is adequate lighting, mark the edge of stairs with red reflective tape, and use nonskid mats and grab bars in the bathroom. Pets who may run underfoot should wear a bell to announce their movements. Older persons may have additional ideas to prevent falls, especially if they have fallen in the past. It is important to include the patient and family in the plan.

3. Many nurses are uncomfortable recommending exercise because they fear the older person will fall, suffer injury, or not take their suggestion seriously. A regular, moderate exercise program is crucial for maintaining cardiovascular conditioning and strength. Walking, swimming, and stretching are all appropriate activities for older people. Chair exercise can be recommended for older persons with balance problems or those confined to

wheelchairs. Urge your patients to see their primary healthcare provider for assessment of exercise ability if you are in doubt. Call your local YMCA and see if they have exercise classes for older people. Sit in on one. You may be pleasantly surprised.

Chapter 19

1. Many older people are overweight, do not exercise, and have other risk factors for the development of type 2 DM. They may be unwilling to discuss lifestyle modification if they are overwhelmed and intimidated by all the changes they will need to make. When educating older patients about lifestyle modification, try to begin with one or two simple suggestions. They will be more likely to come back for a second appointment.

2. Remember that you are a role model for your older patients. Try to maintain your own health and wellness as a good example.

3. Educate your colleagues about the importance of the thyroid in the regulation and maintenance of many of the body's activities and metabolic processes. When the older patient complains of vague signs and symptoms, it will become your habit to suspect the thyroid as the underlying cause.

4. Reorganizing your life to deal with type 1 DM is difficult. It involves regularly checking blood glucose, watching your diet and nutrition, calculating insulin doses, recognizing and managing signs and symptoms of hypoglycemia, and carrying syringes, insulin, lancets, and a glucose monitor with you at all times. Many people will be overwhelmed and frightened. By understanding these fears, you will be in a better position to support and counsel your patients.

5. Some of your colleagues may feel that genetics is more important than lifestyle; others may feel that lifestyle is the key determinant. Either way, it is crucial to consider both factors. Patients have the power to modify their lifestyles, but genetic risks are nonmodifiable. Urge your patients to change the things that can be changed.

Chapter 20

1. Many older people feel embarrassed and defer scheduling a sigmoidoscopy or colonoscopy because of their fears. Urge them to speak with others who have had the procedure and can reassure them. Even if your patient refuses the first request for a colonoscopy, try again. Over time your patient may come to realize the importance of this lifesaving procedure.

2. Because some lifestyle modifications that are associated with GI problems relate to food and food consumption habits, it is sometimes difficult to motivate older people to change. Referral to a dietitian or nutritionist who can make practical suggestions and encourage healthy food choices can be beneficial. When older patients engage in lifestyle modification and enjoy improvement of GI symptoms, they may be motivated to engage in further healthy habits such as increasing consumption of fluids and healthy foods and getting regular exercise.

3. The societal stereotype is that all older persons are bowel obsessed and concerned about constipation. Although this is true for some older persons, many older people do not fit this stereotype. As you work with older people who are excessively concerned with bowel function, try to identify factors in their lifestyle or background that are contributing to the problem. Many times there are contributing factors such as pre-existing illness, medications, or immobility that can be recognized by the nurse rather than attributing the problem to the aging process.

Chapter 21

1. Older patients who are in chronic atrial fibrillation are more at risk for stroke because a thrombus can form in the heart as a result of incomplete emptying of the ventricles. This thrombus can travel to any part of the body and if lodged in the brain can cause a cerebrovascular accident (CVA), brain attack, or stroke. If the use of WARFARIN is indicated, it is necessary to maintain an INR of about 2.5 to 3.0 to prevent stroke.

2. Mr. Thayer is at risk for bleeding from trauma or injury because of his elevated INR. If he is a faller, he should be urged to walk only with assistance and to exercise extreme caution to prevent bleeding and injury. He should avoid all strenuous activities, report any blood in the stool or urine, and avoid vigorous toothbrushing until his INR returns to normal limits.

3. Mr. Thayer should be urged to eat foods high in vitamin K like green leafy vegetables for the next few days. After that, he should eat foods high in vitamin K in a consistent pattern to make titration of his dose of warfarin more stable and consistent.

4. Mr. Thayer, like other older persons with chronic health problems and complicated disease management regimens, may need additional help and support from the interdisciplinary team. Appropriate interventions may include consultation and referral to social workers, nutritionists, and recreational, physical, or occupational therapists. By addressing the patient's problem holistically, the chances of good outcomes and increased quality of life are expanded.

Chapter 22

1. Because there is no one key test or procedure that definitively diagnoses Alzheimer's disease, the diagnosis is a process of exclusion. This process involves eliminating or ruling out all other possible causes of dementia. Families will often exhibit frustration and stress during the period of diagnosis. They may experience relief when the cause of the dementia is known, but feel fear and frustration when told of the devastating diagnosis.

2. Many communities offer support groups sponsored by the Alzheimer's Association. These groups meet regularly and provide information, support, and tips on caring for persons with dementia. Contact the social worker at your clinical agency to find out more about support and resources available in your community.

3. Environmental modifications often can ease agitation and improve the quality of life for older persons with dementia. Many factors in the institutional environment (hospital or long-term care facility) may complicate the care of persons with dementia. Some of these factors include noise, light, waking patients up at night for assessment of vital signs, bathing schedules that may not conform to the best time to approach the patient, and so on. Identifying a few changes to the clinical environment is a good way to begin your professional career.

4. Many nurses would benefit from formal or informal support groups, ongoing professional education (in-service and attendance at professional conferences), training videos, and written materials. It is natural to feel frustration, anger, and other negative feelings when providing care to an older person who may be resistive, hostile, or resentful because of a cognitive impairment. Keep a journal and record the feelings (positive and negative) that you experience when caring for a resistive patient with a cognitive impairment. Share your feelings with a friend, and you may find others experience similar emotional responses. Explore some of the Websites listed in this chapter to identify sources where you can gain valuable practical information to solve clinical problems.

Chapter 23

1. Rheumatoid arthritis requires medications and interventions to relieve pain, prevent further joint destruction, and improve the quality of life. Many of these medications can be toxic to older persons and cause drug interactions when taken with other medications. Careful monitoring of drug levels and ongoing assessment of drug interactions is needed.

2. Many older people are hesitant to discuss sex and sexual behavior with a person of the opposite sex or a younger person. If you sense resistance or embarrassment on the part of older patients, question them as to why they are uncomfortable. If possible, make a referral to someone on your team who may have the skills and experience to work with older persons and teach them safe sex practices. In general, the information you provide to the older person would be similar to the information given to younger patients. They should avoid risky sexual behaviors such as unprotected sexual intercourse and intravenous drug use. Although blood transfusion safety has increased since the 1980s, HIV antibodies in a donor may go undetected if the infected donor has been exposed but has not yet seroconverted (a process that may take up to 6 months). Therefore, many professionals urge autodonation of blood for scheduled surgery.

3. When large numbers of older, frail, and acutely ill persons are placed together in congregate living facilities, drug-resistant bacteria can thrive. Proper sanitation and hand washing are necessary to prevent transmission from person to person, with isolation of those who are at high risk for acquiring infections (patients who are immunosuppressed or have multiple comorbidities) and those who may spread infection (acutely ill with infectious disease such as tuberculosis). Cross-contamination can occur when individuals are transferred for treatment between institutions and are cared for by multiple providers.

4. The main risk factors include inappropriate use of antibiotics (including prescription for viral infections, improper administration and dosing practices, and failure to complete the entire course of treatment); poor hand-washing practices of healthcare workers; use of contaminated equipment between patients, including telephones, blood pressure cuffs, stethoscopes, and eating utensils; exposure to contaminated surfaces, including taking medications dropped on the floor; placing fingers, pens, eyeglasses, hairclips, and so on in the mouth; use of indwelling urinary catheters that encourage development of urinary tract infections; failure to wear gloves or protect clothing when caring for patients who are incontinent; and failure to use aspiration precautions in patients with dysphagia. Develop good habits so that you do not place yourself or your patients at risk for developing nosocomial infections.

Chapter 24

1. Entering a hospital is a stressful situation for any person, regardless of age. Some people are fearful that they

will become a number instead of a person. Taking a few personal items can help strengthen the individual patient's identity and provide a stimulus for conversation with the staff.

2. This exercise may clarify and identify opinions that you and others have about the treatment of patients with cognitive impairment. You may find yourself engaging in this discussion with others many times during your professional career. It is a valuable exercise to learn how to argue your point of view and disagree respectfully with others.

3. Advantages may include improved care by the segregation of older patients on units with specialized resources and caregivers. Disadvantages may include the fact that older people who are not placed on these special units may not enjoy the benefits of specialized care. Segregating older patients on one unit may communicate the unfortunate message that caring for older patients is not a priority on the general units.

4. The most important factor is communication and sharing of crucial information, especially focusing on medications, dosing information, baseline function, food preferences, and advance directives. If there is a close relationship between a nursing home and hospital, the nurses become familiar with one another and will often just pick up the phone and call for information needed to improve the care of the older hospitalized patient.

INDEX

Page numbers followed by italic f *indicate figures and those followed by italic* t *indicate tables or boxes.*

A

Abandonment, 272, 274t. *See also* Elder mistreatment
Abdominal palpation, 664t
ABI (ankle brachial index), 447
Abnormal sleep behaviors, 228. *See also* Sleep disturbances
Abscess, in pneumonia, 506
Absence seizures, 744
Acarbose, 620
Accommodation, 387
Accupril. *See* Quinapril
ACE inhibitors. *See* Angiotensin-converting enzyme (ACE) inhibitors
ACE (acute care of the elderly) units, 806
Acebutolol, for hypertension, 436t
Acetaminophen:
    alcohol use and, 169
    for chronic pain management, 254t
    drug interactions, 170t, 702t
    hemolytic anemia and, 691
    for osteoarthritis, 579
    for pain management during dying process, 305
    toxic effects, 255, 305
Achalasia, 649
Achlorhydria, 112, 643
Acid perfusion tests, 655
Acidosis, blood flow in, 426–27
Acquired active immunity, 756–57
Acquired immunodeficiency syndrome (AIDS). *See* Human immunodeficiency virus
Acquired passive immunity, 757
Actinic damage, 332
Actinic keratosis, 336
Activated partial thromboplastin time, 450t
Active coping, 764
Activity theory, of aging, 20
Actonel. *See* Risedronate
Actos. *See* Pioglitazone
Acute care of the elderly (ACE) units, 806
Acute pain. *See also* Pain; Pain management
    assessment, 258–59
    causes, 258
    treatment, 259, 261
Acute phase reactants, 574
Adalat CC. *See* Nifedipine

Adenocarcinoma:
    colorectal, 667
    gallbladder, 674
    lung, 503
ADEs. *See* Adverse drug events
ADH (antidiuretic hormone), 522
Adjustment disorder, 197
Adjuvant drugs, for pain management, 253–54, 305–6
Adrenergic inhibitors, for hypertension, 436t
Adrenergic receptors, 424
ADRs. *See* Adverse drug reactions
Adult day care, 42–43
Adult protective services (APS), 272, 277t
Adult Treatment Panel (ATP III), 437
Advance directives, 313–16, 720
Advanced practice registered nurse (APRN), 29
Adverse drug events (ADEs), 162, 162t
    causes, 803
    in hospitals, 803
Adverse drug reactions (ADRs). *See also* Medications, side effects
    causes, 161
    definition, 162t, 163t
    monitoring, 178–79
    prevention, 162, 164
    reporting, 163
    symptoms, 161t, 162
Aerophagia, 136, 136t
African Americans:
    asthma in, 466
    chronic obstructive pulmonary disease in, 491
    lung cancer in, 503
    medication effectiveness in, 157
    sickle cell disease in, 694
    tuberculosis in, 500
Afterload, 424
Age-related macular degeneration (ARMD):
    antioxidants and, 124, 392
    characteristics, 390, 391f
    patient education, 391–92
    risk factors, 390–91
    treatment, 391
    vitamins and, 392
Ageism:
    definition, 190
    questionnaire, 4t
Agglutination, 757

Aging:
    attitudes about, 4t
    benefits, 5t
    biological theories
        error theories
            cross-link, 19
            free radical, 19
            somatic DNA damage, 19
            wear and tear, 19
        programmed theories
            endocrine, 19
            immunological, 19, 755–56
            programmed longevity, 18–19
    demographics, 6, 6f
    drug metabolism and, 158–59, 160t
    normal changes, 15–18, 16f, 17f
        cardiovascular system, 427–31, 428f
        cognitive function, 190–92
        contribution to frailty, 790–91t
        eyes, 386–88, 386f, 387t
        gastrointestinal system, 643–46, 645f, 662–63
        genitourinary system, 519f, 521–23, 524f
        hearing, 398–99
        immune system, 761–62, 762t, 763f
        integumentary system, 332–35, 333f, 334f
        memory, 192–93, 192t
        mouth and oral cavity, 366–67, 366f
        musculoskeletal system, 554–56, 555f
        neurological system, 712–13, 714f
        respiratory system, 430–31, 463, 464f
        sleep patterns, 227–29
        smell, 410
        taste, 407
        vision, 387–88, 387t
    nutrition and. *See* Nutrition
    psychological theories
        Erickson's developmental theory, 20
        Jung's theory of individualism, 20
    quiz, 4t
    sociological theories
        activity, 20
        continuity, 20–21
        disengagement, 20
    stereotypes, 3, 5t, 11t
Agitation, 720
Agnosia:
    in Alzheimer's disease, 723
    definition, 279
AIDS. *See* Human immunodeficiency virus